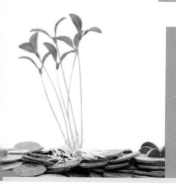
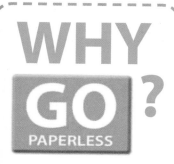
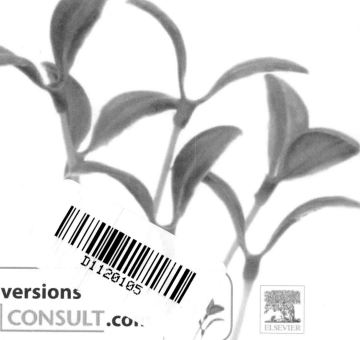

BERNE & LEVY
PHYSIOLOGY

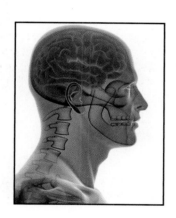

BERNE & LEVY
PHYSIOLOGY

SIXTH EDITION, UPDATED EDITION

EDITORS

Bruce M. Koeppen, MD, PhD

Professor of Medicine and Cell Biology
Dean for Academic Affairs
Departments of Medicine and Cell Biology
University of Connecticut Health Center
Farmington, Connecticut

Bruce A. Stanton, PhD

Professor and Director of the Lung Biology Center
Department of Physiology
Dartmouth School of Medicine
Hanover, New Hampshire

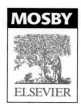

MOSBY

ELSEVIER

MOSBY
ELSEVIER

1600 John F. Kennedy Blvd.
Ste 1800
Philadelphia, PA 19103-2899

BERNE AND LEVY PHYSIOLOGY   ISBN: 978-0-323-07362-2

Copyright © 2010, 2008, 2004, 1998, 1993, 1988, 1983 by Mosby, Inc., an affiliate of Elsevier Inc.

Notice

Knowledge and best practice in this field are constantly changing. As new research and experience broaden our knowledge, changes in practice, treatment and drug therapy may become necessary or appropriate. Readers are advised to check the most current information provided (i) on procedures featured or (ii) by the manufacturer of each product to be administered, to verify the recommended dose or formula, the method and duration of administration, and contraindications. It is the responsibility of the practitioner, relying on their own experience and knowledge of the patient, to make diagnoses, to determine dosages and the best treatment for each individual patient, and to take all appropriate safety precautions. To the fullest extent of the law, neither the Publisher nor the Authors assumes any liability for any injury and/or damage to persons or property arising out of or related to any use of the material contained in this book.

The Publisher

Library of Congress Cataloging-in-Publication Data
Berne & Levy physiology / editors, Bruce M. Koeppen, Bruce A. Stanton. – 6th ed., updated ed.
   p. ; cm.
Includes bibliographical references and index.
ISBN 978-0-323-07362-2
   1. Human physiology.   I. Berne, Robert M., 1918–2001.   II. Koeppen, Bruce M.   III. Stanton, Bruce A.   IV. Title: Berne and Levy physiology.   V. Title: Physiology.
   [DNLM: 1. Physiological Phenomena. QT 104 B5249 2010]
   QP34.5.P496 2010
   612 – dc22

                                                                2009036311

Acquisitions Editor: William Schmitt
Developmental Editor: Andrew Hall
Publishing Services Manager: Linda Van Pelt
Project Manager: Francisco Morales
Design Direction: Steven Stave

Printed in Canada

Last digit is the print number: 9 8 7 6 5 4 3

This updated sixth edition of Physiology *is dedicated to Robert M. Berne (in memoriam) and Matthew N. Levy, the founding editors of this textbook of physiology. Their excellence as scientists and teachers has allowed countless students to learn and appreciate the normal functioning of the human body. We are honored to be able to continue to provide this book as a learning resource for all students of physiology.*

Bruce M. Koeppen, M.D., Ph.D.
Bruce A. Stanton, Ph.D.

Kim E. Barrett, PhD

Professor of Medicine, School of Medicine and Dean
   of Graduate Studies
University of California, San Diego
La Jolla, California
Section VI: Gastrointestinal Physiology

Michelle M. Cloutier, MD

Professor
Department of Pediatrics
University of Connecticut School of Medicine
Farmington, Connecticut
and
Asthma Center
Connecticut Children's Medical Center
Hartford, Connecticut
Section V: The Respiratory System

Bruce M. Koeppen, MD, PhD

Professor of Medicine and Cell Biology
Dean for Academic Affairs
Departments of Medicine and Cell Biology
University of Connecticut Health Center
Farmington, Connecticut
Section I: Cellular Physiology
Section VII: The Renal System

Eric J. Lang, MD, PhD

Associate Professor
Department of Physiology and Neuroscience
New York University School of Medicine
New York, New York
Section II: The Nervous System

Achilles J. Pappano, PhD

Professor
Department of Cell Biology
and
Professor
Calhoun Cardiology Center
University of Connecticut Health Center
Farmington, Connecticut
Section IV: The Cardiovascular System

Helen E. Raybould, PhD

Professor
Department of Anatomy, Physiology, and Cell Biology
University of California-Davis
School of Veterinary Medicine
Davis, California
Section VI: Gastrointestinal Physiology

Kalman Rubinson, PhD

Associate Professor
Department of Physiology and Neuroscience
New York University School of Medicine
New York, New York
Section II: The Nervous System

Bruce A. Stanton, PhD

Professor and Director of the Lung Biology Center
Department of Physiology
Dartmouth Medical School
Hanover, New Hampshire
Section I: Cellular Physiology
Section VII: The Renal System

Roger S. Thrall, PhD

Professor of Medicine
Department of Immunology
University of Connecticut Health Center
Farmington, Connecticut
and
Director of Clinical Research
Department of Research
Hospital for Special Care
New Britain, Connecticut
Section V: The Respiratory System

James M. Watras, PhD

Associate Professor
Department of Cell Biology
University of Connecticut Health Center
Farmington, Connecticut
Section III: Muscle

Bruce A. White, PhD

Professor
Department of Cell Biology
University of Connecticut Health Center
Farmington, Connecticut
Section VIII: The Endocrine and Reproductive Systems

Those who have used this textbook in the past will find many changes in this updated sixth edition; most notable is the use of full-color illustrations and a reorganization of many of the sections. In addition, we welcome a number of new authors to this edition and gratefully acknowledge Drs. Robert Berne, Saul Genuth, Howard Kutchai, Matthew Levy, and William Willis for their contributions to earlier editions. We welcome the following new contributors: Drs. Kalman Rubinson and Eric Lang (nervous system), Dr. Achilles Pappano (cardiovascular system), Drs. Kim Barrett and Helen Raybould (gastrointestinal system), and Dr. Bruce White (endocrine and reproductive systems). Finally, we are pleased that Dr. James Watras (muscle) and Drs. Michelle Cloutier and Roger Thrall (respiratory system) have continued as members of the updated sixth edition team.

As in the previous editions of this textbook, we have attempted to emphasize broad concepts and to minimize the compilation of isolated facts. Each chapter has been altered to make the text as lucid, accurate, and current as possible. We have included both clinical and molecular information in each section. This information is set apart from the main text and serves to provide clinical context and new insights into physiologic phenomena at the cellular and molecular levels. We hope that you find this a valuable addition to the book.

The human body consists of billions of cells that are organized into tissues (e.g., muscle, epithelia, and nervous tissue) and organ systems (e.g., nervous, cardiovascular, respiratory, renal, gastrointestinal, endocrine, and reproductive). For these tissues and organ systems to function properly and thus allow humans to live and carry out daily activities, several general conditions must be met. First and foremost, the cells within the body must survive. Survival requires adequate cellular energy supplies, maintenance of an appropriate intracellular milieu, and defense against a hostile external environment. Once cell survival is ensured, the cell can then perform its designated or specialized function (e.g., contraction by skeletal muscle cells). Ultimately, the function of cells, tissues, and organs must be coordinated and regulated. All of these functions are the essence of the discipline of physiology and are presented throughout this book. What follows is a brief introduction to these general concepts.

Cells need a constant supply of energy. This energy is derived from the hydrolysis of **adenosine triphosphate (ATP)**. If not replenished, the cellular ATP supply would be depleted in most cells in less than 1 minute. Thus, ATP must be continuously synthesized. This in turn requires a steady supply of cellular fuels. However, the cellular fuels (e.g., glucose, fatty acids, and keto-acids) are present in the blood at levels that can support cellular metabolism only for a few minutes. The blood levels of these cellular fuels are maintained through the ingestion of precursors (i.e., carbohydrates, proteins, and fats). In addition, these fuels can be stored and then mobilized when ingestion of the precursors is not possible. The storage forms of these fuels are triglycerides (stored in adipose tissue), glycogen (stored in the liver and skeletal muscle), and protein. The maintenance of adequate levels of cellular fuels in the blood is a complex process involving the following tissues, organs, and organ systems:

- *Liver*: Converts precursors into fuel storage forms (e.g., glucose → glycogen) when food is ingested, and converts storage forms to cellular fuels during fasting (e.g., glycogen → glucose and amino acids → glucose).
- *Skeletal muscle*: Like the liver, stores fuel (glycogen and protein) and converts glycogen and protein to fuels (e.g., glucose) or fuel intermediates (e.g., protein → amino acids) during fasting.
- *Gastrointestinal tract*: Digests and absorbs fuel precursors.
- *Adipose tissue*: Stores fuel during feeding (e.g., fatty acids → triglycerides) and releases the fuels during fasting.
- *Cardiovascular system*: Delivers the fuels to the cells and to and from their storage sites.
- *Endocrine system*: Maintains the blood levels of the cellular fuels by controlling and regulating their storage and their release from storage (e.g., insulin and glucagons).
- *Nervous system*: Monitors oxygen levels and nutrient content in the blood and, in response, modulates the cardiovascular, pulmonary, and endocrine systems and induces feeding and drinking behaviors.

In addition to energy metabolism, the cells of the body must maintain a relatively constant intracellular environment to survive. This includes the uptake of fuels needed to produce ATP, the export from the cell of cellular wastes, the maintenance of an appropriate intracellular ionic environment, the establishment of a resting membrane potential, and the maintenance of a constant cellular volume. All of these functions are carried out by specific membrane transport proteins.

The composition of the extracellular fluid (ECF) that bathes the cells must also be maintained relatively constant. In addition, the volume and temperature of the ECF must be regulated. Epithelial cells in the lungs, gastrointestinal tract, and kidneys are responsible for maintaining the volume and composition of the ECF, while the skin plays a major role in temperature regulation. On a daily basis, H_2O and food are ingested, and essential components are absorbed across the epithelial cells of the gastrointestinal tract. This daily intake of solutes and water must be matched by excretion from the body, thus maintaining **steady-state balance**. The kidneys are critically involved in the maintenance of steady-state balance for water and many components of the ECF (e.g., Na^+, K^+, HCO_3^-, pH, Ca^{++}, organic solutes). The lungs ensure an adequate supply of O_2 to "burn" the cellular fuels for the production of ATP and excrete the major waste product of this process (i.e., CO_2). Because CO_2 can affect the pH of the ECF, the lungs work with the kidneys to maintain ECF pH.

Because humans inhabit many different environments and often move between environments, the body must be able to rapidly adapt to the challenges imposed by changes in ambient temperature and availability of food and water. Such adaptation requires coordination of the function of cells in different tissues and organs as well as their regulation. The nervous and endocrine systems coordinate and regulate cell, tissue, and organ function. The regulation of function can occur rapidly (seconds to minutes), as is the case for levels of cellular fuels in the blood, or over much longer periods of time (days to weeks), as is the case for acclimatization when an individual moves from a cool to a hot environment or changes from a high-salt to a low-salt diet.

The function of the human body represents complex processes at multiple levels. This book explains what is currently known about these processes. Although the emphasis is on the normal function of the human body, discussion of disease and abnormal function is also appropriate, as these often illustrate physiologic processes and principles at the extremes.

The authors for each section have presented what they believe to be the most likely mechanisms responsible for the phenomena under consideration. We have adopted this compromise to achieve brevity, clarity, and simplicity.

We wish to express our appreciation to all of our colleagues and students who have provided constructive criticism during the revision of this book.

Bruce M. Koeppen, MD, PhD
Bruce A. Stanton, PhD

TABLE OF CONTENTS

CELLULAR PHYSIOLOGY

Bruce M. Koeppen and Bruce A. Stanton

CHAPTER 1

Principles of Cell Function

The human body is composed of billions of cells, each with a distinct function. Despite this diversity in cell function, all cells share certain common elements and functions. This chapter provides an overview of these common elements and focuses on the important function of transport of molecules and water into and out of the cell across its plasma membrane.

OVERVIEW OF EUKARYOTIC CELLS

Eukaryotic cells are distinguished by the presence of a membrane-delimited nucleus. With the exception of mature human red blood cells, all cells within the body contain a nucleus. The cell is therefore effectively divided into two compartments: the nucleus and the cytoplasm. The cytoplasm is an aqueous solution containing numerous organic molecules, ions, cytoskeletal elements, and a number of organelles. A brief description of the components of a typical eukaryotic cell follows (Fig. 1-1). Readers who desire a more in-depth presentation of this material are encouraged to consult one of the many cellular and molecular biology textbooks currently available.

Nucleus

The nucleus contains the genome of the cell, which in somatic cells is present on 46 chromosomes, 22 pairs of autosomes, and one pair of sex chromosomes. Both sperm and eggs contain 23 chromosomes, a copy of each autosome and either a male (X) or a female (Y) sex chromosome. The chromosome is a highly ordered structure containing genes (DNA) and associated proteins (i.e., histones). The nucleus also contains the enzymatic machinery for repair of damaged DNA and for its replication, as well as the enzymes needed to transcribe DNA and yield messenger RNA (mRNA).

Plasma Membrane

The plasma membrane surrounds the cell and separates the contents of the cell from the surrounding extracellular fluid. It serves a number of important functions and is described in greater detail later in the chapter.

Mitochondria

It is currently thought that mitochondria evolved from an aerobic prokaryote that lived within primitive eukaryotic cells. Mitochondria synthesize ATP and thus provide the energy needed to power many vital cell functions. They contain their own DNA, which codes for a number of the enzymes needed for oxidative phosphorylation (other mitochondrial enzymes are synthesized in the cytoplasm and imported into the mitochondria), as well as the RNA needed for the transcription and translation of mitochondrial DNA. Mitochondria are composed of two membranes separated by an intermembrane space. The outer mitochondrial membrane lets molecules up to 5 kDa in size cross. Thus, the composition of the intermembrane space is similar to that of cytoplasm with respect to small molecules and ions. The inner membrane is folded into numerous cristae and is the site where ATP is generated through the process of oxidative phosphorylation. The interior of mitochondria (i.e., matrix) contains the enzymes involved in the citric acid cycle and those involved in oxidation of fatty acids. In addition to producing ATP, mitochondria can serve as a site for sequestration of Ca^{++}.

Rough Endoplasmic Reticulum

The rough endoplasmic reticulum (rER) is an extensive membrane network throughout the cytoplasm and is especially well developed in cells that produce and secrete proteins (e.g., pancreatic acinar cell, plasma cell). Attached to the membrane are ribosomes, which when viewed with an electron microscope, impart the "rough" appearance characteristic of this organelle. The rER is the site of translation of mRNA and posttranslational modification of proteins that are destined to be secreted from the cell or are targeted to the plasma membrane or other membranous organelles (e.g., Golgi apparatus, lysosomes).

Golgi Apparatus

Proteins synthesized in the rER are transferred to the Golgi apparatus via coated vesicles. On electron micrographs the Golgi apparatus appears as a stack of flattened membrane sacs. Vesicles from the rER fuse with sacs that are in close proximity to the rER (i.e., the cis-Golgi network). The proteins then traverse through the Golgi membrane sacs, also via coated vesicles, and in this process they may undergo additional post-translational modification (e.g., glycosylation). The Golgi apparatus also sorts the proteins and packages them for delivery to other parts of the cell (e.g., plasma membrane, lysosome, secretory granule). The sorting and packaging of proteins occur in the trans-Golgi network.

Smooth Endoplasmic Reticulum

The smooth endoplasmic reticulum (sER) is devoid of ribosomes and therefore appears "smooth" on electron micrographs. It is a site where many substances are modified and detoxified (e.g., pesticides). Hydrophobic molecules can be converted to water-soluble

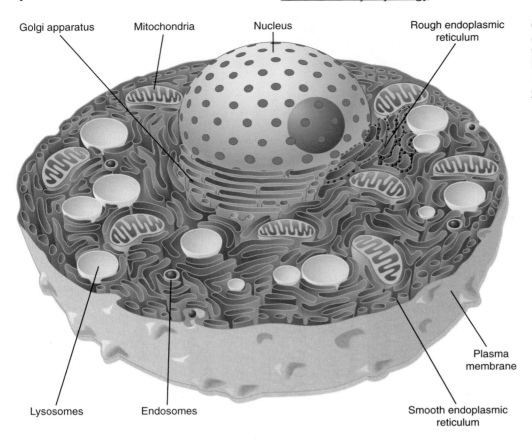

Golgi apparatus Mitochondria Nucleus Rough endoplasmic reticulum

Lysosomes Endosomes Smooth endoplasmic reticulum Plasma membrane

● **Figure 1-1.** Schematic drawing of a eukaryotic cell. The top portion of the cell has been removed to illustrate the nucleus and various intracellular organelles. See text for details.

molecules in the sER, thus facilitating their excretion from the body by the liver and kidneys. The sER is also the site for the synthesis of fats and lipids. For example, the cells of the adrenal gland that secrete the steroid hormone cortisol have an extensive sER. Similarly, the cells within the ovaries and testes that secrete estrogens and testosterone have a well-developed sER. In skeletal and cardiac muscle, the sER, which is called the sarcoplasmic reticulum in these cells, serves to sequester Ca^{++}. Thus, it plays an important role in controlling contraction.

Lysosomes

Lysosomes are part of the endocytic system of the cell (see later) and serve a degradative function. They are membrane-bound organelles with an acidic interior (pH ≈ 4.5), and they contain a number of digestive enzymes (e.g., proteases, nucleases, lipases, glycosidases). Lysosomes degrade material that is brought into the cell via the processes of endocytosis and phagocytosis. They also degrade intracellular organelles, a process called autophagy, and some intracellular proteins. Much of what is degraded is then recycled by the cell. The process of degradation is not random and in a number of instances is targeted. For example, chaperone proteins (e.g., heat shock protein 73) can direct intracellular proteins to the lysosome. In addition, plasma membrane proteins can be targeted for endocytosis and eventual degradation by lysosomes through attachment of specific groups (e.g., ubiquitin) to the protein. These groups act as signals for degradation of the protein.

Proteasomes

Like lysosomes, proteasomes serve a degradative function. However, proteasomes are not membrane bound. They serve to degrade primarily intracellular proteins that have been targeted (e.g., ubiquitinated) for degradation. They may also degrade some membrane-associated proteins.

Free Ribosomes

Ribosomes are located throughout the cytoplasm and are not associated with the endoplasmic reticulum. They translate mRNA for cytosolic proteins, as well as proteins that will neither be secreted from the cell nor incorporated into membrane structures (e.g., mitochondrial enzymes).

Peroxisomes

Peroxisomes (also called microbodies) are membrane-bound organelles that contain various oxidative enzymes (e.g., catalase). These oxidative enzymes can detoxify a number of compounds and oxidize fatty acids. In the liver, peroxisomes metabolize ethanol to acetaldehyde.

Cytoskeleton

The cytoskeleton of the cell consists of actin filaments (also called microfilaments), intermediate filaments, and microtubules. Actin filaments in muscle cells are critical components of the contractile apparatus. In other cells they are involved in locomotion (e.g., macrophages). Actin also makes up the core of microvilli and links the interior of the cell to adjacent cells through some cell junctions (e.g., zonula adherens and zonula occludens). There are several different classes of intermediate filaments, and they can vary by cell type. For example, keratin filaments are found in epithelial cells, whereas neurofilaments are found in neurons. Intermediate filaments are primarily structural in function and can link the interior of the cell to adjacent cells and the surrounding extracellular matrix through desmosomes and hemidesmosomes, respectively. Microtubules serve multiple functions within the cell, including intracellular transport of vesicles, chromosome movement during mitosis and meiosis, and movement of cilia and flagella (e.g., tail of spermatozoa). They are formed from α- and β-tubulin dimers and change length by either adding or removing tubulin dimers. In general, a microtubule-organizing center exists near the cell's nucleus, and microtubules grow out from this center toward the periphery of the cell. As noted, microtubules can move intracellular vesicles within the cell (e.g., transport of neurotransmitter-containing vesicles from the cell body of the neuron down the axon); such movement is driven by motor proteins. One motor protein, **kinesin,** drives transport from the center of the cell toward the periphery, whereas another motor protein, **dynein,** drives movement in the opposite direction. Dynein is the motor protein that drives the movement of both cilia and flagella.

THE PLASMA MEMBRANE

The cells within the body are surrounded by a plasma membrane that separates the intracellular contents from the extracellular environment. Because of the properties of this membrane, in particular, the presence of specific membrane proteins, the plasma membrane is involved in a number of important cellular functions, including

- Selective transport of molecules into and out of the cell, a function carried out by membrane transport proteins
- Cell recognition via cell surface antigens
- Cell communication through neurotransmitter and hormone receptors and signal transduction pathways
- Tissue organization, such as temporary and permanent cell junctions, as well as interaction with the extracellular matrix, through a variety of cell adhesion molecules
- Enzymatic activity
- Determination of cell shape by linking the cytoskeleton to the plasma membrane

Membranes also surround the various organelles within the cell. The organelle membranes not only subdivide the cell into compartments but are also the site of many important intracellular processes (e.g., electron transport by the inner mitochondrial membrane).

In this chapter the structure and function of the plasma membrane of eukaryotic cells is considered. More specifically, the chapter focuses on transport of molecules and water across the plasma membrane. Only the principles of membrane transport are presented here. Additional details as related to specific cells are presented in the various sections and chapters of the book.

Structure and Composition

The plasma membrane of eukaryotic cells consists of a 5-nm-thick lipid bilayer with associated proteins (Fig. 1-2). Some of the membrane-associated proteins are integrated into the lipid bilayer, whereas others are more loosely attached to the inner and outer surfaces of the membrane, often by binding to the integral membrane proteins. Because the lipids and proteins can diffuse within the plane of the membrane and the appearance of the membrane varies regionally as a result of the presence of different membrane proteins, this depiction of the structure of the plasma membrane is often termed the **fluid mosaic model.**

Membrane Lipids

The major lipids of the plasma membrane are **phospholipids** or **phosphoglycerides.** Phospholipids are amphipathic molecules that contain a charged (or polar) hydrophilic head and two (nonpolar) hydrophobic fatty acyl chains (Fig. 1-3). The amphipathic nature of the phospholipid molecule is critical for formation of the bilayer, with the hydrophobic fatty acyl chains forming the core of the bilayer and the polar head groups exposed on the surface.

The majority of membrane phospholipids have a glycerol backbone to which are attached the fatty acyl chains, as well as an alcohol linked to glycerol via a phosphate group. The common alcohols are choline, ethanolamine, serine, inositol, and glycerol. Another important phospholipid, sphingomyelin, has the amino alcohol sphingosine as its backbone instead of glycerol. Table 1-1 lists these common phospholipids. The fatty acyl chains are usually 14 to 20 carbons in length

---

IN THE CLINIC

Microtubules are the target of a number of antitumor drugs (e.g., vincristine and taxol) because disruption of these structures impairs cell division in the highly mitotic tumor cells. Vincristine prevents polymerization of the tubulin dimers and thus prevents the formation of microtubules. As a result, the mitotic spindle cannot form, and the cell cannot divide. Taxol stabilizes the microtubules and thus arrests cells in mitosis.

Kartagener's syndrome is an autosomal recessive disorder in which dynein is missing in cilia and, in males, the flagella of sperm. Accordingly, males with this syndrome are infertile. Because the cilia of the epithelial cells that line the respiratory track work to remove inhaled pathogens, a process termed **mucociliary transport** (see Chapter 20), both men and women with this syndrome are susceptible to repeated lung infections.

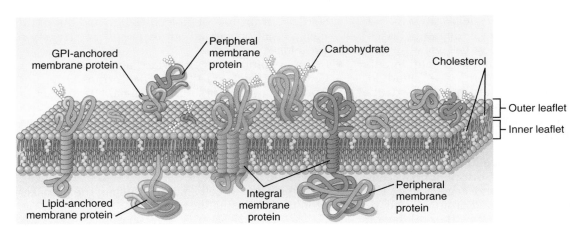

● **Figure 1-2.** Schematic diagram of the cell plasma membrane. Not shown are lipid rafts. See text for details. (Modified from Figure 12-3 in Cooper GM: The Cell—A Molecular Approach, 2nd ed. Washington DC, Sinauer, 2000.)

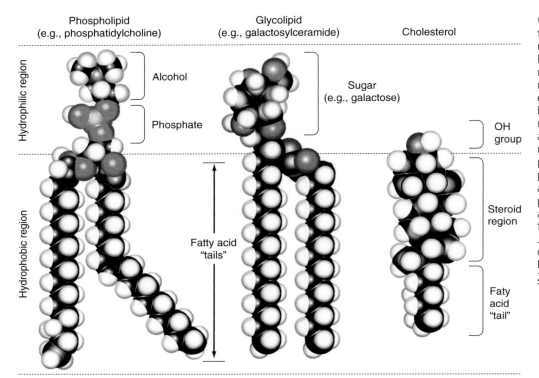

● **Figure 1-3.** Models of the major classes of plasma membrane lipids depicting the hydrophilic and hydrophobic regions of the molecules. The molecules are arranged as they exist in one leaflet of the bilayer. The opposing leaflet is not shown. One of the fatty acyl chains in the phospholipid molecule is unsaturated. The presence of this double bond produces a "kink" in the fatty acyl chain that prevents tight packing of membrane lipids and increases membrane fluidity. (Modified from Hansen JT, Koeppen BM: Netter's Atlas of Human Physiology. Teterboro, NJ, Icon Learning Systems, 2002.)

● **Table 1-1. Plasma Membrane Lipids**

Phospholipid	Leaflet Location
Phosphatidylcholine	Outer
Sphingomyelin	Outer
Phosphatidylethanolamine	Inner
Phosphatidylserine	Inner
Phosphatidylinositol*	Inner

*Involved in signal transduction.

and may be saturated or unsaturated (i.e., contain one or more double bonds).

The phospholipid composition of the membrane varies among different cell types and even between the bilayer leaflets. As summarized in Table 1-1, phosphatidylcholine and sphingomyelin are found predominantly in the outer leaflet of the membrane, whereas phosphatidylethanolamine, phosphatidylserine, and phosphatidylinositol are found in the inner leaflet. As described in detail in Chapter 3, phosphatidylinositol plays an important role in signal transduction, and its location in the inner leaflet of the membrane facilitates this signaling role.

The sterol molecule **cholesterol** is also a critical component of the bilayer (Fig. 1-3). It is found in both leaflets and serves to stabilize the membrane at normal body temperature (37°C). Cholesterol can represent as much as 50% of the lipids found in the membrane. Another minor lipid component of the plasma membrane is **glycolipid.** These lipids, as their name indicates, contain two fatty acyl chains linked to polar head groups that consist of carbohydrates (Fig. 1-3).

As discussed later, one glycolipid, glycosylphosphatidylinositol (GPI), plays an important role in anchoring proteins to the outer leaflet of the membrane. Both cholesterol and glycolipids, like the phospholipids, are amphipathic and orient with their polar groups on the outer surface of the leaflet in which they are located. Their hydrophobic portions are thus located within the interior of the bilayer.

The lipid bilayer is not a static structure. Lipids can freely diffuse within the plane of the membrane. The fluidity of the membrane is determined by temperature and by its lipid composition. As temperature increases, the membrane becomes more fluid. The presence of unsaturated fatty acyl chains in phospholipids and glycolipids also increases membrane fluidity. If a fatty acyl chain is unsaturated, the presence of a double bond introduces a "kink" in the molecule (Fig. 1-3). This kink prevents the molecule from closely associating with surrounding lipids, and as a result membrane fluidity is increased. Some membranes contain lipids (e.g., sphingomyelin and cholesterol) that aggregate into what are called **lipid rafts.** These lipid rafts often have specific proteins associated with them and diffuse in the plane of the membrane as a discrete unit. Lipid rafts appear to serve a number of functions. One important function of these rafts is to segregate signaling mechanisms and molecules.

Membrane Proteins

As much as 50% of the membrane is composed of protein. These membrane proteins are classified as either integral, lipid anchored, or peripheral (Fig. 1-2).

Integral membrane proteins are embedded in the lipid bilayer, where hydrophobic amino acid residues are associated with the hydrophobic fatty acyl chains of the membrane lipids. Many integral membrane proteins span the bilayer and are termed **transmembrane proteins.** Transmembrane proteins have both hydrophobic and hydrophilic regions. The hydrophobic region, often in the form of an α helix with the hydrophobic amino acids facing out, spans the membrane. Hydrophilic amino acid residues are then exposed to the aqueous environment on either side of the membrane. Transmembrane proteins may pass through the membrane multiple times.

Proteins can also be attached to the membrane via **lipid anchors.** The protein is covalently attached to a lipid molecule, which is then embedded in one leaflet of the bilayer. The glycolipid GPI anchors proteins to the outer leaflet of the membrane. Proteins can be attached to the inner leaflet via their N-terminus by fatty acids (e.g., myristate or palmitate) or via their C-terminus by prenyl anchors (e.g., farnesyl or geranylgeranyl).

Peripheral proteins may associate with the polar head groups of the membrane lipids but more commonly bind to integral or lipid-anchored proteins. Peripheral proteins are easily removed from the membrane, whereas integral and lipid-anchored proteins require the use of detergents to isolate them from the membrane.

MECHANISMS OF MEMBRANE TRANSPORT

Intracellular and extracellular fluid is composed primarily of H_2O in which solutes (e.g., ions, glucose, amino acids) are dissolved. The normal function of cells requires continuous movement of water and solutes into and out of the cell. The plasma membrane, with its hydrophobic core, is an effective barrier to the movement of virtually all of these biologically important solutes. It also restricts movement of water across the membrane. With the exception of gases (e.g., O_2 and CO_2) and ethanol, which can diffuse across the lipid bilayer, movement of water and other solutes across the plasma membrane occurs via specific membrane transport proteins.

Membrane Transport Proteins

Table 1-2 lists the major classes of membrane transport proteins, their mode of transport, and the rate at which they transport molecules or ions across the membrane.

Water Channels

Water channels, or **aquaporins (AQPs),** are the main route for water movement into and out of the cell. They are widely distributed throughout the body, although different isoforms are found in different cell types. To date, 12 AQPs have been identified. The amount of H_2O that can enter or leave the cell via AQPs can be regulated by altering the number of AQPs in

---

● AT THE CELLULAR LEVEL

There is a superfamily of membrane proteins that serve as receptors for many hormones, neurotransmitters, and numerous drugs. These receptors are coupled to heterotrimeric G proteins and are termed **G protein–coupled receptors** (see Chapter 3). These proteins span the membrane with seven α-helical domains. The extracellular portion of the protein contains the ligand binding site, whereas the cytoplasmic portion binds to the G protein. This superfamily of membrane proteins makes up the third largest family of genes in humans. Nearly half of all nonantibiotic prescription drugs are targeted toward G protein–coupled receptors.

● **Table 1-2.**

Major Classes of Plasma Membrane Transporters

Class	Transport Mode	Transport Rate
Water channel	Gated*	Up to 10^9 molecules/sec
Ion channel	Gated	10^6-10^8 molecules/sec
Solute carrier	Cycle	10^2-10^4 molecules/sec
ATP dependent	Cycle	10^2-10^4 molecules/sec

*Water channels (i.e., aquaporins) may be continuously open and thus function similar to a pore, which is not gated (e.g., the porins found in the outer membrane of mitochondria). However, the permeability of a water channel can be modified and is therefore listed as gated.

the membrane or by changing their permeability (i.e., gating). Changes in pH have been identified as one factor that can modulate the permeability of AQPs.

Ion Channels

Ion channels are found in all cells and are especially important for the function of excitable cells (e.g., neurons and muscle cells). Ion channels are classified by their selectivity (i.e., the ions that pass through the channel). At one extreme, they can be highly selective by allowing only a specific ion through. At the other extreme, they may be nonselective and allow all or a group of cations or anions through. Channels are also characterized by their conductance, which is typically expressed in picosiemens (pS). The range in conduc-

AQPs are divided into two subgroups. One group is permeable only to water. The second group is permeable not only to water but also to low-molecular-weight substances. Because glycerol can cross the membrane via this later group of AQPs, they are termed **aquaglyceroporins.** AQPs exist in the plasma membrane as a homotetramer, with each monomer functioning as a water channel.

tance is considerable, with some channels having a conductance of only 1 to 2 pS and others having a conductance of greater than 100 pS. For some channels, conductance varies depending on which direction the ion is moving. For example, if the channel has greater conductance when ions are moving into the cell versus out of the cell, the channel is said to be an inward rectifier. Finally, ion channels can be classified by their mechanism of gating. As illustrated in Figure 1-4, ion channels fluctuate between an open state or a closed state, a process called gating. Factors that can control gating include membrane voltage, extracellular agonists or antagonists (e.g., acetylcholine is an extracellular agonist that controls the gating of a cation-selective channel in the motor end plate of skeletal muscle cells—see Chapter 12), intracellular messengers (e.g., Ca^{++}, ATP, cGMP), and mechanical stretch of the plasma membrane. Trans-membrane ion flux can be regulated by changing the number of channels in the membrane or by gating of the channels.

Solute Carriers

Solute carriers represent a large family of membrane transporters, with more than 40 different types (>300 specific transporters) already identified. These carriers are divided into three major functional groups. One group, **uniporters,** transports a single molecule across the membrane. The transporter that brings glucose into the cell (GLUT2) is an important member

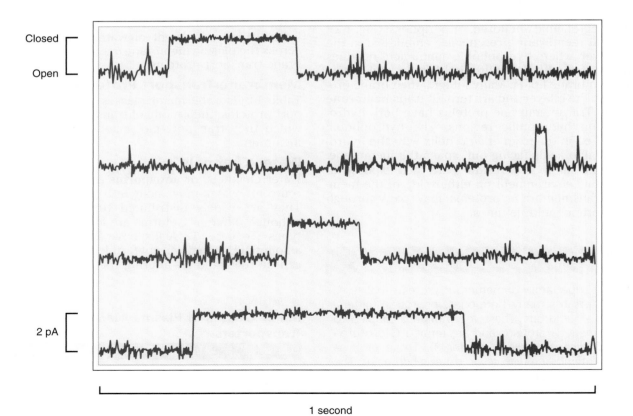

Closed

Open

2 pA

1 second

● Figure 1-4. Recording of current flow through a single K$^+$-selective ion channel. The channel spontaneously fluctuates between an open and closed state. The amplitude of the current is approximately 2 pA (2×10^{-12} amps), or 12.5 million ions cross the membrane per second.

of this group. The second group, **symporters,** couples the movement of two or more molecules/ions across the membrane. As the name implies, the molecules are transported in the same direction. Co-transport is another term used to describe this group of solute carriers. The $1Na^+, 1K^+, 2Cl^-$ symporter found in the kidney (NKCC2), which is critically important for diluting and concentrating urine (see Chapter 33), is an example of a member of this group. The third group, **antiporters,** also couples the movement of two or more molecules/ions across the membrane. However, in this case the molecules/ions are transported in opposite directions. The terms exchangers and counter transporters are also used to describe this group of solute carriers. The Na^+-H^+ antiporter is an example of this group of solute carriers. One isoform (NHE-1) of this antiporter is found in all cells and plays an important role in regulating intracellular pH.

ATP-Dependent Transporters

ATP-dependent transporters, as their name implies, use the energy in ATP to drive the movement of molecules/ions across the membrane. There are two groups of ATP-dependent transporters: **ATPase ion transporters** and **ATP-binding cassette (ABC) transporters.** ATPase ion transporters are subdivided into P-type and V-type ATPases.* P-type ATPases share the feature of being phosphorylated during the transport cycle. Na^+, K^+-ATPase is an important example of a P-type ATPase. With the hydrolysis of each ATP molecule, 3 Na^+ ions are transported out of the cell and 2 K^+ ions into the cell. Na^+, K^+-ATPase is present in all cells and plays a critical role in establishing cellular ion and electrical gradients, as well as maintaining cell volume (see Chapter 2).

V-type H^+-ATPase is found in the membranes of several intracellular organelles (e.g., endosomes, lysosomes) and as a result is also referred to as vacuolar H^+-ATPase. The H^+-ATPase on the plasma membrane plays an important role in urinary acidification (see Chapter 36).

ABC transporters represent a large group of membrane transporters. They are found in both prokaryotic and eukaryotic cells, and they share a common feature of having amino acid domains that bind ATP (i.e., ATP-binding cassette). There are seven subgroups of ABC transporters in humans and more than 40 specific transporters have been identified. They transport a diverse group of molecules/ions, including Cl^-, cholesterol, bile acids, drugs, iron, and organic anions.

AT THE CELLULAR LEVEL

Na^+, K^+-ATPase, also called the Na^+, K^+ pump or just the Na^+ pump, is found in all cells and is responsible for establishing the cellular gradients for Na^+ and K^+. These gradients in turn provide energy for several essential cell functions (see Chapter 2). Na^+, K^+-ATPase is composed of three subunits (α, β, and γ), and the protein exists in the membrane with a stoichiometry of 1α, 1β, 1γ. There are four isoforms of the α subunit and three of the β subunit. The α_1 isoform is the most ubiquitous and is expressed in all cells. The α subunit contains binding sites for Na^+, K^+, and ATP. It is also the subunit that binds cardiac glycosides (e.g., ouabain), which specifically inhibit the enzyme. Although the α subunit is the functional subunit of the enzyme (i.e., it hydrolyzes ATP, binds Na^+ and K^+, and translocates them across the membrane), it cannot function without the β subunit. The β subunit is responsible for targeting the α subunit to the membrane and also appears to modulate the affinity of Na^+, K^+-ATPase for Na^+ and K^+. The γ subunit is a member of a family of proteins called FXYD proteins (so named for the FXYD amino acid sequence found in the protein). There are seven members of this family, and many are associated with Na^+, K^+-ATPase. However, FXYD2 is the isoform referred to as the γ subunit of Na^+, K^+-ATPase. FXYD2 is a small protein (61 amino acids in length) that spans the plasma membrane once. It appears to play a role modulating the affinity of Na^+, K^+-ATPase for Na^+, K^+, and ATP.

IN THE CLINIC

Cystic fibrosis is an autosomal recessive disease characterized by chronic lung infections, pancreatic insufficiency, and infertility in males. Death usually occurs because of respiratory failure. It is most prevalent in the white population, occurring in 1 in 3000 live births, and is the most common lethal genetic disease in this population. It is a result of mutations in a gene on chromosome 7 that codes for an ABC transporter. To date, more than 1000 mutations in the gene have been identified. The most common mutation is deletion of a phenylalanine at position 508 (ΔF_{508}). This deletion results in defective processing of the protein by the endoplasmic reticulum, and as a result the transporter does not reach the plasma membrane. This transporter, called the **cystic fibrosis transmembrane regulator (CFTR),** normally functions as a Cl^- channel and also regulates other membrane transporters (e.g., the epithelial Na^+ channel [ENaC]). Thus, epithelial transport in individuals with cystic fibrosis is defective, which underlies the problems that these patients have. For example, in a normal lung the epithelial cells that line the airway are covered with a layer of mucus that entraps inhaled particulate matter and bacteria. Cilia on the epithelial cells then transport the entrapped material out of the lung, a process termed mucociliary transport (see Chapter 20 for more details). In patients with cystic fibrosis the defective epithelial transport results in thickening of airway mucus, and as a result the cilia cannot transport the entrapped material out of the lung. This in turn leads to recurrent and chronic lung infections. The inflammatory process that accompanies these infections ultimately destroys the lung tissue and causes respiratory failure and death.

---

*F-type ATPases are found in mitochondria and are responsible for ATP synthesis. They are not considered here.

● AT THE CELLULAR LEVEL

The plasma membrane of cells is constantly turning over. As a result, membrane proteins are continuously being replaced. One mechanism by which membrane proteins are "tagged" for replacement is by the attachment of ubiquitin to the cytoplasmic portion of the protein. Ubiquitin is a 76–amino acid protein that is covalently attached to the membrane protein (usually to lysine) by a class of enzymes called ubiquitin protein ligases. One important group of these ligases is the Nedd4/Nedd4-like family. Once a membrane protein is ubiquitinated, it undergoes endocytosis and is degraded either by lysosomes or by proteasomes. Cells also contain deubiquitinating enzymes called DUBs. Thus, the amount of protein in a cell depends on the rate that ubiquitin groups are added by ligases versus the rate that they are removed by DUBs. Ubiquitination of plasma proteins provides one mechanism for regulation of membrane transport by the cell. For example, Na^+ reabsorption by the distal nephron of the kidney is stimulated by the adrenal hormone aldosterone (see Chapters 33 and 34). One of the actions of aldosterone is to inhibit Nedd4-2. This prevents ubiquitination of the Na^+ channel (ENaC) in the apical membrane of epithelial cells in this portion of the nephron. Thus, they are retained for a longer period in the membrane, and as a result more Na^+ enters the cell and is thereby reabsorbed by the nephron.

Table 1-3 is a partial listing of membrane transport proteins that have been well studied and for which much is known about their function (see Fig. 1-5 for some molecular models of membrane transport proteins). Many of these transporters will be considered in greater detail in other chapters.

VESICULAR TRANSPORT

Solute and water can be brought into the cell by the process of **endocytosis** and released from the cell by the process of **exocytosis.** In both processes the integrity of the plasma membrane is maintained, and the vesicles that are formed allow transfer of the contents between cellular compartments. In some cells (e.g., the epithelial cells lining the gastrointestinal tract), endocytosis across one membrane of the cell is followed by exocytosis across the opposite membrane. This allows the transport of substances across the epithelium, a process termed **transcytosis.**

Endocytosis can be subdivided into three mechanisms. The first is **pinocytosis,** which consists of the nonspecific uptake of small molecules and water into the cell. Pinocytosis is a prominent feature of the endothelial cells that line capillaries and is responsible for a portion of the fluid exchange that occurs across blood vessels. A second form of endocytosis allows the internalization of large particles (e.g., bac-

● **Table 1-3.**

Examples of Plasma Membrane Transporters

Water Channels		
Aquaporin (AQP—multiple isoforms)		
Ion Channels		
Na^+		
K^+		Multiple channels exist for each
Ca^{++}		ion listed. They are distinguished
Cl^-	$\rightarrow$	by their selectivity, conductance,
Anion		and mode of regulation (i.e.,
Cation		gating)
Solute Carriers		
Uniport		
Glucose (GLUT2)		
Fructose (GLUT5)		
Urea (UT-A1)		
Fe^{+++} (ferroportin/IREG-1)		
Symport		
$1Na^+$-glucose (SGLT2)		
$2Na^+$-glucose (SGLT1)		
Na^+–amino acid (multiple transporters)		
Na^+-Cl^- (NCC/TSC)		
$1Na^+$, $1K^+$, $2Cl^-$ (NKCC2)		
Na^+-$3HCO_3^-$ (NBC1)		
$3Na^+$-P_i (type IIa phosphate transporter)		
$2Na^+$-$1I^-$ (NIS)		
Na^+–bile acid (NTCP—multiple isoforms)		
$3Na^+$-dicarboxylate (SDCT—multiple isoforms)		
H^+-oligopeptide (PepT and PHT—multiple isoforms)		
H^+-Fe^{+++} (DCT-1)		
K^+-Cl^- (KCC—multiple isoforms)		
Antiport		
Na^+-H^+ (NHE—multiple isoforms)		
Cl^--HCO_3^- (AE-1/band three and pendrin)		
$3Na^+$-Ca^{++} (NCX—multiple isoforms)		
Organic anions (OAT—multiple transporters for different anions)		
Organic cations (OCT and OCTN—multiple isoforms)		
Transport ATPases		
P-Type		
Na^+, K^+-ATPase		
H^+, K^+-ATPase		
H^+, Ca^{++}-ATPase (PMCA)		
V-Type		
H^+-ATPase		
ABC Transporters		
Cystic fibrosis transmembrane regulator (CFTR)		
Multidrug resistance protein (MRP-1)		
Organic anion (MRP-2)		

teria, cell debris). This process is termed **phagocytosis** and is an important characteristic of cells in the immune system (e.g., neutrophils and macrophages). Often but not always, phagocytosis is a receptor-mediated process. For example, macrophages have receptors on their surface that bind the Fc portion of immunoglobulins. When bacteria invade the body, they are often coated with antibody, a process called opsonization. These bacteria then attach to the membrane of macrophages via the Fc portion of the immunoglobulin and are phagocytosed and destroyed inside the cell. The third mechanism is **receptor-mediated endocytosis**, which allows the uptake of specific molecules into the cell. In this form of endocytosis, molecules bind to specific receptors on the surface of the

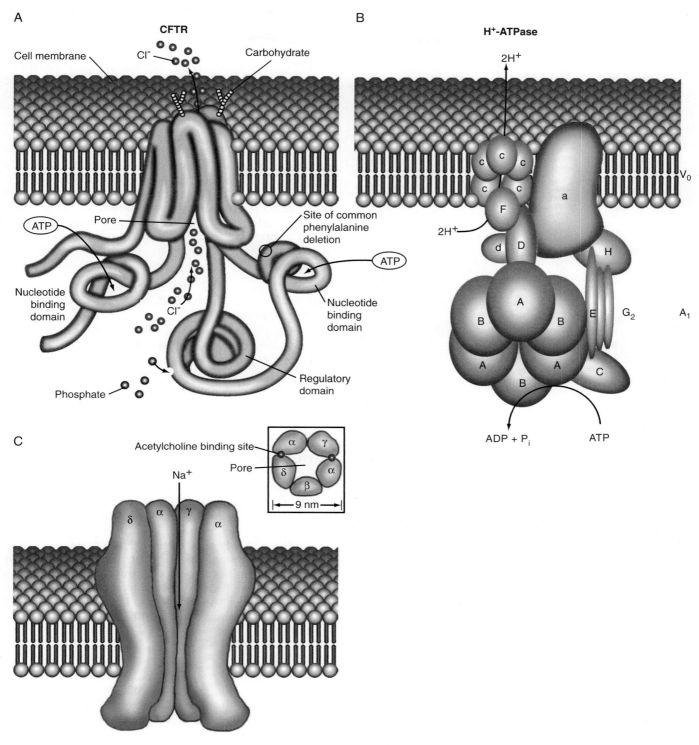

A CFTR

Cell membrane

Cl^-

Carbohydrate

ATP

Pore

Site of common phenylalanine deletion

ATP

Nucleotide binding domain

Cl^-

Nucleotide binding domain

Phosphate

Regulatory domain

B H^+-ATPase

$2H^+$

$2H^+$

V_0

ADP + P_i

ATP

A_1

C

Acetylcholine binding site

Pore

9 nm

Na^+

● **Figure 1-5.** Molecular models of several membrane transport proteins.

cell. Endocytosis involves a number of accessory proteins, including adaptin, clathrin, and the GTPase dynamin (Fig. 1-6).

Exocytosis can be either constitutive or regulated. Constitutive secretion is seen, for example, in plasma cells that are secreting immunoglobulin or in fibroblasts secreting collagen. Regulated secretion occurs in endocrine cells, neurons, and exocrine glandular cells (pancreatic acinar cells). In these cells the secretory product (e.g., hormone, neurotransmitter, or

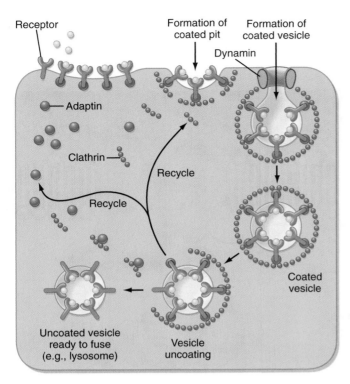

● **Figure 1-6.** Receptor-mediated endocytosis. A receptor on the surface of the cell binds the ligand. A clathrin-coated pit is formed, with adaptin linking the receptor molecules to the clathrin. Dynamin, a GTPase, assists in separation of the endocytic vesicle from the membrane. Once inside the cell, the clathrin and adaptin molecules dissociate and are recycled. The uncoated vesicle is then ready to fuse with other organelles in the cell (e.g., lysosome). (Adapted from Ross MH, Pawlina W: Histology, 5th ed. Baltimore, Lippincott Williams & Wilkins, 2006.)

digestive enzyme), after synthesis and processing in the rER and Golgi apparatus, is stored in the cytoplasm in secretory granules until an appropriate signal for secretion is received. These signals may be hormonal or neural. Once the cell receives the appropriate stimulus, the secretory vesicle fuses with the plasma membrane and releases its contents into the extracellular fluid. Fusion of the vesicle with the membrane is mediated by a number of accessory proteins. One important group is the SNAREs. These membrane proteins help target the secretory vesicle to the plasma membrane. The process of secretion is usually triggered by an increase in intracellular $[Ca^{++}]$. However, two notable exceptions to this general rule exist: renin secretion by juxtaglomerular cells of the kidney is triggered by a decrease in intracellular Ca^{++} (see Chapters 33 and 34), as is the secretion of parathyroid hormone (PTH) by the parathyroid gland (see Chapter 39).

Physiology of Solute and Water Transport

As already noted, the plasma membrane, with its hydrophobic core, is an effective barrier to the movement of virtually all biologically important molecules into or out of the cell. Thus, membrane transport proteins provide the pathway that allows transport to occur. However, the presence of a pathway is not sufficient for transport to occur; an appropriate driving force is also required.

Diffusion

Diffusion is the process by which molecules move spontaneously from an area of high concentration to one of low concentration. Thus, wherever a concentration gradient exists, diffusion of molecules from the region of high concentration to the region of low concentration will dissipate the gradient (as discussed later, establishment of concentration gradients for molecules requires the expenditure of energy). Diffusion is a random process driven by the thermal motion of the molecules. The rate at which a molecule diffuses from point A to point B is quantified by **Fick's first law of diffusion:**

● **Equation 1-1**

$$J = -DA\frac{\Delta C}{\Delta X}$$

where

J = flux or rate of diffusion per unit time
D = diffusion coefficient
A = area across which the diffusion is occurring
ΔC = concentration gradient
ΔX = distance along which the diffusion is occurring

The diffusion coefficient takes into account the thermal energy of the molecule, its size, and the viscosity of the medium through which the diffusion is taking place. For spherical molecules, D is approximated by the **Stokes-Einstein** equation:

● **Equation 1-2**

$$D = \frac{-kT}{6\pi r\eta}$$

where

k = Boltzmann's constant
T = temperature in degrees Kelvin
r = radius of the molecule
η = viscosity of the medium

By inspection of Equations 1-1 and 1-2, it is evident that the rate of diffusion will be faster for small molecules than for large molecules. In addition, diffusion rates are high at elevated temperatures, in the presence of large concentration gradients, and when occurring in a low-viscosity medium. Holding all other variables constant, the rate of diffusion is linearly related to the concentration gradient.

The Fick equation can also be applied to the diffusion of molecules across the plasma membrane. When applied to transport across a membrane, the diffusion coefficient (D) now incorporates the properties of the membrane and especially the ability of the molecule to diffuse through the membrane (i.e., the partition coefficient [β] of the molecule into the membrane). In general, the more lipid soluble the molecule, the larger the partition coefficient and thus the diffusion coefficient, and therefore the rate of diffusion is greater. In this situation, ΔC now represents the concentration gradient across the membrane, A is the membrane area, and ΔX is the thickness of the membrane.

A more useful equation for quantitating the diffusion of molecules across the membrane is

● **Equation 1-3**

$$J = -P(C_i - C_o)$$

where

J = flux or rate of diffusion across the membrane
P = permeability coefficient
C_i = concentration of the molecule inside the cell
C_o = concentration of the molecule outside the cell

This equation is derived from the Fick equation, and P incorporates D, ΔX, and A. P has units of velocity (e.g., cm/sec) and C has the unit mol/cm^3. Thus, the unit of flux is mol/cm^2/sec. Values of P can be obtained experimentally for any molecule and membrane.

As noted, the plasma membrane is an effective barrier to many biologically important molecules. Consequently, diffusion through the lipid phase of the plasma membrane is not an efficient process for movement of these molecules across the membrane. It has been estimated that for a cell 20 μm in diameter with a plasma membrane composed only of phospholipids, dissipation of a urea gradient imposed across the membrane would take about 8 minutes to occur. Similar gradients for glucose and amino acids would take approximately 14 hours to dissipate, whereas ion gradients would take years to dissipate.

The term diffusion is often used to describe the movement of some molecules across the cell membrane. However, it is clear that most biologically important molecules cross the membrane via specific membrane transport proteins (e.g., ion channels and solute carriers) and not by simple diffusion through the membrane. Despite the limitations of using diffusion to describe and understand the transport of many molecules across cell membranes, it is important for comprehending the exchange of gases across the airways of the lung (see Chapter 23), the movement of molecules between cells in the extracellular fluid, and the movement of molecules through the cytoplasm of the cell. For example, one of the physiological responses of skeletal muscle to exercise is the recruitment or opening of capillaries that are not patent at rest. This opening of previously closed capillaries increases capillary density and thereby reduces the diffusion distance between the capillary and the muscle fiber so that O_2 and cellular fuels (e.g., fatty acids and glucose) can be delivered more quickly to the contracting muscle fiber. It has been estimated that in resting muscle the average distance of a muscle fiber from a capillary is 40 μm. However, with exercise this distance decreases to 20 μm or less.

ELECTROCHEMICAL GRADIENT

The **electrochemical gradient** (also called the **electrochemical potential difference**) is used to quantitate the driving force acting on a molecule to cause it to move across a membrane. The electrochemical gradient for any molecule ($\Delta\mu_x$) is calculated as

● **Equation 1-4**

$$\Delta\mu_x = RT\ln\frac{[X]_i}{[X]_o} + z_xFV_m$$

where

R = gas constant
T = temperature in degrees Kelvin
ln = natural logarithm
$[X]_i$ = concentration of X inside the cell
$[X]_o$ = concentration of X outside the cell
z_x = valence of charged molecules
F = Faraday constant
V_m = membrane potential

The electrochemical gradient is a measure of the free energy available to carry out the useful work of transporting the molecule across the membrane. As can be seen, it has two components. One component represents the energy in the concentration gradient for X across the membrane **(chemical potential difference).** The second component **(electrical potential difference)** represents the energy associated with moving charged molecules (e.g., ions) across the membrane when a membrane potential exits (i.e., V_m ≠ 0 mV). Thus, for movement of glucose across a membrane, only the concentrations of glucose inside and outside the cell need be considered. However, move-

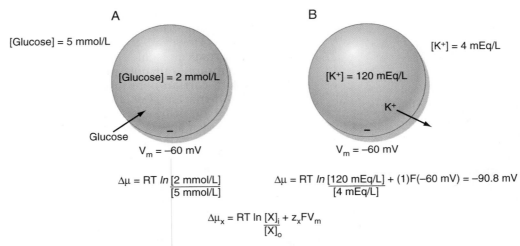

● **Figure 1-7.** Electrochemical gradients and cellular transport of molecules. **A,** Because glucose is uncharged, the electrochemical gradient is determined solely by the concentration gradient for glucose across the cell membrane. As shown, the glucose concentration gradient would be expected to drive glucose into the cell. **B,** Because K^+ is charged, the electrochemical gradient is determined by both the concentration gradient and the membrane voltage (V_m). The energy in the concentration gradient, determined from the Nernst equation, is 90.8 mV (driving K^+ out of the cell). The membrane voltage of −60 mV will drive K^+ into the cell. The electrochemical gradient, or the net driving force, is 30.8 mV, which will drive K^+ out of the cell.

ment of K^+ across the membrane, for example, would be determined by both the concentration of K^+ inside and outside the cell and the membrane voltage (Fig. 1-7).

Equation 1-4 can be used to derive the **Nernst equation** by considering the situation in which the molecule is at equilibrium across the membrane (i.e., $\Delta\mu = 0$).

● **Equation 1-5a**

$$0 = RT\,ln\frac{[X]_i}{[X]_o} + z_x F V_m$$

$$-RT\,ln\frac{[X]_i}{[X]_o} = z_x F V_m$$

$$V_m = -\frac{RT}{z_x F}\,ln\frac{[X]_i}{[X]_o}$$

Alternatively,

● **Equation 1-5b**

$$V_m = \frac{RT}{z_x F}\,ln\frac{[X]_o}{[X]_i}$$

The value of V_m calculated by the Nernst equation represents the equilibrium condition and is referred to as the **Nernst equilibrium potential (E_x).** It should be apparent that the Nernst equilibrium potential quantitates the energy in a concentration gradient and expresses that energy in millivolts. For example, for the cell depicted in Figure 1-7, *B,* the energy in the K^+ gradient (E_K) is 90.8 mV (which causes K^+ to move out of the cell). This is opposite and of greater magnitude than the energy in the membrane voltage ($V_m = -60$ mV), which will cause K^+ to enter the cell. As a

result, the electrochemical gradient is such that the net movement of K^+ across the membrane will be out of the cell. Another way to state this is that the net driving force for K^+ ($V_m - E_K$) is 30.8 mV (which drives K^+ out of the cell).

At body temperature (37°C) and by replacing the natural logarithm with a base 10 logarithm, the Nernst equation can be written as follows:

● **Equation 1-6a**

$$E_x = -\frac{61.5\,mV}{z_x}\,log\frac{[X]_i}{[X]_o}$$

or

● **Equation 1-6b**

$$E_x = \frac{61.5\,mV}{z_x}\,log\frac{[X]_o}{[X]_i}$$

These are the most common forms of the Nernst equation in use. By inspection of these equations it is apparent that for a univalent ion (e.g., Na^+, K^+, Cl^-), a 10-fold concentration gradient across the membrane is equivalent in energy to an electrical potential difference of 61.5 mV and a 100-fold gradient is equivalent to 123 mV. Similarly, for a divalent ion (e.g., Ca^{++}), a 10-fold concentration gradient is equivalent to a 30.7-mV electrical potential difference because z in the above equations is equal to 2.

Active and Passive Transport

When the net movement of a molecule across a membrane occurs in the direction predicted by the electrochemical gradient, the movement is termed **passive**

transport. Thus, for the examples given in Figure 1-7, movement of glucose into the cell and movement of K^+ out of the cell would be considered passive transport. Transport that is passive is sometimes referred to as either "downhill transport" or transport "with the electrochemical gradient." In contrast, if the net movement of a molecule across the membrane is opposite that predicted by the electrochemical gradient, the movement is termed **active transport.** Active transport is sometimes referred to as either "uphill transport" or transport "against the electrochemical gradient."

When considering the various classes of plasma membrane transport proteins, movement of H_2O through water channels is a passive process (see later), as is the movement of ions through ion channels and the transport of molecules via uniporters (e.g., transport of glucose via GLUT1). The ATPase-dependent transporters can use the energy in ATP to drive the active transport of molecules (e.g., Na^+,K^+-ATPase). Because the transport is directly coupled to the hydrolysis of ATP, it is referred to as **primary active transport.** Solute carriers that couple the movement of two or more molecules will often transport one or more molecules against their respective electrochemical gradient by using the energy in the electrochemical gradient of the other molecule or molecules to drive this transport. When this occurs, the molecule or molecules transported against their electrochemical gradient are said to be transported by **secondary active** mechanisms (Fig. 1-8).

OSMOSIS AND OSMOTIC PRESSURE

Movement of water across cell membranes occurs by the process of **osmosis.** The movement of water is passive, with the driving force for this movement being the osmotic pressure difference across the cell membrane. Figure 1-9 illustrates the concept of osmosis and measurement of the osmotic pressure of a solution.

Osmotic pressure is determined solely by the number of molecules in that solution. It is not dependent on such factors as the size of the molecules, their mass, or their chemical nature (e.g., valence). Osmotic pressure (π), measured in atmospheres (atm), is calculated by **van't Hoff's Law** as

● **Equation 1-7**

$$\pi = nCRT$$

where

n = number of dissociable particles per molecule
C = total solute concentration
R = gas constant
T = temperature in degrees Kelvin

● **Figure 1-8.** Examples of several membrane transporters illustrating primary active, passive, and secondary active transport. See text for details.

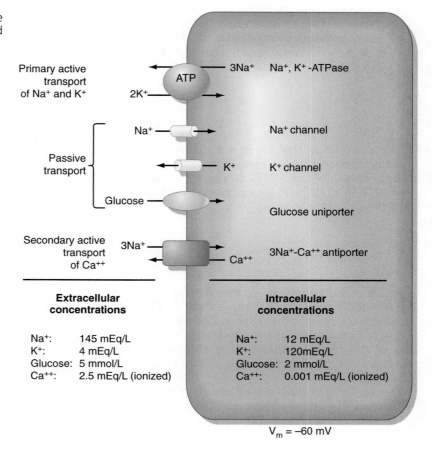

Extracellular concentrations

Na^+:	145 mEq/L
K^+:	4 mEq/L
Glucose:	5 mmol/L
Ca^{++}:	2.5 mEq/L (ionized)

Intracellular concentrations

Na^+:	12 mEq/L
K^+:	120mEq/L
Glucose:	2 mmol/L
Ca^{++}:	0.001 mEq/L (ionized)

$V_m = -60$ mV

● AT THE CELLULAR LEVEL

The epithelial cells that line the gastrointestinal tract (small intestine) and make up the proximal tubule of the kidney transport glucose. In the gastrointestinal tract, glucose is absorbed from ingested food. In the kidney, the proximal tubule reabsorbs the glucose that was filtered at the glomerulus and thereby prevents it from being lost in urine. Uptake of glucose into the epithelial cell from the lumen of the small intestine and from the lumen of the proximal tubule is a secondary active process involving the Na^+-glucose symporters SGLT1 and SGLT2. SGLT2 transports 1 glucose molecule with 1 Na^+ ion, and the energy in the electrochemical gradient for Na^+ (into the cell) is used to drive the secondary active uptake of glucose. Using the equation for calculating the electrochemical gradient, as rearranged below, and assuming a membrane potential (V_m) of −60 mV and a 10-fold $[Na^+]$ gradient across the membrane, an approximate 100-fold glucose gradient could be generated by SGLT2.

$$\frac{[\text{Glucose}]_i}{[\text{Glucose}]_o} = \frac{[Na^+]_o}{[Na^+]_i} \times 10^{-V_m/61.5mV}$$

Thus, if the intracellular [glucose] was 2 mmol/L; the cell could lower the luminal [glucose] to approximately 0.02 mmol/L. However, by increasing the number of Na^+ ions transported with glucose from 1 to 2, SGLT1 can generate a nearly 10,000-fold glucose gradient.

$$\frac{[\text{Glucose}]_i}{[\text{Glucose}]_o} = \left(\frac{[Na^+]_o}{[Na^+]_i}\right)^2 \times 10^{-2V_m/61.5mV}$$

Again, assuming an intracellular [glucose] of 2 mmol/L, SGLT1 could remove virtually all glucose from either the lumen of the small intestine or the lumen of the proximal tubule (i.e., luminal [glucose] of ≈0.0002 mmol/L).

For a molecule that does not dissociate in water, such as glucose or urea, a solution containing 1 mmol/L of these solutes at 37°C can exert an osmotic pressure of 2.54×10^{-2} atm as calculated by Equation 1-7 with the following values:

n = 1
C = 0.001 mol/L
R = 0.082 atm L/mol °K
T = 310°K

Because 1 atm equals 760 mm Hg at sea level, π for this solution can also be expressed as 19.3 mm Hg. Alternatively, osmotic pressure can be expressed in terms of osmolarity (see the following). Thus, regardless of the type of molecules, a solution containing 1 mmol/L of solute exerts an osmotic pressure of 1 mOsm/L.

For molecules that dissociate in a solution, n in Equation 1-7 will have a value other than 1. For example, a 150-mmol/L solution of NaCl has an osmolarity of approximately 300 mOsm/L because each molecule of

NaCl dissociates into an Na^+ and a Cl^- ion (i.e., n = 2).* If dissociation of a molecule into its component ions is not complete, n will not be an integer. Accordingly, the osmolarity of any solution can be calculated as

● **Equation 1-8**

Osmolarity = Concentration × Number
of dissociable particles

mOsm/L = mmol/L × Number of particles/molecule

Osmolarity versus Osmolality

The terms **osmolarity** and **osmolality** are frequently confused and incorrectly interchanged. Osmolarity refers to the osmotic pressure generated by the dissolved solute molecules in 1 L of solvent, whereas osmolality is the osmotic pressure generated by these solute molecules dissolved in 1 kg of solvent. For dilute solutions, the difference between osmolarity and osmolality is insignificant. Measurements of osmolarity are dependent on temperature because the volume of solvent varies with temperature (i.e., the volume is larger at higher temperatures). In contrast, osmolality, which is based on the mass of the solvent, is independent of temperature. For this reason, osmolality is the preferred term for biological systems and is used throughout this book. Osmolality has the units of Osm/kg H_2O. Because of the dilute nature of physiological solutions and because water is the solvent, osmolality is expressed as milliosmoles per kilogram water (mOsm/kg H_2O).

Table 1-4 shows the relationship between molecular weight, equivalence, and osmoles for a number of physiologically significant molecules.

Tonicity

The tonicity of a solution is related to the effect of the solution on the volume of a cell. Solutions that do not change the volume of a cell are said to be **isotonic.** A **hypotonic** solution causes a cell to swell, whereas a **hypertonic** solution causes a cell to shrink. Though related to osmolality, tonicity also takes into consideration the ability of the molecules in solution to cross the cell membrane.

Consider two solutions: a 300-mmol/L solution of sucrose and a 300-mmol/L solution of urea. Both solutions have an osmolality of 300 mOsm/kg H_2O and are therefore said to be **isosmotic** (i.e., they have the same osmolality). When red blood cells, which for the purpose of this example also have an intracellular fluid osmolality of 300 mOsm/kg H_2O, are placed in the two solutions, those in the sucrose solution maintain their normal volume, whereas those placed in urea swell and eventually burst. Thus, the sucrose solution is isotonic and the urea solution is hypotonic. The differential effect of these solutions on red cell volume is related to the permeability of the plasma membrane to sucrose and urea. The red cell membrane contains uniporters for urea. Thus, urea easily crosses the cell membrane (i.e., urea is permeable), driven by the con-

---

*NaCl does not completely dissociate in water. The value for n is 1.88 rather than 2. However, for simplicity the value of 2 is most often used.

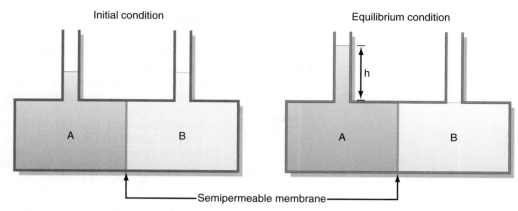

● Figure 1-9. Schematic representation of osmotic water movement and the generation of osmotic pressure. Compartment A and compartment B are separated by a semipermeable membrane (i.e., the membrane is highly permeable to water, but impermeable to solute). Compartment A contains a solute, whereas compartment B contains only distilled water. Over time, water will move by osmosis from compartment B to compartment A. (Note: This water movement is driven by the concentration gradient for water. Because of the presence of solute particles in compartment A, the concentration of water in compartment A is less than that in compartment B. Consequently, water moves across the semipermeable membrane from compartment B to compartment A down its gradient.) This will raise the level of fluid in compartment A and decrease the level in compartment B. At equilibrium, the hydrostatic pressure exerted by the column of water (h) will stop the movement of water from compartment B to compartment A. This pressure will be opposite and equal to the osmotic pressure exerted by the solute particles in compartment A. (Redrawn from Koeppen BM, Stanton BA: Renal Physiology, 4th ed. St. Louis, Mosby, 2006.)

● Table 1-4. Units of Measurement for Physiologically Significant Substances

Substance	Atomic/Molecular Weight	Equivalents/mol	Osmoles/mol
Na^+	23.0	1	1
K^+	39.1	1	1
Cl^-	35.4	1	1
HCO_3^-	61.0	1	1
Ca^{++}	40.1	2	1
Phosphate (P_i)	95.0	3	1
NH_4^+	18.0	1	1
NaCl	58.4	2*	2†
$CaCl_2$	111	4‡	3
Glucose	180		1
Urea	60		1

*One equivalent each from Na^+ and Cl^-.
†NaCl does not dissociate completely in solution. The actual osmoles/mol is 1.88. However, for simplicity, a value of 2 is often used.
‡Ca^{++} contributes two equivalents, as do the $2Cl^-$ ions.

centration gradient (i.e., extracellular [urea] > intracellular [urea]). In contrast, the red cell membrane does not contain sucrose transporters, and sucrose cannot enter the cell (i.e., sucrose is impermeable).

To exert osmotic pressure across a membrane, a molecule must not cross the membrane. Because the red cell membrane is impermeable to sucrose, it exerts an osmotic pressure opposite and equal to the osmotic pressure generated by the contents of the red cell (in this case 300 mOsm/kg H_2O). In contrast, urea is readily able to cross the red blood cell membrane, and it cannot exert an osmotic pressure to balance that generated by the intracellular solutes of the red blood cell. Consequently, sucrose is termed an **effective osmole,** whereas urea is an **ineffective osmole.**

To take into account the effect of a molecule's membrane permeability on osmotic pressure, it is necessary to rewrite Equation 1-7 as

● Equation 1-9

$$\pi = \sigma(nCRT)$$

where σ is the **reflection coefficient** or **osmotic coefficient** and is a measure of the relative ability of the molecule to cross the cell membrane.

For a molecule that can freely cross the cell membrane, such as urea in the aforementioned example, $\sigma = 0$, and no effective osmotic pressure is exerted (i.e., urea is an ineffective osmole for red blood cells). In contrast, $\sigma = 1$ for a solute that cannot cross the cell membrane (i.e., sucrose). Such a substance is said to

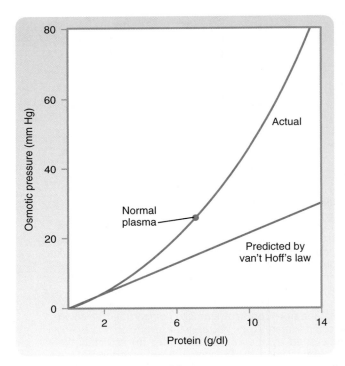

● **Figure 1-10.** Relationship between the concentration of plasma proteins in solution and the osmotic pressure (oncotic pressure) that they generate. Protein concentration is expressed as g/dl. Normal plasma protein concentration is indicated. Note how the actual pressure generated exceeds that predicted by van't Hoff's law. (Redrawn from Koeppen BM, Stanton BA: Renal Physiology, 4th ed. St. Louis, Mosby, 2006.)

be an effective osmole. Many molecules are neither completely able nor completely unable to cross cell membranes (i.e., $0 < \sigma < 1$), and they generate an osmotic pressure that is only a fraction of what is expected from the molecule's concentration in solution.

Oncotic Pressure

Oncotic pressure is the osmotic pressure generated by large molecules (especially proteins) in solution. As illustrated in Figure 1-10, the magnitude of the osmotic pressure generated by a solution of protein does not conform to van't Hoff's law. The cause of this anomalous relationship between protein concentration and osmotic pressure is not completely understood but appears to be related to the size and shape of the protein molecule. For example, the correlation to van't Hoff's law is more precise with small, globular proteins than with larger protein molecules.

The oncotic pressure exerted by proteins in human plasma has a normal value of approximately 26 to 28 mm Hg. Although this pressure appears to be small when considered in terms of osmotic pressure (28 mm Hg ≈ 1.4 mOsm/kg H_2O), it is an important force involved in fluid movement across capillaries (see Chapter 17).

The specific gravity of urine is sometimes measured in clinical settings and used to assess the urine-concentrating ability of the kidney. The specific gravity of urine varies in proportion to its osmolality. However, because specific gravity depends on both the number of molecules and their weight, the relationship between specific gravity and osmolality is not always predictable. For example, patients who have been injected with radiocontrast dye (molecular weight >500 g/mol) for x-ray studies can have high values of urine specific gravity (1.040 to 1.050) even though urine osmolality is similar to that of plasma (e.g., 300 mOsm/kg H_2O).

Specific Gravity

The total concentration of all molecules in a solution can also be measured as **specific gravity**. Specific gravity is defined as the weight of a volume of solution divided by the weight of an equal volume of distilled water. Thus, the specific gravity of distilled water is 1. Because biological fluids contain a number of different molecules, their specific gravities are greater than 1. For example, normal human plasma has a specific gravity in the range of 1.008 to 1.010.

■ KEY CONCEPTS

1. The plasma membrane is a lipid bilayer composed of phospholipids and cholesterol into which a wide range of proteins are embedded. One class of these membrane proteins (membrane transport proteins or transporters) is involved in the selective and regulated transport of molecules into and out of the cell. These transporters include water channels (aquaporins), ion channels, solute carriers, and ATP-dependent transporters.

2. Movement of molecules across the plasma membrane through ion channels via solute carriers is driven by chemical concentration gradients and electrical potential differences (charged molecules only). The electrochemical gradient is used to quantitate this driving force. ATP-dependent transporters use the energy in ATP to transport molecules across the membrane and often establish the chemical and electrical gradients that then drive the transport of other molecules through channels, or via solute carriers. Water movement through aquaporins is driven by an osmotic pressure difference across the membrane.

3. Transport across the membrane is classified as passive or active. Passive transport describes the movement of molecules as expected from the electrochemical gradient for that molecule. Active

transport represents transport against the electrochemical gradient. Active transport is further divided into primary active and secondary active transport. Primary active describes transport directly coupled to the hydrolysis of ATP (e.g., ATP-dependent transporters). Secondary active transport occurs with coupled solute carriers, where passive movement of one or more molecules drives the active transport of other molecules (e.g., Na^+-glucose symporter, Na^+-H^+ antiporter).

CHAPTER 2

Homeostasis of Body Fluids

Normal cellular function requires that the intracellular composition of ions, small molecules, water, pH, and a host of other substances be maintained within a narrow range. This is accomplished by the transport of many substances and water into and out of the cell with the use of membrane transport proteins as described in Chapter 1. In addition, each day food and water are ingested and waste products are excreted from the body. In a healthy individual this occurs without significant changes in either the volume of body fluids or their composition. Such maintenance of steady-state balance, where the volume and composition of body fluids remain constant despite the addition and elimination of water and solutes from the body, to a large degree reflects the function of epithelial cells. These cells, which constitute the interface between the internal environment of the body and the external world, maintain the volume and composition of the fluid bathing all cells (i.e., the **extracellular fluid [ECF]**) constant. The ECF, in turn, helps cell maintain a constant intracellular environment.

The ability of the body to maintain constant volume and composition of the **intracellular fluid (ICF)** and ECF is a complex process that involves all organ systems of the body. Transport by the epithelial cells of the gastrointestinal tract, kidneys, and lungs controls both the intake and excretion of numerous substances and water. The cardiovascular system delivers nutrients to and removes waste products from cells and tissues. Finally, the nervous and endocrine systems provide regulation and integration of these important functions.

To provide background for further study of the organ systems, this chapter presents an overview of the concept of steady-state balance, reviews the normal volume and composition of body fluids, and describes how cells maintain their intracellular composition and volume. Included is a presentation on how cells generate and maintain a membrane potential, which is fundamental to understanding the function of excitable cells (e.g., neurons and muscle cells). Finally, because epithelial cells are so central to the process of regulating the volume and composition of body fluids, the principles of solute and water transport by epithelial cells are reviewed.

CONCEPT OF STEADY-STATE BALANCE

The concept of steady-state balance can be illustrated by considering a river on which a dam is built to create an artificial lake. Each day, water enters the lake from the various streams and rivers that feed it. In addition, water is added by rain and snow. At the same time, water is lost through the spillways of the dam and by the process of evaporation. For the level of the lake to remain constant (i.e., steady-state balance), the rate at which water is added, regardless of the source, must be exactly matched by the amount of water lost, again by whichever route. Because the addition of water and loss by evaporation are not easily controlled, the only way to maintain the amount of the lake constant is to regulate the amount that is allowed through the spillways. For such a system to work, there must be a **"set point,"** or a determination of what the optimal level of water in the lake should be. There must also be some way to measure deviations from the set point, such as a measure of the depth of the lake. Finally, there must be a mechanism, or **"effector,"** that regulates the amount of water that leaves the lake through the spillway. In this example, the dam operator, who controls the spillways, is that effector.

For virtually every substance in the body, the amount or concentration of which must be maintained within a narrow range, there is a set point and mechanism for monitoring deviations from that set point and effector mechanisms to maintain amounts or concentrations of that substance within the body constant, or in steady-state balance.

In keeping with the dam and lake analogy, consider the maintenance of steady-state water balance in humans (see Chapter 34 for details). Each day various volumes of liquid are ingested, and water is produced through cellular metabolism. Importantly, the amount of water added to the body each day is not constant, although it can be regulated to a degree by the thirst mechanism. In addition, water is lost from the body via respiration, sweating, and feces. The amount of water lost by these routes also varies over time, depending on the respiratory rate, physical activity, ambient temperature, and the presence or absence of diarrhea. The only regulated route for excretion of water from the body is the kidneys. The body maintains steady-state water balance by ensuring that the amount of water added to the body each day is exactly balanced by the amount lost or excreted from the body.

The body monitors the amount of water that it contains through changes in the osmolality of ECF. When excess water is added to the body, the osmolality of ECF decreases. Conversely, when excess water is lost from the body, osmolality increases. Cells within the hypothalamus of the brain monitor changes in ECF osmolality around each person's genetically determined set point. When deviations from the set point occur, neural and hormonal signals are activated (i.e., effectors). For example, when ECF osmolality is increased, neural signals are sent to another region of the hypothalamus to stimulate the sensation of thirst. At the same time, antidiuretic hormone (ADH) is secreted from the posterior pituitary and acts on the kidneys to reduce the excretion of water. Thus, water intake is increased at the same time that its loss from the body is reduced, and the osmolality of ECF returns to its set point. When the osmolality of ECF is decreased, thirst is inhibited, as is the secretion of ADH. As a result, intake of water is reduced, and its excretion by the kidneys is increased. Again, these actions return the osmolality of ECF to the set point.

OVERVIEW OF THE INTRACELLULAR AND EXTRACELLULAR COMPARTMENTS

Definitions and Volumes of Body Fluid Compartments

Water makes up approximately 60% of the body's weight, with variability among individuals being a function of the amount of adipose tissue. Because the water content of adipose tissue is lower than that of other tissue, increased amounts of adipose tissue reduce the fraction of total body weight attributable to water. The percentage of body weight attributed to water also varies with age. In newborns it is approximately 75%. This decreases to the adult value of 60% by the age of 1 year.

As illustrated in Figure 2-1, **total body water** is distributed between two major compartments, which are divided by the cell membrane.* The **intracellular fluid** compartment is the larger compartment and contains approximately two thirds of total body water. The remaining third is contained in the **extracellular fluid** compartment. Expressed as percentages of body weight, the volumes of total body water, ICF, and ECF are

Total body water = 0.6 × Body weight
ICF   = 0.4 × Body weight
ECF   = 0.2 × Body weight

The ECF compartment is further subdivided into **interstitial fluid** and **plasma,** which are separated by the capillary wall. The interstitial fluid surrounds the cells in the various tissues of the body and accounts for three fourths of the ECF volume. ECF includes water contained within bone and dense connective tissue, as well as cerebrospinal fluid. Plasma represents the remaining fourth of ECF. Under some pathological conditions, additional fluid may accumulate in what is referred to as a "third space." Third-space col-

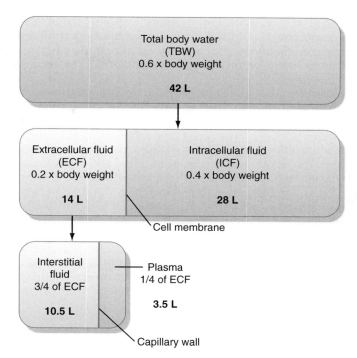

● **Figure 2-1.** Relationship between volumes of the various body fluid compartments. The actual values shown are for an individual weighing 70 kg. (Modified from Levy MN, Koeppen BM, Stanton BA: Berne & Levy's Principles of Physiology, 4th ed. St. Louis, Mosby, 2006.)

● **Table 2-1.**
Ionic Composition of a Typical Cell

	Extracellular Fluid	**Intracellular Fluid**
Na^+ (mEq/L)	135-147	10-15
K^+ (mEq/L)	3.5-5.0	120-150
Cl^- (mEq/L)	95-105	20-30
HCO_3^- (mEq/L)	22-28	12-16
Ca^{++} (mmol/L)*	2.1-2.8 (total) 1.1-1.4 (ionized)	≈10^{-7} (ionized)
P_i (mmol/L)*	1.0-1.4 (total)	
	0.5-0.7 (ionized)	0.5-0.7 (ionized)

*Ca^{++} and P_i ($H_2PO_4^-$/HPO_4^{-2}) are bound to proteins and other organic molecules. In addition, large amounts of Ca^{++} can be sequestered within cells. Large amounts of P_i are present in cells as part of organic molecules (e.g., ATP).

lections of fluid are part of the ECF and include, for example, the accumulation of fluid in the peritoneal cavity **(ascites)** of individuals with liver disease.

Composition of Body Fluid Compartments

Table 2-1 summarizes the composition of the ECF and ICF for a number of important ions and molecules. As discussed in detail later, the composition of ICF is maintained by the action of various specific membrane transport proteins. Principal among these transporters is Na^+,K^+-ATPase, which converts the energy in ATP into ion and electrical gradients, which in turn can be used to drive the transport of other ions and molecules.

---

*In these and all subsequent calculations, it is assumed that 1 L of fluid (e.g., ICF and ECF) has a mass of 1 kg. This allows conversion from measurements of body weight to volume of body fluids.

The composition of the plasma and interstitial fluid compartments of the ECF is similar because they are separated only by the capillary endothelium, a barrier that is freely permeable to ions and small molecules. The major difference between interstitial fluid and plasma is that the latter contains significantly more protein. Although this differential concentration of protein can affect the distribution of cations and anions between these two compartments by the Gibbs-Donnan effect (see later for details), this effect is small, and the ionic composition of interstitial fluid and plasma can be considered to be identical.

Because of its abundance in ECF, Na^+ (and its attendant anions, primarily Cl^- and HCO_3^-) is the major determinant of the osmolality of this compartment. Accordingly, a rough estimate of ECF osmolality can be obtained by simply doubling the sodium concentration $[Na^+]$. For example, if a blood sample is obtained from an individual and the $[Na^+]$ of plasma is 145 mEq/L, its osmolality can be estimated as

● **Equation 2-1**

Plasma osmolality = 2(Plasma $[Na^+]$) = 290 mOsm/kg H_2O

Because water is in osmotic equilibrium across the capillary endothelium and the plasma membrane of cells, measurement of plasma osmolality also provides a measure of the osmolality of the ECF and ICF.

Fluid Exchange between the ICF and ECF

Water moves freely and often rapidly between the various body fluid compartments. Two forces determine this movement: hydrostatic pressure and osmotic pressure. Hydrostatic pressure from pumping of the heart (and the effect of gravity on the column of blood in the vessel) and osmotic pressure exerted by plasma proteins (oncotic pressure) are important determinants of fluid movement across the capillary wall (see Chapter 17). By contrast, because hydrostatic pressure gradients are not present across the cell membrane, only osmotic pressure differences between ICF and ECF cause movement of fluid into and out of cells.

Osmotic pressure differences between ECF and ICF are responsible for movement of fluid between these compartments. Because the plasma membrane of cells contains water channels (aquaporins), water can easily cross the membrane. Hence, a change in the osmolality of either ICF or ECF results in rapid movement (i.e., minutes) of water between these compartments. Thus, except for transient changes, the ICF and ECF compartments are in osmotic equilibrium.

In contrast to water, the movement of ions across cell membranes is more variable from cell to cell and depends on the presence of specific membrane transport proteins (see later). Consequently, as a first approximation, fluid exchange between the ICF and ECF compartments can be analyzed by assuming that appreciable shifts of ions between the compartments do not occur.

A useful approach to understanding the movement of fluids between the ICF and the ECF is outlined in Figure 2-2. To illustrate this approach, consider what

● **Figure 2-2.** Principles for analysis of fluid shifts between ECF and ICF.

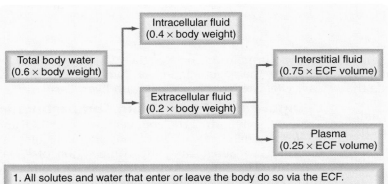

1. All solutes and water that enter or leave the body do so via the ECF.
2. The ICF and ECF are in osmotic equilibrium. Water moves between these compartments only when an osmotic pressure gradient exists.
3. Equilibration of ICF and ECF osmolality occurs primarily by shifts in water and not shifts in solute.

▶ **IN THE CLINIC**

Neurosurgical procedures and cerebrovascular accidents (strokes) often result in the accumulation of interstitial fluid in the brain (i.e., edema) and swelling of neurons. Because the brain is enclosed within the skull, edema can raise intracranial pressure and thereby disrupt neuronal function, eventually leading to coma and death. The blood-brain barrier, which separates the cerebrospinal fluid and brain interstitial fluid from blood, is freely permeable to water but not to most other substances. As a result, excess fluid in brain tissue can be removed by imposing an osmotic gradient across the blood-brain barrier. Mannitol can be used for this purpose. Mannitol is a sugar (molecular weight of 182 g/mol) that does not readily cross the blood-brain barrier and membranes of cells (neurons, as well as other cells in the body). Therefore, mannitol is an effective osmole, and intravenous infusion results in the movement of fluid from brain tissue by osmosis.

happens when solutions containing various amounts of NaCl are added to the ECF.*

Example 1: Addition of Isotonic NaCl to ECF

Addition of an isotonic NaCl solution (e.g., intravenous infusion of 0.9% NaCl, osmolality of ≈290 mOsm/kg H_2O)† to ECF increases the volume of this compartment by the volume of fluid administered. Because this fluid has the same osmolality as ECF and therefore also ICF, there will be no driving force for movement of fluid between these compartments, and the volume of ICF will be unchanged. Although Na^+ can cross cell membranes, it is effectively restricted to the ECF by the activity of Na^+,K^+-ATPase, which is present in the plasma membrane of all cells. Therefore, there is no net movement of the infused NaCl into the cells.

Example 2: Addition of Hypotonic NaCl to ECF

Addition of a hypotonic NaCl solution to ECF (e.g., intravenous infusion of 0.45% NaCl, osmolality of ≈145 mOsm/kg H_2O) decreases the osmolality of this fluid compartment and results in movement of water into the ICF. After osmotic equilibration, the osmolality of ICF and ECF is equal but lower than before the infusion, and the volume of each compartment is increased. The increase in ECF volume is greater than the increase in ICF volume.

Example 3: Addition of Hypertonic NaCl to ECF

Addition of a hypertonic NaCl solution to ECF (e.g., intravenous infusion of 3% NaCl, osmolality of ≈1000 mOsm/kg H_2O) increases the osmolality of this

▶ **IN THE CLINIC**

Fluid and electrolyte disorders are seen commonly in clinical practice (e.g., in patients with vomiting or diarrhea, or both). In most instances these disorders are self-limited, and correction of the disorder occurs without any need for intervention. However, more severe or prolonged disorders may require fluid replacement therapy. Such therapy may be administered orally with special electrolyte solutions, or intravenous fluid may be administered.

Intravenous solutions are available in many formulations. The type of fluid administered to a particular patient is dictated by the patient's need. For example, if an increase in the patient's vascular volume is necessary, a solution containing substances that do not readily cross the capillary wall is infused (e.g., 5% protein or dextran solutions). The oncotic pressure generated by the albumin molecules retains fluid in the vascular compartment and thereby expands its volume. Expansion of ECF is accomplished most often by using isotonic saline solutions (e.g., 0.9% NaCl or lactated Ringer's solution). As already noted, administration of an isotonic NaCl solution does not result in the development of an osmotic pressure gradient across the plasma membrane of cells. Therefore, the entire volume of the infused solution will remain in the ECF. Patients whose body fluids are hyperosmotic need hypotonic solutions. These solutions may be hypotonic NaCl (e.g., 0.45% NaCl or 5% dextrose in water, so-called D5W). Administration of D5W solution is equivalent to the infusion of distilled water because the dextrose is metabolized to CO_2 and water. Administration of these fluids increases the volume of both ICF and ECF. Finally, patients whose body fluids are hypotonic need hypertonic solutions. These are typically NaCl-containing solutions (e.g., 3% and 5% NaCl). These solutions expand the volume of ECF but decrease the volume of ICF. Other constituents, such as electrolytes (e.g., K^+) or drugs, can be added to intravenous solutions to tailor the therapy to the patient's fluid, electrolyte, and metabolic needs.

compartment and results in the movement of water out of cells. After osmotic equilibration, the osmolality of ECF and ICF will be equal but higher than before the infusion. The volume of ECF is increased, whereas that of ICF is decreased.

MAINTENANCE OF CELLULAR HOMEOSTASIS

Normal cellular function requires that the composition of ICF be tightly controlled. For example, the activity of some enzymes is dependent on pH. Therefore, intracellular pH must be regulated. The intracellular ionic composition is similarly held within a narrow range. This is necessary for establishment of the membrane potential, a cell property especially important

---

*Fluids are usually administered intravenously. When electrolyte solutions are infused by this route, there is rapid (i.e., minutes) equilibration between plasma and interstitial fluid because of the high permeability of the capillary wall to water and electrolytes. Thus, these fluids are essentially added to the entire ECF.

†A 0.9% NaCl solution (0.9 g NaCl/100 mL) contains 154 mmol/L of NaCl. Because NaCl does not dissociate completely in solution (i.e., 1.88 Osm/mol), the osmolality of this solution is 290 mOsm/kg H_2O, which is very similar to that of normal ECF.

for the normal function of excitable cells (e.g., neurons and muscle cells) and for intracellular signaling (e.g., intracellular [Ca^{++}]—see Chapter 3). Finally, the volume of cells must be maintained because shrinking or swelling of cells can lead to cell damage or death. Regulation of intracellular composition and cell volume is accomplished through the activity of specific transporters in the plasma membrane of cells. This section reviews the mechanisms by which cells maintain their intracellular ionic environment and membrane potential and control their volume.

Ionic Composition of Cells

The intracellular ionic composition of cells varies from tissue to tissue. For example, the intracellular composition of neurons is different from that of muscle cells, which differs from that of blood cells. Nevertheless, there are similar patterns, and these are presented in Table 2-1. When compared with ECF, ICF is characterized by a low [Na$^+$] and a high [K$^+$]. This is the result of the activity of Na$^+$,K$^+$-ATPase, which transports 3 Na$^+$ ions out of the cell and 2 K$^+$ ions into the cell for each molecule of ATP hydrolyzed. As will be discussed, the activity of Na$^+$,K$^+$-ATPase is not only important for establishing the cellular Na$^+$ and K$^+$ gradients but is also involved in indirectly determining the cellular gradients for many other ions and molecules. Because Na$^+$,K$^+$-ATPase transports three cations out of the cell in exchange for two cations, it is electrogenic and thus contributes to the establishment of membrane voltage (cell interior negative). However, Na$^+$,K$^+$-ATPase typically contributes only a few millivolts to the membrane potential. More importantly, it is the leakage of K$^+$ out of the cell through K$^+$-selective channels that is a major determinant of membrane voltage (see later). Thus, Na$^+$,K$^+$-ATPase converts the energy in ATP into ion gradients (i.e., Na$^+$ and K$^+$) and a voltage gradient (i.e., membrane potential) as a result of leakage of K$^+$ out of the cell driven by the K$^+$ concentration gradient across the membrane ([K$^+$]$_i$ > [K$^+$]$_o$).

The Na$^+$,K$^+$-ATPase–generated ion and electrical gradients are used to drive the transport of other ions and molecules into or out of the cell (Fig. 2-3). For example, as described in Chapter 1, a number of solute carriers couple the transport of Na$^+$ to that of other ions or molecules. The Na$^+$-glucose and Na$^+$–amino acid symporters use the energy in the Na$^+$ electrochemical gradient, directed to bring Na$^+$ into the cell, to drive the secondary active cellular uptake of glucose and amino acids. Similarly, the inwardly directed Na$^+$ gradient drives the secondary active extrusion of H$^+$ from the cell and thus contributes to the maintenance of intracellular pH. The 3Na$^+$-1Ca^{++} antiporter, along with plasma membrane Ca^{++}-ATPase, extrudes Ca^{++} from the cell and thus contributes to maintenance of a low intracellular [Ca^{++}].* Finally, the membrane voltage drives Cl$^-$ out of the cell through Cl$^-$-selective

---

*In muscle cells, where contraction is regulated by the intracellular [Ca^{++}], maintenance of a low intracellular [Ca^{++}] during the relaxed state involves the activity of not only the plasma membrane 3Na$^+$-1Ca^{++} antiporter and Ca^{++}-ATPase but also Ca^{++}-ATPase located in the smooth endoplasmic reticulum (see Chapters 12 to 14). For simplicity Ca^{++}-ATPase refers to the Ca^{++}-H$^+$-ATPase.

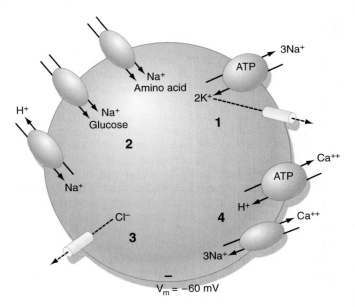

● **Figure 2-3.** Cell model depicting how cellular gradients and the membrane potential (V$_m$) are established. (1) Na$^+$,K$^+$-ATPase decreases intracellular [Na$^+$] and increases intracellular [K$^+$]. Some K$^+$ exits the cell via K$^+$-selective channels and generates the V$_m$ (cell interior negative). (2) The energy in the Na$^+$ electrochemical gradient drives the transport of other ions and molecules via the use of various solute carriers. (3) The V$_m$ drives Cl$^-$ out of the cell through Cl$^-$-selective channels. (4) Ca^{++}-H$^+$-ATPase and the 3Na$^+$-1Ca^{++} antiporter maintain the low intracellular [Ca^{++}].

channels, thus lowering the intracellular concentration below that of the ECF.

Membrane Potential

As described earlier, the Na$^+$,K$^+$-ATPase and K$^+$-selective channels in the plasma membrane are important determinants of the membrane potential (V$_m$) of the cell. For all cells within the body, the resting membrane potential is oriented with the interior of the cell electrically negative with respect to ECF. However, the magnitude of V$_m$ can vary widely.

To understand what determines the magnitude of V$_m$ it is important to recognize that any transporter that transfers charge across the membrane has the potential to influence V$_m$. Such transporters are said to be **electrogenic.** As might be expected, the contribution of various electrogenic transporters to V$_m$ is highly variable from cell to cell. For example, Na$^+$,K$^+$-ATPase transfers one net positive charge across the membrane. However, the direct contribution of Na$^+$,K$^+$-ATPase to the V$_m$ of most cells is only a few millivolts at the most. Similarly, the contribution of other electrogenic transporters, such as the 3Na$^+$-1Ca^{++} antiporter and the Na$^+$-glucose symporter, is minimal. The major determinants of V$_m$ are ion channels. The type (i.e., selectivity), number, and activity (i.e., gating) of these channels determine the magnitude of V$_m$. As described in Chapter 5, rapid changes in ion channel activity underlie the action potential in neurons and other excitable cells such as skeletal and cardiac muscle (see Chapters 12 and 13).

As ions move across the membrane through a channel, they generate a current. As described in Chapter 1, this current can be measured, even at the level of a single channel. By convention, the current generated by the movement of cations into the cell or the movement of anions out of the cell is defined as negative current. Conversely, the movement of cations out of the cell or the movement of anions into the cell is defined as positive current. Also by convention, the magnitude of V_m is expressed with respect to the outside of the cell. Thus, for a cell with a V_m of −80 mV, the interior of the cell is electrically negative with respect to the outside of the cell.

The current carried by ions moving through a channel depends on the driving force for that ion and the conductance of the channel. As described in Chapter 1, the driving force is determined by the energy in the concentration gradient for the ion across the membrane, as calculated by the Nernst equation (E_i), and by V_m.

● **Equation 2-2**

$$\text{Driving force} = V_m - E_i$$

Thus, as defined by **Ohm's law,** the ion current through the channel (I_i) is determined as follows:

● **Equation 2-3**

$$I_i = (V_m - E_i) \times g_i$$

where g_i is the conductance of the channel. For a cell, the conductance of the membrane to a particular ion (g_i) is determined by the number of ion channels in the membrane and the amount of time that each channel is in the open state.

As illustrated in Figure 2-4, V_m is the voltage at which there is no net ion flow into or out of the cell. Thus, for a cell having ion channels selective for Na^+, K^+, and Cl^-,

● **Equation 2-4**

$$I_{Na^+} + I_{K^+} + I_{Cl^-} = 0$$

or

● **Equation 2-5**

$$[(V_m - E_{Na^+}) \times G_{Na^+}] + [(V_m - E_{K^+}) \times G_{K^+}] + [(V_m - E_{Cl^-}) \times G_{Cl^-}] = 0$$

Solving for V_m,

● **Equation 2-6**

$$V_m = E_{Na^+}\frac{G_{Na}}{\Sigma G} + E_{K^+}\frac{G_K}{\Sigma G} + E_{Cl^-}\frac{G_{Cl}}{\Sigma G}$$

where $\Sigma G = G_{Na^+} + G_{K^+} + G_{Cl^-}$

Inspection of Equation 2-6, which is often called the **chord conductance equation,** reveals that V_m will be close to the Nernst potential of the ion to which the membrane has the highest conductance. In Figure 2-4, 80% of the membrane conductance is attributable to K^+; as a result, V_m is close to the Nernst potential for K^+ (E_{K^+}). For most cells at rest, the membrane has high conductance for K^+, and thus V_m approximates E_{K^+}. Moreover, V_m will be greatly influenced by the magnitude of E_{K^+}, which in turn will be greatly influenced by

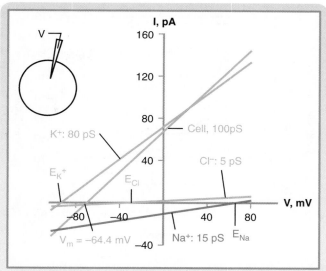

	Intracellular [ ] mEq/L	Extracellular [ ] mEq/L	Nernst potential E_i, mV
Na^+	12	145	66.6
K^+	120	4	−90.8
Cl^-	30	105	−33.5

● **Figure 2-4.** Current-voltage relationship of a hypothetical cell containing Na^+-, K^+-, and Cl^--selective channels. The current-voltage relationship for each ion is shown, as is the relationship for the whole cell. Because 80% of cell conductance is due to K^+, the resting membrane voltage (V_m) of −64.4 mV is close to that of the Nernst equilibrium potential for K^+.

▶ IN THE CLINIC

Changes in extracellular $[K^+]$ can have important effects on excitable cells, especially the heart. A decrease in extracellular $[K^+]$ **(hypokalemia)** hyperpolarizes the V_m of cardiac myocytes and in so doing makes it more difficult to initiate an action potential because a larger depolarizing current is needed to reach threshold (see Chapter 16). If severe, hypokalemia can lead to cardiac arrhythmias and eventually the heart can stop contracting **(asystole).** An increase in extracellular $[K^+]$ **(hyperkalemia)** can be equally deleterious to cardiac function. With hyperkalemia, V_m is depolarized, thus making it easier to initiate an action potential. However, as depolarization of V_m progresses, Na^+ channels, the opening of which initiates the action potential, become inactivated. When this occurs, cardiac arrhythmias develop, and as with hypokalemia, the heart can stop contracting.

changes in $[K^+]$ of the ECF. For example, if intracellular $[K^+]$ is 120 mEq/L and extracellular $[K^+]$ is 4 mEq/L, E_{K^+} has a value of −90.8 mV. If extracellular $[K^+]$ is increased to 7 mEq/L, E_{K^+} would be −79.9 mV. This change in E_{K^+} will **depolarize** V_m (i.e., V_m is less negative). Conversely, if extracellular $[K^+]$ is decreased to 2 mEq/L,

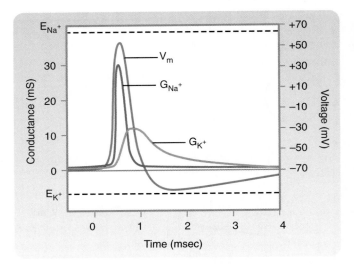

● **Figure 2-5.** Nerve action potential showing the changes in Na^+ (G_{Na^+}) and K^+ (G_{K^+}) conductance and membrane potential (V_m). At rest, the membrane has high K^+ conductance and V_m is near the Nernst equilibrium potential for K^+ (E_{K^+}). With initiation of the action potential there is a large increase in Na^+ conductance of the membrane, and V_m approaches the Nernst potential for Na^+ (E_{Na^+}). The increase in Na^+ conductance is transient, and K^+ conductance then increases above its value before the action potential. This hyperpolarizes the cell as V_m approaches E_{K^+}. As K^+ conductance returns to its baseline value, V_m returns to its resting value of -70 mV. (Modified from Levy MN, Koeppen BM, Stanton BA: Berne & Levy's Principles of Physiology, 4th ed. St. Louis, Mosby, 2006.)

E_{K^+} becomes -109.4 mV, and the V_m **hyperpolarizes** (i.e., V_m is more negative).

Equation 2-6 also defines the limits for the membrane potential. Again looking at the example depicted in Figure 2-4, it is apparent that V_m cannot be more negative than E_{K^+} (-90.8 mV), as would be the case if the membrane were conductive only to K^+. Conversely, V_m could not be more positive than E_{Na^+} (66.6 mV), a condition met if the membrane were conductive only to Na^+. The dependence of V_m on conductance of the membrane to specific ions is the basis by which action potentials in excitable cells are generated (Fig. 2-5). In all excitable cells the membrane at rest is predominantly conductive to K^+, and thus V_m is near E_{K^+}. When an action potential is initiated, Na^+ channels open and the membrane is now predominantly conductive to Na^+. As a result, V_m now approaches E_{Na^+}. The generation of action potentials is discussed in more detail in Chapter 5.

Regulation of Cell Volume

As already noted, changes in cell volume can lead to cell damage and death. Consequently, cells have developed mechanisms to regulate their volume. Most cells are highly permeable to water because of the presence of aquaporins in their plasma membranes. As discussed in Chapter 1, the osmotic pressure gradients across the cell membrane that are generated by effective osmoles will cause water to move either into or out of the cell and result in changes in cell volume.

AT THE CELLULAR LEVEL

Establishment of V_m requires separation of charge across the plasma membrane. However, the number of ions that must move across the membrane is a tiny fraction of the total number of ions in the cell. For example, consider a spherical cell with a diameter of 20 μm and a V_m of -80 mV. Furthermore, assume that the -80 mV is the result of K^+ diffusing out of the cell and that intracellular [K^+] is 120 mEq/L. The amount of K^+ that would have to diffuse out of the cell to establish the -80-mV V_m is then calculated as follows.

First, the charge separation across the membrane needs to be calculated. This is done by knowing that the plasma membrane behaves electrically like a capacitor, the capacitance (C) of which is approximately 1 microfarad/cm^2 (1 μF/cm^2), and

$$C = Q/V_m$$

where Q is charge and has the units of coulombs. Given that the surface area of the cell is $4\pi r^2$, or 1.26×10^{-5} cm^2, the capacitance of the cell is calculated as

$$1 \times 10^{-6}\ F/cm^2 \times 1.26 \times 10^{-5}\ cm^2 = 1.26 \times 10^{-11}\ F$$

Thus, the charge separation across the membrane is calculated as

$$Q = C \times V_m = 1.26 \times 10^{-11}\ F \times 0.08\ volts$$
$$= 1.01 \times 10^{-12}\ coulombs$$

Because 1 mol of K^+ contains 96,480 coulombs, the amount of K^+ that had to diffuse across the membrane to establish the V_m of -80 mV is

$$\frac{1.01 \times 10^{-12}}{96,480\ coulombs/mol} = 1.05 \times 10^{-17}\ mol\ of\ K^+$$

With a cell volume of 4.19×10^{-12} L (volume = $4\pi r^3/3$) and an intracellular [K^+] of 120 mEq/L, the total intracellular [K^+] is

$$4.19 \times 10^{-12} \times 0.12\ mol/L = 5.03 \times 10^{-13}\ mol$$

Thus, the diffusion of 1.05×10^{-17} mol of K^+ out of the cell represents only a 0.002% change in intracellular [K^+]:

$$\frac{1.05 \times 10^{-17}\ mol}{5.03 \times 10^{-13}\ mol} \approx 0.002\%$$

Thus, the intracellular composition of the cell is not appreciably altered by diffusion of K^+ out of the cell.

Thus, cells swell when in hypotonic solutions and shrink when placed in hypertonic solutions (see later). However, even when a cell is placed in an isotonic solution, maintenance of cell volume is an active process requiring the expenditure of ATP and specifically the activity of Na^+,K^+-ATPase.

Isotonic Cell Volume Regulation

The importance of Na^+,K^+-ATPase in isotonic regulation of cell volume can be appreciated by the observation that red blood cells swell when chilled (i.e., reduced ATP synthesis) or when Na^+,K^+-ATPase is inhibited by cardiac glycosides (e.g., ouabain). The necessity for energy expenditure to maintain cell volume in an isotonic solution is a result of the effect of intracellular proteins on the distribution of ions across the plasma membrane, the so-called **Gibbs-Donnan** effect (Fig. 2-6).

The Gibbs-Donnan effect occurs when a membrane separating two solutions is permeable to some but not all the molecules in solution. As noted previously, this effect accounts for the small differences in the ionic composition of plasma versus interstitial fluid. In this case, the capillary endothelium represents the membrane, and the plasma proteins are the molecules whose permeability across the capillary is restricted. For cells, the membrane is the plasma membrane, and the impermeant molecules are the intracellular proteins and organic molecules.

As depicted in Figure 2-6, the presence of impermeant molecules (e.g., protein) in one compartment results over time in the accumulation of permeable molecules/ions in the same compartment. This increases the number of osmotically active particles in the compartment containing the impermeant anions, which in turn increases osmotic pressure, and water enters the compartment. For cells, the Gibbs-Donnan effect would increase the number of osmotically active

particles in the cell and result in cell swelling. However, the activity of Na^+,K^+-ATPase counteracts the Gibbs-Donnan effect by actively extruding cations (3 Na^+ ions are extruded while 2 K^+ ions are brought into the cell). In addition, the K^+ gradient established by Na^+,K^+-ATPase allows for development of the V_m (cell interior negative), which in turn drives Cl^- out of the cell. Thus, through the activity of Na^+,K^+-ATPase the number of intracellular osmotically active particles is reduced from what would occur as a result of the Gibbs-Donnan effect, and cell volume is maintained in isotonic solutions.

Nonisotonic Cell Volume Regulation

Most cells throughout the body are bathed with isotonic ECF, the composition of which is tightly regulated. However, certain regions within the body are not isotonic (e.g., the medulla of the kidney), and with disorders in water balance, the ECF can become either hypotonic or hypertonic. When this occurs, cells will either swell or shrink. Because cell swelling or shrinkage can result in cell damage or death, many cells have mechanisms that limit the degree to which cell volume changes. These mechanisms are particularly important for neurons, where swelling within the confined space of the skull can lead to serious neurological damage.

In general, when a cell is exposed to nonisotonic ECF volume, regulatory responses are activated within seconds to minutes to restore cell volume (Fig. 2-7). In the case of cell swelling, a **regulatory volume decrease (RVD)** response transports osmotically active particles (osmolytes) out of the cell and reduces intracellular osmotic pressure, thereby restoring cell volume to normal. Conversely with cell shrinking, a **regulatory volume increase (RVI)** response transports osmolytes into the cell and raises intracellular osmotic

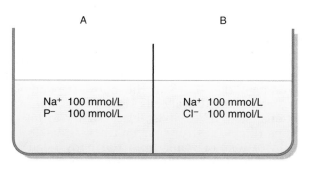

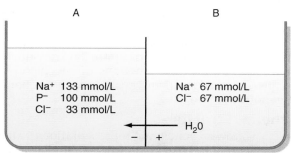

● **Figure 2-6.** The Gibbs-Donnan effect. **Top panel,** Two solutions are separated by a membrane that is permeable to Na^+, Cl^-, and H_2O, but not permeable to protein (P^-). The osmolality of solution A is identical to that of solution B. **Bottom panel,** Cl^- diffuses from solution B to A down its concentration gradient. This causes solution A to become electrically negative with respect to solution B. This membrane voltage then drives the diffusion of Na^+ from solution B to A. The accumulation of additional Na^+ and Cl^- in solution A increases its osmolality and causes water to flow from B to A.

IN THE CLINIC

The ECF of individuals with disorders in water balance may be either hypotonic (positive water balance) or hypertonic (negative water balance). With long-standing positive water balance, for example, as often occurs in individuals with inappropriate secretion of ADH (see Chapter 34), the neurons and glial cells in the brain reduce intracellular osmolytes to minimize cell swelling. If the disturbed water balance is corrected too quickly, the reduced osmolytes within the neurons and glial cells lead to shrinking and damage of the cell. Damage to the glial cells that synthesize myelin within the brain can result in demyelination. This demyelinization response, termed osmotic demyelinization syndrome, can affect any of the white matter of the brain, but especially regions of the pons. These effects are often irreversible. Thus, correction of disorders in water balance is usually accomplished slowly to avoid neurological complications.

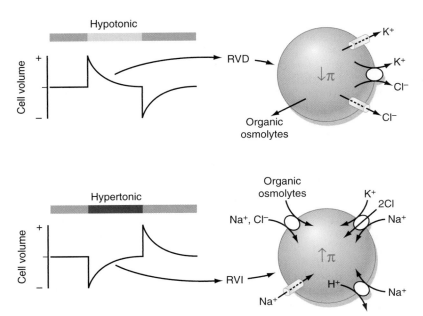

● **Figure 2-7.** Volume regulation of cells in hypotonic and hypertonic media. **Top panel,** When cells are exposed to a hypotonic medium, they swell and then undergo a regulatory volume decrease (RVD). The RVD involves loss of KCl and organic osmolytes from the cell. The reduction in cellular KCl and organic osmolytes decreases intracellular osmotic pressure, water leaves the cell, and the cell returns to near its original volume. **Lower panel,** When cells are exposed to a hypertonic medium, they shrink and then undergo a regulatory volume increase (RVI). During the RVI NaCl and organic osmolytes enter the cell. Na^+,K^+-ATPAse (not depicted) exchanges Na^+ for K^+, so the KCl content of the cell is increased. The increase in cellular KCl and organic osmolytes increases intracellular osmotic pressure and brings water back into the cell, and the cell returns to near its original volume.

pressure, thereby restoring cell volume to normal. These osmolytes include ions and organic molecules such as polyols (sorbitol and myoinositol), methylamines (glycerophosphorylcholine and betaine), and some amino acids (taurine, glutamate, and β-alanine). If exposed to the nonisotonic ECF for an extended period, the cell alters intracellular levels of the organic osmolytes through metabolic processes.

The RVI response results in rapid uptake of NaCl and a number of organic osmolytes. With cell shrinking there is activation of the Na^+-H^+ antiporter (NHE-1), the $1Na^+,1K^+,2Cl^-$ symporter (NKCC1), and a number of cation-selective channels that together bring NaCl into the cell. Na^+,K^+-ATPase then extrudes the Na^+ in exchange for K^+, so ultimately the KCl content of the cell is increased. Several organic osmolyte transporters are also activated by cell shrinkage. These include a $3Na^+,1Cl^-$-taurine symporter, a $3Na^+,2Cl^-$-betaine symporter, a $2Na^+$-myoinositol symporter, and an Na^+–amino acid symporter. These transporters use the energy in the Na^+ and Cl^- gradients to drive the secondary active uptake of these organic osmolytes.

The RVD response results in the loss of KCl and organic osmolytes from the cell. Loss of KCl occurs through the activation of a wide range of K^+-selective, Cl^--selective, and anion channels (the specific channels involved vary depending on the cell), as well as by activation of K^+-Cl^- symporters. Some of the organic osmolytes appear to leave the cell via anion channels (e.g., volume-sensitive organic osmolyte anion channels—VSOAC).

There are several mechanisms involved in activation of these various transporters during the volume regulatory responses. Changes in cell size appear to be monitored by the cytoskeleton, by changes in macromolecular crowding and ionic strength of the cytoplasm, and by channels whose gating is influenced, either directly or indirectly, by stretching of the plasma membrane (e.g., stretch-activated cation channels). A number of second messenger systems may also be involved in these responses (e.g., calmodulin, protein kinase A, and protein kinase C), but the precise mechanisms have not been completely defined.

PRINCIPLES OF EPITHELIAL TRANSPORT

Epithelial cells are arranged in sheets and provide the interface between the external world and the internal environment (i.e., ECF) of the body. Depending on their location, epithelial cells serve several important functions, such as establishing a barrier to microorganisms (lungs, gastrointestinal tract, and skin), prevention of loss of water from the body (skin), and maintenance of a constant internal environment (lungs, gastrointestinal tract, and kidneys). This latter function is a result of the ability of epithelial cells to carry out regulated vectorial transport (i.e., transport from one side of the epithelial cell to the opposite side). In this section the principles of epithelial transport are reviewed. The transport functions of specific epithelial cells are discussed in the appropriate chapters throughout the book.

Epithelial Structure

Figure 2-8 shows a schematic representation of an epithelial cell. The free surface of the epithelial layer is referred to as the apical membrane. It is in contact with the external environment (e.g., air within the alveoli and larger airways of the lung and the contents of the gastrointestinal tract) or with the ECF (e.g., glomerular filtrate in the nephrons of the kidneys and secretions of the ducts of the pancreas or sweat glands). The basal side of the epithelium rests on a basal lamina, which is secreted by the epithelial cells, and this in turn is attached to the underlying connective tissue.

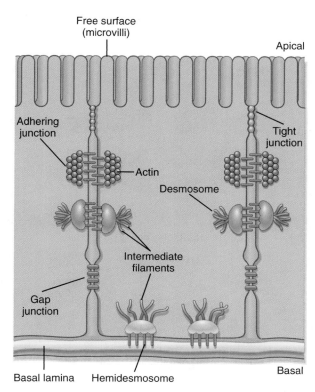

Free surface
(microvilli)

Apical

Adhering
junction

Tight
junction

Actin

Desmosome

Intermediate
filaments

Gap
junction

Basal lamina   Hemidesmosome

Basal

● **Figure 2-8.** Schematic of an epithelial cell illustrating the various adhering junctions. The tight junction separates the apical membrane from the basolateral membrane (see text for details).

AT THE CELLULAR LEVEL

Tight junctions (also called **zonula occludens**) are composed of linear arrays of several integral membrane proteins, including **occludins, claudins,** and several members of the immunoglobulin superfamily. The tight junction complex allows selective diffusion of ions or water, or both, between cells. Junctional proteins (e.g., occludins and claudins) are transmembrane proteins that span the membrane of one cell and link to the extracellular portion of the same molecule in the adjacent cell. Cytoplasmic linker proteins (e.g., ZO-1, ZO-2, and ZO-3) then link the membrane-spanning proteins to the cytoskeleton of the cell. Of these junctional proteins, claudins appear to be important in determining the permeability characteristics of the tight junction. For example, claudin-16 is critical for determining the permeability of the tight junctions to divalent cations in the thick ascending limb of Henle's loop in the kidney. Claudin-4 has been shown in cultured kidney cells to control the permeability of the tight junction to Na^+, whereas claudin-15 determines whether a tight junction is permeable to cations or anions. Thus, the permeability characteristics of the tight junction are determined, at least in part, by the specific claudins expressed by the cells.

Epithelial cells are connected to one another and to the underlying connective tissue by a number of specialized junctions (Fig. 2-8). The **adhering junction, desmosomes,** and **hemidesmosomes** provide mechanical adhesion by linking the cytoskeleton of adjacent cells together. The **gap junction** and **tight junction** play important physiological roles. Gap junctions provide low-resistance connections between cells.* The functional unit of the gap junction is the **connexon.** A connexon is composed of six integral membrane protein subunits called **connexins.** A connexon in one cell is aligned with the connexon in the adjacent cell to form a channel. The channel may be gated and, when open, allows the movement of ions and small molecules between the cells. Because of their low electrical resistance, they effectively couple one cell to the adjacent cell electrically. The tight junction constitutes a pathway for the movement of molecules from one side of the epithelium to the other. This paracellular pathway, as it is called, is described in detail later.

The apical surface of epithelial cells may have specific structural features. One such feature is **microvilli** (Fig. 2-8). Microvilli are small (typically 1 to 2 μm in length), nonmotile projections of the apical plasma membrane that serve to increase surface area. They are commonly seen on cells that must transport large quantities of ions, water, and molecules (e.g., epithelial cells lining the small intestine and cells of the renal proximal tubule). The core of microvilli is composed of actin filaments and a number of accessory proteins (e.g., villin, fimbrin, fascin, and myosin1). This actin core is connected to the cytoskeleton of the cell via the terminal web (a network of actin fibers at the base of the microvilli) and provides structural support for the microvilli. Another surface feature is stereocilia. Stereocilia are long (3 to 5 μm), nonmotile membrane projections that, like microvilli, increase the surface area of the apical membrane. They are found in the epididymis of the testis and the hair cells of the inner ear. Their core contains actin filaments and the accessory proteins erzin and fimbrin. A third apical membrane feature is **cilia.** Cilia may be either motile or nonmotile. Motile cilia contain a microtubule core arranged in a characteristic 9+2 pattern (nine pairs of microtubules around the circumference of the cilium and one pair of microtubules in the center). Dynein is the molecular motor that drives the movement of cilia. Cilia are characteristic features of the epithelial cells that line the respiratory tract. They "beat" in a synchronized manner and serve to transport mucus and inhaled particulates out of the lung, a process termed **mucociliary transport** (see Chapter 25). Nonmotile cilia, also called primary cilia, serve as mechanoreceptors and are involved in determining the left-right asymmetry of organs during embryological development, as well as sensing the flow rate of tubular fluid

*Gap junctions are not limited to epithelial cells. A number of other cells also express this junction (e.g., cardiac myocytes and smooth muscle cells).

in the nephron of the kidneys (see Chapter 33). Only a single primary cilium is found in the apical membrane of the cell. It has a microtubule core (9+0 arrangement) and lacks a molecular motor protein.

The tight junction effectively divides the plasma membrane of epithelial cells into two domains: an apical surface and a basal surface. Because the tight junction is near the apical pole of the cell, the lateral surface of the cell is continuous with the basal surface. Consequently, the term **basolateral membrane** is often used when referring to this surface domain of the epithelial cell. The basolateral membrane of many epithelial cells is folded or invaginated. This is especially so for epithelial cells that have high transport rates. These invaginations serve to increase the membrane's surface area to accommodate the large number of membrane transporters (e.g., Na^+,K^+-ATPase) needed in the membrane.

Vectorial Transport

Because the tight junction divides the plasma membrane into two domains (i.e., apical and basolateral), epithelial cells are capable of vectorial transport, whereby an ion or molecule can be transported from one side of the epithelial sheet to the opposite side (Fig. 2-9). The act of vectorial transport requires that specific membrane transport proteins be targeted to and remain in one or the other of the membrane domains. In the example shown in Figure 2-9, the Na^+ channel is present only in the apical membrane, whereas Na^+,K^+-ATPase and the K^+ channel are confined to the basolateral membrane. The operation of Na^+,K^+-ATPase and leakage of K^+ out of the cell across the basolateral membrane set up a large electrochemical gradient for Na^+ to enter the cell across the apical membrane through the Na^+ channel (intracellular $[Na^+]$ < extracellular $[Na^+]$ and V_m is oriented cell interior negative). The Na^+ is then pumped out of the cell by Na^+,K^+-ATPase, and vectorial transport from the apical side of the epithelium to the basolateral side of the epithelium occurs. Transport from the apical side to the basolateral side of an epithelium is termed **absorption** or **reabsorption.** For example, uptake of nutrients from the lumen of the gastrointestinal tract is termed absorption, and transport of NaCl and water from the lumen of renal nephrons is termed reabsorption. Transport from the basolateral side of the epithelium to the apical side is termed **secretion.**

As noted previously, Na^+,K^+-ATPase and K^+-selective channels play an important role in establishing cellular ion gradients for Na^+ and K^+ and generating V_m. In all epithelial cells, except the choroid plexus,* Na^+,K^+-ATPase is located in the basolateral membrane of the cell. Numerous K^+-selective channels are found in epithelial cells and may be located in either membrane domain. By the establishment of these chemical and voltage gradients, transport of other ions and solutes can be driven (e.g., Na^+-glucose symporter, Na^+-H^+ anti-

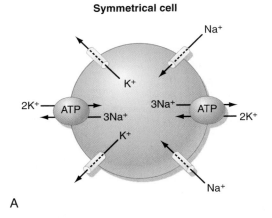

Symmetrical cell

A

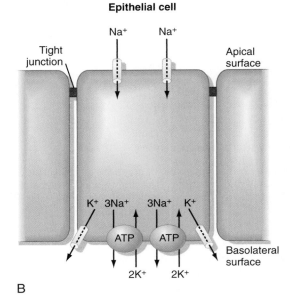

Epithelial cell

B

● **Figure 2-9.** **A,** Symmetrical cells (e.g., red blood cell) have membrane transport proteins distributed over the entire surface of the cell. **B,** Epithelial cells target various membrane transport proteins to either the apical or the basolateral membrane. By confining the transporters to a membrane domain, vectorial transport can occur. In the cell depicted, Na^+ is transported from the apical surface to the basolateral surface.

porter, $1Na^+,1K^+,2Cl^-$ symporter, $1Na^+$-$3HCO_3^-$ symporter). The direction of transepithelial transport (reabsorption or secretion) simply depends on the membrane domain in which the transporter is located. Because of the dependence on Na^+,K^+-ATPase, epithelial transport requires the expenditure of energy. Other ATP-dependent transporters are also involved in epithelial transport, including H^+-ATPase, H^+,K^+-ATPase, and a host of ATP-binding cassette (ABC) transporters such as pGP and MRP2, which transport xenobiotics (drugs), and the cystic fibrosis transmembrane regulator (CFTR).

Solutes and water can be transported across an epithelium by traversing both the apical and basolateral membranes **(transcellular transport)** or by moving between cells across the tight junction **(paracellular**

---

*The choroid plexus is located in the ventricles of the brain and secretes cerebrospinal fluid. Na^+,K^+-ATPase is located in the apical membrane of these cells.

transport). Solute transport via the transcellular route is a two-step process, with the solute molecule being transported across both the apical and basolateral membranes. Uptake into the cell or transport out of the cell may be either a passive or an active process. Typically, one of the steps is passive and the other is active. For the example shown in Figure 2-9, *B,* uptake of Na^+ into the cell across the apical membrane through the Na^+-selective channel is passive and driven by the electrochemical gradient for Na^+. Exit of Na^+ from the cell across the basolateral membrane is achieved by primary active transport via Na^+,K^+-ATPase. Because a transepithelial gradient for Na^+ can be generated by this process (i.e., the $[Na^+]$ in the apical compartment can be reduced below that of the basolateral compartment), the overall process of transepithelial Na^+ transport is said to be active. Any solute that is actively transported across an epithelium must be transported via the transcellular pathway.

Depending on the epithelium, the paracellular pathway is an important route for the transepithelial transport of solute and water. As noted, the permeability characteristics are determined, at least in part, by the specific claudins expressed by the cell. Thus, tight junctions can have low permeability to solutes or water, or to both. Alternatively, tight junctions can have very high permeability. For epithelia in which rates of transepithelial transport are high, the tight junctions typically have high permeability (i.e., are leaky). Examples of such epithelia include the proximal tubule of the renal nephron and the early segments of the small intestine (e.g., jejunum). If the epithelium must establish large transepithelial gradients for solutes or water (or for both), the tight junctions typically have low permeability (i.e., are tight). Examples of this type of epithelium include the collecting duct of the renal nephron and the terminal portion of the colon. In addition, the tight junction may be selective for certain solutes (e.g., selective for cations versus anions).

All solute transport that occurs through the paracellular pathway is passive in nature. The two driving forces for this transport are the transepithelial concentration gradient for the solute and, if the solute is charged, the transepithelial voltage (Fig. 2-10). The transepithelial voltage may be oriented with the apical surface electrically negative with respect to the basolateral surface, as shown in Figure 2-10, or it may be oriented with the apical surface electrically positive with respect to the basolateral surface. The polarity and magnitude of the transepithelial voltage are determined by the specific membrane transporters in the apical and basolateral membranes, as well as by the permeability characteristics of the tight junction.

It is important to recognize that transcellular transport processes set up the transepithelial chemical and voltage gradients, which in turn can drive paracellular transport. This is illustrated in Figure 2-11 for an epithelium that reabsorbs NaCl and for an epithelium that secretes NaCl. In both epithelia, the transepithelial voltage is oriented with the apical surface electrically negative with respect to the basolateral surface. For

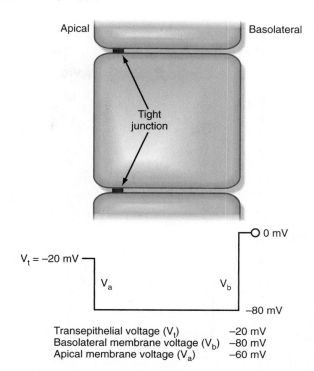

Transepithelial voltage (V_t)	−20 mV
Basolateral membrane voltage (V_b)	−80 mV
Apical membrane voltage (V_a)	−60 mV

● **Figure 2-10.** Electrical profile across an epithelial cell. The magnitude of the membrane voltages and the transepithelial voltage are determined by the various membrane transport proteins in the apical and basolateral membranes (see text for details).

the NaCl-reabsorbing epithelium, the transepithelial voltage is generated by the active transcellular reabsorption of Na^+. This voltage in turn drives Cl^- reabsorption through the paracellular pathway. In contrast, for the NaCl-secreting epithelium, the transepithelial voltage is generated by the active transcellular secretion of Cl^-. Na^+ is then secreted passively via the paracellular pathway.

Transepithelial Water Movement

Water movement across epithelia is passive and driven by transepithelial osmotic pressure gradients. Water movement can occur by a transcellular route involving aquaporins in both the apical and basolateral membranes.* In addition, water may also move through the paracellular pathway. In the NaCl-reabsorbing epithelium depicted in Figure 2-11, *A,* reabsorption of NaCl from the apical compartment lowers the osmotic pressure in that compartment, whereas the addition of NaCl to the basolateral compartment raises the osmotic pressure in that compartment. As a result, a transepithelial osmotic pressure gradient is established that drives the movement of water from the apical to the basolateral compartment (i.e., reabsorption). The opposite occurs with NaCl-secreting epithelium (see Fig. 2-11, *B*), where the transepithelial

---

*Different aquaporin isoforms are often expressed in the apical and basolateral membranes. In addition, multiple isoforms may be expressed in one or more of the membrane domains.

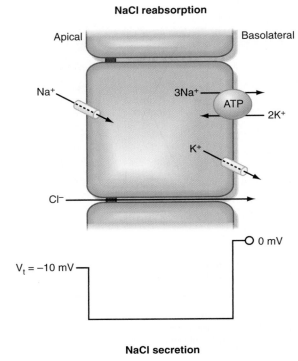

A

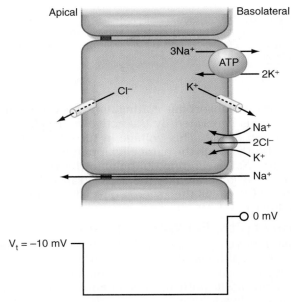

B

● **Figure 2-11.** Role of the paracellular pathway in epithelial transport. **A,** Na⁺ transport through the cell generates a transepithelial voltage that then drives the passive movement of Cl⁻ through the tight junction. NaCl reabsorption results. **B,** Cl⁻ transport through the cell generates a transepithelial voltage that then drives the passive transport of Na⁺ through the tight junction. NaCl secretion results.

secretion of NaCl establishes a transepithelial osmotic pressure gradient that drives water secretion.

In some epithelia (e.g., proximal tubule of the renal nephron), movement of water across the epithelium via the paracellular pathway can drive the movement

of additional solute. This process is termed **solvent drag** and reflects the fact that solutes dissolved in the water will traverse the tight junction with the water.

As is the case with the establishment of transepithelial concentration and voltage gradients, the establishment of transepithelial osmotic pressure gradients requires transcellular transport of solutes by the epithelial cells.

Regulation of Epithelial Transport

Epithelial transport must be regulated to meet the homeostatic needs of the individual. Depending on the epithelium, this regulation involves neural or hormonal mechanisms, or both. For example, the enteric nervous system of the gastrointestinal tract regulates solute and water transport by the epithelial cells that line the intestine and colon. Similarly, the sympathetic nervous system regulates transport by the epithelial cells of the renal nephron. Aldosterone, a steroid hormone produced by the adrenal cortex (see Chapter 42), is an example of a hormone that regulates NaCl transport by the epithelial cells of the colon, renal nephron, and sweat ducts. Epithelial cell transport can also be regulated by locally produced and locally acting substances, a process termed **paracrine regulation.** Regulation of HCl secretion in the stomach by histamine is an example of this process. Cells that are located near the epithelial cells of the stomach release histamine, which then stimulates HCl-secreting cells of the stomach (parietal cells) to secrete HCl.

When acted on by a regulatory signal, the epithelial cell may respond in several different ways, including

- Retrieval of transporters from the membrane by endocytosis or insertion of transporters into the membrane from an intracellular vesicular pool
- Change in the activity of membrane transporters (e.g., channel gating)
- Synthesis of specific transporters

The first two mechanisms can occur quite rapidly (seconds to minutes), whereas the synthesis of transporters takes additional time (minutes to days).

■ KEY CONCEPTS

1. The body maintains steady-state balance for water and a number of important solutes. This occurs when input into the body equals output from the body. For each solute and water there is a normal set point. Deviations form this set point are monitored (i.e., when input ≠ output), and effector mechanisms are activated to restore balance. This balance is achieved by adjusting either intake or excretion of water and solutes so that input and output are again equal.

2. Na⁺,K⁺-ATPase and K⁺-selective channels are critically important in establishing and maintaining intracellular composition, membrane potential (V_m), and cell volume. Na⁺,K⁺-ATPase takes the energy in ATP and converts it into the potential

energy of ion gradients and membrane potential. The ion and electrical gradient thus created are then used to drive the transport of other ions and other molecules, especially by solute carriers (i.e., symporters and antiporters).

3. Epithelial cells constitute the interface between the external world and the internal environment of the body. Vectorial transport of solutes and water across epithelia helps maintain steady-state balance of water and a number of important solutes. Because the external environment constantly changes and dietary intake of food and water is highly variable, transport by epithelia is regulated to meet the homeostatic needs of the individual.

CHAPTER 3

Signal Transduction, Membrane Receptors, Second Messengers, and Regulation of Gene Expression

The human body is composed of billions of cells, each with a distinct function. However, the function of cells is tightly coordinated and integrated by external chemical signals, including hormones, neurotransmitters, growth factors, odorants, and products of cellular metabolism that serve as chemical messengers and provide cell-to-cell communication. Light and mechanical and thermal stimuli are physical external signals that also coordinate cellular function. Chemical and physical messengers interact with receptors located in the plasma membrane, cytoplasm, and nucleus. Interaction of these messengers with receptors initiates a cascade of signaling events that mediate the response to each stimulus. These signaling pathways ensure that the cellular response to external messengers is specific, amplified, tightly regulated, and coordinated. This chapter provides an overview of how cells communicate via external messengers and discusses the receptors and intracellular signaling pathways that process external information into a highly coordinated cellular response. In subsequent chapters, details on signaling pathways in the nervous system, muscle, cardiovascular system, respiratory system, gastrointestinal system, kidneys, and endocrine system will be discussed in greater detail.

CELL-TO-CELL COMMUNICATION

An overview of how cells communicate with each other is presented in Figure 3-1. Cells communicate by releasing extracellular signaling molecules (e.g., **hormones and neurotransmitters**) that bind to **receptor** proteins located in the plasma membrane, cytoplasm, or nucleus. This signal is transduced into the activation, or inactivation, of one or more intracellular messengers by interacting with receptors. Receptors interact with a variety of intracellular signaling proteins, including **kinases, phosphatases,** and GTP-binding proteins **(G proteins).** These signaling proteins interact with and regulate the activity of target proteins and thereby modulate cellular function. Target proteins include, but are not limited to, ion channels and other transport proteins, metabolic enzymes, cytoskeletal proteins, gene regulatory proteins, and

cell cycle proteins that regulate cell growth and division. Signaling pathways are characterized by (1) multiple, hierarchical steps; (2) amplification of the hormone-receptor binding event, which magnifies the response; (3) activation of multiple pathways and regulation of multiple cellular functions; and (4) antagonism by constitutive and regulated feedback mechanisms, which minimize the response and provide tight regulatory control over these signaling pathways. A brief description of how cells communicate follows. Readers who desire a more in-depth presentation of this material are encouraged to consult one of the many cellular and molecular biology textbooks currently available.

Cells in higher animals release hundreds of signaling molecules, including peptides and proteins (e.g., insulin), **catecholamines** (e.g., epinephrine and norepinephrine), **steroid hormones** (e.g., aldosterone, estrogen), **iodothyronines** (e.g., thyroid hormones, including thyroxine [T_4] and triiodothyronine [T_3]), **eicosanoids** (e.g., prostaglandins, leukotrienes, thromboxanes, and prostacyclins), and other small molecules, including amino acids, nucleotides, ions (e.g., Ca^{++}), and gases, such as **nitric oxide** (NO) and carbon dioxide (CO_2), into the extracellular space by the processes of exocytosis and diffusion. Secretion of signaling molecules is cell type specific. For example, beta cells in the pancreas release insulin, which regulates glucose uptake into cells. The ability of a cell to respond to a specific signaling molecule depends on the expression of receptors that bind the signaling molecule with high affinity and specificity. Receptors are located in the plasma membrane, the cytosol, and the nucleus (Fig. 3-2).

Signaling molecules can act over long or short distances and can require cell-to-cell contact or very close cellular proximity (Fig. 3-3). Contact-dependent signaling is important during development and in immune responses. Molecules that are released and act locally are called **paracrine** or **autocrine hormones.** Paracrine signals are released by one type of cell and act on another type; they are usually taken up by target cells or rapidly degraded (within minutes) by enzymes. Autocrine signaling involves the release of a molecule that affects the same cell or other cells

● Figure 3-1. An overview of how cells communicate. A ligand (i.e., hormone or neurotransmitter) binds to a receptor, which may be in the plasma membrane, cytosol, or nucleus. Binding of ligand to a receptor activates intracellular signaling proteins, which interact with and regulate the activity of one or more target proteins to change cellular function. Signaling molecules regulate cell growth, division, and differentiation and influence cellular metabolism. In addition, they modulate the intracellular ionic composition by regulating the activity of ion channels and transport proteins. Signaling molecules also control cytoskeletal-associated events, including cell shape, division, and migration and cell-to-cell and cell-to-matrix adhesion. (Redrawn from Alberts B et al: Molecular Biology of the Cell, 4th ed. New York, Garland Science, 2002.)

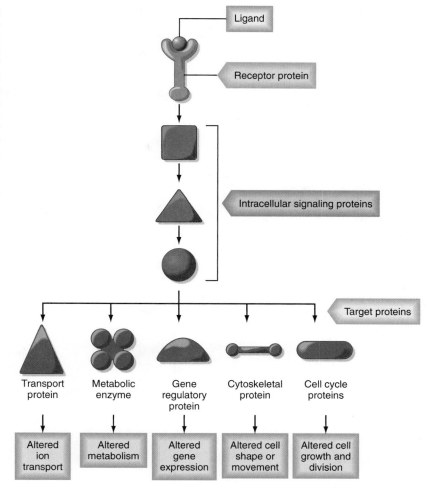

● Figure 3-2. Signaling molecules, especially ones that are hydrophilic and cannot cross the plasma membrane, directly bind to their cognate receptors located in the plasma membrane. Other signaling molecules, including steroid hormones, triiodothyronines, retinoic acids, and vitamin D, bind to carrier proteins in blood and readily diffuse across the plasma membrane, where they bind to cognate so-called nuclear receptors in the cytosol or nucleus. Both classes of receptors, when ligand bound, regulate gene transcription. (Redrawn from Alberts B et al: Molecular Biology of the Cell, 4th ed. New York, Garland Science, 2002.)

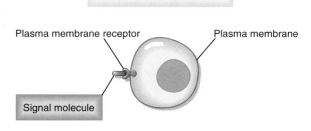

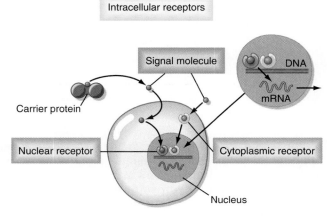

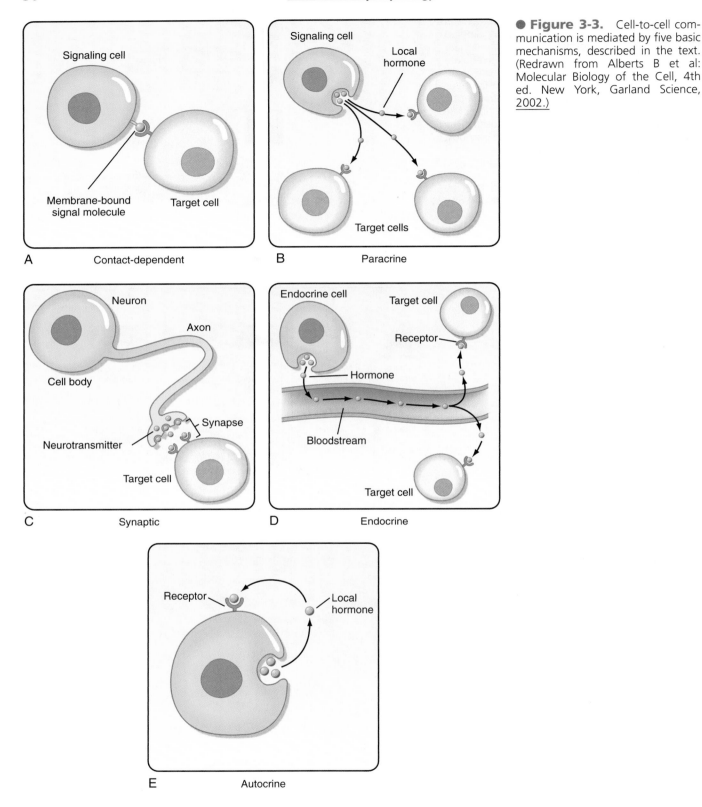

● **Figure 3-3.** Cell-to-cell communication is mediated by five basic mechanisms, described in the text. (Redrawn from Alberts B et al: Molecular Biology of the Cell, 4th ed. New York, Garland Science, 2002.)

of the same type. Synaptic signaling occurs when neurons transmit electrical signals along their axons and release neurotransmitters at synapses that affect the function of other neurons or cells that are distant from the neuron cell body. The physical relationship between the nerve terminal and the target cell ensures that the neurotransmitter is delivered to a specific cell. Details on synaptic signaling are discussed in Chapter 6. Endocrine signals are hormones that are secreted into the blood and are widely dispersed in

● Table 3-1. **Classes of Membrane Receptors**

Receptor Class	Ligand	Signal Transduction Pathway/Target
1. PLASMA MEMBRANE		
A. Ion channel	**Extracellular ligand:** GABA ACh ATP	**Membrane currents:** Cl^- Na^+, K^+, Ca^{++} Ca^{++}, Na^+ K^+
	Intracellular ligand: cAMP cGMP InsP3 Ca^{++}	 Na^+, K^+ Na^+, K^+ Ca^{++} Ca^{++}
B. G protein coupled	**Neurotransmitters Peptides, Odorants, Cytokines, Lipids**	**βγ Subunits activate ion channels α Subunit activates enzymes:** Cyclases that generate cAMP, cGMP, phospholipases that generate IP3 and diacyglycerol, and phospholipases that generate arachidonic acid and its metabolites. **Monomeric G proteins**
C. Catalytic	**ANP Insulin, EGF**	**Receptor guanylyl cyclase Receptor tyrosine kinase**
2. NUCLEAR RECEPTORS	**Steroid hormones:** Mineralocorticoids Glucocorticoids Androgens Estrogens Progestins	**Bind to regulatory sequences in DNA and increase or decrease gene transcription**
	Miscellaneous hormones: Thyroid Vitamin D Retinoic acid Prostaglandins	**Bind to regulatory sequences in DNA and increase or decrease gene transcription**

ACh, acetylcholine; ANP, atrial natriuretic peptide; cAMP, cyclic adenosine monophosphate; cGMP, cyclic guanosine monophosphate; EGF, epidermal growth factor; GABA, γ-aminobutyric acid; InsP3, inositol 1,4,5-triphosphate.

the body. Details on endocrine signaling are discussed in Chapter 37.

In addition to paracrine, autocrine, endocrine, and synaptic signaling, cell-to-cell communication also occurs via the **gap junctions** that form between adjacent cells (see Chapter 2). Gap junctions are specialized junctions that allow intracellular signaling molecules, generally less than 1200 Da in size, to diffuse from the cytoplasm of one cell to an adjacent cell. The permeability of gap junctions is regulated by cytosolic $[Ca^{++}]$, $[H^+]$, and cAMP and by the membrane potential. Gap junctions also allow cells to be electrically coupled, which is vitally important for the coordinated activity of cardiac and smooth muscle cells (see Chapters 13 and 14).

The speed of a response to an extracellular signal depends on the mechanism of delivery. Endocrine signals are relatively slow (seconds to minutes) because time is required for diffusion and blood flow to the target cell, whereas synaptic signaling is extremely fast (milliseconds). If the response involves changes in the activity of proteins in the cell, the response may occur in milliseconds to seconds. However, if the response involves changes in gene expression and the de novo synthesis of proteins, the response may take hours to occur, with days required to achieve a maximal response. For example, the stimulatory effect of aldosterone on sodium transport by the kidney requires days to fully develop (see Chapter 34).

The response to a particular signaling molecule also depends on the ability of the molecule to reach a particular cell, on expression of the cognate receptor (i.e., receptors that recognize a particular signaling molecule or ligand with a high degree of specificity), and on the cytoplasmic signaling molecules that interact with the receptor. Thus, signaling molecules frequently have many different effects that are dependent on the cell type. For example, the neurotransmitter acetylcholine stimulates contraction of skeletal muscle but decreases the force of contraction in heart muscle. This is due to the fact that skeletal muscle and heart cells express different acetylcholine receptors.*

RECEPTORS

All signaling molecules bind to specific receptors that act as signal transducers, thereby converting a ligand-receptor binding event into intracellular signals that affect cellular function. Receptors can be divided into two basic classes based on their structure and mechanism of action: membrane receptors and nuclear receptors (Table 3-1 and Figs. 3-4 and 3-5).

---

*The acetylcholine receptor in skeletal muscle is termed nicotinic because nicotine can mimic this action of the neurotransmitter. In contrast, the acetylcholine receptor in cardiac muscle is termed muscarinic because this effect is mimicked by muscarine, an alkaloid derived from the mushroom *Amanita muscaria.*

Plasma Membrane Receptors

There are four major types of plasma membrane receptors defined by the intracellular signaling pathways that they use: **ion channel–linked receptors, G protein–coupled receptors (GPCRs), catalytic receptors,** and a fourth class of transmembrane receptors that when activated, release transcription factors that undergo proteolytic cleavage and liberate a cytosolic fragment that enters the nucleus and modulates gene expression (Fig. 3-4).

Ion channel–linked receptors, also known as **ligand-gated ion channels,** mediate direct and rapid synaptic signaling between electrically excitable cells (Fig. 3-4, *A*). Neurotransmitters bind to the receptors and either open or close the ion channel, thereby changing the ionic permeability of the plasma membrane and altering the membrane potential. For examples and more details, see Chapter 2.

GPCRs regulate the activity of other proteins, such as enzymes and ion channels (Fig. 3-4, *B*). In this type of receptor the interaction between the receptor and the target protein is mediated by heterotrimeric G proteins, which are composed of α, β, and γ subunits. Stimulation of G proteins by ligand-bound receptors activates or inhibits downstream target proteins that regulate signaling pathways if the target protein is an enzyme or change membrane ion permeability if the target protein is an ion channel.

Catalytic receptors either function as enzymes or are associated with and regulate enzymes (Fig. 3-4, *C*). Most enzyme-linked receptors are protein kinases or are associated with protein kinases, and ligand binding causes the kinases to phosphorylate a specific subset of proteins on specific amino acids, which in turn activates or inhibits protein activity.

Some membrane proteins do not fit the classic definition of receptors, yet they subserve a receptor-like function in that they recognize extracellular signals and transduce the signals into an intracellular second messenger that has a biological effect. For example, on activation by a ligand, some membrane proteins undergo **regulated intramembrane proteolysis (RIP),** which elaborates a cytosolic peptide fragment that enters the nucleus and regulates gene expression (Fig. 3-4, *D*). In this signaling pathway, binding of ligand to a plasma membrane receptor leads to ectodomain shedding, facilitated by members of the metalloproteinase-disintegrin family, and produces a carboxy-terminal fragment that is the substrate for γ-secretase. γ-Secretase induces RIP, thereby releasing an intracellular domain of the protein that enters the nucleus and regulates transcription (Fig. 3-4, *D*). The most well characterized example of RIP is the sterol regulatory element–binding protein (SREB), a transmembrane protein expressed in the membrane of the endoplasmic reticulum. When cellular cholesterol levels are low, SREB undergoes RIP and the proteolytically cleaved fragment is translocated into the nucleus, where it transcriptionally activates genes that promote cholesterol biosynthesis.

Nuclear Receptors

Several classes of small hydrophobic molecules, including steroid hormones, thyroid hormones, retinoids, and vitamin D, are bound to plasma proteins, have a long biological half-life (hours to days), diffuse across the plasma membrane, and bind to nuclear receptors (Fig. 3-5). Some nuclear receptors, such as those that bind cortisol and aldosterone, are located in the cytosol and enter the nucleus after binding to hormone, whereas other receptors, including the thyroid hormone receptor, are bound to DNA in the nucleus, even in the absence of hormone. In both cases, inactive receptors are bound to inhibitory proteins, and binding of hormone results in dissociation of the inhibitory complex. Hormone binding causes the receptor to bind coactivator proteins that activate gene transcription. Once activated, the hormone-receptor complex binds to DNA and regulates the transcription of specific genes. The thyroid hormone-receptor complex binds to DNA complexes adjacent to the genes that the hormone regulates. Activation of specific genes usually occurs in two steps: an early primary response ($\approx$30 minutes), which activates genes that stimulate other genes to produce a delayed (hours to days) secondary response (Fig. 3-5). Each hormone elicits a specific response based on cellular expression of the cognate receptor, as well as cell type–specific expression of gene regulatory proteins that interact with the activated receptor to regulate the transcription of a specific set of genes (see Chapter 37 for more details). In addition to steroid receptors that regulate gene expression, recent evidence suggests that there are also membrane and juxtamembrane steroid receptors that mediate the rapid, nongenomic effects of steroid hormones.

● **Figure 3-4.** Classes of plasma membrane receptors. See text for details. (Redrawn from Alberts B et al: Molecular Biology of the Cell, 4th ed. New York, Garland Science, 2002.)

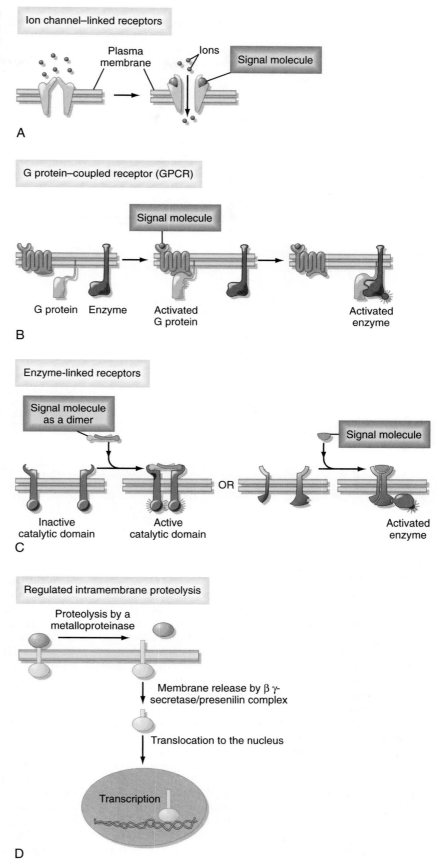

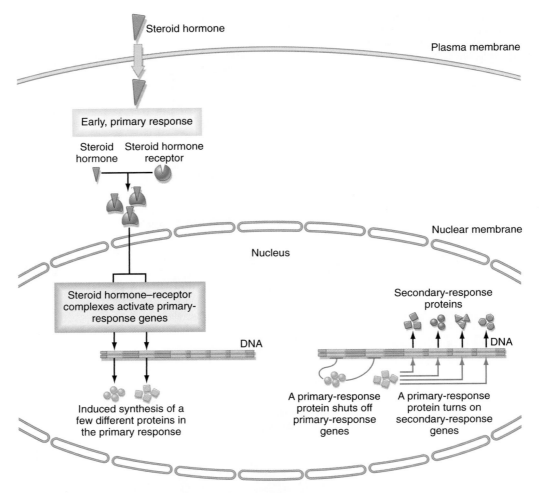

● **Figure 3-5.** Steroid hormones stimulate the transcription of early-response genes and late-response genes. See text for details. (Redrawn from Alberts B et al: Molecular Biology of the Cell, 4th ed. New York, Garland Science, 2002.)

RECEPTORS AND SIGNAL TRANSDUCTION PATHWAYS

Hormones bind to receptors and the signal is translated to effector proteins inside the cell by intracellular signaling proteins. Plasma membrane receptors relay signals via intracellular signaling pathways. Nuclear receptors relay signals primarily through regulation of gene expression. Receptors amplify and integrate signals, as well as down-regulate and desensitize signals, which reduces or terminates the response, even in the presence of hormone.

Intracellular signaling molecules—so-called second messengers (the first messenger of the signal is the ligand that binds to the receptor)—include small molecules such as cAMP, cGMP, Ca^{++}, and diacylglycerol (DAG). Signaling pathways often include dozens of small molecules that form complicated networks within the cell (Fig. 3-6). Some proteins in the intracellular signaling pathways relay the signal by passing the message from one protein to another. Other proteins carry the signal from one region of the cell to another, for example, from the cytosol to the nucleus. Many proteins, usually enzymes or ion channels,

amplify the signal either by producing large amounts of additional signaling molecules or by activating a large number of downstream signaling proteins. Transducer proteins convert the signal into a different form. The enzyme that makes cAMP, **adenylyl cyclase,** transduces a signal (activation of a G protein) and amplifies the signal by generating large amounts of cAMP. Other types of signaling proteins include those that integrate multiple signals.

Intracellular signals also act as **molecular switches:** when a signal is received, they switch from an inactive to an active form or vice versa, until another signaling molecule switches them off. Signaling complexes, composed of multiple proteins that interact physically, enhance the speed, efficiency, and specificity of signaling. Cells can also adjust rapidly to signaling molecules. Cells can respond quickly and in a graded manner to increasing concentrations of hormone, and the effect of a signaling molecule can either be long- or short-lived.

Cells can adjust their sensitivity to a signal by **adaptation** or **desensitization,** whereby prolonged exposure to a hormone decreases the cell's response over

● **Figure 3-6.** Overview of how intracellular signals are amplified and integrated. Signaling pathways often include dozens of small molecules that form complicated networks within the cell. Some signaling proteins relay the signal by passing the message from one protein to another. Other proteins carry the signal from one region of the cell to another. Many proteins amplify the signal either by producing large amounts of additional signaling molecules or by activating a large number of downstream signaling proteins. See text for more details. (Redrawn from Alberts B et al: Molecular Biology of the Cell, 4th ed. New York, Garland Science, 2002.)

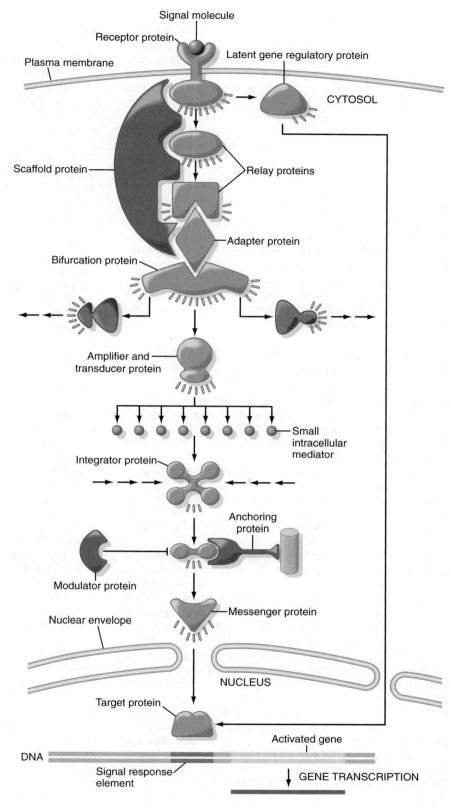

time. Adaptation allows cells to respond to changes in hormone levels rather than to absolute levels. Adaptation is a reversible process that can involve a reduction in the number of receptors expressed in the plasma membrane, inactivation of receptors, and changes in signaling proteins mediating the downstream effect of the receptors.

Table 3-1 summarizes the two general classes of receptors and provides a few examples of the signal transduction pathways associated with each class of receptors.

Ion Channel–Linked Signal Transduction Pathways

This class of receptors transduces a chemical signal into an electrical signal, which elicits a response. For example, activation of the ryanodine receptor (RyR), located in the membrane of the sarcoplasmic reticulum of skeletal muscle, by Ca^{++}, caffeine, ATP, or metabolites of arachidonic acid releases Ca^{++} into the cytosol, which facilitates muscle contraction (see Chapter 12 for details).

G Protein–Coupled Signal Transduction Pathways

G proteins couple to more than 1000 different receptors and thereby mediate the cellular response to an incredibly diverse set of signaling molecules, including hormones, neurotransmitters, peptides, and odorants. G proteins are heterotrimeric complexes composed of three subunits, α, β, and γ. There are 16 α subunits, 5 β subunits and 11 γ subunits. These α, β, and γ subunits can assemble into hundreds of different combinations and thereby interact with a diverse number of receptors and effectors. The assembly of subunits and the association with receptors and effectors depend on the cell type.

An overview of G protein activation and inactivation is illustrated in Figure 3-7. In the absence of ligand, G proteins are inactive and form a heterotrimeric complex in which GDP binds to the α subunit. When a ligand binds to a receptor, the activated receptor interacts with the α, β, γ complex and induces a conformational change that promotes the release of GDP and binding of GTP to the α subunit. Binding of GTP to the α subunit stimulates dissociation of the α subunit from the heterotrimeric complex and results in release of the α subunit from the $\beta\gamma$ dimer, each of which can interact with and regulate downstream effectors such as adenylyl cyclase and phospholipases. G proteins are activated by **guanine nucleotide exchange factors (GEFs),** which facilitate the dissociation of GDP and binding of GTP, and are inactivated by **GTPase-accelerating proteins (GAPS),** which enhance G protein GTPase activity. Activation of downstream effectors by the α subunit and $\beta\gamma$ dimer is terminated when the α subunit hydrolyzes the bound GTP to GDP and P_i. The α subunit bound to GDP reassociates with the $\beta\gamma$ dimer and terminates the activation of effectors. Hydrolysis of GTP by the α subunit is facilitated by a family of proteins known as **RGS proteins** (regulation of G protein **s**ignaling), which facilitate inactivation of signaling.

Another way to terminate signaling through a GPCR involves desensitization and endocytic removal of receptors from the plasma membrane. Binding of hormone to a GPCR increases the ability of **GPCR kinases (GRKs)** to phosphorylate the intracellular domain of GPCRs, which recruits proteins called β-**arrestins** to bind to the GPCR. β-Arrestins inactivate the receptor and promote endocytic removal of the GPCR from the plasma membrane. GRK/β-arrestin inactivation with endocytosis of GPCRs is an important mechanism whereby cells down-regulate (desensitize) a response during prolonged exposure to elevated hormone levels.

Activated α subunits couple to a variety of effector proteins, including adenylyl cyclase, **phosphodiesterases,** and **phospholipases** (A_2, C, and D). A very common downstream effector of G proteins is adenylyl cyclase, which facilitates the conversion of ATP to cAMP (Fig. 3-8, *A*). When a ligand binds to a receptor that interacts with a G protein composed of an α subunit of the α_s class, adenylyl cyclase is activated, thereby increasing cAMP levels and as a result activating **protein kinase A (PKA).** By phosphorylating specific serine and threonine residues on proteins, PKA regulates effector protein activity. In contrast, when a ligand binds to a receptor that interacts with a G protein composed of an α subunit of the α_i class, adenylyl cyclase is inhibited, thereby reducing cAMP levels and consequently reducing PKA levels. cAMP also regulates some effector proteins directly, such as ion-gated channels. cAMP is degraded to AMP by cAMP phosphodiesterases, which are inhibited by caffeine and other methylxanthines. Thus, caffeine can prolong a cellular response mediated by cAMP and PKA. In addition to signaling in the cytoplasm, the catalytic subunit of PKA can enter the nucleus of cells and phosphorylate and activate the transcription factor **cAMP response element–binding (CREB) protein.** Phospho-CREB protein increases the transcription of many genes. Hence cAMP has many cellular effects, including direct and indirect effects mediated by PKA.

G proteins also regulate phototransduction (Fig. 3-8, *B*). In rod cells in the eye, absorption of light by rhodopsin activates the G protein transducin, which via the α_t subunit activates cGMP phosphodiesterase. Activation of this phosphodiesterase lowers the concentration of cGMP and thereby closes a cGMP-activated cation channel. The ensuing change in cation channel activity alters the membrane voltage. The exquisite sensitivity of rods to light—rods can detect a single photon of light—is due to the abundance of rhodopsin in rods and amplification of the signal (a photon of light) by the G protein–cGMP phosphodiesterase–cGMP channel signaling pathway (see Chapter 8 for more details).

G proteins also regulate phospholipases, a family of enzymes that modulate a variety of signaling pathways (Fig. 3-8, *C*). Ligands that activate receptors that are coupled to the α_q subunit stimulate **phospholipase C,**

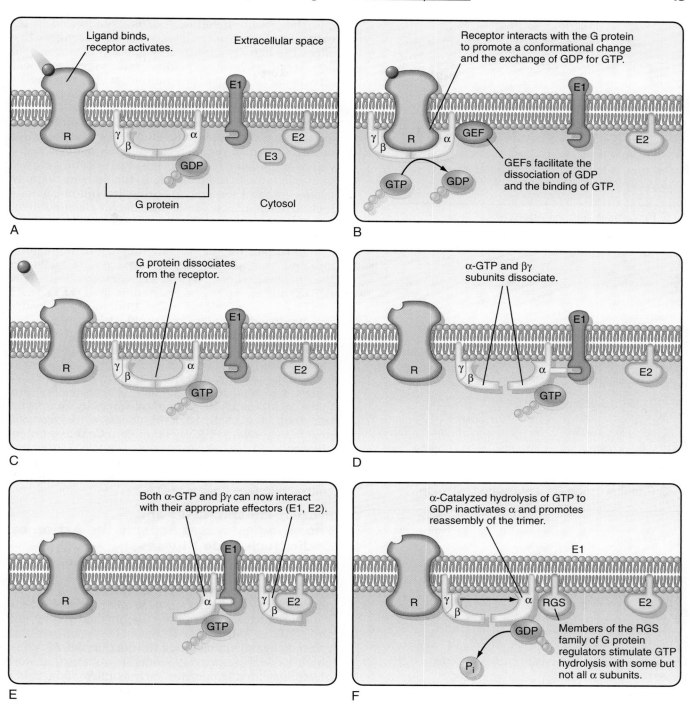

A
Ligand binds, receptor activates.
Extracellular space
E1
R
γ β α
GDP
G protein
Cytosol
E2
E3

B
Receptor interacts with the G protein to promote a conformational change and the exchange of GDP for GTP.
E1
γ β R α GEF
GTP GDP
GEFs facilitate the dissociation of GDP and the binding of GTP.
E2

C
G protein dissociates from the receptor.
E1
R
γ β α
GTP
E2

D
α-GTP and βγ subunits dissociate.
E1
R
γ β α
GTP
E2

E
Both α-GTP and βγ can now interact with their appropriate effectors (E1, E2).
E1
R
α
GTP
γ β E2

F
α-Catalyzed hydrolysis of GTP to GDP inactivates α and promotes reassembly of the trimer.
E1
R
γ β α RGS
GDP
Pi
E2
Members of the RGS family of G protein regulators stimulate GTP hydrolysis with some but not all α subunits.

● **Figure 3-7.** Cycle of heterotrimeric G protein activation and inactivation. The same cycle is involved in the activation and inactivation of small, monomeric G proteins. (Redrawn from Boron W, Boulpaep E: Medical Physiology. Philadelphia, Saunders, 2003.)

an enzyme that converts **phosphatidylinositol 4,5-biphosphate (PIP2)** to **1,4,5-inositol triphosphate (InsP3)** and **DAG** (Fig. 3-8, *C*). InsP3 is a second messenger that diffuses to the endoplasmic reticulum, where it activates a ligand-activated Ca^{++} channel to release Ca^{++} into the cytosol, whereas DAG activates **protein kinase C (PKC),** which phosphorylates effector proteins. As noted earlier, both Ca^{++} and PKC influ-

ence effector proteins, as well as other signaling pathways, to elicit responses.

Ligand binding to GPCRs can also activate **phospholipase A₂,** an enzyme that releases arachidonic acid from membrane phospholipids (Fig. 3-9). **Arachidonic acid** can be released from cells and thereby regulates neighboring cells or stimulates inflammation. It can also be retained within cells, where it is incorporated

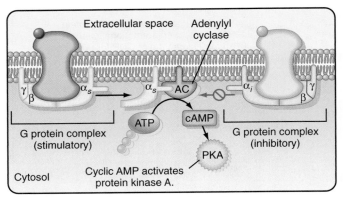

A G Proteins acting via adenylyl cyclase

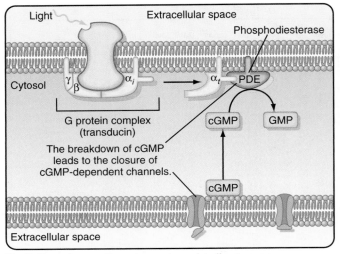

B G Proteins acting via a phosphodiesterase

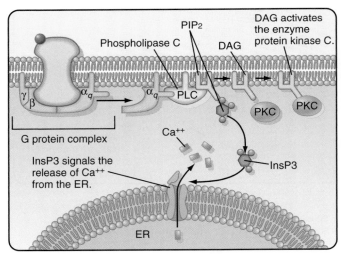

C G Proteins acting via a phospholipase

● **Figure 3-8.** Heterotrimeric G proteins regulate **(A)** adenylyl cyclase and thereby modulate cAMP and PKA levels; **(B)** phosphodiesterases, which modulate cGMP and cAMP levels; and **(C)** phospholipases, which release DAG. In turn, DAG activates PKC and InsP3, which stimulate Ca^{++} release from the endoplasmic reticulum. (Redrawn from Boron W, Boulpaep E: *Medical Physiology*. Philadelphia, Saunders, 2003.)

into the plasma membrane or is metabolized in the cytosol to form intracellular second messengers that affect the activity of enzymes and ion channels (Fig. 3-9). In one pathway, cytosolic **cyclooxygenases** facilitate the metabolism of arachidonic acid to prostaglandins, thromboxanes, and prostacyclins. Prostaglandins mediate aggregation of platelets, cause constriction of the airways, and induce inflammation. Thromboxanes also induce platelet aggregation and constrict blood vessels, whereas prostacyclin inhibits platelet aggregation and dilates blood vessels. In a second pathway of arachidonic acid metabolism, the enzyme 5-lipoxygenase initiates the conversion of arachidonic acid to **leukotrienes,** which participate in allergic and inflammatory responses, including those causing asthma, rheumatoid arthritis, and inflammatory bowel disease. The third pathway of arachidonic acid metabolism is initiated by epoxygenase, an enzyme that facilitates the generation of **hydroxyeicosatetraenoic acid (HETE)** and *cis***-epoxyeicosatrienoic acid (EET).** HETE and EET increase release of Ca^{++} from the endoplasmic reticulum and stimulate cell proliferation.

Ca^{++} is also an intracellular messenger that elicits cellular effects via Ca^{++}-binding proteins, most notably **calmodulin** (CaM). When Ca^{++} binds to CaM, its conformation is altered and the structural change in CaM allows it to bind to and regulate other signaling proteins, including cAMP phosphodiesterase, an enzyme that degrades cAMP to AMP, which is inactive and unable to activate PKA. By binding to **CaM-dependent kinases,** CaM also phosphorylates specific serine and threonine residues in many proteins, including myosin light-chain kinase, which facilitates smooth muscle contraction (see Chapter 14).

Protein Phosphatases and Phosphodiesterases Reverse the Action of Cyclic Nucleotide Kinases

There are two ways to terminate a signal initiated by cAMP and cGMP: enhancing degradation of these cyclic nucleotides by phosphodiesterases and dephosphorylation of effectors by protein **phosphatases.** Phosphodiesterases facilitate the breakdown of cAMP and cGMP to AMP and GMP, respectively, and are activated by ligand activation of GPCRs (Fig. 3-8, *B*). Phosphatases dephosphorylate effector proteins that were phosphorylated by kinases such as PKA. The balance between kinase-mediated phosphorylation and phosphatase-mediated dephosphorylation allows rapid and exquisite regulation of the phosphorylated state and thus the activity of signaling proteins.

Small, Monomeric G Proteins

Low-molecular-weight proteins (monomeric G proteins) also play an important role in many signaling pathways. These monomeric G proteins are composed of a single 20- to 40-kDa protein and are membrane bound because of the addition of lipids posttranslationally. Like heterotrimeric G proteins, their activity depends on the binding of GTP, and they are regulated by GEFs and GAPs. Monomeric G proteins have been classified into five families: Ras, Rho, Rab, Ran, and

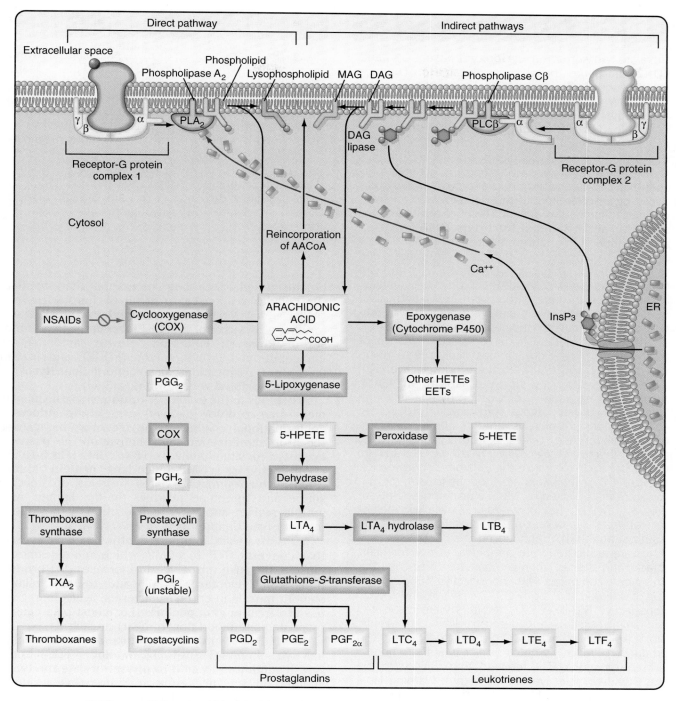

● **Figure 3-9.** Arachidonic acid signaling pathways. See text for details. (Redrawn from Boron W, Boulpaep E: Medical Physiology. Philadelphia, Saunders, 2003.)

Arf. Ras GTPases regulate gene expression and cell proliferation, differentiation, and survival. Rho GTPases regulate actin cytoskeletal organization, cell cycle progression, and gene expression. The Rab GTPase family members regulate intravesicular transport and trafficking of proteins between organelles in the secretory and endocytic pathways. Ran GTPases regulate nucleo-cytoplasmic transport of RNA and proteins. Finally,

Arf GTPase, like Rab GTPases, regulates vesicular transport.

Catalytic Receptor–Linked Signal Transduction Pathways

There are several classes of receptors that have catalytic activity or are intimately associated with proteins that have catalytic activity. Four of these classes will

IN THE CLINIC

There are two isoforms of **cyclooxygenase: COX1** and **COX2,** the genes for which are located on chromosomes 9 and 1, respectively. COX1 is constitutively expressed. When activated in endothelial cells, COX1 facilitates the production of prostacyclins (Fig. 3-9), which inhibit blood clots **(thrombi).** COX1 also facilitates the production of thromboxane A_2, which is prothrombotic (Fig. 3-9). Thus, cardiovascular health depends in part on the balance between prostacyclins generated by endothelial cells and thromboxane A_2, which is produced by vascular smooth muscle cells. COX2 is activated by inflammatory stimuli. Thus, the ability of **nonsteroidal antiinflammatory drugs (NSAIDs)** (e.g., aspirin, ibuprofen, naproxen, acetaminophen, indomethacin) to suppress the inflammatory response is due to inhibition of COX2. Both COX1 and COX2 facilitate the production of prostanoids that protect the stomach. Recent evidence suggests that both COX1 and COX2 must be inhibited to elicit damage to the gastrointestinal tract. Consequently, the negative effects of NSAIDs on the gastric mucosa (e.g., increased incidence of gastrointestinal bleeding) are most likely due to inhibition of COX1 and COX2 by these nonselective COX inhibitors. However, low doses of **aspirin,** an NSAID, reduces thromboxane A_2 production by platelets with little effect on endothelial prostacyclin production. Thus, low-dose aspirin is antithrombotic. Selective COX2 inhibitors (e.g., celecoxib, rofecoxib, lumiracoxib) are very effective in selectively inhibiting COX2 and are used extensively to reduce the inflammatory response. Because COX2 inhibitors are thought to lack the untoward effects elicited by NSAIDs on the gastrointestinal tract, their use has increased dramatically in the last several years. However, in 2005 the Food and Drug Administration (FDA) announced that COX2-selective drugs are associated with an increased risk for heart attacks and strokes when compared with placebo but not when compared with nonselective NSAIDs. The FDA concluded that both COX2-selective and COX2-nonselective NSAID (COX) inhibitors were associated with an increased risk for adverse cardiovascular events, most likely by inhibiting COX2-mediated prostacyclin production, which as noted earlier is antithrombotic. Subsequently, the FDA required that COX2-selective and COX2-nonselective NSAIDs carry a warning label on product packaging highlighting the potential for the increased risk for adverse cardiovascular events. In addition, although much evidence suggests that COX2-selective inhibitors do not cause gastrointestinal bleeding, recent evidence led the FDA to also require the pharmaceutical industry to add to the warning label on COX2-selective drugs a caution about the potential for increased risk for gastrointestinal bleeding. The cardiovascular risks associated with COX2-selective inhibitors continue to be a topic of debate and intensive research.*

*See also Mitchell JA, Warner TD: COX isoforms in the cardiovascular system: Understanding the activities of non-steroidal anti-inflammatory drugs. Nat Rev Drug Discov 5:75-86, 2006.

AT THE CELLULAR LEVEL

Ras GTPases are involved in many signaling pathways that control cell division, proliferation, and death. Many Ras family proteins are **oncogenic** (cancer causing), whereas others appear to act as tumor suppressors. Mutations in Ras genes that inhibit GTPase activity, as well as overexpression of Ras proteins as a result of transcriptional activation, lead to continuous cell proliferation, a major step in the development of cancer in many organs, including the pancreas, colon, and lung. In addition, mutations in and overexpression of GEFs, which facilitate exchange of GTP for GDP, and GAPs, which accelerate GTP hydrolysis, may also be oncogenic.

be discussed, including receptors that mediate the cellular responses to atrial natriuretic peptide (ANP) and NO **(receptor guanylyl cyclases);** transforming growth factor-β (TGF-β) **(receptor threonine/serine kinases);** epidermal growth factor (EGF), platelet-derived growth factor (PDGF), and insulin **(receptor tyrosine kinases);** and interleukins **(tyrosine kinase–associated receptors)** (Fig. 3-10).

ANP binds to the extracellular domain of the plasma membrane receptor guanylyl cyclase and induces a conformational change in the receptor that causes receptor dimerization and activation of guanylyl cyclase, which metabolizes GTP to cGMP (Fig. 3-10, *A*). cGMP activates **cGMP-dependent protein kinase (PKG),** which phosphorylates proteins on specific serine and threonine residues. In the kidney, ANP inhibits sodium and water reabsorption by the collecting duct (see Chapter 34).

NO activates a soluble receptor guanylyl cyclase that converts GTP to cGMP, which relaxes smooth muscle. Because nitroglycerin increases NO production, which increases cGMP and thereby relaxes smooth muscle in coronary arteries, it has long been used to treat **angina pectoris** (i.e., chest pain caused by inadequate blood flow to heart muscle).

The TGF-β receptor is a threonine/serine kinase that has two subunits (Fig. 3-10, *B*). Binding of TGF-β to the type II subunit induces it to phosphorylate the type I subunit on specific serine and threonine residues, which in turn phosphorylates other downstream effector proteins on serine and threonine residues and thereby elicits a cellular response.

There are two classes of tyrosine kinase receptors. Nerve growth factor (NGF) receptors are a typical example of one class (Fig. 3-10, *C*). Ligand binding to two NGF receptors facilitates their dimerization and activation of tyrosine kinase activity. Activation of the insulin receptor, which is tetrameric and composed of two α and two β subunits, by insulin is an example of the other type of tyrosine kinase receptor. Binding of insulin to the α subunits produces a conformational change that facilitates interaction between the two α and β pairs. Binding of insulin to its receptor causes

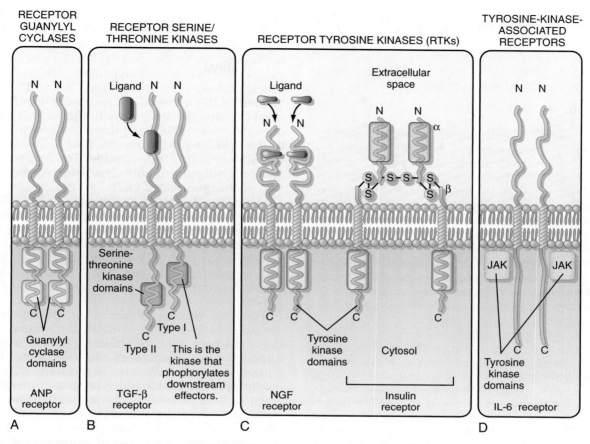

● **Figure 3-10.** Four types of catalytic receptors are illustrated in this figure. See text for details. (Redrawn from Boron W, Boulpaep E: Medical Physiology. Philadelphia, Saunders, 2003.)

autophosphorylation of tyrosine residues in the catalytic domains of the β subunits, and the activated receptor then phosphorylates cytoplasmic proteins to initiate its cellular effects.

The fourth class of catalytic receptors includes the tyrosine-associated receptors, which have no intrinsic kinase activity but associate with proteins that have tyrosine kinase activity, including tyrosine kinases of the **Src family** and **Janus family (JAK)** (Fig. 3-10, *D*). Receptors in this class bind several cytokines, including interleukin-6, and erythropoietin. Tyrosine kinase–associated receptor subunits assemble into homodimers (αα), heterodimers (αβ), or heterotrimers (αβγ) when ligand binds. Subunit assembly enhances the binding of tyrosine kinases, which induces kinase activity and thereby phosphorylates tyrosine residues on the kinases, as well as on the receptor.

REGULATION OF GENE EXPRESSION BY SIGNAL TRANSDUCTION PATHWAYS

Steroid and thyroid hormones, cAMP, and receptor tyrosine kinases are transcription factors that regulate gene expression and thereby participate in signal transduction pathways. This section discusses the regulation of gene expression by steroid and thyroid hormones, cAMP, and receptor tyrosine kinases.

Nuclear Receptor–Linked Signal Transduction Pathways

The family of nuclear receptors includes more than 30 genes and has been divided into two subfamilies based on structure and mechanism of action: (1) steroid hormone receptors and (2) receptors that bind retinoic acid, thyroid hormones (iodothyronines), and vitamin D. When ligands bind to these receptors, the ligand-receptor complex activates transcription factors that bind to DNA and regulate the expression of genes (Figs. 3-2, 3-5, and 3-6).

The location of nuclear receptors varies. Glucocorticoid and mineralocorticoid receptors are located in the cytoplasm, where they interact with chaperones (i.e., heat shock proteins) (Fig. 3-2). Binding of hormone to these receptors results in a conformational change that causes chaperones to dissociate from the receptor, thereby uncovering a nuclear localization motif that facilitates translocation of the hormone-bound receptor complex to the nucleus. Estrogen and progesterone receptors are located primarily in the nucleus, and thyroid hormone and reti-

► IN THE CLINIC

The significance of signaling pathways in medicine is illustrated by the following short list of popular drugs that act by regulating signaling pathways.

- **Aspirin,** the first pharmaceutical (1899), inhibits COX1 and COX2.
- **β-Adrenergic receptor agonists and antagonists** are used to treat a variety of medical conditions. β_1-Agonists increase cardiac contractility and heart rate in patients with low blood pressure. β_2-Agonists dilate bronchi and are used to treat asthma and chronic obstructive lung disease. By contrast, β-adrenergic antagonists are used to treat patients with hypertension, angina, cardiac arrhythmias, and congestive heart failure (see Chapter 18).
- **Fluoxetine (Prozac)** is an antidepressant medication that inhibits reuptake of the neurotransmitter serotonin into the presynaptic cell, which results in enhanced activation of serotonin receptors (see Chapter 6).
- Several monoclonal antibodies are used to treat cancer caused by the activation of growth factor receptors in cancer cells. For example, **trastuzumab (Herceptin)** is a monoclonal antibody used to treat women with metastatic breast cancer who overexpress **HER2/neu,** a member of the EGF receptor family that stimulates cell growth and differentiation. **Cetuximab (Erbitux)** and **bevacizumab (Avastin)** are monoclonal antibodies that are used to treat metastatic colorectal cancer and head and neck cancer. These antibodies bind to and inhibit the EGF receptor and thereby inhibit EGF-induced cell growth in cancer cells.
- Drugs that inhibit cGMP-specific phosphodiesterase type 5, such as **sildenafil (Viagra), Cialis (tadalafil),** and **Levitra (vardenafil),** prolong the vasodilatory effects of NO and are used to treat patients with erectile dysfunction and pulmonary arterial hypertension.

noic acid receptors are located in the nucleus bound to DNA (Fig. 3-2).

When activated by hormone binding, nuclear receptors bind to specific DNA sequences in the regulatory regions of responsive genes called **hormone response elements.** Ligand-receptor binding to DNA causes a conformational change in DNA that initiates transcription. Nuclear receptors also regulate gene expression by acting as transcriptional repressors. For example, glucocorticoids suppress the **transcription activator protein-1 (AP-1)** and **nuclear factor κB (NF-κB),** which stimulate the expression of genes that cause inflammation. By this mechanism glucocorticoids reduce inflammation.

As noted previously, cAMP is an important second messenger. In addition to its importance in activating

PKA, which phosphorylates specific serine and threonine residues on proteins, cAMP stimulates the transcription of many genes, including those that code for hormones, including somatostatin, glucagon, and vasoactive intestinal polypeptide (Fig. 3-6). Many genes activated by cAMP have a **cAMP response element (CRE)** in their DNA. Increases in cAMP stimulate PKA, which translocates to the nucleus, where it phosphorylates **CREB** and thereby increases its affinity for **CREB-binding protein (CBP).** The CREB-CBP complex activates transcription. The response is terminated when PKA phosphorylates a phosphatase that dephosphorylates CREB.

Many growth factors, including EGF, PDGF, NGF, and insulin, bind to and activate receptors that have tyrosine kinase activity. Activation of tyrosine kinases initiates a cascade of events that enhance the activity of the small GTP-binding protein Ras, which in a series of steps and intermediary proteins leads to transcriptional activation of genes that stimulate cell growth.

Tyrosine kinase–associated receptors, as noted earlier, are activated by a variety of hormones, including cytokines, growth hormone, and interferon. Although these receptors do not have tyrosine kinase activity, they are associated with **Janus family proteins (JAK),** which do have tyrosine kinase activity. Once activated, hormone tyrosine kinase–associated receptors activate JAK, which phosphorylates latent transcription factors called **signal transducers and activators of transcription (STATs).** When phosphorylated on tyrosine residues, STATs dimerize and then enter the nucleus and regulate transcription.

■ KEY CONCEPTS

1. The function of cells is tightly coordinated and integrated by external chemical signals, including hormones, neurotransmitters, growth factors, odorants, and products of cellular metabolism, that serve as chemical messengers and provide cell-to-cell communication. Chemical and physical signals interact with receptors located in the plasma membrane, cytoplasm, and nucleus. Interaction of these signals with receptors initiates a cascade of events that mediate the response to each stimulus. These pathways ensure that the cellular response to external signals is specific, amplified, tightly regulated, and coordinated.

2. G protein–coupled receptors interact with and regulate ion channels; adenylyl cyclase and the cAMP-PKA signaling pathway; phosphodiesterases, which also regulate cAMP and cGMP signaling pathways; and phospholipases, which regulate the production of prostaglandins, prostacyclins, and thromboxanes. Monomeric G proteins regulate many cellular processes, including gene expression, actin cyto-

skeleton organization, cell cycle progression, and intracellular vesicular transport.

3. There are four subtypes of catalytic receptors that mediate the cellular response to a wide variety of hormones, including ANP, NO, TGF-β, PDGF, insulin, and interleukins.

4. There are two types of nuclear receptors: one type that in the absence of ligand is located in the cytoplasm and when bound to ligand translocates to the nucleus, and another class that permanently resides in the nucleus. Both classes of receptors regulate gene transcription.

THE NERVOUS SYSTEM

Kalman Rubinson and Eric J. Lang

CHAPTER 4

The Nervous System: Introduction to Cells and Systems

The nervous system is a communications and control network that allows an organism to interact in appropriate ways with its environment. The environment includes both the external environment (the world outside the body) and the internal environment (the components and cavities of the body). The nervous system can be divided into central and peripheral parts, each with further subdivisions. The peripheral nervous system (PNS) provides an interface between the environment and the central nervous system (CNS). It includes sensory (or primary afferent) neurons, somatic motor neurons, and autonomic motor neurons. Autonomic motor neurons are discussed in Chapter 11.

The general functions of the nervous system include sensory detection, information processing, and the expression of behavior. Other systems, such as the endocrine and immune systems, share some of these functions, but the nervous system is specialized for them.

Sensory detection is the process whereby neurons transduce environmental energy into neural signals. Sensory detection is accomplished by special neurons called sensory receptors. Various forms of energy can be sensed, including mechanical, light, sound, chemical, thermal, and in some animals, electrical.

Information processing, including learning and memory, depends on intercellular communication in neural circuits. The mechanisms involve both electrical and chemical events. Information processing includes the following:

1. Transmission of information via neural networks
2. Transformation of information by recombination with other information (neural integration)
3. Perception of sensory information
4. Storage and retrieval of information (memory)
5. Planning and implementation of motor commands
6. Thought processes and conscious awareness
7. Learning
8. Emotion and motivation

Behavior consists of the totality of the organism's responses to its environment. Behavior may be covert, as in cognition, but animals can only overtly express behavior with a motor act (such as a muscle contraction) or an autonomic response (such as glandular release). In humans, language constitutes a particularly important set of behaviors, and plays a role in the processing and storage of information. Learning and memory are special forms of information processing that permit behavior to change appropriately in response to previously experienced environmental challenges.

CELLULAR COMPONENTS OF THE NERVOUS SYSTEM

The nervous system is made up of cells, connective tissue, and blood vessels. The major cell types are **neurons** (nerve cells) and **neuroglia** ("nerve glue"). Neurons are anatomically and physiologically specialized for communication and signaling, and these properties are fundamental to function of the nervous system. Traditionally, neuroglia, or just glia, are characterized as supportive cells that sustain neurons both metabolically and physically, as well as isolate individual neurons from each other and help maintain the internal milieu of the nervous system.

Neurons

The functional unit of the nervous system is the neuron (Fig. 4-1), and neural circuits are made up of synaptically interconnected neurons. Neural activity is generally coded by sequences of action potentials propagated along axons in the neural circuits (see Chapter 5). The coded information is passed from one neuron to the next by synaptic transmission (see Chapter 6). In synaptic transmission, the action potentials that reach a presynaptic ending usually trigger the release of a chemical neurotransmitter. The neurotransmitter can either excite the postsynaptic cell (possibly to discharge one or more action potentials), inhibit the activity of the postsynaptic cell, or influence the action of other axon terminals.

The typical neuron consists of a cell body, or soma, with a variable number of branch-like dendrites and a single process, the axon, that extend from the soma. The cell body (perikaryon, soma) of the neuron contains the nucleus and nucleolus of the cell and also possesses a well-developed biosynthetic apparatus for manufacturing membrane constituents, synthetic enzymes, and other chemical substances needed for the spe-cialized functions of nerve cells. The neuronal biosynthetic apparatus includes Nissl bodies, which are stacks of rough endoplasmic reticulum, and a

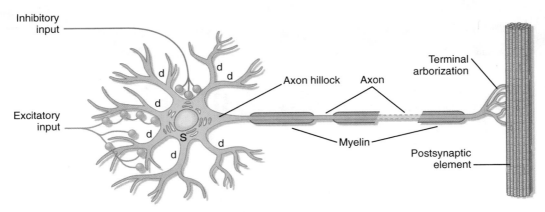

● **Figure 4-1.** Schematic diagram of an idealized neuron and its major components. Most afferent input from axons of other cells terminates in synapses on the dendrites (d), although some may terminate on the soma (S). Excitatory terminals tend to terminate more distally on dendrites than inhibitory ones do, which often terminate on the soma. (Redrawn from Williams PL, Warwick R: Functional Neuroanatomy of Man. Edinburgh, Churchill Livingstone, 1975.)

prominent Golgi apparatus. The soma also contains numerous mitochondria and cytoskeletal elements, including neurofilaments and microtubules. In contrast to most cells in the body, neurons have an enormous variety of shapes and sizes. Neurons with similar morphologies often characterize specific regions of the CNS. Morphological variation is produced by differences in the branching pattern of dendrites and the axon.

Dendrites are tapering and branching extensions of the soma and generally convey information toward the cell body. A neuron's branched set of dendrites is termed its dendritic tree. In some neurons the dendrites are longer than 1 mm, and they may account for more than 90% of the surface area. The proximal dendrites (near the cell body) contain Nissl bodies and parts of the Golgi apparatus. However, the main cytoplasmic organelles in dendrites are microtubules and neurofilaments. Because the dendrites are the major area that receives synaptic input from other neurons, the shape and size of the dendritic tree, as well as the population and distribution of channels in the dendritic membrane, are important determinants of how the synaptic input will affect the neuron. Synaptic input to dendrites can be passively conducted to the cell body, but these signals usually diminish as they pass to the soma and, in large cells, would have little influence on it. However, the dendrites of large neurons may have active zones, often using Ca^{++}-dependent, voltage-dependent channels, that can produce voltage spikes important in the integration of multiple synaptic input to a single neuron (see Chapter 6).

The axon is an extension of the cell that conveys the output of the cell to the next neuron or, in the case of a motor neuron, to a muscle. In general, each neuron has only one axon, and it is usually of uniform diameter. The length and diameter of axons vary with the neuronal type. Some axons do not extend much beyond the length of the dendrites, whereas others may be a meter or more long. Axons may have orthogonal branches en passant, but they often end in a spray of

branches called terminal arborization (Fig. 4-1). The size, shape, and organization of the terminal arborization determine which other cells it will contact. The axon arises from the soma (or sometimes from a proximal dendrite) in a specialized region called the axon hillock. The axon hillock and axon differ from the soma and proximal dendrites in that they lack rough endoplasmic reticulum, free ribosomes, and Golgi apparatus. The axon hillock is usually the site where action potentials are generated because it has a high concentration of the necessary channels (see Chapters 5 and 6). Because the soma is the metabolic engine for the axon, it is only reasonable that a large soma is required to support large, long axons and that very small neurons are associated with short axons. Thus, axons not only transmit information in neural circuits but also convey chemical substances toward or away from the synaptic terminals by axonal transport. For this reason also, axons degenerate when disconnected from the cell body.

Axonal Transport

Most axons are too long to allow efficient movement of substances from the soma to the synaptic endings by simple diffusion. Membrane and cytoplasmic components that originate in the biosynthetic apparatus of the soma must be distributed to replenish secreted or inactivated materials along the axon and, especially, to the presynaptic elements at the terminal end. A special transport mechanism called axonal transport accomplishes this distribution (Fig. 4-2).

Several types of axonal transport exist. Membrane-bound organelles and mitochondria are transported relatively rapidly by fast axonal transport. Substances that are dissolved in cytoplasm, such as proteins, are moved by slow axonal transport. In mammals, fast axonal transport proceeds as rapidly as 400 mm/day, whereas slow axonal transport occurs at about 1 mm/day. Synaptic vesicles, which travel by fast axonal transport, can travel from the soma of a motor neuron in the spinal cord to a neuromuscular junction in a

● **Figure 4-2.** Axonal transport has been proposed to depend on the movement of transport filaments. Energy is required and is supplied by glucose. Mitochondria control the level of cations in the axoplasm by supplying ATP to the ion pumps. An important cation for axonal transport is Ca⁺⁺. Transport filaments move along the cytoskeleton (microtubules [M] or neurofilaments [NF]) by means of cross-bridges. Transported components attach to the transport filaments. CaBP, Ca⁺⁺-binding protein; NF, neurofilaments.

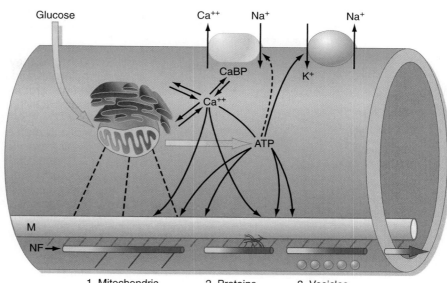

1. Mitochondria   2. Proteins   3. Vesicles

person's foot in about 2.5 days. In comparison, the movement of some soluble proteins over the same distance can take nearly 3 years.

Axonal transport requires metabolic energy and involves calcium ions. Microtubules provide a system of guide wires along which membrane-bound organelles move (Fig. 4-2). Organelles attach to microtubules through a linkage similar to that between the thick and thin filaments of skeletal muscle fibers. Ca⁺⁺ triggers movement of the organelles along the microtubules. Special microtubule-associated motor proteins called kinesin and dynein are required for axonal transport.

Axonal transport occurs in both directions. Transport from the soma toward the axonal terminals is called anterograde axonal transport. This process involves kinesin, and it allows the replenishment of synaptic vesicles and enzymes responsible for the synthesis of neurotransmitters in synaptic terminals. Transport in the opposite direction, which is driven by dynein, is called retrograde axonal transport. This process returns recycled synaptic vesicle membrane to the soma for lysosomal degradation.

THE SUPPORTIVE MATRIX OF THE CENTRAL NERVOUS SYSTEM

The local environment of most CNS neurons is controlled such that neurons are normally protected from extreme variations in the composition of the extracellular fluid that bathes them. This control is provided by the buffering functions of neuroglia, regulation of the CNS circulation, the presence of a blood-brain barrier, and exchange of substances between the cerebrospinal fluid (CSF) and extracellular fluid of the CNS.

Neuroglia

The major nonneuronal cellular elements of the nervous system are the neuroglia (Fig. 4-3), or sup-

▶ IN THE CLINIC

Certain viruses and toxins can be conveyed by axonal transport along peripheral nerves. For example, herpes zoster, the virus of chickenpox, invades dorsal root ganglion cells. The virus may be harbored by these neurons for many years. However, eventually, the virus may become active because of a change in immune status. The virus may then be transported along the sensory axons to the skin, causing shingles, a very painful disease. Another example is the axonal transport of tetanus toxin. *Clostridium tetani* bacteria may grow in a dirty wound, and if the person had not been vaccinated against tetanus toxin, the toxin can be transported retrogradely in the axons of motor neurons. The toxin can escape into the extracellular space of the spinal cord ventral horn and block the synaptic receptors for inhibitory amino acids. This process can result in tetanic convulsions.

portive cells. Neuroglial cells in the human CNS outnumber neurons by an order of magnitude: there are about 10^{13} neuroglia and 10^{12} neurons.

Neuroglia do not participate directly in the short-term communication of information through the nervous system, but they do assist in that function. For example, some types of neuroglial cells take up neurotransmitter molecules and in this manner directly influence synaptic activity. Others provide many axons with myelin sheaths that speed up the conduction of action potentials along axons (see Chapter 5) and thereby allow some axons to communicate rapidly over relatively long distances.

Neuroglial cells in the CNS include astrocytes and oligodendroglia (Fig. 4-3) and, in the PNS, Schwann cells and satellite cells. Microglia and ependymal cells are also considered to be central neuroglial cells.

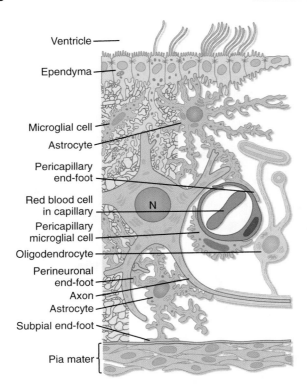

Ventricle

Ependyma

Microglial cell

Astrocyte

Pericapillary
end-foot

Red blood cell
in capillary

Pericapillary
microglial cell

Oligodendrocyte

Perineuronal
end-foot

Axon

Astrocyte

Subpial end-foot

Pia mater

N

● **Figure 4-3.** Schematic representation of nonneural elements in the CNS. Two astrocytes are shown ending on a neuron's soma and dendrites. They also contact the pial surface or capillaries, or both. An oligodendrocyte provides the myelin sheaths for axons. Also shown are microglia and ependymal cells. N, neuron. (Redrawn from Williams PL, Warwick R: *Functional Neuroanatomy of Man.* Edinburgh, Churchill Livingstone, 1975.)

Astrocytes (named for their star shape) help regulate the microenvironment of the CNS. Their processes contact neurons and surround groups of synaptic endings, isolating them from adjacent synapses and the general extracellular space. Astrocytes also have foot processes that contact the capillaries and connective tissue at the surface of the CNS, the pia mater (Fig. 4-3). These foot processes may help mediate the entry of substances into the CNS. Astrocytes can actively take up K^+ ions and neurotransmitter substances, which they metabolize, biodegrade, or recycle. Thus, astrocytes serve to buffer the extracellular environment of neurons with respect to both ions and neurotransmitters. The cytoplasm of astrocytes contains glial filaments, which provide mechanical support for CNS tissue. After injury, the astrocytic processes that contain these glial filaments hypertrophy and form a glial "scar."

Many axons are surrounded by a myelin sheath, which is a spiral multilayered wrapping of glial cell membrane (Fig. 4-4; see also Fig. 4-1). In the CNS, myelinated axons are ensheathed by the membranes of oligodendroglia (Fig. 4-4, *A*), and unmyelinated axons are bare. In the PNS, unmyelinated axons are surrounded by Schwann cells (Fig. 4-4, *C*), whereas myelinated axons are ensheathed by multiply wrapped

AT THE CELLULAR LEVEL

Astrocytes are coupled to each other by gap junctions such that they form a syncytium through which small molecules and ions can redistribute along their concentration gradients or by current flow. When normal neural activity gives rise to a local increase in extracellular $[K^+]$, this coupled network can enable the spatial redistribution of K^+ over a wide area via current flow in many astrocytes.

Under conditions of hypoxia, such as might be associated with ischemia secondary to blockage of an artery (i.e., a stroke), $[K^+]$ in the extracellular space of a brain region can increase by a factor of as much as 20. This will depolarize neurons and synaptic terminals and result in the release of transmitters such as glutamate, which will cause further release of K^+ from neurons. The additional release only exacerbates the problem and can lead to neuronal death. Under such conditions, local astroglia will probably take up the excess K^+ by K^+-Cl^- symport rather than by spatial buffering because the elevation in extracellular $[K^+]$ tends to be widespread rather than local.

membranes of Schwann cells, much as the oligodendroglia ensheath central axons. One major distinction is that many central axons can be myelinated by a single oligodendroglial cell, whereas in the periphery, each Schwann cell myelinates only one axon. Myelin increases the speed of action potential conduction, in part by restricting the flow of ionic current to small unmyelinated portions of the axon between adjacent sheath cells, the nodes of Ranvier (Fig. 4-4, *B*; see also Chapter 5).

Satellite cells encapsulate dorsal root and cranial nerve ganglion cells and regulate their microenvironment in a fashion similar to that used by astrocytes.

Microglia are latent phagocytes. When the CNS is damaged, microglia help remove the cellular products of the damage. They are assisted by neuroglia and by other phagocytes that invade the CNS from the circulation.

Ependymal cells form the epithelium lining the ventricular spaces of the brain that contain CSF. Many substances diffuse readily across the ependyma, which lies between the extracellular space of the brain and the CSF. CSF is secreted in large part by specialized ependymal cells of the choroid plexuses located in the ventricular system.

Most neurons in the adult nervous system are postmitotic cells (although some stem cells may also remain in certain sites in the brain). Many glial precursor cells are present in the adult brain, and they can still divide and differentiate. Thus, the cellular elements that give rise to most intrinsic brain tumors in the adult brain are the glial cells. For example, brain tumors can be derived from astrocytes (which vary in malignancy from the slowly growing astrocytoma to the rapidly fatal glioblastoma multiforme), from oligodendroglia (oligodendroglioma), or from ependymal cells (ependymoma). Meningeal cells can also give rise to slowly growing tumors (meningiomas) that compress brain tissue, as Schwann cells do (e.g., "acoustic schwannomas," which are tumors formed by Schwann cells of the eighth cranial nerve). In the brain of infants,

neurons that are still dividing can sometimes give rise to neuroblastomas (e.g., of the roof of the fourth ventricle) or retinoblastomas (in the eye).

The Blood-Brain Barrier

Movement of large molecules and highly charged ions from blood into the brain and spinal cord is severely restricted. The restriction is at least partly due to the barrier action of the capillary endothelial cells of the CNS and the tight junctions between them. Astrocytes may also help limit the movement of certain substances. For example, astrocytes can take up potassium ions and thus regulate $[K^+]$ in the extracellular space. Some pharmaceutical agents, such as penicillin, are removed from the CNS by transport mechanisms.

THE CENTRAL NERVOUS SYSTEM

The CNS, among other functions, gathers information about the environment from the PNS; processes this information and perceives part of it; organizes reflex and other behavioral responses; is responsible for cognition, learning, and memory; and plans and executes voluntary movements. The CNS includes the spinal cord and the brain (Fig. 4-5).

All vertebrate nervous systems begin as an invagination of a longitudinal groove in a thickened ectodermal plate, the neural plate. Closure of the neural groove

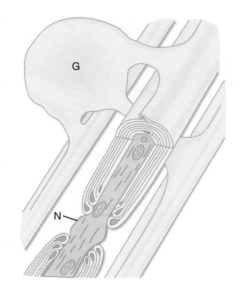

A

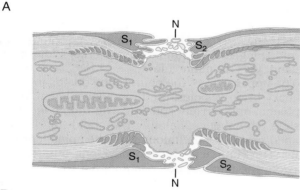

B

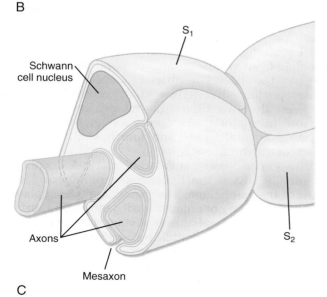

C

> ### IN THE CLINIC
>
> The blood-brain barrier can be disrupted by pathology of the brain. For example, brain tumors may allow substances that are otherwise excluded to enter the brain from the circulation. Radiologists can exploit this by introducing a substance into the circulation that normally cannot penetrate the blood-brain barrier. If the substance can be imaged, its leakage into the region occupied by the brain tumor can be used to demonstrate the distribution of the tumor.

● **Figure 4-4.** Myelin sheaths of axons. **A,** Myelinated axons in the CNS. A single oligodendrocyte (G) emits several processes, each of which winds in a spiral fashion around an axon to form the myelin sheath. The axon is shown in cutaway. The myelin from a single oligodendrocyte ends before the next wrapping from another oligodendrocyte. The bare axon between segments is the node of Ranvier (N). Conduction of action potentials is saltatory down the axon, skipping from node to node. **B,** Myelinated axon in the PNS shown in a longitudinal view. The node of Ranvier (N) is shown between adjacent sheaths formed by two Schwann cells (S_1 and S_2). (Redrawn from Patton HD et al: Introduction to Basic Neurology. Philadelphia, Saunders, 1976.) **C,** Three-dimensional impression of the appearance of a bundle of unmyelinated axons enwrapped by Schwann cells. The cut face of the bundle is seen to the left. One of the three unmyelinated axons is represented as protruding from the bundle. A mesaxon is shown as the continuity of the outer Schwann cell membrane to that surrounding the axon. To the right, the adjacent nerve segment with its Schwann cell is depicted.

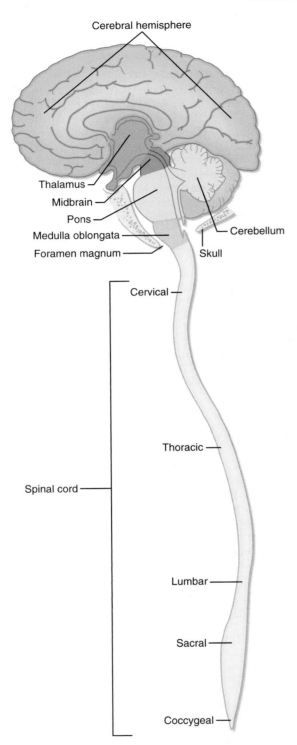

● **Figure 4-5.** Schematic of the major components of the CNS as shown in a longitudinal midline view. (From Haines DE [ed]: Fundamental Neuroscience for Basic and Clinical Applications, 3rd ed. Philadelphia, Churchill Livingstone, 2006.)

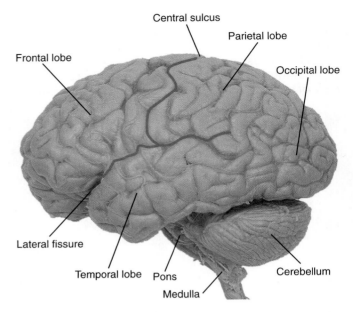

● **Figure 4-6.** Lateral view of the human brain showing the left cerebral hemisphere, cerebellum, pons, and medulla. Note the division of the lobes of the cerebrum (frontal, parietal, occipital, and temporal) and the two major fissures (lateral and central). (From Nolte J, Angevine J: The Human Brain in Photographs and Diagrams, 2nd ed. St Louis, Mosby, 2000.)

crest is the source of cells in the dorsal root and autonomic ganglia, Schwann cells, Merkel's disks, and melanocytes, to name a few.

The upper part of the neural tube dilates into three primary brain vesicles, the rhombencephalon, mesencephalon, and prosencephalon. The rhombencephalic vesicle (rhombencephalon = rhomboid- or diamond-shaped brain) is continuous with the spinal cord caudally. The rhombencephalon develops into a caudal portion, the medulla oblongata, and a rostral portion that includes the pons and cerebellum. The mesencephalon becomes the midbrain. Above, the prosencephalon develops into the diencephalon (thalamus and hypothalamus), and the telencephalon (cerebrum) most rostrally. The spaces in these vesicles become the fluid-filled ventricles and cerebral aqueduct. The largest, the lateral ventricles, develop inside the telencephalon; the narrow third ventricle remains between the two halves of the diencephalon. The narrow lumen of the mesencephalon becomes the cerebral aqueduct, and the fourth ventricle is the space of the rhombencephalon.

The enormous expansion of the telencephalon eventually covers the thalamus, midbrain, and portions of the cerebellum. The expanding telencephalon takes on a shape not unlike a boxing glove. The surface area of the telencephalon is divided into five deeply furrowed lobes named after the overlying bones of the skull: the frontal, parietal, temporal, and occipital lobes (Fig. 4-6). The right and left cerebral hemispheres are connected across the midline by a massive bundle of axons, the corpus callosum (Figs. 4-7, *A* and 4-9).

results in the formation of a hollow neural tube that is bordered dorsolaterally by columns of neural crest. The ectoderm closes over the invaginated neural tube to form the skin of the back. The neural tube subsequently develops into the CNS, whereas the neural

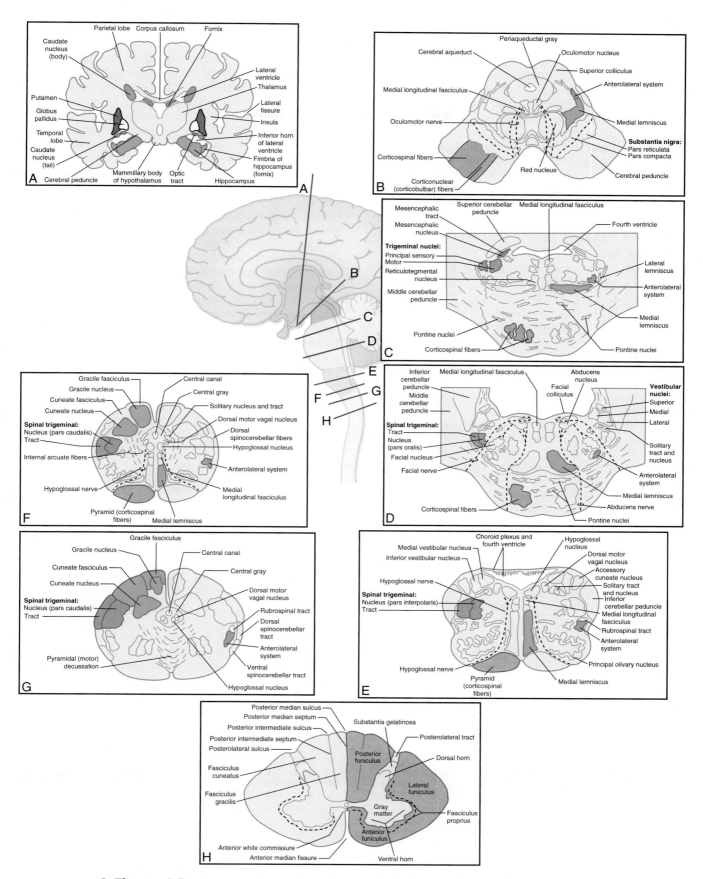

● **Figure 4-7.** Representative sections through the brain at various levels, with the major landmarks labeled. **A,** Cerebrum and thalamus; **B,** midbrain; **C,** upper pons; **D,** lower pons; **E,** upper medulla; **F,** lower medulla; **G,** junction of the medulla and spinal cord; **H,** cervical spinal cord.

Expansion of the frontal, parietal, and temporal lobes buries and isolates the insula, hence its name, deep within the lateral fissure (Fig. 4-7A).

The spinal cord (lower part of Fig. 4-5) can be subdivided into a series of regions, each composed of a number of segments named for the vertebrae where their nerve roots enter or leave: 8 cervical, 12 thoracic, 5 lumbar, 5 sacral, and 1 coccygeal. Each portion maintains its tubular appearance, although its lumen, the spinal canal, may not remain patent (Fig. 4-7, *H*).

The major functions of the different parts of the CNS are listed in Table 4-1.

Cellular Circuitry in the Central Nervous System

Sensory receptors can be classified in terms of the type of energy that they transduce (e.g., photoreceptors transduce light, mechanoreceptors transduce displacement and force) or according to the source of the input (e.g., exteroceptors signal external events, proprioceptors signal the position of a body part with respect to space or another body part). Primary afferent neurons are connected peripherally to sensory receptors, which are specialized structures that transduce changes in environmental energy. In general, that information is transmitted to the CNS by trains of action potentials in primary afferent neurons. The cell bodies of primary afferent neurons are located in dorsal root and cranial nerve ganglia. Each primary afferent neuron has two types of processes: (1) a peripheral process that extends distally within a peripheral nerve to reach the appropriate sensory receptors and (2) a central process that enters the CNS through a dorsal root or a cranial nerve (Fig. 4-8).

In the CNS, axons often travel in bundles or tracts. The names applied to tracts usually describe their origin and termination. For example, the spinocerebellar tract conveys information from the spinal cord to the cerebellum. The term **pathway** is similar to tract but is generally used to suggest a particular function (e.g., the auditory pathway: a series of neuron-to-neuron links, across several synapses, that convey and process auditory information).

Behavior is expressed by movement brought about through the contraction of muscle fibers or by the release of chemical compounds from glands. These events are triggered by the activation of motor neurons, the term applied to cells whose axons leave the CNS to affect the periphery. For example, a motor unit can be regarded as the basic unit of movement, and it consists of an α motor neuron, its axon, and all the skeletal muscle fibers that it supplies. A given α motor neuron (and its motor unit) may participate in a variety of reflexes and in voluntary movement as it responds to the central neurons and pathways that synapse on it. Because the α motor neuron (in mammals) and its axon represent the only means of communication between the nervous system and the muscle, these motor neurons have been termed the final common pathway. They are also sometimes referred to as "lower motor neurons" to distinguish them from the central "upper motor neurons," which synapse on them via various central pathways.

Regions of the CNS containing high concentrations of axon pathways (and very few neurons) are called **white matter** because the axonal myelin sheaths of the axons are highly refractive to light. Regions containing high concentrations of neurons and dendrites are, by contrast, called **gray matter.** Axons are also present in

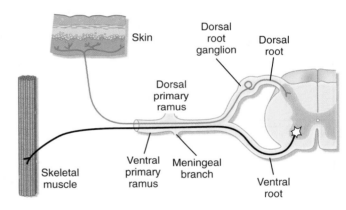

● **Figure 4-8.** Diagram of the spinal cord, spinal roots, and spinal nerve. A primary afferent neuron is shown with its cell body in the dorsal root ganglion and its central and peripheral processes distributed, respectively, to the spinal cord gray matter and to a sensory receptor in the skin. An α motor neuron is shown to have its cell body in the spinal cord gray matter and to project its axon out the ventral root to innervate a skeletal muscle fiber.

● **Table 4-1. Parts and Functions of the Central Nervous System**

Region	Nerves (Input/Output)	General Functions
Spinal cord	Dorsal/ventral roots	Sensory input, reflex circuits, somatic and autonomic motor output
Medulla	Cranial nerves VIII-XII	Cardiovascular and respiratory control, auditory and vestibular input, brainstem reflexes
Pons	Cranial nerves V-VIII	Respiratory/urinary control, control of eye movement, facial sensation/motor control
Cerebellum	Cranial nerve VIII	Motor coordination, motor learning, equilibrium
Midbrain	Cranial nerves III-IV	Acoustic relay and mapping, control of the eye (including movement, lens and pupillary reflexes), pain modulation
Thalamus	Cranial nerve II	Sensory and motor relay to the cerebral cortex, regulation of cortical activation, visual input
Hypothalamus		Autonomic and endocrine control, motivated behavior
Basal ganglia		Shape patterns of thalamocortical motor inhibition
Cerebral cortex	Cranial nerve I	Sensory perception, cognition, learning and memory, motor planning and voluntary movement, language

gray matter. Gray matter has a much higher metabolic rate than white matter does and consequently is more highly vascularized. A group of neurons in the CNS is called a **nucleus,** similar to what would be called a ganglion outside the CNS. When neurons are organized into layers, they may form a **cortex.** The most prominent cortex covers the entire surface of the cerebral hemispheres, where its structural variation reflects the general functional organization of the cerebrum (see Fig. 10-3).

Cerebrospinal Fluid

CSF fills the ventricular system, a series of interconnected spaces within the brain, and the subarachnoid space directly surrounding the brain. The volume of CSF within the cerebral ventricles is approximately 30 mL, and that in the subarachnoid space is about 125 mL. Because about 0.35 mL of CSF is produced each minute, CSF is turned over more than three times daily. The intraventricular CSF reflects the composition of the brain's extracellular space via free exchange across the ependyma, and the brain "floats" in the subarachnoid CSF to minimize the effect of external mechanical forces.

CSF is formed largely by the choroid plexuses, which contain ependymal cells specialized for trans-port. The choroid plexuses are located in the lateral, third, and fourth ventricles (Fig. 4-9). The lateral ventricles are situated within the two cerebral hemispheres. They connect with the third ventricle through the interventricular foramina (of Monro). The third ventricle lies in the midline between the diencephalon on the two sides. The cerebral aqueduct (of Sylvius) traverses the midbrain and connects the third ventricle with the fourth ventricle. The fourth ventricle is interposed between the pons and medulla below and the cerebellum above. The central canal of the spinal cord continues caudally from the fourth ventricle, although in adult humans the canal is not generally patent.

CSF escapes from the ventricular system through three apertures (the medial aperture of Magendie and the two lateral apertures of Luschka) located in the roof of the fourth ventricle. After it leaves the ventricular system, CSF circulates through the subarachnoid space that surrounds the brain and spinal cord. Regions where these spaces are expanded are called subarachnoid cisterns. An example is the lumbar cistern, which surrounds the lumbar and sacral spinal roots below the level of termination of the spinal cord. The lumbar cistern is the target for lumbar puncture, a procedure used clinically to sample CSF. A large part

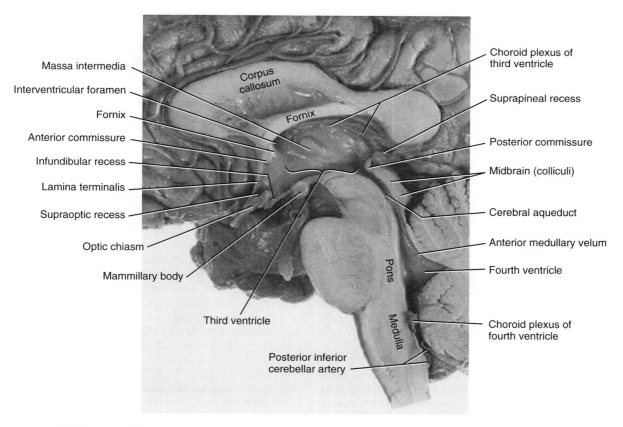

● **Figure 4-9.** Midsagittal view of the brain showing the third and fourth ventricles, the cerebral aqueduct of the midbrain, and the choroid plexus. The CSF formed by the choroid plexus in the lateral ventricles enters this circulation via the interventricular foramen. Note also the location of the corpus callosum and other commissures. (From Haines DE [ed]: Fundamental Neuroscience for Basic and Clinical Applications, 3rd ed. Philadelphia, Churchill Livingstone, 2006.)

of CSF is removed by bulk flow through the valvular arachnoid granulations into the dural venous sinuses in the cranium.

Because the extracellular fluid within the CNS communicates with the CSF, the composition of the CSF is a useful indicator of the composition of the extracellular environment of neurons in the brain and spinal cord. The main constituents of CSF in the lumbar cistern are listed in Table 4-2. For comparison, the concentrations of the same constituents in blood are also given. CSF has a lower concentration of K^+, glucose, and protein but a greater concentration of Na^+ and Cl^-

● Table 4-2.
Constituents of Cerebrospinal Fluid and Blood

Constituent	Lumbar CSF	Blood
Na^+ (mEq/L)	148	136-145
K^+ (mEq/L)	2.9	3.5-5
Cl^- (mEq/L)	120-130	100-106
Glucose (mg/dL)	50-75	70-100
Protein (mg/dL)	15-45	6.8×10^3
pH	7.3	7.4

From Willis WD, Grossman RG: Medical Neurobiology, 3rd ed. St Louis, Mosby, 1981.

than blood does. Furthermore, CSF contains practically no blood cells. The increased concentration of Na^+ and Cl^- enables CSF to be isotonic to blood.

The pressure in the CSF column is about 120 to 180 mm H_2O when a person is recumbent. The rate at which CSF is formed is relatively independent of the pressure in the ventricles and subarachnoid space, as well as systemic blood pressure. However, the absorption rate of CSF is a direct function of CSF pressure.

NERVOUS TISSUE REACTIONS TO INJURY

Injury to nervous tissue elicits responses by neurons and neuroglia. Severe injury causes cell death. Except in specific instances, once a neuron is lost, it cannot be replaced because neurons are postmitotic cells.

Degeneration
When an axon is transected, the soma of the neuron may show chromatolysis, or "axonal reaction." Normally, Nissl bodies stain well with basic aniline dyes, which attach to the RNA of ribosomes (Fig. 4-10, *A*). After injury to the axon (Fig. 4-10, *B*), the neuron

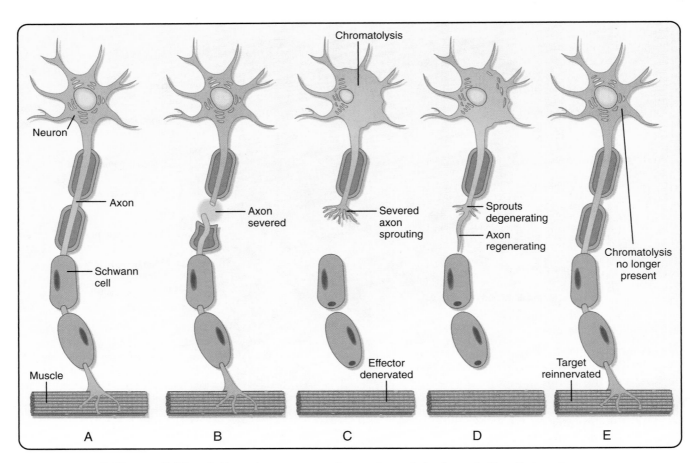

● **Figure 4-10.** **A,** Normal motor neuron innervating a skeletal muscle fiber. **B,** A motor axon has been severed, and the motor neuron is undergoing chromatolysis. **C,** This is associated in time with sprouting and, in **D,** with regeneration of the axon. The excess sprouts degenerate. **E,** When the target cell is reinnervated, chromatolysis is no longer present.

attempts to repair the axon by making new structural proteins, and the cisterns of the rough endoplasmic reticulum become distended with the products of protein synthesis. The ribosomes appear to be disorganized, and the Nissl bodies are stained weakly by basic aniline dyes. This process, called chromatolysis, alters the staining pattern (Fig. 4-10, *C*). In addition, the soma may swell and become rounded, and the nucleus may assume an eccentric position. These morphological changes reflect the cytological processes that accompany increased protein synthesis.

Because it cannot synthesize new protein, the axon distal to the transection dies (Fig. 4-10, *C*). Within a few days, the axon and all the associated synaptic endings disintegrate. If the axon had been a myelinated axon in the CNS, the myelin sheath would also fragment and eventually be removed by phagocytosis. However, in the PNS the Schwann cells that had formed the myelin sheath remain viable, and in fact they undergo cell division. This sequence of events was originally described by Waller and is called wallerian degeneration.

If the axons that provide the sole or predominant synaptic input to a neuron or to an effector cell are interrupted, the postsynaptic cell may undergo transneuronal degeneration and even death. The best known example of this is atrophy of skeletal muscle fibers after their innervation by motor neurons has been interrupted. If only one or a few axons are removed, the other surviving axons may sprout additional terminals, thereby taking up the synaptic space of the damaged axons and increasing their influence on the postsynaptic cell.

Regeneration

In the PNS, after an axon is lost through injury, many neurons can regenerate a new axon. The proximal stump of the damaged axon develops sprouts (Fig. 4-10, *C*), these sprouts elongate, and they grow along the path of the original nerve if this route is available (Fig. 4-10, *D*). The Schwann cells in the distal stump of the nerve not only survive the wallerian degeneration but also proliferate and form rows along the course previously taken by the axons. Growth cones of the sprouting axons find their way along these rows of Schwann cells, and they may eventually reinnervate

the original peripheral target structures (Fig. 4-10, *E*). The Schwann cells then remyelinate the axons. The rate of regeneration is limited by the rate of slow axonal transport to about 1 mm/day.

In the CNS, transected axons also sprout. However, proper guidance for the sprouts is lacking, in part because the oligodendroglia do not form a path along which the sprouts can grow. This limitation may be a consequence of the fact that a single oligodendroglial cell myelinates many central axons, whereas a single Schwann cell provides myelin for only a single axon in the periphery. In addition, different chemical signals may affect peripheral and central attempts at regeneration differently. Another obstacle to CNS regeneration is the formation of a glial scar by astrocytes.

Trophic Factors

A number of proteins are now known to affect the growth of axons and maintenance of synaptic connections. The best studied of these substances is nerve growth factor (NGF). NGF was initially thought to enhance the growth and maintain the integrity of many neurons of neural crest origin, including small dorsal root ganglion cells and autonomic postganglionic neurons. However, NGF also affects some neurons in the CNS.

Many other growth factors have also been described, including the brain-derived growth factors neurotrophin 3, neurotrophin 4, neurotrophin 5, and ciliary neurotrophic factor. Some of these factors affect the growth of large dorsal root ganglion cells or motor neurons.

A large assortment of molecular factors play roles in the differentiation, growth, and migration of neurons to their proper locations in the PNS and CNS, and another large contingent influences the growth and guidance of axons as they extend from neurons to reach their proper synaptic targets. Prenatal and perinatal disruption of these factors secondary to genetic or environmental influences can result in malformations, ectopic locations, and errors in circuitry that can be associated with functional deficits from the punctate (e.g., loss of a single function) to the global (e.g., mental retardation). Known environmental influences include radiation, chemical exposure, maternal alcohol consumption, and malnutrition.

■ KEY CONCEPTS

1. General functions of the nervous system include excitability, sensory detection, information processing, and behavior. Different types of neurons are specialized for different functions.

2. The CNS includes the spinal cord and brain. The brain includes the medulla, pons, cerebellum, midbrain, thalamus, hypothalamus, basal ganglia, and cerebral cortex.

3. The PNS includes primary afferent neurons and the sensory receptors that they innervate, somatic motor neurons, and autonomic neurons.

4. The neuron is the functional unit of the nervous system. Neurons contain a nucleus and nucleolus, Nissl bodies (rough endoplasmic reticulum), Golgi apparatus, mitochondria, neurofilaments, and microtubules.

5. Information is conveyed through neural circuits by action potentials in the axons of neurons and by synaptic transmission between axons and the dendrites and somas of other neurons or between axons and effector cells.

6. Sensory receptors include exteroceptors, interoceptors, and proprioceptors. Stimuli are environmental events that excite sensory receptors, responses are the effects of stimuli, and sensory transduction is the process by which stimuli are detected.

7. Sensory receptors can be classified in terms of the type of energy they transduce or according to the source of the input. Central pathways are usually named by their origin and termination or for the type of information conveyed. The motor neuron is the only means of communication between the CNS and effectors, like muscles and glands. It is often referred to as "the final common pathway" as it is the only way for the CNS to express its operations as behavior.

8. Chemical substances are distributed along the axons by fast or by slow axonal transport; the direction of axonal transport may be anterograde or retrograde.

9. Neuroglial cells include astrocytes (regulate the CNS microenvironment), oligodendroglia (form CNS myelin), Schwann cells (form PNS myelin), ependymal cells (line the ventricles), and microglia (CNS macrophages). Myelin sheaths increase the conduction velocity of axons.

10. Choroid plexuses form CSF. CSF differs from blood in having a lower concentration of K^+, glucose, and protein and a higher concentration of Na^+ and Cl^-; CSF normally lacks blood cells.

11. The extracellular fluid composition of the CNS is regulated by CSF, the blood-brain barrier, and astrocytes.

12. Damage to the axon of a neuron causes an axonal reaction (chromatolysis) in the cell body and Wallerian degeneration of the axon distal to the injury. Regeneration of PNS axons is more likely than regeneration of CNS axons.

13. The growth and maintenance of axons are affected by trophic factors such as nerve growth factor.

CHAPTER 5

Generation and Conduction of Action Potentials

An **action potential** is a rapid, all-or-none change in the membrane potential followed by a return to the resting membrane potential.

- Voltage-dependent ion channels in the plasma membrane are the basis for action potentials.
- An action potential is propagated with the same shape and size along the entire length of an axon.
- Action potentials are usually initiated at the axon hillock of the axon.
- The action potential is the basis of the signal-carrying ability of nerve cells.
- The patterns of conducted action potentials encode the information conveyed by nerve cells.

This chapter describes how action potentials are generated and conducted. Within this general discussion, the influence of axon geometry, ion channel distribution, and myelin is discussed and explained. The ways in which information is encoded by the frequency and pattern of action potentials in individual cells and in groups of nerve cells are also presented. Finally, because the nervous system provides important information about the external world through specific sensory receptors, the general principles of sensory transduction and coding are reviewed. More detailed information on these sensory mechanisms and systems is provided in other chapters.

MEMBRANE POTENTIALS

Observations of Membrane Potentials

All cells, including neurons, have a resting potential that is typically around −70 mV, as detailed in Chapter 1. One of the signature features of neurons is their ability to change their membrane potential rapidly in response to an appropriate stimulus, and the most significant of these responses is the action potential. Our current knowledge about the ionic mechanisms of action potentials comes from experiments with many species. One of the most studied, however, is the squid because the large diameter (up to 0.5 mm) of the squid giant axon makes it a convenient model for electrophysiological research with intracellular electrodes. When a microelectrode (tip diameter <0.5 µm) is inserted through the plasma membrane of the squid giant axon, a potential difference is observed between the tip of the microelectrode inside the cell and an electrode placed outside the cell. The internal electrode is approximately 70 mV negative with respect to the external electrode. This 70-mV potential difference is the **resting membrane potential** of the axon. By convention, membrane potentials are expressed as the intracellular potential minus the extracellular potential; therefore, the resting potential of squid giant axons, as well as many mammalian neurons, is about −70 mV. In the absence of perturbing influences, the resting membrane potential remains at −70 mV.

The Passive Response

Figure 5-1 illustrates the results of an experiment in which the membrane potential of an axon is perturbed by passing rectangular pulses of **depolarizing** or **hyperpolarizing** current across the plasma membrane. The injection of positive charge, which changes the membrane potential from −70 mV to −60 mV, is depolarizing because it makes the cell more positive (i.e., decreases the potential difference across the cell membrane). Conversely, a change in the membrane potential from −70 mV to −80 mV as a result of the injection of negative charge increases the polarization of the membrane; this change in potential is called hyperpolarization. The more current that passes across the plasma membrane, the larger the change in the membrane potential.

Note that although the current is injected as rectangular pulses, with vertical rising and falling edges, the shape of the membrane response to small-amplitude current pulses has a slower rise and fall. For hyperpolarizing and small-amplitude depolarizing current pulses, the rise and fall in the membrane voltage response has an exponential shape because the membrane is responding to the current as would a passive RC circuit. That is, the stimulus causes no change in membrane resistance or capacitance, and thus the time course of the rise and fall simply reflects the time required to discharge or charge the membrane capacitance. Recall that because there is an excess of negative ions inside the axon in comparison to outside, those negative ions will attract some positive ions to the outside of the membrane. These charges remain separated from each other by the cell membrane, similar to the storage of charge in a capacitor. Thus, at least in this passive domain, the membrane response to electrical stimuli closely follows the

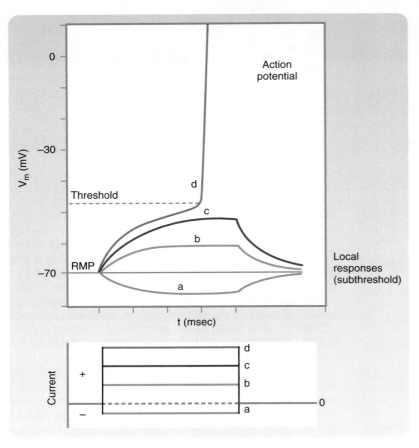

● **Figure 5-1.** Responses of an axon to rectangular pulses of hyperpolarizing (a) or depolarizing (b to d) current. The change in transmembrane current and potential as recorded by an intracellular electrode is shown as a function of time. Note that when stimulated to threshold (d), the axon fires an action potential. For clarity, only the rising phase of the action potential is shown. RMP, resting membrane potential. (Redrawn from Blankenship J: Neurophysiology. Philadelphia, Mosby, 2002.)

same laws that govern an electric circuit composed of a resistor and capacitor connected in parallel.

When current pulses that elicit only passive responses are passed across the plasma membrane, the size of the potential change recorded depends on the distance of the recording electrode from the point of passage of the current (Fig. 5-2). The closer the recording electrode to the site of current passage, the larger and steeper the potential change. The magnitude of the potential change decreases exponentially with distance from the site of passage of the current, and the potential change is said to reflect **passive** or **electrotonic conduction.** Such changes do not spread very far along the membrane before they become insignificant. As shown in Figure 5-2, an electrotonically conducted signal dies away over a distance of a few millimeters. The distance over which the potential change decreases to 1/e (37%) of its maximal value is called the **length constant** or **space constant** (e is the base of natural logarithms and is equal to 2.7182). A length constant of 1 to 3 mm is typical for mammalian axons.

The length constant can be related to the electrical properties of the axon via cable theory because nerve fibers have many of the properties of an electrical cable. In a perfect cable, the insulation surrounding the core conductor prevents all loss of current to the surrounding medium so that a signal is transmitted along the cable with undiminished strength. If we

compare an unmyelinated (see later) nerve fiber with an electrical cable, the plasma membrane equates to the insulation and the cytoplasm to the core conductor, but the plasma membrane is not a perfect insulator. Thus, the spread of signals depends on the ratio of the **membrane resistance (r_m)** and the **axial resistance of the axonal cytoplasm (r_a).** The higher the ratio of r_m to r_a, the less current lost across the plasma membrane per unit of axonal length, the better the axon can function as a cable, and the longer the distance that a signal can be transmitted electrotonically without significant decrement. A useful analogy is to think of the axon as a garden hose with holes poked in it. The more holes in the hose, the more water will leak out along its length (analogous to more loss of current when r_m is low) and the less water delivered to its nozzle.

Based on cable theory, the length constant can be related to axonal resistance and is equal to $\sqrt{r_m/r_a}$. By using this relationship we can determine how changes in axonal diameter will affect the length constant and hence how the decay of electrotonic potentials will vary. An increase in diameter of the axon will reduce both r_a and r_m. However, r_m is inversely proportional to diameter (because it is related to the circumference of the axon), whereas r_a varies inversely to the diameter squared (because it is related to the cross-sectional area of the axon). Thus, r_a decreases more rapidly than r_m does as axonal

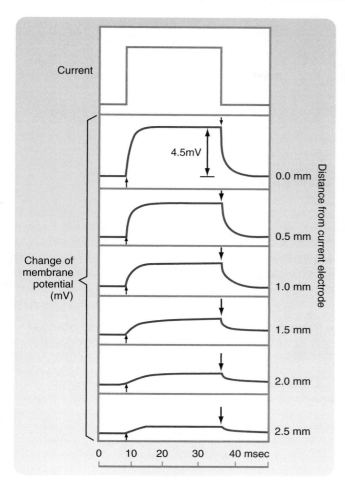

● Figure 5-2. Responses of an axon of a shore crab to a subthreshold rectangular current pulse by an extracellular electrode applied closely to its surface and located at different distances from the current-passing electrode. As the recording electrode is moved farther from the point of stimulation, the response of the membrane potential is slower and smaller. (Redrawn from Hodgkin AL, Rushton WAH: Proc R Soc ser B 133:444–479, 1946.)

diameter increases, and therefore the length constant increases (Fig. 5-3).

Membrane capacitance is a major factor that shapes the time course of passive responses. To depolarize an adjacent portion of axon, the injected depolarizing positive charges must draw the inner negative charges from the membrane and thereby free the external positive charges (Fig. 5-4). The time that this process takes increases with the amount of axon membrane to be depolarized.

The Local (Subthreshold) Response

If a somewhat larger depolarizing current pulse is applied to a small portion of the membrane of an axon (Fig. 5-1, c), the voltage response no longer looks like that of a passive RC circuit (e.g., the tail does not decay exponentially). The shape is altered because the stimulus has changed the membrane potential sufficiently to cause the opening of significant numbers of voltage-sensitive Na^+ channels (see later). Opening of these channels changes the membrane's resistance

and allows Na^+ to enter, driven by its electrochemical gradient. This entry of positive charge enhances the depolarization by adding to the current pulse. The resulting depolarization is called a **local** or **subthreshold response.** The local response results from active changes in membrane properties (specifically, r_m), which distinguishes it from the passive electrotonic response. Nevertheless, it is not self-regenerating and does not propagate down the axon but, again, decreases in amplitude with distance. The change in membrane properties is insufficient for what is needed to generate an action potential.

SUPRATHRESHOLD RESPONSE: THE ACTION POTENTIAL

Somewhat larger local responses are observed with still larger depolarizing current pulses until a **threshold membrane potential** is reached at which a different sort of response, the **action potential** (or **spike**), occurs (Fig. 5-5; see also Fig. 5-1, d). For example, the threshold value for the squid giant axon is near –55 mV. When the membrane potential exceeds this value, an action potential is triggered. Thus, the threshold can be defined as the membrane voltage at which there is a 50:50 chance of generating an action potential.

The action potential differs from the subthreshold and passive responses in three important ways: (1) it is a much larger response in which the polarity of the membrane potential actually overshoots (the cell interior becomes positive with respect to the exterior), (2) the action potential is propagated down the entire length of the nerve fiber, and (3) the action potential is propagated without decrement (i.e., it maintains its size and shape as it is regenerated along the axon). In addition, when a stimulus even larger than the threshold stimulus is applied, the action potential remains the same and does not increase with greater stimulus strength. A stimulus either produces a full-sized action potential or fails to do so. For this reason, the action potential is described as an **all-or-none response.**

Action potentials can be generated in other parts of the nerve cell membrane, but their most prominent role is signal conduction along the axon. When the membrane is depolarized to threshold, the depolarization becomes explosive (Fig. 5-5). The depolarization completely depolarizes the membrane and even overshoots such that the membrane potential reverses from negative to positive. The peak of the action potential approaches +50 mV. The membrane potential then returns toward the resting membrane potential almost as rapidly as it was depolarized. After repolarization, a variable hyperpolarization occurs that is known as the **afterhyperpolarization.** The action potential's depolarization has a duration of 1 to 2 msec, but the hyperpolarizing afterpotential can persist from a few to 100 msec, depending on the particular type of neuron.

Ionic Basis of Action Potentials

An action potential is the result of successive, rapid, and transient changes in plasma membrane conduc-

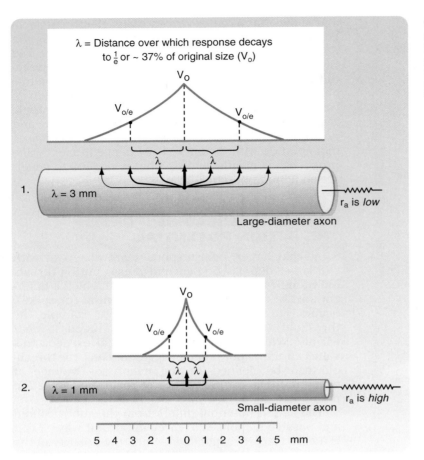

● **Figure 5-3.** Comparison of the length constant, λ, in relation to axon diameter. Note that the increase in diameter is associated with a decrease in r_i and an increase in the length constant. (Redrawn from Blankenship J: Neurophysiology. Philadelphia, Mosby, 2002.)

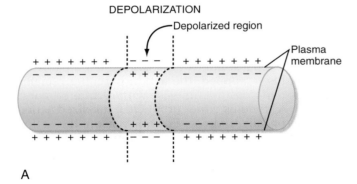

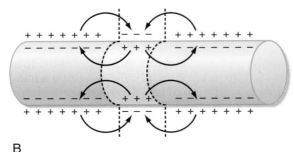

● **Figure 5-4.** Mechanism of electrotonic spread of depolarization. **A,** The reversal of membrane polarity that occurs with local depolarization. **B,** The local currents that flow to depolarize adjacent areas of the membrane and allow conduction of the depolarization.

tance to sodium and potassium ions. In the squid giant axon, the resting membrane potential (V_m) is about −70 mV, and the equilibrium potential of K^+ (E_K) is about −100 mV. An increase in g_K would therefore hyperpolarize the membrane, whereas a decrease in g_K would tend to depolarize the membrane (see Chapter 2). Conversely, an increase in g_{Na} would cause depolarization and, if of sufficient magnitude, even a reversal in membrane polarity because E_{Na} is about +65 mV in the squid giant axon.

As with the resting membrane potential, the action potential depends on the opposing tendencies of (1) the Na^+ gradient to bring the resting membrane potential toward the equilibrium potential for Na^+ and (2) the K^+ gradient to bring the resting membrane potential toward the equilibrium potential for K^+. The relationship between potential, conductance, and ion current during an action potential includes the following (Fig. 5-6):

1. A rapid increase in g_{Na} and I_{Na} during the early phase of the action potential causes the membrane potential to move toward the equilibrium potential for Na^+ (+65 mV). The peak of the action potential does not reach +65 mV because the Na^+ channels quickly inactivate, thereby reducing g_{Na} and I_{Na}, and because the slower increase in g_K and I_K provides mounting opposition to depolarization.

2. The rapid return of the membrane potential toward the resting potential is caused by the continuing

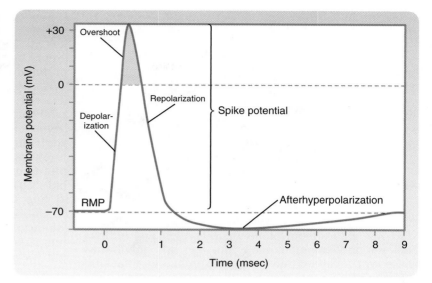

● **Figure 5-5.** Components of the action potential with respect to time and voltage. Note that the time scale for the first few milliseconds has been expanded for clarity. RMP, resting membrane potential. (Redrawn from Blankenship J: Neurophysiology. Philadelphia, Mosby, 2002.)

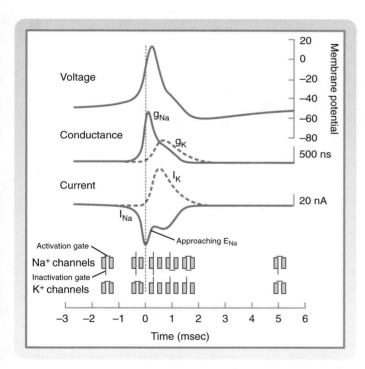

● **Figure 5-6.** The action potential and the conductance and currents that underlie the action potential with respect to time. Note that the increased conductance for Na⁺ (and its inward flow) is associated with the rising phase of the action potential, whereas the slower increase in conductance for K⁺ (and its outward flow) is associated with repolarization of the membrane and with afterhyperpolarization. The reduction in I_{Na} before the peak of the action potential (even though G_{Na} is still high) is due to inactivation of the Na⁺ channels. (Redrawn from Squires LR et al: Fundamental Neuroscience, 2nd ed. San Diego, CA, Academic Press, 2002.)

increase in g_K, as well as by the decrease in g_{Na}. The result is that the membrane potential is driven toward E_K.

3. During the hyperpolarizing afterpotential, the membrane potential is actually more negative than the resting potential because g_{Na} has returned to baseline levels but g_K remains elevated. Thus, the resting membrane potential is pulled even closer to the K⁺ equilibrium potential (–100 mV), and the membrane remains hyperpolarized as long as g_K remains elevated.

Ion Channels and Gates

Early studies on the mechanism underlying action potentials proposed that ion currents pass through separate Na⁺ and K⁺ channels, each with distinct characteristics, in the plasma membrane. Subsequent research has supported this interpretation. The amino acid sequences of the channel proteins and many of the functional and structural characteristics of the channels are now known in detail.

The structure of a voltage-gated Na⁺ channel (Fig. 5-7) consists of a single α subunit in association with a β₁ and a β₂ subunit. The α subunit has four repeated motifs of six transmembrane helices that surround a central ion channel or pore. The channel's walls are partly formed by the number 6 helices in each motif. The functional channels of most voltage-gated K⁺ channels are comprised of four separate subunits, each consisting of a polypeptide with six membrane-spanning segments and similar to the motifs which make up the single α subunit of the Na⁺ channel.

Another important characteristic of some channels such as those that underlie the action potential is that they are gated by change in voltage (i.e., they are voltage-gated channels). The gates sense the potential across the membrane and then act to either open or close the channel according to the membrane potential. The gates are formed by groups of charged

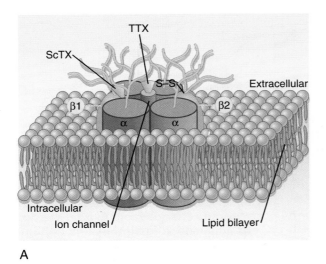

A

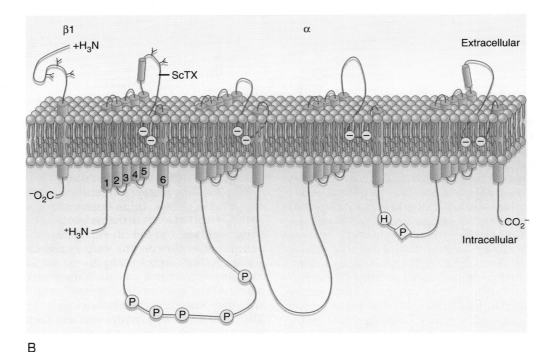

B

● **Figure 5-7.** Three-dimensional model of the voltage-gated Na^+ channel. **A,** The large cylinders represent the four α subunits and the two β subunits with the receptor sites for α scorpion toxin (ScTX) and tetrodotoxin (TTX) indicated. **B,** The β1 subunit and an α subunit are shown with their transmembrane helices. (Redrawn from Squires LR et al: Fundamental Neuroscience, 2nd ed. San Diego, CA, Academic Press, 2002.)

amino acid residues, and the voltage dependence of the Na^+ and K^+ channel gates can account for the complex changes in g_{Na} and g_K that occur during an action potential.

Behavior of Individual Ion Channels during the Action Potential

One way to study the behavior of individual ion channels and how they contribute to the membrane potential is to incorporate either purified ion channel proteins or bits of nerve membrane into planar lipid bilayers separating two aqueous compartments. Electrodes placed in the aqueous compartments can then be used to monitor or impose currents and voltages across the membrane. Another way to study individual ion channels involves the use of **patch electrodes.** A fire-polished microelectrode is placed against the surface of a cell, and suction is applied to the electrode. A high-resistance seal is formed around the tip of the electrode (Fig. 5-8, *A*). The sealed patch elec-

AT THE CELLULAR LEVEL

Knowledge of the molecular structure of channels has increased our understanding of the basis of their properties. For example, most channels are highly selective for a particular ion. First, by lining the channel walls with either positive or negative charges, one can exclude either cations or anions; however, most channels are also differentially permeable to different ions of the same charge. This further selectivity appears to be the result of requiring ions to become dehydrated as they pass through the narrowest part of a channel, known as the **selectivity filter.** Ions in solution are hydrated (are surrounded by a shell of H_2O molecules), and the radius of this hydration shell is different for each type of ion. In Na^+ and K^+ channels, to make dehydration energetically possible, negatively polarized amino acid substituents of a particular geometry line the pore of the channel and substitute for the water molecules. Such substitution, however, requires close matching of the filter's size to the ion's hydration shell. Because each ion has a different-sized shell, a particular channel will best allow passage of one particular ionic species.

AT THE CELLULAR LEVEL

Tetrodotoxin (TTX), one of the most potent poisons known, specifically blocks the Na^+ channel. TTX binds to the extracellular side of the sodium channel (see Fig. 5-7, *A*). **Tetraethylammonium (TEA$^+$),** another poison, blocks K^+ channels. TEA$^+$ enters the K^+ channel from the cytoplasmic side and blocks the channel because TEA is unable to pass through it. The ovaries of certain species of puffer fish, also known as blowfish, contain TTX. Raw puffer fish is a highly prized delicacy in Japan. Connoisseurs of puffer fish enjoy the tingling numbness of the lips caused by the minuscule quantities of TTX present in the flesh. Sushi chefs who are trained to remove the ovaries safely are licensed by the government to prepare puffer fish. Despite these precautions, several people die each year as a result of eating improperly prepared puffer fish.

Saxitoxin is another blocker of Na^+ channels that is produced by the reddish dinoflagellates that are responsible for so-called red tides. Shellfish eat the dinoflagellates and concentrate saxitoxin in their tissues. A person who eats these shellfish may experience life-threatening paralysis within 30 minutes after the meal.

trode can then be used to monitor the activity of whatever channels happen to be trapped inside the seal. Under ideal conditions only one or only a few ion channels of a single type may be present in either the planar membrane or the membrane patch. The ion channels spontaneously oscillate between conductance states: an open state and a closed state. In the

case of voltage-gated channels, the time spent in a particular state will be a probabilistic function of the membrane potential.

The action potential starts with a rapid increase in Na^+ conductance (g_{Na}; Fig. 5-6). This increase in Na^+ conductance reflects the opening of thousands of Na^+ channels in response to the depolarization (thus, it is inferred that Na^+ channels have a gate that opens in response to depolarization). The open channels allow the influx of Na^+ ions, and the effect of this current is to depolarize the membrane further. Note that this is a positive feedback loop that accounts for the explosive nature of the action potential: the Na^+ current depolarizes the membrane, which causes more Na^+ channels to open, which in turn increases the Na^+ current. In sum, the voltage-dependent opening of Na^+ channels and the depolarizing action of the Na^+ current explain the rising phase of the action potential.

The falling phase of the action potential is the result of two processes: a reduction in g_{Na} and an increase in g_K. A decrease in g_{Na} results from repolarizing the membrane because of the voltage dependence of the Na^+ channel gate, but if the membrane is experimentally fixed at a depolarized level, Na^+ conductance still rapidly drops to zero. This behavior led to the idea that Na^+ channels have a second gate, called the inactivation gate, that closes with increasing probability as the membrane is depolarized. In sum, the presence of two gates ensures that a depolarization will always produce a transient increase in g_{Na} (see Fig. 5-6).

When the transient increase in g_{Na} is over, the resting g_K (i.e., the leak channels) will allow a current that repolarizes the membrane. In some axons the change in g_{Na} against a fixed g_K explains the entire action potential. In many other cases, however, voltage-gated K^+ channels also contribute. Voltage-gated K^+ channels have only a single gate that opens with depolarization. When the membrane depolarizes during an action potential, many of these K^+ channels open, and the result is an increase in g_K, which allows a K^+ current to flow. The K^+ current, flowing opposite the Na^+ current, causes repolarization of the membrane. Because voltage-gated K^+ channels do not close immediately upon repolarization, the overall membrane conductance to K^+ is higher at the end of the action potential than it was just before its initiation. This means that the membrane potential will become closer to the Nernst potential for K^+ and is the basis of the afterhyperpolarization that follows a spike. Note that the membrane potential then returns to its original resting value as the voltage-gated K^+ channels close. Also note that the K^+ channels close as a result of the voltage becoming negative again rather than an inactivation process. Indeed, if one voltage-clamps the membrane at a depolarized level, g_K will remain elevated.

Voltage Inactivation
Explosive depolarization of the action potential can occur only if a critical number of Na^+ channels are recruited. In response to membrane depolarization,

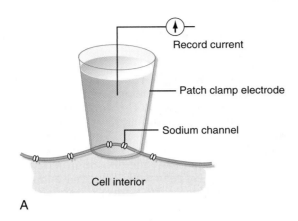

A

● **Figure 5-8.** **A,** A patch electrode is sealed to a small area of membrane to record the ionic currents that flow through the small number of ion channels that are isolated in the electrode patch. **B,** Record of (1) a depolarizing voltage pulse applied to patch, (2) multiple records indicating current flow through individual channels, and (3) the summed current response from many trials. (Redrawn from Blankenship J: Neurophysiology. Philadelphia, Mosby, 2002.)

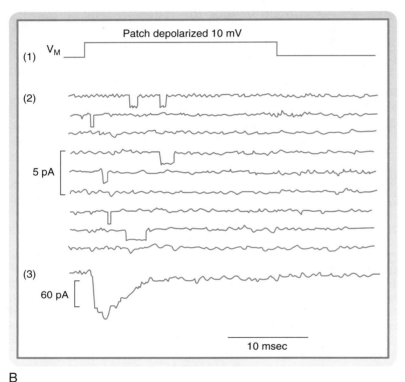

B

g_{Na} first increases and then, a short time later, decreases. The initial increase in g_{Na} is due to the activation gates of Na^+ channels opening in response to the transmembrane voltage. The decrease in g_{Na} is caused by closing of the channels' inactivation gates, which respond more slowly to transmembrane voltage but, once closed, cannot reopen until the membrane is repolarized to near the normal resting membrane potential. Thus, if a cell is partly depolarized, the pool of noninactivated Na^+ channels is reduced; consequently, a stimulus may not be able to recruit a sufficient number of Na^+ channels to generate an action potential. This is a result of voltage inactivation of some of the Na^+ channels.

Accordingly, when a nerve is depolarized slowly, the normal threshold may be passed without an action potential being fired; this phenomenon is called **accommodation.** Na^+ and K^+ channels are both involved in accommodation. If the depolarization is slow enough, the critical number of open Na^+ channels required to trigger the action potential may never be attained because of inactivation. In addition, K^+ channels open slowly in response to the depolarization. The increased g_K tends to oppose depolarization of the membrane, thus making it still less likely to fire an action potential.

Refractory Periods

During much of the action potential the cell is completely refractory to further stimulation. When a cell is refractory, it is unable to fire a second action potential no matter how strongly it is stimulated. This unresponsive state is called the **absolute refractory period** (Fig. 5-9). The cell is refractory because a large fraction of its Na^+ channels are voltage inactivated and cannot be reopened until the membrane is repolarized. In this

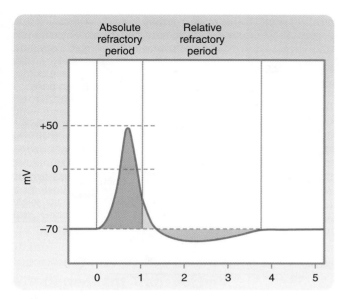

● **Figure 5-9.** Absolute and relative refractory periods of the action potential. The horizontal scale is in milliseconds.

state the critical number of Na+ channels required to produce an action potential cannot be recruited.

During the latter part of the action potential, the cell is able to fire a second action potential, but a stronger than normal stimulus is required. This period is called the **relative refractory period.** Early in the relative refractory period, before the membrane potential has returned to the resting potential level, some Na+ channels are still voltage inactivated. Therefore, a stronger than normal stimulus is required to open the critical number of Na+ channels needed to trigger an

action potential. Throughout the relative refractory period, conductance to K+ is elevated, which opposes depolarization of the membrane. This increase in K+ conductance also contributes to the refractoriness and, because of the relatively slow response of the K+ channels, to its extension in time.

CONDUCTION OF ACTION POTENTIALS

A fundamental activity of neurons is to transmit nerve impulses in the form of action potentials. The axons of motor neurons of the ventral horn of the spinal cord conduct action potentials from the cell body of the neuron to skeletal muscle fibers in the body, and the length of the axon may be longer than 1 m.

Conduction of an action potential along an axon is based on local current flow, just as occurs in electrotonic conduction of subthreshold potential changes. Thus, many of the same factors that govern the velocity of electrotonic conduction also determine the speed of propagation of action potentials.

Action Potential as a Self-Reinforcing Signal

Conduction with decrement will not get a signal from one end of an axon to the other unless the axon is very short. For example, in the retina of the eye, the distance from one neuron to the next is so small that electrotonic conduction is sufficient. Axons elsewhere can be up to 1 m or more in length, and therefore most are many times longer than their length constants. For an electrical impulse to travel the full length of these cells with undiminished strength, the action potential regenerates itself as it is conducted along the fiber. The action potential can be said to be **propagated,** as well as conducted.

Propagation involves the generation of "new" action potentials as they spread along the length of the cell. As seen in Figure 5-4, conduction of the local response occurs via local circuit currents. If instead of a subthreshold local response the instigating stimulus generates an action potential, the explosive depolarization should provide sufficient inward current flow to bring the areas on either side to threshold and generate action potentials. These areas could then provide the local current flow to bring still more distant areas to threshold so that they in turn generate action potentials. In short, propagation involves recurring cycles of depolarization to provide sufficient local current flow for generation of an action potential in an adjacent region of the cell membrane. Thus, the action potential is conducted down the axon, with "new" action potentials being generated along its length. In this way the action potential propagates over long distances while retaining the same size and shape.

Note that as shown in Figure 5-4, the action potential can be generated by a depolarization in the middle of an axon and would be conducted in both directions simultaneously. However, in the nervous system, action potentials are first generated at the axon hillock (i.e., where the axon is attached to the neuron cell body) and conducted to the terminal end. The reason that the axon hillock is the first site of generation of an action potential is that it is invested with a high density of voltage-gated Na⁺ channels, thus giving its membrane the lowest threshold in the cell. In addition, the action potential's refractory periods are also responsible for ensuring that conduction is usually unidirectional. Because the action potential is generated first at the axon hillock, any propagating action potential in the middle of the axon cannot generate another in the direction of the cell body since the immediately preceding portions are refractory.

Because the shape and size of the action potential are relatively constant, only variations in the number or frequency of action potentials can be used as the "code" for transmission of information along axons (see later). The maximal frequency is limited by the duration of the absolute and relative refractory periods (Fig. 5-9) and rarely exceeds 1000 spikes per second in large mammalian nerves. This also means that a single axon cannot convey adequate coded information about events that occur more frequently than it can conduct action potentials. For example, signaling of high-frequency sounds may require the combined activity of several neurons.

Effect of Fiber Diameter on Conduction Velocity

In nonmyelinated fibers, conduction velocity is proportional to the square root of the diameter. This effect is related to the longitudinal resistance. As the diameter of a fiber increases, r_i decreases with the square of the diameter and r_m increases only linearly with diameter. As a result, there is much less resistance to conduction while the membrane is only slightly leakier. This effectively increases the length constant, and thus the action potential will be conducted faster along fibers with large diameters (Fig. 5-3).

However, increasing the diameter also increases the surface area of the plasma membrane over which inner negative and outer positive charges are held to each other. Discharging this increased capacitance tends to slow conduction and mitigate the increase in conduction velocity gained by increasing diameter (Fig. 5-10).

Myelination

The speed of conduction in a nerve fiber is determined by the electrical properties of the cytoplasm and the plasma membrane that surrounds the fiber, as well as by its geometry. In vertebrates, many nerve fibers are coated with **myelin,** and such fibers are said to be myelinated. Myelin consists of the plasma membranes of **Schwann cells** (located in the peripheral nervous system) or **oligodendroglia** (located in the central nervous system [CNS]), which wrap around and insulate the nerve fiber (Fig. 5-11, *A* and *B*). The myelin sheath consists of several to more than 100 layers of glial cell plasma membrane. Gaps occur in the myelin sheath every 1 to 2 mm. These gaps are known as **nodes of Ranvier** and are about 1 μm wide. For all but the smallest diameter axons, a myelinated axon

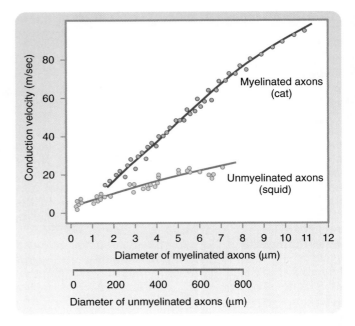

● **Figure 5-10.** Conduction velocities of myelinated and unmyelinated axons as functions of axon diameter. Myelinated axons are from cat saphenous nerve at 38°C. Unmyelinated axons are from squid at 20°C to 22°C. Note that myelinated axons have greater conduction velocities than unmyelinated axons that are 100 times greater in diameter. (Based on data from Gasser HS, Grundfest H: Am J Physiol 127:393, 1939 [myelinated axons]; and Pumphrey RJ, Young JZ: J Exp Biol 15:453, 1938 [unmyelinated axons].)

has much greater conduction velocity than an unmyelinated fiber of the same caliber does because the myelin sheath increases the length constant of the axon, decreases the capacitance of the axon membrane, and restricts the generation of action potentials to the nodes of Ranvier. In short, myelination greatly alters the electrical properties of the axon.

The many wrappings of membrane around the axon increase the effective membrane resistance so that r_m/r_i and thus the length constant are much greater. This increased membrane resistance means that less of the conducted signal is lost through the membrane and the amplitude of a conducted signal decreases less with distance along the axon.

In addition, the thicker myelin-wrapped membrane enforces a much larger separation between the inside and outside of the axon such that the charges across it are much less tightly bound to each other. Because the effect of membrane capacitance is to slow the rate at which the membrane potential can be changed, this reduced capacitance of myelinated axons means that the depolarization occurs more rapidly. For all these reasons, conduction velocity is greatly increased by myelination, and the current generated at one node of Ranvier is conducted at great speed to the next (Fig. 5-12).

The Na⁺ channels that bring about generation of the action potential are highly concentrated at the nodes of Ranvier and are not found between them. Thus, the

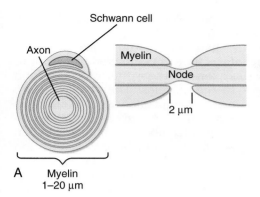

Schwann cell

Axon

Myelin

Node

2 μm

A   Myelin
1–20 μm

● **Figure 5-11.** **A,** Schematic drawings, in cross section and longitudinal section through a node of Ranvier, of a Schwann cell wrapped around an axon to form myelin. Note that the axon is exposed to the extracellular space only at the node of Ranvier. **B,** View of two nodes and the intervening internode of myelin. (Redrawn from Squires LR et al: Fundamental Neuroscience, 2nd ed. San Diego, CA, Academic Press, 2002.) **C,** Saltatory conduction in a myelinated axon with a plot of the action potential location along the axon vs. time. Note the short time taken for the action potential to traverse the large distance between nodes (shallow sloped lines on the plot) due to the high resistance and low capacitance of the internodal region. In contrast, the action potential slows as it crosses each node (steep sloped line segments). (Redrawn from Blankenship J: Neurophysiology. Philadelphia, Mosby, 2002.)

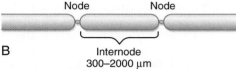

Node   Node

B   Internode
300–2000 μm

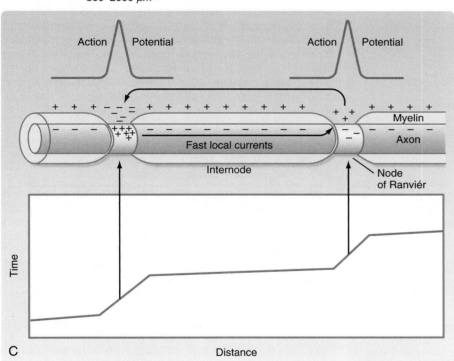

C

action potential is regenerated only at the nodes of Ranvier (1 to 2 mm apart) rather than being regenerated continuously along the fiber, as is the case in an unmyelinated fiber. Resistance to the flow of ions across the many layers that make up the myelin sheath is so high that transmembrane currents are effectively restricted to the short stretches of naked plasma membrane that occur at the nodes of Ranvier (Fig. 5-11, *C*). Therefore, the action potential is regenerated at each successive node. The local currents entering the node are almost entirely conducted from one node to the next node, bringing it to threshold in about 20 μsec! Thus, the action potential appears to "jump"

from one node of Ranvier to the next, and the process is called **saltatory** (from the Latin word *saltare*, to leap) **conduction**.

Functional Consequences of Myelination

Although our nerve fibers are much smaller in diameter than squid giant axons, our axons conduct at comparable or even faster speeds because of myelination. The unmyelinated squid giant axon has a 500-μm diameter, which results in it having a conduction velocity of about 20 m/sec (Fig. 5-10). However, unmyelinated mammalian nerve fibers, which have diameters under

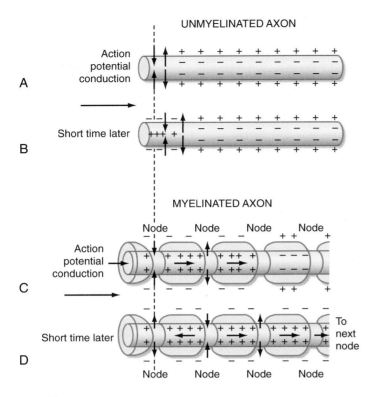

UNMYELINATED AXON

A — Action potential conduction

B — Short time later

MYELINATED AXON

Node   Node   Node   Node

C — Action potential conduction

D — Short time later   To next node

Node   Node   Node   Node

● **Figure 5-12.** Comparison of action potential conduction in an unmyelinated axon and a myelinated axon. At the initial time (**A** and **C**), an action potential is being generated at the left side of each axon. Note that the inward current in the unmyelinated axon (**A**) is depolarizing an adjacent portion, whereas the inward current in the myelinated axon (**C**) is depolarizing the next node. At the second instant in time (**B** and **D**), the action potential in the unmyelinated axon has been generated in the adjacent portion while the action potential in the myelinated axon (**D**) has been generated at subsequent nodes and is already depolarizing the last node to the right. (Redrawn from Castro A et al: Neuroscience: An Outline Approach. Philadelphia, Mosby, 2002.)

2 µm have conduction velocities less than 2 m/sec. With such slow conduction velocity, reflex withdrawal of the foot from a sharp object would take at least 2 seconds as the information is conducted from foot to spinal cord by this axon and the withdrawal command conducted back to the muscles. The myelin sheath that surrounds many mammalian nerve fibers is responsible for the greatly increased conduction velocity over that of unmyelinated fibers of similar diameter. A 10-µm myelinated fiber would have a conduction velocity in the range of 50 m/sec, more than twice that of the 500-µm squid giant axon. The high conduction velocity permits reflexes that are fast and also supports efficient and complex mental processing.

The action potentials of myelinated axons do not have a hyperpolarizing afterpotential or extended relative refractory period because they lack K^+ channels at their nodes. This increases the rate at which these fast-conducting axons can fire. Myelinated axons are also more metabolically efficient than unmyelinated axons. Na^+,K^+-ATPase extrudes the Na^+ that enters and reaccumulates the K^+ that leaves the cell during action potentials. In myelinated axons, ionic currents are restricted to the small fraction of the membrane surface at the nodes of Ranvier. For this reason, far fewer ions traverse a unit length of fiber membrane, and much less ion pumping—and energy expenditure—is required to maintain the gradients.

▶ IN THE CLINIC

An action potential can be recorded with a microelectrode without penetrating the axon by placing two spaced electrodes on its surface and comparing the electrical charge at each point. An electrode located where there is an action potential would be somewhat negative in comparison to an electrode where there is no action potential (Fig. 5-12). As the action potential is conducted to the second electrode, the polarity of the recording reverses. This technique is used clinically to assess nerve function. Peripheral nerves and many central pathways consist of a population of axons of various diameter, some of which are myelinated and some are not. Consequently, action potentials travel at different velocities in the individual axons. As a result, a recording from such a nerve with external electrodes does not show a single synchronous peak but a series of peaks that vary in time (reflecting the conduction velocity of groups of axons) and in size (reflecting the number of axons in each velocity group). This is called a **compound action potential,** and its shape bears a striking resemblance to curves of Figure 5-13, which show the distribution of axons' size in particular nerves. The clinical value of such a recording is its ability, in certain disease states, to reveal the dysfunction of a particular group of axons associated with specific functions, as well as the noninvasive nature of the technique because it can be done with skin surface electrodes (Table 5-1).

▶ IN THE CLINIC

In some diseases known as **demyelinating disorders,** the myelin sheath deteriorates. In **multiple sclerosis,** scattered progressive demyelination of axons in the CNS results in loss of motor control. The neuropathy common in severe cases of diabetes mellitus is caused by the demyelination of peripheral axons. When myelin is lost, the length constant, which is dramatically increased by myelination, becomes much shorter. Hence, the action potential loses amplitude as it is electrotonically conducted from one node of Ranvier to the next. If demyelination is sufficiently severe, the action potential may arrive at the next node of Ranvier with insufficient strength to fire an action potential. The axon may then fail to propagate action potentials.

● **Table 5-1.**

Correlation of Axon Groups, as Revealed by Compound Action Potential Recordings, with Their Functional Properties

Electrophysiologic Classification of Peripheral Nerves	Classification of Afferent Fibers ONLY (Class/Group)	Fiber Diameter (mm)	Conduction Velocity (m/sec)	Receptor Supplied
Sensory Fiber Type				
Aα	Ia and Ib	0.13-20	0.80-120	Primary muscle spindles, Golgi tendon organ
Aβ	II	0.16-12	0.35-75	Secondary muscle spindles, skin mechanoreceptors
Aδ	III	0.11-51	0.15-30	Skin mechanoreceptors, thermal receptors, nociceptors
C	IV	0.2-1.5	0.5-2	Skin mechanoreceptors, thermal receptors, nociceptors
Motor Fiber Type				
Aα	N/A	0.12-20	0.72-120	Extrafusal skeletal muscle fibers
Aγ	N/A	0.12-8.2	0.12-48	Intrafusal muscle fibers
B	N/A	0.21-33	0.86-18	Preganglionic autonomic fibers
C	N/A	0.2-2	0.5-2	Postganglionic autonomic fibers

From Haines DE (ed): Fundamental Neuroscience for Basic and Clinical Applications, 3rd ed. Philadelphia, Churchill Livingstone, 2006.

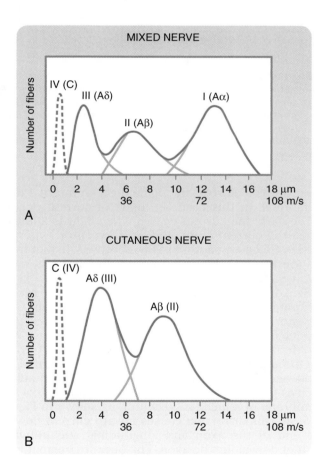

● **Figure 5-13.** The distribution of axons, by size and conduction velocity, in a mixed nerve **(A)** and a cutaneous nerve **(B)** in response to electrical stimulation. Note the increased number of small-diameter fibers and the absence of Aα fibers in the cutaneous nerve. (From Haines DE [ed]: Fundamental Neuroscience for Basic and Clinical Applications, 3rd ed. Philadelphia, Churchill Livingstone, 2006.)

SENSORY TRANSDUCTION AND CODING

As already discussed, the mechanism for the generation of action potentials is depolarization of the axon hillock of the axon. However, for the nervous system to receive input, it must be stimulated by the application of energy, and this energy must be transduced into a neural event (i.e., the action potential discussed earlier). The parameters of the energy (e.g., its intensity and duration) are then encoded into patterns of action potentials conducted over one or more axons.

Stimulation is the action of environmental energy through activation of one or more sensory receptors. A **stimulus** is the environmental event that excites sensory receptors, which then provide information about the stimulus to the CNS. The **response** to the stimulus is the effect that the stimulus has on the organism. Responses can be recognized at several levels, including (1) receptor potentials in the sensory receptors; (2) transmission of action potentials along axons in sensory pathways; (3) synaptic events in central neural networks; and (4) motor activity triggered by sensory stimulation, which is ultimately observed as behavior. The process that enables a sensory receptor to respond usefully to a stimulus is called **sensory transduction.**

Environmental events that involve sensory transduction can be mechanical, thermal, chemical, or other forms of energy; the type of transduction depends on the sensory apparatus that serves as a transducer. Although humans cannot sense electrical or magnetic fields, other animals can respond to such stimuli. For example, many fish have electroreceptors, and various fish and birds use the earth's magnetic field to orient themselves during migration.

Figure 5-14 shows three examples of how stimuli can alter the membrane properties of the specific sensory receptor neurons that transduce such stimuli (details for each of these examples are found in other chapters). Figure 5-14, *A*, illustrates how a **chemoreceptor,** such as we use for taste and smell, might respond when a chemical stimulant reacts with receptor

CHEMORECEPTOR

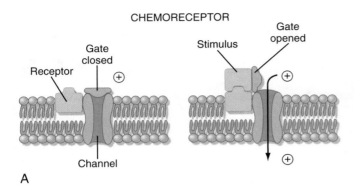

A

MECHANORECEPTOR

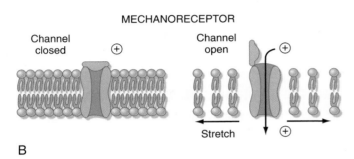

B

PHOTORECEPTOR

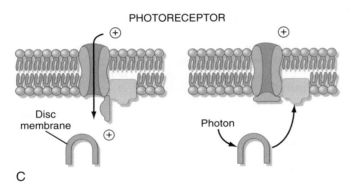

C

● **Figure 5-14.** Conceptual models of transducer mechanisms in three types of receptors. **A,** Chemoreceptor; **B,** mechanoreceptor; **C,** photoreceptor.

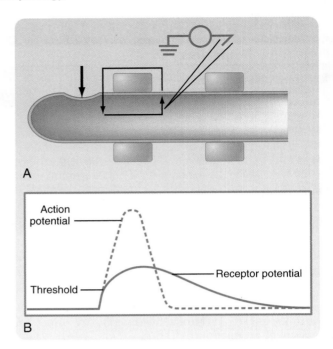

● **Figure 5-15.** **A,** Current flow _(small arrows)_ produced by stimulation of a mechanoreceptor at the site indicated by the large arrow. An intracellular recording electrode is placed at the first node of Ranvier. **B,** The receptor potential produced by the current and an action potential that would be superimposed on the receptor potential if it exceeds threshold at the first node of Ranvier.

molecules on the plasma membrane of the sensory receptor. (Note the distinction between a sensory receptor, which includes one or more cells, and a receptor molecule, which is a protein inserted into the membrane of a cell.) Binding of the chemical stimulant to the receptor molecule opens an ion channel, which enables the influx of an ionic current that depolarizes the sensory receptor cell. (This is similar to what is described for ligand-gated channels in Chapter 6.) In Figure 5-14, _B,_ the ion channel of a **mechanoreceptor,** such as found in the skin, opens in response to the application of a mechanical force along the membrane, and this allows an influx of current to depolarize the sensory receptor. In Figure 5-14, _C,_ the ion channel of a retinal **photoreceptor** cell (so called because it responds to light) is open in the dark and closed when

a photon is absorbed by pigment on an internal disc membrane. In this case, an influx of current occurs in the dark; the current ceases when light is applied. When the current stops, the photoreceptor hyperpolarizes. (Because capture of the photon is distant from the ion channel that it influences, this process must involve a "second messenger" mechanism.)

Sensory transduction generally produces a **receptor potential** in the primary afferent neuron. The receptor potential is usually a depolarizing event that results from inward current flow, which brings the membrane potential of the sensory receptor toward the threshold needed to trigger an action potential, as explained earlier. For example, a mechanical stimulus, such as pressure on the skin of a finger, can distort the membrane of a mechanoreceptor, as shown in Figure 5-15, _A._ This distortion causes inward current flow at the end of the axon and longitudinal and outward current flow along the axon. The outward current produces a depolarization (the receptor potential) that might exceed the threshold for an action potential (Fig. 5-15, _B_). If so, the action potential will travel along this primary afferent fiber to the CNS and signal sensory information. There can be variations on this theme in which the primary afferent fiber terminates on a separate, peripherally located sensory receptor cell. For example, in the **cochlea,** primary afferent fibers end on **hair cells.** Sensory transduction in such sense organs is made more complex by this arrangement. In photoreceptors, moreover, the receptor potential is hyperpolarizing, as mentioned earlier, and interruption of the dark current is the signal event. Information about each of these mechanisms is discussed in Chapter 8.

A **stimulus threshold** is defined by the weakest stimulus that can be reliably detected. For detection, a stimulus must produce receptor potentials that are large enough to activate one or more primary afferent fibers. Weaker intensities of stimulation can produce subthreshold receptor potentials; however, such stimuli would not excite central sensory neurons and thus could not be detected. Furthermore, the number of primary afferent neurons that need to be excited for sensory detection depends on the requirements for **spatial** and **temporal summation** in the pathway (see Chapter 6).

Adaptation, a change in the way that a receptor responds to sequential or prolonged stimulation, is a characteristic property of sensory receptors that makes them better suited to signal particular kinds of sensory information. For example, slowly adapting receptors in the skin produce a repetitive discharge in response to a prolonged stimulus. However, rapidly adapting receptors produce only a few spikes at the onset (or offset) of the same stimulus. Figure 5-16 shows the responses of three types of receptors to slow deflection of the skin graphed at the bottom. The functional implication is that different temporal features of a stimulus can be signaled by receptors with different adaptation rates.

Receptive Fields

The relationship between the location of a stimulus and activation of particular sensory neurons is a major

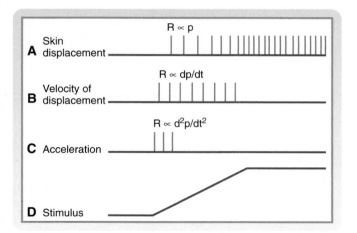

● **Figure 5-16.** Responses of slowly and rapidly adapting mechanoreceptors to displacement of the skin. **A** to **C** are the discharges of primary afferent fibers during a ramp-and-hold stimulus shown in **D. A** shows the response of a slowly adapting receptor that signals the magnitude and duration of displacement. **B** shows the response of a rapidly adapting receptor whose output signals the velocity of displacement. **C** shows the response of a different rapidly adapting receptor that responds to acceleration. R, response; p, displacement; t, time.

theme in sensory physiology. The receptive field of a sensory neuron is the region that when stimulated, affects the behavior of the neuron. For example, a sensory receptor might be activated by indentation of only a small area of skin. That area is the **excitatory receptive field** of the sensory receptor. A neuron in the CNS might be excited by stimulation of a receptive field several times as large as that of a sensory receptor because it may receive information from many sensory receptors, each with a slightly different receptive field. The receptive field of that CNS neuron is the sum of the receptive fields of the sensory receptors that influence it. The location of the receptive field is determined by the location of the sensory transduction apparatus responsible for signaling information about the stimulus to the sensory neuron.

Generally, the receptive fields of sensory receptors are excitatory. However, a central sensory neuron can have either an excitatory or an inhibitory receptive field or, indeed, a complex receptive field that includes areas that excite it and areas that inhibit it. Examples of such complex receptive fields will be discussed in Chapters 7 and 8.

Sensory Coding

Sensory neurons encode stimuli. In the process of sensory transduction, one or more aspects of the stimulus must be encoded in a way that can be interpreted by the CNS. The encoded information is an abstraction based on (1) which sensory receptors are activated, (2) the responses of sensory receptors to the stimulus, and (3) information processing in the sensory pathway. Some of the aspects of stimuli that may be encoded include the **sensory modality, spatial location, threshold, intensity, frequency,** and **duration.** Other aspects of stimuli that are encoded are presented in relation to particular sensory systems in later chapters.

A **sensory modality** is a readily identified class of sensation. For example, sustained mechanical stimuli applied to the skin result in sensations of touch or pressure, and transient mechanical stimuli may evoke sensations of flutter or vibration. Other cutaneous modalities include cold, warmth, and pain. Vision, audition, position, taste, and smell are examples of noncutaneous sensory modalities. The encoding of sensory modality is done by labeled-line sensory channels in most sensory systems and derives from the specific sensory receptors at its beginning. For example, the visual pathway includes photoreceptors, neurons in the retina, the lateral geniculate nucleus of the thalamus, and the visual areas of the cerebral cortex (see Chapter 8). The normal means of activating the visual system is light striking the retina. However, mechanical (e.g., by pressure on the eyeball) or electrical stimulation of neurons in the visual pathway also produces a visual sensation. Thus, neurons of the visual system can be regarded as a labeled line, which when activated by whatever means, causes a visual sensation.

The **spatial location** of a stimulus is signaled by activation of the particular population of sensory neurons whose receptive fields are affected by the stimulus. The information may be encoded in the CNS by a neural map. For example, a **somatotopic map** is formed by arrays of neurons in the somatosensory cortex that receive information from corresponding locations on the body surface (see Chapter 7). In the visual system, points on the retina are represented by neuronal arrays that form **retinotopic maps** (see Chapter 8). In the auditory system the frequency of sounds is represented in **tonotopic maps** (see Chapter 8). In some cases an inhibitory receptive field or a contrasting border between an excitatory and an inhibitory receptive field can have localizing value. Resolution of two different adjacent stimuli may depend on the excitation of partially separate populations of neurons and on inhibitory interactions.

Stimulus intensity may be encoded in a number of ways. Because action potentials have a uniform magnitude, some sensory neurons encode intensity by their frequency of discharge. The relationship between stimulus intensity and response can be plotted as a stimulus-response function. For many sensory neurons, the stimulus-response function approximates an exponential curve with an exponent less than, equal to, or greater than 1. Stimulus-response functions with fractional exponents characterize many mechanoreceptors. **Thermoreceptors,** which detect changes in temperature, have linear stimulus-response curves (exponent of 1). **Nociceptors,** which detect painful stimuli, may have linear or positively accelerating stimulus-response functions (i.e., the exponent for these curves is 1 or greater). The positively accelerating stimulus-response functions of nociceptors help explain the urgency that is experienced as the pain sensation increases.

Another way in which stimulus intensity is encoded is by the number of sensory receptors that are activated. A stimulus at the threshold for perception may activate just one or just a few primary afferent neurons of an appropriate class, whereas a strong stimulus of the same type may excite many similar receptors. Central sensory neurons that receive input from this particular class of sensory receptor would be more powerfully activated as more primary afferent neurons discharge. Greater activity in central sensory neurons is perceived as a stronger stimulus.

Stimuli of different intensities may also activate different sets of sensory receptors. For example, a weak mechanical stimulus applied to the skin might activate only mechanoreceptors, whereas a strong mechanical stimulus might activate both mechanoreceptors and nociceptors. In this case the sensation evoked by the stronger stimulus would be more intense, and the quality perceived would be different.

Stimulus frequency can sometimes be encoded by action potentials whose interspike intervals correspond exactly to the intervals between stimuli (e.g., at intervals corresponding to that of a low-frequency vibration). In other cases, a given neuron may discharge at intervals that are multiples of the interstimulus interval. Clearly, a discharge rate cannot unambiguously signal both frequency and intensity in the same system.

Another method for encoding information is to encode the communicated information into structured patterns of nerve impulse trains. Several different types of nerve impulse codes have been proposed. A commonly used code depends on the mean discharge frequency. For example, in many sensory systems, increases in the intensity of a stimulus cause a greater frequency of discharge of the sensory neurons. Other candidate codes depend on the time of firing, the temporal pattern, and the duration of bursts.

Stimulus duration may be encoded in slowly adapting sensory neurons by the duration of enhanced firing. The beginning and end of a stimulus may be signaled by transient discharges of rapidly adapting sensory receptors (Fig. 5-16).

■ KEY CONCEPTS

1. The action potential is generated by the rapid opening and subsequent voltage inactivation of voltage-dependent Na^+ channels and the delayed opening and closing of voltage-dependent K^+ channels.

2. Ion channels are integral membrane proteins that have ion-selective pores. Different regions of an ion channel protein act as gates to activate and inactivate the channel. An ion channel typically has two states: high conductance (open) and zero conductance (closed). The channel oscillates randomly between the open and closed states. For a voltage-dependent channel, the fraction of time that the channel spends in the open state is a function of the transmembrane potential difference.

3. Local circuit currents produce electrotonic conduction. Both subthreshold signals and action potentials are conducted along the length of a cell by local circuit currents. The action potential is propagated rather than merely being conducted; it is regenerated as it moves along the axon. In this way an action potential remains the same size and shape as it is conducted.

4. Voltage inactivation of Na^+ channels and membrane hyperpolarization due to slow closure of K^+ channels are the major factors determining the absolute and relative refractory periods that limit the maximum firing rate of action potentials.

5. The propagation velocity is determined by the electrical properties of the axon. A large-diameter axon has faster propagation velocity.

6. Myelination dramatically increases the conduction velocity of a nerve axon. Because myelin increases membrane resistance and lowers membrane capacitance, an action potential is conducted very rapidly from one node of Ranvier to the next. Since it takes much longer to generate an action potential at each node than it does for the action potential to be

conducted between nodes, the action potential appears to jump from node to node; this form of conduction is called saltatory conduction.

7. Receptor potentials are changes in membrane potential that result from transduction of a sensory stimulus. Receptor adaptation is a mechanism for signaling the temporal features of a stimulus.

8. The receptive field of a receptor or any central neuron is that area of the periphery that affects its activity. The specific type of energy that stimulates a response in the receptor cell defines the modality of the sensory pathway. Timing, duration, and patterns of action potentials encode stimulus intensity, frequency, and duration.

CHAPTER 6

Synaptic Transmission

Synaptic transmission is the major process by which electrical signals are transferred between cells within the nervous system (or between neurons and muscle cells or sensory receptors). Within the nervous system, synaptic transmission is usually conceived of as an interaction between two neurons that occurs in a point-to-point manner at specialized junctions called synapses. Two main classes of synapses are distinguished: electrical and chemical. However, as the list of chemical neurotransmitters has grown and as understanding of their mechanisms of action has increased, the definition and conception of what constitutes synaptic transmission has had to be refined and expanded. We no longer think of synaptic transmission as a process that involves only neurons, but now realize that glia form an important element of the synapse and that signaling occurs between neurons and glia. Moreover, in many cases neurotransmitter released at a synapse will act over a widespread territory rather than just at the synapse from which it is released. Thus, we must either generalize the definition of synaptic transmission or consider classically defined synaptic transmission as but one of several mechanisms by which cells in the nervous system communicate with each other. In this chapter we first describe the classic conception of synaptic transmission (electrical and chemical) and then introduce some of the nontraditional neurotransmitters and discuss how they have forced modifications in our conception of chemical communication between cells in the nervous system.

ELECTRICAL SYNAPSES

Although their existence in the mammalian central nervous system (CNS) has been known for a long time, electrical synapses, or gap junctions, between neurons were thought to be of relatively little importance for the functioning of the adult mammalian CNS. Only recently has it become apparent that these synapses are quite common and that they may underlie important neuronal functions.

An electrical synapse is effectively a low-resistance pathway between cells that allows current to flow directly from one cell to another and, more generally, allows the exchange of small molecules between cells. Electrical synapses are present in the CNS of animals from invertebrates to mammals. They are present

between glial cells, as well as between neurons. Electrical coupling of neurons has been demonstrated for most brain regions, including the inferior olive, cerebellum, spinal cord, neocortex, thalamus, hippocampus, olfactory bulb, retina, and striatum.

A gap junction is the morphological correlate of an electrical synapse (see also Chapter 1). These junctions are plaque-like structures in which the plasma membranes of coupled cells become closely apposed (the intercellular space narrows to approximately 3 nm) and filled with electron-dense material (Fig. 6-1). Freeze-fracture electron micrographs of gap junctions display regular arrays of intramembrane particles that correspond to proteins that form the intercellular channels connecting the cells. The typical channel diameter is large (1 to 2 nm), thus making it permeable not only to ions but also other small molecules up to approximately 1 kDa in size.

Electrical synapses are fast (essentially no synaptic delay) and bidirectional (i.e., current generated in either cell can flow across the gap junction to influence the other cell). In addition, they act as **low-pass filters.** That is, slow electrical events are much more readily transmitted than are fast signals such as action potentials. One important role for neuronal gap

● AT THE CELLULAR LEVEL

Each gap junction channel is formed by two hemichannels (called connexons), one contributed by each cell. Each connexon, in turn, is a hexamer of connexin protein subunits, which are encoded for by a gene family of at least 21 different members in mammals. (Recently, a second family of proteins that form gap junctions, the pannexins, has also been identified.) Gap junctions formed by different connexins have distinct biophysical properties (gating and conductance) and cellular distributions. Although at least 10 connexin types are expressed in the CNS, connexin 36 (connexins are named according to their molecular weight; thus, the number refers to the approximate molecular weight of the connexin in kilodaltons) is the major neuronal connexin in the adult CNS. Other connexin types found in the CNS form gap junctions between glial cells or are primarily expressed transiently during development.

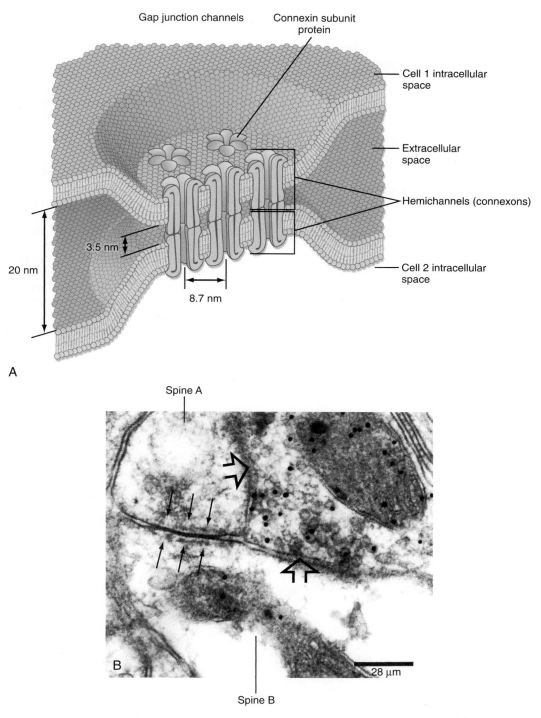

● **Figure 6-1.** Gap junction structure. **A,** Schematic view of the gap junction showing narrowing of the intercellular space to 3.5 nm at the junction. The gap junction has multiple channels, with each channel formed by two connexon hemichannels. Each connexon in turn comprises six connexin subunits. **B,** Electron micrograph of part of a complex synaptic arrangement called a glomerulus that is found in the inferior olive and some other CNS regions. Two dendritic spines are coupled by a gap junction *(small black arrows)*. An axon terminal packed with synaptic vesicles fills the upper right part of the panel. Large arrowheads point to the electron-dense material that marks the active zone. Black dots are immunogold labeling for GABA, thus identifying this terminal as GABAergic. (From De Zeeuw CI, Lang EJ, Sugihara I, et al: J Neurosci 16:3420, 1996. Copyright 1996 by the Society for Neuroscience.)

junctions appears to be synchronization of network activity. For example, the activity of inferior olivary neurons is normally synchronized but becomes uncorrelated when pharmacological blockers of gap junctions are injected into the inferior olive. It also appears that the patterns of electrical coupling by gap junctions may be highly specific. For example, neocortical interneurons almost exclusively couple to interneurons of the same type. This specific gap junction–coupling pattern suggests that multiple, independent, electrically coupled networks of interneurons may coexist across the neocortex.

Finally, although electrical synapses are generally regarded as relatively simple and static in comparison to chemical synapses, they may actually be fairly dynamic entities. For example, the properties of electrical synapses can be modulated by several factors, including voltage, intracellular pH, and [Ca^{++}]. Moreover, they are subject to regulation by G protein–coupled receptors, and the connexins contain sites for phosphorylation. These factors can change the coupling between cells by causing changes in single-channel conductance, the formation of new gap junctions, or removal of existing ones.

CHEMICAL SYNAPSES

Chemical synaptic transmission was first demonstrated between the vagus nerve and the heart by a simple experiment by Otto Loewi. The vagus nerve of a frog was stimulated to slow the heart rate down while the solution perfusing the heart was collected. This solution was then used to perfuse a second heart, whose beating slowed on being perfused. The chemical responsible was found to be acetylcholine, which we now know is also a neurotransmitter at the neuromuscular junction and at synapses in the peripheral and central nervous systems.

Unlike the situation at electrical synapses, at chemical synapses there is no direct communication between the cytoplasm of the two cells. Instead, the cell membranes are separated by a synaptic cleft of some 20 μm, and interaction between the cells occurs via chemical intermediaries known as **neurotransmitters.** Chemical synapses are generally unidirectional, and thus one can refer to the presynaptic and postsynaptic elements that are diagrammed in Figure 6-2. The **presynaptic** element is often the terminal portion of an axon and is packed with small vesicles whose exact shape and size

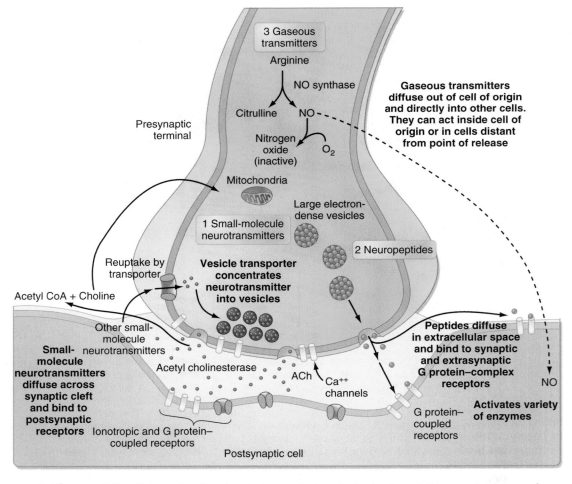

● **Figure 6-2.** Schematic of a chemical synaptic terminal releasing all three main classes of neurotransmitter. For each, the mechanisms of release, sites of action, and mechanisms for termination of activity are shown. Real synapses release transmitter from one or more classes.

vary with the neurotransmitter that they contain. In addition, the presynaptic membrane apposed to the **postsynaptic** element has regions, known as active zones, of electron-dense material that corresponds to the proteins involved in transmitter release (Fig. 6-1, *B*). Moreover, mitochondria and rough endoplasmic reticulum are typically found in the presynaptic terminal. The postsynaptic membrane is also characterized by electron-dense material, which in this case corresponds to the receptors for the neurotransmitter.

Chemical synapses occur between different parts of neurons. Traditionally, focus has been placed on synapses formed by an axon onto the dendrites or soma of a second cell (**axodendritic** or **axosomatic synapses**), and our description will be based primarily on such synapses. However, there are many additional types of chemical synapses, such as **axoaxonic** (axon to axon), **dendrodendritic** (dendrite to dendrite), and **dendrosomatic** (dendrite to soma). Furthermore, complex synaptic arrangements are possible, such as mixed synapses, in which cells form both electrical and chemical synapses with each other; serial synapses, in which an axoaxonic synapse is made onto the axon terminal and influences the efficacy of that terminal's synapse with yet a third element; and reciprocal synapses, in which both cells can release transmitter to influence the other. Figure 6-1, *B*, shows a complex synaptic arrangement, called a glomerulus, that involves both chemical and electrical synapses among the participating elements.

Much of what we know about chemical synapses comes from the study of two classic preparations, the frog neuromuscular junction (the synapse from a motor neuron onto the muscle) and the squid giant synapse (the synapse from a second-order neuron onto third-order neurons that innervate the muscle of the squid's mantle; i.e., the motor neurons, which are the cells whose axons were used to characterize the conductances underlying the action potential [see Chapter 5]). The principles governing transmission at these synapses mostly apply to synapses within the mammalian CNS as well, at least with regard to synapses using what are called the "classic" neurotransmitters (see the section Neurotransmitters). Thus, much of the following discussion will be based on results from these two preparations; however, some differences in CNS synapses will also be pointed out.

Synaptic transmission at a chemical synapse may be summarized as follows. Synaptic transmission is initiated by arrival of the action potential at the presynaptic terminal. The action potential depolarizes the terminal, which causes Ca^{++} channels to open. The subsequent rise in $[Ca^{++}]$ within the terminal triggers the fusion of vesicles containing neurotransmitter with the plasma membrane. The transmitter is then expelled into the synaptic cleft, diffuses across it, and binds to specific receptors on the postsynaptic membrane. Binding of transmitter to receptors then causes the opening (or less often, the closing) of ion channels in the postsynaptic membrane, which in turn results in changes in the potential and resistance of the postsynaptic membrane that alter the excitability of the

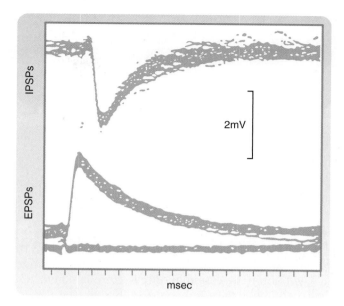

● **Figure 6-3.** IPSPs and EPSPs recorded with a microelectrode in a cat spinal motor neuron in response to stimulation of appropriate peripheral afferent fibers. Forty traces are superimposed. Note that these IPSPs are hyperpolarizing, but in some cases IPSPs can be depolarizing—see text for an explanation. (Redrawn from Curtis DR, Eccles JC: J Physiol 145:529, 1959.)

cell. The changes in membrane potential of the postsynaptic cell are termed **excitatory** and **inhibitory postsynaptic potentials** (**EPSPs** and **IPSPs**) (Fig. 6-3), depending on whether they increase or decrease, respectively, the cell's excitability, which can be defined as its probability of firing action potentials. The transmitter acts for only a very short time (milliseconds) because reuptake and degradation mechanisms rapidly clear the transmitter from the synaptic cleft.

The succeeding sections will amplify specific points of this summary. However, it is worth mentioning at this point that some of the nonclassic types of neurotransmitters (e.g., neuropeptides and gaseous neurotransmitters such as nitric oxide) and the discovery of **metabotropic receptors** have required modifications of several aspects of this basic conception (a metabotropic receptor does not contain an ion channel but, instead, is coupled to a G protein that initiates second messenger cascades that can ultimately affect ion channels, whereas an **ionotropic receptor** contains the ion channel as an integral part of itself). Some of the differences between classic and peptide transmitters are listed in Table 6-1. More details on the properties of peptide and gaseous transmitters are provided in the relevant parts of the Neurotransmitters section of this chapter, and metabotropic receptors are covered in the Receptors section.

Calcium Entry Is the Signal for Transmitter Release

Depolarization of the presynaptic membrane by the action potential causes voltage-gated Ca^{++} channels to

● **Table 6-1.**

Distinctions between Classic Nonpeptide Neurotransmitters and Peptide Neurotransmitters

Nonpeptide Transmitters	Peptide Transmitters
Synthesized and packaged in the nerve terminal	Synthesized and packaged in the cell body; transported to the nerve terminal by fast axonal transport
Synthesized in active form	Active peptide formed when it is cleaved from a much larger polypeptide that contains several neuropeptides
Usually present in small, clear vesicles	Usually present in large, electron-dense vesicles
Released into a synaptic cleft	May be released some distance from the postsynaptic cell. There may be no well-defined synaptic structure
Action of many terminated because of uptake by presynaptic terminals via Na^+-powered active transport	Action terminated by proteolysis or by the peptide diffusing away
Typically, action has short latency and short duration (msec)	Action may have long latency and may persist for many seconds

open, which makes it possible for Ca^{++} to flow into the terminal and trigger the release of transmitter. However, Ca^{++} will enter the terminal only if there is a favorable electrochemical gradient to do so. Recall that it is the combination of the concentration and voltage gradients that determines the direction of ion flow through open channels. Extracellular $[Ca^{++}]$ is high relative to intracellular $[Ca^{++}]$, which favors entry into the terminal; however, during the peak of the action potential, the membrane potential is positive, and the voltage gradient opposes the entry of Ca^{++} because of its positive charge. Thus, at the peak of the action potential, relatively little Ca^{++} enters the terminal because although the membrane is highly permeable to Ca^{++}, the overall driving force is small. In fact, by using a voltage clamp, one can experimentally make the membrane potential positive and equal to the Nernst equilibrium potential for Ca^{++}. If this is done, no Ca^{++} will enter the terminal despite Ca^{++} channels being open, and as a result no transmitter is released and no postsynaptic response is observed. This voltage is known as the **suppression potential.** If the membrane potential is rapidly made negative again (because of either the end of the action potential or by adjusting the voltage clamp), Ca^{++} rushes into the terminal as a result of the large driving force (which arises instantaneously on repolarization) and the high membrane permeability to Ca^{++} (which remains high because it takes the Ca^{++} channels several milliseconds to close in response to the new membrane potential), thereby resulting in release of transmitter and a postsynaptic response (Fig. 6-4).

Synaptic Vesicles and the Quantal Nature of Transmitter Release

How neurotransmitter is stored and how it is released are questions fundamental to synaptic transmission. Answering these questions began with two observations. The first was the discovery of small round or irregularly shaped organelles known as synaptic vesicles in presynaptic terminals by electron microscopy (Fig. 6-2). The second observation came from recordings of postsynaptic responses at the neuromuscular junction. Normally, an action potential in a motor neuron causes a large depolarization in the postsynaptic muscle, termed an **end plate potential (EPP),** which is equivalent to an EPSP in a neuron. However, under conditions of low extracellular $[Ca^{++}]$, the EPP amplitude is reduced (because the presynaptic Ca^{++} current is reduced, leading to a smaller rise in intracellular $[Ca^{++}]$ and transmitter release is proportional to $[Ca^{++}]$). In this condition, the EPP is seen to fluctuate among discrete values (Fig. 6-5). Moreover, small, spontaneous depolarizations of the postsynaptic membrane, termed **miniature end plate potentials (mEPPs),** are observable. The amplitude of the mEPP (≤ 1 mV) corresponds to that of the smallest EPP evoked under low $[Ca^{++}]$, and the amplitudes of other EPPs were shown to be integral multiples of the mEPP amplitude; thus, it was natural to propose that each mEPP corresponded to the release of transmitter from a single vesicle and that EPPs represented the combined simultaneous release of transmitter from many vesicles.

This linking of mEPPs and vesicles implies that each mEPP is caused by the action of many molecules of neurotransmitter binding to postsynaptic receptors. The alternative that each mEPP could be caused by a single transmitter molecule binding to and opening a single postsynaptic receptor was rejected, in part because responses smaller in amplitude than mEPPs could be generated experimentally by directly applying dilute solutions of acetylcholine to the muscle. In fact, mEPPs were calculated to be caused by the action of approximately 10,000 molecules, which corresponds well to estimates of the number of neurotransmitter molecules contained within a single vesicle.

Many additional studies have confirmed the vesicle hypothesis of neurotransmitter release. For example, biochemical studies have shown that neurotransmitter is concentrated in vesicles, and fusion of vesicles to the plasma membrane and their depletion in the terminal cytoplasm after action potentials have been shown with electron microscopic techniques.

Molecular Apparatus Underlying Vesicular Release

The small vesicles that contain nonpeptide neurotransmitters can fuse with the presynaptic membrane only at specific sites, called active zones. To become competent to fuse with the presynaptic membrane at an active zone, a small vesicle must first dock at the active zone. It must then undergo a priming process

● Figure 6-4. Presynaptic Ca⁺⁺ current and its relationship to the postsynaptic response. **A,** Schematic of a squid giant synapse preparation. Electrodes 1 and 2 are used to voltage-clamp the presynaptic terminal and record its voltage and current. Note that TTX and TEA were present to block Na⁺ and K⁺ conductance, in order to isolate the Ca⁺⁺ conductance. Electrode 3 records the membrane potential of the postsynaptic axon. The presynaptic terminal was voltage-clamped to increasingly more depolarized levels *(blue traces)*. With a small depolarization **(B),** a small Ca⁺⁺ current starts shortly after the voltage step, continues to grow for the duration of the step (on current), and then decays exponentially after its termination (off or tail current). A larger voltage step **(C)** increases both the on and the off components of the Ca⁺⁺ current, and now distinct on and off responses are observed in the postsynaptic response. **D,** The voltage step is to the Nernst potential for Ca⁺⁺, so there is no Ca⁺⁺ current during the step, but a large tail current and off response are observed. TTX-tetrodotoxin; TEA, tetraethyl ammonium. (Based on data of Llinas R, et al: Biophys J 33:323–351, 1981.)

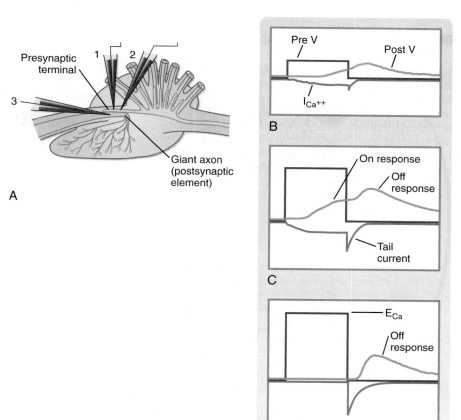

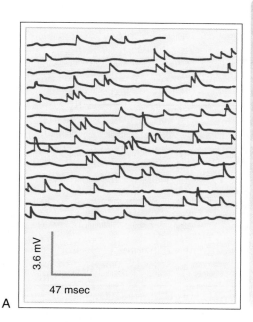

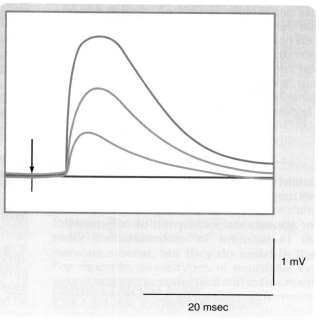

● Figure 6-5. **A,** Spontaneous mEPPs recorded at a neuromuscular junction in a fiber of frog extensor digitorum longus. **B,** EPPs evoked by nerve stimulation under low-[Ca⁺⁺] conditions, which reduce the probability of transmitter release. The small-amplitude EPPs evoked under these conditions vary in amplitude in a step-like manner, where the size of the step is equal to the smallest EPP, which in turn equals the size of the mEPPs (note that in these conditions the stimulus often fails to evoke any response, as indicated by a flat response). (**A,** Data from Fatt P, Katz B: Nature 166:597, 1950; **B,** data from Fatt P, Katz B: J Physiol 117:109, 1952.)

before the vesicle can fuse and release its transmitter into the synaptic cleft in response to an increase in local cytoplasmic [Ca^{++}]. On the order of 25 proteins may play roles in docking, priming, and fusion. Some of these proteins are cytosolic, whereas others are proteins of the vesicle membrane or the presynaptic plasma membrane. The functions of most of these proteins are incompletely understood; however, knowledge of the molecular details of transmitter release has increased dramatically in recent years.

As with other exocytotic processes, neurotransmitter release involves **SNARE** (**s**oluble *N*-ethyl maleimide-**s**ensitive factor **a**ttachment protein **r**eceptor) proteins: v-SNARES in the vesicle membrane and t-SNARES on the (target) presynaptic plasma membrane. Zipper-like interactions between **synaptobrevin** (a v-SNARE) and **syntaxin** and **SNAP-25** (two t-SNARES) bring the vesicle membrane and the presynaptic plasma membrane close together before fusion. The SNARE proteins are targets for various **botulinum toxins,** which disrupt synaptic transmission, thus demonstrating their critical role in this process. Nevertheless, they do not bind Ca^{++}, so another protein must be the Ca^{++} sensor that triggers the actual fusion event. Although several proteins in the terminal do bind Ca^{++}, **synaptotagmin** is almost certainly the Ca^{++} sensor.

Calcium channels are located in the active zone membrane at sites adjacent to the docked vesicles. When they open, a small area of high [Ca^{++}], which lasts for less than a millisecond and is termed a micro-domain, is created at the active zone. This local high concentration allows the rapid binding of Ca^{++} to a protein called synaptotagmin, and it is thought that this binding causes a conformational change in synaptotagmin that triggers the fusion event of a docked vesicle. Indeed, the time from Ca^{++} influx to vesicle fusion is about 0.2 msec.

Synaptic Vesicles Are Recycled

During synaptic transmission, vesicles must fuse with the plasma membrane to release their contents into the synaptic cleft. However, there must be a reverse process; otherwise, not only would it be hard to sustain the vesicle population, but the presynaptic membrane's surface area would also grow with each bout of synaptic transmission, and its molecular content and functionality would likewise change (because, as just discussed, the protein content of the vesicle membrane is distinct from that of the terminal membrane).

There appear to be two distinct mechanisms by which vesicles are retrieved after release of their neurotransmitter content (Fig. 6-6). One mechanism is the endocytotic pathway commonly found in most cell types. Coated pits are formed in the plasma membrane, which then pinch off to form coated vesicles within the cytoplasm of the presynaptic terminal. These vesicles then lose their coat and undergo further transformations (i.e., acquire the correct complement

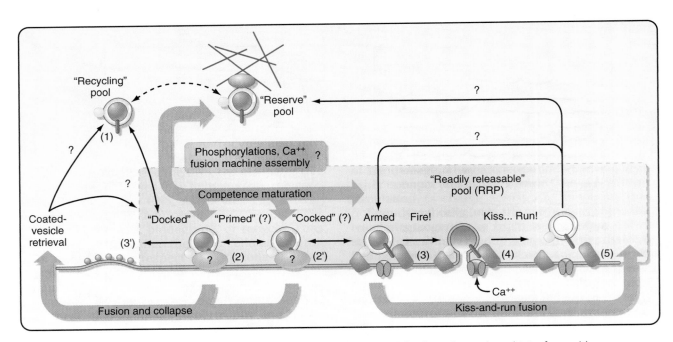

● **Figure 6-6.** Vesicle recycling pathways. Synaptic vesicles have been thought to fuse with the membrane while emptying their contents and then be recycled by forming clathrin-coated pits that are endocytosed to form coated vesicles (1 → [2 or 2'] → 3' → 1). An alternative pathway that may allow more rapid recycling of vesicles has been proposed. This pathway, called "kiss and run," involves only transient fusion of the vesicle to the presynaptic membrane to form a pore through which the vesicle contents may be emptied, followed by detachment of the vesicle from the membrane (1 → 2 → 3 → 4 → 5 → 1). (Redrawn from Valtorta F, Meldolesi J, Fesce R: Trends Cell Biol 11:324, 2001.)

of membrane proteins and be refilled with neurotransmitter) to become once again synaptic vesicles ready for release.

Recently, evidence for a second, more rapid recycling mechanism has been obtained (Fig. 6-6). It involves transient fusion of the vesicle to the synaptic membrane and has been called "kiss and run." In this case, fusion of the vesicle with the synaptic membrane leads to the formation of a pore through which the transmitter is expelled, but there is no wholesale collapse of the vesicle into the membrane. Instead, the duration of the fusion is very brief, after which the vesicle detaches from the plasma membrane and reseals itself. Thus, the vesicle membrane retains its molecular identity. Its contents can then simply be replenished, thereby making the vesicle ready for use again.

The relative importance of these two mechanisms is still being debated. However, at central synapses, which tend to be small and contain relatively few vesicles in comparison to the neuromuscular junction, the rapid time course of the kiss-and-run mechanism may help avoid the problem of vesicle depletion and the consequent failure of synaptic transmission during periods of high activity (many neurons in the CNS can show sustained firing rates of several hundred hertz, and a few types of neuron can fire at rates of approximately 1000 Hz).

Postsynaptic Potentials

When an action potential triggers release of neurotransmitter from a motor neuron, an EPP is generated in the muscle. More generally, at excitatory synapses throughout the nervous system, action potentials trigger EPSPs in the postsynaptic cell. In both cases there is a depolarization of the membrane that increases the excitability of the cell (i.e., makes it more likely to fire an action potential or, if it is already active, increases the firing rate). The EPP is so large that under normal circumstances it depolarizes the sarcolemma well above the action potential threshold and thus always triggers a spike leading to contraction of the muscle cell. This is an example of a synapse with a high (>1) **safety factor** (ratio of synaptic potential to the amplitude needed to reach threshold), which makes sense for the neuromuscular junction because each muscle cell is contacted by only a single motor neuron and if that motor neuron is firing, the nervous system has basically made the decision to contract that muscle. In contrast, most neurons receive thousands of excitatory synapses from many different cells. Here, each synapse generates a small EPSP, and thus it takes the summed EPSPs of multiple active synapses to trigger an action potential in the postsynaptic neuron.

In both situations the basic process leading to the EPSP is the same: the neurotransmitter binds to receptors in the postsynaptic cell that open channels to allow an inward current to flow, which in turn leads to depolarization of the membrane. These channels are termed ligand gated because their opening and closing are primarily controlled by the binding of neurotrans-

mitter. This mechanism can be contrasted with the channels underlying the action potential, which open and close in response to changes in membrane potential. However, there are some channels, most notably the NMDA (N-methyl-D-aspartate) channel, that are both ligand and voltage gated.

It is also worth noting here that the preceding description and what follows in this section refer to what happens when neurotransmitter binds to receptors in which the ion channel is part of the receptor itself. These receptors are referred to as ionotropic receptors and underlie what is now called "fast" synaptic transmission. There is also "slow" synaptic transmission, mediated by what are called metabotropic receptors, in which the receptor and ion channel are not part of the same molecule and binding of neurotransmitter to the receptor initiates biochemical cascades that lead to much slower responses (see the section Receptors for details). Despite the differing time courses, many of the same basic principles apply to both types of synaptic potential.

Once the EPSP channels are open, the direction of current flow through them is determined by the electrochemical driving force for the permeant ions. It turns out that the pores of most channels that underlie EPSPs are relatively large and therefore allow passage of most cations with similar ease. As an example, consider the acetylcholine-gated channel that is opened at the neuromuscular junction. Na^+ and K^+ are the major cations present (Na^+ extracellularly and K^+ intracellularly); therefore, the net current through the channel is approximately the sum of the Na^+ and K^+ currents ($I_{net} = I_{Na} + I_K$). Recall that the current through a channel from a particular ion is dependent on two factors: the conductance of the channel to the ion and the driving force on the ion. This relationship is expressed by the equation

● **Equation 6-1**

$$I_x = g_x \times (V_m - E_x)$$

where g_x is the conductance of the channel to ion x, V_m is the membrane potential, and E_x is the Nernst equilibrium potential for ion x. In this case g_x is similar for Na^+ and K^+, so the main determinant of net current is the relative driving forces ($V_m - E_x$). If the membrane is at its resting potential (typically around −70 mV), there is a strong driving force ($V_m - E_{Na}$) for Na^+ to enter the cell because this potential is far from the Na^+ Nernst potential (about +55 mV), whereas there is only a small driving force for K^+ to leave the cell because V_m is close to the K^+ Nernst potential (about −90 mV). Thus, if acetylcholine-gated channels open when the membrane is at its resting potential, a large inward Na^+ current and a small outward K^+ current will flow through the acetylcholine channel, thereby resulting in a net inward current, which acts to depolarize the membrane.

The net inward current that results from opening such channels is called the **excitatory postsynaptic current (EPSC).** Figure 6-7, *A*, contrasts the time course of the EPSC and the resulting EPSP for fast synaptic transmission. The EPSC is much shorter ($\approx$1 to 2 msec

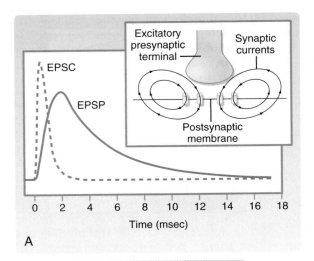

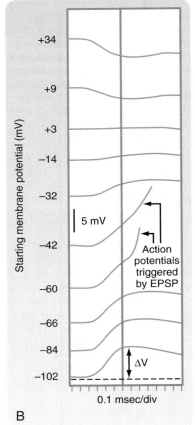

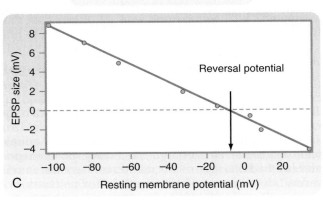

● **Figure 6-7.**   Properties of EPSPs. **A,** Time course of a fast EPSP compared with that of the underlying EPSC. In many cases, such as this one, the EPSC is much shorter than the EPSP; however, sometimes the EPSC can have a fairly extensive tail. **B,** Intracellularly recorded EPSPs at different levels of depolarization. EPSPs were evoked in motor neurons by stimulation of Ia afferents. The number to the left of each trace indicates the membrane potential induced by injection of current through the electrode. At initial membrane potentials of −42 and −60 mV, the EPSP triggered an action potential. At more depolarized levels, Na⁺ channels are inactivated, so no spike occurs. **C,** To determine the EPSP reversal potential, the initial membrane potential is plotted against the size of the EPSP (ΔV). This EPSP reversed at −7 mV. (**A,** Data from Curtis DR, Eccles JC: J Physiol 145:529, 1959; **B,** data from Coombs JS et al: J Physiol 130:374, 1955.)

in duration) and corresponds to the time that the channels are actually open. The short duration of the EPSC is due to the fact that the released neurotransmitter remains in the synaptic cleft for only a short while before being either enzymatically degraded or taken up by either glia or the presynaptic terminal. Binding and unbinding of a neurotransmitter to its receptor take place rapidly, so once its concentration falls in the cleft, the postsynaptic receptor channels rapidly close as well and terminate the EPSC. Note how the end of the EPSC corresponds to the peak of the EPSP, which is followed by a long tail. The duration of the tail and the rate of the decay in EPSP amplitude reflect the passive membrane properties of the cell (i.e., its RC properties). In slow synaptic transmission, the duration of the EPSP reflects the activation and deactivation of biochemical processes more than the membrane properties. The long duration of even fast EPSPs is functionally important because it allows EPSPs to overlap and thereby summate. Such summation is central to the integrative properties of neurons (see the later section Synaptic Integration).

Normally, an EPSP depolarizes the membrane, and if this depolarization reaches threshold, an action potential is generated. However, consider what happens if the channels underlying the action potential are blocked and the membrane of the postsynaptic cell is experimentally depolarized by injecting current through an intracellular electrode. Because the membrane potential is now more positive, the driving force for Na⁺ is decreased and that for K⁺ increased. If the synapse is activated at this point, the net current through the receptor channel (the EPSC) will be smaller because of changes in the relative driving force. This implies that if the membrane potential is depolarized enough, there will be a point at which the Na⁺ and K⁺ currents through the channel are equal and opposite and thus there is no net current and no EPSP. If the membrane is depolarized beyond this point, there is a net outward current through the receptor channels, and the membrane will hyperpolarize (i.e., the EPSP will be negative). Thus, the potential at which there is no EPSP (or EPSC) is known as the **reversal**

potential. For excitatory synapses, the reversal potential is usually around 0 mV (±10 mV), depending on the synapse (Fig. 6-7, *B* and *C*).

It is worth noting that a reversal potential is a key criterion for demonstrating the chemical-gated as opposed to the voltage-gated nature of a synaptic response because currents through voltage-gated channels do not reverse, except at the Nernst potential of the ion for which they are selective (and then only if the channel is open at that potential). Consequently, beyond a certain membrane potential, no current will flow through voltage-gated channels because they will be closed. In contrast, ligand-gated channels can be opened at any membrane potential and thus can always have a net current flow through them, except at one specific voltage, the reversal potential.

IPSPs, like EPSPs, are triggered by the binding of neurotransmitter to receptors on the postsynaptic membrane and typically involve an increase in membrane permeability as a result of the opening of ligand-gated channels. They differ in that IPSP channels are permeable to only a single ionic species, either Cl^- or K^+. Thus, IPSPs will have a reversal potential equal to the Nernst potential of the ion carrying the underlying current. Typically, the Nernst potential for these ions is somewhat negative relative to the resting potential, so when IPSP channels open, there is an outward flow of current through them that results in hyperpolarization of the membrane (Fig. 6-3).

However, in some cells, activation of an inhibitory synapse may produce no change in potential (if the membrane potential equals the Nernst potential for Cl^- or K^+) or may actually result in a small depolarization. Nevertheless, in both these cases, the reversal potential for the IPSP is still negative with regard to the threshold for eliciting an action potential (otherwise it would increase the probability of the cell spiking and by definition be an EPSP). It may seem counterintuitive that something that depolarizes the membrane can still be considered inhibitory, but if it decreases the probability of spiking, then it is indeed inhibitory. A further explanation is given in the next section.

In sum, starting from the resting membrane potential, EPSPs are always depolarizing, IPSPs can be either depolarizing or hyperpolarizing, and a hyperpolarizing potential is always an IPSP. Thus, the key distinction between inhibitory and excitatory synapses (and IPSPs and EPSPs) is how they affect the probability of the cell firing an action potential: EPSPs increase the probability, whereas IPSPs decrease the probability.

SYNAPTIC INTEGRATION

The overall effect of a particular synapse is dependent on its location. To understand this concept fully, we must first recall that action potentials are typically generated at the axon hillock of the cell because it has the highest density of voltage-gated Na^+ channels and therefore the lowest threshold for initiation of a spike. Thus, it is the summed amplitudes of the synaptic potentials at this point, the axon hillock, that is critical

for the decision to spike. EPSPs generated by synapses close to the axon hillock (i.e., synapses onto the soma or proximal dendrites) will result in a larger depolarization at the hillock than will EPSPs generated by synapses on distal dendrites (Fig. 6-8, *A*, single action potential in axon 1 versus 2). Remember that the cell membrane is leaky and synaptic currents are generated locally at the synapse, so even if two synapses generate a local EPSC of the same size, less of the initial current will arrive at the axon hillock from the more distal synapse than from the more proximal one, thereby resulting in the generation of a smaller EPSP at the axon hillock by the distal synapse (see discussion of length constant in Chapter 5). Thus, the synapse's spatial location in the dendritic tree is an important determinant of its efficacy.

As already mentioned, EPSPs generated by most CNS synapses, even those in favorable positions (i.e., close to the axon hillock), are too small by themselves

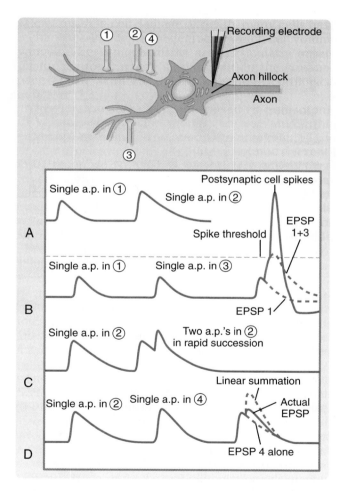

● **Figure 6-8.** Synaptic integration of EPSPs recorded at axon hillock. **A,** Comparison of EPSPs evoked by proximal versus distal synapses (1 versus 2). **B,** Example of a spatial summation response evoked by synapses that are electrically independent of each other (1 and 3). **C,** Temporal summation. The postsynaptic response to two spikes in the same axon occurs in rapid succession (axon 2). **D,** Sublinear summation of two synapses located near each other (2 and 4). a.p., action potential.

to reach the spiking threshold in the postsynaptic cell. An action potential will result only when the summed excitation from multiple inputs reaches threshold. For example, in Figure 6-8, suppose axon 1 fires an action potential. This results in an EPSP that depolarizes the cell but is too small to reach threshold. Now suppose that axon 1 fires an action potential followed by an action potential in axon 3 some time later. Each of the resulting EPSPs is too small to reach threshold, but, instead, if they occur within a short enough time of each other, their effect can be additive, as shown in Figure 6-8, *B.* The combined amplitude may then reach threshold and lead to spiking of the cell. The ability of such asynchronous EPSPs to summate is known as **temporal summation.** The fact that EPSPs have a long time course (when compared with action potentials or the underlying EPSCs) facilitates this type of synaptic integration. Temporal summation can also occur when the same synapse is activated multiple times in rapid succession because axons can fire action potentials at rates well over 100 Hz; in this situation, successive EPSPs will be less than 10 msec apart and therefore overlap and summate (Fig. 6-8, *C*).

The example of temporal summation between two synapses just presented also illustrates the principle of **spatial summation,** which refers to the fact that synaptic potentials generated throughout the soma and dendrites interact. Interestingly, the nature of this interaction depends on the relative locations of the two synapses. In the foregoing example, the combined EPSP was approximately the linear summation of the two individual EPSPs evoked by action potentials in axons 1 and 3. This is the case when two synapses are far apart. If the two synapses are close together, such as for axons 2 and 4 (Fig. 6-8, *D*), the summation becomes less than linear because of what is known as a **shunting effect.** That is, when synapse 2 is active, channels are opened in the cell membrane, which means that it is more leaky. Therefore, when synapse 4 is also active, more of its EPSC will be lost (shunted) through the dendritic membrane, and less current will be left to travel down the dendrite to the axon hillock. The result is that synapse 4 causes a smaller EPSP at the hillock than it would have generated in isolation. Nevertheless, the combined EPSP is still larger than an EPSP caused by either synapse 2 or 4 alone.

Where do IPSPs fit into synaptic integration? In many cases one can think of them as negative EPSPs. Thus, whereas EPSPs add together to help bring the membrane potential up to and beyond the spiking threshold, IPSPs subtract from the membrane potential to make it more negative and therefore further from threshold. In deciding whether to spike, a cell adds up the ongoing EPSPs and subtracts the IPSPS to determine whether the sum reaches threshold. As with an EPSP, the efficacy of an IPSP varies with its location.

In addition to subtracting algebraically from the membrane potential, IPSPs exert an inhibitory action via the shunting mechanism, just as was described earlier for EPSPs. That is, while the IPSP channels are open, they make the membrane very leaky (i.e., lower its resistance) and thereby reduce the size of EPSPs, thus making them less effective. This shunting mechanism explains how IPSPs that do not change the membrane potential—or even those that slightly depolarize it—can still decrease the excitability of the cell. An alternative way to look at this effect is to view each synapse as a device that tries to bring the membrane potential to its own equilibrium potential. Because this potential is below the action potential threshold in the case of IPSPs, it makes it harder for the cell to spike.

Thus far the interaction of synaptic potentials has been presented under the assumption that the postsynaptic cell membrane is passive (i.e., it acts as though it were simply resistors and capacitors in parallel with each other). However, recent evidence has made it clear that the dendrites and somas of most, if not all, neurons contain active elements (i.e., gated channels) that can amplify and alter EPSPs and IPSPs. For example, distal EPSPs can have a larger than expected effect because of voltage-gated Na^+ or Ca^{++} channels that are activated by the EPSP and that, in turn, boost its amplitude or even generate propagated dendritic action potentials. Another example is Ca^{++}-activated K^+ channels that are present in the dendrites of some neurons. These channels are activated by the influx of Ca^{++} either through synaptic channels or via dendritic voltage-gated Ca^{++} channels opened by EPSPs and can cause long-lasting hyperpolarizations that effectively make the cell inexcitable for tens to hundreds of milliseconds. As a final example, there are some Ca^{++} channels that underlie a low-threshold Ca^{++} spike. These channels are normally inactive at resting membrane potentials, but the hyperpolarization that results from a large IPSP can de-inactivate them and allow them to open (and produce a spike) after termination of the IPSP. In this case "inhibition" actually increases the cell's excitability. In sum, synaptic integration is a highly complex, nonlinear process. Nevertheless, the basic principles just described remain at its core.

MODULATION OF SYNAPTIC ACTIVITY

Integration of synaptic input by a postsynaptic neuron, as described in the previous section, represents one aspect of the dynamic nature of synaptic transmission. A second dynamic aspect is that the strength of individual synapses can vary as a function of their use or activity. That is, a synapse's current functional state reflects, to some extent, its history.

Activation of a synapse typically produces a response in the postsynaptic cell (i.e., a postsynaptic potential) that will be roughly the same each time, assuming that the postsynaptic cell is in a similar state. Certain patterns of synaptic activation, however, result in changes in the response to subsequent activation of the synapse. Such use-related changes may remain for short (milliseconds) or long (minutes to days) durations and may be either a potentiation or suppression of the synapse's strength. These changes probably underlie cognitive abilities, such as learning and memory. Thus, the processes by which activity results in changes in a synapse's efficacy are a critical feature of synaptic transmission.

Paired-Pulse Facilitation

When a presynaptic axon is stimulated twice in rapid succession, it is often found that the response evoked by the second stimulus is larger in amplitude than the one evoked by the first (Fig. 6-9). This increase is known as **paired-pulse facilitation (PPF).** If one plots the relative size of the two postsynaptic potentials (PSPs) (i.e., the responses) as a function of the time between two stimuli, the amount of increase in the second PSP will be seen to depend on the time interval. Maximal facilitation occurs at around 20 msec, followed by a gradual reduction in facilitation as the interstimulus interval continues to increase; with intervals of several hundred milliseconds, the two PSPs are equal in amplitude and no facilitation is observed. Thus, PPF is a relatively rapid, but short-lasting change in synaptic efficacy.

Posttetanic Potentiation

Posttetanic potentiation is similar to PPF; however, in this case the responses are compared before and after stimulation of the presynaptic neuron tetanically (tens to hundreds of stimuli at a high frequency). Such a tetanic stimulus train causes an increase in synaptic efficacy, known as posttetanic potentiation (Fig. 6-9, *C*). Posttetanic potentiation, like facilitation, is an enhancement of the postsynaptic response, but it lasts longer: tens of seconds to several minutes after the cessation of tetanic stimulation.

Numerous experiments have shown that PPF and posttetanic potentiation are the result of changes in the presynaptic terminal and do not generally involve a change in the sensitivity of the postsynaptic cell to transmitter. Rather, the repeated stimulation leads to an increased number of quanta of transmitter being released. This increase is thought to be due to residual amounts of Ca^{++} that remain in the presynaptic terminal after each stimulus and help potentiate subsequent release of transmitter. However, the exact mechanism or mechanisms by which this residual Ca^{++} enhances release is not yet clear. The residual Ca^{++} does not, however, appear to act simply by binding to the same sites as the Ca^{++} that enters at the active zone and directly triggers vesicle fusion in response to the action potential.

Synaptic Depression

Use of a synapse can also lead to a short-term depression in its efficacy. Most commonly, the postsynaptic cell at such a fatigued or depressed synapse responds normally to transmitter applied from a micropipette; hence, as was the case for PPF and posttetatic

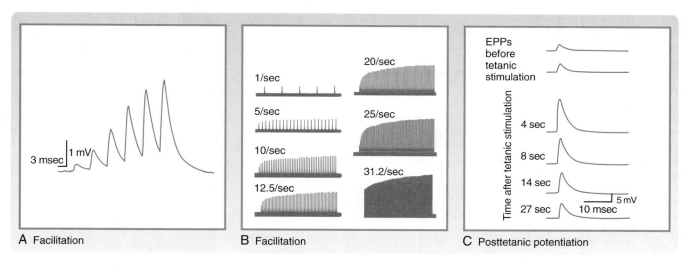

● **Figure 6-9.**   **A,** Facilitation at a neuromuscular junction. EPPs at a neuromuscular junction in toad sartorius muscle were elicited by successive action potentials in the motor axon. Neuromuscular transmission was depressed by 5 mM Mg⁺⁺ and 2.1 mM curare so that action potentials did not occur. **B,** EPPs at a frog neuromuscular junction elicited by repetitively stimulating the motor axon at different frequencies. Note that facilitation failed to occur at the lowest frequency of stimulation (1/sec) and that the degree of facilitation increased with increasing frequency of stimulation in the range of frequency used. Neuromuscular transmission was inhibited by bathing the preparation in 12 to 20 mM Mg⁺⁺. **C,** Posttetanic potentiation at a frog neuromuscular junction. The top two traces indicate control EPPs in response to single action potentials in the motor axon. Subsequent traces indicate EPPs in response to single action potentials after tetanic stimulation (50 impulses/sec for 20 seconds) of the motor neuron. The time interval between the end of tetanic stimulation and the single action potential is shown on each trace. The muscle was treated with tetrodotoxin to prevent the generation of action potentials. (**A,** Redrawn from Belnave RJ, Gage PW: J Physiol 266:435, 1977; **B,** redrawn from Magelby KL: J Physiol 234:327, 1973; **C,** redrawn from Weinrich D: J Physiol 212:431, 1971.)

potentiation, the change is presynaptic. In general, the depression is thought to reflect depletion of the number of releasable presynaptic vesicles. Thus, short-term depression of synaptic transmission is most often and most easily seen at synapses in which the probability of release after a single stimulus is high and under conditions that favor release (i.e., high [Ca^{++}]). A postsynaptically related cause of synaptic depression can be desensitization of the receptors in the postsynaptic membrane.

Both potentiation and depressive processes can occur at the same synapse. So in general, the type of modulation observed will depend on which process dominates. This, in turn, can reflect stimulus parameters, local ionic conditions, and the properties of the synapse. In particular, synapses have different baseline probabilities for releasing vesicles. Synapses with a high release probability will be more likely to show poststimulus depression, whereas those with low release probability are less likely to deplete their vesicle store and thus can be facilitated more easily. Sometimes mixed responses can occur. For example, during a tetanic stimulus train a synapse may show a depressed response, but after the train the synapse can show posttetanic facilitation once the vesicles are recycled.

Presynaptic Receptors Can Modulate Transmitter Release

Just as the postsynaptic membrane contains receptors for neurotransmitters, so does the presynaptic membrane. When these presynaptic receptors bind neurotransmitter, they cause events that can modulate subsequent release of transmitter by the terminal. There are several sources of transmitter that binds to presynaptic receptors: it can be the transmitter released by the terminal itself (i.e., self-modulation, in which case the receptors are referred to as autoreceptors), it can be released by another presynaptic terminal that synapses onto the terminal (a serial synapse), or it can be a nonsynaptically acting neurotransmitter (see the section Neurotransmitters).

Presynaptic receptors can be either ionotropic or metabotropic. In the latter case, recall that their action will be relatively slow in onset and long in duration and the effect will depend on the specific second messenger cascades that are activated. Such cascades can ultimately regulate presynaptic voltage-gated Ca^{++} and K$^+$ channels and other presynaptic proteins and thereby alter the probability of vesicle release.

In contrast, activation of presynaptic ionotropic receptors will directly alter the electrical properties of the presynaptic terminal and cause rapid transient (millisecond time scale) changes in the probability of vesicle release (although they too can have much longer lasting effects). Binding of an ionotropic receptor will open channels in the presynaptic terminal and thereby alter the amount of transmitter released by an action potential.

Presynaptic inhibition refers to occasions when binding of presynaptic receptors leads to a decrease in release of transmitter, and it can be the result of one

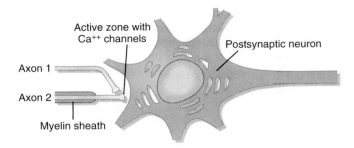

● **Figure 6-10.** Presynaptic inhibition. Active regeneration of action potentials in axon 2 ends at the last node. The action potential is then passively conducted into the terminal. Axon 1 makes an axoaxonic synapse with axon 2. Activation of this synapse reduces conduction of the action potential in axon 2 to the active zone of its synaptic terminal by mechanisms described in the text. This reduces the opening of voltage-gated Ca^{++} channels and therefore release of neurotransmitter.

or more mechanisms (Fig. 6-10). First, opening of channels decreases membrane resistance and creates a current shunt. The shunt acts to divert the current associated with the action potential from the active zone membrane and thereby lessens the depolarization of the active zone, which results in less activation of Ca^{++} channels, less Ca^{++} entry, and less release of transmitter. A second mechanism is the change in membrane potential caused by the opening of presynaptic ionotropic channels. If a small depolarization is the result, there will be inactivation of Na$^+$ channels and thereby lessening of the action potential–associated current and transmitter release. Presynaptic γ-aminobutyric acid A receptors (GABA$_A$) occur in the spinal cord and mediate presynaptic inhibition by these mechanisms. They control Cl$^-$ channels. Generally, opening of Cl$^-$ channels generates a hyperpolarization. However, in the presynaptic terminal, the [Cl$^-$] gradient is such that Cl$^-$ flows out of the cell and generates a small depolarization. This depolarization is small enough that it does not cause significant opening of voltage-gated Ca^{++} channels; otherwise, it would increase release of transmitter (presynaptic facilitation). In fact, there are other receptors that control cation channels and create large depolarizations, thereby increasing the release of transmitter. In addition, presynaptic nicotinic acetylcholine receptors control a cation channel that is permeable to Ca^{++}. By allowing additional entry of Ca^{++}, these receptors increase the release of transmitter from the terminal.

Long-Term Changes in Synaptic Strength

Repetitive stimulation of certain synapses in the brain can also produce more persistent changes in the efficacy of transmission at these synapses, a process called **long-term potentiation** or **long-term depression**. Such changes can persist for days to weeks and are believed to be involved in the storage of memories.

The increased synaptic efficacy that occurs in long-term potentiation probably involves both presynaptic (greater transmitter release) and postsynaptic (greater sensitivity to transmitter) changes, in contrast to the short-term changes that involve changes only in presynaptic function. Entry of calcium into the postsynaptic region is an early step required for initiating the changes that result in long-term enhancement of the response of the postsynaptic cell to neurotransmitter. Entry of calcium occurs through NMDA and some AMPA (α-amino-3-hydroxy-5-methyl-4-isoxazole propionic acid) receptors (classes of glutamate receptors; see the section Receptors). Entry of Ca^{++} is believed to activate Ca^{++}-calmodulin kinase II, a multifunctional protein kinase that is present in very high concentrations in postsynaptic densities. In the presence of high $[Ca^{++}]$, this kinase can phosphorylate itself and thereby become active. Calcium-calmodulin kinase II is believed to phosphorylate proteins that are essential for the induction of long-term potentiation. Long-term potentiation may also have an anatomic component. After appropriate stimulation of a presynaptic pathway, the number of dendritic spines and the number of synapses on the dendrites of postsynaptic neurons may increase rapidly. Changes in the presynaptic nerve terminal may also contribute to long-term potentiation. The postsynaptic neuron may release a signal (nitric oxide has been suggested) that enhances release of transmitter by the presynaptic nerve terminal.

NEUROTRANSMITTERS

Neurotransmitters are the substances that mediate chemical signaling between neurons. For a substance to be considered a neurotransmitter, it must meet several generally recognized criteria. First, the substance must be demonstrated to be present in the presynaptic terminal and the cell must be able to synthesize the substance. It should be released on depolarization of the terminal. Finally, there should be specific receptors for it on the postsynaptic membrane. This last criterion is certainly true for substances that act as synaptic transmitters, but if we want to be inclusive and include substances that act over widespread territories rather than just at a single synapse, the last criterion needs to be relaxed to include situations in which receptors are located at sites outside the synapse. Neurotransmission has been suggested as a general term to describe both synaptic and nonsynaptic signaling between cells.

More than 100 substances have been identified as potential neurotransmitters because they have met some (hence the "potential" qualifier) or all of these criteria. These substances can be subdivided into three major categories: small-molecule transmitters, peptides, and gaseous transmitters. The small-molecule neurotransmitters may be further subdivided into acetylcholine, amino acids, biogenic amines, and purines. The first three groups of small-molecule transmitters contain what are considered the classic neurotransmitters. Remaining transmitters are substances that are more recent additions to the list of neurotransmitters, although many of them have been known as biologically important molecules in other contexts for a long time.

Small-Molecule Neurotransmitters
Acetylcholine

In the peripheral nervous system, acetylcholine is the transmitter at neuromuscular junctions, at sympathetic and parasympathetic ganglia, and of the postganglionic fibers from all parasympathetic ganglia and a few sympathetic ganglia. It is also a transmitter within the CNS, most prominently of neurons in some brainstem nuclei, in several parts of the basal forebrain (septal nuclei and nucleus basalis) and basal ganglia, and in the spinal cord (e.g., motor neuron axon collaterals). Cholinergic neurons from the basal forebrain areas project diffusely throughout the neocortex and to the hippocampus and amygdala, and they have been implicated in memory functions. Indeed, degeneration of these cells occurs in Alzheimer's disease, a form of dementia in which memory function is gradually and progressively lost.

Acetylcholine is synthesized from acetyl coenzyme A and choline by the enzyme choline acetyltransferase, which is located in the cytoplasm of cholinergic

> ### IN THE CLINIC

A number of drugs, known as **anticholinesterases,** interfere with acetylcholinesterase and thereby prolong the action of acetylcholine at its synapses. Such drugs include insecticides and chemical warfare agents, as well as some therapeutic drugs, such as those used to treat myasthenia gravis. Myasthenia gravis is an autoimmune disease in which antibodies bind to acetylcholine receptors at the neuromuscular junction, thereby disrupting their functionality and causing them to be more rapidly degraded. This reduction in receptors leads to severe weakness and ultimately paralysis. The weakness is characterized by rapid tiring of the muscle with repeated use. Rapid tiring occurs because the number of presynaptic vesicles available for release drops during the high-frequency train of motor neuron action potentials that generates such contractions. Normally, because of the high safety factor of the neuromuscular junction, smaller but still suprathreshold EPPs would still be generated and maintain muscle contraction during repeated use, but in people with myasthenia gravis, the safety factor is so reduced by the loss of acetylcholine receptors that the decrease in release of acetylcholine with repeated activity leads to EPPs that fail to trigger spikes and thus muscular contraction fails. Standard treatments include anticholinesterases, which allow a greater concentration of acetylcholine to partially overcome the deficit caused by the reduced number of functional postsynaptic receptors, and immunosuppressive therapies and plasma exchange, which reduce levels of autoantibodies against the acetylcholine receptor. These therapies are all relatively nonspecific and can therefore have many side effects. Potential future therapies are being developed and include inducing tolerance to the acetylcholine receptor and selective destruction of the B cells that make antibodies against the receptor.

presynaptic terminals. After synthesis, acetylcholine is concentrated in vesicles. After release, the action of acetylcholine is terminated by the enzyme acetylcholinesterase, which is highly concentrated in the synaptic cleft. Acetylcholinesterase hydrolyzes acetylcholine into acetate and choline. The choline is then taken up by an Na^+ symporter in the presynaptic membrane for the resynthesis of acetylcholine. The extracellular enzymatic degradation of acetylcholine is unusual for a neurotransmitter inasmuch as the synaptic action of other classic neurotransmitters is terminated via reuptake by a series of specialized transporter proteins.

Amino Acids

A variety of amino acids function as neurotransmitters. The three most important are glutamate, glycine, and GABA.

Glutamate is the neurotransmitter at the overwhelming majority of excitatory synapses throughout the CNS. Despite its ubiquity, it was initially difficult to identify specific neurons as glutamatergic because glutamate is present in all cells; it has a key role in multiple metabolic pathways, and it is a precursor to GABA, the major inhibitory neurotransmitter. Nevertheless, experimental results have now clearly established glutamate as the major excitatory CNS neurotransmitter. When applied to cells, it causes depolarization and is released from neurons, and specific receptors and transporters for it have been identified.

In addition to being the main excitatory neurotransmitter, glutamate is a potent neurotoxin at high concentrations. Thus, strict limitation of glutamate's activity after its release from the presynaptic terminal is necessary, not only to allow normal synaptic transmission but also to prevent cell death. This task is accomplished by specialized membrane transporter proteins (Fig. 6-11 and box, At the Cellular Level).

GABA and **glycine** act as inhibitory neurotransmitters. GABA is the major inhibitory transmitter throughout the nervous system. GABA is produced from glutamate by a specific enzyme (glutamic acid decarboxylase) that is present only in neurons that use GABA as a transmitter. Thus, experimentally, it is possible to identify cells as inhibitory GABA-ergic neurons by using antibodies to this enzyme to mark them (immunolabeling). Many local interneurons are GABA-ergic. In addition, several brain regions contain large numbers of GABA-ergic projection neurons. The most notable are the spiny neurons of the striatum and the Purkinje cells of the cerebellar cortex. The inhibitory nature of Purkinje cells was especially surprising because they represent the entire output of the cerebellar cortex, and thus cerebellar cortical activity basically functions to suppress the activity of its downstream targets (cerebellar and vestibular nuclei).

Glycine functions as an inhibitory neurotransmitter in a much more restricted territory. Glycinergic synapses are predominantly found in the spinal cord, where they represent approximately half of the inhibitory synapses. They are likewise present in the lower brainstem, cerebellum, and retina in significant numbers. Interestingly, glycine also has another synaptic function. At excitatory NMDA-type glutamate receptors, glycine must also be bound for the ion channel to open. Thus, it acts as a cotransmitter at these synapses. It was generally thought that under physiological conditions the extracellular glycine concentration was high enough that the glycine binding sites of the NMDA channel were always saturated, but recent results suggest that this may not always be true, which implies that fluctuations in glycine levels may also be an important modulator of NMDA-mediated synaptic transmission.

After GABA and glycine are released from the presynaptic terminal, they are taken back up into the nerve terminal and neighboring glia by high-affinity Na^+-Cl^-–coupled membrane transporters. These Na^+-Cl^- transporters are part of a superfamily of transporters that also includes those for the biogenic amine neurotransmitters, but it is distinct from those for glutamate. Transport of the neurotransmitter into the cell is accomplished by symport with two Na^+ and one Cl^- ion. There are four GABA transporters (GAT1 to GAT4), which are found on neurons and glia, the exact distribution varying by subtype. There are two main glycine transporters, GlyT1 and GlyT2. GlyT1 is found predominantly on astrocytes and is present throughout the CNS. In contrast, GlyT2 is located on glycinergic nerve terminals and is largely restricted to the spinal cord, brainstem, and cerebellum.

Biogenic Amines

Many of the neurotransmitters in this category may be familiar because they have roles outside the nervous system, often as hormones. Among the amines known to act as neurotransmitters are **dopamine, norepinephrine** (noradrenaline), **epinephrine** (adrenaline), **serotonin** (5-hydroxytryptamine [5-HT]), and **histamine.** Dopamine, norepinephrine, and epinephrine are catecholamines, and they share a common biosynthetic pathway that starts with the amino acid tyrosine. Tyrosine is converted to L-dopa by the enzyme tyrosine hydroxylase. L-Dopa is then converted to dopamine by dopa-decarboxylase. In dopaminergic neurons, the pathway stops here. In noradrenergic neurons, another enzyme, dopamine β-hydroxylase, converts dopamine to norepinephrine. Epinephrine is obtained by adding a methyl group to norepinephrine via phenylethanolamine-*N*-methyl transferase. In serotoninergic neurons, serotonin is synthesized from the essential amino acid tryptophan. Tryptophan is first converted to 5-hydroxytryptophan by tryptophan 5-hydroxylase, which is then converted to serotonin by aromatic L-amino acid decarboxylase. Finally, in histaminergic neurons the conversion of histidine to histamine is catalyzed by histidine decarboxylase.

Removal of synaptically released biogenic amines is generally accomplished by reuptake into glia and neurons via transporters belonging to the Na^+-Cl^-–dependent transporter family. The catecholamines are then degraded by two enzymes, monoamine oxidase and catechol *O*-methyltransferase.

Within the CNS, nerve cells that use biogenic amines as neurotransmitters are primarily found within one

AT THE CELLULAR LEVEL

At least five transporters (called EAAT1 to EAAT5, where EAAT stands for excitatory amino acid transporter) that carry glutamate across the plasma membrane have been identified. They are all part of the Na^+-K^+–dependent family of transporters. Inward movement of each glutamate molecule is driven by the cotransport of three Na^+ ions and one H^+ ion and the countertransport of one K^+ ion out of the cell (Fig. 6-11B). In addition, the transporter has Cl^- conductance, although passage of Cl^- ions is not stoichiometrically linked to glutamate transport. Glutamate transporters are found on both neurons and glia. However, the transporters differ in their regional and cellular distribution and in their pharmacological and biophysical properties. For example, EAAT2 is found on glia and is generally responsible for more than 90% of glutamate uptake from the extracellular space. The glu-tamate taken up into glial cells by EAAT2 is eventually returned to the presynaptic terminal by the glutamate-glutamine cycle (Fig. 6-11). Inside glial cells glutamate is converted to glutamine. Glutamine is then transported out of the glial cell and back into the presynaptic terminal, where it is subsequently converted back to glutamate. Glutamate inside the presynaptic terminal is packaged into synaptic vesicles by a second set of glutamate transporters known as **vGLUTs (vesicular glutamate transporters)**, which are present in the membrane of glutamatergic vesicles. Transport of glutamate into synaptic vesicles by vGLUT is driven by the countertransport of H^+ ions, the electrochemical gradient for which having been established by an H^+-ATPase in the vesicle membrane.

● **Figure 6-11.** Glutamate transport cycle. **(A)** A schematic shows the fate of glutamate released from a presynaptic terminal. Distinct glutamate transporters exist on the presynaptic and postsynaptic cell membranes for reuptake. In addition, glial cells take up glutamate and convert it to glutamine. The glutamine is then released and taken into the presynaptic terminal, where it is converted back to glutamate before being repackaged into synaptic vesicles. **(B)** Schematic of transporter showing direction of ion flow associated with the movement of glutamate across the membrane.

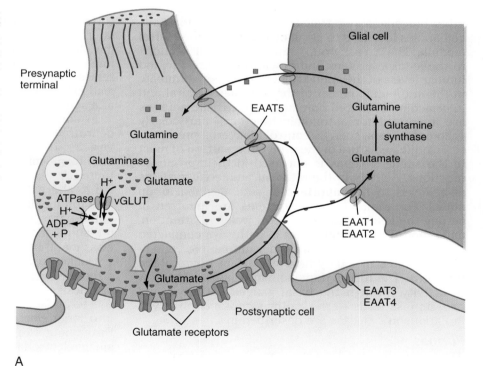

A

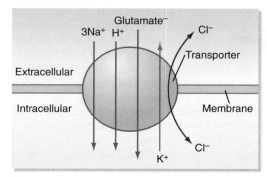

B

of a few brainstem nuclei, most of which project rather diffusely throughout large areas of the brain. Noradrenergic neurons are primarily found in the locus coeruleus and nucleus subcoeruleus, which are located near each other in the dorsal part of the rostral pons. The neurons of the locus coeruleus project throughout the entire brain. Targets of the nucleus subcoeruleus are more limited, but still widespread and include the pons, medulla, and spinal cord. (Norepinephrine is also important in the peripheral nervous system because it is used by postganglionic sympathetic cells.) Serotoninergic fibers arise from a series of nuclei located at the midline of the brainstem, known as the raphe nuclei. Similar to the noradrenergic fibers, serotoninergic fibers are distributed throughout most of the brain and spinal cord. Dopaminergic fibers arise from two main brainstem regions: the substantia nigra pars compacta, which projects to the striatum, and the ventral tegmental area, which projects more widely to the neocortex and subcortical areas. Histaminergic neurons are located within the tuberomammillary nucleus of the hypothalamus but project diffusely throughout the CNS. Finally, adrenergic neurons are relatively few in number when compared with the other biogenic amine transmitters, but they too have cell bodies localized to small cell groups in the rostral medulla. The largest group, termed C1, has projections to the locus coeruleus and down to the thoracic and lumbar levels of the spinal cord, where they terminate in the autonomic nuclei of the intermediolateral and intermediomedial cell columns. Thus, these neurons are important for autonomic functions, particularly vasomotor ones, such as control of arterial pressure.

The diffuse nature of the projection pattern of most of the amine systems is mirrored in their proposed functions. Activity in the different aminergic systems is believed to be important in setting global brain states. For example, these systems are involved in setting the level of arousal (sleep, waking), attention, and mood. Their involvement in pathways connected with the hypothalamus and other autonomic centers also indicates that they have important homeostatic functions. The role of dopamine in balancing the flow of activity through the basal ganglia pathways and how its loss leads to the motor symptoms observed in Parkinson's disease are described in Chapter 9.

Purines

ATP has the potential to act as a transmitter or cotransmitter at synapses in the peripheral and central nervous systems. ATP is found in all synaptic vesicles and thus is coreleased during synaptic transmission. ATP has its own receptors, which like standard neurotransmitters, are coupled to ion channels, but it can also modify the action of other neurotransmitters with which it is coreleased, including norepinephrine, serotonin, glutamate, dopamine, and GABA. Glial cells may also release ATP after certain types of stimulation. Once released, ATP is broken down by ATPases and 5-nucleotidase to **adenosine,** which can be taken up again by the presynaptic terminal.

Peptides

Peptide neurotransmitters consist of chains of between 3 and about 40 amino acids. Studies of neuropeptides focused on the hypothalamus for many years. However, it is now clear that neuropeptides are released by neurons and act on receptors throughout the CNS and thus are a fundamental mechanism of neurotransmission throughout the CNS. To date, more than 100 neuropeptides have been identified. They can be classified into several functional groups, as shown in Table 6-2, which lists some of the known neuropeptides. It is now clear that many neurons that release classic neurotransmitters also release neuropeptides. As detailed later, understanding the interaction between coexisting classic and peptide transmitters has become an important area of research. In addition to being coreleased with another transmitter, neuropeptides can also function as the sole or primary neurotransmitter at a synapse.

In some ways neuropeptides are like the classic neurotransmitters: they are packaged into synaptic vesicles, their release is dependent on Ca^{++}, and they bind to specific receptors on target neurons. However, there are also significant differences, ones that have led to alternative names for the intercellular communication mediated by neuropeptides, such as nonsynaptic, parasynaptic, and volume transmission. Table 6-1 summarizes some of these differences between classic and peptide neurotransmitters.

Unlike classic neurotransmitters, which are synthesized at the presynaptic terminal, neuropeptides are synthesized at the cell body and then transported to the terminal (Fig. 6-2). Neuropeptides are packaged into large electron-dense vesicles that are scattered throughout the presynaptic terminal rather than in small electron-lucent vesicles docked at the active zone, where small-molecule transmitters are stored. (In neurons that make multiple neuropeptides, the various peptides are costored in the same vesicles.) Neuropeptide receptors are not confined to the synaptic region, and in general, peptide action is not limited by reuptake mechanisms.

Each of these differences has functional implications. For example, the separate storage of peptide and nonpeptide transmitters immediately raises the question of whether the two transmitters are coreleased or differentially released in response to particular stimulation patterns.

In fact, differential release of peptide and classic transmitters from the same cell has been demon-

---

> ▶ **IN THE CLINIC**
>
> Hyperactivity of dopaminergic synapses may be involved in some forms of psychosis. **Chlorpromazine** and related antipsychotic drugs inhibit dopamine receptors on postsynaptic membranes and thus diminish the effects of dopamine released from presynaptic nerve terminals. Overdoses of such antipsychotic drugs can produce a temporary parkinsonian-like state.

● Table 6-2.   Some Neuroactive Peptides

Hypothalamic Hormones

Corticotropin-releasing hormone (CRH)

Growth hormone–releasing hormone (GHRH)

Luteinizing hormone–releasing hormone (LHRH)

Oxytocin

Somatostatin

Thyrotropin-releasing hormone (TRH)

Vasopressin

NPY-Related Peptides

Neuropeptide Y

Opioid Peptides

Dynorphin

Methionine enkephalin

Leucine enkephalin

Tachykinins

Neurokinin α

Neurokinin β

Neuropeptide K

Substance P

VIP-Glucagon Family

Glucagon-like peptide 1

Peptide histidine-leucine

Pituitary adenylyl cyclase–activating peptide (PACAP)

Vasoactive intestinal polypeptide (VIP)

Others

Adrenocorticotropic hormone (ACTH)

Brain natriuretic peptide

Cholecystokinin (CCK)

Galanin

Hypocretins/orexins

Neurotensin

Motilin

Insulin

α-Melanocyte–stimulating hormone (α-MSH)

Neurotensin

Prolactin-releasing peptide

Secretoneurin

Urocortin

strated for several types of neurons and is probably a result of the differences in vesicle storage described earlier. Because of their proximity to the active zones, nonpeptide vesicles can be released rapidly (<1 msec) in response to single action potentials as a result of localized influx of Ca^{++}. Thus, low-frequency stimulation of the cell causes just the release of nonpeptide transmitter. In contrast, with higher-frequency stimulation of the presynaptic neuron, there is a more global increase in $[Ca^{++}]$ throughout the nerve terminal that leads to release of neuropeptide, as well as neurotransmitter.

When neuropeptides are coreleased with other transmitters, they may act synergistically or antagonistically. For example, in the spinal cord, **tachykinins** and **calcitonin gene–related peptide (CGRP)** act synergistically with glutamate and with **substance P** to enhance the action of serotonin. Conversely, tachykinins and CGRP antagonize norepinephrine's action at other synapses. The interactions, however, are not simply a one-to-one synergism or antagonism at a particular synapse because of the differing temporal and spatial profiles of the action of peptides versus classic transmitters. In particular, the slower release and lack of rapid reuptake mean that neuropeptides can act for long durations, diffuse over a region of brain tissue, and affect all cells in that region (that have the appropriate receptors) rather than just acting at the specific synapse at which it was released. In fact, studies have shown that there is often a spatial mismatch between the presynaptic terminals that contain a particular neuropeptide and the sites of the receptors for that peptide. In sum, peptides released from a particular synapse probably affect the local neuronal population as a whole, whereas the coreleased classic transmitters act in more of a point-to-point manner.

Opioid Peptides

Opiates are drugs derived from the juice of the opium poppy. Compounds that are not derived from the opium poppy but that exert direct effects by binding to opiate receptors are called **opioids** and form a clinically and functionally important class of neuropeptides. Operationally, opioids are defined as compounds whose effects are stereospecifically antagonized by a morphine derivative called naloxone.

The three major classes of endogenous opioid peptides in mammals are **enkephalins, endorphins,** and **dynorphins.** Enkephalins are the simplest opioids; they are pentapeptides. Dynorphin and the endorphins are somewhat longer peptides that contain one or the other of the enkephalin sequences at their N-terminal ends.

Opioid peptides are widely distributed in neurons of the CNS and intrinsic neurons of the gastrointestinal tract. The endorphins are discretely localized in particular structures of the CNS, whereas the enkephalins and dynorphins are more widely distributed. Opioids inhibit neurons in the brain involved in the perception of pain. Indeed, opioid peptides are among the most potent analgesic (pain-relieving) compounds known, and opiates are used therapeutically as powerful analgesics. They exert their analgesic effect by binding to specific opiate receptors.

Substance P

Substance P is a peptide consisting of 11 amino acids. It is present in specific neurons in the brain, in primary sensory neurons, and in plexus neurons in the wall of the gastrointestinal tract. The wall of the gastrointestinal tract is richly innervated with neurons that form networks or plexuses (see also Chapter 32). The intrinsic plexuses of the gastrointestinal tract exert primary control over its motor and secretory activities. These enteric neurons contain many of the neuropeptides, including substance P, that are found in the brain and spinal column. Substance P is involved in pain transmission and has a powerful effect on smooth muscle.

Substance P is probably the transmitter used at synapses made by primary sensory neurons (their cell bodies are in the dorsal root ganglia) with spinal interneurons in the dorsal horn of the spinal column, and thus it is an example of a peptide acting as a primary transmitter at a synapse. Enkephalins act to decrease the release of substance P at these synapses and thereby inhibit the pathway for pain sensation at the first synapse in the pathway.

Gas Neurotransmitters

This is the newest category of neurotransmitter to be defined and stretches the usual definition of synaptic transmission even further than neuropeptides do. Gas neurotransmitters are neither packaged into synaptic vesicles nor released by exocytosis. Instead, gas neurotransmitters are highly permeant and simply diffuse from synaptic terminals to neighboring cells after synthesis, their synthesis being triggered by depolarization of the nerve terminal (the influx of Ca^{++} activates synthetic enzymes). Moreover, there are no specific reuptake mechanisms, nor do they undergo enzymatic destruction, so their action appears to be ended by diffusion or binding to superoxide anions or various scavenger proteins. Both **nitric oxide (NO)** and **carbon monoxide (CO)** are examples of gaseous neurotransmitters. NO is a transmitter at synapses between inhibitory motor neurons of the enteric nervous system and gastrointestinal smooth muscle cells (see Chapter 32). NO also functions as a neurotransmitter in the CNS. The enzyme NO synthase catalyzes the production of NO as a product of the oxidation of arginine to citrulline. This enzyme is stimulated by an increase in cytosolic $[Ca^{++}]$.

In addition to serving as a neurotransmitter, NO functions as a cellular signal transduction molecule both in neurons and in nonneuronal cells (such as vascular smooth muscle; see Chapter 14). One way that NO functions as a signal transduction molecule is by regulating **guanylyl cyclase,** the enzyme that produces **cGMP** from **GTP.** NO binds to a heme group in soluble guanylyl cyclase and potently stimulates the enzyme. Stimulation of this enzyme leads to an elevation in cGMP in the target cell. The cGMP can then influence multiple cellular processes.

NEUROTRANSMITTER RECEPTORS

The multitude of neurotransmitters used in the nervous system provides it with a specific and flexible interneuronal communications system. These characteristics are even further enhanced by the variety of receptors for each neurotransmitter. Receptors for a particular neurotransmitter were traditionally distinguished primarily by pharmacological differences in their sensitivity to particular agonists and antagonists. For example, acetylcholine receptors were split into **muscarinic** and **nicotinic** classes, depending on whether they bind muscarine or nicotine. Similarly, glutamate receptors were split into three main groups according to their sensitivity to the agonists NMDA, kainic acid, or AMPA. Though useful, this classification scheme has several limitations: some receptors fail to be activated by agonists, and it fails to disclose all the various receptor subtypes for a particular transmitter. Over the past 15 years or so, molecular biological

approaches have been used to identify and sequence the receptor genes for many of the known neurotransmitters. It is thought that we now have a relatively complete catalog of the genes for these receptors. What this work has revealed is that there is a tremendous diversity of actual and potential receptor subtypes that are or could be used by the nervous system. Moreover, knowledge of the gene sequences has enabled an understanding of the relationship of different receptor proteins to each other and to other important proteins. This knowledge, combined with the results of biochemical, crystallographic, and other types of studies, has led to a much deeper understanding of the structural and functional workings of receptor proteins. In particular, various receptors can be grouped into families based on gene sequences, and members of each family share various structural and functional features.

Neurotransmitter receptors are members of one of two large groups or families of proteins: ligand-gated ion channels, also known as ionotropic receptors, and G protein–coupled receptors, also referred to as metabotropic receptors (Fig. 6-12, *A* and *B*). Almost all classic neurotransmitters and neuropeptides have at least one metabotropic-type receptor. Many of the classic neurotransmitters also have at least one ionotropic receptor. Ionotropic receptors are protein complexes that both have an extracellular binding site for the transmitter and form an ion channel (pore) through the cell membrane. The receptor is made up of several protein subunits, usually three to five, each of which typically has a series of membrane-spanning domains, some of which contribute to the wall of the ion channel. Binding of the neurotransmitter alters (usually increases) the probability of the ion channel being in the open state and thus typically results in postsynaptic events that are rapid in both onset and decay, with a duration of several milliseconds. Ionotropic receptors underlie fast synaptic EPSPs and IPSPs, as described earlier.

⬤ AT THE CELLULAR LEVEL

The ionotropic receptors can be divided into several superfamilies. Members of the cys-loop superfamily have peptide subunits that have an N-terminal extracellular domain that contains a loop delimited by cysteine residues. This family includes the ionotropic receptors for acetylcholine, serotonin, GABA, and glycine. In addition to their family-defining cysteine loop, these receptors share the following common features: they are pentamers, with each peptide subunit having four transmembrane domains; the neurotransmitter binds to the N-terminal domain; and the second transmembrane domains are thought to form the wall of the ion pore.

Ionotropic glutamate and ATP receptors form two other ionotropic receptor superfamilies; the details for each are given in the later corresponding sections. Transient receptor potential channels, which are important for transduction of pain and thermal sensations, form yet another family (see Chapter 7).

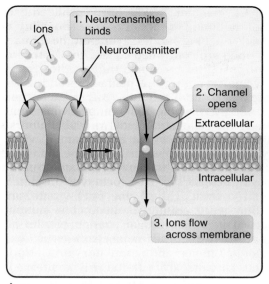

A Ligand-gated ion channels (ionotropic)

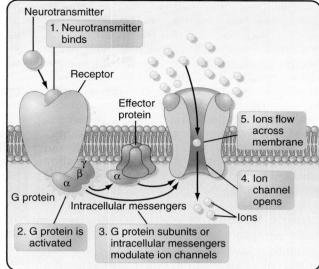

B G protein–coupled receptors (metabotropic)

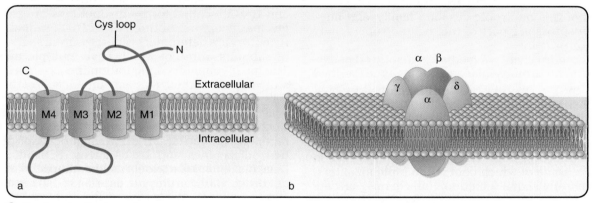

C Cys-loop family channels

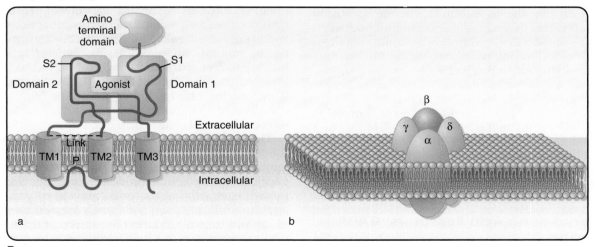

D Glutamate channels

● **Figure 6-12.** Neurotransmitter receptors. The basic structure and mechanism of action are shown for ligand-gated ion channels (ionotropic receptors) **(A)** and G protein–coupled (metabotropic) receptors **(B)**. Detailed structures of cys-loop and glutamate ionotropic receptors are shown in **C** and **D,** respectively. Cys-loop receptors include ionotropic receptors for GABA, glycine, serotonin, and acetylcholine. Note the differing membrane topologies of the individual subunits of these two classes of receptors: four transmembrane domains for cys-loop receptors and three plus a pore loop for glutamate receptors. Pore loops form the internal wall of the glutamate channel, whereas transmembrane domain 2 forms the internal wall of cys-loop receptors. (**A** and **B**, From Purves D, Augustine GJ, Fitzpatrick D, Neuroscience, 2nd ed. Sunderland, MA, Sinauer Associates, 2001.)

Metabotropic receptors are not ion channels. Instead, they are protein monomers that have an extracellular binding site for a particular transmitter and an intracellular site for binding a G protein. Binding of the receptor leads to activation of a G protein, which is the first step in a signal transduction cascade that alters the function of an ion channel in the postsynaptic membrane. In contrast to ionotropic receptors, metabotropic receptors mediate postsynaptic phenomena that have a slow onset and that may persist from hundreds of milliseconds to minutes. Because of the various biochemical cascades that they initiate, they have great potential to cause changes in the neuron beyond just generating a postsynaptic potential.

Acetylcholine Receptors

Acetylcholine receptors were originally classified on a pharmacological basis (being sensitive to nicotine or muscarine) into two major groups. This grouping corresponds to groupings based on structural and molecular biological studies. Nicotinic receptors are members of the ionotropic cys-loop family, and muscarinic receptors are part of the metabotropic family of receptor proteins.

The nicotinic receptors mediate synaptic transmission at the neuromuscular junction, as described earlier; however, nicotinic receptors are also present within the CNS. The nicotinic receptor contains a relatively nonselective cationic channel, so binding of acetylcholine produces an EPSP. Being members of the cys-loop family, acetylcholine receptors are pentamers constructed from a series of subunit types called α, β, γ, δ, ϵ, some of which contain multiple members. At the neuromuscular junction the channel is constructed from 2α, β, δ, ϵ, whereas in the CNS, the composition is typically 3α, 2β. Furthermore, the junctional receptors all use the α_1 subunit, whereas centrally located receptors use one of the α subunits between α_2 and α_{10}. As noted, the differing subunits result in receptors with differing pharmacological sensitivities and channel kinetics and selectivity.

There are five known muscarinic subtypes of acetylcholine receptors (M_1 to M_5). All are metabotropic receptors; however, they are coupled to different G proteins and can thus have distinct effects on the cell. M_1, M_3, and M_5 are coupled to pertussis toxin–insensitive G proteins, whereas M_2 and M_4 are coupled to pertussis toxin–sensitive G proteins. Each set of G proteins is coupled to different enzymes and second messenger pathways (see Chapter 3 for details of these pathways).

Inhibitory Amino Acid Receptors: GABA and Glycine

As noted, the most common inhibitory synapses in the CNS use either glycine or GABA as their transmitter. Glycine-mediated inhibitory synapses predominate in the spinal cord, whereas GABAergic synapses make up the majority of inhibitory synapses in the brain.

Both glycine and GABA (GABA$_A$ and GABA$_C$) have ionotropic receptors that are members of the cys-loop family, thus sharing a number of characteristics, as already described. In addition, each of these receptors has a Cl$^-$ channel, which opens while the receptor portion is bound. Therefore, the probability of these channels opening and the average time that a channel stays open are controlled by the concentration of the neurotransmitter for which the receptor is specific.

Glycine receptors are pentamers and may be heteromers of α and β subunits (3:2 ratio) or homomers. Interestingly, the molecular composition appears to be related to its cellular location, with heteromers located postsynaptically and homomers located extrasynaptically. The β subunit seems to bind to an intracellular scaffold protein called gephyrin that appears to help localize receptors to the postsynaptic site. The α subunit contains the glycine binding site, and there are four genes coding for distinct α subunits (and splice variants of each). Each variant results in a receptor having distinct conductance, kinetics, agonist and antagonist affinity, and modulatory sites. Intriguingly, subunit variants are differentially expressed during development and in different brain regions.

GABA has two separate ionotropic receptors (GABA$_A$ and GABA$_C$) coded for by distinct sets of genes. Like glycine receptors, both control a Cl$^-$ channel. GABA$_A$ receptors are heteromers generated from seven classes of subunits, three of which have multiple members. The most common configuration is α_1, β_2, γ_2 in a 2:2:1 stoichiometry, which may account for 80% of the receptors; however, many other heteromers are found in the brain. As with glycine, different subunits confer distinct properties on the receptor. For example, GABA$_A$ receptors are the targets of two major classes of drugs: benzodiazepines and barbiturates. Benzodiazepines (e.g., diazepam) are widely used antianxiety and relaxant drugs. Barbiturates are used as sedatives and anticonvulsants. Both classes of drugs bind to distinct sites on the α subunits of GABA$_A$ receptors and enhance opening of the receptors' Cl$^-$ channels in response to GABA. The sedative and anticonvulsant actions of benzodiazepines appear to be mediated by receptors with the α_1 subunit, whereas the anxiolytic effects reflect binding to receptors with the α_2 subunit. GABA$_C$ receptors are structurally similar to GABA$_A$ receptors but have a distinct pharmacological profile (e.g., they are not affected by benzodiazepines) and are coded for by a separate set of genes (ρ_1, ρ_2, and ρ_3).

The GABA$_B$ receptor is a metabotropic receptor. Binding of GABA to this receptor activates a heterotrimeric GTP-binding protein (G protein; see Chapter 3), which leads to activation of K$^+$ channels and hence hyperpolarization of the postsynaptic cell, as well as inhibition of Ca^{++} channels (when located presynaptically) and thus a reduction in release of transmitter.

Excitatory Amino Acid Receptors: Glutamate

Glutamate has both ionotropic and metabotropic receptors. Based on pharmacological properties and subunit composition, several distinct ionotropic receptor subtypes are recognized: AMPA, kainate, and NMDA. Overall, there are 18 known genes that code for glutamate subunits for the ionotropic glutamate receptors. However, the genes are divided into several families (AMPA, kainate, NMDA, and δ) that essentially correspond to the pharmacological subtypes of receptors. Each glutamate receptor is a tetramer. Thus, there is a certain correspondence between the genes and the receptor types that are formed. For example, AMPA receptors are formed from GluR1 to GluR4 subunits, kainate receptors require either KA1 or KA2 and GluR5 to GluR7 subunits, and NMDA receptors all have NR1 subunits plus some combination of NR2 and NR3 subunits. As was mentioned for the other receptors, the various receptor properties vary with subunit composition. Ionotropic glutamate receptors are excitatory and contain a cationic-selective channel. Thus, all the channels are permeable to Na^+ and K^+, but only a subset allow Ca^{++} to pass.

AMPA and kainate receptors behave as classic ligand-gated channels, as already discussed; on binding of glutamate to the receptor, the channel opens and allows current to flow, thereby generating an EPSP. NMDA channels are different. First, they require binding of both glutamate and glycine to open. Second, they display voltage sensitivity as a result of Mg^{++} blockade of the channel. That is, at resting (or more negative) membrane potentials, a Mg^{++} ion blocks the entrance to the channel so that even when glutamate and glycine are bound, no current flows through the channel. However, if the cell is depolarized (either experimentally by injection of current through a recording electrode or by other EPSPs), the Mg^{++} block is relieved and current can flow through the channel. A further interesting feature of NMDA channels is that they are generally permeable to Ca^{++}, which can act as a second messenger. The combination of voltage sensitivity and Ca^{++} permeability of the NMDA channels has led to hypotheses concerning their role in learning and memory-related functions (see Chapter 10).

Eight genes coding for metabotropic glutamate receptors have been identified and classified into three groups. Group I receptors are found postsynaptically, whereas groups II and III are found presynaptically. These receptors generate slow EPSPs, but probably at least as importantly, they trigger second messenger cascades (see Chapter 3).

Purine (ATP) Receptors

Purines have two receptor families: an ionotropic (P2X) and a metabotropic (P2Y) family. There are seven identified P2X subunit types that form channels, and they represent their own superfamily of ligand-gated channels. Each subunit has only two transmembrane domains, with the loop between these two domains located extracellularly and containing the ATP binding site. The receptors are heterotrimers or homotrimers or hexamers. In general, these receptors form a cationic channel that is permeable to Na^+, K^+, and Ca^{++}. The distribution of subunits in the brain varies significantly, with some subunits having a widespread distribution (P2X$_2$) and others being quite limited (P2X$_3$ is present mostly on cells involved in pain-related pathways).

Metabotropic purine receptors are coded for by 10 genes, but only six are expressed in the human CNS.

They have the typical features of G protein–coupled receptors and are known to activate K^+ currents and modulate both NMDA and voltage-gated Ca^{++} currents. An interesting localization distinction between P2X and P2Y receptors is that although both are present on neurons, the latter dominates on astrocytes.

Finally, in addition to the P2X and P2Y receptors, which respond to ATP, there are adenosine receptors that respond to the adenosine that is released after the enzymatic breakdown of ATP. These receptors are located presynaptically and act to inhibit synaptic transmission by inhibiting influx of Ca^{++}.

Biogenic Amine Receptors: Serotonin, Dopamine, Noradrenaline, Adrenaline, Histamine

With the exception of one class of serotonin receptors (5-HT$_3$), which are part of the cys-loop ionotropic family, the receptors for the various biogenic amines are all metabotropic-type receptors. Thus, these neurotransmitters tend to act on relatively long time scales by generating slow synaptic potentials and by initiating second messenger cascades. Agonists and blockers of many of these receptors are important clinical tools for treating various neurological and psychiatric disorders. The role of different dopamine receptors in basal ganglia disorders will be covered in the motor systems (Chapter 9).

Neuropeptide Receptors

As is the case with the biogenic amines, receptors for the various peptides are essentially all of the metabotropic type and are coupled to G proteins that mediate effects via second messenger cascades. It is worth mentioning again that studies consistently show a mismatch between the locations of terminals containing a particular peptide and the receptors for it. Thus, these receptors are often activated by neurotransmitter diffusing through the extracellular space rather than at synapses. This implies that these receptors will experience much lower concentrations of agonist, and indeed, they are more sensitive to their agonists.

Gas Neurotransmitter Receptors

Unlike the other neurotransmitters that were covered, NO and CO do not bind to receptors. One way that they do affect cell activity is to activate enzymes involved in second messenger cascades, such as guanylyl cyclase. In addition, NO has been shown to modify the activity of other proteins, such as NMDA receptors and the Na^+,K^+-ATPase pump, by nitrosylating them.

■ KEY CONCEPTS

1. Both electrical and chemical synapses are important means of cellular communication in the mammalian nervous system.

2. Electrical synapses directly connect the cytosol of two neurons and allow rapid bidirectional current flow between neurons. They act as low-pass filters.

3. Gap junctions are the morphological correlate of electrical synapses. Gap junctions contain channels formed by hemichannels called connexons. Connexons are formed by proteins called connexins.

4. Standard chemical synaptic transmission involves the release of transmitter from a presynaptic terminal, diffusion of transmitter across a synaptic cleft, and binding of the transmitter to receptors on the apposed postsynaptic membrane.

5. Entry of calcium into the presynaptic terminal triggers the release of neurotransmitter. Release of neurotransmitter is quantal, as first demonstrated by the recording of mEPPs at the frog neuromuscular junction.

6. Transmitter is packaged into synaptic vesicles in the presynaptic terminal. The vesicles are the quantal elements. That is, the release of transmitter from one vesicle causes a mEPP at the neuromuscular junction or, equivalently, one mPSP at a central synapse.

7. Many proteins are involved in priming, docking, and fusion of synaptic vesicles. Synaptotagmin is the Ca^{++} sensor for triggering vesicle fusion.

8. Excitatory and inhibitory synapses increase or decrease, respectively, the probability that the postsynaptic neuron will spike.

9. The reversal potential is the membrane potential at which net current flow through a ligand-gated channel reverses. Excitatory synapses generate depolarizing potentials (EPSPs) that have reversal potentials positive to the spike threshold, most often as a result of the opening of nonselective cation channels.

10. Inhibitory synapses generate IPSPs that have reversal potentials more negative than the spike threshold, but not necessarily negative to the resting potential. Inhibitory synapses can decrease spike probability by two mechanisms: hyperpolarization of the membrane and a decrease in the input resistance of the neuron leading to a shunt of synaptic currents.

11. The process by which a neuron decides to fire an action potential as a result of its inputs is referred to as synaptic integration. The summation of EPSPs and IPSPs can be highly nonlinear and depends on many factors, including the geometry of the dendritic tree, location of the synaptic inputs relative to the axon hillock, and the passive (RC) and active membrane properties of the cell.

12. The efficacy of synaptic transmission depends on the timing and frequency of action potentials in the presynaptic neuron. Facilitation, posttetanic potentiation, and long-term potentiation are examples of increased efficacy of synaptic transmission in response to previous multiple stimulations of a synapse. Long-term depression is an example of reduced efficacy resulting from previous activation of the synapse.

13. The nervous system uses hundreds of neurotransmitters. Neurotransmitters can be subdivided into a few broad functional classes: small-molecule transmitters (acetylcholine, amino acids, biogenic amines, and purines), peptides, and gases (CO, NO). The action of a neurotransmitter depends on its postsynaptic receptors. Most nongaseous transmitters have both ionotropic and metabotropic receptors.

14. Small-molecule transmitters act locally, mainly across a single synapse, and their duration of action is limited by reuptake and enzymatic degradation. Peptides can diffuse from their presynaptic release site and thus have the potential to affect all cells within a local region. Gaseous transmitters are free to diffuse from their release site.

15. Ionotropic receptors contain an ion channel whose state (open versus closed) is gated by the binding of neurotransmitter to the receptor. Metabotropic receptors activate second messengers on binding neurotransmitter.

16. Many synapses can release multiple types of transmitters, and which ones they release depends on the activity pattern of the terminal. Coreleased transmitters may function independently or act synergistically or antagonistically.

CHAPTER 7

The Somatosensory System

The somatosensory system provides information to the central nervous system (CNS) about the state of the body and its contact with the world. It does so by using a variety of sensory receptors that transduce mechanical (pressure, stretch, and vibrations) and thermal energies into electrical signals. These electrical signals are called generator, or receptor, potentials and occur in the distal ends of axons of first-order somatosensory neurons, where they trigger action potential trains that reflect information about the characteristics of the stimulus. The cell bodies of these neurons are located in dorsal root (Fig. 7-1, *A*; see Fig. 4-8) and cranial nerve ganglia.

Each ganglion cell gives off an axon that after a short distance, divides into a peripheral process and a central process. The peripheral processes of the ganglion cells coalesce to form peripheral nerves. A purely sensory nerve will have only axons from such ganglion cells; however, mixed nerves, which innervate muscles, will contain both afferent (sensory) fibers and efferent (motor) fibers. At the target organ, the peripheral process of an afferent axon divides repeatedly, with each terminal branch ending as a sensory receptor. In most cases, the free nerve ending by itself forms a functional receptor, but in some, the nerve ending is encapsulated by accessory cells, and the entire structure (axon terminal plus accessory cells) forms the receptor.

The central axonal process of the ganglion cell either enters the spinal cord via a dorsal root or enters the brainstem via a cranial nerve. A central process typically gives rise to numerous branches that may synapse with a variety of cell types, including second-order neurons of the somatosensory pathways. The terminal location of these central branches varies depending on the type of information being transmitted. Some terminate at or near the segmental level of entry, whereas others project to brainstem nuclei.

Second-order neurons that are part of the pathway for the perception of somatosensory information project to specific thalamic nuclei, where the third-order neurons reside. These neurons in turn project to the primary somatosensory cortex (S-I). Within the cortex, somatosensory information is processed in S-I and in numerous higher-order cortical areas. Somatosensory information is also transmitted by other second-order neurons to the cerebellum for use in its motor coordination function.

The organization of the somatosensory system is quite distinct from that of the other senses, which has both experimental and clinical implications. In particular, other sensory systems have their receptors localized to a single organ, where they are present at high density (e.g., the eye for the visual system). In contrast, somatosensory receptors are distributed throughout the body (and head). In addition, the other senses convey their information to the brain via a single nerve bundle (or in one case, via two to three nerves), whereas somatosensory information arrives via spinal dorsal roots and cranial nerves (primarily the trigeminal).

SUBDIVISIONS OF THE SOMATOSENSORY SYSTEM

The somatosensory system receives three broad categories of information based on the distribution of its receptors. Its **exteroceptive** division is responsible for providing information about contact of the skin with objects in the external world, and a variety of cutaneous mechanoceptive, nociceptive (pain), and thermal receptors are used for this purpose. Understanding this division will be the main focus of this chapter. The **proprioceptive** component provides information about body and limb position and movement and relies primarily on receptors found in the joints, muscles, and tendons. Because these receptors initiate pathways that in part are intimately involved in the control of movement, they will be discussed in Chapter 9; however, the ascending central pathways that originate with them and that underlie conscious and unconscious proprioceptive functions will be covered later in this chapter. Finally, the **enteroceptive** division has receptors for monitoring the internal state of the body and includes mechanoreceptors that detect distention of the gut or fullness of the bladder.

The somatosensory pathways can also be classified by the type of information that they carry. Two broad functional categories are recognized, each of which subsumes several somatosensory submodalities. **Fine discriminatory touch** sensations include light touch, pressure, vibration, flutter (low-frequency vibration), and stretch or tension. The second major functional group of sensations is that of **pain and temperature.** Submodalities here include both noxious and innocu-

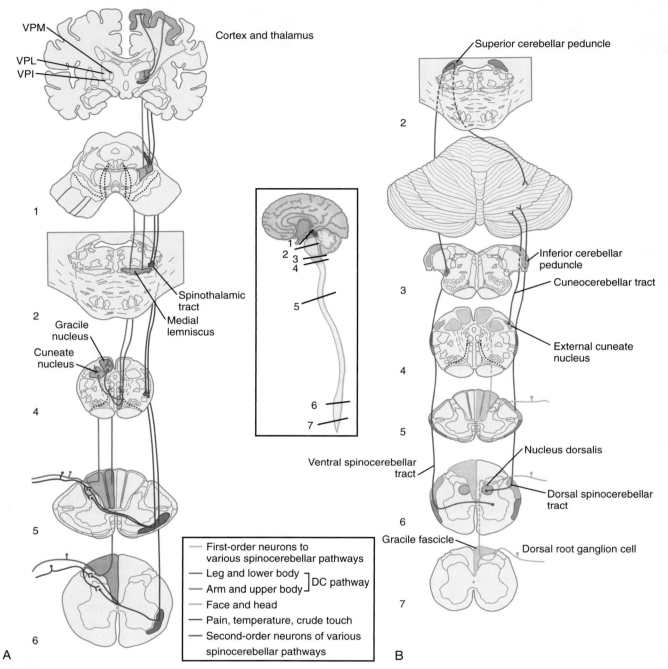

● **Figure 7-1.** Ascending somatosensory pathways from the body. **A,** First-, second-, and third-order neurons are shown for the two main pathways conveying cutaneous information from the body to the cerebral cortex: the dorsal column/medial lemniscal and the spinothalamic pathways. Note that the axon of the second-order neuron crosses the midline in both cases, so sensory information from one side of the body is transmitted to the opposite side of the brain, but the levels in the neuraxis at which this takes place are distinct for each pathway. Homologous central pathways for the head originate in the trigeminal nucleus and are described in text, but they are not illustrated for clarity. **B,** Major spinocerebellar pathways carrying tactile and proprioceptive information to the cerebellum from the upper and lower parts of the body. Again, pathways from the head originate in the trigeminal nuclei but are not shown for clarity. A midsagittal view of the nervous system shows the levels of the spinal and brainstem cross sections in panels **A** and **B.**

> ### ► IN THE CLINIC
>
> The sensory functions of various cutaneous sensory receptors have been studied in human subjects with a technique known as **microneurography,** in which a fine metal microelectrode is inserted into a nerve trunk in the arm or leg to record the action potentials from single sensory axons. When a recording can be made from a single sensory axon, the receptive field of the fiber is mapped. Most of the various types of sensory receptors that have been studied in experimental animals have also been found in humans with this technique.
>
> After the receptive field of a sensory axon has been characterized, the electrode can be used to stimulate the same sensory axon. In these experiments the subject is asked to locate the perceived receptive field of the sensory axon, which turns out to be identical to the mapped receptive field.

ous cold and warm sensations and mechanical and chemical pain. Itch is also closely related to pain and appears to be carried by particular fibers associated with the pain system.

Of great importance experimentally, the afferent fibers that convey these somatosensory submodalities to the CNS are different sizes. Recall that the compound action potential recorded from a peripheral nerve (Table 5-1) consists of a series of peaks, thus implying that the diameters of axons in a nerve are grouped rather than being uniformly distributed. Information about tactile sensations is carried primarily by large-diameter myelinated fibers in the Aα and Aβ classes, whereas pain and temperature information travels via small-diameter, lightly myelinated (Aδ) and unmyelinated (C) fibers. It is possible to block or selectively stimulate a class of axons of particular size, thereby allowing study of the different somatosensory submodalities in isolation.

Innervation of the Skin
Low-Threshold Mechanosensory

The skin is an important sensory organ and, not surprisingly, is richly innervated with a variety of afferents. We first consider the afferent types related to fine or discriminatory touch sensations. These afferents are related to what are called low-threshold mechanoreceptors. Nociceptor and thermoceptor innervation will be considered separately in a later section of this chapter.

To study the responsiveness of tactile receptors, a small-diameter rod or wire is used to press on a localized region of skin. With this technique, two basic types of responses may be seen when recording sensory afferent fibers: fast-adapting (FA) and slow-adapting (SA) responses (Fig. 7-2). They are present in similar quantities. FA fibers will show a short burst of action potentials when the rod first pushes down on the skin, but then they will cease firing despite contin-

ued application of the rod. They may also burst at the cessation of the stimulus (i.e., when the rod is lifted off). In contrast, SA units will start firing action potentials (or increase their firing rate) at the onset of the stimulus and continue to fire until the stimulus ends (Fig. 7-2).

Both the FA and SA afferent classes can be subdivided on the basis of other aspects of their receptive fields, where **receptive field** is defined as the region of skin from which stimuli can evoke a response (i.e., change the firing of the afferent axon). Type 1 units have small receptive fields with well-defined borders. Particularly for glabrous skin (i.e., hairless skin, such as on the palms of the hands and soles of the feet), the receptive field has a circular or ovoid shape, within which there is relatively uniform and high sensitivity to stimuli that decreases sharply at the border (Fig. 7-3). Type 1 units, particularly SA1 units, respond best to edges. That is, a larger response is elicited from them when the edge of a stimulus cuts through their receptive field than when the entire receptive field is indented by the stimulus.

Type 2 units have wider receptive fields with poorly defined borders and only a single point of maximal sensitivity, from which there is a gradual reduction in sensitivity with distance (Fig. 7-3). For comparison, a type 1 unit's receptive field typically will cover approximately four papillary ridges in the fingertip, whereas a type 2 unit will have a receptive field that covers most or all of a finger.

Receptive Field Properties

Thus, four main classes of low-threshold mechanosensitive afferents have been identified physiologically (FA1, FA2, SA1, and SA2). Peripherally, these axons may terminate as either free nerve endings or within a capsule made up of supporting cells.

For glabrous skin, the four afferent classes have been associated with four specific types of histologically identified receptor capsules whose locations and physical structure help explain the firing properties of these sensory afferents. FA1 afferents terminate in **Meissner's corpuscles,** whereas SA1 afferents terminate in **Merkel's disks.** In both cases the capsule is located relatively superficially, either in the basal epidermis (Merkel) or just below the epidermis (Meissner) (Fig. 7-2). These capsules are small and oriented to detect stimuli pressing down on the skin surface just above them, thus allowing SA1 and FA1 afferents to have small receptive fields. For glabrous skin, SA2 afferents terminate in **Ruffini's endings** and FA2 afferents end in **Pacinian corpuscles.** Both these receptors lie deeper in the dermis and connective tissue and therefore are sensitive to stimuli applied over much larger territory. Both Pacinian and Meissner's capsules act to filter out slowly changing or steady stimuli, thus making these afferents selectively sensitive to changing stimuli.

For hairy skin, the relationship between receptors and afferent classes is similar to that of glabrous skin. SA1 and SA2 fibers connect to Merkel's and Ruffini's endings, the same as for glabrous skin. Pacinian cor-

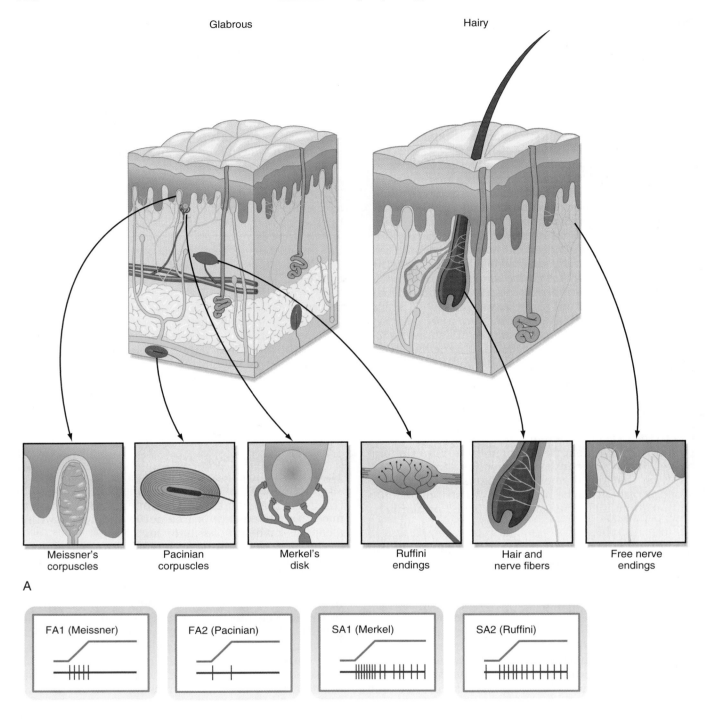

Glabrous

Hairy

| Meissner's corpuscles | Pacinian corpuscles | Merkel's disk | Ruffini endings | Hair and nerve fibers | Free nerve endings |

A

FA1 (Meissner)

FA2 (Pacinian)

SA1 (Merkel)

SA2 (Ruffini)

B

● **Figure 7-2.** Cutaneous mechanoreceptors and the response patterns of associated afferent fibers. **A,** Schematic views of glabrous (hairless) and hairy skin showing the arrangement of the various major mechanoreceptors. **B,** Firing patterns of the different cutaneous low-threshold mechanosensitive afferent fibers that innervate the various encapsulated receptors of the skin. (Traces in **B** are based on data from Johansson RS, Vallbo ÅB: Trends Neurosci 6:27, 1983.)

● **Figure 7-3.** Receptive field characteristics for type 1 and type 2 sensory afferents. Plots in the top row show the threshold level of force needed to evoke a response as a function of the distance across the receptive field. Receptive field size is shown on the hand below each plot. (Data from Johansson RS, Vallbo ÅB: Trends Neurosci 6:27, 1983.)

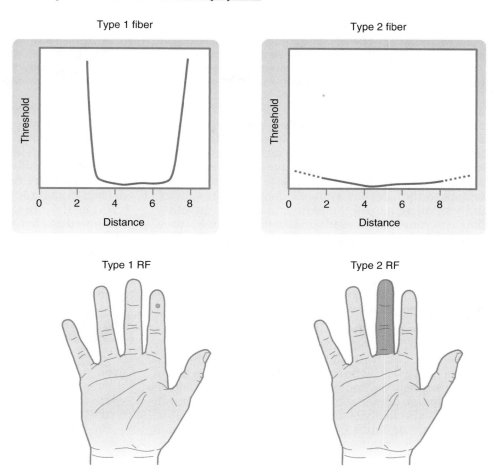

puscles also underlie the properties of FA2 afferents; however, they are not found in hairy skin but, instead, are located in deep tissues surrounding muscles and blood vessels. There is not an exact analogue to the FA1 afferents. Rather, there are **hair units,** which are afferents whose free endings wrap around hair follicles (Fig. 7-2). Each such hair unit will connect with about 20 hairs to produce a large ovoid or irregularly shaped receptive field. These units are extremely sensitive to movement of even a single hair. There are also **field units** that respond to touch of the skin, but unlike FA1 units, they have large receptive fields.

Several psychophysical and neural coding questions can be related to the receptive field properties and sensitivities of the various categories of afferents. For example, is the threshold of perception of tactile stimuli due to the sensitivity of the peripheral receptors or to central processes? In fact, by using microneurography, it is possible to show that a single spike in an FA1 afferent from the finger can be perceived, thus indicating that the receptors limit the sensitivity; however, for other skin regions, perception is more dependent on central factors such as attention.

An important behavioral and clinical measure of somatosensory function is spatial acuity or two-point discrimination. Clinically, a doctor will apply two needle-like points simultaneously to the skin of a patient. The patient will generally perceive the points

as two distinct stimuli as long as they are farther apart than some threshold distance, which varies across the body. The best discrimination (shortest threshold distance) is at the fingertips. Type 1 units underlie spatial acuity, which is not surprising given the smaller receptive fields of type 1 units than type 2 units; moreover, the threshold distance for a region of skin is most closely related to its density of type 1 units because these units have similarly sized receptive fields throughout the glabrous skin but their density falls off from fingertip to palm to forearm and this fall-off correlates with the rise in threshold distance. Note that this variation in innervation density also matches the overall sensitivity of different skin regions to cutaneous stimuli.

The relationship of the firing rates in the various afferent classes to perceived stimulus quality is another important issue that has been addressed with microneurographic techniques. When a single SA fiber is stimulated with brief current pulses such that each pulse triggers a spike, a sensation of steady pressure is felt at the receptive field area of that fiber. As pulse frequency is intensified, an increase in pressure is perceived. Thus, the firing rate in SA fibers codes for the force of the tactile stimulus. As another example, when an FA fiber is repetitively stimulated, a sensation of tapping results first, and as the frequency of the stimulus is increased, the sensation turns to one of vibration. Interestingly, in neither case does the stimulus change its qualitative character, for example, to a feeling of pain, as long as the stimulus activates only a particular fiber class. This is evidence that pain is a distinct submodality that uses a set of fibers distinct from those used by low-threshold mechanoreceptors.

These findings illustrate an important principle of sensory systems called **labeled line.** The idea is that the quality (i.e., modality) of a particular sensation results from the fact that it is conveyed to the CNS by a specific set of afferents that have a distinct set of targets in the nervous system. Alterations in activity in these afferents will therefore change only quantitative aspects of the sensation. As will be seen in more detail later, the various somatosensory submodalities (i.e., information arising from FA and SA mechanoreceptors, proprioceptors, and nociceptors) appear to use relatively separate dedicated cell populations, even at relatively high levels of the CNS, such as the thalamus and primary somatosensory cortex.

Innervation of the Body

Axons of the peripheral nervous system (PNS) enter or leave the CNS through the **spinal roots** (or through cranial nerves). The dorsal root on one side of a given spinal segment is composed entirely of the central processes of dorsal root ganglion cells. The ventral root consists chiefly of motor axons, including α motor axons, γ motor axons (see Chapter 9), and at certain segmental levels, autonomic preganglionic axons (see Chapter 11).

The pattern of innervation is determined during embryological development. In adults, a given dorsal root ganglion supplies a specific cutaneous region, which is called a **dermatome.** Many dermatomes become distorted during development, chiefly because

of rotation of the upper and lower extremities as they are formed, but also because humans maintain an upright posture. However, the sequence of dermatomes can readily be understood if depicted on the body of a person in a quadrupedal position (Fig. 7-4).

Although a dermatome receives its densest innervation from the corresponding spinal cord segment, collaterals of afferent fibers from the adjacent spinal segments also supply the dermatome. Thus, transection of a single dorsal root causes little sensory loss in the corresponding dermatome. Anesthesia of any given dermatome requires the interruption of several adjacent dorsal roots.

Within the dorsal roots, fibers are not randomly distributed. Rather, the large myelinated primary afferent fibers assume a medial position in the dorsal root, whereas the fine myelinated and unmyelinated fibers are more lateral. The large, medially placed afferent fibers enter the dorsal column, where they bifurcate to form rostrally and caudally directed branches.

▶ IN THE CLINIC

A common disease that illustrates the dermatomal organization of the dorsal roots is **shingles.** Shingles is the result of reactivation of the herpes zoster virus, which typically causes chickenpox during the initial infection. During the initial infection the virus infects dorsal root ganglion cells, where it can remain latent for years to decades. When the virus reactivates, the cells of that particular dorsal root ganglion become infected, and the virus travels along the peripheral axon branches and gives rise to a painful or itchy rash that is confined to one side of the body (ends at the midline) in a dermatomal or belt-like distribution.

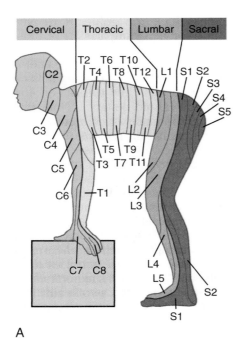

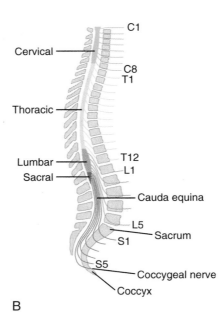

● **Figure 7-4. A,** Dermatomes represented on a drawing of a person assuming a quadrupedal position. **B,** Sagittal view of the spinal cord showing the origin of nerves corresponding to each of the dermatomes shown in **A.**

A   B

These branches give off collaterals that terminate in the several neighboring segments. The rostral branch also ascends to the medulla as part of the **dorsal column–medial lemniscus pathway.** The axonal branches that terminate locally in the spinal cord gray matter transmit sensory information to neurons in the dorsal horn and also provide the afferent limb of reflex pathways (see Chapter 9).

Innervation of the Face

The arrangement of primary afferent fibers that supply the face is comparable to that of fibers that supply the body and is provided for primarily by fibers of the **trigeminal nerve.** Peripheral processes of neurons in the trigeminal ganglion pass through the ophthalmic, maxillary, and mandibular divisions of the trigeminal nerve to innervate dermatome-like regions of the face. These fibers carry both tactile information and pain and temperature information. The trigeminal nerve also innervates the teeth, the oral and nasal cavities, and the cranial dura mater.

The central processes of trigeminal ganglion cells enter the brainstem at the midpontine level, which also corresponds to the level of the chief sensory trigeminal nucleus (nucleus of cranial nerve V). Some axons terminate in this nucleus (primarily large-caliber axons carrying the information needed for fine discriminative touch), whereas others (intermediate- and small-caliber axons that carry information about touch, as well as pain and temperature) form the spinal trigeminal tract, which descends through the medulla just lateral to the spinal trigeminal nucleus. As the tract descends, axons peel off and synapse in the nucleus.

Proprioceptive information is also conveyed via the trigeminal nerve; however, in this unique case, the cell bodies of the first-order fibers are located within the CNS in the mesencephalic portion of the trigeminal nucleus. The central processes of these neurons terminate in the motor trigeminal nucleus (to subserve segmental reflexes equivalent to the segmental spinal cord reflexes—see Chapter 9), the reticular formation, and the chief sensory trigeminal nucleus.

Central Somatosensory Pathways for Discriminatory Touch and Proprioception

As may already be clear, information related to the different somatosensory submodalities travels, to a large extent, via separate pathways up the spinal cord and brainstem. For example, from the body, fine discriminatory touch information is conveyed by the dorsal column–medial lemniscus pathway, whereas pain, temperature, and crude touch information is conveyed by the **anterolateral system.**

Proprioceptive information is transmitted by yet another route that partially overlaps with the dorsal column–medial lemniscal pathway. Note, however, that this functional segregation is not absolute, so, for example, there can be some recovery of discriminative touch ability after a lesion of the dorsal columns. The anterolateral system will be discussed in the section on pain because it is the critical pathway for that information. Here, the central pathways for discriminatory touch and proprioception are considered in detail.

Dorsal Column–Medial Lemniscus Pathway

This pathway is shown in its entirety in Figure 7-1, *A.* The dorsal columns are formed by ascending branches of the large myelinated axons of dorsal root ganglion cells (the first-order neurons). These axons enter at each spinal segmental level and travel rostrally up to the caudal medulla to synapse in one of the dorsal column nuclei: the nucleus gracilis, which receives information from the lower part of the body and leg, and the nucleus cuneatus, which receives information from the upper part of the body and arm. Note that in the dorsal columns and across the dorsal column nuclei there is a somatotopic representation of the body, with the legs represented most medially, followed by the trunk and then the upper limb. This somatotopy is a consequence of newly entering afferents being added to the lateral border of the dorsal funiculus as the spinal cord is ascended. Such somatotopic maps are present at all levels in the somatosensory system, at least through the primary sensory cortices.

The dorsal column nuclei are located in the medulla and contain the second-order neurons of the pathway for discriminatory touch sensation. These cells respond similarly to the primary afferent fibers that synapse on them (see the earlier description of afferent types). The main differences between the responses of dorsal column neurons and primary afferent neurons are as follows: (1) dorsal column neurons have larger receptive fields because multiple primary afferent fibers synapse on a given dorsal column neuron, (2) dorsal column neurons sometimes respond to more than one class of sensory receptor because of the convergence of several different types of primary afferent fibers on the second-order neurons, and (3) dorsal column neurons often have inhibitory receptive fields that are mediated through local interneurons.

The axons of dorsal column nuclear projection neurons exit the nuclei and are referred to as the internal arcuate fibers as they sweep ventrally and then medially to cross the midline at the same medullary level as the nuclei (Fig. 4-7, *F*). Immediately after crossing the midline, these fibers form the medial lemniscus, which projects rostrally to the thalamus. Knowledge of this decussation level is clinically important because damage to the dorsal column–medial lemniscal pathway below this level, which includes all of the spinal cord, will produce loss of fine somatosensory discriminatory abilities on the same, or ipsilateral, side of the lesion, whereas lesions above this level will produce contralateral deficits. Moreover, because there is a clear somatotopic arrangement of fibers in the medial lemniscus, localized lesions cause selective loss of fine-touch sensations limited to specific body regions.

The third-order neurons of the pathway are located in the **ventral posterior lateral (VPL) nucleus of the thalamus** and project to somatosensory areas of the cerebral cortex (Fig. 7-5).

The dorsal column–medial lemniscus pathway conveys information about fine-touch and vibratory sensations. This information is critical for many of the discriminatory tactile abilities that we have. For example, spatial acuity is lowered by damage to this pathway, and the ability to identify objects by their shape and texture can be lost by damage to this pathway. Clinically, one may test for impaired graphes-

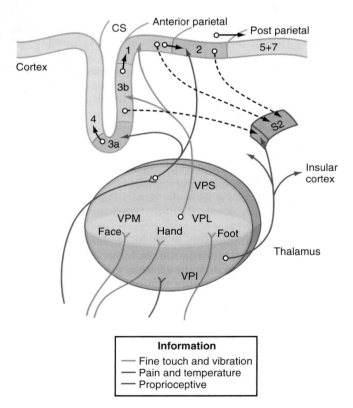

● **Figure 7-5.** Diagram of connections from the somatosensory receiving nuclei of the thalamus to the somatosensory cortex of the parietal lobe. Note the parallel flow of different types of somatosensory information through the thalamus and onto the cortex. CS, central sulcus; S1 and S2 are primary and secondary somatosensory areas, respectively. Note: collectively areas 3a, 3b, 1, and 2 are referred to as S1.

thesia, or the ability to recognize letters or numbers traced on the skin, or for loss of the ability to tell the direction of a line drawn across the skin. Importantly, some tactile function remains even after complete loss of the dorsal columns, and awareness and localization of nonnoxious tactile stimuli can still occur. Thus, at least some of the information carried by the dorsal column pathway is also conveyed by additional ascending pathways. In contrast to the severe deficits in discriminatory touch sensation, cutaneous pain and temperature sensations are unaffected by lesions of the dorsal columns. However, visceral pain is substantially diminished by damage to this pathway.

Trigeminal Pathway for Fine-Touch Sensation from the Face

Primary afferent fibers that supply the face, teeth, oral and nasal cavities, and cranial meninges synapse in several brainstem nuclei, including the main sensory nucleus and the spinal nucleus of the trigeminal nerve.

The pathway through the main sensory nucleus resembles the dorsal column–medial lemniscus pathway. This sensory nucleus relays tactile information to the contralateral **ventral posterior medial (VPM) thalamic nucleus** by way of the **trigeminothalamic tract.** Third-order neurons in the VPM nucleus project to the facial area of the somatosensory cortex.

Spinocerebellar and Proprioceptive Pathways

Proprioceptors provide information about the positions and movement of parts of the body. In addition to being used for local reflexes (see Chapter 9), this information has two main targets, the cerebellum and the cerebral cortex. The cerebellum uses this information for its motor coordination functions. The information sent to the cortex is the basis for conscious awareness of our body parts (e.g., the position of our hand), which is referred to as kinesthesia.

The major pathways by which somatosensory information is brought to the cerebellum are shown in Figure 7-1, *B*. These pathways carry both cutaneous and proprioceptive information to the cerebellum. For the trunk and lower part of the leg, the pathway starts with dorsal root ganglion cells whose axons synapse in (nucleus dorsalis) **Clarke's column.** The cells of Clarke's column send their axons into the ipsilateral lateral funiculus to form the **dorsal spinocerebellar tract,** which enters the cerebellum via the inferior cerebellar peduncle. The **ventral spinocerebellar tract** also provides somatosensory input from the lower limb to the cerebellum. Note the double decussation of the ventral spinocerebellar pathway (one decussation at the spinal cord levels and a second one in the cerebellar white matter). This double crossing highlights the general rule that each half of the cerebellum is functionally related to the ipsilateral side of the body.

To provide proprioceptive information from the lower limb to the cerebral cortex, the main axons of the dorsal spinocerebellar tract give off a branch in the medulla that terminates in nucleus z, which is just rostral to the nucleus gracilis. The axons of cells from **nucleus z** then form part of the internal arcuate fibers and medial lemniscus and ascend to the VPL nucleus of the thalamus.

The ascending somatosensory pathways to the cerebellum for the upper limb are simpler than those from the lower limb (Fig. 7-1, *B*). The route to the cerebellum starts with dorsal root ganglion fibers from the cervical spinal levels that ascend in the cuneate fasciculus to the external cuneate nucleus. The axons of the external cuneate then form the cuneocerebellar tract, which enters the cerebellum via its inferior peduncle.

The route to the cerebral cortex for proprioceptive information from the upper limb is identical to that for discriminative touch: the dorsal column–medial lemniscal pathway, with a synapse in the cuneate nucleus and then in the VPL nucleus of the thalamus.

For the head, proprioceptive input is carried by cells of the mesencephalic nucleus of the trigeminal nerve. Recall that the neurons in this nucleus are actually the cell bodies of the primary afferents that innervate stretch receptors in the muscles of mastication and in other muscles of the head. The central processes of these neurons project to the trigeminal motor nucleus for local reflexes or to the nearby reticular formation. Axons from these reticular formation neurons join the trigeminothalamic tract, which terminates in the VPM of the thalamus. There are also trigeminocerebellar pathways for conveying somatosensory (tactile and proprioceptive) information from the head to the cerebellum.

THALAMIC AND CORTICAL SOMATOSENSORY AREAS
Thalamus
The ventroposterior nuclear complex of the thalamus represents the main termination site for ascending somatosensory information in the diencephalon. It consists of two major nuclei, the VPL and VPM, and a smaller nucleus called ventral posterior inferior (VPI) (Fig. 7-5). The medial lemniscus forms the main input to the VPL nucleus, and the equivalent trigeminothalamic tract from the main sensory nucleus of the trigeminal nerve forms the main input to the VPM nucleus. These nuclei also receive weaker input from the spinothalamic or equivalent trigeminothalamic tracts, respectively. The VPI nucleus receives input from the spinothalamic tract.

Single-unit recordings from the ventroposterior complex of nuclei have shown that the responses of many of the neurons in these nuclei to stimuli resemble those of first- and second-order neurons in the ascending tracts. The receptive fields of thalamic cells are small, but somewhat larger than those of primary afferent fibers. Moreover, the responses may be dominated by a particular type of sensory receptor. For example, VPL and VPM nuclei have cells whose receptive fields typically reflect input either from one type of cutaneous receptor (FA or SA) or from proprioceptive receptors, as expected from their dominant medial lemniscal input. In contrast, cells of the VPI and posterior nuclei show responses to activation of nociceptors, the main input to the spinothalamic pathway.

Thalamic neurons often have inhibitory, as well as excitatory, receptive fields. The inhibition may actually take place in the dorsal column nuclei or in the dorsal horn of the spinal cord. However, inhibitory circuits are also situated within the thalamus. The VPL and VPM nuclei contain inhibitory interneurons (in primates, but not in rodents), and some of the inhibitory interneurons in the reticular nucleus of the thalamus project into the VPL and VPM nuclei. The inhibitory neurons intrinsic to the VPL and VPM nuclei and in the reticular nucleus use γ-aminobutyric acid (GABA) as their inhibitory neurotransmitter.

One difference between neurons in the VPL and VPM nuclei and sensory neurons at lower levels of the somatosensory system is that thalamic neuron excitability depends on the stage of the sleep-wake cycle and on the presence or absence of anesthesia. During a state of drowsiness or during barbiturate anesthesia, thalamic neurons tend to undergo an alternating sequence of excitatory and inhibitory postsynaptic potentials. The alternating bursts of discharges in turn intermittently excite neurons in the cerebral cortex. Such patterns of excitation and inhibition result in an α rhythm or in spindling on the electroencephalogram. This alternation of excitatory and inhibitory postsynaptic potentials during these two states may reflect the level of excitation of thalamic neurons by excitatory amino acids that act at NMDA and non-NMDA receptors. It may also reflect inhibition of the thalamic neurons by recurrent pathways through the reticular nucleus.

Thalamic neuron receptive fields are on the side of the body contralateral to the neuron, and the receptive field locations vary systematically across the ventroposterior nuclear complex. That is, the VPL and VPM nuclei are somatotopically organized such that the lower limb is represented most laterally and the upper limb most medially in the VPL nucleus and the head is represented even more medially in the VPM nucleus. Moreover, the fact that thalamic neurons often receive input from only one class of receptor suggests that there are multiple somatotopic maps laid out across the ventroposterior nuclear complex. That is, there appear to be separate somatotopic maps for SA, FA, and proprioceptive and pain sensations laid out across the ventroposterior nuclear complex.

These maps are not randomly interspersed. As already mentioned, pain sensation is largely mapped across the VPI nucleus. In addition, the cutaneous receptors appear to drive cells located in a central "core" region of the VPL-VPM complex, whereas proprioceptive information is directed to cells that form a "shell" (VPS) around this core. This parallel flow of information into thalamus and then onto the cortex is diagramed in Figure 7-5.

The spinothalamic tract also projects to other thalamic regions, including the posterior nucleus and the central lateral nucleus of the intralaminar complex of the thalamus. The intralaminar nuclei of the thalamus are not somatotopically organized, and they project diffusely to the cerebral cortex, as well as to the basal ganglia (see Chapter 9). The projection of the central lateral nucleus to the S-I cortex may be involved in arousal of this part of the cortex and in selective attention.

Somatosensory Cortex

Third-order sensory neurons in the thalamus project to the somatosensory cortex. The details of this projection pattern are shown in Figure 7-5. The main somatosensory receiving areas of the cortex are called the S-I and S-II areas. The S-I cortex (or primary somatosensory cortex) is located on the postcentral gyrus, and the S-II cortex (secondary somatosensory cortex) is in the superior bank of the lateral fissure (Fig. 7-5).

As previously discussed, the S-I cortex, like the somatosensory thalamus, has a somatotopic organization. The S-II cortex also contains a somatotopic map, as do several other less understood areas of the cortex. In the S-I cortex, the face is represented in the lateral part of the postcentral gyrus, above the lateral fissure. The hand and the rest of the upper extremity are represented in the dorsolateral part of the postcentral gyrus and the lower extremity on the medial surface of the hemisphere. A map of the surface of the body and face of a human on the postcentral gyrus is called a **sensory homunculus.** The map is distorted because the volume of neural tissue devoted to a body region is proportional to the density of its innervation. Thus, in humans, the perioral area, the thumb, and other digits take up a disproportionately large expanse of cortex relative to their size.

The sensory homunculus is an expression of place coding of somatosensory information. A locus in the S-I cortex encodes the location of a somatosensory stimulus on the surface of the body or face. For example, the brain knows that a certain part of the body has been stimulated because certain neurons in the postcentral gyrus are activated.

The S-I cortex has several morphological and functional subdivisions, and each subdivision has a somatotopic map. These subdivisions were originally described by Brodmann, and they were based on the arrangements of neurons in the various layers of the cortex, as seen in Nissl-stained preparations. The subdivisions are therefore known as Brodmann areas 3a, 3b, 1, and 2 (see Chapter 10). Cutaneous input dominates in areas 3b and 1, whereas muscle and joint input (proprioceptive) dominates in areas 3a and 2. Thus, separate cortical zones are specialized for the processing of tactile and proprioceptive information (Fig. 7-5).

Within any particular area of S-I cortex, all the neurons along a line perpendicular to the cortical surface have similar response properties and receptive fields. The S-I cortex is thus said to have a columnar organization. A comparable columnar organization has also been demonstrated for other primary sensory receiving areas, including the primary visual and auditory cortices (see Chapter 8). Nearby cortical columns in the S-I cortex may process information for different sensory modalities. For example, the cutaneous information that reaches one cortical column in area 3b may come from FA mechanoreceptors, whereas the information that reaches a neighboring column might originate from SA mechanoreceptors.

Besides being responsible for the initial processing of somatosensory information, the S-I cortex also begins higher-order processing, such as feature extraction. For example, certain neurons in area 1 respond preferentially to a stimulus that moves in one direction across the receptive field, but not in the opposite direction (Fig. 7-6). Such neurons presumably contribute to the perceptual ability to recognize the direction of an applied stimulus and could help detect slippage of an object being grasped by the hand.

Effects of Lesions of the Somatosensory Cortex

A lesion of the S-I cortex in humans produces sensory changes similar to those produced by a lesion of the somatosensory thalamus. However, usually only a part of the cortex is involved, and thus the sensory loss may be confined, for example, to the face or to the leg, depending on the location of the lesion with respect to the sensory homunculus. The sensory modalities most affected are discriminative touch and position sense. Graphesthesia and stereognosis (i.e., the ability to recognize objects, such as coins and keys, as they are handled) are particularly disturbed. Pain and thermal sensation may be relatively unaffected, although loss of pain sensation may follow cortical lesions. Conversely, cortical lesions can result in a central pain state that resembles thalamic pain (see below).

PAIN AND TEMPERATURE SENSATION

The sensations of pain and temperature are related and often grouped together because they are mediated by overlapping sets of receptors and are conveyed by the same types of fibers in the PNS and the same pathways in the CNS. One consequence of these labeled lines is that pain sensations, in particular, are not due to stronger activation of touch pathways, as might naively be thought. This difference is borne out experimentally because if SA afferents, for example, are stimulated more and more frequently, the sensation of tactile pressure becomes stronger, but not painful.

Nociceptors and Primary Afferents

The axons that carry painful and thermal sensations are members of the relatively slowly conducting Aδ and C classes. However, not all Aδ and C axons carry pain and temperature information; some respond to light touch in a manner similar to what was described for low-threshold mechanoreceptors.

Unlike the case for low-threshold mechanoreceptors in which morphologically distinct receptors correspond to response properties, the Aδ and C axons conveying pain and temperature information appear to originate mostly as "free nerve endings." (This descrip-

● **Figure 7-6.** Feature extraction by cortical neurons. The responses were recorded from a neuron in the somatosensory cortex of a monkey. The direction of a stimulus was varied, as shown by the arrows in the drawing. Note that the responses were greatest when the stimulus moved in the direction from UW to RF and least from RW to UF. F, fingers; R, radial side; U, ulnar side; W, wrist. (From Costanzo RM, Gardner EP: J Neurophysiol 43:1319, 1980.)

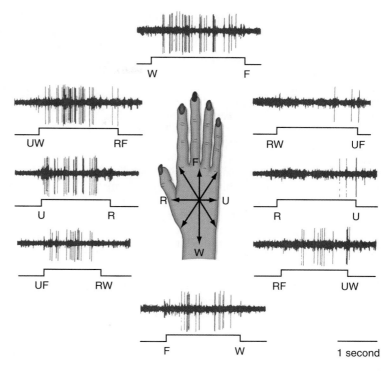

tion is not entirely accurate because the endings are mostly, but not entirely, covered by Schwann cells.) Despite the lack of distinct morphological specialization associated with their endings, Aδ and C axons constitute a heterogeneous population that is differentially sensitive to a variety of tissue-damaging or thermal stimuli (or both). This ability to sense tissue-damaging stimuli (mechanical, thermal, or chemical) is mediated by what are called **nociceptors.** These receptors share some features with low-threshold mechanoreceptors but are distinct in many ways, such as the ability to become sensitized (see later). Indeed, there appear to be a significant number of C fibers that are silent or unresponsive to any stimuli until first sensitized.

The first functional distinction that may be made in the pain system is between Aδ and C axons. Aδ axons conduct signals faster than C fibers do and are thought to underlie what is called **first pain,** whereas C fibers are responsible for **second pain.** Thus, after a damaging stimulus, one first feels an initial sharp, pricking, highly localized sensation (first pain), followed by a duller, more diffuse, burning sensation (second pain). Experiments in which Aδ or C fibers were selectively activated demonstrated that activity in Aδ fibers produces sensations similar to first pain and that activity in C fibers produces second pain–like sensations.

Each fiber class, in turn, forms a heterogeneous group with regard to sensitivity to stimuli. Thus, afferents are classified according to both size and their sensitivity to mechanical, thermal, and chemical stimuli. Fibers may have a low or high threshold to mechanical stimulation or be completely insensitive to it. Thermal sensitivity has been classified as responsiveness to warmth, noxious heat, cool, and noxious

cold. Note that 43°C and 15°C are the approximate limits above and below which, respectively, thermal stimuli are sensed as painful. Chemical sensitivity to a variety of irritating compounds has been tested, including capsaicin (found in chili peppers), mustard oil, and acids.

Afferent fibers may be sensitive to one or more types of stimuli and have been named accordingly. For example, C fibers sensitive only to high-intensity (damaging) mechanical stimuli are called C mechanosensitive fibers, whereas those sensitive to heat and mechanical stimuli are labeled C mechanoheat-sensitive fibers (also called polymodal fibers). Other identified fiber types include Aδ and C cold-sensitive, Aδ mechanosensitive, and mechanoheat-sensitive fibers. Thus, there is quite a variety of afferent types; however, the most common afferent type is the C polymodal fiber, which accounts for nearly half of the cutaneous C fibers. Surprisingly, the second most common type is the mechanoheat-insensitive afferent (i.e., an afferent that is not sensitive to noxious stimuli until sensitized—see later).

Because all these fibers begin as free nerve endings, their distinct sensitivities must be the result of distinct membrane receptors. These proteins, however, have been difficult to identify, in large part because the low density of receptors makes purification of these proteins difficult (contrast single nerve endings scattered within a patch of skin to the numbers of rod cell outer segments in the retina, each of which is packed with discs filled with rhodopsin molecules). Nevertheless, over the past decade or so potential candidates have been identified via a variety of approaches. The receptor that binds capsaicin (the molecule in chili peppers responsible for their spiciness) has been identified, and either it or one of a family of related proteins has been found to be expressed in populations of dorsal root ganglion cells. These proteins belong to the **TRP (transient receptor potential)** protein family and are currently the most likely candidates for being the transducers of thermal sensations.

It is important to note that many ion channels (and other proteins, e.g., enzymes) are sensitive to temperature; however, in the case of TRP channels, temperature is acting directly as the gating mechanism. The temperatures at which specific TRP channels are active are indicated by arrows in Figure 7-7, where the direction of each arrow indicates which temperatures cause greater activation. For comparison, Figure 7-7 also plots the firing rates of several thermosensitive fibers as a function of temperature. Note how the response ranges of the afferents can overlap with those of the heat-sensitive channels. The cold fibers, however, show firing over a wider range than any one TRP channel does. One possible explanation for this discrepancy is that dorsal root ganglion cells may express multiple classes of TRP, which would enable

them to respond over a wider range of physiological temperatures.

The transducer proteins for noxious mechanical stimulation have not been definitively identified in humans; however, at least some are likely to be homologues of proteins identified in *Caenorhabditis elegans* that belong to the **DEG/ENaC (degenerin/epithelial Na⁺ channel)** family. These are Na⁺ channels that are not voltage gated but are blocked by amiloride. The exact transduction mechanism is not known; however, two hypotheses are that the channel senses and is gated by tension in the cell membrane and that the channel is attached to the cytoskeleton intracellularly and fibers of the extracellular matrix and senses tension via these connections.

As with the low-threshold mechanoreceptors for innocuous touch sensations, activation of the various

---

● AT THE CELLULAR LEVEL

Members of the TRP protein family were first identified in *Drosophila* and were found to be part of the phototransduction process in *Drosophila* photoreceptors. Thus, the name (TRP) refers to the fact that a mutation in the gene leads to a transient depolarizing response to a light stimulus instead of the normal sustained response. On the basis of sequence homology, a number of genes encoding TRP proteins have been found in mammals (27 in humans alone), which are currently divided into seven subfamilies. TRP channels are cation permeable and have a structure similar to voltage-gated K⁺ channels. They are homotetramers or heterotetramers. Each subunit has six transmembrane domains. TRP proteins appear to have a variety of functions (e.g., phototransduction, chemotransduction, and mechanotransduction) and are expressed in a number of cell types. Those listed in Table 7-1 appear to act as temperature sensors with distinct thermal sensitivities that span the range of physiologically relevant temperatures.

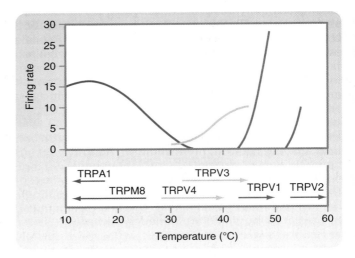

● **Figure 7-7.** Temperature dependence of firing rates in different thermosensitive afferents. Below the firing curves are shown the ranges over which the different TRP channels are activated. The direction of increasing activation is indicated by arrow in each case. Note how in some cases the range over which an afferent is active corresponds well to the activation range of a single TRP channel, thus suggesting that the afferent would need to express only a single type of channel. In other cases, the afferent firing range suggests that multiple TRP channels would be needed to underlie the complete responsiveness of the afferent.

● **Table 7-1 TRP Family Proteins Involved in Thermal Transduction**

Receptor Protein	Threshold or Temperature Range for Activation (°C)	Other Characteristics
TRPV1	>42	Activated by capsaicin
TRPV2	>52	
TRPV3	34-38	Activated by camphor
TRPV4	27-40	
TRPM8	<25	Activated by menthol
TRPA1	<18	Activated by mustard oil

The fourth letter in the name identifies the subfamily and was chosen because of the first member of the subfamily identified: V, vanilloid; M, melastatin; A, ankyrin-like. Each of the proteins listed is expressed in at least some dorsal root ganglion cells, but they are also expressed in other cell types.

nociceptor transduction proteins leads to a generator potential that causes spiking of the afferent, which transmits information to the CNS. In addition, activation of nociceptors also leads to the local release of various chemical compounds, including **tachykinins (substance P [SP])** and **calcitonin gene–related protein (CGRP)**. These substances and others released from the damaged cells cause neurogenic inflammation (edema and redness of the surrounding skin).

In addition to causing a local reaction, these substances may serve to activate the insensitive or silent nociceptors mentioned earlier such that they can henceforth respond to any subsequent damaging stimuli. Sensitization of silent nociceptors has been suggested to underlie *allodynia* (elicitation of painful sensations by stimuli that were innocuous before an injury) and *hyperalgesia* (increase in the level of pain felt to already painful stimuli).

Spinal Cord Gray Matter and Trigeminal Nucleus

The central portion of the Aδ and C axons carrying pain and temperature information from the body terminates in the dorsal horn of the spinal cord. The Aδ fibers target lamina I, V, and X of the gray matter, whereas the C fibers terminate in lamina I and II. The distinct termination patterns of the Aδ and C fibers in the spinal cord suggest that the messages they are carrying to the CNS are kept separated, and this is consistent with our ability to feel two distinct types of pain.

The primary afferent termination patterns in the spinal cord are also important because they may help determine the possible interactions that pain fibers can have with other afferents and with descending control systems (see later). Indeed, the **gate control theory of pain** refers to the phenomenon that innocuous stimuli, such as rubbing a hurt area, can block or reduce painful sensations. Such stimulation activates the large-diameter (Aα and Aβ) fibers, and their activity leads to release of GABA and other neurotransmitters by interneurons within the dorsal horn. GABA then acts by both presynaptic and postsynaptic mechanisms to shut down the activity of spinothalamic tract cells. Presynaptically, GABA activates both GABA$_A$ and GABA$_B$ receptors, which leads to partial depolarization of the presynaptic terminal and blocking of Ca^{++} channels, respectively. Both actions will decrease release of transmitter by the afferent terminal and thereby lessen excitation of the tract cell (see Chapter 6 section on presynaptic inhibition).

Nociceptive and thermoreceptive information that originates from regions of the head is processed in a fashion similar to that for the trunk and limbs. The primary afferent fibers of nociceptors and thermoreceptors in the head enter the brainstem through the trigeminal nerve (some also enter through the facial, glossopharyngeal, and vagus nerves). Of note, the trigeminal distribution includes both tooth and headache pain. These fibers then descend through the brainstem to the upper cervical spinal cord via the spinal tract of the trigeminal nerve. Some mechano-

receptive afferent fibers also join the spinal tract of the trigeminal nerve. Axons in the spinal tract synapse on second-order neurons in the spinal nucleus of the trigeminal nerve.

Central Pain Pathways

The central pain pathways include the spinothalamic, spinoreticular, and spinomesencephalic tracts. The **spinothalamic tract** is the most important sensory pathway for somatic pain and thermal sensations from the body (Fig. 7-1, *A*). It also contributes to tactile sensation. The spinothalamic tract originates from second-order neurons located in the spinal cord (primarily laminae I and IV to VI). The axons of these cells cross to the opposite side of the cord at or near to their level of origin. They then ascend to the brain in the ventral part of the lateral funiculus and subsequently through the brainstem to the thalamus, where they terminate on third-order neurons, as described earlier. Spinothalamic cells conveying pain and temperature target the VPI portion of the ventroposterior complex (although some also end in the VPL), the posterior nucleus, and the intralaminar nuclei of the thalamus. Nociceptive signals are then forwarded to several cortical areas, including not only the somatosensory cortex but also cortical areas that are involved in affective responses, such as the cingulate gyrus and the insula, which have limbic system functions (Fig. 7-5).

Most spinothalamic tract cells receive excitatory input from nociceptors in the skin, but many can also be excited by noxious stimulation of muscle, joints, or viscera. Few receive input only from viscera. Effective cutaneous stimuli include noxious mechanical, thermal (hot or cold), and chemical stimuli. Thus, different spinothalamic tract cells respond in a manner appropriate for signaling noxious, thermal, or mechanical events.

Some nociceptive spinothalamic tract cells receive convergent excitatory input from several different classes of cutaneous sensory receptors. For example, a given spinothalamic neuron may be activated weakly by tactile stimuli but more powerfully by noxious stimuli (Fig. 7-8). Such neurons are called wide–dynamic range cells because they are activated by

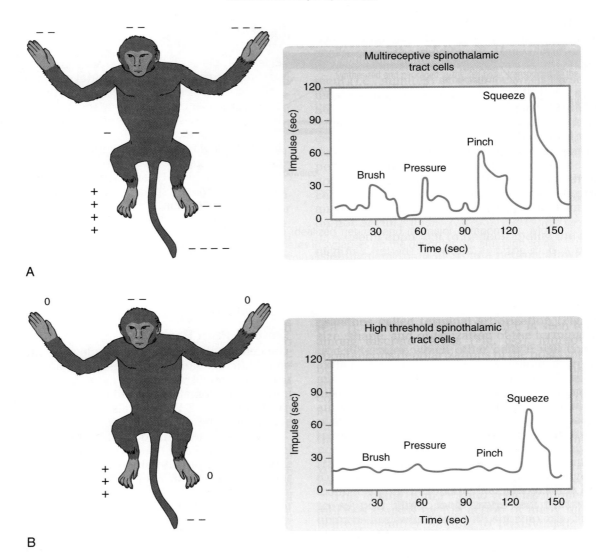

● **Figure 7-8.** **A,** Responses of a wide–dynamic range or multireceptive spinothalamic tract cell. **B,** Responses of a high-threshold spinothalamic tract cell. The figures indicate the excitatory (plus signs) and inhibitory (minus signs) receptive fields. The graphs show the responses to graded intensities of mechanical stimulation. Brush stimulus is a camel's hair brush repeatedly stroked across the receptive field. Pressure is applied by attachment of an arterial clip to the skin. This is a marginally painful stimulus to a human. Pinch is achieved by attachment of a stiff arterial clip to the skin and is distinctly painful. Squeeze is applied by compressing a fold of skin with forceps and is damaging to the skin.

stimuli with a wide range of intensities. Wide–dynamic range neurons signal mainly noxious events; weak responses to tactile stimuli appear to be ignored by the higher centers. However, in certain pathological conditions, these neurons may be sufficiently activated by tactile stimuli to evoke a sensation of pain, possibly as a result of activity in sensitized afferents that were previously silent. This would explain some pain states in which the activation of mechanoreceptors causes pain (mechanical allodynia). Other spinothalamic tract cells are activated only by noxious stimuli. Such neurons are often called high-threshold or nociceptive-specific cells (Fig. 7-8, *B*).

Because cells signaling visceral input also typically convey information from cutaneous receptors, the brain may misidentify the source of the pain. This phenomenon is called **referred pain.** A typical example is when the heart muscle becomes ischemic and pain is felt in the chest wall and left arm.

Neurotransmitters released by **nociceptive afferents** that activate spinothalamic tract cells include the excitatory amino acid glutamate and any of several peptides, such as SP, CGRP, and vasoactive intestinal polypeptide (VIP). Glutamate appears to act as a fast transmitter by its action on non-NMDA excitatory amino acid receptors. However, with repetitive stimulation, glutamate can also act through NMDA receptors. Peptides appear to act as neuromodulators. For example, through a combined action with an excitatory amino acid such as glutamate, SP can produce a long-lasting increase in the responses of spinothalamic tract cells; this enhanced responsiveness is called central sensitization. CGRP seems to increase release of SP and prolong the action of SP by inhibiting its enzymatic degradation.

Spinothalamic tract cells often have inhibitory receptive fields. Inhibition may result from weak mechanical stimuli, but usually the most effective inhibitory stimuli are noxious ones. The nociceptive inhibitory receptive fields may be very large and may include most of the body and face (Fig. 7-8, *A*). Such receptive fields may account for the ability of various physical manipulations, including transcutaneous electrical nerve stimulation and acupuncture, to suppress pain. Neurotransmitters that can inhibit spinothalamic tract cells include the inhibitory amino acids GABA and glycine, as well as monoamines and the endogenous opioid peptides.

Spinoreticular tract neurons frequently have large, sometimes bilateral receptive fields, and effective stimuli include noxious ones. These dorsal horn neurons target multiple regions in the medullary and pontine reticular formation. The reticular formation, which projects to the intralaminar complex of the thalamus and then to wide areas of the cerebral cortex, is involved in attentional mechanisms and arousal (see Chapter 10). The reticular formation also gives rise to descending reticulospinal projections, which contribute to the descending systems that control transmission of pain.

Many cells of the **spinomesencephalic tract** respond to noxious stimuli, and the receptive fields may be small or large. The terminations of this tract are in several midbrain nuclei, including the periaqueductal gray, which is an important component of the endogenous analgesia system. Motivational responses may also result from activation of the periaqueductal gray matter. For example, stimulation in the periaqueductal gray matter can cause vocalization and aversive behavior. Information from the midbrain is relayed not only to the thalamus but also to the amygdala, a part of the limbic system. This provides one of several pathways by which noxious stimuli can trigger emotional responses.

Pain and temperature information originating from the face and head is conveyed along analogous ascending central pathways, as is such information from the body. Neurons in the spinal trigeminal nucleus transmit pain and temperature information to specific nuclei (VPM, VPI) of the contralateral thalamus via the ventral trigeminothalamic tract, which runs in close association with the medial lemniscus. The spinal nucleus also projects to the intralaminar complex and other thalamic nuclei in a fashion similar to that of the spinothalamic tract. The thalamic nuclei in turn project to the somatosensory cerebral cortex for sensory discrimination of pain and temperature and to other cor-

tical regions responsible for motivational-affective responses.

Effects of Interruption of the Spinothalamic Tract and Lesions of the Thalamus on Somatosensory Sensation

When the spinothalamic tract and accompanying ventral spinal cord pathways are interrupted, both the sensory-discriminative and the motivational-affective components of pain are lost on the contralateral side of the body. This result motivated development of the surgical procedure known as anterolateral cordotomy, which was used to treat pain in many individuals, especially those suffering from cancer. This operation is now used infrequently because of improvements in drug therapy and because pain often returns months to years after an initially successful cordotomy. Return of pain may reflect either an extension of the disease or the development of a central pain state. In addition to the loss of pain sensation, anterolateral cordotomy produces loss of cold and warmth sensation on the contralateral side of the body. Careful testing may reveal a minimal tactile deficit as well, but the intact sensory pathways of the dorsal part of the spinal cord provide sufficient tactile information that any loss caused by interruption of the spinothalamic tract is insignificant.

Destruction of the VPL or VPM nuclei diminishes sensation on the contralateral side of the body or face. The sensory qualities that are lost reflect those that are transmitted mainly by the dorsal column–medial lemniscus pathway and its trigeminal equivalent. The sensory-discriminative component of pain sensation is also lost. However, the motivational-affective component of pain is still present if the medial thalamus is intact. Presumably, pain persists because of the spinothalamic and spinoreticulothalamic projections to this part of the thalamus. In some individuals, a lesion of the somatosensory thalamus results in a central pain state known as thalamic pain. However, pain that is indistinguishable from thalamic pain can also be produced by lesions in the brainstem or cortex.

Neuropathic Pain

Pain sometimes occurs in the absence of nociceptor stimulation. This type of pain is most likely to occur after damage to peripheral nerves or to parts of the CNS that are involved in transmitting nociceptive information. Pain caused by damage to neural structures is called neuropathic pain. Neuropathic pain states include peripheral neuropathic pain, which may follow damage to a peripheral nerve, and central neuropathic pain, which sometimes occurs after damage to CNS structures.

Examples of pain secondary to damage to a peripheral nerve are causalgia and phantom limb pain. Causalgia may develop after traumatic damage to a peripheral nerve. Even though evoked pain is reduced, severe pain may develop in the area innervated by the damaged nerve. This pain may be very difficult to treat, even with strong analgesic drugs. The pain is caused in part by spontaneous activity that develops in dorsal root ganglion cells; such activity may be attributed to up-regulation of Na^+ channels. In some cases the pain seems to be maintained by sympathetic neural activity because a sympathetic nerve block may alleviate the pain. Sympathetic involvement may relate to the sprouting of damaged sympathic postganglionic axons into the dorsal root ganglia, and it may be accompanied by up-regulation of adrenoreceptors in primary afferent neurons. Phantom limb pain follows traumatic amputation in some individuals. Such phantom pain is clearly not caused by the activation of nociceptors in the area in which pain is felt because these receptors are no longer present.

Lesions of the thalamus or at other levels of the spinothalamocortical pathway may cause central pain, which is a severe, spontaneous pain. However, interruption of the nociceptive pathway by the same lesion may simultaneously prevent or reduce the pain evoked by peripheral stimulation. The mechanism of such trauma-induced pain caused by neural damage is poorly understood. The pain appears to depend on changes in the activity and response properties of more distant neurons in the nociceptive system.

CENTRIFUGAL CONTROL OF SOMATOSENSATION

Sensory experience is not just the passive detection of environmental events. Instead, it more often depends on exploration of the environment. Tactile cues are sought by moving the hand over a surface. Visual cues result from scanning targets with the eyes. Thus, sensory information is often received as a result of activity in the motor system. Furthermore, transmission in pathways to the sensory centers of the brain is regulated by descending control systems. These systems allow the brain to control its input by filtering the incoming sensory messages. Important information can be attended to and unimportant information can be ignored.

The tactile and proprioceptive somatosensory pathways are regulated by descending pathways that originate in the S-I and motor regions of the cerebral cortex. For example, cortical projections to the dorsal column nuclei help control the sensory input that is transmitted by the dorsal column–medial lemniscus pathway.

Of particular interest is the descending control system that regulates the transmission of nociceptive information. This system presumably suppresses excessive pain under certain circumstances. For example, it is well known that soldiers on the battlefield, accident victims, and athletes in competition often feel little or no pain at the time that a wound occurs or a bone is broken. At a later time, pain may develop and become severe. Although the descending regulatory system that controls pain is part of a more general centrifugal control system that modulates all

forms of sensation, the pain control system is so important medically that it is distinguished as a special system called the **endogenous analgesia system.**

Several centers in the brainstem and pathways descending from these centers contribute to the endogenous analgesia system. For example, stimulation in the midbrain periaqueductal gray, the locus coeruleus, or the medullary raphe nuclei inhibits nociceptive neurons at the spinal cord and brainstem level, including spinothalamic and trigeminothalamic tract cells (Fig. 7-9, *A*). Other inhibitory pathways originate in the sensorimotor cortex, the hypothalamus, and the reticular formation.

The endogenous analgesia system can be subdivided into two components: one component uses endogenous **opioid** peptides as neurotransmitters and the other does not. Endogenous opioids are neuropeptides that activate one of several types of opiate receptors. Some of the endogenous opioids include enkephalin, dynorphin, and β-endorphin. Opiate analgesia can generally be prevented or reversed by the narcotic antagonist naloxone. Therefore, naloxone is frequently used to determine whether analgesia is mediated by an opioid mechanism.

The opioid-mediated endogenous analgesia system can be activated by the exogenous administration of morphine or other opiate drugs. Thus, one of the oldest medical treatments of pain depends on the triggering of a sensory control system. Opiates typically inhibit neural activity in nociceptive pathways. Two sites of action have been proposed for opiate inhibition, presynaptic and postsynaptic (Fig. 7-9, *B*). The presynaptic action of opiates on nociceptive afferent terminals is thought to prevent the release of excitatory transmitters such as SP. The postsynaptic action of opiates produces an inhibitory postsynaptic potential. How can an inhibitory neurotransmitter activate descending pathways? One hypothesis is that the descending analgesia system is under tonic inhibitory control by inhibitory interneurons in both the midbrain and the medulla. The action of opiates would inhibit the inhibitory interneurons and thereby disinhibit the descending analgesia pathways.

Some endogenous analgesia pathways operate by neurotransmitters other than opioids and thus are unaffected by naloxone. One way of engaging a nonopioid analgesia pathway is through certain forms of stress. The analgesia thus produced is a form of stress-induced analgesia.

Many neurons in the raphe nuclei use serotonin as a neurotransmitter. Serotonin can inhibit nociceptive neurons and presumably plays an important role in the endogenous analgesia system. Other brainstem neurons release catecholamines, such as norepinephrine and epinephrine, in the spinal cord. These catecholamines also inhibit nociceptive neurons; therefore, catecholaminergic neurons may contribute to the endogenous analgesia system. Furthermore, these monoamine neurotransmitters interact with endogenous opioids. Undoubtedly, many other substances are involved in the analgesia system. In addition, there

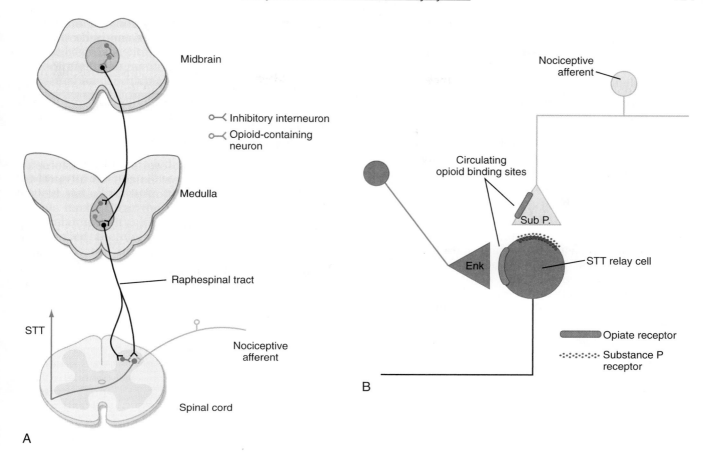

● **Figure 7-9.** **A,** Some of the neurons thought to play a role in the endogenous analgesia system. Neurons in the midbrain periaqueductal gray activate the raphespinal tract, which in turn inhibits nociceptive spinal neurons, such as those of the spinothalamic tract (STT). Interneurons containing opioid substances are involved in the system at each level. **B,** Possible presynaptic and postsynaptic sites of action of enkephalin (Enk). The presynaptic action might prevent the release of substance P (Sub P.) from nociceptors. (Redrawn from Henry JL. In Porter R, O'Connor M [eds]: Ciba Foundation Symposium 91. London, Pitman, 1982.)

is evidence for the existence of endogenous opiate antagonists that can prevent opiate analgesia.

■ KEY CONCEPTS

1. Sensory neurons have cell bodies in sensory nerve ganglia: (1) dorsal root ganglia for neurons innervating the body and (2) cranial nerve ganglia for neurons innervating the face, oral and nasal cavities, and dura, except for proprioceptive neurons, which are in the trigeminal mesencephalic nucleus. They connect peripherally to a sensory receptor and centrally to second-order neurons in the spinal cord or brainstem.

2. Skin contains low-threshold mechanoreceptors, thermoreceptors, and nociceptors. Muscle, joints, and viscera have mechanoreceptors and nociceptors. Low-threshold mechanoreceptors may be rapidly or slowly adapting. Thermoreceptors include cold and warm receptors. Aδ and C nociceptors detect noxious mechanical, thermal, and

chemical stimuli and may be sensitized by release of chemical substances from damaged cells. Peripheral release of substances, such as peptides, from nociceptors themselves may contribute to inflammation.

3. Large primary afferent fibers enter the dorsal funiculus through the medial part of the dorsal root; collaterals synapse in the deep dorsal horn, intermediate zone, and ventral horn. Small primary afferent fibers enter the spinal cord through the lateral part of the dorsal root; collaterals synapse in the dorsal horn.

4. Ascending branches of large primary afferent fibers synapse on second-order neurons in the dorsal column nuclei. These second-order neurons project in the medial lemniscus to the contralateral thalamus and synapse on third-order neurons of the VPL nucleus. The equivalent trigeminal pathway is relayed by the main sensory nucleus to contralateral VPM nucleus.

5. The dorsal spinal cord pathways signal the sensations of flutter-vibration, touch-pressure, and proprioception. They also contribute to visceral sensation, including visceral pain.

6. The spinothalamic tract includes nociceptive, thermoreceptive, and tactile neurons; its cells of origin are mostly in the dorsal horn, and the axons cross, ascend in the ventrolateral funiculus, and synapse in the VPL, VPI, and posterior and intralaminar nuclei of the thalamus. The equivalent trigeminal pathway is relayed by the spinal trigeminal nucleus and projects to the contralateral VPM and intralaminar nuclei.

7. The spinothalamic relay in the VPL, VPM, and VPI nuclei helps account for the sensory-discriminative aspects of pain. Parallel nociceptive pathways in the ventrolateral funiculus are the spinoreticular and spinomesencephalic tracts; these tracts and the spinothalamic projection to the medial thalamus contribute to the motivational-affective aspects of pain.

8. Referred pain is explained by convergent input to spinothalamic tract cells from the body wall and from viscera.

9. The VPL and VPM nuclei are somatotopically organized and contain inhibitory circuits. These nuclei contain multiple somatotopic maps, one for each somatosensory submodality. The somatosensory cortex includes the S-I and S-II regions; these regions are also somatotopically organized.

10. The S-I cortex contains columns of neurons with similar receptive fields and response properties. Some S-I neurons are involved in feature extraction.

11. Transmission in somatosensory pathways is regulated by descending control systems. The endogenous analgesia system regulates nociceptive transmission, and it uses transmitters such as endogenous opioid peptides, norepinephrine, and serotonin.

CHAPTER 8

The Special Senses

The evolution of vertebrates shows a trend called **cephalization** in which special sensory organs develop in the heads of animals, along with the corresponding development of the brain. These special sensory systems, which include the visual, auditory, vestibular, olfactory, and gustatory systems, detect and analyze light, sound, and chemical signals in the environment, as well as signal the position and movement of the head. The stimuli detected and transduced by these systems are most familiar to us when they provide conscious awareness of our environment, but they are equally important as sensory input for reflexive and subconscious behavior.

THE VISUAL SYSTEM

Vision is one of the most important special senses in humans and, along with audition, is the basis for most human communication. The visual system detects and interprets electromagnetic waves between 400 and 750 nm long, which constitutes **visible light.**

The eye can distinguish two aspects of light, its **brightness** (or luminance) and its **wavelength** (or color). Light enters the eye and impinges on **photoreceptors** in a specialized sensory epithelium, the **retina.** The photoreceptors include rods and cones. **Rods** have high sensitivity for detecting low light intensities but do not provide well-defined visual images, nor do they contribute to color vision. Rods operate best under conditions of reduced lighting **(scotopic vision).** **Cones,** by contrast, are not as sensitive to light as rods are and thus operate best under daylight conditions **(photopic vision).** Cones are responsible for high visual acuity and color vision.

Information processing within the retina is performed by **retinal interneurons,** and the output signals are carried to the brain by the axons of **retinal ganglion cells.** The axons travel in the **optic nerves;** there is a partial crossing in the optic chiasm that results in all input from one side of the visual space being directed to the opposite side of the brain. Posterior to the **optic chiasm,** the axons of retinal ganglion cells pass through the **optic tracts** and synapse in nuclei of the brain. The main visual pathway in humans is through the **lateral geniculate nucleus (LGN)** of the thalamus. This nucleus projects through the visual radiation to the visual cortex. Other visual pathways project to the **superior colliculus, pretectum,** and **hypothalamus,** and these structures participate in orientation of the eyes, control of pupil size, and circadian rhythms, respectively.

Structure of the Eye

The wall of the eye is composed of three concentric layers (Fig. 8-1). The outer layer, or the fibrous coat, includes the transparent **cornea,** with its epithelium, and the opaque **sclera.** The middle layer, or vascular coat, includes the iris and the choroid. The **iris** contains both radially and circularly oriented smooth muscle fibers, which make up the pupillary dilator and sphincter muscles. The **choroid** is rich in blood vessels that support the outer layers of the retina, and it also contains pigment. The innermost layer of the eye is the retina, which is embryologically derived from the diencephalon and is therefore part of the central nervous system (CNS). The functional part of the retina covers the entire posterior aspect of the eye except for the optic nerve head or **optic disc,** which is where the optic nerve axons leave the retina. Because there are no receptors at this location, it is often referred to as the anatomic "blind spot" (Fig. 8-1).

A number of functions of the eyes are under muscular control. Externally attached extraocular muscles aim the eyes toward an appropriate visual target (see Chapter 9). These muscles are innervated by the **oculomotor (cranial nerve [CN] III), trochlear (CN IV),** and **abducens (CN VI)** nerves. Several muscles are also found within the eye (intraocular muscles). The **muscles in the ciliary body** control lens shape and thereby the focus of images on the retina. The **pupillary dilator** and **sphincter** muscles allow the iris to control the amount of light entering the eye, similar to the diaphragm of a camera. The dilator is activated by the sympathetic nervous system, whereas the sphincter and ciliary muscles are controlled by the parasympathetic nervous system (through the oculomotor nerve) (see Chapter 11).

Light enters the eye through the cornea and passes through a series of transparent fluids and structures that are collectively called the **dioptric media.** These fluids and structures consist of the cornea, aqueous humor, lens, and vitreous humor. The aqueous humor, located in the **anterior** and **posterior chambers** and the vitreous humor in the space behind the lens,

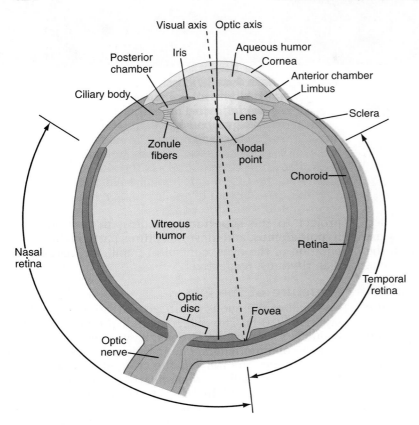

Visual axis   Optic axis

Posterior chamber   Iris   Aqueous humor   Cornea

Ciliary body   Anterior chamber   Limbus

Zonule fibers   Lens   Sclera

Nodal point

Choroid

Vitreous humor

Retina

Nasal retina

Temporal retina

Optic disc   Fovea

Optic nerve

● **Figure 8-1.** View of a horizontal section of the right eye. (Redrawn from Wall GL: The Vertebrate Eye and Its Adaptive Radiation. Bloomfield Hills, MI, Cranbrook Institute of Science, 1942.)

IN THE CLINIC

If aqueous humor is not absorbed adequately, intraocular pressure increases, a condition known as **glaucoma.** An increase in intraocular pressure can cause blindness by impeding blood flow to the retina. In addition, cloudiness or objects floating (floaters or "mouches volantes") in the vitreous humor can disrupt the light path to the retina and distort clear vision.

respectively, help maintain the shape of the eye. The **aqueous humor** is secreted by the epithelium of the **ciliary body** into the posterior chamber of the eye. It then circulates through the pupil and into the anterior chamber, where it is drained into the venous system by the **canal of Schlemm.** Aqueous humor pressure, which is normally less than 22 mm Hg, determines the pressure within the eye. The **vitreous humor** is a gel composed of extracellular fluid that contains collagen and hyaluronic acid; unlike aqueous humor, however, it turns over very slowly.

Normally, light from a visual target is focused sharply on the retina by the cornea and lens, which bend or refract the light. The cornea is the major refractive element of the eye, with a refractive power of 43 diopters* (D). However, unlike the cornea, the

lens can change shape and vary its refractive power between 13 and 26 D. Thus, the lens is responsible for adjusting the optical focus of the eye. **Suspensory ligaments** (or **zonule fibers**), which attach to the wall of the eye at the ciliary body (Fig. 8-1), hold the lens in place. When the muscles in the ciliary body are relaxed, the tension exerted by the suspensory ligaments flattens the lens. When the ciliary muscles contract, the tension on the suspensory ligaments is reduced; this process allows the somewhat elastic lens to assume a more spherical shape. The ciliary muscles are activated by the parasympathetic nervous system (via the oculomotor nerve).

In this way the lens allows the eye to focus on, or accommodate to, either near or distant objects. For instance, when light from a distant visual target enters a normal eye (one with a relaxed ciliary muscle), the target is in focus on the retina. However, if the eye is directed at a nearby visual target, the light is initially focused behind the retina (i.e., the image at the retina is blurred) until accommodation occurs. The ciliary muscle contracts and the zonule fibers relax; the image is sharpened when the convexity of the lens increases as a result of these muscular changes.

Although the optic axis of the human eye passes through the nodal point of the lens and reaches the retina at a point between the fovea and the optic disc (Fig. 8-1), the eye is directed by the oculomotor system to a point, called the **fixation point,** on the visual target. Light from the fixation point passes along the optic axis, and is focused on the **fovea.** Light from the

---

*A diopter describes the refractile power of a lens and equals the reciprocal of the focal length of the lens in meters.

remainder of the visual target falls on the retina surrounding the fovea.

Proper focus of light on the retina depends not only on the lens but also on the iris, which also adjusts the amount of light that can enter the eye. In this respect

As an individual ages, the elasticity of the lens gradually declines. As a result, accommodation of the lens for near vision becomes progressively less effective, a condition called **presbyopia.** A young person can change the power of the lens by as much as 14 D. However, by the time that a person reaches 40 years of age, the amount of accommodation halves, and after 50 years it decreases to 2 D or less. Presbyopia can be corrected by convex lenses.

Defects in focus are caused by a discrepancy between the size of the eye and the refractive power of the dioptric media. For example, in **myopia** (near-sightedness), the images of distant objects are focused in front of the retina. Concave lenses correct this problem. Conversely, in **hypermetropia** (far-sightedness), the images of distant objects are focused behind the retina; this problem can be corrected with convex lenses. In **astigmatism,** an asymmetry exists in the radii of curvature of different meridians of the cornea or lens (or sometimes of the retina). Astigmatism can often be corrected with lenses that possess appropriately matched radii of curvature.

the iris acts like the diaphragm in a camera, which also controls the depth of field of the image and the amount of spherical aberration produced by the lens. When the pupil is constricted, the depth of field is increased, and the light is directed through the central part of the lens, where spherical aberration is minimal. Pupillary constriction occurs reflexively when the eye accommodates for near vision or adapts to bright light, or both. Thus, when a person reads or does other fine visual work, the quality of the image is improved by having adequate light.

Retina

Layers of the Retina

The 10 layers of the retina are shown in Figure 8-2. The retina begins with the **pigmented epithelium** (layer 1), which is just inside the choroid. The pigment cells have tentacle-like processes that extend into the **photoreceptor layer** (layer 2) and surround the outer segments of the rods and cones. These processes prevent transverse scatter of light between photoreceptors. In addition, they serve a mechanical function in maintaining contact between layers 1 and 2 so that the pigmented epithelium can (1) provide nutrients and remove waste from the photoreceptors; (2) phagocytose the ends of the outer segments of the rods, which are continuously shed; and (3) reconvert metabolized photopigment into a form that can be reused after it is transported back to the photoreceptors.

Light rays that originate from different parts of the visual target map onto the photoreceptor array of

● **Figure 8-2.** Layers of the retina. Light impinging on the retina comes from the top of the figure and passes through all the superficial layers to reach the photoreceptor rods and cones.

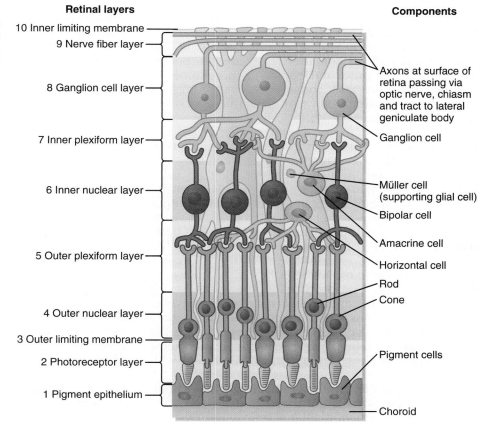

Retinal layers

10 Inner limiting membrane
9 Nerve fiber layer
8 Ganglion cell layer
7 Inner plexiform layer
6 Inner nuclear layer
5 Outer plexiform layer
4 Outer nuclear layer
3 Outer limiting membrane
2 Photoreceptor layer
1 Pigment epithelium

Components

Axons at surface of retina passing via optic nerve, chiasm and tract to lateral geniculate body
Ganglion cell
Müller cell (supporting glial cell)
Bipolar cell
Amacrine cell
Horizontal cell
Rod
Cone
Pigment cells
Choroid

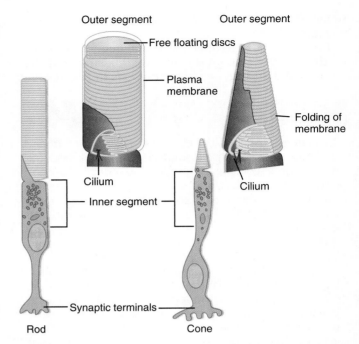

● Figure 8-3. Rods and cones. The drawings at the bottom show the general features of a rod and a cone. The insets show the outer segments.

layer 2 in a point-to-point fashion. Retinal glial cells, known as **Müller cells,** play an important role in maintaining the internal geometry of the retina. Müller cells are oriented radially, parallel to the light path through the retina. The outer ends of Müller cells form tight junctions with the inner segments of the photoreceptors. The numerous connections made between Müller cells and the inner segments give the appearance of a continuous layer, the **outer limiting membrane** (layer 3 of the retina).

Inside the external limiting membrane is the **outer nuclear layer** (layer 4 of the retina) that contains the cell bodies and nuclei of the rods and cones. The next layer of the retina (layer 5) is called the **outer plexiform layer.** It contains synapses between the photoreceptors and retinal interneurons, including the bipolar cells and horizontal cells, whose cell bodies are found in the **inner nuclear layer** (layer 6 of the retina). This layer also contains the cell bodies of other retinal interneurons (the amacrine and interplexiform cells) and the Müller cells.

The next layer is the inner plexiform layer (layer 7 of the retina). It contains synapses between the retinal neurons of the inner nuclear layer, including the bipolar and amacrine cells, and the ganglion cells. Layer 8 of the retina is the **ganglion cell layer.** As previously mentioned, the ganglion cells are the output cells of the retina; it is their axons that transmit visual information to the brain. These axons form the **optic fiber layer** (layer 9 of the retina), pass along the vitreous surface of the retina while avoiding the fovea, and enter the optic disc, where they leave the eye in the optic nerve. The portions of the ganglion cell axons that are in the optic fiber layer remain unmyelinated, but the axons become myelinated after they reach the optic disc. The lack of myelin where the axons cross the retina is a specialization that helps permit light to pass through the inner retina with minimal distortion.

The innermost layer of the retina is the **inner limiting membrane** (layer 10 of the retina). This layer is formed by the end-feet of Müller cells.

Structure of Photoreceptors: Rods and Cones

Each rod or cone photoreceptor cell is composed of a cell body (in layer 4), an inner segment and an outer segment that extend into layer 2, and a synaptic terminal that projects into layer 5 (Fig. 8-3). The outer segments of cones are not as long as those of rods, and they contain stacks of disc membranes formed by infoldings of the plasma membrane. The outer segments of rods are longer, and the stacks of membrane discs float freely in the outer segment after having disconnected from the plasma membrane when formed at the base. Both sets of discs are rich in photopigment molecules, but the greater photopigment density of rods partly accounts for their greater sensitivity to light. A single photon can elicit a rod response, whereas several hundred photons may be required for a cone response.

The inner segments of the photoreceptors are connected to the outer segments by a modified cilium that contains nine pairs of microtubules, but it lacks the two central pairs of microtubules found in most cilia. The inner segments contain a number of organelles, including numerous mitochondria.

The photopigment is synthesized in the inner segment and incorporated into the membranes of the outer segment. In rods, the pigment is inserted into new membranous discs, which are then displaced distally until they are eventually shed at the apex of the outer segment. There, they are phagocytozed by cells of the pigmented epithelium. This process determines the rod-like shape of the outer segments of rods. In cones, the photopigment is inserted randomly into the membranous folds of the outer segment, and shedding, comparable to that seen in rods, does not take place.

Regional Variations in the Retina

The **macula lutea** is the area of central vision and is characterized by a slight thickening and a pale color. The thickness is due to the high concentration of photoreceptors and interneurons, which are needed for high-resolution vision. The pale color is a consequence of the fact that both optic nerve fibers and blood vessels are routed around it.

The fovea, which is a depression in the macula lutea, is the region of the retina that has the very highest visual resolution. Correspondingly, the image from the fixation point is focused on the fovea. The retinal layers in the foveal region are unusual because several of them appear to be pushed aside into the surrounding macula. Because light can reach the foveal photoreceptors without having to pass through the inner layers of the retina, both image distortion and light loss are minimized. The fovea has cones with unusually long and thin outer segments. This cone shape permits high packing density. In fact, cone density is maximal in the fovea, and this high density provides for high visual resolution, as well as high quality of the image (Fig. 8-4).

The optic disc lacks photoreceptors and therefore lacks photosensitivity. Thus, the optic disc is a "blind spot" in the visual surface of the retina. A person is normally unaware of the blind spot, both because the corresponding part of the visual field can be seen by the contralateral eye and because of the psychological process in which incomplete visual images tend to be completed perceptually.

Visual Transduction

Light energy must be absorbed for it to be detected by the retina. Light absorption is accomplished by the visual pigments, which are located in the outer segments of the rods and cones. The pigment found in the outer segments of rods is **rhodopsin,** or visual purple (so named because it has a purple appearance after green or blue light have been absorbed), and it absorbs light best at a wavelength of 500 nm. Three variants of visual pigment are found in cones, and these cone pigments absorb best at 419 nm (blue), 533 nm (green), or 564 nm (red). However, the absorption spectrum of visual pigments is broad so that they overlap considerably (Fig. 8-5).

● **Figure 8-4.** This graph plots the density of cones and rods as a function of retinal eccentricity from the fovea. Note that cone density peaks at the fovea, rod density peaks at about 20 degrees eccentricity, and no photoreceptors are found at the optic disc. (Data from Cornsweet TN: Visual Perception. New York, Academic Press, 1970.)

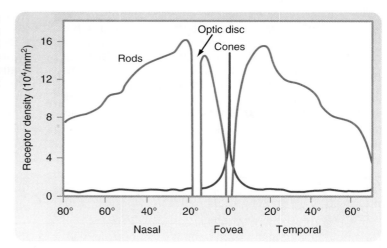

● **Figure 8-5.** The spectral sensitivity of the three types of cone pigments in the human retina is shown. Note that the curves overlap and that the so-called blue and red cones actually absorb maximally in the violet and yellow range, respectively. (Data from Squire LR et al [eds]: Fundamental Neuroscience. San Diego, CA, Academic Press, 2002.)

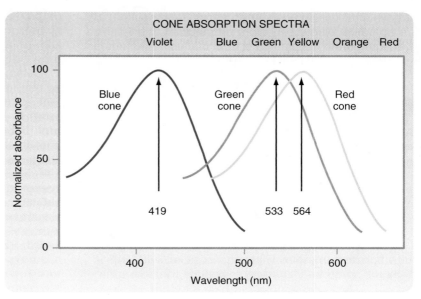

Rhodopsin is formed when a retinal isomer, 11-*cis* retinal, is combined with a glycoprotein known as opsin. When rhodopsin absorbs light, it is "boosted" to a higher energy state. This boost causes a series of chemical changes that lead to isomerization of 11-*cis* retinal to all-*trans* retinal, release of the bond with opsin, and conversion of retinal to retinol. Separation of all-*trans* retinal from opsin causes bleaching of the visual pigment; that is, the pigment loses its purple color.

In darkness, photoreceptors are slightly depolarized (around −40 mV) because cGMP-gated Na⁺ channels (Fig. 8-6, *A*) in their outer segments are open, thereby increasing g_{Na} and driving the membrane potential toward the Na⁺ equilibrium potential. This net influx of Na⁺ results in a continuous current, called the dark current. As a consequence of this constant depolarization, the neurotransmitter glutamate is tonically released at the rod cell's synapses. Intracellular [Na⁺] is kept at a steady-state level by the pumping action of Na⁺,K⁺-ATPase.

When light is absorbed, the photoisomerization of rhodopsin activates a G protein called **transducin** (Fig. 8-6, *B*). This G protein, in turn, activates **cyclic guanosine monophosphate phosphodiesterase,** which is associated with the rhodopsin-containing discs, hydrolyzes cGMP to 5′-GMP, and lowers the cGMP concentration in the rod cytoplasm. The reduction in cGMP leads to closing of the cGMP-gated Na⁺ channels, hyperpolarization of the photoreceptor membrane, and a reduction in the release of transmitter. Thus, cGMP acts as a "second messenger" to translate reception of a photon by the photopigment into a change in membrane potential.

IN THE CLINIC

As mentioned, the axons of retinal ganglion cells cross the retina in the optic fiber layer (layer 9) and enter the optic nerve at the optic disc. Axons in the optic fiber layer pass around the macula and fovea, as do the blood vessels that supply the inner layers of the retina. The optic disc can be visualized on physical examination with an **ophthalmoscope.** The normal optic disc has a slight depression in its center. Changes in the appearance of the optic disc are important clinically. For example, the depression may be exaggerated by loss of ganglion cell axons **(optic atrophy),** or the optic disc may protrude into the vitreous space because of edema **(papilledema)** caused by increased intracranial pressure.

AT THE CELLULAR LEVEL

Rhodopsin contains a chromophore, called retinal, that is the aldehyde of **retinol,** or vitamin A. Retinol is derived from carotenoids, such as β-carotene, the orange pigment found in carrots. Like other vitamins, retinol cannot be synthesized by humans; instead, it is derived from food sources. Individuals with a severe vitamin A deficiency suffer from "night blindness," a condition in which vision is defective in low light situations.

● **Figure 8-6.** **A,** Drawing of a rod. The flow of current in the dark is indicated, as well as the Na⁺ pump. **B,** Sequence of the second messenger events that follow the absorption of light. cGMP, cyclic guanosine monophosphate; GC, guanylate cyclase; GTP, guanosine triphosphate; PDE, phosphodiesterase; Rh, rhodopsin; T, transducin.

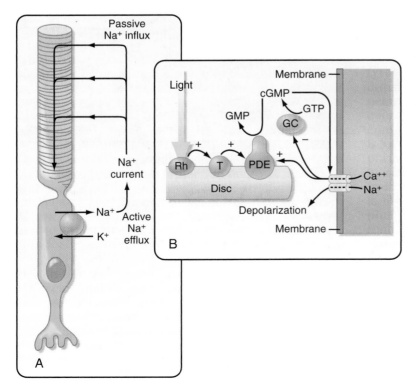

The extraordinary sensitivity of rods, which can signal the capture of a single photon, is enhanced by an amplification mechanism such that photoactivation of only one rhodopsin molecule can activate hundreds of transducin molecules. In addition, each phosphodiesterase molecule hydrolyzes thousands of cGMP molecules per second. Similar events occur in cones, but the membrane hyperpolarization occurs much more quickly than in rods, and requires thousands of photons.

Thus, in all photoreceptors, capture of light energy leads to (1) hyperpolarization of the photoreceptor and (2) a reduction in the release of transmitter. Note that with the very short distance between the site of transduction and the synapse, this transmitter modulation is accomplished without the generation of an action potential.

Visual Adaptation

Adaptation permits the retina to adjust its sensitivity to large changes in ambient lighting, such as you experience when entering a darkened movie theater or, later, leaving to encounter afternoon sunlight. **Light adaptation** is associated with a reduction in the amount of rhodopsin and the resulting reduced photosensitivity. In bright light, 11-*cis* retinal is isomerized into the all-*trans* form, which then splits from the opsin. To regenerate the rhodopsin, the all-*trans* retinal is transported to the retinal pigmented cell layer to be reduced to retinol, isomerized, and esterified back to 11-*cis* retinal. It is then transported back to the photoreceptor layer, taken up by outer segments, and recombined with opsin to regenerate the rhodopsin. Light adaptation, which occurs rapidly, within seconds, favors cone vision because the rhodopsin in rods bleaches (separates from its opsin) more readily than the cone pigments do.

The regeneration of photopigment is also involved in **dark adaptation,** a process that results in an increase in visual sensitivity. Cones adapt more rapidly to darkness than rods do, but their adapted threshold is relatively high. Thus, cones do not function when the ambient light level is low. By contrast, rods adapt to darkness slowly, as their sensitivity increases. Within 10 minutes in a dark room, rod vision is more sensitive than cone vision.

Dark adaptation is very familiar to moviegoers, who must wait several minutes after entering the darkened theater before they can see an empty seat. Although the theater is dark and rod vision is operative, visual acuity is low and colors are not distinguished (this is called scotopic vision). When the movie is projected, however, cone function resumes (this is called photopic vision), and visual acuity and color vision are restored.

Color Vision

The three visual pigments in the cone outer segments have opsins that differ from the opsin found in rhodopsin. As a result of these differences, the three types of cone pigments absorb light best at different wavelengths. Although the cone pigments have maximum efficiency closer to violet, green, and yellow wavelengths, they are referred to as blue, green, and red pigments, respectively (Fig. 8-5).

According to the **trichromacy theory,** these differences in absorption efficiency are presumed to account for color vision because a suitable mixture of three colors can produce any other color. However, a neural system must also exist for the analysis of color brightness because the amount of light absorbed by a visual pigment, as well as the subsequent response of the cell, depends on both the wavelength and the intensity of the light (Fig. 8-5). Two or three of the cone pigments may absorb a particular wavelength of light, but the amount absorbed by each will differ according to their efficiencies at that wavelength. If the intensity of the light is increased (or decreased), all will absorb more (or less), but the ratio of absorption among them will remain constant. Consequently, there must be a neural mechanism to compare the absorption of light of different wavelengths by the different types of cones for the visual system to distinguish different colors. At least two different kinds of cones are required for color vision. The presence of three kinds decreases the ambiguity in distinguishing colors when all three absorb light, and it ensures that at least two types of cones will absorb most wavelengths of visible light.

The **opponent process theory** is based on observations that certain pairs of colors seem to activate opposing neural processes. Green and red are opposed, as are yellow and blue, as well as black and white. For example, if a gray area is surrounded by a green ring, the gray area appears to acquire a reddish color. Furthermore, a greenish red or a bluish yellow color does not exist. These observations are supported by findings that neurons activated by green are inhibited by red. Similarly, neurons excited by blue may be inhibited by yellow. Neurons with these characteristics are found both in the retina and at higher levels of the visual pathway and seem to serve to increase our ability to see the contrast between opposing colors.

Retinal Circuitry

A diagram of the basic circuitry of the retina is shown in Figure 8-7. Photoreceptors (R) synapse on the dendrites of bipolar cells (B) and horizontal cells (H) in the outer plexiform layer. The horizontal cells make

> ### IN THE CLINIC

Observations on color blindness are consistent with the trichromacy theory. In color blindness, a genetic defect (sex-linked recessive), one or more cone mechanisms are lost. Normal people are trichromats because they have three cone mechanisms. Individuals who have lost one of the cone mechanisms are called dichromats. When the long-wavelength cone mechanism is lost, the resulting condition is called protanopia; loss of the medium-wavelength system causes deuteranopia; and loss of the short-wavelength system causes tritanopia. Monochromats have lost two or more cone mechanisms.

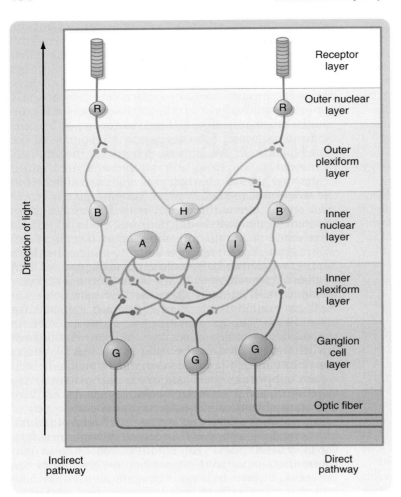

● **Figure 8-7.** Basic retinal circuitry. The arrow at the left indicates the direction of light through the retina. A, amacrine cells; B, bipolar cells; G, ganglion cells; H, horizontal cells; I, interplexiform cells; R, photoreceptors.

reciprocal synaptic connections with photoreceptor cells, are electrically coupled to other horizontal cells, and receive input from interplexiform cells (I). Bipolar cells synapse on the dendrites of ganglion cells (G) and on the processes of amacrine cells (A) in the inner plexiform layer. Amacrine cells connect with ganglion cells, other amacrine cells, and interplexiform cells.

Several features of this circuitry are noteworthy. Input to the retina is provided by light striking the photoreceptors. The output is carried by axons of the retinal ganglion cells to the brain. Information is processed within the retina by the interneurons. The most direct pathway through the retina is from a photoreceptor to a bipolar cell and then to a ganglion cell (Fig. 8-7). More indirect pathways that provide for intraretinal signal processing involve photoreceptors, bipolar cells, amacrine cells, and ganglion cells, as well as horizontal cells to provide lateral interactions between adjacent pathways. Interplexiform cells allow interactions to occur from the inner to the outer retina.

Contrasts in Rod and Cone Pathway Functions

Rod and cone pathways have several important functional differences, based partly on differences in their phototransduction mechanisms and partly on retinal circuitry. As described previously, rods have more

photopigment and a better signal amplification system than cones do, and there are many more rods than cones. Thus, rods function better in dim light (scotopic vision), and loss of rod function results in night blindness. In addition, all rods contain the same photopigment, so they cannot signal color differences. Furthermore, because many rods converge onto individual bipolar cells, thereby resulting in very large receptive fields, rods cannot provide high-resolution vision. Finally, in bright light most rhodopsin is bleached, so rods no longer function under photopic conditions.

Cones have a higher threshold to light and thus are not activated in dim light after dark adaptation. However, they operate very well in daylight. They provide high-resolution vision because only a few cones converge onto individual bipolar cells in the cone pathways. Moreover, no convergence occurs in the fovea where the cones make one-to-one connections to bipolar cells. As a result of the reduced convergence, cone pathways have very small receptive fields and can resolve stimuli that originate from sources very close to each other. Cones also respond to sequential stimuli with good temporal resolution. Finally, cones have three different cone photopigments. Thus, they can discriminate relative spectral content independent of absolute intensity and therefore provide for color vision. Loss of cone function results in functional blindness; rod vision is not sufficient for normal visual requirements.

Synaptic Interactions

The distances between retinal components are short. Hence, modulated transmitter release and postsynaptic potentials are sufficient for most of the activity in retinal circuits, and action potentials are not required in most of the interneurons. Only the ganglion cells and some amacrine cells generate action potentials. It is unclear why amacrine cells have action potentials, but ganglion cells must generate them to transmit information over the relatively long distance from the retina to the brain.

Although receptor potentials in photoreceptors are hyperpolarizing, synaptic potentials in the retina can be either hyperpolarizing or depolarizing. Hyperpolarizing events reduce neurotransmitter release from the synaptic terminals of a retinal interneuron,

whereas depolarizing events increase neurotransmitter release.

Receptive Field Organization

The receptive field of an individual photoreceptor is small and circular. Light in the receptive field will hyperpolarize the photoreceptor cell and cause it to release less neurotransmitter. The receptive fields of photoreceptors and retinal interneurons determine the receptive fields of the retinal ganglion cells onto which their activity converges. The characteristics of the receptive fields of retinal ganglion cells constitute an important step in visual information processing because it is this processed information about visual events that is conveyed to the brain.

A bipolar cell that receives input from a photoreceptor can have either of two types of receptive fields, as shown in Figure 8-8. Both are described as having a center-surround organization in which the light that

● **Figure 8-8.** The receptive fields of on-center (**A**) and off-center (**F**) bipolar and ganglion cells. **B** and **G** show the responses of these ganglion cells to central (*upper record*) and peripheral (*lower record*) spots. Also shown are responses to central (**C** and **H**), surround (**D** and **G**), and diffuse whole field (**E** and **J**) Illumination in their receptive fields. The on-center and off-center bipolar cells providing input to these ganglion cells have similar receptive fields, but wheras ganglion cells increase or decrease their spike frequency, bipolar cells depolarize or hyperpolarize, without generating action potentials. (Redrawn from Squire LR et al [eds]: Fundamental Neuroscience. San Diego, CA, Academic Press, 2002.)

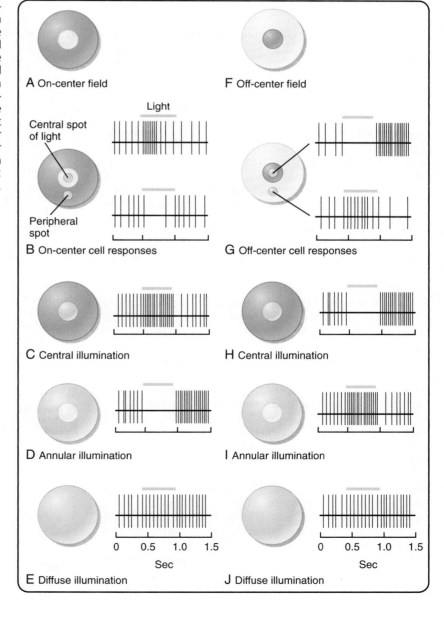

strikes the central region of the receptive field either excites or inhibits the cell, whereas the light that strikes the annular region that surrounds the central portion has the converse effect. The receptive field with a centrally located excitatory region surrounded by an inhibitory annulus is called an **on-center, off-surround receptive field** (Fig. 8-8, *A*). Bipolar cells with such a receptive field are described as "on" bipolars. The other type of receptive field has an **off-center, on-surround** arrangement, which characterizes "off" bipolars (Fig. 8-8, *F*).

The receptive fields of bipolar cells depend on input from photoreceptors and from horizontal cells. The neurotransmitter used in the retinal pathway from photoreceptor cells to bipolar cells and to horizontal cells is the excitatory amino acid glutamate. Excitatory amino acids depolarize "off" bipolar cells, as well as horizontal cells, through the activation of ionotropic glutamate receptors. These are called "off" bipolars because when light is removed from the receptive field center, the photoreceptor is depolarized and releases more glutamate to depolarize the bipolar cell. In contrast, "on" bipolar cells have metabotropic glutamate receptors that close their Na^+ channels, and thus "on" bipolars are depolarized by turning the light on because the reduced release of glutamate results in more influx of Na^+.

In other words, if the neurotransmitter tonically released by the photoreceptor hyperpolarizes the bipolar cell, absorption of light will hyperpolarize the photoreceptor and thereby reduce its release of the neurotransmitter; the "on" bipolar cell will be depolarized (disinhibited) and thus excited. On the other hand, the neurotransmitter tonically released by the photoreceptor depolarizes the "off" bipolar cell, and it will be hyperpolarized (disfacilitated) by central illumination.

The central property of bipolar cell receptive fields is due to only a few directly connected photoreceptors. The antagonistic surround response is due to light impinging on adjacent photoreceptors, which changes the activity of horizontal cells. This pathway through the horizontal cells results in a response that is opposite in sign to that produced directly by the photoreceptors that mediate the center response. The basis for this is that horizontal cells, like "off" bipolars, are hyperpolarized in the light and, because they are electrically coupled to each other by gap junctions, have very large receptive fields. Darkness in the periphery of a bipolar cell's receptive field (such as an annulus that does not affect the photoreceptors to which it is directly connected) will depolarize neighboring photoreceptors and horizontal cells. Depolarized horizontal cells release GABA onto central (and peripheral) photoreceptor terminals, reducing their release of glutamate. Thus, when a darkness surrounds central illumination, there is increased excitation of **on-center** bipolars. There is a complementary effect on **off-center** bipolars when a bright annulus surrounds a central dark spot (Fig. 8-8).

Bipolar cells may not respond at all to large or diffuse areas of illumination, covering both the receptors that cause the surround response and those responsible for the center response because of the opposing actions from the center and surround. Thus, bipolar cells may not signal changes in the intensity of light that strikes a large area of the retina. On the other hand, a small spot of light moving across the receptive field may sequentially and dramatically alter the activity of the bipolar cell as the light crosses the receptive field from surround to center and then back again to surround. This demonstrates that bipolar cells respond best to the local contrast of stimuli and function as contrast detectors.

Amacrine cells receive input from different combinations of on-center and off-center bipolar cells. Thus, their receptive fields are mixtures of on-center and off-center regions. There are many different types of amacrine cells, and they may use at least eight different neurotransmitters. Accordingly, the contributions of amacrine cells to visual processing are complex.

Ganglion cells may receive dominant input from bipolar cells, dominant input from amacrine cells, or mixed input from amacrine and bipolar cells. When amacrine cell input dominates, the receptive fields of ganglion cells tend to be diffuse, and they are either excitatory or inhibitory. Most ganglion cells are dominated by bipolar cell input and have a center-surround organization, similar to that of bipolar cells (Fig. 8-8).

P, M, and W Cells

Experiments have shown that in primates, retinal ganglion cells can be subdivided into three general types called **P cells, M cells,** and **W cells.** P and M cells are fairly homogeneous groups, whereas W cells are heterogeneous. P cells are so named because they project to the parvocellular layers of the LGN, whereas M cells project to the magnocellular layers of the LGN. P and M cells have center-surround receptive fields; hence, they are presumably controlled by bipolar cells. W cells may also have center-surround receptive fields, but many have large, diffuse receptive fields (which corresponds to extensive dendritic fields) and slowly conducting axons, and they respond poorly to visual stimuli. They are probably influenced chiefly through amacrine cell pathways, but less is known of them than of M and P cells.

Several of the physiological differences among these cell types correspond to morphological differences (Table 8-1). For example, P cells have small receptive

● **Table 8-1.**
Properties of Retinal Ganglion Cells

Properties	P Cells	M Cells	W Cells
Cell body and axon	Medium sized	Large	Small
Dendritic tree	Restricted	Extensive	Extensive
Receptive field			
Size	Small	Medium	Large
Organization	Center-surround	Center-surround	Diffuse Poorly responsive
Adaptation	Tonic	Phasic	
Linearity	Linear	Nonlinear	
Wavelength	Sensitive	Insensitive	Insensitive
Luminance	Insensitive	Sensitive	Sensitive

fields (which corresponds to smaller dendritic trees) and more slowly conducting axons than M cells do. In addition, P cells show a linear response in their receptive field; that is, they respond with a sustained, tonic discharge of action potentials to maintained light but do not signal shifts in the pattern of illumination as long as the overall level of illumination is constant. Thus, a small object entering a P cell's central receptive field will change its firing, but continued movement within the field will not be signaled. P cells respond differently to different wavelengths of light. Because there are blue, green, and red cones, many combinations of color properties are possible, but in fact P cells have been shown to have only opposing responses to red and green or to blue and yellow (a combination of red and green). They may have center-surround antagonism in which one color excites the center while the other inhibits the surround (or vice versa), or one color might excite the entire receptive field while another inhibits it (e.g., R+G− describes a cell that is excited by red and inhibited by green). These mechanisms can greatly reduce the ambiguity of color detection caused by the overlap in cone color sensitivity and may provide a substrate for the opponency process observations.

M cells, on the other hand, respond with phasic bursts of action potentials to the redistribution of light, such as would be caused by the movement of an object within their large receptive fields. M cells are not sensitive to differences in wavelength but are more sensitive to luminance than P cells are.

Thus, the output of the retina consists primarily of ganglion cell axons from (1) sustained, linear P cells with small receptive fields that convey information about color, form, and fine details and (2) phasic, nonlinear M cells with larger receptive fields that convey information about illumination and movement. Both come in on-center and off-center varieties.

The Visual Pathway

Retinal ganglion cells transmit information to the brain by way of the optic nerve, optic chiasm, and optic tract. Figure 8-9 shows the relationships between a visual target (*arrow*), the retinal images of the target in the two eyes, and the projections of retinal ganglion cells to the two hemispheres of the brain. The eyes and the optic nerves, chiasm, and tract are viewed from above.

The visual target, an arrow, is in the visual fields of both eyes (Fig. 8-9) and, in this case, is so long that it extends into the monocular segments of each retina (i.e., one end of the target can be seen only by one eye and the other end only by the other eye). The shaded circle at the center of the target shows the fixation point. The image of the target is reversed on the retinas by the lens system. The left half of the visual target is

● **Figure 8-9.** Relationships between a visual target, images on the retinas of the two eyes, and projections of the ganglion cells carrying visual information about these images. The image is so large that it extends into the monocular segments of the eyes where the image is seen in only one eye. Note that all the information about the left visual field of both eyes is conveyed to the right side of the brain and all the information about the right visual field is conveyed to the left side.

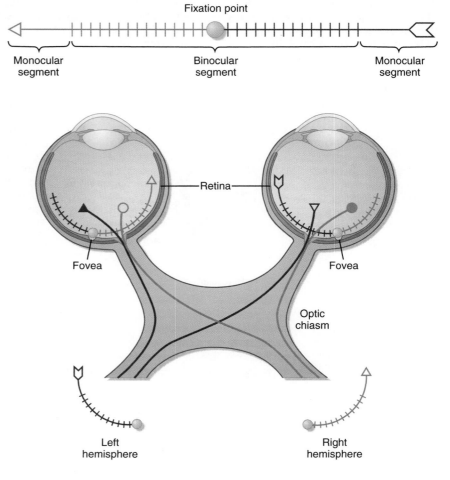

imaged on the nasal retina of the left eye and the temporal retina of the right eye. Thus, the left visual field is seen by the left nasal retina and the right temporal retina. Similarly, the right half of the visual target is imaged on and seen by the left temporal retina and the right nasal retina. There is also an inversion in the vertical axis, with the upper visual field imaged on the lower retina and vice versa.

The projections of retinal ganglion cells may be uncrossed or crossed, depending on the location of the ganglion cell in the retina (Fig. 8-9). Axons from the temporal portion of each retina pass through the optic nerve, the lateral side of the optic chiasm, and the ipsilateral optic tract and terminate ipsilaterally in the brain. Axons from the nasal portion of each retina pass through the optic nerve, cross to the opposite side in the optic chiasm, and then pass through the contralateral optic tract to end in the contralateral side of the brain. This arrangement results in the representation of objects in the left field of vision in the right side of the brain and those in the right field of vision in the left side of the brain (Fig. 8-10).

Retinal ganglion cell axons can synapse in several nuclei of the brain, but the main target for vision is the **lateral geniculate nucleus (LGN)** of the thalamus. The LGN in turn projects to the **primary visual cortex** or **striate cortex** by way of the **visual radiation.** The visual radiation fans out, and the fibers carrying information derived from the lower half of the appropriate hemiretinas (and therefore the contralateral upper visual field) project to the **lingual gyrus,** which lies on the medial surface of the occipital lobe, just below the calcarine fissure. Axons in the visual radiation that represent the contralateral lower visual field project to the adjacent **cuneus gyrus,** which lies just above the calcarine fissure. Together, the portions of these two gyri that line and border the calcarine fissure constitute the primary visual cortex (or area 17) (Fig. 8-10).

In addition, the representation of the macula occupies the most posterior and largest part of both gyri, with progressively more peripheral retina projected to

IN THE CLINIC

Interruption of the visual pathway at any level will cause a defect in the appropriate part of the visual field (Fig. 8-9). For example, a tiny lesion in the retina would result in a blind spot **(scotoma)** in that eye, whereas a similar lesion in the striate cortex would produce corresponding scotomas in both eyes. Interruption of the optic nerve on one side produces blindness in that eye. Damage to the optic nerve fibers as they cross in the optic chiasm results in loss of vision in both temporal fields of vision; this condition is known as **bitemporal hemianopsia** and occurs because the crossing fibers originate from ganglion cells in the nasal halves of each retina. A lesion of the entire optic tract, LGN, visual radiation, or visual cortex on one side causes **homonymous hemianopsia,** which is loss of vision in the entire contralateral visual field. Partial lesions result in partial visual field defects. For example, a lesion in the lingual gyrus causes an upper **homonymous quadrantanopsia,** which in this case is loss of vision in the contralateral, upper visual field.

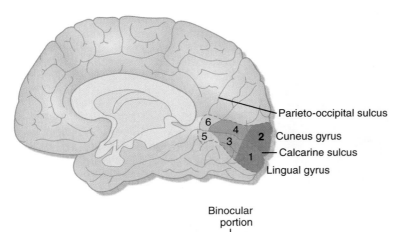

● **Figure 8-10.** The left visual field is relayed, via the LGN and visual radiation to the primary visual cortex of the right hemisphere, as a point-to-point retinotopic map. The representation of each part of visual space is proportional to the number of afferent axons with receptive fields in that part of space. As a result, the area of macular representation (near the occipital pole) is larger than that for the rest of the binocular and monocular fields. Note that the lower half of the field is represented in the cuneus gyrus above the calcarine fissure and the upper half of the field in the lingual gyrus below the fissure. (Redrawn from Purves D et al [eds]: Neuroscience, 3rd ed. Sunderland, MA, Sinauer, 2004.)

more anterior parts of these gyri. Overall, there is an orderly mapping of retinal loci across the surface of the striate cortex.

Lateral Geniculate Nucleus

The LGN is a layered structure. The first two layers, which contain large neurons, are called the magnocellular layers. The other four layers are the parvocellular layers. There is a point-to-point projection from the retina to the LGN. The LGN thus has a retinotopic map. Cells that represent a particular retinal location are aligned along projection lines that can be drawn across the layers of the LGN.

The projection from each eye is distributed to three of the layers of the LGN, one of the magnocellular layers (layers 1 and 2 get M cell input) and two parvocellular layers (layers 3 to 6 get P cell input). Color-coded ganglion cells project to groups of cells between the major layers, the intralaminar zones. Thus, the properties of LGN neurons are very similar to those of retinal ganglion cells. For example, LGN neurons can be classified as P or M cells, and they have on-center or off-center receptive fields.

The LGN also receives input from the visual areas of the cerebral cortex, the thalamic reticular nucleus, and several nuclei of the brainstem reticular formation. The activity of LGN projection neurons is inhibited by interneurons both in the LGN and in the thalamic reticular nucleus. These cells use γ-aminobutyric acid (GABA) as their inhibitory neurotransmitter. In addition, the activity of LGN neurons is influenced by corticofugal pathways and by brainstem neurons that use monoamine transmitters. These control systems filter visual information and may be important for selective attention.

Striate Cortex

The geniculostriate pathway ends chiefly in layer 4 of the striate cortex (Fig. 8-11), with the M and P cells segregated into separate sublayers 4Cα and 4Cβ, respectively, while the projection from the intralaminar LGN terminates in so-called blobs in layers 2 and 3. Similarly, axons that represent one eye or the other terminate within layer 4C in alternate patches that define ocular dominance columns. Cortical neurons in such a column respond preferentially to input from one eye. Near the border between two **ocular dominance columns,** neurons respond about equally to input from the two eyes.

Like the LGN, the striate cortex contains a retinotopic map (actually, two interlaced retinotopic maps, one for each eye). The macula is represented by a relatively large region in comparison to the remainder of the retina. The macular representation extends forward from the occipital pole for about a third the length of the striate cortex (Fig. 8-10).

The receptive fields of neurons in the striate cortex, aside from the monocular cells in layer 4C, are more complex than those of LGN neurons. Neurons in other layers may be binocular and respond to stimulation of both eyes, although the input from one eye often dominates (see Chapter 10). In addition, cortical neurons outside layer 4C often show **orientation selectivity** (i.e., they respond best when the stimulus, such as a bar or an edge, is oriented and positioned in a particular way) (Fig. 8-12). These "simple cells" appear to be responding as though they received input from cells whose concentric center-surround receptive fields were arranged such that their "on" centers were aligned in a row flanked by antagonistic regions. "Complex" cortical neurons are similar to "simple" cells in that they are orientation specific, but instead of having flanking excitatory and inhibitory zones, they respond best to a particular stimulus orientation anywhere in their receptive field. They may also display **direction selectivity;** that is, they may respond when the stimulus is moved in one direction but not when it is moved in the opposite direction (Fig. 8-12). The receptive field of a "complex" cell may be thought of as a composite of adjacent "simple" cells with similar orientation selectivity. Because such neurons in a particular zone of the cortex all tend to have the same orientation selectivity, they are considered to form an orientation column (Fig. 8-13).

However, this classification does not take into account the separate P and M cell pathways. Presumably, parallel P and M cell pathways contribute to the complexity of visual cortical organization. Cortical receptive field organization may depend on both serial and parallel processing.

Stereopsis is defined as binocular depth perception and appears to be dependent on slight differences in the retinal images formed in the two eyes. Such disparities give different perspectives that lead to visual cues about depth. Stereopsis is useful only for relatively nearby objects. Such perception must be a cortical function because it depends on convergent input

● **Figure 8-11.** Diagram of visual information flow into the visual cortex from the LGN and its projection to extrastriate cortex, superior colliculus (SC), and back to the LGN. M, magnocellular path; P, parvocellular path. (Redrawn from Squire LR et al [eds]: Fundamental Neuroscience. San Diego, CA, Academic Press, 2002.)

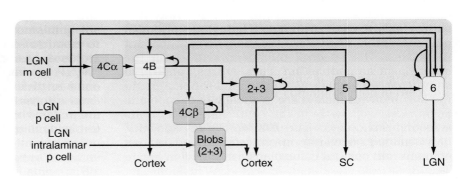

● **Figure 8-12.** Simple and complex receptive fields in the visual cortex can be generated from multiple inputs with concentric fields. **A** and **B** represent on-center and off-center input. If three on-center cells (**A**) with adjacent receptive fields converged onto one cortical neuron (**E**), that neuron, a simple cell, would respond best to a long bar stimulus at a specific location and orientation (**C**). For three off-center inputs (**B**), the resulting receptive field is shown in **D.** The convergence of multiple simple cells onto another cortical neuron (**F**) would result in a complex cell that responds best to a bar stimulus with a specific orientation that can be placed anywhere within its receptive field. (Redrawn from Squire LR et al [eds]: Fundamental Neuroscience. San Diego, CA, Academic Press, 2002.)

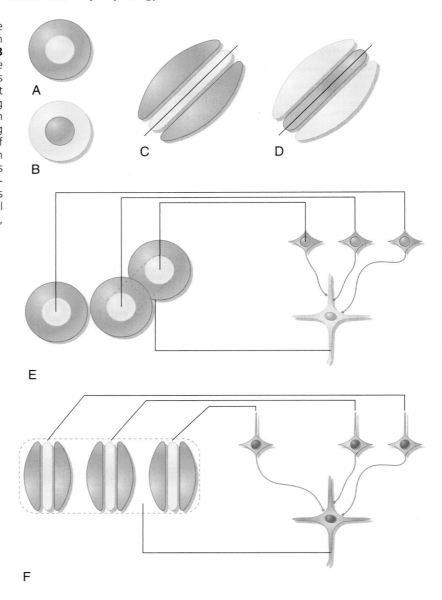

from the two eyes. Depth cues are also available when a single eye is used. For example, the brain interprets distance according to the relative size of familiar objects.

As already discussed, color vision may depend on the presence in the retina of three different types of cones, as well as neurons in the visual pathway that show spectral opposition. Retinal ganglion cells, LGN neurons, and some P cells display spectral opponent properties. The spectral opponent neurons in the striate cortex are found in cortical "blobs," and these show double-opponency in which both the center and the surround respond antagonistically to two colors. Such a cell with R+G− in the center and R−G+ in its surround is shown in Figure 8-13, *A.* The relationships between the ocular dominance and orientation columns and cortical color blobs are shown in Figure 8-13, *B.*

Extrastriate Visual Cortex

In animal studies, at least 25 different visual areas have been identified in the cerebral cortex, in addition to the striate cortex (area 17 or V1). The extrastriate areas include several different parallel visual processing pathways. The P pathway originates with P cells and functions in the recognition of form and color. Structures in the P pathway include LGN layers 3 to 6, layer 4Cb of the striate cortex, V4 (Brodmann's area 19), and several areas in the inferotemporal region (Fig. 8-14). Processing of form includes recognition of complex visual patterns, such as faces. Color information is processed separately from form. The M pathway originates with M cells and functions in motion detection and control of eye movement. Cortical structures in the M pathway include layers 4B and 4Ca of the striate cortex and areas MT (medial temporal) and MST (medial superior temporal) on the lateral aspect

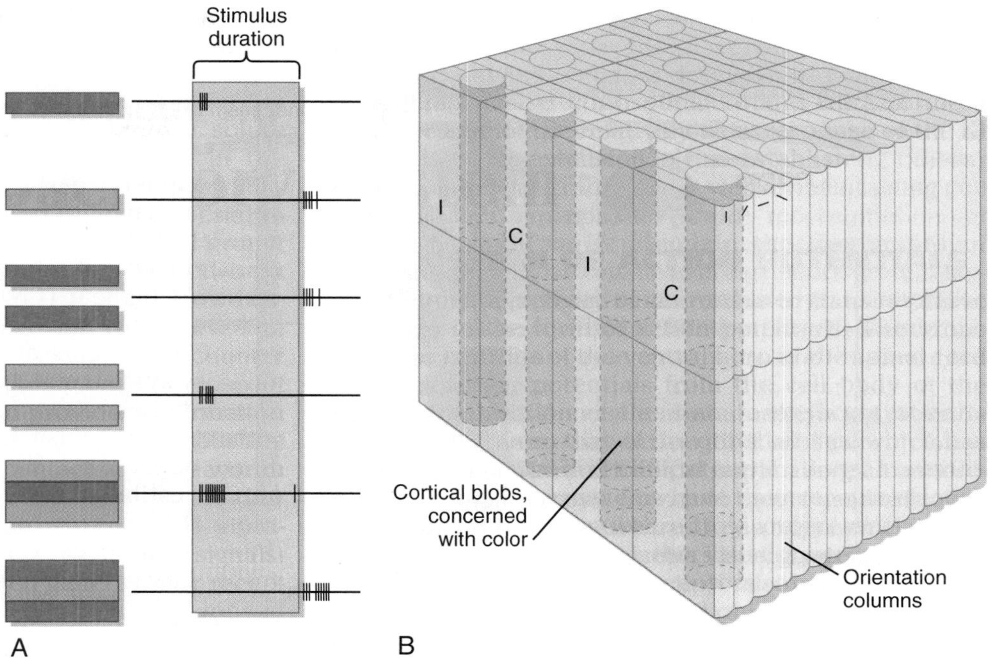

● **Figure 8-13.** **A,** The receptive field and responses of a double-opponent neuron in the striate cortex that responds to various combinations of red and green bars. The best "on" response is to a red bar flanked by two green bars. **B,** Diagram of the columnar arrangement of the visual cortex. Ocular dominance columns are indicated by I (for ipsilateral) and C (for contralateral). Orientation columns are indicated by the smaller columns marked with short bars at various angles. The cortical blobs contain neurons like that of **A** and have spectral opponent receptive fields.

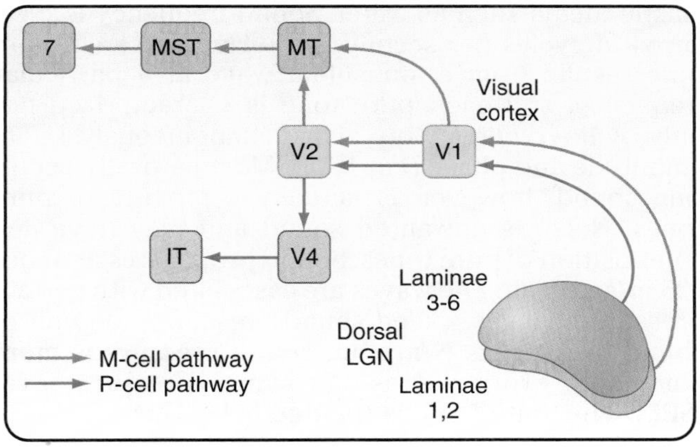

● **Figure 8-14.** Distribution of P and M cell influences on different areas of the visual cortex. IT, inferotemporal area; MST, medial superior temporal; MT, medial temporal; V1, striate cortex; V2, V4, higher-order visual areas.

of the temporal lobe, as well as area 7a of the parietal lobe (Fig. 8-14). Both P and M pathways contribute to depth perception.

The separation of M and P pathways from the retina through the thalamus and all the cortical regions raises the issue of how all the parts are combined to account for the clear, coherent images of events, objects, and persons that we perceive. It seems unlikely that all the components that represent a percept, such as recognizing a face and then identifying it as belonging to a familiar person, are somehow converged onto a single neuron that will recognize it. The process by which we achieve this "binding" of disparate elements into a percept is unclear, but one working hypothesis is that it may be accomplished by the temporal synchronization of many anatomically distributed neural events.

IN THE CLINIC

Lesions of the extrastriate visual cortex can produce various deficits. Bilateral lesions of the inferotemporal cortex can result in cortical color blindness **(achromatopsia)** or in an inability to recognize faces, even of close members of the family **(prosopagnosia).** A lesion in area MT or MST can interfere with motion detection and eye movements.

Other Visual Pathways

Superior Colliculus

The superior colliculus of the midbrain is a layered structure. The three most superficial layers are involved exclusively in visual processing, whereas the deeper layers have multimodal input from the somatosensory and auditory systems, as well as the visual system, particularly from cortical areas involved in eye movement (see Chapter 9).

Neurons in the superficial layers of the superior colliculus receive a projection from retinal ganglion cells and are organized into a retinotopic map. Collicular neurons are particularly sensitive to rapid stimulus motion in a particular direction. Most of the cells have binocular input, but they lack orientation selectivity. The ganglion cells include both W and M cells (but not P cells), and they are located chiefly in the contralateral nasal retina. Neurons in the superficial layers of the superior colliculus also receive a projection from the visual cortex, including the striate cortex. The cortical loop involves neurons activated by M cells. The superficial layers of the superior colliculus, in turn, project to several thalamic nuclei (pulvinar, LGN), and they are connected directly and indirectly to large areas of posterior parietal, temporal, and occipital cortex, including visual cortex.

The deep layers of the superior colliculus receive connections from the somatosensory and auditory pathways, in addition to visual input from the superficial layers. Thus, the deep layers of the superior colliculus contain overlaid somatotopic and retinotopic maps, as well as a map of sound in space. For example, an area that receives information about the contralateral visual field will also receive information about sounds that originate from the contralateral auditory space, as well as information about somatic stimuli applied to the contralateral surface of the body. Moreover, the deep layers of the superior colliculus contain a motor map that controls eye and head position. For instance, activation of neurons in the superior colliculus by a visual target causes movement of the eyes to center the visual target on the fovea. In this way the superior colliculus is involved in reflex responses to the appearance of a novel or threatening object in the visual field. Similarly, a sound or a sudden contact with the body will elicit appropriate eye and head movement to enable visualization of the source of the stimulus. The descending pathways include connections to the oculomotor system and to the spinal cord through the tectospinal tract. See Chapter 9 for information on the role of the superior colliculus in eye movements.

Another retinal projection is to the **pretectum,** which bilaterally activates parasympathetic preganglionic neurons in the **Edinger-Westphal nucleus** that cause pupillary constriction in the pupillary light reflex. The pretectal areas are also interconnected through the posterior commissure, and thus the reflex causes both ipsilateral (direct) and contralateral (consensual) pupillary constriction when a light is shown in one eye.

The visual pathways also include connections to nuclei that serve functions other than vision. For example, a retinal projection to the **suprachiasmatic nucleus** of the hypothalamus controls circadian rhythmicity.

THE AUDITORY AND VESTIBULAR SYSTEMS

The peripheral parts of the auditory and vestibular systems share components of the bony and membranous labyrinths, use hair cells as mechanical transducers, and transmit information to the CNS through the vestibulocochlear (CN VIII) nerve. However, the CNS processing and sensory functions of the auditory and vestibular systems are distinct. The function of the auditory system is to transduce sound. This allows us to recognize environmental cues and to communicate with other organisms. The most complex auditory functions are those involved in language. The function of the vestibular system is to provide the CNS with information related to the position and movements of the head in space. Control of eye movement by the vestibular system is discussed in Chapter 9.

Audition
Sound
Sound is produced by compression and decompression waves that are transmitted in air or in other elastic media such as water. Sound frequency is measured in cycles per second, or **hertz (Hz).** Each pure tone results from a sinusoidal wave at a particular frequency, and each pure tone is characterized not only by its frequency but also, instantaneously, by its amplitude and phase (Fig. 8-15). Most naturally occurring sound, however, is actually a mixture of pure tones. **Noise** is unwanted sound and may have any composition of pure tones. Sound propagates at about 335 m/sec in air. The waves are associated with certain pressure changes, called sound pressure. The unit of sound pressure is N/m^2, but sound pressure is more commonly expressed as the **sound pressure level (SPL).** The unit of SPL is the **decibel (dB):**

● **Equation 8-1**

$$SPL = 20 \log P/P_R$$

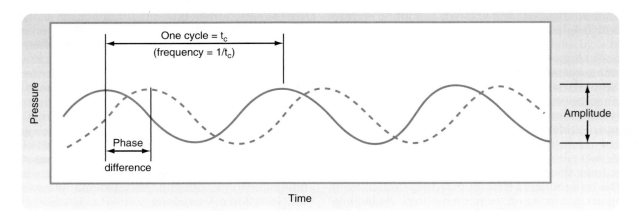

● **Figure 8-15.** Two pure tones are shown by the solid and dashed lines. Frequency is determined from the wavelength as indicated. Amplitude is the peak-to-peak change in sound pressure. Both tones have the same frequency and amplitude but differ in phase.

where P is sound pressure and P_R is a reference pressure (0.0002 dyne/cm², the absolute threshold for human hearing at 1000 Hz). A sound with intensity 10 times greater would be 20 dB; one 100 times greater would be 40 dB.

The normal young human ear is sensitive to pure tones with frequencies that range between about 20 and 20,000 Hz. The threshold for detection of a pure tone varies with its frequency (Fig. 8-16). The lowest thresholds for human hearing are for pure tones around 3000 Hz. The threshold at these frequencies is approximately –3 to –5 dB, as compared with the reference 0 dB at 1000 Hz. According to this scale, normal speech has an intensity of about 65 dB. The main frequencies used in speech fall in the range of 300 to 3500 Hz. Sounds that exceed 100 dB can damage the peripheral auditory apparatus, and those higher than 120 dB can cause pain and permanent damage. As people age, their thresholds at high frequencies rise, thereby reducing their ability to hear such tones, a condition called **presbycusis.**

The Ear
The peripheral auditory apparatus is the ear, which can be subdivided into the external ear, the middle ear, and the inner ear (Fig. 8-17).

External Ear. The external ear includes the pinna and the external auditory meatus (auditory canal). The auditory canal contains glands that secrete **cerumen,** a waxy protective substance. The pinna helps direct sounds into the auditory canal and plays a role in sound localization. The auditory canal transmits the sound pressure waves to the tympanic membrane. In humans, the auditory canal has a resonant frequency of about 3500 Hz, and this frequency contributes to the low threshold sensitivity in that range.

Middle Ear. The external ear is separated from the middle ear by the **tympanic membrane** (Fig. 8-17, *A*). The middle ear contains air. A chain of ossicles connect the tympanic membrane to the oval window, an opening into the inner ear. Adjacent to the oval window is the round window, another membrane-covered opening between the middle and inner ear (Fig. 8-17, *A* and *B*).

The ossicles include the **malleus,** the **incus,** and the **stapes.** The stapes has a footplate that inserts into the oval window. Behind the oval window is a fluid-filled component of the inner ear, the **vestibule.** It is continuous with a tubular structure known as the **scala vestibuli.** Inward movement of the tympanic membrane by a sound pressure wave causes the chain of ossicles to push the footplate of the stapes into the oval window (Fig. 8-17, *B*). This movement of the stapes footplate in turn displaces the fluid within the scala vestibuli. The pressure wave that ensues within the fluid is transmitted through the **basilar membrane** of the **cochlea** to the **scala tympani** (see later), and it causes the round window to bulge into the middle ear.

The tympanic membrane and the chain of ossicles serve as an impedance-matching device. The ear must detect sound waves traveling in air, but the neural transduction mechanism depends on movement in the fluid-filled cochlea, where acoustic impedance is much higher than that of air. Therefore, without a special device for impedance matching, most sound reaching the ear would simply be reflected, as are voices from shore when you are swimming under water. Impedance matching in the ear depends on (1) the ratio of the surface area of the large tympanic membrane to

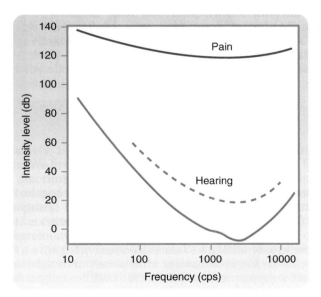

● **Figure 8-16.** Sound threshold intensities at different frequencies. The bottom curve indicates the absolute intensity needed to detect a sound. The dashed curve is the threshold for functional hearing. The top curve indicates levels at which sound is felt as painful.

IN THE CLINIC

The middle ear also serves other functions. Two muscles are found in the middle ear: the tensor tympani attached to the malleus and the stapedius attached to the stapes. When these muscles contract, they damp movements of the ossicles and decrease the sensitivity of the acoustic apparatus. This action can protect the acoustic apparatus against damaging sounds that can be anticipated. However, a sudden explosion can still damage the acoustic apparatus because reflex contraction of the middle ear muscles does not occur quickly enough. The chamber of the middle ear connects to the pharynx through the eustachian tube. Pressure differences between the external and middle ear can be equalized through this passage. If fluid collects in the middle ear, such as during an infection, the eustachian tube may become blocked. The resulting pressure difference between the external and middle ear can produce painful displacement of the tympanic membrane and, in extreme cases, by rupture of the tympanic membrane. Unequalized pressure changes as a result of flying or diving can also cause discomfort.

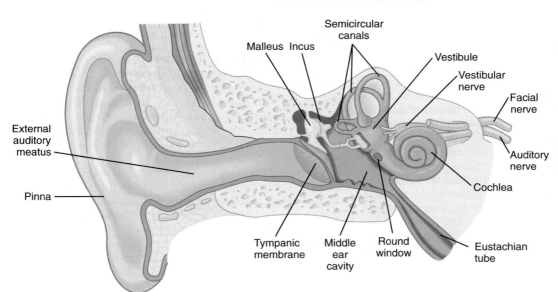

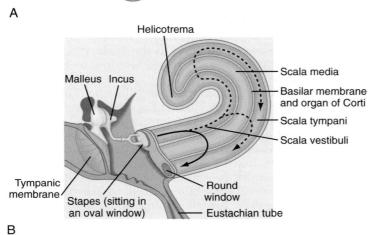

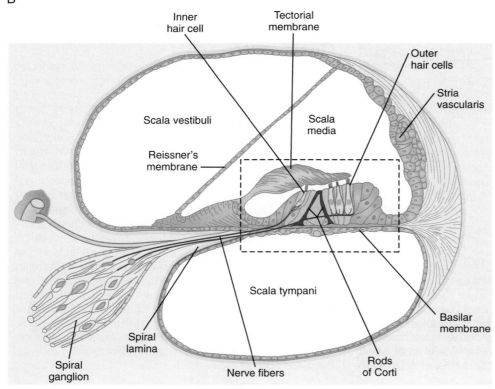

● **Figure 8-17.** Ear and cochlear structure. **A,** Location of the right human cochlea in relation to the vestibular apparatus and middle and external ears. **B,** Relationships between the outer, middle, and inner ear spaces, with the cochlea unrolled for clarity. **C,** Drawing of a cross section through the cochlea. The organ of Corti (Fig. 8-18, **A** and **B**) is outlined.

A

B

C

that of the smaller oval window and (2) the mechanical advantage of the lever system formed by the ossicle chain. This impedance matching is sufficient to increase the efficiency of energy transfer by nearly 30 dB in the range of hearing from 300 to 3500 Hz.

Inner Ear. The inner ear includes the bony and membranous labyrinths. The bony labyrinth is a complex, but continuous series of spaces in the temporal bone of the skull, whereas the membranous labyrinth consists of a series of soft tissue spaces and channels lying inside the bony labyrinth. The cochlea and the vestibular apparatus are formed from these structures.

The cochlea is a spiral-shaped organ (Fig. 8-17, *A* and *B*). In humans, the spiral consists of 2¾ turns from a broad base to a narrow apex, although its internal lumen is small at the base and wide at the top. The apex of the cochlea faces laterally (Fig. 8-17, *A*). The bony core around which the cochlea coils is the **modiolus.**

The bony labyrinth component of the cochlea is subdivided into several chambers. The vestibule is the space facing the oval window (Fig. 8-17, *A*). Continuous with the vestibule is the scala vestibuli, a spiral-shaped chamber that extends to the apex of the cochlea, where it meets and merges with the **scala tympani** at the **helicotrema.** The scala tympani is another spiral-shaped space that winds back down the cochlea to end at the round window (Fig. 8-17, *B*). Separating the two, except at the helicotrema, is the scala media enclosed in the membranous labyrinth.

The **scala media,** or **cochlear duct** (Fig. 8-17, *B* and *C*), is a membrane-bound spiral tube that extends 35 mm along the cochlea, between the scala vestibuli and scala tympani. One wall of the scala media is formed by the **basilar membrane,** another by **Reissner's membrane,** and the third by the **stria vascularis** (Fig. 8-17, *C*).

The spaces within the cochlea are filled with fluid. The fluid in the bony labyrinth, including the scala vestibuli and scala tympani, is **perilymph,** which closely resembles cerebrospinal fluid. The fluid in the membranous labyrinth, including the scala media, is endolymph, which is very different from perilymph. **Endolymph** contains high $[K^+]$ (about 145 mM) and low $[Na^+]$ (about 2 mM) and has a high positive potential (about +80 mV) with respect to the perilymph. As a result, a very large potential gradient (about 140 mV) exists across the membranes of the hair cell cilia that extend into the endolymph. (These hair cells, which are the sensory receptors for sound, are discussed in more detail later.) Endolymph is secreted by the stria vascularis and is drained through the endolymphatic duct into the dural venous sinuses.

The neural apparatus responsible for transduction of sound is the **organ of Corti** (Fig. 8-17, *C*), which is located within the cochlear duct. It lies on the basilar membrane and consists of several components, including three rows of **outer hair cells,** a single row of **inner hair cells,** a gelatinous **tectorial membrane,** and a number of types of supporting cells. The organ of Corti

in humans contains 15,000 outer and 3500 inner hair cells. The **rods of Corti** help provide a rigid scaffold. Located on the apical surface of the hair cells are stereocilia, which can be described as nonmotile cilia that contact the tectorial membrane.

The organ of Corti is innervated by nerve fibers that belong to the cochlear division of the eighth cranial nerve. The 32,000 auditory afferent fibers in humans originate in sensory ganglion cells in the **spiral ganglion,** which is located within the modiolus. These nerve fibers penetrate the organ of Corti and terminate at the base of the hair cells (see Fig. 8-17, *C* and 8-18). About 90% of the fibers end on inner hair cells, and the remainder end on outer hair cells. Thus, in this arrangement about 10 afferent fibers supply each inner hair cell, whereas other afferent fibers diverge to supply about five outer hair cells each. The inner hair cells clearly provide most of the neural information about acoustic signals that the CNS uses for hearing. The function of the outer hair cells is less clear.

In addition to afferent fibers, the organ of Corti is supplied by efferent fibers, most of which terminate on the outer hair cells. These cochlear efferents originate in the superior olivary nucleus of the brainstem and are often called **olivocochlear fibers.** The length of the outer hair cells varies; this characteristic suggests that changes in outer hair cell length may affect the sensitivity, or "tuning," of the inner hair cells. The cochlear efferent fibers may control outer hair cell length. Such a mechanism could conceivably influence the sensitivity of the cochlea and the way that the brain recognizes sound. Other efferent fibers that end on cochlear afferent fibers may be inhibitory, and they may help improve frequency discrimination.

Sound waves are transduced by the organ of Corti. Sound waves that reach the ear cause the tympanic membrane to oscillate, and these oscillations are transmitted to the scala vestibuli by the ossicles. This creates a pressure difference between the scala vestibuli and the scala tympani (Fig. 8-17, *B*) that serves to displace the basilar membrane and, with it, the organ of Corti (Fig. 8-18, *A* and *B*). Because of the shear forces set up by the relative displacement of the basilar and tectorial membranes, the stereocilia of the hair cells bend. Upward displacement bends the stereocilia toward the tallest cilium (away from the modiolus),

> ### ▶ IN THE CLINIC

A common cause of deafness is the destruction of hair cells by loud sounds. Hair cells can be destroyed, for example, by exposure to industrial noise or by listening to loud music. Typically, hair cells in certain parts of the cochlea are selectively damaged, and thus hearing may be lost over a discrete frequency range. Presbycusis, or the loss of high-frequency hearing with age, is probably increased by the loss of hair cells because of long-term noise exposure in urban environments.

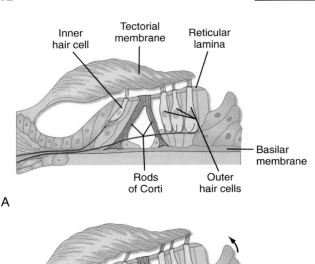

A

B

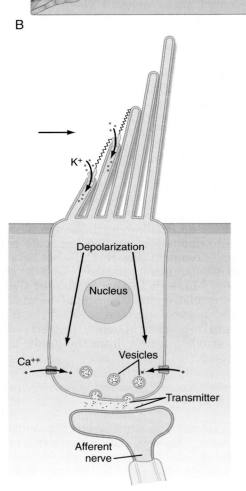

C

which depolarizes the hair cells; downward deflection bends the stereocilia in the opposite direction, which hyperpolarizes the hair cells.

Sound Transduction

In view of the wide range of frequencies and amplitudes of sound stimuli, it is no surprise that hair cell transduction must provide for a fast response. The fast response to deflection of the cilia is based on direct opening of ion channels by "tip links" that connect the tip of each stereocilium with the shaft of the next taller one (Fig. 8-18, *C*). With deflection, the tip links are subjected to a lever action that transiently opens the channels, permits the entry of K^+ (because of the high $[K^+]$ and high potential in endolymph), and depolarizes the hair cell. Several mechanisms have been proposed to account for the equally important rapid adaptation necessary for a high-frequency response. A "spring" response by the tip links would allow the attachment point of the tip link to be moved along the stereocilium's shaft to reset the mechanical leverage of the tip link. In addition, it has been observed that Ca^{++} can enter and bind to the open channel, change it to require greater opening force, and thereby reduce the statistical probability of opening.

The potential gradient that induces movement of ions into hair cells includes both the resting potential of the hair cells and the positive potential of the endolymph. As noted previously, the total gradient across the apical membrane of hair cells is about 140 mV. Therefore, a change in membrane conductance in the apical membranes of hair cells results in a rapid current flow that produces the receptor potential in these cells. This current flow can be recorded extracellularly as a **cochlear microphonic potential,** an oscillatory event that has the same frequency as the acoustic stimulus. The cochlear microphonic potential represents the sum of the receptor potentials of a number of hair cells.

Hair cells, like retinal photoreceptors, release an excitatory neurotransmitter (probably glutamate) when depolarized. The transmitter produces a generator potential in the cochlear afferent nerve fibers with which the hair cell synapses. In summary, sound is transduced when oscillatory movements of the basilar membrane cause transient changes in the transmembrane voltage of the hair cells and, consequently, the generation of action potentials in cochlear afferent nerve fibers. The activity of a large number of cochlear afferent fibers can be recorded extracellularly as a compound action potential.

● **Figure 8-18.** **A** and **B,** Detail of the area indicated in Figure 8-17, **C,** showing the organ of Corti and demonstrating how movement of the basilar membrane will cause the stereocilia to bend because of shear forces produced by relative displacement of the hair cells and the tectorial membrane. **C,** Diagram of a hair cell with tip-link connections between the hair cell cilia to demonstrate how shear forces open mechanoreceptor channels.

However, not all the cochlear afferent fibers discharge in response to a particular sound frequency. One factor that influences which afferent fibers discharge is their location along the organ of Corti. The location of an afferent fiber is important because for any given sound frequency, there is a site of maximum displacement as the pressure wave travels along the basilar membrane (Fig. 8-19). The location varies because the width and tension along the basilar membrane vary with distance from the base.

On the basis of these differences in width and tension, investigators originally concluded that different parts of the basilar membrane have different resonance frequencies. For example, the basilar membrane is about 100 μm wide at the base and 500 μm wide at the apex. It also has higher tension at the base. Thus, the base was predicted to vibrate at higher frequencies than the apex, as do the shorter strings of musical instruments. However, experiments have shown that the basilar membrane moves as a whole in traveling waves (Fig. 8-19). Movements of the basilar membrane are maximal nearer the base of the cochlea during high-frequency tones and maximal nearer the apex during low-frequency tones.

In effect, the basilar membrane serves as a frequency analyzer; it distributes the stimulus along the organ of Corti so that different hair cells will respond differentially to particular frequencies of sound. This is the basis of the **place theory of hearing.** In addition, hair cells located at different places along the organ of Corti are tuned to different frequencies because of differences in their stereocilia and biophysical properties. As a result of these factors, the basilar membrane and organ of Corti have a so-called tonotopic map (Fig. 8-20).

Cochlear Nerve Fibers

Transmitter release by hair cells in the organ of Corti causes action potentials in the primary afferent fibers of the cochlear nerve. These afferents of the vestibulocochlear nerve (CN VIII) are bipolar cells with a myelin sheath around the cell bodies, as well as around the axons. Their cell bodies are in the spiral ganglion, their peripheral processes end on hair cells, and their central processes terminate in the cochlear nuclei of the brainstem.

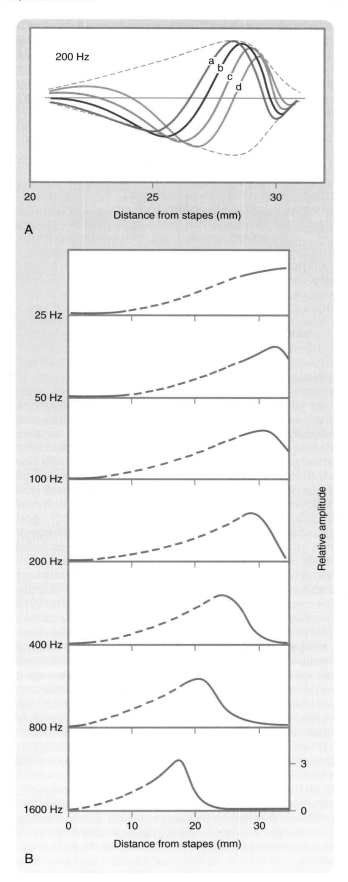

● **Figure 8-19.** Different frequencies of sound result in different amplitudes of displacement of the basilar membrane at different sites along the organ of Corti. **A,** Traveling wave produced in the basilar membrane by a sound of 200 Hz. The curves at a, b, c, and d represent displacement of the basilar membrane at different times, and the dashed line is the envelope formed by the peaks of the wave at different times. Maximum deflection occurs at about 29 mm from the oval window. **B,** Envelopes of traveling waves produced by several frequencies of sound. Note that the maximum displacement varies with frequency and is closest to the stapes when the frequency is highest. (Redrawn from von Bekesy G: Experiments in Hearing. New York, McGraw-Hill, 1960.)

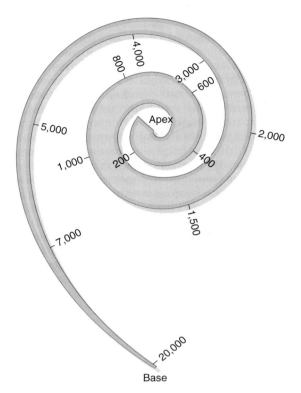

● **Figure 8-20.** Layout of the tonotopic map of the cochlea. (Redrawn from Stuhlman O: An Introduction to Biophysics. New York, John Wiley & Sons, 1943.)

Characteristic Frequencies. A cochlear afferent fiber discharges maximally when stimulated by a particular sound frequency called the **characteristic frequency** of that fiber. The characteristic frequency can be determined from a tuning curve for the fiber (Fig. 8-21). A **tuning curve** plots the threshold for activation of the nerve fiber by different sound frequencies. Typically, tuning curves are sharp near the characteristic frequency, but they broaden at high sound pressure levels. Tuning curves can have excitatory and inhibitory areas (Fig. 8-21, *A*). The sharpness of the excitatory regions may reflect inhibitory processes.

Encoding. The different features of an acoustic stimulus are encoded in the discharges of cochlear nerve fibers. Duration is signaled by the duration of activity; intensity is signaled both by the amount of neural activity and by the number of fibers that discharge. For low-frequency sounds, the frequency is signaled by the tendency of an afferent fiber to discharge in phase with the stimulus (**phase locking,** Fig. 8-22, *A*). Phase locking can also occur for sounds with periods shorter than the absolute refractory period of the afferent fiber. If the tone is much more than 1 kHz, a single fiber cannot discharge with every cycle. The CNS can detect higher-frequency information, however, from the activity of a population of afferent fibers, each of which discharges in phase with the stimulus and which, as a group, signal the frequency of the stimulus (Fig. 8-22, *B*). This observation is the basis of the **frequency theory of hearing.**

For still higher frequencies (>5000 Hz), the place theory must dominate, with the CNS interpreting sounds that activate afferent fibers supplying hair cells near the base of the cochlea as being of high frequency. Thus, both the place and the frequency theories are required to explain the frequency coding of sound **(duplex theory)** across the entire range from 20 to 20,000 Hz.

Central Auditory Pathway

Cochlear afferent fibers synapse on neurons of the dorsal and ventral cochlear nuclei. These neurons give rise to axons that contribute to the central auditory pathways. Some of the axons from the cochlear nuclei cross to the contralateral side and ascend in the **lateral lemniscus,** the main ascending auditory tract. Others connect with various ipsilateral or contralateral nuclei, such as the **superior olivary nuclei,** which project through the ipsilateral and contralateral lateral lemnisci. Each lateral lemniscus ends in an **inferior colliculus.** Neurons of the inferior colliculus project to the **medial geniculate nucleus** of the thalamus, which gives rise to the auditory radiation. The auditory radiation ends in the **auditory cortex** (areas 41 and 42), located in the transverse temporal gyri in the temporal lobe.

● **Figure 8-21.** Tuning curves of neurons in the auditory system. Tuning curves can be considered as receptive field plots. **A,** Tuning curve with excitatory (E) and inhibitory (I) regions. **B,** Tuning curves for cochlear nerve fibers *(upper left),* neurons in the inferior colliculus *(upper right),* trapezoid body *(lower left),* and medial geniculate nucleus *(lower right).* (**A,** Redrawn from Arthur RM et al: J Physiol [Lond] 212:593, 1971; **B,** redrawn from Katsui Y. In Rosenblith WA [ed]: Sensory Communication. Cambridge, MA, MIT Press, 1961.)

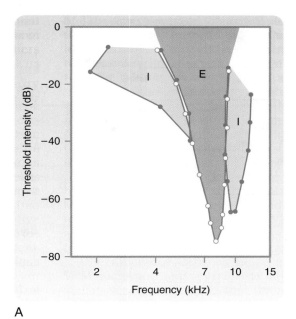

A

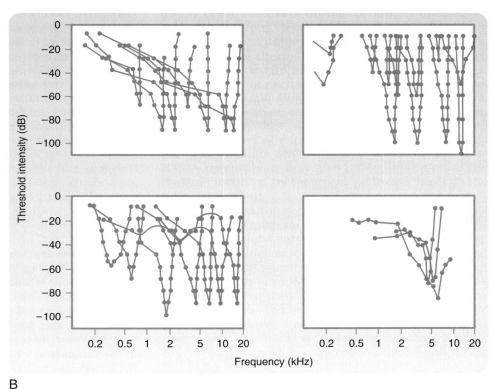

B

Functional Organization of the Central Auditory System

Receptive Fields and Tonotopic Maps. The responses of neurons in several structures that belong to the auditory system can be described by **tuning curves** (Fig. 8-21, *B*). By plotting the distribution of the characteristic frequencies of neurons within a nucleus or in the auditory cortex, a **tonotopic map** may be revealed in which neurons are ordered by their "best" frequencies. Tonotopic maps have been found in the cochlear nuclei, superior olivary complex, inferior colliculus, medial geniculate nucleus, and auditory cortex. A given auditory structure may, in fact, contain several tonotopic maps.

Binaural Interactions. Most auditory neurons at levels above the cochlear nuclei respond to stimulation of either ear (i.e., they have **binaural receptive fields**). Binaural receptive fields contribute to sound localization. A human can distinguish sounds originating from sources separated by as little as 1 degree.

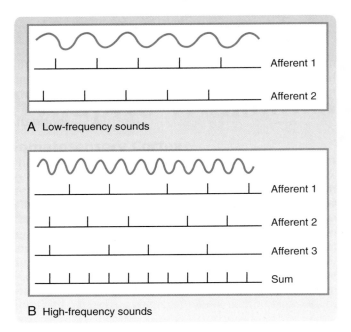

A Low-frequency sounds

B High-frequency sounds

● **Figure 8-22.** **A,** At low frequencies, individual auditory afferents can respond at each cycle to the signal frequency. **B,** At higher frequencies, each afferent generates an action potential only at certain cycles, limited by its maximum firing frequency. However, the overall population of afferents can still signal stimulus frequency by their aggregate firing frequency.

The auditory system uses several clues to judge the origin of sounds, including differences in the time (or phase) of arrival of the sound at the two ears and differences in sound intensity on the two sides of the head.

These factors provide information about the location of a sound by influencing the activity of neurons in the superior olivary complex. For example, neurons in the medial superior olivary nucleus have medial and lateral dendrites. The synapses on the medial dendrites are largely excitatory, and they originate from the contralateral ventral cochlear nucleus. Those on the lateral dendrites are mostly inhibitory and come from the ipsilateral ventral cochlear nucleus. Differences in the phase of the sound reaching the two ears affect the strength and timing of the excitation and inhibition reaching a particular medial olivary neuron. The activity of that neuron can then provide information about sound localization. The lateral superior olivary nucleus uses differences in the sound intensity that reaches the two ears to provide information about the source of the sound.

Cortical Organization. Several features of the primary auditory cortex resemble those of other primary sensory areas. Not only are sensory maps, in this case tonotopic maps, present in the auditory cortex, but this cortical region also performs feature extraction. Neurons in the primary auditory cortex form **isofrequency columns** (in which the neurons in the column have the same characteristic frequency), and they also form alternating columns, known as summation and suppression columns. Neurons in **summation columns** are more responsive to binaural

than to monaural input. Neurons in **suppression columns** are less responsive to binaural than to monaural stimulation, and accordingly, the response to one ear is dominant. Some neurons are selective for the direction of frequency change.

Bilateral lesions of the auditory cortex have some effect on the ability to distinguish the frequency or intensity of different sounds, and the ability to localize sound and to understand speech is reduced. Unilateral lesions, however, have little effect, especially if the nondominant (for language) hemisphere is involved (see Chapter 10). Evidently, frequency discrimination depends on activity at lower levels of the auditory pathway, possibly the inferior colliculus.

Auditory Testing

As already discussed, unilateral deafness can be caused by damage to the peripheral auditory apparatus or to the cochlear nuclei, but not by other CNS lesions. A discrete loss of hearing for particular frequencies can result from damage to a part of the organ of Corti (e.g., by exposure to intense sound, such as particularly loud music or industrial noise). The degree of deafness can be quantified for different frequencies by audiometry. In audiometry, each ear is presented with tones of different frequencies and intensities. An **audiogram** is plotted to show the thresholds of each ear for representative frequencies of sound. Comparison with the audiogram of normal individuals shows the auditory deficit (in decibels). The pattern of deficit aids in diagnosis of the cause of the hearing loss.

Two simple tests are often used clinically to distinguish the most important types of deafness: **conduction loss** and **sensorineural loss.** Conduction hearing loss occurs in disorders of the external ear (e.g., ear canal blocked by cerumen) or middle ear (e.g., rupture of the eardrum). Sensorineural hearing loss reflects disorders of the inner ear, the cochlear nerve, or central connections.

The **Weber test** is used to evaluate the magnitude of conduction hearing loss. In this test the base of a vibrating tuning fork is placed against the middle of the forehead and the subject is asked to localize the sound. Normally, the sound is not localized to a particular ear. However, if the person has conductive hearing loss (e.g., because of a punctured tympanic membrane, fluid in the middle ear, otosclerosis, or loss of continuity of the ossicular chain), the sound is localized to the deaf ear because it is conducted to the cochlea through bone. The sound is also conducted to the cochlea of the undamaged ear, but bone-conducted sound does not activate the organ of Corti as well as sound conducted normally through the tympanic membrane and ossicle chain. One reason why the sound in the Weber test is not localized to the normal ear may be that hearing in the normal ear is inhibited by the ambient sound level **(auditory masking).** Conversely, in subjects with sensorineural hearing loss (e.g., because of damage to the organ of Corti, the cochlear nerve, or the cochlear nuclei), the sound is localized to the normal side.

In the **Rinne test,** a vibrating tuning fork is placed against the mastoid process, and the subject is asked to indicate when the sound dies out. The tuning fork is then held near the external auditory meatus. In normal subjects the sound is again heard because the sound is more effectively transmitted to the cochlea in air (i.e., air conduction>bone conduction). If the conduction mechanism is damaged, the sound is not heard when the tuning fork is held near the external auditory meatus. Bone conduction in this case is better than air conduction. If the hearing loss is sensorineural, the sound is heard again when the tuning fork is placed by the external auditory meatus because with sensorineural hearing loss, the inner ear and cochlear nerve are less able to transmit impulses regardless of whether the sound vibrations reach the cochlea via air or bone. Thus, because air conduction is more effective than bone conduction, the bone conduction pattern seen with sensorineural hearing loss is the same as in a normal ear.

The Vestibular System

The vestibular system detects angular and linear accelerations of the head. Signals from the vestibular system trigger head and eye movements to stabilize the visual image on the retina and allow the body to make adjustments in posture that maintain balance. The following description of the vestibular system emphasizes the sensory aspects of vestibular function, and it introduces the central vestibular pathways. The role of the vestibular apparatus in motor control is discussed in Chapter 9.

The Vestibular Apparatus

Structure of the Vestibular Labyrinth. The vestibular apparatus, like the cochlea, consists of a component of the membranous labyrinth located within the bony labyrinth. The vestibular apparatus on each side is composed of three **semicircular canals** and two **otolith organs** (Fig. 8-23; see also Fig. 8-17, *A*). These structures are surrounded by perilymph and contain endolymph. The semicircular canals include the **horizontal, superior,** and **posterior** canals. The otolith organs include the **utricle** and the **saccule.** A swelling called an **ampulla** is found on each semicircular canal where it joins the utricle. The semicircular canals all connect with the utricle. The utricle joins the saccule through the ductus reuniens. The endolymphatic duct originates from the **ductus reuniens,** and it ends in the **endolymphatic sac.** The saccule connects with the cochlea, through which endolymph (produced by the stria vascularis of the cochlea) can reach the vestibular apparatus.

The three semicircular canals on one side are matched with corresponding coplanar semicircular canals on the other side. The horizontal canals on each side of the head correspond, as do the superior canal on one side and the posterior canal on the other side (Fig. 8-23, *B*). This arrangement allows the sensory epithelia, in corresponding pairs of canals on the two sides, to cooperate in sensing movement of the head in all planes. An important feature of the horizontal canals is that they are in the horizontal plane with respect to the horizon if the head is first tilted down 30 degrees. The utricle is oriented nearly horizontally; the saccule is oriented vertically.

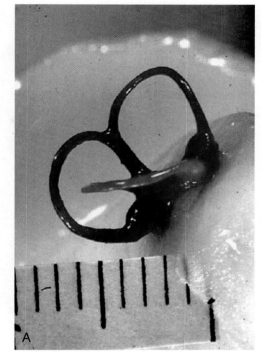

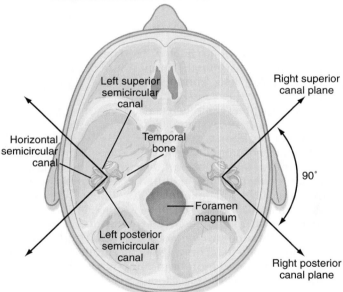

● **Figure 8-23.** **A,** Lateral view of the right semicircular canals of a Rhesus monkey dissected after filling with plastic. Scale in mm. (Courtesy of Dr. John Simpson, New York University School of Medicine.) **B,** View of the base of the skull showing the orientation of structures of the inner ear. Coplanar pairs of semicircular canals include the horizontal canals, as well as the superior and contralateral posterior canals. (Redrawn from Haines DE [ed]: Fundamental Neuroscience for Basic and Clinical Applications, 3rd ed. Philadelphia, Churchill Livingstone, 2006.)

The ampulla of each of the semicircular canals contains a sensory epithelium. The sensory epithelium in a semicircular canal is called a **crista ampullaris,** or **ampullary crest** (Fig. 8-24). An ampullary crest consists of a ridge that is covered by epithelium in which

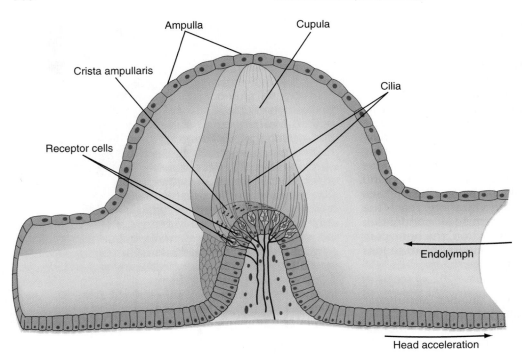

Ampulla   Cupula

Crista ampullaris

Cilia

Receptor cells

Endolymph

Head acceleration

● **Figure 8-24.** Drawing of an ampullary crest inside an ampulla. The stereocilia and the kinocilium of each hair cell extend into the cupula, which extends across the entire cross section of the ampulla.

there are vestibular hair cells. These hair cells are innervated by primary afferent fibers of the vestibular nerve, which is a subdivision of the eighth cranial nerve.

Like cochlear hair cells, each vestibular hair cell contains a set of stereocilia on its apical surface. However, unlike cochlear hair cells, vestibular hair cells also contain a large single kinocilium. The cilia on ampullary hair cells are embedded in a gelatinous structure called the cupula. The cupula crosses the ampulla and occludes its lumen completely. Movement of endolymph, produced by angular acceleration of the head in the plane of the canal, deflects the cupula and consequently bends the cilia on the hair cells. The cupula has the same specific gravity as endolymph, and thus it is unaffected by linear acceleratory forces, such as that exerted by gravity.

The sensory epithelia of the otolith organs are called the **macula utriculi** and the **macula sacculi** (Fig. 8-25). The hair cells are embedded in the epithelium that overlies each macula. As in the ampullary crests, the stereocilia and kinocilia of the macula project into a gelatinous mass. However, the gelatinous mass in the macula contains numerous otoliths ("ear stones") composed of calcium carbonate crystals. Together, the gelatinous mass and its otoliths are known as an **otolithic membrane.** The otoliths increase the specific gravity of the otolithic membrane to about twice that of the endolymph. Hence, the otolithic membrane tends to move when subjected to acceleration, whether linear, such as that produced by gravity, or angular, particularly when the center of rotation is outside the head.

Innervation of Sensory Epithelia of the Vestibular Apparatus. The cell bodies of the primary afferent fibers of the vestibular nerve are located in Scarpa's ganglion. The neurons are bipolar, and their cell bodies, as well as axons, are myelinated. The vestibular nerve gives off separate branches to each of the sensory epithelia. The vestibular nerve is accompanied by the cochlear and facial nerves as it enters the internal auditory meatus of the skull.

Vestibular Transduction

Like cochlear hair cells, vestibular hair cells are functionally polarized, and the transduction mechanism is presumed to be similar. When the stereocilia are bent toward the longest cilium (in this case, the **kinocilium**), conductance of the apical membrane increases for cations, and the vestibular hair cell is depolarized (Fig. 8-26). Conversely, when the cilia are bent away from the kinocilium, the hair cell is hyperpolarized. The hair cell releases an excitatory neurotransmitter (either glutamate or aspartate) tonically, so the afferent fiber on which it synapses has a resting discharge. When the hair cell is depolarized, more transmitter is released, and the discharge rate of the afferent fiber increases. Conversely, when the hair cell is hyperpolarized, less transmitter is released, and the firing rate of the afferent fiber slows or stops.

Semicircular Canals. Angular accelerations of the head produce minute movement of the endolymph in relation to the head (Fig. 8-27). This happens because the inertia of the endolymph causes it to shift in relation to the wall of the membranous labyrinth. This lag distorts the cupula, causes the cilia to bend, and consequently changes the discharge rates of the

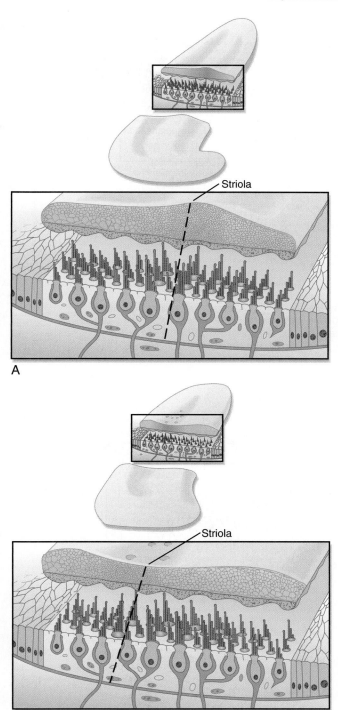

Striola

A

Striola

B

● **Figure 8-25.** Structure of the otolith organs. The saccule is shown in **A** and the utricle in **B**. (Redrawn from Lindeman HH: Adv Otorhinolaryngol 20:405, 1973.)

be exemplified by the activity that originates from the horizontal canals. Figure 8-27 shows the horizontal canals and utricle, as seen from above. The hair cells in these canals are polarized toward the utricle. Thus, movement of the endolymph and cilia toward the utricle increases the discharge rate of the afferent fibers, and conversely, movement of the endolymph and cilia away from the utricle reduces the discharge rate.

In Figure 8-27, the head is rotated to the left. As acceleration to the left begins, inertia causes the endolymph in the horizontal canals to increase pressure toward the right. This bends the cilia on hair cells of the ampulla of the left horizontal canal toward the utricle and bends the cilia of the right canal away from the utricle. These actions increase the firing rate in the afferent fibers on the left and decrease the firing rate of the afferent fibers on the right. At a constant velocity of rotation (i.e., no acceleration), there would be no force on either cupula, and therefore the hair cells of both canals would be firing as at rest and at the same rate. However, when the indicated rotation is stopped, the inertia of the endolymph creates a force on both cupulas, but in the opposite direction. This results in an increase in the discharge rate of afferent fibers on the right side and a decrease in the discharge rate on the left. This postrotatory effect is of functional and clinical significance.

Otolith Organs. The hair cells in the otolith organs, unlike those in the ampullary crests, are not all oriented in the same direction. Instead, they are oriented with respect to a ridge, called the **striola,** along the otolith organ (Fig. 8-25). In the utricle the hair cells on either side of the striola are polarized toward the striola, whereas in the saccule they are polarized away from the striola. Because the striola in each otolith organ is curved, there are hair cells with all orientations in the plane of the organ (Fig. 8-28). When the head is tilted so that gravity produces a different linear acceleration, the otolithic membranes shift and the cilia of the hair cells bend in a new way. This bending of the cilia of the hair cells changes the pattern of input from the otolith organs to the CNS. Similarly, a linear acceleration caused by other forces, such as might occur in a

vestibular afferent fibers. All the cilia in a given ampullary crest are oriented in the same direction. In the horizontal canal, the cilia are oriented toward the utricle, and in the other ampullae they are oriented away from the utricle.

The way in which angular acceleration of the head affects the discharge of vestibular afferent fibers can

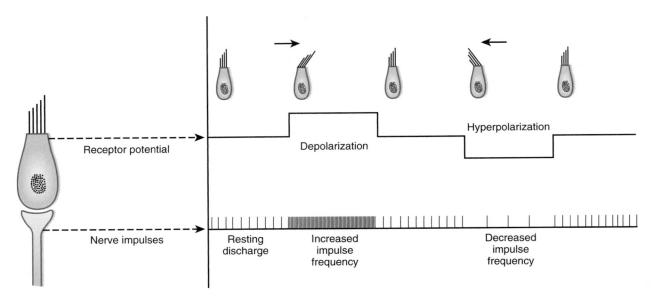

● **Figure 8-26.** Functional polarization of vestibular hair cells. When the stereocilia are bent toward the kinocilium, the hair cell is depolarized and the afferent fiber is excited. When the stereocilia are bent away from the kinocilium, the hair cell is hyperpolarized and the afferent discharge slows or stops. (Redrawn from Kandel ER, Schwartz JH: Principles of Neural Science. New York, Elsevier, 1981.)

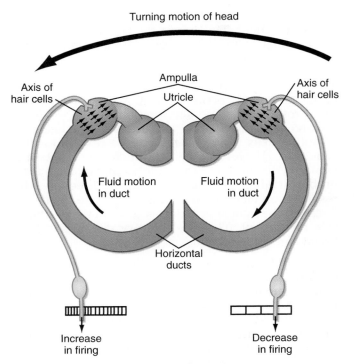

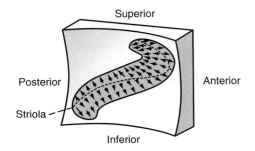

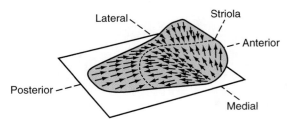

● **Figure 8-27.** Effect of head movement to the left on the activity of vestibular afferent fibers supplying hair cells in the horizontal semicircular canals. Small arrows in the ampulla indicate the functional polarity of the hair cells. The large curved arrow, top, indicates movement of the head; smaller curved arrows indicate relative movement of the endolymph.

● **Figure 8-28.** Functional polarization of hair cells in the otolith organs. **A,** The saccule. **B,** The utricle. The striola in each case is indicated by the dotted line. (Redrawn from Spoendlin HH. In Wolfson RJ [ed]: The Vestibular System and Its Diseases. Philadelphia, University of Pennsylvania Press, 1966.)

fall or the angular acceleration when turning a car around a curve (angular accelerations have linear centripetal and instantaneous tangential components), will also affect output from the otolith organs.

Central Vestibular Pathways

The vestibular afferent fibers project to the brainstem through the vestibular nerve. As previously mentioned, the cell bodies of these afferent fibers are located in Scarpa's ganglion. The afferent fibers terminate in the **vestibular nuclei,** (Fig. 4-7, *D* to *E*), which are located in the rostral medulla and caudal pons. Afferent fibers from different parts of the vestibular apparatus end in different vestibular nuclei and also give off collaterals to the **cerebellum.**

The vestibular nuclei give rise to various projections, including projections through the **medial longitudinal fasciculus** (Fig. 4-7, *B* to *E*) to the oculomotor nuclei. Therefore, it is not surprising that the vestibular nuclei exert powerful control over eye movements (the **vestibuloocular reflex**). Other projections give rise to the **lateral** and **medial vestibulospinal tracts,** which provide, respectively, for the activation of trunk and neck muscles and thereby contribute to equilibrium and to head movements **(vestibulocolic reflex).** There are vestibular projections to the cerebellum, the reticular formation, and the contralateral vestibular complex, as well as to the thalamus. The latter mediate conscious sensation of vestibular activity. Vestibular reflexes and clinical tests of vestibular function are described in Chapter 9.

THE CHEMICAL SENSES

The senses of **gustation** (taste) and **olfaction** (smell) depend on chemical stimuli that are present either in food and drink or in the air. In the evolution of humans, these chemical senses did not have the survival value of some of the other senses, but they contribute considerably to quality of life and are important stimulants of digestion. In other animals, the chemical senses have greater survival value, and their activation evokes a number of social behaviors, including mating, territoriality, and feeding.

Taste

The stimuli that we know as tastes or flavors are actually mixtures of five elementary taste qualities: salty, sweet, sour, bitter, and umami. Taste stimuli that are particularly effective in eliciting these sensations are, respectively, sodium chloride, sucrose, hydrochloric acid, quinine, and monosodium glutamate. Umami has been described as a proteinaceous, meaty flavor.

Taste Receptors

The sensation of taste depends on the activation of chemoreceptors located in taste buds. A taste bud consists of a group of 50 to 150 receptor cells, as well as supporting cells and basal cells (Fig. 8-29, *A*). The chemoreceptor cells synapse at their bases with primary afferent nerve fibers. Two types of chemoreceptor cells can be distinguished by differences in

their synaptic vesicle content: one type has dense core vesicles, whereas the other has clear round vesicles. The apices of the cells have microvilli that extend toward a taste pore. Chemoreceptor cells live only about 10 days. They are continuously replaced by new chemoreceptor cells that differentiate from basal cells located near the base of the taste bud.

Chemoreceptor molecules, each specialized for one type of taste stimulus, sit on the microvilli of chemoreceptor cells and detect stimulatory molecules that diffuse into the taste pore from the overlying fluid layer. Part of this fluid originates from glands adjacent to the taste buds. Some stimuli can pass directly into the cell to depolarize it (Na^+ and H^+ for salty and sour) or open cation channels to generate a receptor potential (also salty and sour), whereas others (sucrose, quinine, and glutamate for sweet, bitter, and umami) activate a second messenger that can either open cation channels or directly activate intracellular Ca^{++} stores (Fig. 8-29, *B*). In each case, depolarization of the receptor evokes a generator potential that results in the release of an excitatory neurotransmitter and, consequently, action potentials in the primary afferent nerve fiber that are transmitted to the CNS.

Coding of taste, however, is not based entirely on the selectivity of the chemoreceptors for the different primary qualities because each cell responds to a range of stimuli, though most intensely to one. Since most natural flavors have chemicals that effect responses from a number of chemoreceptors, recognition of taste quality appears to depend on the patterned input from a population of chemoreceptors, each responding differentially to the components of the stimulus. The intensity of the stimulus is reflected in the total amount of activity evoked.

Distribution and Innervation of Taste Buds

Taste buds are located on different types of taste papillae found on the tongue, palate, pharynx, and larynx. Types of taste papillae include **fungiform** and **foliate papillae** on the anterior and lateral aspects, respectively, of the tongue and **circumvallate papillae** on the base of the tongue (Fig. 8-29, *C*). The latter may contain several hundred taste buds. The tongue in humans may have several thousand taste buds. The sensitivity of different regions of the tongue for different taste qualities varies only slightly because taste buds responding to each type of flavor are widely distributed. The taste buds are innervated by three cranial nerves. The chorda tympani branch of the **facial nerve** (CN VII) supplies taste buds on the anterior two thirds of the tongue, and the **glossopharyngeal nerve** (CN IX) supplies taste buds on the posterior third of the tongue (Fig. 8-29, *C*). The **vagus nerve** (CN X) supplies a few taste buds in the larynx and upper esophagus.

Central Taste Pathways

The cell bodies of taste fibers in cranial nerves VII, IX, and X are located in the **geniculate, petrosal,** and **nodose ganglia,** respectively. The central processes of the afferent fibers enter the medulla, join the solitary tract, and synapse in the **nucleus of the solitary**

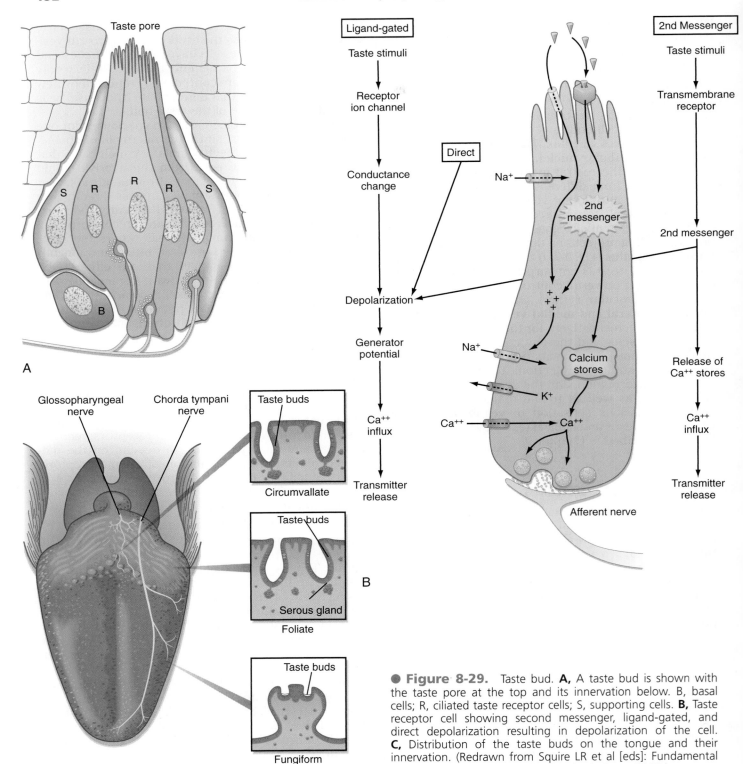

A

B

C

● Figure 8-29. Taste bud. **A,** A taste bud is shown with the taste pore at the top and its innervation below. B, basal cells; R, ciliated taste receptor cells; S, supporting cells. **B,** Taste receptor cell showing second messenger, ligand-gated, and direct depolarization resulting in depolarization of the cell. **C,** Distribution of the taste buds on the tongue and their innervation. (Redrawn from Squire LR et al [eds]: Fundamental Neuroscience. San Diego, CA, Academic Press, 2002.)

tract (Fig. 4-7, *D–F*). In some animals, including several rodent species, the second-order taste neurons of the solitary nucleus project rostrally to the ipsilateral parabrachial nucleus. The parabrachial nucleus then projects to the small-celled (parvocellular) part of the **ventroposterior medial** (VPMc) nucleus of the thala-

mus. In monkeys, the solitary nucleus projects directly to the VPMc nucleus. The VPMc nucleus is connected to two different gustatory areas of the cerebral cortex, one in the face area of the S1 cortex and the other in the insula. An unusual feature of the central gustatory pathway is that it is predominantly an

● **Figure 8-30.** Olfactory chemoreceptors and supporting cells. (Redrawn from de Lorenzo AJD. In Zotterman Y [ed]: Olfaction and Taste. Elmsford, NY, Pergamon, 1963.)

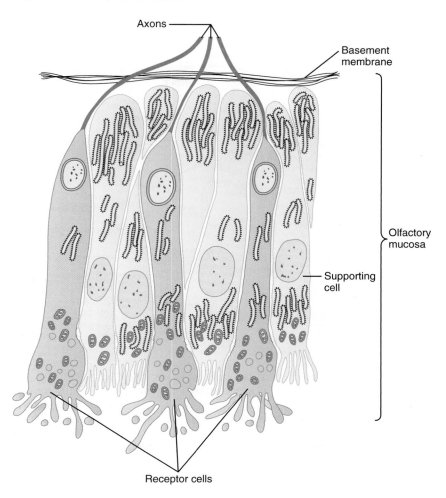

Axons

Basement membrane

Olfactory mucosa

Supporting cell

Receptor cells

uncrossed pathway (unlike the central somatosensory, visual, and auditory pathways, which are predominantly crossed).

Olfaction

The sense of smell is much better developed in animals **(macrosmatic animals)** than in humans and other primates **(microsmatic animals).** The ability of dogs to track other animals on the basis of odor is legendary, as is the use of **pheromones** by insects to attract mates. However, olfaction contributes to our emotional life, and odors can effectively call up memories. In addition, it helps us avoid consuming spoiled food and lets us detect dangerous situations, for example, the strong odorant added to odorless, colorless natural gas.

Olfactory Receptors

The olfactory chemoreceptor cells are located in the **olfactory mucosa,** a specialized part of the nasopharynx. Olfactory chemoreceptors are bipolar nerve cells (Fig. 8-30). The nonmotile cilia on the apical surface of these cells contain chemoreceptors that detect odorant chemicals dissolved in the overlying mucus layer. From the basal surface, the cell gives off an unmyelinated axon that joins other **olfactory nerve filaments** and penetrates the base of the skull through openings in the **cribriform plate** of the ethmoid bone. These olfactory nerves synapse in the **olfactory bulb,** a portion of the cerebral hemisphere of the brain located at the base of the cranial cavity, just below the frontal lobe (Fig. 8-31).

Humans have about 10 million olfactory chemoreceptors. Like taste cells, olfactory chemoreceptors have a short life span (about 60 days), and they are also continuously replaced. However, olfactory

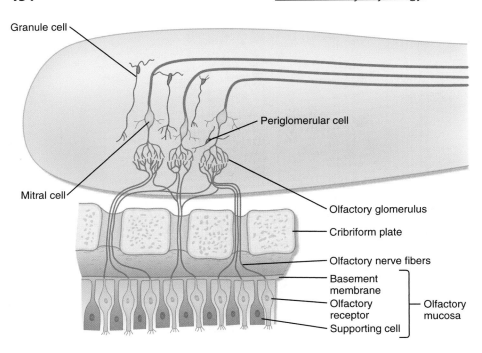

Granule cell

Periglomerular cell

Mitral cell

Olfactory glomerulus

Cribriform plate

Olfactory nerve fibers

Basement membrane

Olfactory receptor

Supporting cell

Olfactory mucosa

● **Figure 8-31.** Drawing of a sagittal section through an olfactory bulb showing terminations of the olfactory chemoreceptor cells in the olfactory glomerulus and the intrinsic neurons of the olfactory bulb. The axons of the mitral cells are shown exiting in the olfactory tract to the right. (Modified from House EL, Pansky B: A Functional Approach to Neuroanatomy, 2nd ed. New York, McGraw-Hill, 1967.)

receptor cells are true neurons and, as such, are the only neurons that are continuously regenerated throughout life.

Odorant molecules are introduced to the olfactory mucosa by ventilatory air currents or from the oral cavity during feeding. Sniffing increases the influx of odorants. The odorants are temporarily bound in mucus to an olfactory binding protein that is secreted by a gland in the nasal cavity.

Odor has more primary qualities than taste does. As many as 1000 different odor receptors are coded in the human genome, and although we probably have only about 350 functional types, they represent the largest population of G protein–coupled receptors in the genome. The olfactory mucosa also contains somatosensory receptors of the trigeminal nerve. When performing clinical tests of olfaction, it is necessary to avoid activating these somatosensory receptors with thermal or noxious stimuli, such as the ammonia used in "smelling salts."

Olfactory coding resembles taste coding in that most natural odors consist of molecules that excite olfactory chemoreceptors of more than one odorant class. Coding for a particular perceived odor depends on the responses of many olfactory chemoreceptors, and the strength of the odorant is represented by the overall amount of afferent neural activity.

Central Pathways

The initial relay of the olfactory pathway is located in the olfactory bulb, which is a specialized portion of the cerebral cortex. It contains **mitral cells** and interneurons **(granule cells; periglomerular cells)** (Fig. 8-31). The dendrites of mitral cells are long, and they branch to form the postsynaptic components of the olfactory glomeruli. The olfactory afferent fibers that reach the olfactory bulb from the olfactory mucosa

ramify as they approach the olfactory glomeruli and synapse on the dendrites of mitral cells. Each glomerulus is the target of thousands of olfactory afferents, each of which share the same type of olfactory receptor. This is all the more remarkable because olfactory receptor cells are being regenerated continuously and new axons must therefore navigate their way to a correct glomerulus. The granule and periglomerular cells are inhibitory interneurons. They form **dendrodendritic reciprocal synapses** with the dendrites of mitral cells. Activity in a mitral cell depolarizes the inhibitory cells that synapse with it, and they in turn release GABA, an inhibitory neurotransmitter, back into the original and adjacent glomeruli. Because each glomerulus is specialized by being the target of specific olfactory afferents for a unique combination of odor qualities, this appears to be a way of enhancing stimulus contrast, much the way horizontal cells do in the retina. In addition, it provides a mechanism for adaptation to continuous stimulation.

The axons of mitral cells leave the olfactory bulb and enter the olfactory tracts. From here, the olfactory connections become highly complex. Within the olfactory tracts is a nucleus, called the **anterior olfactory nucleus,** that receives input from the olfactory bulb and projects to the contralateral olfactory bulb through the **anterior commissure.** As each olfactory tract approaches the base of the brain, it splits into the **lateral** and **medial olfactory striae.** Axons of the lateral olfactory stria synapse in the primary olfactory cortex, which includes the **prepiriform cortex** (and, in many animals, the piriform lobe). The medial olfactory stria includes projections to the **amygdala,** as well as to the basal forebrain. These structures are portions of, or directly connected to, the limbic system (see Chapters 10 and 11).

> **IN THE CLINIC**

Olfaction is not generally examined in a routine neurological examination. However, smell can be tested by having the patient inhale and identify an odorant. One nostril should be examined at a time while the other nostril is occluded. Strong odorants, such as ammonia, should be avoided because they also activate trigeminal nerve fibers. Smell sensation can be lost **(anosmia)** after a basal skull fracture or after damage to one or both olfactory bulbs or tracts by a tumor (such as an **olfactory groove meningioma**). An aura of a disagreeable odor, often the smell of burning rubber, occurs during **uncinate fits,** which are epileptic seizures that originate in the medial temporal lobe.

Note that the olfactory pathway is the only sensory system that does not have an obligatory synaptic relay in the thalamus before reaching the cortex. However, olfactory information does reach the mediodorsal nucleus of the thalamus, and it is then transmitted to the prefrontal and orbitofrontal cortex. The functional roles of olfaction, in addition to the conscious perception of odor, include providing much of the subtleties of taste by enhancing the narrow range of gustatory receptors with the wide repertoire of olfactory receptors. In addition, via its intimate connections with limbic and, by extension, hypothalamic structures, it provides input to subconscious mechanisms related to emotions, memory, and sexual behavior.

■ KEY CONCEPTS

1. Light enters the eye through the cornea and lens and is focused on the retina, which lines the back of the eye. The cornea is the most powerful refractive surface, but the lens has a variable power that allows images of near objects to be focused on the retina. The iris regulates depth of field and the amount of illumination that enters the eye.

2. The outer segments of the photoreceptor cells transduce light. Photoreceptors synapse on retinal bipolar cells, which in turn synapse on other interneurons and on ganglion cells. The ganglion cells project to the brain through the optic nerve. The optic disc, where the optic nerve leaves the retina, contains no photoreceptors and is therefore a blind spot. The portion of the retina with the highest degree of spatial resolution is the fovea and the surrounding macula.

3. Rod photoreceptors have high sensitivity, no color discrimination, and function best under low light levels. Cone photoreceptors have lower sensitivity but higher spatial resolution. Color vision relies on the three types of cones having different spectral sensitivities.

4. Bipolar cells and many ganglion cells have receptive fields with an on-center/off-surround or off-center/on-surround organization. The horizontal cells mediate the center-surround antagonism. Photoreceptor, bipolar, and horizontal cells modulate their membrane potential in response to stimulation, but ganglion cells generate action potentials.

5. The axons of ganglion cells in the temporal retina project to the brain ipsilaterally; those in the nasal retina cross in the optic chiasm. The result is that, because the lens inverts the image that falls on the retina, each side of the visual field, from both eyes, is projected to the contralateral side of the brain. In the lateral geniculate nucleus (LGN) of the thalamus, the input from each eye terminates in separate layers, and the M ganglion cells (sensitive to motion) and P ganglion cells (sensitive to detail and color) project to separate layers as well.

6. The LGN projects to primary visual (striate) cortex via the visual radiation and terminates largely in layer 4, where there is an orderly retinotopic map. Within the map, information from one or the other eye terminates at adjacent points to create ocular dominance columns that extend vertically in the cortex. Striate cortical neurons outside of layer 4 respond best to bars or edges oriented in a particular way. Cells that prefer a particular stimulus orientation are grouped in orientation columns.

7. The many cortical extrastriate visual areas have different functions. Some in the inferotemporal cortex are influenced chiefly by P cells, and they function in form detection, color vision, and face discrimination. M cells influence regions of the middle temporal and parietal cortex, which function in motion detection and the control of eye movements.

8. A pure tone is characterized in terms of its amplitude, frequency, and phase. Natural sounds are combinations of pure tones. Sound pressure is measured in decibels (dB), relative to a reference level.

9. The pinna and auditory canal convey airborne sound waves to the tympanic membrane. The three small bones (ossicles) of the middle ear transmit the vibrations of the tympanic membrane to the oval window of the fluid-filled inner ear. Hearing is most sensitive at about 3000 Hz because of the dimensions of the auditory canal and the mechanics of the ossicles.

10. The cochlea of the inner ear has three main compartments: the scala vestibuli, the scala tympani, and the scala media (cochlear duct). The cochlear duct is bounded on one side by the basilar membrane, on which lies the organ of Corti, the sound transduction mechanism.

11. When the basilar membrane oscillates in response to pressure waves introduced into the scala vestibuli at the oval window, the stereocilia of the hair cells of the organ of Corti are subjected to shear

forces, which open mechanoreceptor channels. This results in a membrane conductance change that creates a generator potential in cochlear nerve fibers.

12. High-frequency sounds best activate the hair cells near the base of the cochlea, and low-frequency sounds activate cells near the apex. Such a tonotopic organization is also found in central auditory structures, including the cochlear nuclei, superior olivary complex, inferior colliculus, medial geniculate nucleus, and primary auditory cortex.

13. Auditory processing at many sites in the central auditory pathway contributes to sound localization, frequency and intensity analysis, and speech recognition.

14. The vestibular apparatus is part of the inner ear. It includes three semicircular canals (horizontal, superior, and posterior) and two otolith organs (utricle and saccule) on each side. These transduce, respectively, angular and linear accelerations of the head. The three semicircular canals are mutually orthogonal, so they can resolve angular acceleration of the head about any axis of rotation.

15. In each semicircular canal, there are sensory hair cells whose cilia extend into a cupula, which blocks the cross section of the endolymph-filled canal. Angular head acceleration displaces the endolymph and the cupula, bending the cilia. If the stereocilia bend toward the kinocilium, the hair cell is depolarized, causing an increase in the firing rate in the afferent fiber.

16. In the otolith organs, the cilia project into an otolithic membrane. Acceleration of the head, such as with linear movement or change in position with respect to gravity, displaces the otolithic membrane (because of the mass of the otoliths) and changes the firing patterns of the hair cells, depending on their orientation.

17. Central vestibular pathways include afferent connections to the vestibular nuclei and the cerebellum. Activation of the vestibular afferents is detected by the brain as head acceleration or position change and is relayed via the vestibular nuclei to pathways that mediate compensatory eye movements, neck movements, and adjustments to posture.

18. Taste buds contain chemoreceptor cells arranged around a taste pore. Taste buds are located on several kinds of papillae on the tongue and in the pharynx and larynx. Five types of taste-receptor cells detect the five elementary qualities of taste: salty, sweet, sour, bitter, and umami. Complex flavors are signaled by patterned population codes using multiple classes of receptor and by central correlation with accompanying olfactory input.

19. Afferent taste fibers synapse in the nucleus of the solitary tract. The thalamic relay is to a part of the VPM nucleus, and the taste-receiving areas are located in the S-I cortex and the insula.

20. Odors are detected by olfactory chemoreceptor cells, which are continuously regenerated in the olfactory mucosa. These cells are true neurons, which are endowed with a wide array of G protein–coupled receptors that permit the detection of hundreds of odor molecules.

21. Individual olfactory axons project to olfactory glomeruli, specific for each stimulus type, in the olfactory bulb. They synapse on the dendrites of mitral cells, which have reciprocal synapse with inhibitory interneurons. This synaptic organization in the glomerulus underlies stimulus adaptation and contrast enhancement.

CHAPTER 9

Organization of Motor Function

Movements are the major way that we interact with the world. Most of our activities, whether running, reaching, eating, talking, writing, or reading, ultimately involve motor acts. Thus, motor control is a major task of the nervous system, and from an evolutionary perspective, it is probably the reason that nervous systems first arose. Not surprisingly, a large amount of the nervous system is devoted to motor control, which can be defined as the generation of signals to coordinate contraction of the musculature of the body and head either to maintain a posture or to make a movement (transition between two postures).

Given that large amounts of the nervous system are involved in motor control, it follows that damage or diseases of the nervous system often result in motor abnormalities. Conversely, particular motor symptoms help determine the location of the damaged or malfunctioning region, thus making assessment of motor function an important clinical tool for doctors.

In this chapter each major nervous system area involved in motor control will be described, starting with the spinal cord and then proceeding to the brainstem, cerebral cortex, cerebellum, and basal ganglia. Eye movement will be discussed at the end of the chapter because of the specialized circuits involved in their generation. Although each area will be described separately, it is important to keep in mind that they are highly interdependent and that most movements result from the coordinated action of multiple brain regions. For example, even spinal reflexes, which are mediated by local circuits in the cord, can be modified by descending motor commands, and virtually all voluntary movements are generated by activation of the spinal cord circuitry (or analogous brainstem nuclei for muscles in the head and face).

PRINCIPLES OF SPINAL CORD ORGANIZATION

The spinal cord has several levels of organization, including segmental organization, which will be our initial focus. Segmental organization refers to the fact that there are basic circuits and connections that take place at each level of the spinal cord and that are largely confined to a single or several neighboring segments. The basic spinal reflexes (i.e., the myotactic, inverse myotactic, and flexion reflexes) are mediated by such circuits. However, superimposed on this seg-

mental organization is the propriospinal system, which is a series of neurons whose axons run up and down the spinal cord to connect the different levels of the cord to one another. This system allows the coordination of activity at different spinal levels, which is important for behavior involving forelimbs and hind limbs, such as locomotion. Finally, there are descending motor (and ascending sensory) tracts that interact with these spinal circuits. These motor pathways carry signals related to voluntary movement, but they are also important for the more automatically (or non-consciously) controlled aspects of motor function, such as the setting of muscle tone (the resting resistance of muscles to changes in length).

Somatic Motor Neurons

Contractions of skeletal muscle fibers are responsible for movement of the body. Skeletal muscle fibers are innervated by large neurons, called α **motor neurons,** in the ventral horn of the spinal cord or in cranial nerve nuclei. These neurons are large, multipolar neurons that range in size up to 70 μm in diameter (Fig. 4-10, *A*). Their axons leave the spinal cord through the ventral roots and from the brainstem via several cranial nerves. The motor axons are distributed to the appropriate skeletal muscles through peripheral nerves, and they terminate with synapses, called **neuromuscular junctions** or **end plates,** on skeletal muscle fibers.

A given skeletal muscle is supplied by a group of α motor neurons located in a **motor nucleus.** In the ventral horn, a motor nucleus is typically a sausage-shaped array of motor neurons that extend over several spinal cord segments.

A **motor unit** is an α motor neuron and all of the skeletal muscle fibers that its axon supplies. Each skeletal muscle fiber in mammals is supplied by just one α motor neuron. However, a given α motor neuron may innervate a variable number of skeletal muscle fibers; the number depends on how fine a control of the muscle is required. For highly regulated muscles, such as the eye muscles, an α motor neuron may supply only a few skeletal muscle fibers. However, in a proximal limb muscle, such as the quadriceps femoris, a single α motor neuron may innervate thousands of skeletal muscle fibers.

The motor unit can be regarded as the basic unit of movement. When an α motor neuron discharges under normal circumstances, all the muscle fibers of the motor unit contract. A given α motor neuron may participate in a variety of reflexes and in voluntary movement. Because decisions about whether the synaptic input from various sources will cause particular muscle fibers to contract are made at the level of the α motor neuron (in mammals), these motor neurons have been termed the **final common pathway.**

Another type of motor neuron is called the γ **motor neuron.** γ Motor neurons are smaller than α motor neurons; they have a soma diameter of about 35 μm. The γ motor neurons that project to a particular muscle are located in the same motor nucleus as the α motor neurons that supply that muscle. γ Motor neurons do not supply ordinary skeletal muscle fibers. Instead, they synapse on specialized striated muscle fibers, the **intrafusal muscle fibers,** that are found within muscle spindles (see later).

The skeletal muscle fibers that belong to a given motor unit are called a muscle unit. All the muscle fibers in a muscle unit are of the same histochemical type (i.e., they are all either slow twitch [type I] or fast twitch [type IIA or IIB]). For an in-depth presentation of muscle fiber types, see Chapter 12.

The first motor units to be activated, either by voluntary effort or during reflex action, are those with the smallest motor axons; these motor units generate the smallest contractile force and allow the initial contraction to be finely graded. As more motor units are recruited, motor neurons with progressively larger axons become involved, and they generate progressively larger amounts of tension. This orderly recruitment of motor units is called the **size principle** because the motor units are recruited in order of motor neuron axon size. The size principle depends on the fact that small motor neurons are activated more easily than large motor neurons. Recall that if an excitatory synapse is active, it will open channels in the postsynaptic membrane and cause an excitatory postsynaptic current (EPSC). The same size EPSC will generate a larger potential change at the axon hillock of a small motor neuron than it will at a larger motor neuron, simply as a consequence of Ohm's law ($V = IR$) and the fact that smaller motor neurons have higher membrane resistance than larger motor neurons do. Thus, recalling that excitatory postsynaptic potentials (EPSPs) in the central nervous system (CNS) are small and need to summate to reach threshold for triggering spikes, it is easy to see that as the level of synaptic bombardment rises, the resulting depolarization will reach spiking threshold in smaller motor neurons first, assuming the same level of bombardment. As the size principle is usually obeyed, this assumption generally appears to hold; however, there can be exceptions, and in these cases one assumes that the descending motor pathways must provide differing levels of synaptic drive to the different sized motor neurons.

Autonomic motor neurons are discussed in Chapter 11.

Spinal Reflexes

A reflex is a relatively predictable, involuntary, and stereotyped response to an eliciting stimulus. Because of these properties, spinal reflexes have been used to identify and classify spinal cord neurons, determine their connectivity, and study their response properties. Thus, knowledge of spinal reflexes is essential for understanding spinal cord function.

The basic circuit that underlies a reflex is called a **reflex arc.** A reflex arc can be divided into three parts: an afferent limb (sensory receptors and axons) that carries information to the CNS, a central component (synapses and interneurons within the CNS), and an efferent limb (motor neurons) that causes the motor response. The knee jerk response to tapping on the patellar tendon with a reflex hammer by a doctor is a common example of a spinal reflex and illustrates the various components of the definition. The tap on the tendon actually causes brief stretching of the quadriceps muscle (eliciting stimulus) and thus activates sensory receptors (Ia fibers in muscle spindles). Activation of sensory receptors causes an excitatory signal to be sent to the spinal cord to activate motor neurons that go back to the quadriceps and cause it to contract, thereby resulting in a kick (stereotyped response). The person feels the kicking motion but has no sense that it was generated by himself or herself (involuntary). In this case, the afferent limb is represented by the Ia fibers and the efferent limb by the motor neurons. The central portion of this arc is minimal (a synapse from the Ia afferents onto the motor neurons), but in most reflexes it is more complex and can involve multiple types of interneurons.

It is the predictable linking of stimulus and response that makes reflexes a useful tool both for clinicians and for neuroscientists trying to understand spinal cord function. However, one danger to avoid is think-

▶ IN THE CLINIC

A clinically useful way to monitor the activity of motor units is **electromyography.** An electrode is placed within a skeletal muscle to record the summed action potentials of the skeletal muscle fibers of a muscle unit (see Fig. 12-7). If no spontaneous activity is noted, the patient is asked to contract the muscle voluntarily to increase the activity of motor units in the muscle. As the force of voluntary contraction increases, more motor units are recruited. In addition to the recruitment of more motor neurons, contractile strength increases with increases in the rate of discharge of the active α motor neurons. Electromyography is used for various purposes. For example, the conduction velocity of motor axons can be estimated by measuring the difference in latency of motor unit potentials when a peripheral nerve is stimulated at two sites separated by a known distance. Another use is to observe fibrillation potentials that occur when muscle fibers are denervated. Fibrillation potentials are spontaneously occurring action potentials in single muscle fibers. These spontaneous potentials contrast with motor unit potentials, which are larger and have a longer duration because they represent the action potentials in a set of muscle fibers that belong to a motor unit.

ing that a particular neuron's function is solely participation in a particular reflex because these same neurons are the targets of descending motor pathways and thus are involved in generating voluntary movement. Indeed, many of these neurons are active even when the afferent leg of their reflex arc is silent. One such example is the interneurons of the flexion reflex arc because they are also part of the central pattern generator for locomotion.

Later in this section we will discuss three well-known spinal reflexes because they illustrate important aspects of spinal cord circuitry and function and because of their behavioral and clinical importance. However, you should be aware that there are a number of additional reflexes that are mediated by spinal circuits (e.g., see micturition reflex, Fig. 11-3).

Sensory Receptors Responsible for Eliciting Spinal Reflexes

Each spinal reflex is elicited by the activation of one or more classes of sensory receptors. In the following section, two receptor types, muscle stretch receptors (muscle spindles) and Golgi tendon organs, are described in detail because these receptors are important both for spinal reflexes and as a source of the proprioceptive information that gives us an awareness of our limbs and helps guide voluntary movement.

The Muscle Spindle

Muscle spindles are found in almost all skeletal muscles and are particularly concentrated in muscles that exert fine motor control (e.g., the small muscles of the hand and eye).

Structure of the Muscle Spindle. As its name implies, a muscle spindle is a spindle or fusiform-shaped organ composed of a bundle of specialized muscle fibers richly innervated both by sensory and by motor axons (Fig. 9-1). A muscle spindle is about 100 μm in diameter and up to 10 mm long. The innervated part of the muscle spindle is encased in a connective tissue capsule. Muscle spindles lie between

regular muscle fibers and are typically located near the tendinous insertion of the muscle. The distal ends of the spindle are attached to the connective tissue within the muscle (endomysium). Thus, muscle spindles lie in parallel with the regular muscle fibers. This arrangement has important functional implications, as will be made clear later.

The muscle fibers within the spindle are called **intrafusal fibers** to distinguish them from the regular or extrafusal fibers that make up the bulk of the muscle. Individual intrafusal fibers are much narrower than extrafusal fibers and do not run the length of the muscle. Thus, they are too weak to contribute significantly to muscle tension or to directly cause changes in the overall length of the muscle by their contraction.

Morphologically, two types of intrafusal muscle fibers are found within muscle spindles: **nuclear bag** and **nuclear chain fibers** (Fig. 9-1, *B*). These names are derived from the arrangement of nuclei in the fibers. Nuclear bag fibers are larger than nuclear chain fibers, and their nuclei are bunched together like a bag of oranges in the central, or equatorial, region of the fiber. In nuclear chain fibers, the nuclei are arranged in a row. Functionally, nuclear bag fibers are divided into two types: bag1 and bag2. As detailed later, bag2 fibers are functionally similar to chain fibers.

The neural innervation of an intrafusal fiber differs significantly from that of an extrafusal fiber, which is innervated by a single motor neuron. Intrafusal fibers are multiply innervated and receive both sensory and motor innervation. The sensory supply includes a single group Ia afferent and a variable number of group II afferent fibers (Fig. 9-1, *B*). Group Ia fibers belong to the largest-diameter class of sensory nerve fibers and conduct at 72 to 120 m/sec; group II fibers are intermediate in size and conduct at 36 to 72 m/sec. A group Ia afferent fiber forms a primary ending consisting of a spiral-shaped terminal composed of branches of the group Ia fiber on each of the intrafusal muscle fibers. Thus, terminals of primary endings are found on both

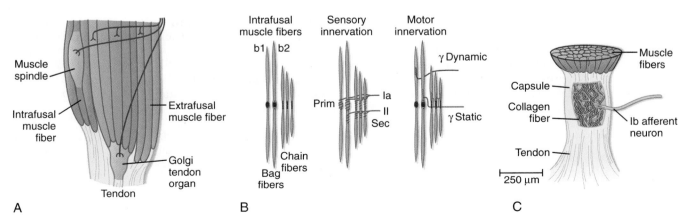

● **Figure 9-1.** Muscle proprioceptors. Skeletal muscles contain sensory receptors embedded within the muscle (spindles) and within their tendons (Golgi tendon organs). **A,** Schematic of a muscle showing the arrangement of a spindle in parallel with extrafusal muscle fibers and a tendon organ in series with muscle fibers. **B,** Structure and motor and sensory innervation of a muscle spindle. **C,** Structure and innervation of a tendon organ.

types of nuclear bag fibers and on nuclear chain fibers. The group II afferent fiber forms a secondary ending, which is found on nuclear chain and bag2 fibers, but not on bag1 fibers. The primary and secondary endings have mechanosensitive channels that are sensitive to the level of tension on the intrafusal muscle fiber.

The motor supply to a muscle spindle consists of two types of γ motor axons (Fig. 9-1, *B*). Dynamic γ motor axons end on nuclear bag1 fibers, and static γ motor axons end on nuclear chain and bag2 fibers.

Muscle Spindles Detect Changes in Muscle Length. Muscle spindles respond to changes in muscle length because they lie in parallel with the extrafusal fibers and therefore will also be stretched or shortened along with the extrafusal fibers. Because intrafusal fibers, like all muscle fibers, display spring-like properties, a change in their length will change the tension that they are under, and this change is sensed by mechanoreceptors of the Ia and II spindle afferents.

Figure 9-2 shows the changes in activity of the afferent fibers of a muscle spindle when the muscle is stretched. It is clear that Ia and II fibers respond differently to stretch. Group Ia fibers are sensitive both to the amount of muscle stretch and to its rate, whereas group II fibers respond chiefly to the amount of stretch. Thus, when a muscle is stretched to a new longer length, group II firing will increase in proportion to the amount of stretch (Fig. 9-2, *left*), and when the muscle is allowed to shorten, its firing rate will decrease proportionately (Fig. 9-2, *right*). Group Ia fibers show this same **static-type response,** and thus under steady-state conditions (i.e., constant muscle length), their firing rate will reflect the amount of muscle stretch, similar to that of group II fibers. However, while muscle length is changing, group Ia firing also reflects the rate of stretch or shortening that the muscle is undergoing. Its activity overshoots during muscle stretch and undershoots (and possibly ceases) during muscle shortening. These are called **dynamic responses.** This dynamic sensitivity also means that the activity of group Ia fibers is much more sensitive to transient stretches, such as shown in the middle diagrams of Figure 9-2. In particular, the tap profile is what occurs when a doctor uses a reflex hammer to hit the muscle tendon and thereby cause a brief stretching of the attached muscle. The change in muscle length is too brief for changes in group II firing to occur, but because the magnitude of the rate of change (slopes of the tap

profile) is so high with this stimulus, large dynamic responses are elicited in the group Ia fibers. Thus, the functionality of reflex arcs involving Ia afferents is what is being assessed by using a reflex hammer to tap on tendons.

γ Motor Neurons Adjust the Sensitivity of the Spindle. Up to this point we have described only how muscle spindles behave when there are no changes in γ motor neuron activity. The efferent innervation of muscle spindles is extremely important, however, because it determines the sensitivity of muscle spindles to stretch. For example, in Figure 9-3, *A*, the activity of a muscle spindle afferent is shown during a steady stretch. When the extrafusal portion of the muscle contracts (Fig. 9-3, *B*), the muscle spindle is unloaded by the resultant shortening of the muscle, and the muscle spindle afferent may stop discharging and thus become insensitive to further changes in muscle length. However, this unloading of the spindle can be counteracted if γ motor neurons are simultaneously stimulated. Such stimulation causes the intrafusal muscle fibers of the spindle to shorten along with the extrafusal muscle fibers (Fig. 9-3, *C*). Actually, only the two polar regions of the intrafusal muscle contract; the equatorial region, where the nuclei are located, does not contract because it has little contractile protein. As a result, when the polar regions contract, the equatorial region elongates and regains its sensitivity. Conversely, when a muscle relaxes and thus elongates, a concurrent decrease in γ motor neuron activity will allow the intrafusal fibers to relax as well and thereby prevent the tension on the central portion of the intrafusal fiber from reaching a level at which firing of the afferents is saturated. Thus, the γ motor neuron system allows the muscle spindle to operate over a wide range of muscle lengths while retaining high sensitivity to small changes in length.

Descending motor commands from the brain typically activate α and γ motor neurons simultaneously and thus cause a synchronous contraction of extrafusal and intrafusal muscle fibers. This co-contraction means that as the muscle shortens from the contraction of extrafusal fibers, the polar regions of the intrafusal fibers also shorten, thereby maintaining relatively constant tension on the equatorial portion and thus the sensitivity of the spindle apparatus.

As mentioned earlier, there are two types of γ motor neurons—dynamic and static (Fig. 9-1). Dynamic γ

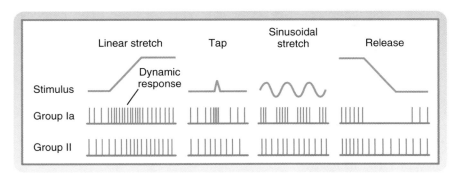

● **Figure 9-2.** Responses of a primary ending (Ia) and a secondary ending (II) to changes in muscle length. Note the difference in dynamic and static responsiveness of these endings. The waveforms at the top represent the changes in muscle length. The middle and bottom rows show the discharges of a group Ia and II fiber, respectively, during the various changes in muscle length.

● **Figure 9-3.** The activity of γ motor neurons can counteract the effects of unloading on the discharge of a muscle spindle afferent. **A,** The activity of a muscle spindle afferent is shown during steady stretch. **B,** α Motor neuron stimulation at time t = 0 msec causes contraction of the extrafusal fibers, which leads to muscle shortening and increased muscle tension, but unloading of the tension across the muscle spindle, which in turn induces the afferent to stop firing. Upon relaxation the muscle returns to its original length and tension is restored on the intrafusal fibers, causing the return of activity in the Ia afferent. **C,** Coactivation of α and γ motor neurons causes shortening of both extrafusal and intrafusal fibers. Thus, there is no unloading of the spindle, and the afferent maintains its spontaneous activity. (Redrawn from Kuffler SW, Nicholls JG: From Neuron to Brain. Sunderland, MA, Sinauer, 1976.)

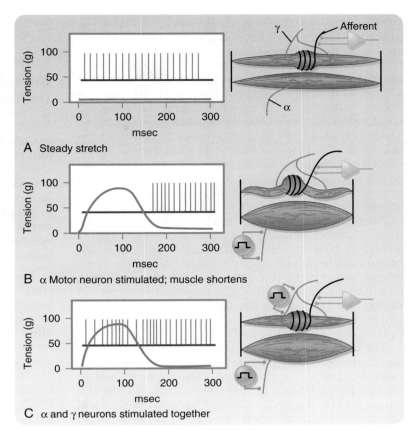

A Steady stretch

B α Motor neuron stimulated; muscle shortens

C α and γ neurons stimulated together

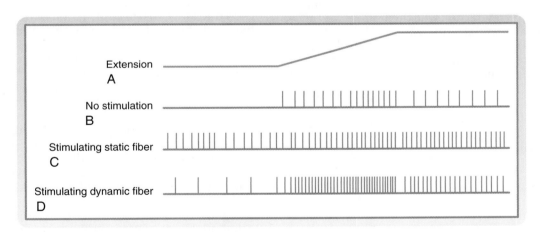

● **Figure 9-4.** Effects of static and dynamic γ motor neurons on the responses of a primary ending to muscle stretch. The upper trace, **A,** is the time course of the stretch. **B** shows the discharge of group Ia fibers in the absence of γ motor neuron activity. In **C,** a static γ motor axon was stimulated, and in **D,** a dynamic γ motor axon was stimulated. (Redrawn from Crowe A, Matthews PBC: J Physiol 174:109, 1964.)

motor axons end on nuclear bag1 fibers, and static γ motor axons synapse on nuclear chain and bag2 fibers. Thus, when a dynamic γ motor neuron is activated, the response of the group Ia afferent fiber is enhanced, but the activity of the group II afferents is unchanged; when a static γ motor neuron discharges, the responsiveness of the group II afferents and the static response siveness of the group Ia afferents are increased. The effects of stimulating the static and dynamic fibers on a group Ia afferent's response to stretch is illustrated in Figure 9-4. Descending pathways can preferentially influence dynamic or static γ motor neurons and thereby alter the nature of reflex activity in the spinal cord.

Golgi Tendon Organ

A second type of mechanosensitive receptor associated with skeletal muscle is the Golgi tendon organ (Fig. 9-1). A Golgi tendon organ is innervated from the terminals of group Ib afferent fibers. The diameter of a Golgi tendon organ is about 100 μm and its length is about 1 mm. A group Ib fiber has a large diameter and conducts in the same velocity range as a group Ia fiber. The terminals of a Ib fiber are wrapped about bundles of collagen fibers in the tendon of a muscle (or in tendinous inscriptions within the muscle). Thus, the sensory ending is arranged in series with the muscle, in contrast to the parallel arrangement of the muscle spindle.

Because of their in-series relationship to the muscle, Golgi tendon organs can be activated either by muscle stretch or by contraction of the muscle. In both cases, however, the actual stimulus sensed by the Golgi tendon organ is the force that develops in the tendon to which it is linked. Thus, the response to stretch is the result of the spring-like nature of the muscle (i.e., by Hooke's law, the force on a spring is proportional to how much it is stretched).

The distinction between the responsiveness of the muscle spindles and Golgi tendon organs can be made clear by comparing the firing patterns of Ia and Ib fibers when a muscle is stretched and then held at a longer length (Fig. 9-5). The Ia fiber's firing rate will maintain its increase until the stretch is reversed. In contrast, the Ib fiber will show an initial large increase in firing, reflecting the increased tension on the muscle caused by the stretch, but will then show a gradual return toward its initial firing rate as the tension on the muscle is lowered because of cross-bridge recycling and the resultant lengthening of the sarcomeres. Therefore, Golgi tendon organs signal force, whereas

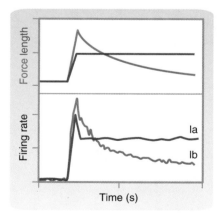

● **Figure 9-5.** Changes in group Ia and Ib firing rates when muscle is stretched to a new length as indicated in the top graph _(blue line)._ After a transient burst, the firing rate of the Ia fiber remains constant at a new higher level that is proportional to the increase in length _(lower graph, blue line)._ In contrast, the Ib unit shows an initial rapid increase in firing followed by a slow decrease back toward its original level _(bottom graph, red line)_ and has a firing profile that matches the tension level in the muscle caused by the stretch _(top graph, red line)._

spindles signal muscle length. Further evidence of this distinction is that Ib firing correlates with force level during isometric contraction even though muscle length, and therefore Ia activity, are unchanged.

The Myotatic or Stretch Reflex

The stretch reflex is key for the maintenance of posture and helps overcome unexpected impediments during a voluntary movement. Changes in the stretch reflex are involved in actions commanded by the brain, and pathological alterations in this reflex are important signs of neurological disease. The phasic stretch reflex occurs in response to rapid, transient stretches of the muscle, such as those elicited by a doctor using a reflex hammer or by an unexpected impediment to an ongoing movement. The tonic stretch reflex occurs in response to a slower or steady stretch applied to the muscle.

The Phasic (or Ia) Stretch Reflex. The phasic stretch reflex is elicited by the primary endings of the muscle spindles. The reflex arc responsible for the phasic stretch reflex is shown in Figure 9-6. A group Ia afferent fiber from a muscle spindle in the rectus femoris muscle is shown to branch as it enters the gray matter of the spinal cord. It will form excitatory synapses directly (monosynaptically) on virtually all α motor neurons that supply the same (also known as the homonymous) muscle and with many of its synergists, such as the vastus intermedius muscle in this case, which also acts to extend the leg at the knee. If the excitation is powerful enough, the motor neurons discharge and cause a contraction of the muscle. Note that the Ia fibers do not contact the γ motor neurons, possibly to avoid a positive-feedback loop situation. This selective targeting of α motor neurons is exceptional in that most other reflex and descending pathways will target both α and γ motor neurons.

Other branches of group Ia fibers end on a variety of interneurons; however, one type, the reciprocal Ia inhibitory interneuron (black cell in Fig. 9-6), is particularly important with regard to the stretch reflex. These interneurons are identifiable because they are the only inhibitory interneurons that receive input from both the Ia afferents and **Renshaw cells** (see Fig. 9-11). They end on α motor neurons that innervate the antagonist muscles, in this case the hamstring muscles, including the semitendinosus muscle, which act to flex the knee.

The organization of the stretch reflex arc guarantees that one set of α motor neurons is activated and the opposing set is inhibited. This arrangement is known as **reciprocal innervation.** Although many reflexes involve such reciprocal innervation, this type of innervation is not the only possible organization of a motor control system, and indeed, descending motor pathways can override such patterns.

The stretch reflex is quite powerful, in large part because of its monosynaptic nature. The power of this reflex also derives from the essentially maximal convergence and divergence that exist in this pathway, which is not apparent from the circuit diagrams, such as Figure 9-6, that are typically used to illustrate reflex

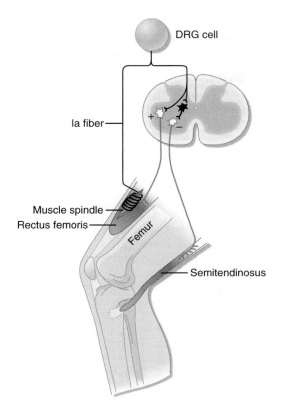

● Figure 9-6. Reflex arc of the stretch reflex. The pathway back to the Rectus femoris in this arc contains a single synapse within the CNS; hence, it is a monosynaptic reflex. The interneuron, shown in black, is a group Ia inhibitory interneuron.

pathways. That is, each Ia fiber will contact virtually all homonymous α motor neurons, and each such α motor neuron will receive input from every spindle in that muscle. Although its monosynaptic nature makes the Ia reflex rapid and powerful, it also means that there is relatively little opportunity for direct control of activity flow through its reflex arc. The CNS overcomes this problem by controlling muscle spindle sensitivity via the γ motor neuron system.

The Tonic Stretch Reflex. The tonic stretch reflex can be elicited by passively bending a joint. This reflex circuit includes both group Ia and group II afferent fibers from muscle spindles. Group II fibers make monosynaptic excitatory connections with α motor neurons, but they also excite them through disynaptic and polysynaptic pathways. Normally, there is ongoing activity in the Ia and II afferents that helps maintain a baseline firing of α motor neurons; therefore, the tonic stretch reflex contributes to muscle tone. Its activity also contributes to our ability to maintain a posture. For example, if the knee of a soldier standing at attention begins to flex because of fatigue, the quadriceps muscle will be stretched, a tonic stretch reflex will be elicited, and the quadriceps will contract more, thereby opposing the flexion and restoring the posture.

▶ IN THE CLINIC

Hyperactive stretch reflexes can lead to tremors and clonus. Although the negative-feedback action of the stretch reflex should help stabilize the limb, the conduction delay between the initiating stimulus (muscle stretch) and the response (muscle contraction) can cause it to be a source of instability resulting in rhythmic movements such as tremors and clonus. Clonus is elicited by a sustained stretch of a muscle in a person who has spinal cord damage. Normally, an imposed sustained stretch on a muscle will elicit an increase in Ia and II activity, which after a delay will cause a contraction in the muscle that opposes the stretch but does not completely return the muscle to its initial length because the gain of the stretch reflex is much less than 1.* This partial compensation, in turn, will lead to a decrease in Ia and II activity, which causes the limb to lengthen again, but not fully. This lengthening will once again increase Ia and II activity, and so on. The delay is key in setting up this oscillation because it leads to the feedback signal continuing even after the muscle has compensated and thus results in an overcompensation that leads to the next overcorrection. However, because the reflex gain is normally much less than 1, this oscillation dies out quickly (the overcompensation gets smaller and smaller), and the muscle comes to rest at an intermediate length. In contrast, when descending motor pathways are damaged, the resulting changes in spinal cord connectivity and increases in neuronal excitability result in a hyperactive reflex (which is equivalent to raising the gain close to 1). In this case, the successive overcompensations are much larger, and an overt but transient oscillation can be observed (clonus). If the gain equals 1, the clonus does not die out but rather persists for as long as the initial stretch stimulus is maintained.

*In general, gain of a system is defined as its output for a given input. Here, the input to the system is the imposed stretch, and the output is movement caused by the stretch reflex–evoked contraction.

The foregoing discussion suggests that stretch reflexes can act like a negative-feedback system to control muscle length. By following the stretch reflex arc, it is possible to see that changes in its activity will act to oppose changes in muscle length from a particular equilibrium point. For example, if the muscle's length is increased, there will be an increase in Ia and II firing, which will excite homonymous α motor neurons and lead to contraction of the muscle and reversal of the stretch. Similarly, passive shortening of the muscle will unload the spindles and lead to a decrease in the excitatory drive to the motor neurons and thus relaxation of the muscle. So how are we able to rotate our joints? It is partly because the γ motor neurons are coactivated during a movement and thereby shift the equilibrium point of the spindle and partly because the gain or strength of the reflex is low enough that other input to the motor neuron can override the stretch reflex.

Inverse Myotatic or Ib Reflex

Just as the stretch reflex can be thought of as a feedback system to regulate muscle length, the inverse myotactic, or Ib, reflex can be thought of as a feedback system to help maintain force levels in a muscle. Using the upper part of the leg as an example, the Ib reflex arc is shown in Figure 9-7. In this example the receptor organs are Golgi tendon organs of the rectus femoris muscle. The afferent fibers branch as they enter the spinal cord and end on interneurons. There are no monosynaptic connections to α motor neurons. Rather, the Ib afferents synapse onto two classes of interneurons: interneurons that inhibit α motor neurons that supply the homonymous muscle, in this case the rectus femoris, and excitatory interneurons that activate α motor neurons to the antagonist (semitendinosus). Because there are two synapses in series in the CNS, this is a disynaptic reflex arc. Given these connections, Ib activity should have the opposite action of the Ia stretch reflex during passive stretch of the muscle, which explains this reflex's other name, the inverse myotactic reflex. However, functionally, the two reflex arcs can act synergistically, as the following example shows. Recall that the Golgi tendon organs monitor force levels across the tendon that they supply. If during maintained posture, such as standing at attention, knee extensors, such as the rectus femoris muscle, begin to fatigue, the force in the patellar tendon will decline. The decline in force will reduce the activity of Golgi tendon organs in this tendon. Because the Ib reflex normally inhibits the α motor neurons to the rectus femoris muscle, reduced activity of the Golgi tendon organs will enhance the excitability of (i.e., disinhibit) the α motor neurons and thereby help reverse the decrease in force caused by the fatigue. Simultaneously, bending of the knee will stretch the knee extensors and activate the Ia fibers, which will then excite the same α motor neurons. Thus, coordinated action of both muscle spindle and Golgi tendon organ afferent fibers is needed to cause greater contraction of the rectus femoris muscle and maintenance of the posture.

Flexion Reflexes and Locomotion

The flexion reflex starts with activation of one or more of a variety of sensory receptors, including nociceptors, whose signals can be carried to the spinal cord via a variety of afferents, including group II and III fibers, collectively called the **flexion reflex afferents (FRAs).** In flexion reflexes, afferent volleys (1) cause excitatory interneurons to activate the α motor neurons that supply the flexor muscles in the ipsilateral limb and (2) cause inhibitory interneurons to inhibit the α motor neurons that supply the antagonistic extensor muscles (Fig. 9-8). This pattern of activity causes one or more joints in the stimulated limb to flex. In addition, commissural interneurons evoke the opposite pattern of activity in the contralateral side of the spinal cord (Fig. 9-8), which results in extension of the opposite limb, the **crossed extension reflex.** For our lower limbs (or in quadrupeds for both forelimbs

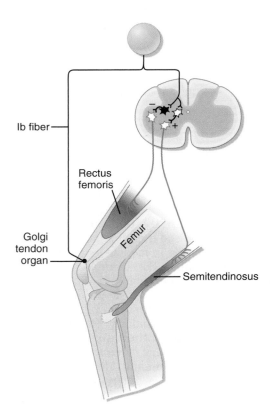

● **Figure 9-7.** Reflex arc of the inverse myotatic reflex. The interneurons include both excitatory *(clear)* and inhibitory *(black)* interneurons. This is an example of a disynaptic reflex.

Labels on figure: Ib fiber; Rectus femoris; Golgi tendon organ; Femur; Semitendinosus

IN THE CLINIC

After damage to the descending motor pathways, hyperactive stretch reflexes may result in spasticity, in which there is large resistance to passive rotation of the limbs. In this condition it may be possible to demonstrate what is called the **clasp-knife reflex.** When spasticity is present, attempts to rotate a limb about a joint will initially meet high resistance. However, if the applied force is increased, there will come a point at which the resistance suddenly dissipates and the limb rotates easily. This change in resistance is caused by reflex inhibition. The Ib reflex arc suggests that rising activity in this pathway could underlie the sudden release of resistance, and indeed, the clasp-knife reflex was once attributed to the activation of Golgi tendon organs when these receptors were thought to have a high threshold to muscle stretch. However, the tendon organs have since been shown to be activated at very low levels of force and are no longer thought to cause the clasp-knife reflex. It is now thought that this reflex is caused by the activation of other high-threshold muscle receptors that supply the fascia around the muscle. Signals from these receptors cause the activation of interneurons that lead to inhibition of the homonymous motor neurons.

● **Figure 9-8.** The reflex arc of the flexion reflex. Black interneurons are inhibitory and clear ones are excitatory. FRA, flexion reflex afferent.

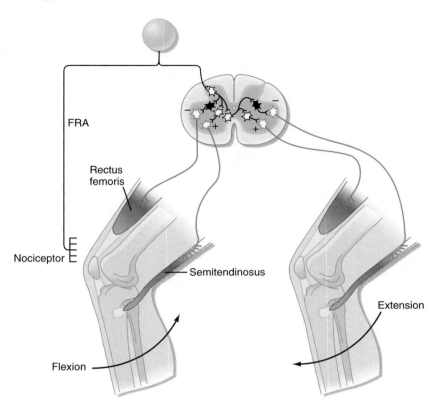

FRA

Rectus femoris

Nociceptor

Semitendinosus

Extension

Flexion

and hind limbs), the crossed extension part of the reflex helps in maintaining balance by enabling the contralateral limb to be able to support the additional load that is transferred to it when the flexed limb is lifted.

Because flexion typically brings the affected limb in closer to the body and away from a painful stimulus, flexion reflexes are a type of withdrawal reflex. In Figure 9-8, the neural circuit of the flexion reflex is shown for neurons that affect only the knee joint. Actually, however, considerable divergence of the primary afferent and interneuronal pathways occurs in the flexion reflex. In fact, all the major joints of a limb (e.g., hip, knee, and ankle) may be involved in a strong flexor withdrawal reflex. Details of the flexor withdrawal reflex vary, depending on the nature and location of the stimulus. This variability in flexion reflex is called the local sign. Flexor withdrawal reflexes also occur in areas other than the limbs; for example, visceral disease may cause contractions of muscles in the chest wall or abdomen and thereby decrease the mobility of the trunk.

The interneurons subserving flexion reflexes also appear to be part of the **central pattern generator (CPG)** for generating locomotion and thus are an example of how the reflex circuits are used for multiple purposes. A CPG is a set of neurons and circuits capable of generating the rhythmic activity that underlies motor acts, even in the absence of sensory input. Using the FRA interneurons as an example, one can see that activation of the FRA interneurons leads to a pattern of flexor excitation and extensor inhibition on one side and the converse pattern on the opposite side and that if the FRA interneurons on each side of the spinal cord alternated in being active, a stepping pattern would emerge. That is, walking motion is the result of alternately activating flexors and extensors in each leg such that activation of the flexors (and extensors) in the two legs occurs out of phase with each other, exactly what would be produced by alternately activating the FRA interneurons on each side. Note that such a rhythmic activity pattern in the FRA circuits is not dependent on activity from the FRAs themselves (e.g., they could be activated by descending pathways from the brain).

To show that these circuits are actually involved in generating the locomotion rhythm, spinal cord preparations were made that showed spontaneous locomotion (i.e., if the brainstem is transected and weight is supported, the spinal cord circuits can generate activity that causes the limbs to generate a normal locomotion sequence.) In one such preparation, the electromyogram from the flexors and extensors of a limb were recorded and the FRAs then stimulated to see the effect on locomotion rhythm (Fig. 9-9). Before any stimulus, a spontaneous alternating pattern of flexor and extensor electromyographic (EMG) activity exists. If the FRAs were not involved in the locomotion circuit or at least were not a critical part of the circuits responsible for generating the rhythm (Fig. 9-9, *B*), we would expect the stimulus to produce only a transient response (i.e., a single EMG response of the flexors and brief inhibition of the extensors) and have no long-term effect on this pattern. Such a transient response is observed (Fig. 9-9, *A;* EMG records just after the stimulus). However, the stimulus also causes a permanent,

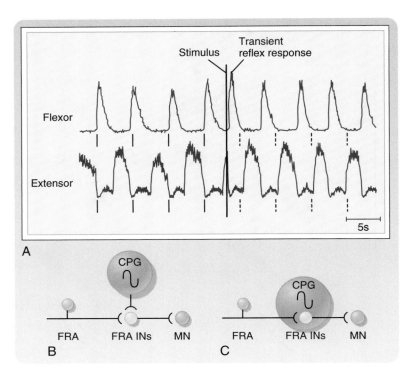

● **Figure 9-9.** Phase reset of locomotion rhythm by FRA stimulation helps identify neuronal components of the underlying central pattern generator (CPG). **A,** EMG records from knee flexor and extensor muscles. Note the rhythmic alternating pattern before application of the stimulus. The solid vertical lines below each trace indicate the times at which flexor contraction is initiated. The dashed vertical lines indicate the times at which flexor contraction would have been initiated if the stimulus caused no lasting effect on the rhythmic pattern. **B** and **C,** Two possible models for the CPG underlying the locomotor rhythm seen in **A. B** does not include the FRA interneurons in the CPG, whereas **C** does. The data shown in **A** support the model shown in **C.** (Data from Hultborn H et al: Ann N Y Acad Sci 860:70, 1998.)

approximately 180-degree phase shift in locomotor rhythm, as can be seen by comparing the times of contractions before and after the stimulus. The dashed vertical lines indicate the times at which a flexor EMG response would be expected if the stimulus had produced no phase shift from the EMG activity pattern; before the stimulus, each vertical line is aligned with the onset of a flexor EMG burst, whereas after the stimulus, each vertical line occurs at the end of the flexor burst. Therefore, we can conclude that the stimulus affected the locomotor CPG itself and that the FRA interneurons are a critical part of this CPG (Fig. 9-9, _C_).

A second important point illustrated by this experiment is that the locomotion CPG (and CPGs generally) can be influenced by strong afferent activity. The afferent influence ensures that the pattern generator adapts to changes in the terrain as locomotion proceeds. Such changes may occur rapidly during running, and locomotion must then be adjusted to ensure proper coordination.

Determining Spinal Cord Organization by Using Reflexes

As already discussed, divergence is an important aspect of reflex pathways. Convergence is another important organizational feature of reflex arcs. Convergence is defined as the termination of several neurons on one other neuron. For example, all group Ia afferent fibers from the muscle spindles of a particular hind limb muscle synapse onto any given α motor neuron to that muscle. Convergent input can be demonstrated by using the phenomenon of **spatial facilitation,** which is illustrated in Figure 9-10.

In this example, a monosynaptic reflex is elicited by electrical stimulation of the group Ia fibers in each of two branches of a muscle nerve (Fig. 9-10, _A_). The reflex response is characterized by recording the discharges of α motor axons from the appropriate ventral root (as a compound action potential). When muscle nerve branch A is stimulated, a small compound action potential is recorded as reflex A. Similarly, when muscle nerve branch B is stimulated, reflex B is recorded. Figure 9-10, _B,_ depicts the motor neurons contained within the motor nucleus. The discharge zones (pink colored areas) enclose α motor neurons that are activated above threshold when each muscle nerve branch is stimulated separately. Thus, two α motor neurons spike when each muscle nerve branch is stimulated alone (an additional seven motor neurons in the subliminal fringe are excited, but not sufficiently to trigger spikes). When the two nerves are stimulated at the same time, a much larger reflex discharge is recorded (see recordings at the right of Fig. 9-10, _B_). As the figure demonstrates, this reflex represents the discharge of seven α motor neurons: the four that spiked after the singular stimulation of each nerve (two per nerve) and three additional α motor neurons (located in the facilitation zone) that are made to discharge only when the two muscle nerves are stimulated simultaneously because they lie in the subliminal fringe for both nerves.

A similar effect could be elicited by repetitive stimulation of one of the muscle nerves, provided that the stimuli occur close enough together that some of the excitatory effect of the first volley still persists after the second volley arrives. This effect is called **tempo-**

● **Figure 9-10. A,** Arrangement for using electrically evoked afferent volleys and recordings from motor axons in a ventral root to study reflexes. **B,** Experiment in which combined stimulation of two muscle nerves resulted in spatial summation. In **C,** the combined volleys caused occlusion. (Redrawn from Eyzaguirre C, Fidone SJ: Physiology of the Nervous System, 2nd ed. Chicago, Mosby–Year Book, 1975.)

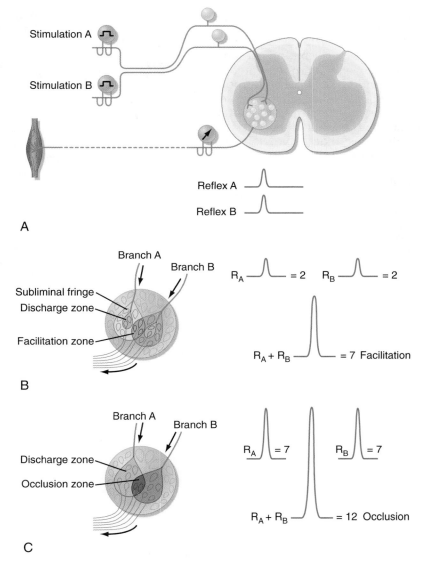

ral summation. Both spatial summation and temporal summation depend on the properties of the EPSPs evoked in α motor neurons by the group Ia afferent fibers (see Fig. 6-8).

If a volley in one of the two muscle nerves in Figure 9-10 reaches the motor nucleus at a time when the motor neurons are highly excitable, the reflex discharge will be relatively large (see Fig. 9-10, *C*). A similar volley in the other muscle nerve might also produce a large reflex response. However, when the two muscle nerves are excited simultaneously, the reflex can be less than the sum of the two independently evoked reflexes if the cells reaching threshold to activation of either of the two nerves alone overlap significantly. In this case, each afferent nerve activates 7 α motor neurons, but the volleys in the two nerves together cause only 12 motor neurons to discharge. This phenomenon is called **occlusion.**

The phenomena of spatial and temporal summation and occlusion can also be used to demonstrate interactions between spinal cord neurons and the various reflex circuits. To start, a monosynaptic reflex discharge can be evoked by stimulating the group Ia afferent fibers in a muscle nerve. This tests the reflex excitability of a population of α motor neurons. The discharges of either extensor or flexor α motor neurons can be recorded by choosing the proper muscle nerve to be stimulated. Other kinds of afferent fibers are then stimulated along with the homonymous Ia afferent from the muscle to see whether the response to the Ia stimulation changes. For example, stimulation of group Ia afferent fibers in the nerve to the antagonist muscles produces inhibition of the response to the homonymous Ia stimulation (which is mediated by what is called the reciprocal Ia inhibitory interneuron). Alternatively, if the small afferent fibers of a cutaneous nerve are stimulated to evoke a flexion reflex, the responses to Ia stimulation of the α motor neurons that innervate the extensor muscles will be inhibited (and those of α motor neurons that innervate flexor muscles will be potentiated). As a final example, stimulation of a ventral root causes inhibition of Ia responses and inhibits the reciprocal Ia inhibition. Because the ventral root contains only motor neuron axons, this result implies the presence of axon collaterals that excite inhibitory interneurons that feed back onto the same motor neuron population (Fig. 9-11). These interneurons are named Renshaw cells. Because ventral root stimulation also inhibits the Ia inhibition of antagonist motor neurons, but no other classes of interneurons, the reciprocal Ia interneurons can be uniquely identified by their being inhibited by ventral root stimulation (and activated by Ia stimulation).

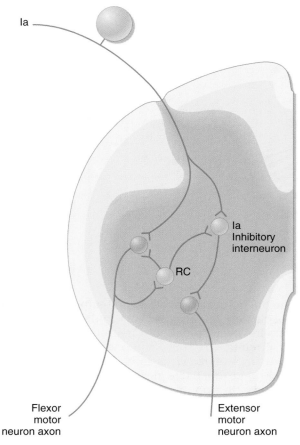

● **Figure 9-11.** Renshaw cell (RC) connections with motor neurons and Ia inhibitory interneurons. The circuits shown mediate Ia reciprocal inhibition of antagonist muscles (in this case an extensor) and inhibition of this reciprocal inhibition by Renshaw cells. Note that there are equivalent Renshaw cells and Ia inhibitory interneurons associated with extensor motor neurons and Ia input from spindles in extensor muscles, but they are not shown for simplicity. Orange cells are inhibitory and blue and green ones are excitatory.

Topographic Organization of the Ventral Horn

Up to this point we have considered the functional organization of the spinal cord, largely without regard to its physical (i.e., anatomic) instantiation. We now turn to this aspect of spinal cord organization by discussing the organization of the ventral horn and in particular the topographic arrangement of the motor neurons contained therein. This topography has functional implications for how the descending motor tracts interact with the spinal cord machinery that we have been discussing.

Spinal cord motor neurons are organized topographically in rostrocaudally running columns in the ventral horn (Fig. 9-12). Motor neurons that supply the axial musculature form a column of cells that extends the length of the spinal cord. In the cervical and lumbosacral enlargements, these cells are located in the most medial part of the ventral horn. Motor neurons that supply the limb muscles form columns that extend for several segments in the lateral part of the ventral horn in the cervical and lumbosacral enlargements. Motor neurons to muscles of the distal part of the limb are located most laterally, whereas those that innervate more proximal muscles are located more medially. Motor neurons to flexors are dorsal to those that innervate extensors. Note that the α and γ motor neurons to a given muscle are found intermixed within the same motor neuron column.

The interneurons that connect with the motor neurons in the enlargements are also topographically organized. In general, interneurons that supply the limb muscles are located mainly in the lateral parts of the deep dorsal horn and the intermediate region that lies between the dorsal and ventral horns. Those that supply the axial muscles, however, are located in the medial part of the ventral horn. These interneurons receive synaptic connections from primary afferent fibers and from the axons of pathways that descend from the brain, and thus are both part of spinal reflex arcs and descending motor control pathways.

An important aspect of interneuronal systems is that the laterally placed interneurons project ipsilaterally to motor neurons that supply the distal or the proximal limb muscles, whereas the medial interneurons project bilaterally. This arrangement of the lateral interneurons allows the limbs to be controlled independently. In contrast, the bilateral arrangement of the medial interneurons allows bilateral control of motor neurons to the axial muscles to provide postural support to the trunk and neck.

DESCENDING MOTOR PATHWAYS

Classification of Descending Motor Pathways

Pyramidal versus Extrapyramidal Pathways

Descending motor pathways were traditionally subdivided into **pyramidal tract** and **extrapyramidal pathways.** This terminology reflects a clinical dichotomy

● **Figure 9-12.** Musculotopic organization of motor neurons in the ventral horn of the spinal cord. **A,** Schematic of the cervicothoracic spinal cord and associated cross sections, showing the locations of motor neurons that innervate a flexor *(blue dots)* and an extensor *(red dots)*. **B,** Spinal cord cross section with locations of different muscles represented by a drawing of the arm. (Redrawn from Purves D et al [eds]: Neuroscience, 3rd ed. Sunderland, MA, Sinauer, 2004.)

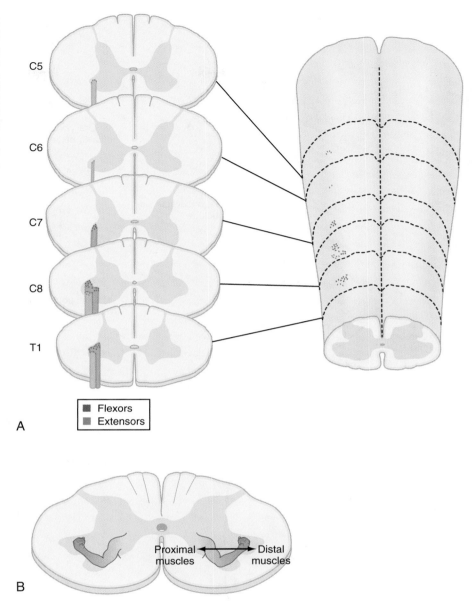

C5
C6
C7
C8
T1

■ Flexors
■ Extensors

A

Proximal muscles ←→ Distal muscles

B

between pyramidal tract disease and extrapyramidal disease. In pyramidal tract disease, the **corticospinal,** or pyramidal, tract is interrupted. The signs of this disease were originally attributed to the loss of function of the pyramidal tract (so named because the corticospinal tract passes through the medullary pyramid). However, in many cases of pyramidal tract disease, the functions of other pathways are also altered, and most pyramidal tract signs (see the later section Motor Deficits Caused by Lesions of Descending Motor Pathways) appear to not be caused by loss of the corticospinal tract or at least require damage to additional motor pathways. The term extrapyramidal is even more problematic. Thus, this classification system is not used in this book.

Lateral versus Medial Motor Systems

Another way of classifying the motor pathways is based on their sites of termination in the spinal cord

and the consequent differences in their roles in the control of movement and posture. The **lateral pathways** terminate in the lateral portions of the spinal cord gray matter (Fig. 9-13). The lateral pathways can excite motor neurons directly, although interneurons are their main target. They influence reflex arcs that control fine movement of the distal ends of limbs, as well as those that activate supporting musculature in the proximal ends of limbs. The **medial pathways** end in the medial ventral horn on the medial group of interneurons (Fig. 9-13). These interneurons connect bilaterally with motor neurons that control the axial musculature and thereby contribute to balance and posture. They also contribute to the control of proximal limb muscles. In this book we use the lateral/medial terminology to classify the descending motor pathways. However, even this scheme is not perfect, partly because although motor neuron cell bodies form localized columns, motor neuron dendritic trees

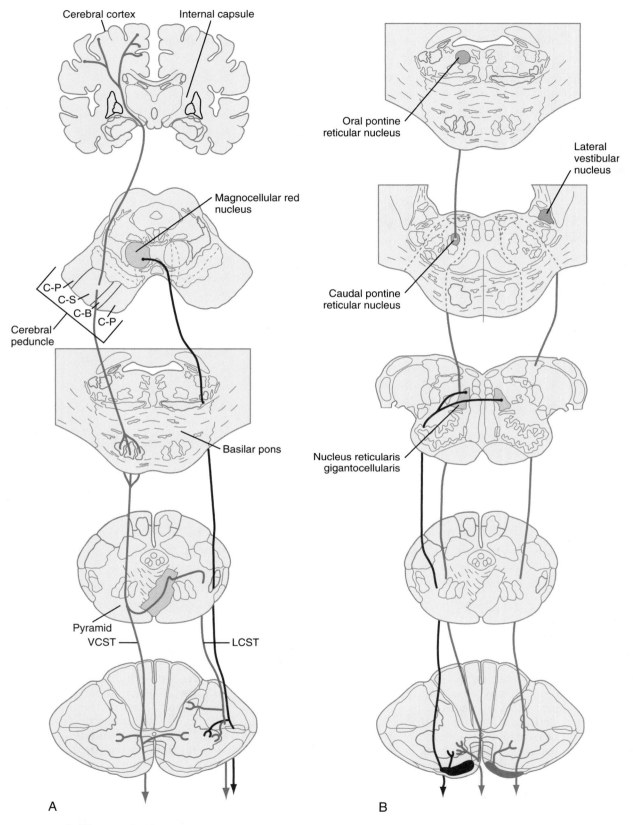

● **Figure 9-13.** Descending motor pathways. Major pathways connecting the cortical and brainstem motor areas to the spinal cord are shown. **A,** Lateral system pathways, corticospinal *(red)* and rubrospinal *(blue)* pathways. Note that the ventral corticospinal pathway is part of the medial system, but is shown in **A** for simplicity. **B,** Medial system pathways, medullary *(blue)* and pontine *(green)* reticulospinal and lateral vestibulospinal *(red)* pathways. C-B, corticobulbar; C-P, corticopontine; C-S, corticospinal; LCST, lateral corticospinal tract; VCST, ventral corticospinal tract.

are rather large and typically span most of the ventral horn. Thus, any motor neuron can potentially receive input from so-called medial or lateral system pathways.

The Lateral System
Lateral Corticospinal and Corticobulbar Tracts
The corticospinal and corticobulbar tracts originate from a wide region of the cerebral cortex. This region includes the primary motor, premotor, supplementary, and cingulate motor areas of the frontal lobe and the somatosensory cortex of the parietal lobe. The cells of origin of these tracts include both large and small pyramidal cells of layer V of the cortex, including the **giant pyramidal cells of Betz.** Although Betz cells are a defining feature of the motor cortex, they represent a small minority (< 5%) of the cells that contribute to these tracts, in part because they are found only in the primary motor cortex, and even here they represent a minority of the cells contributing to the tract. These tracts leave the cortex and enter the internal capsule, then traverse the midbrain in the cerebral peduncle, pass through the basilar pons, and emerge as the pyramids on the ventral surface of the medulla (Fig. 9-13, *A*). The corticobulbar axons leave the tract as it descends the brainstem and terminate in the various cranial nerve motor nuclei. The corticospinal fibers continue caudally, and in the most caudal region of the medulla, about 90% of them cross to the opposite side. They then descend in the contralateral lateral funiculus as the lateral corticospinal tract. The lateral corticospinal axons terminate at all spinal cord levels, primarily on interneurons, but also on motor neurons. The remaining uncrossed axons continue caudally in the ventral funiculus on the same side as the ventral corticospinal tract, which belongs to the medial system. Many of these fibers ultimately decussate at the spinal cord level at which they terminate.

The lateral corticospinal tract is a relatively minor tract in lower mammals but becomes quantitatively and functionally very important in primates and in humans in particular, where it contains over 1 million axons. This number still represents a relatively small proportion of the outflow from the cortex because there are approximately 20 million axons in the cerebral peduncles. Nevertheless, the corticospinal pathway is critical for the fine independent control of finger movement inasmuch as isolated lesions of the corticospinal tract typically lead to a permanent loss of this ability, even though there is often recovery of other movement abilities with such lesions. Indeed, in primates, corticospinal synapses directly onto motor neurons are particularly prevalent for the motor neurons controlling finger muscles and are probably the basis of our ability to make independent, finely controlled finger movements.

The corticobulbar tract, which projects to the cranial nerve motor nuclei, has subdivisions that are comparable to the lateral and ventral corticospinal tracts. For example, part of the corticobulbar tract ends contralaterally in the portion of the facial nucleus that supplies muscles of the lower part of the face and in the hypoglossal nucleus. This component of the corticobulbar tract is organized like the lateral corticospinal tract. The remainder of the corticobulbar tract ends bilaterally.

Rubrospinal Tract
This tract originates in the magnocellular portion of the red nucleus, which is located in the midbrain tegmentum. These fibers decussate (cross) in the midbrain, descend through the pons and medulla, and then take up a position just ventral to the lateral corticospinal tract in the spinal cord. They preferentially affect motor neurons controlling distal musculature, similar to the corticospinal fibers. Red nucleus neurons receive input from the cerebellum and from the motor cortex, thus making this an area of integration of activity from these two motor systems.

The Medial System
The ventral corticospinal tract and much of the corticobulbar tract can be regarded as medial system pathways. These tracts end on the medial group of interneurons in the spinal cord and on equivalent neurons in the brainstem. The axial muscles are controlled by these pathways. These muscles often contract bilaterally to provide postural support or some other bilateral function, such as swallowing or wrinkling of the brow.

Other medial system pathways originate in the brainstem. These include the pontine and medullary reticulospinal tracts, the lateral and medial vestibulospinal tracts, and the tectospinal tract.

Pontine and Medullary Reticulospinal Tracts
The cells that give rise to the pontine reticulospinal tract are in the medial pontine reticular formation. The tract descends in the ventral funiculus, and it ends on the ipsilateral medial group of interneurons. Its function is to excite motor neurons to the proximal extensor muscles to support posture.

The medullary reticulospinal tracts arise from neurons of the medial medulla, in particular the nucleus gigantocellularis. The tracts descend bilaterally in the ventral lateral funiculus, and they end mainly on interneurons associated with medial motor neuron cell groups. The function of the pathway is mainly inhibitory.

Lateral and Medial Vestibulospinal Tracts
The lateral vestibulospinal tract originates in the lateral vestibular nucleus, also known as Deiter's nucleus. This tract descends ipsilaterally through the ventral funiculus of the spinal cord and ends on interneurons associated with the medial motor neuron groups. The lateral vestibulospinal tract excites motor neurons that supply extensor muscles of the proximal part of the limb that are important for postural control. In addition, this pathway inhibits flexor motor neurons because it also excites the reciprocal Ia interneurons that receive Ia input from extensor muscles, which therefore inhibits flexor motor neurons. The excitatory input to the lateral vestibular nucleus is from both the semicircular canals and the otolith organs, whereas

the inhibitory input is from the Purkinje cells of the anterior vermis region of the cerebellar cortex. An important function of the lateral vestibulospinal tract is to assist in postural adjustments after angular and linear accelerations of the head.

The medial vestibulospinal tract originates from the medial vestibular nucleus. This tract descends in the ventral funiculus of the spinal cord to the cervical and midthoracic levels, and it ends on the medial group of interneurons. Sensory input to the medial vestibular nucleus from the labyrinth is chiefly from the semicircular canals. This pathway thus mediates adjustments in head position in response to angular acceleration of the head.

The Tectospinal Tract

The tectospinal tract originates in the deep layers of the superior colliculus. The axons cross to the contralateral side, just below the periaqueductal gray matter. They then descend in the ventral funiculus of the spinal cord to terminate on the medial group of interneurons in the upper cervical spinal cord. The tectospinal tract regulates head movement in response to visual, auditory, and somatic stimuli.

Monoaminergic Pathways

In addition to the lateral and medial systems, less specifically organized systems descend from the brainstem to the spinal cord. These include several pathways that use monoamines as synaptic transmitters.

The locus coeruleus and the nucleus subcoeruleus are nuclei located in the rostral pons, and they are composed of norepinephrine-containing neurons. These nuclei project widely throughout the CNS and their projection to the spinal cord travels in the lateral funiculus. Their terminals are on interneurons and motor neurons. The dominant effect of the pathway is inhibitory.

The raphe nuclei of the medulla also project widely throughout the CNS and give rise to several raphe-spinal pathways. Many of the raphe-spinal cells contain serotonin. Terminals on dorsal horn interneurons are inhibitory, whereas terminals on motor neurons are excitatory. The dorsal horn projection may help reduce nociceptive transmission (Fig. 7-9), whereas the ventral horn projection may enhance motor activity.

In general, the monoaminergic pathways may alter the responsiveness of spinal cord circuits, including the reflex arcs. In this respect, they induce widespread changes in excitability rather than discrete movements or specific changes in behavior.

Motor Deficits Caused by Lesions of Descending Motor Pathways

A common cause of motor impairment in humans is interruption of the cerebral cortical efferent fibers in the internal capsule; such interruptions occur in capsular strokes. The resulting disorder is often termed a **pyramidal tract syndrome,** or **upper motor neuron disease,** although these names are misnomers. Motor changes characteristic of this disorder include (1) increased phasic and tonic stretch reflexes (spasticity); (2) weakness, usually of the distal muscles, especially the finger muscles; (3) pathological reflexes,

including the **sign of Babinski** (dorsiflexion of the big toe and fanning of the other toes when the sole of the foot is stroked); and (4) a reduction in superficial reflexes, such as the abdominal and cremasteric reflexes. It is important to emphasize that if only the corticospinal tract is interrupted, as can occur with a lesion of the medullary pyramid, most of these signs are absent. In this situation, the most prominent deficits are weakness of the distal muscles, especially those of the fingers, and a Babinski sign. Spasticity does not occur, but instead muscle tone may actually decrease. Evidently, spasticity requires the disordered function of other pathways, such as the reticulospinal tracts, as would occur after loss of the descending cortical influence to the brainstem nuclei of origin of these tracts.

The effects of interruption of the medial system pathways are quite different from those produced by corticospinal tract lesions. The main deficits associated with medial system interruption are an initial reduction in the tone of postural muscles and loss of righting reflexes. Long-term effects include locomotor impairment and frequent falling. However, manual manipulation of objects is perfectly normal.

The Decerebrate Preparation

The decerebrate preparation has been useful for experimentally investigating how various descending pathways interact with the spinal cord circuitry. Surgical decerebration is achieved either by transecting the midbrain, often at an intercollicular level, or by occluding the blood vessels feeding this area. In the latter case, the anterior vermis of the cerebellum is also lesioned, an important distinction. With the intercollicular transection, some descending pathways, such as those originating in the cerebral cortex, are interrupted, whereas others, such as those originating in the brainstem, remain intact.

However, remember that the corticospinal tract is only a minor component of the cortical descending fibers. Many other cortical fibers project to locations throughout the brainstem, including the nuclei of origin for the medial descending pathways. Loss of these cortical control systems results in altered activity in the intact descending pathways. As a result, animals show hypertonia and suppression of some spinal reflexes, such as the flexion reflex, and exaggeration of others, such as the stretch reflex, a condition called **decerebrate rigidity.** Decerebrate animals maintain a posture that has been called **exaggerated standing.** Human patients with brainstem damage may also develop a decerebrate state that has many of the same reflex features as animal preparations. The prognosis in such patients is poor if signs of decerebration appear.

Loss of descending control on the reticular formation results in increased activity in the pontine reticulospinal pathway and decreased activity in the medullary reticulospinal pathway. This increase and decrease in activity, respectively, produce increased excitation and decreased inhibition (disinhibition) of the motor neurons, which explains the observed rigidity. Interestingly, this hypertonia can be relieved by cutting the dorsal roots, thus indicating that the reticulospinal tracts have a major effect on γ motor neurons, whose activity alters muscle stiffness only by increasing muscle spindle sensitivity and thereby causes increased activity in the Ia and II afferents that innervate the α motor neurons.

When vessel occlusion is used to generate the decerebrate state, the lateral vestibulospinal tract becomes hyperactive because of damage to Purkinje cells in the anterior vermis of the cerebellum, which provide the major inhibitory projection to the lateral vestibular nucleus. Interestingly, this hypertonia is not lost after transection of the dorsal roots, which implies that the lateral vestibulospinal tract is acting to a significant extent directly on the α motor neurons (either monosynaptically or via interneurons).

BRAINSTEM CONTROL OF POSTURE AND MOVEMENT

The importance of motor control pathways that originate in the brainstem is evident from observations of the extensor hypertonus and increased phasic stretch reflexes that occur in decerebrate animals. Particular brainstem systems have been identified that influence posture and locomotion. Brainstem circuits are also critically involved in the control of eye movement; these circuits are discussed in a separate section at the end of the chapter.

Postural Reflexes

Several reflex mechanisms are evoked when the head is moved or the neck is bent. There are three types of postural reflexes: vestibular reflexes, tonic neck reflexes, and righting reflexes. The sensory receptors responsible for these reflexes include the vestibular apparatus (see Chapter 8), which is stimulated by head movement, and stretch receptors in the neck.

The **vestibular reflexes** constitute one class of postural reflex. Rotation of the head activates sensory receptors of the semicircular canals (see Chapter 8). In addition to generating eye movement, the sensory input to the vestibular nuclei results in postural adjustments. Such adjustments are mediated by commands transmitted to the spinal cord through the lateral and medial vestibulospinal tracts and the reticulospinal tracts. The lateral vestibulospinal tract activates extensor muscles that support posture. For instance, if the head is rotated to the left, postural support is increased on the left side. This increased support prevents the subject from falling to the left as the head rotation continues. Any disease that eliminates labyrinthine function in the left ear will cause the person to tend to fall to the left. Conversely, a disease that irritates (stimulates) the left labyrinth will cause the person to tend to fall to the right. The medial vestibulospinal tract causes contractions of neck muscles that oppose the induced movement **(vestibulocollic reflex).**

Tilting the head also changes the linear acceleration on individual hair cells of the otolith organs of the vestibular apparatus. The resulting changes in hair cell activity can produce eye movement and postural adjustment. For example, tilting the head and body forward (without bending the neck and consequently without evoking the tonic neck reflexes) in a quadruped, such as a cat, results in extension of the forelimbs and flexion of the hind limbs. This vestibular action tends to restore the body toward its original orientation. Conversely, if the head and body are tilted backward (without bending the neck), the forelimbs flex and the hind limbs extend. Otolithic organs also contribute to the **vestibular placing reaction.** If an animal, such as a cat, is dropped, stimulation of the utricles leads to extension of the forelimbs in preparation for landing.

The **tonic neck reflexes** are another type of positional reflex. These reflexes are activated by the muscle spindles found in neck muscles. These muscles contain the largest concentration of muscle spindles of any muscle in the body. If the neck is bent (without tilting the head), the neck muscle spindles evoke tonic neck reflexes without interference from the vestibular system. When the neck is extended, the forelimbs extend and the hind limbs flex. The opposite effects occur when the neck is flexed. Note that these effects are opposite those evoked by the vestibular system. Furthermore, if the neck is bent to the left, the extensor muscles in the limbs on the left contract more, and the flexor muscles in the limbs on the right side relax.

The third class of postural reflex is the **righting reflexes.** These reflexes tend to restore an altered position of the head and body toward normal. The receptors responsible for righting reflexes include the vestibular apparatus, the neck stretch receptors, and mechanoreceptors of the body wall.

Brainstem Control of Locomotion

The spinal cord contains neural circuits that serve as **central pattern generators** for locomotion, as discussed earlier. These CPG circuits produce very regular rhythmic output that characterizes stereotyped behavior, such as walking. The irregularities of real-world environments, however, often require modification of this stereotyped output (e.g., if you are walking and see a hole in the floor where you are about to step, you can extend the forward swing of your leg past the hole onto solid ground beyond it).

Such modifications can be the result of sensory input to the spinal cord, as was shown in Figure 9-9, where stimulation of FRA fibers in a peripheral nerve caused a phase shift in the locomotor pattern. They can also be the result of descending commands along the motor pathways discussed earlier. In this case, sensory data (e.g., visual) can be used by the brain to make anticipatory modifications in CPG activity so that potential obstacles can be avoided. In addition, we can voluntarily control activation, or shutdown, of the CPG (i.e., deciding consciously when to start and stop walking). Such voluntary regulation of spinal CPGs originates in the cerebral cortex; however, much of the cortical influence on locomotion appears to be mediated via projections to brainstem regions known as locomotor regions. A locomotor region can be defined as a brain area that when stimulated, leads to sustained locomotion.

There are several such locomotor regions in the brainstem, and they are located at different levels ranging from the subthalamus to the medulla and are connected with each other. The best known is the **midbrain locomotor region,** which is thought to organize commands to initiate locomotion. It is located in the midbrain at the level of the inferior colliculus. Voluntary activity that originates in the motor cortex can trigger locomotion by the action of corticobulbar fibers projecting to the midbrain locomotor region. The commands are relayed through the reticular formation and then to the spinal cord via the reticulospinal tracts.

Motor Control by the Cerebral Cortex

Thus far in this chapter, emphasis has been placed on reflexes and relatively automatic types of movement. We will now discuss the neural basis for more complex, goal-directed voluntary movement. Such movement often varies when repeated and is frequently initiated as a result of cognitive processes rather than in direct response to an external stimulus. Thus, it requires the participation of motor areas of the cerebral cortex.

Let us first consider what is necessary to generate a voluntary movement. For example, to make a reaching movement with your arm, you must first identify the target (or goal) and locate it in external space. Next, a limb trajectory must be determined based on an internal representation of your arm and, in particular, your hand relative to the target. Finally, a set of forces necessary to generate the desired trajectory must be computed. This process is often thought of as a series of transformations between coordinate systems. For example, the location of a visually identified target is measured in a retinotopic space, but its location is perceived in an external or world space (i.e., the position of a nonmoving target is perceived as stable, even when the eye, and thus the target's image on the retina, changes). Next, calculation of a trajectory would involve a body- or hand-centered system, and finally, forces must ultimately be computed in a muscle-based reference frame.

These steps form a linear sequence, and traditionally it was thought that a hierarchy of motor areas carried out the successive steps. For example, the target of the movement was thought to be identified by pooling sensory information in the **posterior parietal cerebral cortex** (Fig. 9-14, *A*). This information would then be transmitted to the supplementary motor and premotor areas, where a motor plan is

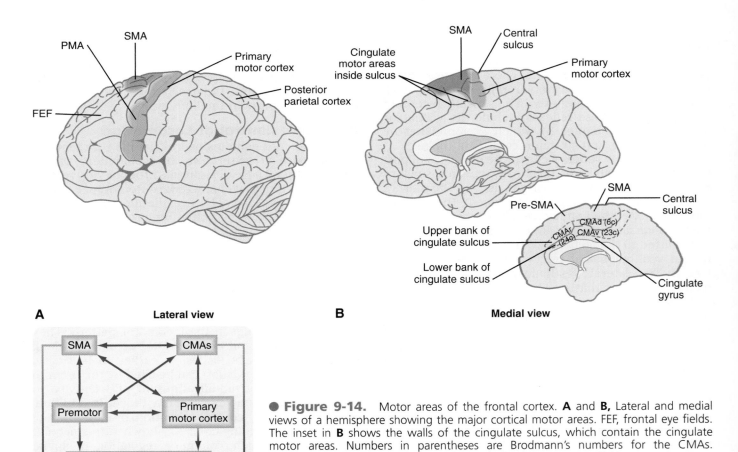

● **Figure 9-14.** Motor areas of the frontal cortex. **A** and **B,** Lateral and medial views of a hemisphere showing the major cortical motor areas. FEF, frontal eye fields. The inset in **B** shows the walls of the cingulate sulcus, which contain the cingulate motor areas. Numbers in parentheses are Brodmann's numbers for the CMAs. **C,** Diagram showing interconnections of the motor areas. PMA, premotor area; SMA, supplementary motor area; CMA, cingulate motor area.

developed and then forwarded to the primary motor cortex, whose activity would be related to the final execution stage (e.g., generation of appropriate force levels). The motor cortex would then transmit commands, via the descending pathways discussed earlier, to the spinal cord and brainstem motor nuclei.

Although there is significant evidence in support of this hierarchical view of the generation of voluntary movement by the cortical motor system, more recent results have suggested a different conception, namely, that the various motor areas should be thought of as forming a parallel distributed network rather than a strict hierarchy (Fig. 9-14, _C_). For example, each cortical motor area makes its own significant contribution to the descending motor pathways, with the primary motor cortex contributing only about half the fibers in the corticospinal tract that arise from the frontal lobe. Moreover, the various motor areas are all bidirectionally connected to each other, and the single-unit recording studies described later suggest that each of the areas plays a role in several of the stages of planning and executing a movement. This debate forms one of the themes of the following discussion because in its various guises, the distributed network versus hierarchical organization debate has been ongoing for decades and will probably continue for some time.

Cortical Motor Areas

The motor areas in the cerebral cortex were originally defined on the basis of experiments in which electrical stimuli applied to the cortex evoked discrete, contralateral movement. Movement, however, can also be evoked when other cortical areas are stimulated more intensely. Thus, motor areas are defined as those from which movement can be evoked by the lowest stimulus intensity. On the basis of these stimulation studies, the effects produced by lesions, anatomic experiments, electrophysiological recordings, and modern imaging studies in humans, several "motor" areas of the cerebral cortex have been recognized (Fig. 9-14), including the **primary motor cortex** in the precentral gyrus, the **premotor area** just rostral to the primary motor cortex, the **supplementary motor cortex** on the medial aspect of the hemisphere, and three **cingulate motor areas** located on the walls of the cingulate sulcus in the frontal lobe. There are also cortical regions scattered across all cortical lobes whose activity is related specifically to eye movement (see the section Eye Movement).

Somatotopic Organization of Cortical Motor Areas
Primary Motor Cortex

The primary motor cortex (or just motor cortex) can be defined as the region of cortex from which movements are elicited with the least amount of electrical stimulation. It is essentially congruent with Brodmann's cytoarchitectonic area 4 (Fig. 10-3). In humans it is located on the parts of the precentral gyrus that form the rostral wall of the central sulcus and the caudal half of the apex of the gyrus. Based on initial mapping studies, which were done with surface stimu-

lation, the motor cortex was described as having a topographic organization that parallels that of the somatosensory cortex. The face, body, and upper limb were represented on the lateral surface with the face located inferiorly, near the lateral fissure, the torso most superiorly, and the lower extremity mostly on the medial aspect of the hemisphere. This somatotopic organization is often represented as a figurine or in a graphic form called a **motor homunculus** (Fig. 9-15, _A_). The distortion of the various body parts in the homunculus indicates approximately how much of the cortex is devoted to their motor control. This simple homunculus was likened to a piano keyboard and fit well with traditional conceptions of the motor cortex being the final cortical stage and acting as a relay for sending motor commands to the spinal cord.

Beginning in the 1960s and 1970s, mapping studies began using microelectrodes inserted to the deep, or output, layers of the cortex to apply stimuli. With this technique, called **intracortical microstimulation (ICMS),** much lower stimulus intensities could be used to evoke movements and thus allowed higher-resolution mapping of the motor cortex, which revealed a much more complex topography than was previously imagined (Fig. 9-15, _C_). Movement about each joint was found to be evoked by many noncontiguous columns throughout wide regions of the motor cortex. Thus, cell columns related to movement about a particular joint are actually interspersed among columns that control movement about many other joints. In sum, although the motor cortex may have large subdivisions corresponding to a limb or the head, within each such area there is a complex intermingling of cell columns that control the muscles within that body part.

Such mixing of cell columns makes functional sense because most movement requires the coordinated action of muscles throughout a limb and most connectivity in the cortex is localized (i.e., axon collaterals that connect different cell columns are primarily confined to a 1- to 3-mm region surrounding the column from which they originate). Thus, by having multiple cell columns that control movement about a joint and intermixing them with columns controlling movement about other joints, multijoint movement can be generated as a whole.

Although the somatotopy of the motor cortex is in part anatomically determined by the topography of the corticospinal pathway, it is also a dynamic map. Axon collaterals link the different cell columns, so activity in one column could potentially lead to movement about multiple joints. In fact, this can happen, but these intercolumnar connections are modulated by inhibitory GABAergic interneurons. This was shown by locally blocking GABA in one region of the motor cortex and then stimulating the neighboring region. Before the block, stimuli evoked contractions of one set of muscles, but once inhibition was blocked, contractions were also evoked in muscles controlled by the region that was no longer inhibited (Fig. 9-16). Functional connections between cell columns can be controlled on a millisecond time scale, and depending

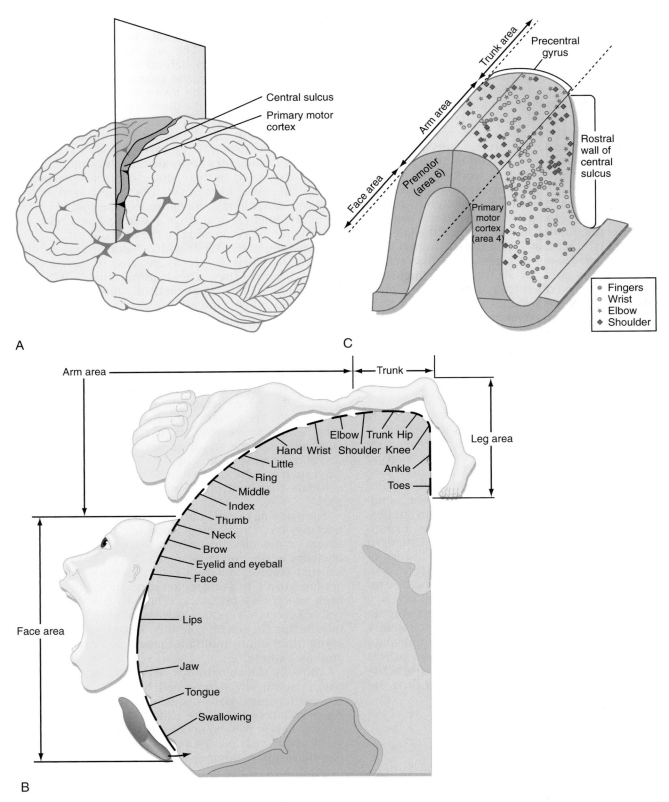

Central sulcus

Primary motor cortex

Trunk area

Precentral gyrus

Arm area

Rostral wall of central sulcus

Face area

Premotor (area 6)

Primary motor cortex (area 4)

- Fingers
- Wrist
- Elbow
- Shoulder

A

C

Arm area — Trunk

Elbow Trunk Hip

Hand Wrist Shoulder Knee

Leg area

Little

Ring

Ankle

Middle

Toes

Index

Thumb

Neck

Brow

Eyelid and eyeball

Face

Face area

Lips

Jaw

Tongue

Swallowing

B

● **Figure 9-15.** Traditional and modern views of motor cortex musculotopic organization. **A,** Lateral view of the cerebrum showing a plane of section through the precentral gyrus (primary motor cortex) to obtain the section shown in **B. B,** Classic view of motor cortex musculotopy. **C,** Modern view of motor cortex organization in which each body part is represented multiple times across several discrete regions.

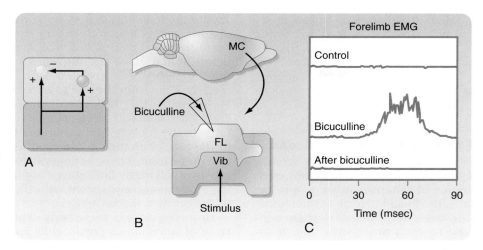

● **Figure 9-16.** Dynamic nature of a motor cortex musculotopic map. Inhibitory GABAergic interneurons play an important role in shaping motor responses to stimulation of each region of the motor cortex. **A,** Schematic showing excitatory connections between two regions of primary motor cortex and local inhibitory neurons within a single region. **B,** Schematic of a rat brain indicating motor cortex regions where electrical stimuli were applied to evoke movements (Vib region) and bicuculline was applied to block GABAergic synapses (in the FL region). FL, forelimb; HL, hind limb; Vib, vibrissa. **C,** FL EMG records showing response to stimulation of the Vib region before, during the application of bicuculline, and after washing it out. Note that Vib stimulation evoked vibrissae movement in all conditions but evoked forelimb movement only when inhibitory interneurons were blocked. (Data from Jacobs K, Donoghue J: Science 251:944, 1991.)

on their state, the somatotopic map can be radically changed. Longer-term plastic changes are also known to occur; for example, the use (or disuse) of a body part can affect the size of its representation.

Supplementary Motor Area

The supplementary motor area (SMA) is located mainly on the medial surface of the hemisphere, just anterior to the primary motor cortex, and corresponds to the medial portion of Brodmann's area 6 (Fig. 9-14). It is subdivided into two regions: the more posterior part is referred to as the SMA proper (or just SMA), and the anterior portion is called the pre-SMA. The SMA proper is similar to the other motor areas already listed: it contains a complete somatotopic map, it contributes to the corticospinal tract, and it is interconnected with the other motor areas. In contrast, the pre-SMA is not strongly connected with the other motor areas and spinal cord but rather is connected to the prefrontal cortex.

The results of stimulation studies show that as in the motor cortex, there is a complete somatotopic map in the SMA. Stimulation of the SMA can evoke isolated movement about single joints, similar to that after stimulation of the motor cortex, but higher-intensity and longer-duration stimulation is necessary; moreover, the evoked movements are often more complex than those evoked by stimulation of the motor cortex. However, longer-duration stimulation of the primary motor cortex can also evoke complex, apparently purposeful movement sequences, so the distinction is not absolute. In addition, stimulation of the SMA can produce vocalization or complex postural movements,

but it can also have the opposite result, namely, a temporary arrest of movement or speech. Removal of the supplementary motor cortex retards movement of the opposite extremities and may result in forced grasping movements with the contralateral hand.

Premotor Area

This area lies rostral to the primary motor cortex and is contained in Brodmann's area 6 on the lateral surface of the brain (Fig. 9-14). It can be distinguished from the primary motor cortex by the higher stimulus intensities needed to evoke movement. The premotor area has been divided into two functionally distinct subdivisions: dorsal and ventral. Like the motor cortex, both subdivisions are somatotopically organized and both contribute to the corticospinal tract. The dorsal division (PMd) contains a relatively complete map representing the leg, trunk, arm, and face. In contrast, the somatotopic map of the ventral division (PMv) is mostly limited to the arm and face, with only a small leg representation. Thus, the PMv appears to be specialized for control of upper limb and head movement. A second difference between the subdivisions is that PMd contains a large representation of the proximal muscles, whereas PMv has a large representation of the distal muscles.

Cingulate Motor Areas

These motor areas are located within the cingulate sulcus at approximately the same anterior-posterior level as the SMA. There are three cingulate motor areas (dorsal, ventral, and rostral) (Fig. 9-14, *B*). Each contains a somatotopic map and contributes to the corticospinal tract. Microstimulation in these areas evokes movement similar to that evoked by motor cortex stimulation, except that once again, higher stimulus intensities are needed. Single-cell recordings during movements have shown that the spontaneous activity of neurons in the cingulate motor areas is related to the preparation and execution of movements.

Connections of the Cortical Motor Areas

The motor areas of the cortex receive input from a number of sources, cortical and subcortical; however, the single largest source of synapses in an area is the area itself, specifically, the local intrinsic connections. Second, all the motor areas described earlier are bidirectionally connected to each other with high topographic specificity (Fig. 9-14, C). For example, the arm regions of the primary motor cortex and the cingulate motor areas project to each other. Sensory information comes from ascending pathways that relay in the thalamus. This information can reach the motor cortex directly from the thalamus or indirectly by way of the somatosensory cortex. Both somatosensory information and visual information are conveyed to the motor areas from the posterior parietal cortex. The motor areas of the cortex also receive information through circuits that interconnect them with the other major brain regions involved in motor control, namely, the cerebellum and basal ganglia. These two structures project to distinct parts of the thalamus (the ventral lateral [VL] and ventral anterior [VA] nuclei), which then project to the cortical motor areas.

The output of the cortical motor areas to the spinal cord and brainstem is conducted through several descending pathways. These pathways include not only direct projections through the corticospinal and corticobulbar tracts (to the cranial nerve nuclei) but also indirect projections to the red nucleus and to various nuclei in the reticular formation. Descending projections from these brainstem sites were reviewed earlier (see the section Descending Motor Pathways). Control of head and neck muscles is mediated by projections to the various cranial nerve nuclei. The motor regions also project to the cerebellum and basal ganglia, thus completing neuroanatomic loops with these structures. The major connection to the cerebellum is via the corticopontine projections to the basilar pontine nuclei, which in turn project to the cerebellum. In addition, the cortical motor areas project, mostly via disynaptic pathways that synapse in the midbrain, to the inferior olive, another important precerebellar nucleus. The cortical motor regions project directly to the striatum of the basal ganglia. Finally, there are major projections to the thalamus by which the cortex regulates the information that it receives.

Activity of Motor Cortex Cells

The role of individual motor cortex neurons in the control of movement has been extensively investigated in trained monkeys. In these experiments, discharges from a neuron in the primary motor cortex are recorded during the execution of a previously learned simple movement, such as wrist flexion, made immediately in response to a sensory cue (Fig. 9-17). Motor cortex neurons were found to change their firing rates before initiation of the movement, and the onset of this change was correlated with the reaction time (i.e., the time from the cue to onset of the movement). Moreover, in this task the change in firing of motor cortex neurons was often correlated to the contractile force of the muscle that generates the movement and to the rate of change in force rather than to the position of the joint. These findings suggest that these cells are involved in the final stages of planning and executing movements, consistent with the hierarchical view of the cortical motor areas.

However, even in these early experiments, the firing rates of some motor cortex cells appeared to relate to earlier planning stages. Moreover, even when a monkey was trained to withhold the movement for a certain period after the cue, the firing rates of motor cortex neurons still changed despite the absence of any movement. Such "set-related" activity has been amply confirmed in a variety of other tasks and suggests that motor cortex activity may be involved in the earlier planning stages along with activity in other motor areas of the cortex. It also suggests the possibility that other, perhaps subcortical, systems may be needed to generate a trigger signal for the initiation of movement.

Subsequent studies have used tasks in which animals were trained to move a manipulandum (a device with a handle to hold and a small circle on the end) to capture lighted targets on a surface in front of them (Fig. 9-18, A). These experiments demonstrated that cells in the arm region of the motor cortex showed changes in their firing rates to movement in many different directions and thus were described as broadly tuned (Fig. 9-18, B). That is, a cell that showed a maximal increase for movement in one particular direction, called its preferred direction, would also show somewhat smaller increases or even decreases for movement in other directions (Fig. 9-18, C). Moreover, the preferred directions of the different cells were uniformly distributed across all 360 degrees of possible movement directions. These results implied that a particular cell is probably involved in most arm movements, but they also raised the problem of how precise movements could be made with such broadly tuned cells. It was suggested that although changes in the activity of individual cells could not precisely predict or specify the direction of the upcoming movement, the net activity of the population could. To test this idea, models were made in which the activity of each cell is represented as a vector (Fig. 9-18, D). The direction of each cell vector is determined by the preferred direction of the cell, and the magnitude of the vector for a particular movement is proportional to the firing rate of the cell during the time preceding the movement. The individual cell vectors (Fig. 9-18, D, black lines) from hundreds of cells can then be vectorially summed to get a resultant or population vector (Fig. 9-18, D, red lines) that accurately predicts the upcoming movement.

One of the difficulties in assessing the relationship between firing of cortical cells and various movement

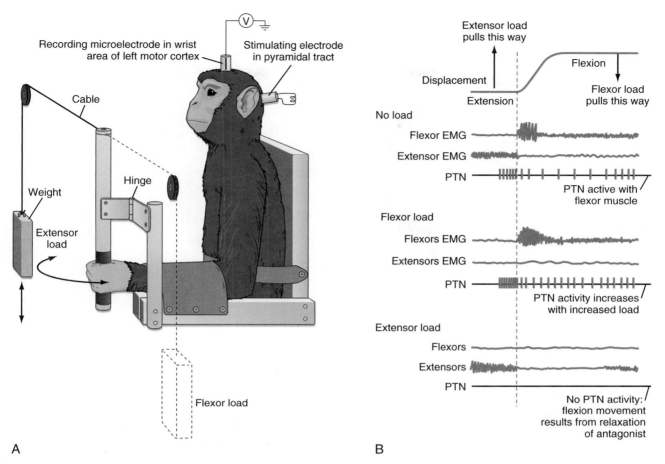

● Figure 9-17. **A,** Experimental arrangement for recording from a corticospinal neuron while a monkey performs trained wrist movements. The stimulation electrode is used to elicit antidromic spikes that are used to identify the motor cortex neuron specifically as a pyramidal tract neuron. Stimuli are not applied while the monkey is performing movements. **B,** The pyramidal tract neuron (PTN) discharges before the onset of movement or EMG activity when flexors need to generate force (no load and flexor load conditions). Moreover, the firing rate is correlated with the level of flexor force that is needed. In the extensor load condition, flexors do not need to contract to generate movement, and thus there is no activity in this PTN. The top trace shows wrist movement, which is essentially identical for all three experimental conditions. Thus this cell's activity encodes force magnitude and direction, but not displacement. Figure based on work of Evarts and colleagues.

parameters, such as force, velocity, displacement, and target location, is that these parameters are normally correlated with each other. Thus, variations of the tasks described earlier have been used to decorrelate these various parameters (e.g., using weights to vary the force needed to make a movement without changing the displacement as illustrated in Fig. 9-17, *A,* or rotating the starting position of the wrist so that different muscles are required to generate the same trajectory in external space). The results of these experiments showed that the activity of motor cortex cells may be related to each of the various motor planning stages. Furthermore, the activity of a single cell may correlate with one parameter initially and then switch as the time for onset of movement approaches.

Activity in Other Cortical Motor Areas

Activity in the premotor and supplementary motor areas is in many ways similar to that in the primary motor cortex. Cells in these areas show activity related to upcoming movement, and the activity is correlated

with movement parameters, such as displacement, force, and target location, just as primary motor cortex activity can be, consistent with the distributed network view of the cortical motor areas. There do, however, appear to be some real differences between the areas as well, although these differences may be more quantitative than qualitative. For example, a higher percentage of cells in the premotor and supplementary motor areas show activity related to earlier motor planning stages than do cells in the primary motor cortex. In addition, the premotor and supplementary motor areas can be distinguished from each other by the apparently greater involvement of the premotor area in movements made to external cues (such as in the task shown in Fig. 9-18) and the greater involvement of the supplementary motor area in movements made in response to internal cues (i.e., self-initiated). Recent research has also revealed that each of these areas is functionally heterogeneous and can therefore be further subdivided; however, such details are beyond the present scope.

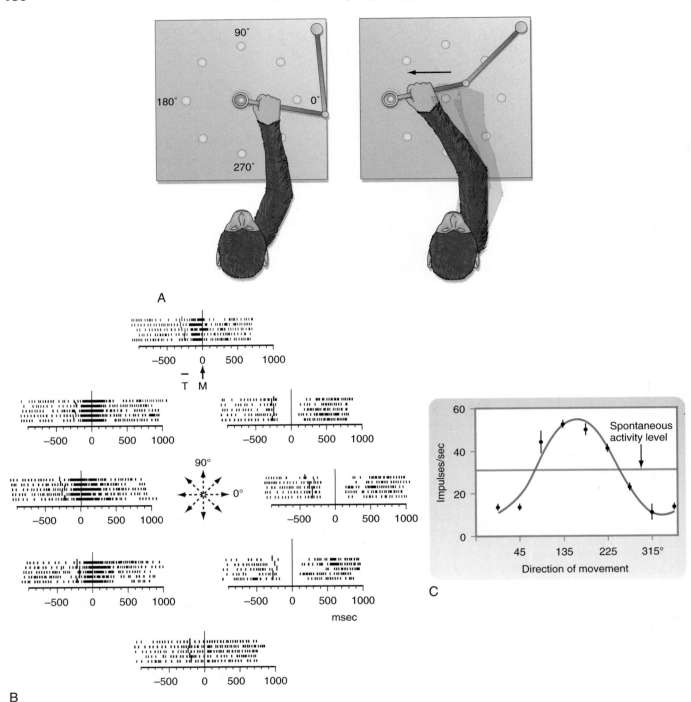

● **Figure 9-18.** **A,** Experimental setup in which a monkey holds onto the arm of the apparatus and captures light spots with the distal end of the arm. The monkey first captures the central light spot and then captures whichever of the surrounding targets that becomes illuminated. **B,** Raster plots showing the activity of one motor cortex cell during movement in eight different directions. T indicates the time at which the target light turns on, whereas M indicates the time at the onset of movement, which is at the center of each raster. Each mark on a raster represents a spike of a motor cortex cell, and each row of marks shows the cell's activity during one trial. **C,** Cosine function was fit to the firing level as a function of the direction of movement. The horizontal bar indicates the average spontaneous firing rate in the absence of an upcoming movement. Note that for most directions, the activity in the periods just before and during movement changes significantly from baseline.

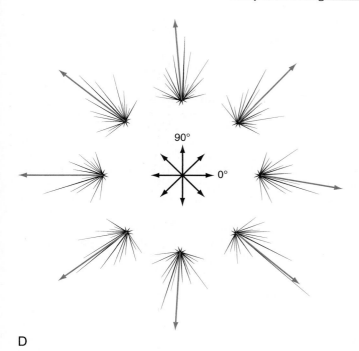

D

● **Figure 9-18, cont'd D,** Vector model of population activity in the motor cortex. Black lines are individual cell vectors. When all of them are summed for a particular direction of movement, the resulting population vector *(red)* points in essentially the direction of the upcoming movement. (**B** and **C,** Modified from Georgopoulos AP et al: J Neurosci 2:1527, 1982; **D,** modified from Georgopoulos AP et al. In Massion J et al [eds]: Neuronal coding of motor performance. Exp Brain Res Suppl 7:327, 1983.)

MOTOR CONTROL BY THE CEREBELLUM

Overview of the Role of the Cerebellum in Motor Control

More than 100 years ago, scientists showed that damage to the cerebellum led to deficits in motor coordination. That is, damage or loss of the cerebellum does not lead to paralysis, loss of sensation, or an inability to understand the nature of a task, but rather it leads to an inability to perform movements well. Yet it has been hard to define the cerebellum's precise role or roles in generating movement despite, paradoxically, also having more detailed knowledge of its deceptively simple anatomic and physiological organization than any other CNS region. The cerebellum is proposed to play a critical role in the learning and execution of both voluntary and certain reflex movements. However, hypotheses about these roles face significant challenges that prevent their current acceptance. Here, the behavioral effects of damaging the cerebellum are presented, followed by a description of its connectivity, both intrinsic and with the rest of the CNS, and then finally its activity.

Behavioral Consequences of Cerebellar Damage

Damage to the cerebellum impairs motor function on the ipsilateral side of the body. This reflects a double crossing of most cerebellar-related output as it travels

to the motor neurons. The first crossing typically occurs in the cerebellar efferent pathway, whereas the second crossing takes place in the descending motor pathways. For example, the cerebellum projects to the contralateral motor cortex, via the thalamus, and the corticospinal pathway recrosses the midline at the lower medulla.

The specific motor deficits that result from cerebellar lesions depend on which functional component of the cerebellum is most affected. If the flocculonodular lobe is damaged, the motor disorders resemble those produced by a lesion of the vestibular apparatus; such disorders include difficulty in balance and gait and often nystagmus. If the vermis is affected, the motor disturbance affects the trunk, and if the intermediate region or hemisphere is involved, motor disorders occur in the limbs. The part of the limbs affected depends on the site of damage; hemispheric lesions affect the distal muscles more than paravermal lesions do.

Types of motor dysfunction in cerebellar disease include disorders of coordination, equilibrium, and muscle tone. Incoordination is called **ataxia** and is often expressed as **dysmetria,** a condition in which errors in the direction and force of movement prevent a limb from being moved smoothly to a desired position. Ataxia may also be expressed as **dysdiadochokinesia,** in which rapid alternating supination and pronation of the arm is difficult to execute. When more complicated movement is attempted, **decomposition of movement** occurs, in which the movement is accomplished in a series of discrete steps rather than as a smooth sequence. An **intention tremor** appears when the subject is asked to touch a target; the affected hand (or foot) develops a tremor that increases in magnitude as the target is approached. When equilibrium is disturbed, impaired balance may be seen, and the individual tends to fall toward the affected side and may walk with a wide-based stance (gait ataxia). Speech may be slow and slurred, a defect called **scanning speech.** Muscle tone may be diminished **(hypotonia),** except for lesions of the anterior vermis (see earlier section on decerebrate rigidity); the diminished tone may be associated with a **pendular knee jerk.** This can be demonstrated by eliciting a phasic stretch reflex of the quadriceps muscle by striking the patellar tendon. The leg continues to swing back and forth because of the hypotonia, in contrast to the highly damped oscillation in a normal person.

These disorders reflect, in part, abnormal timing of muscle contractions. Normally, limb movements involve precisely timed EMG bursts in both agonist and antagonist muscles. There is an initial agonist burst followed by a burst in the antagonist and, finally, a second agonist burst. With cerebellar damage, the relative timing of these bursts is abnormal (Fig. 9-19).

Cerebellar Organization

The cerebellum ("little brain") is located in the posterior fossa of the cranium, just below the occipital lobe, and is connected to the brainstem via three cerebellar peduncles (superior, middle, and inferior). From the outer surface, only the cortex is visible. Deep to the

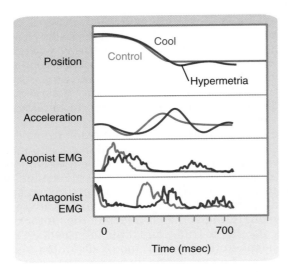

● Figure 9-19. Disruption of cerebellar activity alters the timing of EMG responses during movement. The cerebellar nuclei were cooled to block their functioning temporarily while monkeys performed movements about their elbow. Loss of cerebellar activity disrupts the relative timing of agonist and antagonist EMG bursts. This leads to abnormal acceleration of the limb and a movement trajectory that overshoots the target position (hypermetria). (Data from Flament D, Hore J: J Neurophysiol 55:1221, 1986.)

cortex is the white matter of the cerebellum, and buried within the white matter are the four cerebellar nuclei: proceeding medially to laterally, the fastigial, globose, emboliform, and dentate nuclei. The middle two nuclei are often grouped together and referred to as the interpositus nucleus. For the most part, cerebellar afferents to the cortex and nuclei enter the cerebellum via the inferior and middle peduncles, and efferents from the cerebellar nuclei leave via the superior peduncle.

The cerebellar cortex is subdivided into three rostrocaudally arranged lobes: the **anterior lobe,** the **posterior lobe,** and the **flocculonodular lobe** (Fig. 9-20, *A*). The cerebellar lobes are separated by two major fissures, the **primary fissure** and the **posterolateral fissure,** and each lobe is made up of one or more **lobules.** Each lobule of the cerebellar cortex is composed of a series of transverse folds called **folia.**

The cerebellar cortex has also been divided into longitudinal compartments (Fig. 9-20, *B* and *C*). Initially, the cerebellar cortex was divided into three such compartments: the vermis, which lies on the midline; the paravermis, which lies adjacent to both sides of the vermis; and the lateral hemispheres. These regions have now been subdivided into many further compartments on the basis of **myeloarchitectonics** (patterns of axonal bundles in the white matter) and the expression patterns of specific molecules, such as aldolase C. Although the functional significance of these compartments is not fully known, the topography of cerebellar afferents, specifically the olivocerebellar system, is precisely aligned with them, and the receptive field properties of cerebellar Purkinje cells also tend to follow this organizational scheme.

Cerebellar Cortex
Afferent Systems
There are two major cerebellar afferent systems: mossy fibers and climbing fibers. Mossy fibers are named for their distinctive appearance in the cerebellar cortex: as a mossy fiber courses through the granule layer, on occasion it swells and sends out a bunch of short twisty branchlets. These entities are called rosettes and are points of synaptic contact between these fibers and neurons in the granule cell layer. Mossy fibers arise from many sources, including the spinal cord (the spinocerebellar pathways), dorsal column nuclei, trigeminal nucleus, nuclei in the reticular formation, primary vestibular afferents, vestibular nuclei, cerebellar nuclei, and the basilar pontine nuclei. The details of mossy fiber projection patterns are beyond the scope of the present chapter; however, several general points are worth noting:

1. Mossy fibers are excitatory.
2. They convey exteroceptive and proprioceptive information from the body and head and form at least two somatotopic maps of the body across the cerebellar cortex. However, similar to what was described for the motor cortex, these maps are fractured in the sense that contiguous body regions are not necessarily represented on contiguous areas of the cerebellar cortex; rather, the maps are complicated mosaics.
3. Mossy fibers conveying vestibular-related information are restricted to the flocculonodular lobe and regions of the vermis. This sometimes leads to the flocculonodular lobe and regions of the vermis being referred to as the vestibulocerebellum. However, these same regions also receive mossy fibers conveying a variety of other information (e.g., visual, neck, oculomotor), so their function is not exclusively vestibular.
4. The single largest source of mossy fibers comes from the basilar pontine nuclei, which serve to relay information from areas throughout much of the cerebral cortex.
5. Mossy fibers enter the cerebellum via all three cerebellar peduncles and provide collaterals to the cerebellar nuclei before heading up to the cortex. In sum, via the mossy fiber system, the cerebellum receives a wide variety of sensory information, as well as descending motor–related activity.

In contrast to the diverse origins of mossy fibers, climbing fibers all originate from a single nucleus: the inferior olive, which is located in the rostral medulla, just dorsal and lateral to the pyramids. The olivary neurons are almost all projection cells whose axons leave the nucleus without giving off collaterals and then cross the brainstem to enter the cerebellum primarily via the inferior cerebellar peduncle. Like mossy fibers, olivocerebellar axons are excitatory and send collaterals to the cerebellar nuclei as they ascend through the cerebellar white matter to the cortex. In the cerebellar cortex, olivocerebellar axons may synapse with basket, stellate, and Golgi cells but form a special synaptic

● **Figure 9-20.** Anatomic divisions of the cerebellum. **A,** Midsagittal view showing folding of the cortex into lobe, lobules, and folia. **B,** Schematic view of an unfolded ferret cerebellar cortex to illustrate earlier compartmentation schemes for subdividing the cerebellar cortex into three (vermis, paravermis, and hemisphere) and then seven longitudinally running zones. Light yellow colored portion of each hemisphere indicates an area for which no data were available.

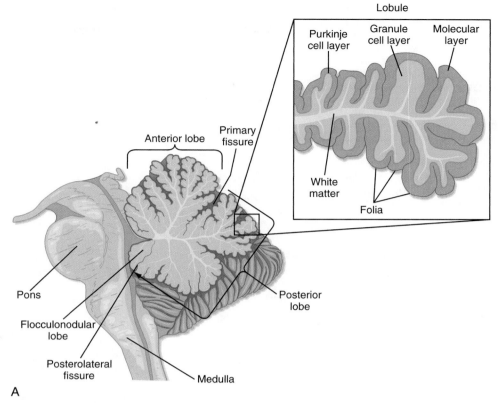

A

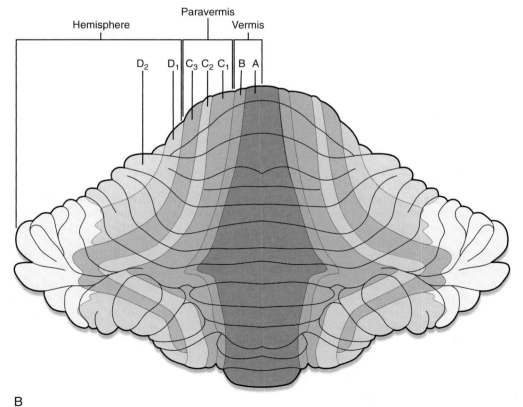

B

● **Figure 9-20, cont'd**
C, Schematic of an unfolded rat cerebellum showing its subdivision into well over 20 compartments based on staining for molecular markers, in this case zebrin II (aldolase C). Letters and numbers on the right half of the cerebellum indicate the zebrin compartment number. Roman numerals down the center indicate cerebellar lobules. Names on left hemisphere indicate names of cerebellar lobules. CP, copula pyramis; Cr, crus; DPFL, dorsal paraflocculus; FL, flocculus; Par, paramedian; pf, primary fissure; Sim, simplex; VPFL, ventral paraflocculus. (**B,** Modified from Voogd J. In Neurobiology of Cerebellar Evolution and Development. Chicago, American Medical Association, 1969; **C,** courtesy of Dr. Izumi Sugihara.)

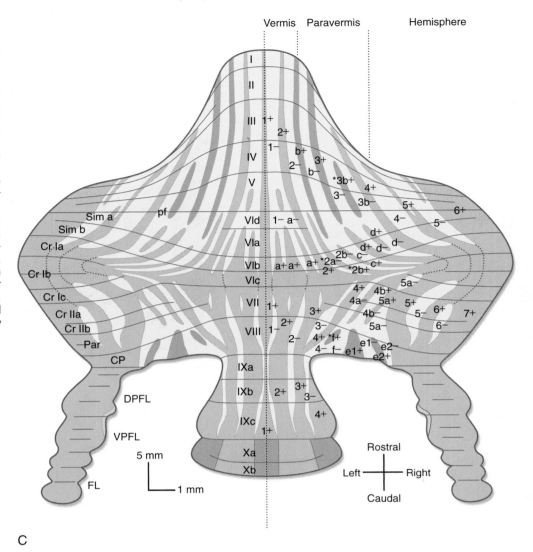

C

arrangement with Purkinje cells. Each Purkinje cell receives input from only a single climbing fiber, which "climbs" up its proximal dendrites and makes hundreds of excitatory synapses. Note, the terminal portion of the olivocerebellar axon is referred to as a climbing fiber. Conversely, each olivary axon will branch to form about 10 to 15 climbing fibers.

The inferior olive is a distinctive brain region for several reasons. As already noted, its neurons are virtually all projection cells, so there is little local chemical synaptic interaction between the cells. Instead, olivary neurons are electrically coupled to each other by gap junctions. In fact, the olive has the highest density of neuronal gap junctions in the CNS. This allows olivary neurons to have synchronized activity that gets transmitted to the cerebellum. Afferents to the olive may be divided into two main classes, excitatory input, which arises from many regions throughout the CNS, and inhibitory GABAergic input from the cerebellar nuclei and a few brainstem nuclei. Although these afferents can modulate the firing rates of olivary neurons (as is typical in most brain regions), the mem-

brane conductance of olivary neurons limits this modulation to a range of a few hertz and endows these neurons with the potential to be intrinsic oscillators. Instead of just modulating firing rates, olivary afferent activity acts to modify the effectiveness of the electrical coupling between olivary neurons and thus changes the patterns of synchronous activity delivered to the cerebellum. Afferent activity may also modulate expression of the oscillatory potential of olivary neurons. Thus, the inferior olive appears to be organized to generate patterns of synchronous activity across the cerebellar cortex. The functional significance of these patterns remains controversial. One hypothesis is that they provide a gating signal for synchronizing motor commands to various muscle combinations.

Cellular Elements and Efferents of the Cortex
Despite its enormous expansion throughout vertebrate evolution, the basic anatomic organization of the cerebellar cortex has remained nearly invariant. The circuitry is also among the most regular and stereo-

typed of any brain region. The cerebellar cortex contains eight different neuronal types: Purkinje cells, Golgi cells, granule cells, Lugaro cells, basket cells, stellate cells, unipolar brush cells, and candelabrum cells. These cells are found in all regions of the cerebellar cortex, with the exception of unipolar brush cells, which are limited mainly to cerebellar areas receiving vestibular input (i.e., the flocculonodular lobe). These eight cell types are distributed among the three layers that make up the cerebellar cortex of higher vertebrates. The outer or superficial layer is the **molecular layer** (Fig. 9-20, *A*). **Stellate and basket cells** are found here. The deepest layer is the **granule cell layer.** This layer has the highest cellular density in the nervous system and contains granule, **Golgi,** and **unipolar brush cells.** Separating the molecular and granule cell layers is the **Purkinje cell layer,** formed by Purkinje cell somata, which are arranged as a one-cell-thick sheet of cells. **Candelabrum cells** are also located in this layer. **Lugaro cells** are situated slightly deeper at the upper border of the granule cell layer.

The sole efferent from the cortex is the Purkinje cell axon, which also has local collaterals and is GABAergic and inhibitory. Thus, the remaining seven cell types are local interneurons. Of these, the stellate, basket, Golgi, Lugaro, and candelabrum cells are also inhibitory GABAergic neurons, whereas the granule and unipolar brush cells are excitatory.

Microcircuitry of the Cortex

The dendrites, axons, and patterns of synaptic connections of most neurons within the cerebellar cortex are organized with respect to the transverse (short) and longitudinal (long) folial axes (Fig. 9-21). In the vermis, where the folia run perpendicular to the sagittal plane, these axes lie in the sagittal and coronal planes, respectively. In the hemispheres, where the folia are oriented at various angles with respect to the sagittal plane, this correspondence is lost, and the local folial axes must then serve as the reference axes.

The Purkinje cell dendritic tree is the largest in the CNS. It extends from the Purkinje cell layer through the molecular layer to the surface of the cerebellar cortex and for several hundred microns along the transverse axis of the folium, but only 30 to 40 µm in the longitudinal direction. Thus, it is like a flat pancake that lies in a plane parallel to the transverse folial axis. Accordingly, a set of Purkinje cell dendritic trees can be thought of as a stack of pancakes, with the stack running along the longitudinal folial axis.

The dendritic trees of the molecular layer interneurons (stellate and basket cells) are oriented similar to the Purkinje cell dendritic tree, although they are much less extensive. The axons of stellate and basket cells run transversely across the folium and form synapses with Purkinje cells. Stellate and basket cells synapse onto Purkinje cell dendrites. In addition, basket cells make synapses on the Purkinje cell soma and form a basket-like structure around the base of the soma, which gives the basket cell its name.

Granule cells are small neurons with four to five short unbranched dendrites, each ending in a claw-like expansion that synapses with a mossy fiber rosette and with terminals from Golgi cell axons in a complex arrangement known as a glomerulus. The axons of granule cells ascend through the Purkinje cell layer to the molecular layer, where they bifurcate and form

●**Figure 9-21.**   Three-dimensional view of the cerebellar cortex showing some of the cerebellar neurons. The cut face at the left is along the long axis of the folium; the cut face at the right is at right angles to the long axis. BC, basket cell; CF, climbing fiber; CN, cerebellar nuclear cell; GC, Golgi cell; Glm, glomerulus; GrC, granule cell; MF, mossy fiber; PC, Purkinje cell; PF, parallel fiber; SC, stellate cell.

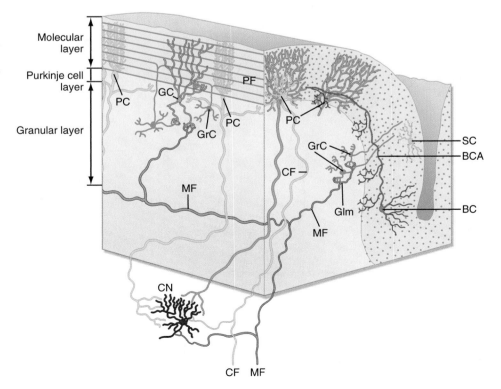

parallel fibers. The parallel fibers run parallel to the cerebellar surface along the longitudinal axis of the folium (perpendicular to the planes of the Purkinje, stellate, and basket cell dendritic trees) and form excitatory synapses with the dendrites of the Purkinje, Golgi, stellate, and basket cells.

The orthogonal relationship between the parallel fibers and the dendritic trees of the Purkinje cells and molecular layer interneurons (basket and stellate cells) has significant functional consequences. This arrangement allows maximal convergence and divergence to occur. A single parallel fiber, which can be up to 6 mm long, will pass through more than 100 Purkinje cell dendritic trees (and also interneuron dendrites); however, it has the chance to make only one or two synapses with any particular cell because it crosses through the short dimension of the dendritic tree. Conversely, a given Purkinje cell receives synapses from about 200,000 parallel fibers. Thus, a beam of parallel fibers can be excited experimentally, which will excite a row of Purkinje cells and interneurons that are in line with this beam (Fig. 9-22). In addition, because the axons of the interneurons run perpendicular to the parallel fibers, this beam of excitation will be flanked by inhibition. Although this classic electrophysiological experiment clearly demonstrates the functional connectivity of the cerebellar cortex, whether such beams of excitation occur normally remains a controversial question.

The Golgi cells are inhibitory interneurons in the granule cell layer. The geometry of their axonal and dendritic arbors is an exception to the orthogonal and planar organization of the cortex in that their dendrites and axons carve out roughly conical territories. One can think of it as two cones, tip to tip, where the soma is at the point at which the two cone tips meet. The dendritic tree forms the upper cone, which often extends into the molecular layer, and the axon forms the lower one. Golgi cells are excited by mossy and climbing fibers and by granule cell axons (parallel fibers) and inhibited by basket, stellate, and Purkinje cell axon collaterals. They in turn inhibit granule cells. Thus, they participate in both feedback (when excited by parallel fibers) and feedforward (when excited by mossy fibers) inhibitory loops that control activity in the mossy fiber–parallel fiber pathway to the Purkinje cell.

Lugaro cells have fusiform somata from which emerge two relatively unbranched dendrites, one from each side, that run along the transverse folial axis for several hundred microns, usually just under the Purkinje cell layer. Purkinje cell axon collaterals provide the main input to these neurons, with granule cell axons adding a minor input. The axon terminates

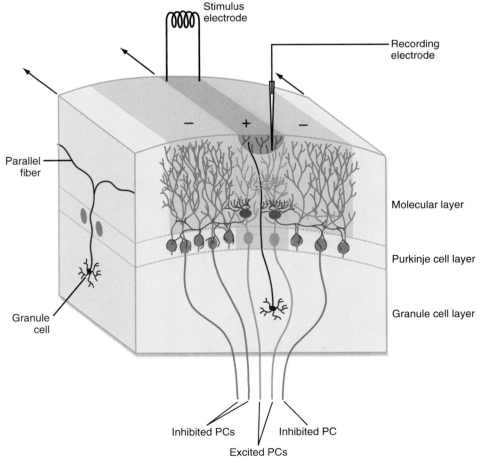

● **Figure 9-22.** Functional connectivity of the cerebellar cortex. The geometry of the cerebellar cortical circuits makes electrophysiological determination of the functional connectivity of the cellular elements possible. The figure shows a classic paradigm in which stimulation of the cerebellar cortex activates a beam of parallel fibers *(brown)*. Recordings from the stellate and basket cells *(green cells)* and Purkinje cells (PCs) *(orange cells)* in line with this beam show that they are excited by the parallel fibers. In contrast, Purkinje cells located rostral or caudal to the beam receive only inhibition *(purple areas)* as a result of the perpendicular spatial relationship of the parallel fibers and the stellate and basket cell axons.

mainly in the molecular layer on basket, stellate, and possibly Purkinje cells. Thus, these cells appear to sample the activity of Purkinje cells and provide both positive-feedback signals (they inhibit the interneurons that inhibit Purkinje cells) and negative-feedback signals (they directly inhibit the Purkinje cell).

Unipolar brush cells have only a single dendrite that ends as a tight bunch of branchlets that resemble a brush. These cells receive excitatory input from mossy fibers and inhibitory input from Golgi cells. It is thought that they synapse with granule and Golgi cells, which would make these cells an excitatory feedforward link in the mossy fiber–parallel fiber pathway.

Candelabrum cells are GABAergic cells located in the Purkinje layer. Their dendrites and axons terminate in the molecular layer, where the axonal arborization pattern resembles a candelabrum.

Cerebellar Nuclei

The cerebellar nuclei are the main targets of the cerebellar cortex. This projection is topographically organized such that each longitudinal strip of cortex targets a specific region of the cerebellar nuclei. The gross pattern is that the vermis projects to the fastigial and vestibular nuclei, the paravermal region projects to the interpositus, and the lateral hemisphere projects to the dentate nucleus.

The cerebellar nuclear neurons in turn provide the output from the cerebellum to the rest of the brain (with the primary exception of Purkinje cells that project to the vestibular nuclei). In discussing the output of the cerebellar nuclei, it is useful to group the nuclear cells according to whether they are GABAergic because the GABAergic cells project back to the inferior olive and form a negative-feedback loop to one of the cerebellum's principal afferent sources. It is important to note that GABAergic cells project to the specific part of the inferior olive from which they receive input and from which their overlying longitudinal strip of cortex receives climbing fibers. Thus, the cerebellar cortex, cerebellar nuclei, and inferior olive are functionally organized as a series of closed loops. The non-GABAergic, excitatory nuclear cells project to a variety of targets from the spinal cord to the thalamus. In general, each nucleus gives rise to crossed ascending and descending projections that leave the cerebellum via the superior cerebellar peduncle. The fastigial nucleus also gives rise to significant uncrossed fibers, as well as a second crossed projection called the uncinate or hook bundle that leaves via the inferior cerebellar peduncle.

Although there are differences in the specific targets of each nucleus, in general, the ascending cerebellar projections target midbrain structures, such as the red nucleus and superior colliculus, and the VL nucleus of the thalamus, which connects to the primary motor cortex and thereby links the cerebellum to motor areas of the cerebrum. (The cerebral motor areas are likewise linked to the cerebellum by multiple pathways, including ones that relay in the basilar pons and inferior olive.) The descending fibers target mainly the basilar pontine nuclei, inferior olive, and several reticular nuclei. In addition, there is a small cerebellospinal pathway that arises principally from the fastigial nucleus. Finally, the fastigial nucleus has significant projections to the vestibular nuclei.

Activity of Purkinje Cells in the Cerebellar Cortex in the Context of Motor Coordination

Mossy fiber input to the cerebellar cortex, via their excitation of granule cells, causes a Purkinje cell to discharge single action potentials, referred to as simple spikes (Fig. 9-23). The spontaneous simple spike firing rate is typically around 20 to 50 Hz but can vary widely (from 0 to > 100 Hz), depending on the relative balance of excitation from parallel fiber input and inhibition from cerebellar cortex interneurons. Thus, this activity reflects the state of the cerebellar cortex.

In contrast, a climbing fiber discharge causes a high-frequency burst of action potentials, called a complex spike (Fig. 9-23), in an all-or-none manner because of the massive excitation that is provided by the single climbing fiber to a Purkinje cell. This excitation is so powerful that there is essentially a one-to-one relationship between climbing fiber discharge and a complex spike. Thus, complex spikes essentially override what is happening at the cortex level and reflect the state of the inferior olive. The average firing rate of a spontaneous complex spike is only about 1 Hz.

Because the climbing fibers generate complex spikes at such a low frequency, they do not substan-

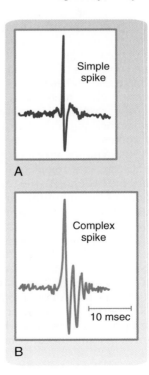

● **Figure 9-23.** Responses of a Purkinje cell to excitatory input recorded extracellularly. **A,** Granule cells, via their ascending axons and parallel fibers, excite Purkinje cells and trigger simple spikes. **B,** Climbing fiber activity leads to high-frequency (≈500 Hz) bursts of two to four spikes known as complex spikes in Purkinje cells.

tially change the average firing rates of Purkinje cells, and consequently, it is commonly argued that they have no direct role in shaping the output of the cerebellar cortex and are therefore not involved in ongoing motor control. Instead, it is commonly thought that their function is to alter the responsiveness of Purkinje cells to parallel fiber input. In particular, under certain circumstances, complex spike activity produces a prolonged depression in parallel fiber synaptic efficacy, termed **LTD** (long-term depression). This phenomenon is the proposed mechanism by which climbing fibers act in motor-learning hypotheses. Such hypotheses typically state that the parallel fiber system, and hence simple spikes, are involved in generating ongoing movement and, when there is a mismatch between the intended and actual movement, this error activates the inferior olive and complex spikes result, which then lead to LTD of the active parallel fiber synapses. This adjustment in synaptic weight will change the motor output in the future. If this change results in a properly executed movement, activation of the inferior olive will not occur and the motor program will be unchanged, but if there is still an error, the olivocerebellar system will trigger additional complex spikes that will cause further changes in synaptic efficacy, and so on. Major challenges to this view are that motor learning can occur when LTD is chemically blocked and that learned behavior can remain after removal of portions of the cerebellum where the memory is supposedly stored.

An alternative view is that the olivocerebellar system is directly involved in motor control (note that this does not preclude a role in motor learning as well) and, in particular, helps in the timing of motor commands. This view follows from the types of motor deficits observed in cerebellar damage and makes use of the special properties of the inferior olive mentioned earlier, namely, that it can generate rhythmic synchronous complex spike discharges across populations of Purkinje cells. These complex spikes would then produce synchronized inhibitory postsynaptic currents (IPSPs) on cerebellar nuclear neurons as a result of the convergence present in the Purkinje cell axon to the cerebellar nuclear projection. Because of the membrane properties of cerebellar nuclear neurons, these synchronized IPSPs could have a qualitatively different effect on nuclear cell firing than would the IPSPs caused by more numerous, but asynchronous simple spikes. Specifically, they could trigger rebound bursts in the nuclear cells that would then be transmitted to other motor systems as a gating signal. In fact, voluntary movements appear to be composed of a series of periodic accelerations that reflect a central oscillatory process. However, whether the olivocerebellar system helps time motor commands requires further evidence.

MOTOR CONTROL BY THE BASAL GANGLIA

The basal ganglia are the deep nuclei of the cerebrum. In association with other nuclei in the diencephalon

and midbrain, the basal ganglia differ from the cerebellum in the way that they regulate motor activity. Unlike the cerebellum, the basal ganglia do not receive input from the spinal cord, but they do receive direct input from the cerebral cortex. The main action of basal ganglia is on the motor areas of the cortex by way of the thalamus. In addition to their role in motor control, the basal ganglia contribute to affective and cognitive functions. Lesions of the basal ganglia produce abnormal movement and posture.

Organization of the Basal Ganglia and Related Nuclei

The basal ganglia include the **caudate nucleus,** the **putamen,** and the **globus pallidus** (Fig. 9-24). The term **striatum,** derived from the striated appearance of these nuclei, refers only to the caudate nucleus and putamen. The striations are produced by the fiber bundles formed by the anterior limb of the internal capsule as it separates the caudate nucleus and putamen. The globus pallidus typically has two parts, an **external segment** and an **internal segment.** The combination of putamen and globus pallidus is often referred to as the **lentiform nucleus.**

Associated with the basal ganglia are several thalamic nuclei. These include the **ventral anterior (VA)** and **ventral lateral (VL) nuclei** and several components of the intralaminar complex. Other associated nuclei are the **subthalamic nucleus** of the diencephalon and the **substantia nigra** of the midbrain (Fig. 9-24). The substantia nigra ("black substance") derives its name from its content of melanin pigment. Many of the neurons in the **pars compacta** of this nucleus contain melanin, a byproduct of dopamine synthesis. The other subdivision of the substantia nigra is the **pars reticulata.** This structure can be regarded as an extension of the internal segment of the globus pallidus because these nuclei have an identical origin and similar connections.

Connections and Operation of the Basal Ganglia

Neurons of the striatum begin to discharge before movement occurs. This sequence suggests that these neurons help select the movement that is to be made. Activity in the putamen is related to the occurrence of movement of the body, whereas activity in the caudate nucleus is related to eye movement.

With the exception of the primary visual and auditory cortices, most regions of the cerebral cortex project topographically to the striatum. An important component of the cortical input to the striatum originates in the motor cortex. The corticostriatal projection arises from neurons in layer V of the cortex. The neurons appear to use glutamate as their excitatory neurotransmitter. The striatum then influences neurons in the VA and VL nuclei of the thalamus by two pathways, direct and indirect (Fig. 9-25, *A*). The thalamic neurons in turn excite neurons of the motor areas of the cerebral cortex.

● **Figure 9-24.** Components of basal ganglia and other closely associated brain regions. The main components of the basal ganglia are the caudate, putamen, globus pallidus, and substantia nigra pars reticulata. The motor loop of the basal ganglia connects with motor areas in the frontal cortex, the VA and VL thalamic nuclei, and the superior colliculus. Input from the substantia nigra pars compacta is critical for normal basal ganglia function. GPe, external segment of globus pallidus; GPi, internal segment of globus pallidus.

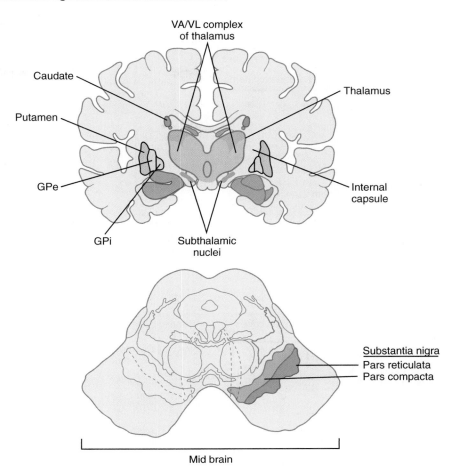

Direct Pathway

The overall action of the direct pathway through the basal ganglia to motor areas of the cortex is to enhance motor activity. In the direct pathway, the striatum projects to the internal segment of the globus pallidus (GPi). This projection is inhibitory, and the main transmitter is GABA. The GPi projects to the VA and VL nuclei of the thalamus. These connections also use GABA and are inhibitory. The VA and VL nuclei send excitatory connections to the prefrontal, premotor, and supplementary motor cortex. This input to the cortex influences motor planning, and it also affects the discharge of corticospinal and corticobulbar neurons.

The direct pathway appears to function as follows. Neurons in the striatum have little background activity, but during movement they are activated by their input from the cortex. In contrast, neurons in the GPi have a high level of background activity. When the striatum is activated, its inhibitory projections to the globus pallidus slow the activity of pallidal neurons. However, the pallidal neurons themselves are inhibitory, and they normally provide tonic inhibition of neurons in the VA and VL nuclei of the thalamus. Therefore, activation of the striatum causes **disinhibi-**

tion of neurons of the VA and VL nuclei. When disinhibited, the VA/VL neurons increase their firing rates, exciting their target neurons in the motor areas of the cerebral cortex. Because the motor areas evoke movement by activating α and γ motor neurons in the spinal cord and brainstem, the basal ganglia can regulate movement by enhancing the activity of neurons in the motor cortex.

Indirect Pathway

The overall effect of the indirect pathway is to reduce the activity of neurons in motor areas of the cerebral cortex. The indirect pathway involves inhibitory connections from the striatum to the external segment of the globus pallidus (GPe), which in turn sends an inhibitory projection to the subthalamic nucleus and to GPi. The subthalamic nucleus then sends an excitatory projection back to the GPi (Fig. 9-25, A).

In this pathway, pallidal neurons in the external segment are inhibited by the GABA released from striatal terminals in the globus pallidus. The GPe normally releases GABA in the subthalamic nucleus and thereby inhibits the subthalamic neurons. Therefore, striatal inhibition of the GPe results in the disinhibition of neurons of the subthalamic nucleus. The subthalamic

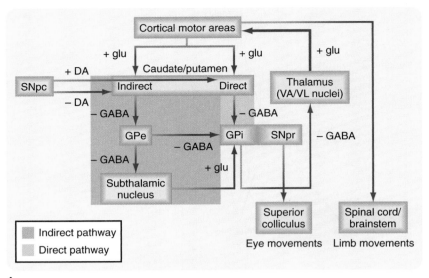

● **Figure 9-25.** Functional connectivity of the basal ganglia for motor control. **A,** Connections between various basal ganglia components and other associated motor areas. The excitatory cortical input to the caudate and putamen influences output from the GPi and SNpr via a direct and an indirect pathway. Note that the two inhibitory steps in the indirect pathway mean that activity through this pathway has an effect on basal ganglia output to the thalamus and superior colliculus opposite that of the direct pathway. Note that DA is a neuromodulator that acts on D_1 and D_2 receptors on striatal neurons participating in the direct and indirect pathways, respectively. **B,** Changes in activity flow that occur in Parkinson's disease in which the SNpc is degenerated. **C,** Changes in activity flow in Huntington's disease in which inhibitory control of the GPe is lost. Plus (+) and minus (−) symbols, respectively, indicate the excitatory or inhibitory nature of a synaptic connection. DA, dopamine; glu, glutamate; GPe, GPi, globus pallidus external and internal; SNpc, SNpr, substantia nigra pars compacta and pars reticulata; VA/VL, ventral anterior and ventral lateral nuclei of the thalamus.

A

B Parkinson's disease (hypokinetic)

C Huntington's disease (hyperkinetic)

neurons are normally active, and they excite neurons in the GPi by releasing glutamate. When the neurons of the subthalamic nucleus become more active because of disinhibition, they release more glutamate in the GPi. This transmitter excites neurons in the GPi and consequently activates inhibitory projections that affect the VA and VL thalamic nuclei. The activity of the thalamic neurons consequently decreases, as does the activity of the cortical neurons that they influence.

The direct and indirect pathways thus have opposing actions; an increase in the activity of either one of these pathways might lead to an imbalance in motor control. Such imbalances, which are typical of basal ganglion diseases, may alter the motor output of the cortex.

Actions of Neurons in the Pars Compacta of the Substantia Nigra on the Striatum

Dopamine is the neurotransmitter used by neurons of the pars compacta of the substantia nigra. In the nigrostriatal pathway, release of dopamine has an overall excitatory action on the direct pathway and an inhibitory action on the indirect pathway. This is, however, a modulatory type of effect. That is, dopamine is apparently causing its action not by generating postsynaptic potentials but rather by altering the striatal cells' response to other transmitters. The different actions on the direct and indirect pathways result from different types of dopamine receptors being expressed by the spiny projection cells of the striatum that contribute to the direct and indirect pathways. D_1 receptors are found on striatal cells that form the direct pathway by projecting to the GPi, whereas D_2 receptors are found on striatal cells that participate in the indirect pathway and project to the GPe. The overall consequence of dopamine release in both cases is facilitation of activity in the motor areas of the cerebral cortex.

Subdivision of the Striatum into Striosomes and Matrix

On the basis of the associated neurotransmitters, the striatum has been subdivided into zones called **striosomes** and **matrix.** The cortical projections related to motor control end in the matrix area. The limbic system projects to the striosomes. Striosomes are thought to synapse in the pars compacta of the substantia nigra and to influence the dopaminergic nigrostriatal pathway.

Role of the Basal Ganglia in Motor Control

The basal ganglia mainly influence the motor cortex. Therefore, the basal ganglia have an important influence on the lateral system of motor pathways. Such an influence is consistent with some of the movement disorders observed in diseases of the basal ganglia. However, the basal ganglia must additionally regulate the medial motor pathways because diseases of the basal ganglia can also affect the posture and tone of proximal muscles.

The deficits seen in the various basal ganglia diseases include abnormal movement **(dyskinesia),** increased muscle tone **(cogwheel rigidity),** and slowness in initiating movement **(bradykinesia).** Abnormal movement includes tremor, **athetosis, chorea, ballism,** and **dystonia.** The tremor of basal ganglion disease is a "pill-rolling," 3-Hz tremor that occurs when the limb is at rest. Athetosis consists of slow, writhing movement of the distal parts of the limbs, whereas chorea is characterized by rapid, flicking movement of the extremities and facial muscles. Ballism is associated with violent, flailing movement of the limbs (ballistic movement). Finally, dystonic movement is slow trunk movement that distorts body positions.

Parkinson's disease is a common disorder characterized by tremor, rigidity, and bradykinesia. This disease is caused by loss of neurons in the pars compacta of the substantia nigra. Consequently, the striatum suffers a severe loss of dopamine. Neurons of the locus coeruleus and the raphe nuclei, as well as other monoaminergic nuclei, are also lost. The loss of dopamine diminishes the activity of the direct pathway and increases the activity of the indirect pathway (Fig. 9-25, *B*). The net effect is an increase in the activity of neurons in the internal segment of the globus pallidus. This results in greater inhibition of neurons in the VA and VL nuclei and less pronounced activation of the motor cortical areas. The consequence is slowed movement (bradykinesia).

Before the dopaminergic neurons are completely lost, administration of L-DOPA can relieve some of the motor deficits in Parkinson's disease. L-DOPA is a precursor of dopamine, and it can cross the blood-brain barrier. Currently, the possibility of transplanting dopamine-synthesizing neurons into the striatum is being explored. Future research will no doubt focus on the potential for human embryonic stem cells to play such a therapeutic role.

Another basal ganglion disturbance is Huntington's disease, which results from a genetic defect that involves an autosomal dominant gene. This defect leads to the preferential loss of striatal GABAergic and cholinergic neurons that project to the GPe as part of the indirect pathway (and also degeneration of the cerebral cortex, with resultant dementia). Loss of inhibition of the GPe presumably leads to diminished activity of neurons in the subthalamic nucleus (Fig. 9-25, *C*). Hence, the excitation of neurons of the GPi would be reduced. This will disinhibit neurons in the VA and VL nuclei. The resulting enhancement of activity in neurons in the motor areas of the cerebral cortex may help explain the choreiform movements of Huntington's disease. The rigidity in Parkinson's disease may in a sense be the opposite of chorea because overtreatment of patients with Parkinson's disease with L-DOPA can result in chorea.

Hemiballism is caused by a lesion of the subthalamic nucleus on one side of the brain. In this disorder, involuntary, violent flailing movements of the limbs may occur on the side of the body contralateral to the lesion. Because the subthalamic nucleus excites neurons of the GPi, a lesion of the subthalamic nucleus would reduce the activity of these pallidal neurons. Therefore, neurons in the VA and VL nuclei of the thalamus would be less inhibited, and the activity of neurons in the motor cortex would be increased.

In all these basal ganglia disorders, the motor dysfunction is contralateral to the diseased component. This is understandable because the main final output of the basal ganglia to the body is mediated by the corticospinal tract.

Differences between the Basal Ganglia and Cerebellar Motor Loops

The organization of the motor loops that connect the basal ganglia and cerebellum with the motor regions of the cerebral cortex differs in several ways. The basal ganglia receive input from most areas of the cerebral cortex, whereas input to the cerebellum from the cerebral cortex is more restricted. Output from the basal ganglia is also more widespread and reaches the prefrontal cortex, as well as all the premotor areas. The cerebellar circuit influences only the premotor and motor cortex. Finally, the basal ganglia do not receive somatosensory information from ascending pathways in the spinal cord, and they have few connections with the brainstem. In contrast, the cerebellum is the target of several somatosensory pathways, and it has rich connections with brainstem nuclei.

EYE MOVEMENT

Eye movement has a number of features that distinguish it from other motor behavior. When compared with the movement that limbs, with their multiple joints and muscles, can perform, eye movement is relatively simple. For example, each eye is controlled by only three agonist-antagonist muscle pairs: the medial and lateral recti, the superior and inferior recti, and the superior and inferior obliques. These muscles allow the eye to rotate about three axes. Assuming that the head is in an upright position, the axes are the vertical axis, a horizontal axis that runs left to right, and the torsional axis (which is directed along the axis of sight). The medial and lateral recti control movement about the vertical axis; the other four muscles generate movement about the horizontal and torsional axes. Another simplifying feature is that there are no external loads to be compensated for. Furthermore, eye movement appears to be separable into a few distinct types, with each type being controlled by its own specialized circuitry. Thus, eye movement offers a number of advantages as a model system for studying motor control. Moreover, deficits in eye movement provide important clinical clues to the diagnosis of neurological problems. We first review the different eye movement types and then discuss the neural circuitry underlying their generation.

Types of Eye Movement
Vestibuloocular Reflex

Eye movement probably first evolved to hold the eye still, in contrast to limb movement, where one typi-cally wants to generate movement with respect to the external world. The reason is that visual acuity degrades rapidly when there is eye movement relative to the external world (i.e., the visual scene slips across the retina). A major cause of such slippage is movement of the head. The vestibuloocular reflex (VOR) is one of the main mechanisms by which head movement is compensated in order to allow a stable visual scene to be maintained on the retina.

To maintain a stable visual scene on the retina, the VOR produces movement of the eyes that is equal and opposite the movement of the head. This reflex is initiated by stimulation of the receptors (hair cells) in the vestibular system (see Chapter 8). Recall that the vestibular organs are sensitive to head acceleration, not visual cues, and thus the VOR occurs in both the light and dark. Functionally, it is what is called an open loop system in that it generates an output (eye movement) in response to a stimulus (head acceleration), but its immediate behavior is not regulated by feedback about the success or failure of its output. It is worth noting, however, that in the light at least, any failure by the VOR to match eye and head rotation will result in what is called retinal slip (i.e., slip of the visual image across the retina), and this error signal can be fed back to the VOR circuits by other neuronal pathways and over time can lead to adjustments in the strength of the VOR to eliminate the error. This adaptation of the VOR is a major model for studying plasticity in the brain.

As stated, acceleration signals initiate the VOR. The output of the VOR, however, must be a change in eye position in the orbit. Thus, the problem to be solved by the nervous system is to translate the acceleration signals sensed by the vestibular organs into correct positional signals for the eyes. Mathematically, this can be thought of as a double integration. The first integration is done by the vestibular receptor apparatus because although the hair cells respond to head acceleration, the signals in the vestibular afferents are proportional to head velocity (at least for most stimuli that are encountered physiologically). The second integration, from velocity to position, occurs in the CNS in circuits described later.

The head can move in six different ways, often referred to as six degrees of freedom: three translational and three rotational. To compensate for these different types of movement, there are both translational and angular VORs, as well as separate subsystems for handling movement about different directions (e.g., rotation about a vertical or a horizontal axis).

Optokinetic Reflex

The optokinetic reflex (OKR) is a second mechanism by which the nervous system stabilizes the visual scene on the retina, and it often works in conjunction with the VOR. Whereas the VOR is activated only by head motion, the OKR is activated by movement of the visual scene, whether caused by motion of the scene itself or by head motion. That is, the sensory stimulus for this reflex is slip of the visual scene on the retina as detected by motion-sensitive retinal ganglion cells. An example of the former is when you are sitting in a train and a train on the adjacent track begins moving, your eyes rotate to keep the image of the neighboring car stable. This often leads to a sensation that you are moving (this is not entirely surprising because OKR circuits feed into the same circuits as used by the vestibular system).

The OKR can work in conjunction with the VOR to stabilize the visual image and is particularly important for maintaining a stable image when head movements are slow because the VOR works poorly in these conditions. In addition, as mentioned earlier, the VOR circuits by themselves act in an open loop mode and thus have no way to correct errors or calibrate their performance (i.e., detect a mismatch between head and eye rotation). The OKR allows for corrections and for calibration by triggering mechanisms to adjust the sensitivity of the VOR. Such mismatches occur as the head grows during childhood or when one puts on glasses.

Saccades

In animals whose eyes have a fovea, it becomes particularly advantageous to be able to move the eye with respect to the world (i.e., the main visual scene) so that objects of importance can be focused onto the fovea and scrutinized with this high-resolution part of the retina. Two classes of eye movement underlie this ability: saccadic and smooth pursuit. Movements that bring a particular region of the visual world onto the fovea are called saccades. For example, to read this sentence you are making a series of saccades to bring successive words onto your fovea to be read. However, even afoveate animals make saccades, and thus saccades may also be used to rapidly scan the visual environment.

Saccades are extremely rapid eye movements. In humans, eye velocity during a saccade can reach 800 degrees/sec, as compared with movement velocity of less than 10 degrees/sec generated in response to typical VOR and OKR stimuli (velocities of up to ≈120 degrees/sec can be produced by OKR stimuli in humans; however, they are still much slower than the maximal saccade velocities). Saccades can be made voluntarily or reflexively. Moreover, although they are usually made in response to visual targets, they can also be made toward auditory or other sensory cues, in the dark, or toward memorized targets.

Interestingly, visual processing appears to be suppressed just before and during saccades, particularly in the magnocellular visual pathway that is concerned with visual motion. This phenomenon is known as saccadic suppression and may function to prevent sensations of sudden, rapid movement of the visual world that would result during a saccade in the absence of such suppression. The mechanisms underlying saccadic suppression are not fully known, but in areas of the cortex related to visual processing, the responsiveness of the cells to visual stimuli is reduced and altered during saccades.

Smooth Pursuit

Once a saccade has brought a moving object of interest onto the fovea, the smooth pursuit system allows us to keep it stable on the fovea despite its continued motion. This ability appears to be limited to primates and allows prolonged continuous observation of a moving object. Note that in some respects, smooth pursuit might seem similar to the OKR, and in fact there may not be an absolute dividing line because as the target size grows, the distinction between target and background is lost; however, for small moving targets, smooth pursuit requires suppression of the OKR. You can see the effect of this suppression by moving your finger back and forth in front of this text while tracking it with your eyes. Your finger will be in focus while the words on this page will be part of the background scene and will become illegible as they slip along your retina.

Nystagmus

When there is a prolonged OKR or VOR stimulus (e.g., if you keep turning in one direction), these reflexes will initially counterrotate the eyes in an attempt to maintain a stable image on the retina, as described earlier. However, with a prolonged stimulus, the eyes will reach their mechanical limit, no further compensation will be possible, and the image will begin to slip on the retina. To avoid this situation, a fast saccade-like movement of the eyes occurs in the opposite direction, essentially resetting the eyes to begin viewing the visual scene again. Then the slow OKR- or VOR-induced counterrotation will start anew. This alternation of slow and fast movement in opposite directions is nystagmus and can be displayed on a nystagmogram (Fig. 9-26). Thus, nystagmus can be defined as oscillatory or rhythmic movements of the eye in which there is a fast and a slow phase. The nystagmus is named according to the direction of the fast phase, because it is more easily observed.

In addition to being induced physiologically by VOR or OKR stimuli, nystagmus can result from damage to the vestibular circuits, either in the periphery (e.g., VIII nerve) or centrally (e.g., vestibular nuclei), and can be a useful diagnostic symptom.

Vergence

Conjugate eye movement is movement of both eyes in the same direction and in an equal amount. Such

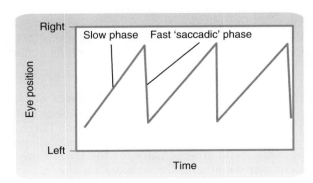

● **Figure 9-26.** Nystagmogram showing eye movements that occur during nystagmus. The plot shows a left nystagmus because the fast phase is directed toward the left (downward on the graph).

coordination allows a target to be maintained on both fovea during eye movement and is necessary to maintain binocular vision without experiencing diplopia (double vision). However, when objects are close (< 30 m), maintaining a target on both fovea requires eye movement that is no longer identical. Such disjunctive or vergence movements are also necessary for fixation of both eyes on objects that are approaching or receding. During convergence movements, accommodation of the lens for near vision and pupillary constriction also occur. In sum, the stimuli for vergence movements are diplopia and blurry images.

Neural Circuitry and Activity Underlying Eye Movement
Motor Neurons of the Extraocular Muscles

Three cranial nerve nuclei supply the extraocular muscles: oculomotor, trochlear, and abducens nuclei. Note that we will sometimes refer to these three nuclei collectively as the oculomotor nuclei; however, the context should make clear whether we mean the specific nucleus or all three. Motor neurons for the ipsilateral medial and inferior recti, ipsilateral inferior oblique, and contralateral superior rectus muscles reside in the oculomotor nucleus; those for the contralateral superior oblique muscle reside in the trochlear nucleus; and those for the ipsilateral lateral rectus muscle are located in the abducens nucleus. These motor neurons form some of the smallest motor units (1:10 nerve-to-muscle ratio), consistent with the very fine control needed for precise eye movement.

An important point regarding motor neurons to the extraocular muscles is that most have spontaneous activity when the eye is in the primary position (looking straight ahead) and their firing rate correlates with eye position and velocity. This spontaneous activity allows the antagonist muscle pairs to act in a push-pull fashion, which increases the responsiveness of the system. That is, as motor neurons innervating one muscle are activated and cause increased contraction, those to its antagonist are inhibited and lead to relaxation.

In addition to motor neurons, the abducens nuclei have internuclear neurons. These neurons project, via the medial longitudinal fasciculus, to medial rectus motor neurons in the contralateral oculomotor nucleus. As we will see, this projection facilitates the coordinated action of the medial and lateral recti that is needed for conjugate movements, such as occur in the VOR.

Circuits Underlying the Vestibuloocular Reflex

The VOR acts to counter head motion by causing rotation of the eyes in the opposite direction. There are separate circuits for rotational and translational movement of the head. The sensors for the former are the semicircular canal, and the sensors for the latter are the otoliths (the utricle and saccule). The circuits for the angular VOR are more straightforward (but still complex!), so we will focus on these pathways to illustrate how this reflex works; however, the basic scheme is the same: vestibular afferents go to vestibular nuclei,

the vestibular nuclei in turn project to the various oculomotor nuclei, and motor neurons in the oculomotor nuclei give rise to axons that innervate the extraocular muscles. What varies are the specific vestibular and oculomotor nuclei that are involved.

Focusing on the angular VOR pathways, the pathway for generating horizontal eye movement originates in the horizontal canals, and the analogous one for vertical movement originates in the anterior and posterior canals. Figure 9-27, *A*, shows the basic circuit for the horizontal VOR. Note that only the major central circuits originating in the left horizontal canal and vestibular nuclei are shown; however, mirror image pathways arise from the right canal and vestibular nuclei. Vestibular afferents involved in the horizontal VOR pathway primarily synapse in the medial vestibular nucleus, which projects to the abducens nucleus bilaterally; inhibitory neurons project ipsilaterally and excitatory ones project contralaterally. Control of the medial rectus muscle is achieved by abducens internuclear neurons that project from the abducens to the part of the oculomotor nucleus controlling the medial rectus muscle. Note the double crossing of this pathway, which results in aligning of the responses of functional synergists (e.g., the left medial rectus with the right lateral rectus).

The vertical VOR pathway primarily involves the superior vestibular nucleus, which has direct bilateral projections to the oculomotor nucleus.

Consider what happens in the horizontal canal pathway when there is head rotation to the left as shown in Figure 9-27, *B*. Leftward head rotation would cause the visual image to slip to the right. However, compensation by the VOR will be triggered by depolarization of the hair cells of the left canal in response to the angular acceleration (Fig. 8-27). The depolarized hair cells will cause increased activity in the left vestibular afferents and thereby excite neurons of the left medial vestibular nucleus. These include excitatory neurons that project to the contralateral abducens nucleus and synapse with both motor neurons and internuclear neurons. Excitation of the motor neurons will lead to contraction of the right lateral rectus and rotation of the right eye to the right, whereas excitation of the internuclear neurons of the right abducens nucleus will lead to excitation of the medial rectus motor neurons in the left oculomotor nucleus, thus causing the left eye to rotate to the right as well.

If we now follow the pathway starting with the inhibitory vestibular neurons that project from the left medial vestibular nucleus to the ipsilateral abducens nucleus, we can see that the activity of these cells leads to inhibition of motor neurons to the left lateral rectus and motor neurons to the right medial rectus (the latter via internuclear neurons to the right oculomotor nucleus). Consequently, these muscles will relax, thereby facilitating rotation of the eyes to the right. Thus, the eye is being pulled by the increased tension of one set of muscles and "pushed" by the release of tension in the antagonist set of muscles.

Note that the mirror image pathways originating from the right canal have been left out of Figure 9-27

● **Figure 9-27.** Circuits underlying the horizontal vestibuloocular reflex (VOR). **A,** The vestibular nuclei receive excitatory input from the horizontal canal afferents and project to the abducens (VI) nucleus. The VI nucleus innervates the lateral rectus and projects to the contralateral oculomotor (III) nucleus, which controls the medial rectus. Excitatory neurons are shown in red, inhibitory ones in blue. Note that only the major pathways originating in the left vestibular nuclei are shown. For clarity, only the beginnings of mirror image pathways from the right vestibular nuclei are shown *(dotted lines).* **B,** Flow of activity in the VOR circuitry induced by leftward head rotation. Increased soma size and axonal thickness indicate increased activity; thinner axons indicate decreased activity in comparison to levels at rest (**A**). Note that leftward rotation causes both an increase in activity of the left vestibular afferents and a decrease in activity of the right ones. MLF, medial longitudinal fasciculus. Vestibular nuclei: I, inferior; L, lateral; M, medial; S, superior.

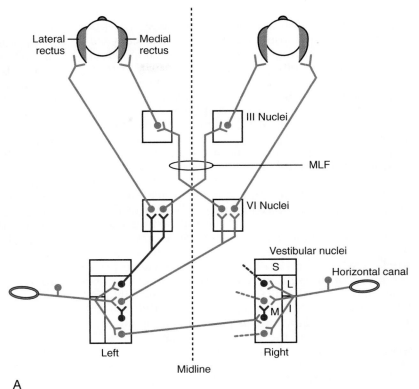

A

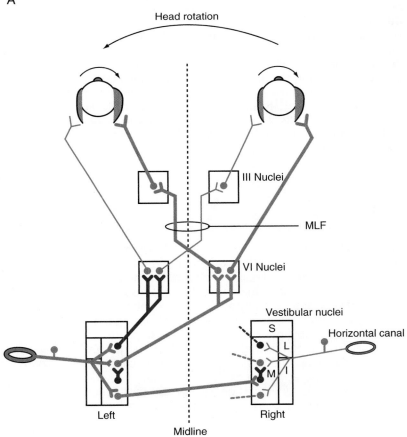

B

for clarity, but the changes in activity through them with leftward head rotation would be exactly the opposite, and thus they would function synergistically with those that are shown. As an exercise the reader should work out the resulting changes in activity through these circuits. Remember that leftward head rotation hyperpolarizes the hair cells of the right canal, thereby leading to a decrease in right vestibular afferent activity and disfacilitation of the right vestibular nuclear neurons.

Now, consider the commissural fibers that connect the two medial vestibular nuclei. These fibers are excitatory but end on local inhibitory interneurons of the contralateral vestibular nucleus and thus inhibit the projection neurons of that nucleus. This pathway reinforces the actions of the contralateral vestibular afferents on their target vestibular nuclear neurons. In our example, commissural cells in the left vestibular nucleus will be activated and therefore cause active inhibition of the right medial vestibular nuclei projection neurons, which reinforces the disfacilitation caused by the decrease in right afferent activity. In fact, this commissural pathway is powerful enough to modulate the activity of the contralateral vestibular nuclei even after unilateral labyrinthectomy, which destroys the direct vestibular afferent input to these nuclei.

Finally, it is important to note that superimposed on the brainstem circuits is the cerebellum. Parts of the vermis and flocculonodular lobe receive primary vestibular afferents or secondary vestibular afferents (axons of the vestibular nuclear neurons), or both, and in turn project back to the vestibular nuclei directly and via a disynaptic pathway involving the fastigial nucleus. The exact role of these cerebellar circuits in generating the VOR is much debated, but they are critical inasmuch as damage to them leads to abnormal eye movement, such as spontaneous nystagmus, and other symptoms of vestibular dysfunction.

Circuits Underlying the Optokinetic Reflex

The stimulus eliciting the OKR is visual (retinal slip), so photoreceptors are the start of the reflex arc. Key brainstem centers for this reflex lie in the tegmentum and pretectal region of the rostral midbrain. They are the nucleus of the optic tract (NOT) and a group of nuclei collectively known as the accessory optic nuclei (AON). Direction-selective, motion-sensitive retinal ganglion cells are a major afferent source carrying visual information to these nuclei. In addition, input comes from primary and higher-order visual cortical areas in the occipital and temporal lobes. These latter afferent sources become particularly important in primates and humans. Cells of the NOT and AON have large receptive fields, and their responses are selective for the direction and speed of movement of the visual scene. Interestingly, the preferred directions of movement of the NOT/AON cells correspond closely to motion caused by rotation about axes perpendicular to the semicircular canals, thereby facilitating coordination of the VOR and OKR to produce stable retinal

> ### IN THE CLINIC
>
> Clinical testing of labyrinthine function is done either by rotating the patient in a Bárány chair to activate the labyrinths in both ears or by introducing cold or warm water into the external auditory canal of one ear **(caloric test).** When a person is rotated in a Bárány chair, nystagmus develops during the rotation. The direction of the fast phase of the nystagmus is in the same direction as the rotation. When the rotation of the chair is halted, nystagmus develops in the opposite direction (postrotatory nystagmus) because stopping a rotation is equivalent to accelerating in the opposite direction.
>
> The caloric test is more useful because it can distinguish between malfunction of the labyrinths on the two sides. The head is bent backward about 60 degrees so that the two horizontal canals are essentially vertical. If warm water is introduced into the left ear, the endolymph in the outer portion of the loop of the left semicircular canal tends to rise as the specific gravity of the endolymph decreases because of heating. This sets up a convection flow of endolymph, and as a result, the kinocilia of the left ampullary crest hair cells are deflected toward the utricle, the same as if there was head rotation to the left, the discharge of the afferents that supply this canal increases, and nystagmus occurs with the fast phase toward the left. The nystagmus produces a sense that the environment is spinning to the right, and the subject tends to fall to the right. The opposite effects are produced if cold water is placed in the ear. A mnemonic expression that can help in remembering the direction of the nystagmus in the caloric test is COWS ("cold opposite, warm same"). In other words, cold water results in a fast phase of nystagmus toward the opposite side, and warm water causes a fast phase toward the same side.

> ### IN THE CLINIC
>
> When a labyrinth is irritated in one ear, as in **Ménière's disease,** or when a labyrinth is rendered nonfunctional, as may happen as a result of head trauma or disease of the labyrinth, the signals transmitted through the VOR pathways from the two sides become unbalanced. Vestibular nystagmus can then result. For example, irritation of the labyrinth of the left ear can increase the discharge of afferents that supply the left horizontal semicircular duct. The signal produced resembles that normally generated when the head is rotated to the left. Because the stimulus is ongoing, a left nystagmus results, with a slow phase to the right (caused by the VOR pathway) and a fast phase to the left. Destruction of the labyrinth in the right ear produces effects similar to those induced by irritation of the left labyrinth. Interestingly, the nystagmus is temporary, thus showing the ability of these circuits to adapt over time.

images. The efferent connections of these nuclei are numerous and complex and not fully understood. There are polysynaptic pathways to the oculomotor and abducens nuclei and monosynaptic input to the vestibular nuclei, which allows interaction with the VOR. There are projections to various precerebellar nuclei, including the inferior olive and basilar pontine nuclei. These pathways then loop through the flocculus and back to the vestibular nuclei. In sum, via several pathways operating in parallel, activity ultimately arrives at the various oculomotor nuclei whose motor neurons are activated, and proper counterrotation of the eyes results.

Circuits Underlying Saccades

Saccades are generated in response to activity in the superior colliculus or the cerebral cortex (frontal eye fields and posterior parietal areas). Activity in the superior colliculus is related to computation of the direction and amplitude of the saccade. Indeed, the deep layers of the superior colliculus contain a topographic motor map of saccade locations. From the superior colliculus, information is forwarded to distinct sites for control of horizontal and vertical saccades, referred to as the horizontal and vertical gaze centers, respectively. The horizontal gaze center consists of neurons in the paramedian pontine reticular formation (PPRF), in the vicinity of the abducens nucleus (Fig. 9-28, *A*). The vertical gaze center is located in the reticular formation of the midbrain, specifically, the rostral interstitial nucleus of the medial longitudinal fasciculus and the interstitial nucleus of Cajal. Because the circuitry and operation of the horizontal gaze center are better understood than those of the vertical gaze center, it is discussed here in detail. However, cells showing similar activity patterns have been described in the vertical gaze center.

Figure 9-28, *A* is an overview of the neural circuitry by which saccades are generated, and Figure 9-28, *B* shows the activity of certain types of neurons found in the gaze center that are responsible for horizontal saccades. Each horizontal gaze center has excitatory burst neurons that project to motor neurons in the ipsilateral abducens nucleus and to the internuclear neurons (which will excite medial rectus motor neurons in the contralateral oculomotor nucleus). It also has inhibitory burst neurons that inhibit the contralateral abducens. These burst neurons are capable of extremely high bursts of spikes (up to 1000 Hz). Moreover, the gaze center has neurons showing tonic activity and burst-tonic activity.

Normally, both inhibitory and excitatory burst neurons are inhibited by omnipause neurons located in the nucleus of the dorsal raphe. When a saccade is to be made, activity from the frontal eye fields or the superior colliculus, or both, leads to inhibition of the omnipause cells and excitation of the burst cells on the contralateral side. The resulting high-frequency bursts in the excitatory burst neurons provide a powerful drive to motor neurons of the ipsilateral lateral rectus and contralateral medial rectus (Fig. 9-28, *A*) while at the same time, inhibitory burst neurons permit

relaxation of the antagonists. The initial bursts of these neurons allow strong contraction of the appropriate extraocular muscles, which overcomes the viscosity of the extraocular muscle, and permits rapid movement to occur.

Circuits Underlying Smooth Pursuit

Smooth pursuit involves tracking a moving target with one's eyes (Fig. 9-29). Visual information about target velocity is processed in a series of cortical areas, including the visual cortex in the occipital lobe, several temporal lobe areas, and the frontal eye fields. It should be noted that in the past it was thought that the frontal eye fields were related only to control of saccades, but evidence has recently shown that there are distinct regions within the frontal eye fields dedicated to either saccade production or smooth pursuit. Indeed, there may be two distinct cortical networks, each specialized for one of these types of eye movement. Cortical activity from multiple cortical areas is

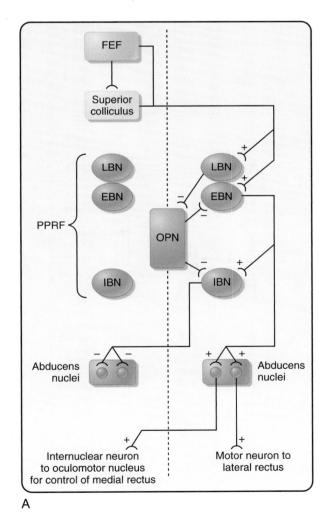

● **Figure 9-28.** Horizontal saccade pathways. **A,** Circuit diagram of the major pathways. EBN, excitatory burst neuron; FEF, frontal eye field; IBN, inhibitory burst neuron; LBN, long lead burst neuron; OPN, omnipause neuron; PPRF, paramedian pontine reticular formation.

Continued

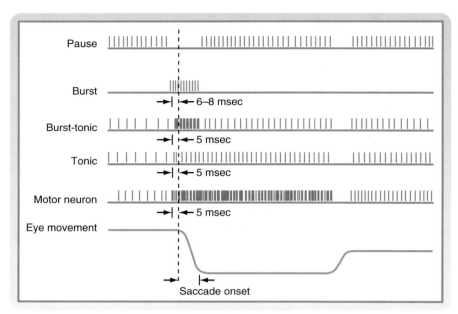

● **Figure 9-28, cont'd** **B,** Firing patterns of some of the neurons involved in making saccades. Excitation of burst neurons of the right horizontal gaze center causes abducens motor neurons on the right and medial rectus motor neurons on the left to be activated. The ascending pathway to the oculomotor nucleus is through the medial longitudinal fasciculus. The left horizontal gaze center is simultaneously inhibited.

B

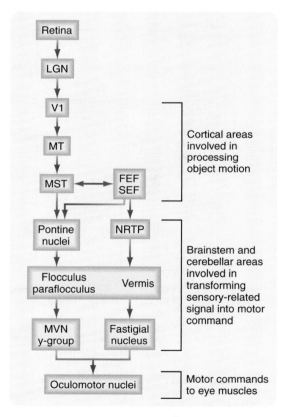

● **Figure 9-29.** Smooth pursuit pathways. The stimulus for smooth pursuit eye movement is a moving visual target. This causes activity to flow through the circuitry diagramed in the figure and leads to maintenance of the fovea on the target. FEF, frontal eye field; LGN, lateral geniculate nucleus; MVN, medial vestibular nucleus; NRTP, nucleus reticularis tegmenti pontis; SEF, supplementary eye field; V1, primary visual cortex. MT and MST are higher-order visual association areas.

fed to the cerebellum via parts of the pontine nuclei and nucleus reticularis tegmenti pontis. Specific areas in the cerebellum, namely, parts of the posterior lobe vermis, the flocculus, and the paraflocculus, receive this input and in turn project to the vestibular nuclei. From the vestibular nuclei, activity can then be forwarded to the oculomotor, abducens, and trochlear nuclei, as was described for the VOR earlier.

Circuits Underlying Vergence

The neural circuits underlying vergence movements are not well known. There are premotor neurons (neurons that feed onto motor neurons) located in the brainstem areas surrounding the various oculomotor nuclei. In some cortical visual areas and the frontal eye fields there are neurons whose activity is related to the disparity of the image on the two retinas or varies during vergence movements. How vergence signals in these cortical areas feed into the brainstem premotor neurons is not clear. The cerebellum also appears to play a role in vergence movements because cerebellar lesions impair this type of eye movement.

■ KEY POINTS

1. α Motor neurons innervate the extrafusal skeletal muscle fibers. A motor unit is a single α motor neuron and all the muscle fibers with which it synapses. Motor unit size varies greatly among muscles; small motor units allow finer control of muscle force.

2. The size principle refers to the orderly recruitment of α motor neurons according to their size, from smallest to largest. Because smaller motor neurons connect to weaker motor units, the relative fineness of motor control is similar for weak and strong contractions.

3. A reflex is a simple, stereotyped motor response to a stimulus. A reflex arc includes the afferent fibers, interneurons, and motor neurons responsible for the reflex.

4. Muscle spindles are complex sensory receptors found in skeletal muscle. They lie parallel to extrafusal muscle fibers, and they contain nuclear bag and nuclear chain intrafusal muscle fibers. By being in parallel to the main muscle, the spindle can detect changes in muscle length.

5. Group Ia afferent fibers form primary endings on nuclear bag1, bag2, and chain fibers, and group II fibers form secondary endings on nuclear chain and bag2 fibers.

6. Primary endings demonstrate both static and dynamic responses that signal muscle length and rate of change in muscle length. Secondary endings demonstrate only static responses and signal only muscle length.

7. γ Motor neurons innervate the intrafusal muscle fibers associated with muscle spindles. Contraction of intrafusal fibers does not directly cause significant changes in muscle tension or length; however, γ motor neurons, by adjusting the level of tension in these fibers, influence the sensitivity of the muscle spindle to stretch.

8. Golgi tendon organs are located in the tendons of muscles and are thus arranged in series with the muscle. They are supplied by group Ib afferent fibers. Their in-series relationship means that tendon organs can detect the force level generated by the muscle, whether it is due to passive stretch or to active contraction of the muscle.

9. The phasic stretch (or myotactic) reflex includes (1) a monosynaptic excitatory pathway from group Ia muscle spindle afferent fibers to α motor neurons that supply the same and synergistic muscles and (2) a disynaptic inhibitory pathway to antagonistic motor neurons.

10. The inverse myotatic reflex is evoked by Golgi tendon organs. Afferent volleys in group Ib fibers from a given muscle cause disynaptic inhibition of α motor neurons to the same muscle, and they excite α motor neurons to antagonist muscles.

11. The flexion reflex is an important protective response because it acts to withdraw a limb from damaging stimuli. The reflex is evoked by volleys in afferent fibers that supply various receptors, particularly nociceptors. Via polysynaptic pathways, these volleys cause excitation of flexor motor neurons and inhibition of extensor motor neurons ipsilaterally. Concurrently, the opposite pattern of action (inhibition of flexor and excitation of extensor motor neurons) occurs contralaterally, and is referred to as the crossed extension reflex.

12. Descending pathways can be subdivided into (1) a lateral system, which ends on motor neurons to limb muscles and on the lateral group of interneu-rons, and (2) a medial system, which ends on the medial group of interneurons.

13. The lateral system includes the lateral corticospinal tract and part of the corticobulbar tract. These pathways influence the contralateral motor neurons that supply the musculature of the limbs, especially of the digits, and the muscles of the lower part of the face and the tongue.

14. The medial system includes the ventral corticospinal, lateral and medial vestibulospinal, reticulospinal, and tectospinal tracts. These pathways mainly affect posture and provide the motor background for movement of the limbs and digits.

15. Locomotion is triggered by commands relayed through the midbrain locomotor center. However, central pattern generators formed by spinal cord circuits and influenced by afferent input provide for the detailed organization of locomotor activity.

16. Voluntary movements depend on interactions among motor areas of the cerebral cortex, the cerebellum, and the basal ganglia.

17. Motor areas of the cerebral cortex are arranged as a parallel distributed network, with each contributing to the various descending motor pathways. The areas primarily involved in body and head movement include the primary motor cortex, the premotor area, the supplementary motor cortex, and the cingulate motor areas. The frontal eye fields are important for eye movement and help initiate voluntary saccades.

18. Individual corticospinal neurons discharge before voluntary contractions of related muscles occur. The discharges are typically related to contractile force rather than to joint position. However, the activity of an individual neuron may encode different parameters of a movement at different times relative to the execution of that movement.

19. The population activity of motor cortex neurons can be used to predict the direction of upcoming movements.

20. The cerebellum influences the rate, range, force, and direction of movements. It also influences muscle tone and posture, as well as eye movement and balance.

21. The intrinsic circuitry of the cerebellum is remarkably uniform. Differences in function of different parts of the cerebellum arise as a result of differing afferent sources and efferent targets.

22. Traditionally, the cerebellum was divided into three zones on the basis of afferent types: vestibulocerebellum, spinocerebellum, and corticocerebellum. Although these names are still used, the basis for them is now known to not be strictly correct.

23. Modern anatomic and physiological techniques indicate that the cerebellar cortex may be divided

into tens of functionally distinct longitudinally running compartments.

24. Most of the input to the cerebellum is through pathways that end as mossy fibers. Mossy fibers excite granule cells, which in turn can evoke single action potentials, called simple spikes, in Purkinje cells.

25. The inferior olive projections to the cerebellum end as climbing fibers and are the only source of them. Each Purkinje cell receives massive input from just one climbing fiber. As a result, each climbing fiber discharge produces a high-frequency burst of two to four action potentials, known as a complex spike, in the Purkinje cell.

26. Although complex spike activity is relatively rare in comparison to simple spike activity, complex spikes are precisely synchronized across populations of Purkinje cells, and because of the convergence of these cells onto cerebellar nuclear neurons, this synchronization may allow complex spike activity to significantly affect cerebellar output. Synchronization of complex spikes is the result of electrical coupling of inferior olivary neurons by gap junctions.

27. The basal ganglia include several deep telencephalic nuclei (including the caudate nucleus, putamen, and globus pallidus). The basal ganglia interact with the cerebral cortex, subthalamic nucleus, substantia nigra, and thalamus.

28. Activity transmitted from the cerebral cortex through the basal ganglia can either facilitate or inhibit the thalamic neurons that project to motor areas of the cortex, depending on the balance between direct and indirect basal ganglia pathways. When there is an imbalance of these two pathways, hyperkinetic or hypokinetic disorders occur.

29. Some types of eye movement help stabilize the visual world. This is critical because visual acuity drops dramatically when the visual world moves, or slips, across the retina. Vestibuloocular and optokinetic movements help stabilize the visual world on the retina by compensating for movement of the head or external world (or both). Smooth pursuit movements allow tracking of a visual target so that it remains foveated.

30. Saccades act to move a part of the visual scene that is of interest to the fovea, the retinal area of highest acuity, for detailed inspection.

31. There are specialized circuits and areas in the brainstem for control of vertical and horizontal eye movements. These areas are used both by the cortex (when voluntary eye movements are made) and by the sensory input that initiates reflexive eye movement.

CHAPTER 10

Higher Functions of the Nervous System

Interactions between different parts of the cerebral cortex and between the cerebral cortex and other parts of the brain are responsible for many of the higher functions that characterize humans. The neural basis for some of these higher functions is discussed in this chapter.

THE CEREBRAL CORTEX

The cerebral cortex in humans occupies a volume of about 600 cm³ and has a surface area of 2500 cm². The surface of the cortex is highly convoluted and folded into ridges known as **gyri.** Gyri are separated by grooves called **sulci** (if shallow) or **fissures** (if deep). This folding greatly increases the surface area of cortex that can be fit into the limited and fixed volume that exists within the skull. Indeed, most of the cortex cannot be seen from the brain surface because of this folding.

The cerebral cortex can be divided into the left and right hemispheres and subdivided into a number of lobes (Fig. 10-1), including the **frontal, parietal, temporal,** and **occipital lobes.** These lobes are named for the overlying bones of the skull. The frontal and parietal lobes are separated by the central sulcus; they are separated from the temporal lobe by the lateral fissure. The occipital and parietal lobes are separated (on the medial surface of the hemisphere) by the parietooccipital fissure (Fig. 10-1). Buried within the lateral fissure is another lobe, the **insula** (Fig. 4-7A). The **limbic lobe** is formed by the cortex on the medial aspect of the hemisphere that borders on the brainstem. Part of the limbic lobe, the **hippocampal formation,** is folded into the **parahippocampal gyrus** of the temporal lobe and cannot be seen from the surface of the brain.

Activity in the two hemispheres of the cerebral cortex is coordinated by interconnections through the cerebral commissures. The bulk of the neocortex on the two sides is connected through the massive **corpus callosum** (Fig. 10-1). Parts of the temporal lobes connect through the anterior commissure, and the hippocampal formations on the two sides communicate through the hippocampal commissure (which is formed between the fornices on the two sides as they approximate each other at the back of the septum pellucidum and pass under the corpus callosum).

Functions of the Lobes of the Cerebral Cortex

Some specific functions of the cerebral cortex can be associated with different lobes of the cerebral hemispheres.

Frontal Lobe

One of the main functions of the **frontal lobe** is motor behavior. As discussed in Chapter 9, the motor, premotor, cingulate motor, and supplementary motor areas are located in the frontal lobe, as is the frontal eye field. These areas are crucial for planning and executing motor behavior. **Broca's area,** essential for the generation of speech, is located in the inferior frontal gyrus of the dominant hemisphere for human language (almost always the left hemisphere, as explained later). In addition, the prefrontal cortex in the rostral part of the frontal lobe plays a major role in personality and emotional behavior.

Bilateral lesions of the prefrontal cortex may be produced either by disease or by surgically induced frontal lobotomy. Such lesions produce deficits in attention, difficulty in planning and problem solving, and inappropriate social behavior. Aggressive behavior is also reduced, and the motivational-affective component of pain is lost, although pain sensation remains. Frontal lobotomies are rarely performed today because improved drug therapies have become available for mental illness and chronic pain.

Parietal Lobe

The **parietal lobe** contains the **somatosensory cortex** and the adjacent **parietal association cortex** (see Chapter 7). This lobe is involved in the processing and perception of sensory information. Connections with the frontal lobe allow somatosensory information to affect voluntary motor activity. Visual information from the occipital lobe reaches the parietal association cortex and the frontal lobe, where it also helps guide voluntary movements. Somatosensory information can also be transferred to language centers, such as Wernicke's area, in the dominant hemisphere, as described later. The parietal lobe in the nondominant hemisphere is involved in determining spatial context, as shown by the effects of specific lesions (see Chapters 7 and 9).

Occipital Lobe

The primary function of the **occipital lobe** is visual processing and perception (see Chapter 8). Connec-

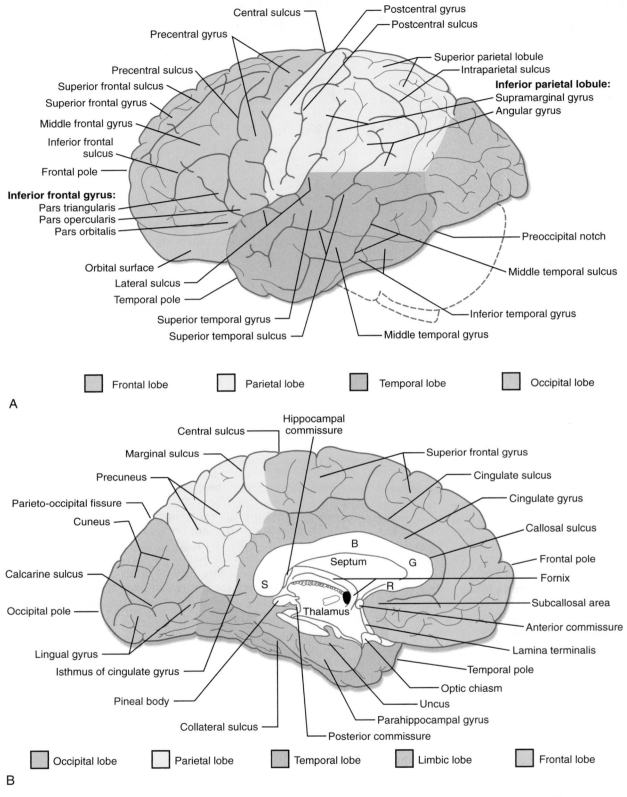

● Figure 10-1. Lateral and medial views of the left hemisphere of the human cerebrum with the major features labeled and the lobes indicated by color. R, G, B, and S indicate, respectively, the rostrum, genu, body, and splenium of the corpus callosum. (From Haines DE [ed]: Fundamental Neuroscience for Basic and Clinical Applications, 3rd ed. Philadelphia, Churchill Livingstone, 2006.)

tions to the frontal eye fields affect eye movements, and a projection to the midbrain assists in the control of convergent eye movements, pupillary constriction, and accommodation, all of which occur when the eyes adjust for near vision.

Temporal Lobe

The **temporal lobe** has many different functions. One of these functions is hearing, which depends on processing and perception of information related to sounds (see Chapter 8). Another function is processing of vestibular information. Several visual areas have been discovered in the temporal lobe; hence, this lobe is also involved in higher-order visual processing (see Chapter 8). For example, the infratemporal cortex, on its inferior surface, is involved in the recognition of faces. In addition, Meyer's loop, which forms part of the optic pathway, passes through the temporal lobe. Therefore, temporal lobe lesions can damage vision in part of the visual fields. Similarly, some of Wernicke's area, essential for the understanding of language, lies in the posterior region of the temporal lobe.

The medial temporal lobe belongs to the limbic system, which participates in emotional behavior and regulates the autonomic nervous system (see Chapter 11). The hippocampal formation is involved in learning and memory (see later).

Neocortical Layering and Subdivisions

The cerebral cortex can be subdivided phylogenetically into the **archicortex, paleocortex,** and **neocortex.** In humans, 90% of the cortex is neocortex.

The different phylogenetic subdivisions of the cerebral cortex can be recognized on the basis of their layering pattern. The neocortex is generally character- ized by the presence of six cortical layers (Fig. 10-2). In contrast, the archicortex has only three layers and the paleocortex has four to five layers.

Cell Types in the Neocortex

A number of different cell types have been described in the neocortex (Fig. 10-2). **Pyramidal cells** are the most abundant cell type and account for approximately 75% of neocortical neurons. **Stellate cells** and various other types of nonpyramidal cells make up the balance. Pyramidal cells have a large triangular cell body, a long apical dendrite directed toward the cortical surface, and several basal dendrites. The axon emerges from the cell body opposite the apical dendrite, and those from the larger pyramidal cells project into the subcortical white matter. The axon may give off collaterals as it descends through the cortex. Pyramidal cells use an excitatory amino acid (glutamate or aspartate) as their neurotransmitter. Stellate cells, often called **granule cells,** are interneurons. They have a small soma and numerous branched dendrites, although many will have an apical dendrite and thus look like small pyramidal cells. Some are excitatory interneurons; these cells are abundant in layer IV of the cortex (see below). Their axons remain in the same cortical region and frequently ascend into the upper cortical layers. Other stellate cells are inhibitory interneurons that use γ-aminobutyric acid (GABA) as their neurotransmitter.

Cytoarchitecture of Cortical Layers

Each of the six layers of the neocortex has a characteristic cellular content (Fig. 10-2). Layer I (molecular layer) has few neuronal cell bodies; instead, it contains mostly axon terminals and synapses on dendrites. Layer II (external granular layer) contains mostly stellate cells. Layer III (external pyramidal layer) consists mostly of small pyramidal cells. Layer IV (internal granular layer) contains mostly stellate cells, including the excitatory type. Layer V (internal pyramidal layer) is dominated by large pyramidal cells. These cells are the main source of cortical efferents to most subcortical regions. Layer VI (multiform layer) contains pyramidal, fusiform, and other types of cells. This layer is also an important origin of cortical efferents, those that target thalamic nuclei.

Cortical Afferent and Efferent Fibers

Thalamocortical afferent fibers from thalamic nuclei that have specific (topographically mapped) cortical projections end chiefly in layers III, IV, and VI. Neurons in other thalamic nuclei (particularly those relaying input from the reticular formation) project diffusely and terminate in layers I and VI.

Several nonthalamic, diffusely projecting nuclei (including the basal nucleus of Meynert, the locus coeruleus, and the dorsal raphe nucleus) project to all cortical layers. These projections, along with those projecting from the thalamus to layers I and VI, modulate cortical activity globally, perhaps in conjunction with changes in state (e.g., sleep or waking).

> ### ▶ IN THE CLINIC
>
> The functions of the different lobes of the cerebral cortex have been defined both from the effects of lesions produced by disease or by surgical interventions to treat disease in humans and from experiments on animals. In another approach, the physical manifestations of **epileptic seizures** have been correlated with the brain locations that give rise to seizures **(epileptic seizure foci).** For example, epileptic foci in the motor cortex cause movements on the contralateral side; the exact movements relate to the somatotopic location of the seizure focus. Seizures that originate in the somatosensory cortex cause an **epileptic aura** in which a touch sensation is perceived. Similarly, seizures that start in the visual cortex cause a visual aura (scintillations, colors), those in the auditory cortex cause an auditory aura (humming, buzzing, ringing), and those in the vestibular cortex cause a feeling of spinning. Complex behavior results from seizures that originate in the temporal lobe association areas; in addition, a malodorous aura may be perceived if the olfactory cortex is involved **(uncinate fit).**

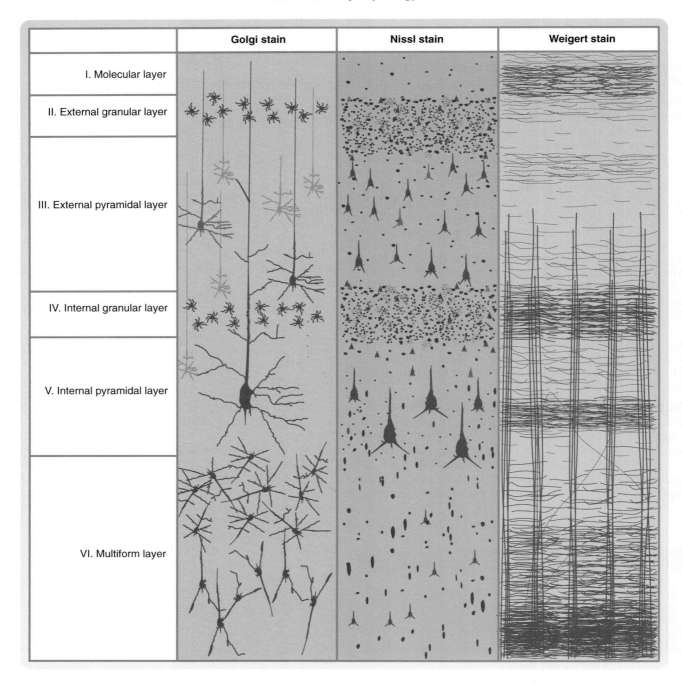

	Golgi stain	Nissl stain	Weigert stain
I. Molecular layer			
II. External granular layer			
III. External pyramidal layer			
IV. Internal granular layer			
V. Internal pyramidal layer			
VI. Multiform layer			

● **Figure 10-2.** A small area of neocortex stained by three different methods. The Nissl stain *(center)* shows the cell bodies of all neurons and reveals how different types are distributed among the six layers. The Golgi stain *(left)* shows only a sample of the neuronal population but reveals details of their dendrites. The Weigert stain for myelin *(right)* demonstrates vertically oriented bundles of axons entering and leaving the cortex and horizontally coursing fibers that interconnect neurons within a layer. (From Brodmann K: Vergleichende Lokalisation lehre der Grosshirnrinde in ihren prinzipien Dargestellt auf Grund des Zellenbaues. Leipzig, Germany, JA Barth, 1909.)

The cortical efferent axons originate from pyramidal cells. The pyramidal cells of layers II and III project to other cortical areas, either ipsilaterally or contralaterally, via the corpus callosum. The pyramidal cells of layer V project in many descending pathways and have synaptic targets in the spinal cord, brainstem, striatum, and thalamus. The pyramidal cells of layer VI form corticothalamic projections to the thalamic nuclei with specific cortical projections. Reciprocal thalamocortical and corticothalamic interconnections are likely to make important contributions to the electroencephalogram (EEG) (see later).

Regional Variations in Neocortical Structure

On the basis of differences in cytoarchitecture, a number of subdivisions of the neocortex can be recognized. Most of the cortex is composed of six readily distinguishable layers. The primary and premotor areas are sometimes said to be **agranular cortex.** This is a misnomer because all cortical areas, including these motor areas, have similar percentages of pyramidal and nonpyramidal cells ($\approx$75% versus 25%). However, in the frontal motor areas, the nonpyramidal cell bodies do not group in a manner that leads to the formation of distinct "granular" layers. Moreover, local inhibitory interneurons play an important role in somatotopic organization of the primary motor cortex (see Chapter 9).

The primary motor cortex, in fact, is characterized by the presence of the largest pyramidal neurons in the cortex, called **Betz cells.** These enormous cells have axons that contribute to the corticospinal tracts and whose soma size (diameter >150 µm) is necessary for the metabolic maintenance of so much axoplasm. (Note that most corticospinal axons are from other pyramidal cells because Betz cell axons account for less than 5% of all corticospinal fibers.)

Another type of cortex has a very prominent layer IV and thus is called **granular cortex.** Dominated as it is by the stellate cells seen in layer IV of Figure 10-2, it is specialized for processing afferent input. Therefore, this kind of cortex is found in the primary sensory receiving areas: the somatosensory cortex (S-I), the primary auditory cortex, and the primary visual (striate) cortex. The striate cortex is given its name because of a particularly prominent horizontal sheet of axons in layer IV known as the **stripe of Gennari.**

Most of the other regions of cortex show less dramatic variations and often seem to grade from one type of layer morphology to the next as one looks at adjacent areas of cortex. On the basis of such an extensive cytoarchitectural analysis, Brodmann divided the cortex into 52 discrete areas (Fig. 10-3). Commonly referred to areas include **Brodmann's areas 3, 1,** and **2** (the S-I cortex of the postcentral gyrus); **area 4** (the primary motor cortex of the precentral gyrus); **area 6** (the premotor and supplementary motor cortex); **areas 41** and **42** (the primary auditory cortex on the superior temporal gyrus); and **area 17** (the primary visual cortex mostly on the medial surface of the occipital lobe). Detailed studies have confirmed that the Brodmann areas are, in fact, distinctly different, both with respect to their interconnections and with respect to their functions, but more recent work has shown that there is some plasticity, both in the size of the areas and in their internal organization (see later).

Archicortex and Paleocortex

About 10% of the human cerebral cortex is archicortex and paleocortex. The archicortex has a three-layered structure; the paleocortex has four to five layers. The paleocortex is located at the border between the archicortex and neocortex.

Hippocampal Formation

In humans the hippocampal formation is part of the archicortex. It is folded into the temporal lobe and can be viewed only when the brain is dissected. The hippocampal formation consists of several parts, including the hippocampus (Ammon's horn or cornu ammonis), the dentate gyrus, and the subiculum. These divisions are well demarcated in a cross section through the hippocampal formation (Fig. 10-4).

The hippocampus has three layers: the molecular, pyramidal cell, and polymorphic layers. They resemble layers I, V, and VI in the neocortex. The folding of the hippocampus imparts an inverted appearance because the white matter is at the surface of the lateral ventricle (Fig. 10-4). The white matter covering the hippocampus is called the **alveus,** which contains hippocampal afferent and efferent fibers. The axons in the alveus continue into a nerve fiber bundle called the **fimbria;** the fimbria is continuous with the fornix.

The hippocampal formation receives its main neural input from the entorhinal cortex of the parahippocampal gyrus. Important, generally reciprocal connections are formed between the pyramidal cells of the hippocampus and (1) the septal nuclei and mammillary body by way of the fornix and (2) the contralateral hippocampal formation by way of the fornix and the hippocampal commissure. The hippocampus is a major component of Papez's circuit (see Fig. 11-6).

HIGHER FUNCTIONS OF THE NERVOUS SYSTEM

The Electroencephalogram

An **EEG** is a recording of neuronal electrical activity that can be made from the cerebral cortex via electrodes placed on the skull. In an **electrocorticogram,** electrical activity of the cortex is recorded via electrodes placed on the surface of the brain. These are both called **field potentials** because they detect the electrical field generated by large groups of relatively distant neurons. The EEG waves are derived from the excitatory and inhibitory synaptic potentials that occur in cortical neurons as a result of thalamocortical and other input, and they are produced chiefly by extracellular currents that flow across the cortex during the generation of synaptic potentials in the pyramidal cells. The potentials recorded as the EEG are relatively large (around 100 µV) and reflect the activity of many pyramidal cells, which are arranged with their apical dendrites aligned in parallel to form a dipole sheet. One pole of this sheet is oriented toward the cortical surface and the other toward the subcortical white matter. Note that the sign of an EEG wave does not in itself indicate whether pyramidal cells are being excited or inhibited. For instance, a negative EEG potential may be generated at the surface of the skull (or cortex) by excitation of apical dendrites or by inhibition near the somas. Conversely, a positive EEG wave can be produced by inhibition of apical dendrites or by excitation near the somas.

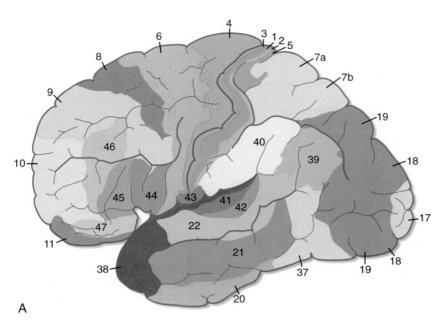

A

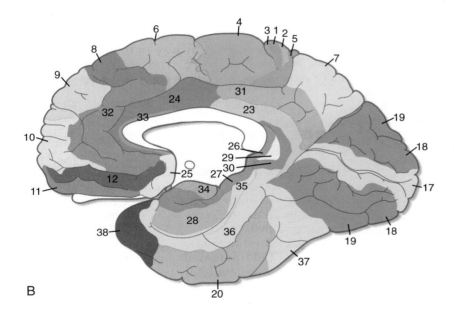

B

● **Figure 10-3.** Brodmann's areas in the human cerebral cortex. (Redrawn from Crosby EC et al: Correlative Anatomy of the Nervous System. New York, Macmillan, 1962.)

Although a brief EEG wave is sometimes referred to as a **spike,** this term does not refer to action potentials because the extracellular currents associated with action potentials are too small, fast, and asynchronous to be recorded with EEG electrodes.

In human studies, the EEG is recorded from a grid of standard recording sites. Thus, EEGs can be recorded from approximately the same sites at different times from one individual or from analogous sites in different subjects. The EEG is an important diagnostic tool in clinical neurology and is particularly useful in patients with epilepsy.

A normal EEG consists of waves of various frequencies. The dominant frequencies depend on several factors, including the state of wakefulness, the age of

the subject, the location of the recording electrodes, and the absence or presence of drugs or disease. When a normal awake adult is relaxed with the eyes closed, the dominant frequencies of the EEG recorded over the parietal and occipital lobes are about 8 to 13 Hz, the **alpha rhythm.** If the subject is asked to open his eyes, the EEG becomes less synchronized and the dominant frequency increases to 13 to 30 Hz, which is called the **beta rhythm.** The **delta** (0.5 to 4 Hz) and **theta** (4 to 7 Hz) **rhythms** are observed during sleep (see the following discussion) (Fig. 10-5).

Evoked Potentials

An EEG change that can be elicited by a stimulus is called a **cortical evoked potential**. A cortical evoked

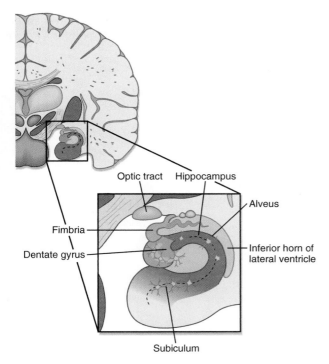

Optic tract   Hippocampus

Alveus

Fimbria

Inferior horn of
lateral ventricle

Dentate gyrus

Subiculum

● **Figure 10-4.** The hippocampal formation is found on the medial aspect of the temporal lobe, and it protrudes into the inferior horn of the lateral ventricle. Its major components are the hippocampus, the dentate gyrus, and the subiculum, all of which are three-layered archicortex. The fimbria is the major output pathway from the hippocampal region to the mammillary body and the septal nuclei.

potential is best recorded from the part of the skull located over the cortical area being activated. For example, a visual stimulus results in an evoked potential that can be recorded best over the occipital bone, whereas a somatosensory evoked potential is recorded most effectively near the junction of the frontal and parietal bones. Evoked potentials reflect the activity in large numbers of cortical neurons. They may also reflect activity in subcortical structures.

Evoked potentials are small in comparison to the size of the EEG waves. However, their apparent size can be enhanced by a process called **signal averaging.** In this process, the stimulation is repeated and EEGs are recorded during each trial and are electronically averaged. With each repetition of the stimulus, the evoked potential occurs at a fixed interval after the stimulus. When the records are averaged, the other components of the EEG, which have a random temporal association with the stimulus, cancel each other, whereas the evoked potentials sum. In signal averaging, evoked potentials are electronically averaged. The random temporal association of the EEG waves with the stimulus results in their cancellation, whereas the evoked potentials sum.

Sleep-Wake Cycle

Sleep and wakefulness are among the many functions of the body that show **circadian** (about 1 day) periodicity. The sleep-wake cycle has an endogenous period-

icity of about 25 hours, but it normally becomes entrained to the day-night cycle. However, the entrainment can be disrupted when the subject is isolated from the environment or shifts time zones (jet lag).

Characteristic changes in the EEG can be correlated with changes in the behavioral state during the sleep-wake cycle. **Beta wave** activity (15 to 40 Hz) dominates in an awake, aroused individual. The EEG is said to be **desynchronized;** it displays low-voltage, high-frequency activity. In relaxed individuals with their eyes closed, the EEG is dominated by **alpha waves** (8 to 12 Hz) (Fig. 10-5). A person falling asleep passes sequentially through four stages of **slow-wave sleep** (called stages 1 through 4) over a period of 30 to 45 minutes (Fig. 10-5). In stage 1, alpha waves are interspersed with lower-frequency waves (3 to 7 Hz) called **theta waves.** In stage 2, the EEG slows further, but the slow-wave activity is interrupted by **sleep spindles,** which are bursts of activity at 12 to 14 Hz, and by large **K complexes** (large, slow potentials). Stage 3 sleep is associated with **delta waves,** (0.5 to 2 Hz), and with occasional sleep spindles. Stage 4 is characterized by delta waves without spindles.

During slow-wave sleep the muscles of the body relax, but the posture is adjusted intermittently. The heart rate and blood pressure decrease and gastrointestinal motility increases. The ease with which individuals can be awakened decreases progressively as they pass through these sleep stages. As individuals awaken, they pass through the sleep stages in reverse order.

About every 90 minutes slow-wave sleep changes to a different form of sleep, called **rapid eye movement (REM)** sleep. In REM sleep, the EEG again becomes desynchronized. The low-voltage, fast activity of REM sleep resembles that seen in the EEG from an aroused subject (Fig. 10-5, *bottom trace*). The similarity of the EEG to that of an awake individual and the difficulty awaking the person have suggested the term **paradoxical sleep** for this type of sleep. Muscle tone is completely lost, but phasic contractions occur in a number of muscles, most notably the eye muscles. The resulting rapid eye movements are basis of the name for this type of sleep. Many autonomic changes also take place. Temperature regulation is lost, and meiosis occurs. Penile erection may occur during this type of sleep. Heart rate, blood pressure, and respira-

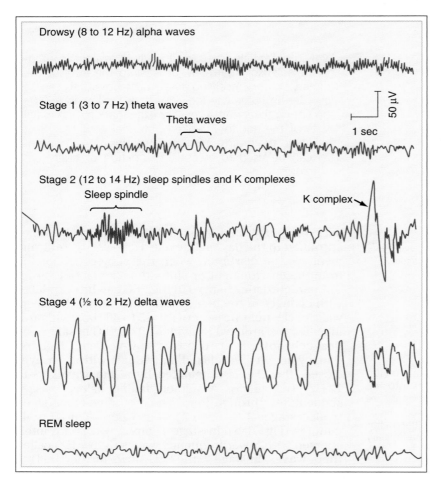

Drowsy (8 to 12 Hz) alpha waves

Stage 1 (3 to 7 Hz) theta waves

Theta waves

50 μV

1 sec

Stage 2 (12 to 14 Hz) sleep spindles and K complexes

Sleep spindle

K complex

Stage 4 (½ to 2 Hz) delta waves

REM sleep

● **Figure 10-5.** EEG during drowsiness and stages 1, 2, and 4 of slow-wave (non–rapid eye movement [non-REM]) sleep and REM sleep. (Modified from Shepherd GM: Neurobiology. London, Oxford University Press, 1983.)

IN THE CLINIC

The purpose of sleep is still unclear. However, it must have a high value because so much of life is spent in sleep and lack of sleep can be debilitating. Medically important disorders of the sleep-wake cycle include **insomnia, bed-wetting, sleepwalking, sleep apnea, and narcolepsy.**

tion change intermittently. Several episodes of REM sleep occur each night. Although it is difficult to arouse a person from REM sleep, internal arousal is common. Most dreaming occurs during REM sleep.

The proportion of slow-wave (non-REM) to REM sleep varies with age. Newborn children spend about half of their sleep time in REM sleep, whereas the elderly have little REM sleep. About 20% to 25% of the sleep of young adults is REM sleep.

The mechanism of sleep is incompletely understood. Stimulation in the brainstem reticular formation in a large region known as the **reticular activating system** causes arousal and low-voltage, fast EEG activity. Sleep was once thought to be caused by a reduced level of activity in the reticular activating system.

However, substantial data, including the observations that anesthesia of the lower brainstem results in arousal and that stimulation in the medulla near the nucleus of the solitary tract can induce sleep, suggest that sleep is an active process. Investigators have tried to relate sleep mechanisms to brainstem networks that use particular neurotransmitters, including serotonin, norepinephrine, and acetylcholine, because manipulations of the levels of these transmitters in the brain can affect the sleep-wake cycle. However, a detailed neurochemical explanation of the neural mechanisms of sleep is not yet available.

The source of circadian periodicity in the brain appears to be the suprachiasmatic nucleus of the hypothalamus. This nucleus receives projections from the retina, and its neurons seem to form a biological clock that adapts to the light-dark cycle. Destruction of the suprachiasmatic nucleus disrupts a number of biological rhythms, including the sleep-wake cycle.

Cerebral Dominance and Language

While right-handedness represents a sensorimotor dominance of the left hemisphere and left-handedness represents a sensorimotor dominance of the right hemisphere, the left cerebral hemisphere is the **dominant hemisphere** for language in over 90% of both right- and left-handed people. This dominance has been demonstrated (1) by the effects of lesions of the

IN THE CLINIC

The EEG becomes abnormal in a variety of pathological circumstances. For example, during coma the EEG is dominated by delta activity. **Brain death** is defined by a maintained flat EEG.

Epilepsy commonly causes EEG abnormalities. There are several forms of epilepsy, and examples of EEG patterns from some of these types of epilepsy are shown in Figure 10-6. Epileptic seizures can be either partial or generalized.

One form of partial seizures originates in the motor cortex and results in localized contractions of contralateral muscles. The contractions may then spread to other muscles; such spread follows the somatotopic sequence of the motor cortex (see Chapter 9). This stereotypical progression is called a **Jacksonian march.** Complex partial seizures (which may occur in **psychomotor epilepsy**) originate in the limbic structures of the temporal lobe and result in illusions and semipurposeful motor activity. During and between focal seizures, scalp recordings may reveal EEG spikes (Fig. 10-6, *C* and *D*).

Generalized seizures involve wide areas of the brain and loss of consciousness. Two major types are **petit mal** and **grand mal seizures.** In petit mal epilepsy, consciousness is lost transiently (typically for less than 15 seconds), and the EEG displays **spike and wave activity** (Fig. 10-6, *B*). In grand mal seizures, consciousness is lost for a longer period, and the individual may fall to the ground if standing when the seizure starts. The seizure begins with a generalized increase in muscle tone **(tonic phase),** followed by a series of jerky movements **(clonic phase).** The bowel and bladder may be evacuated. The EEG shows widely distributed seizure activity (Fig. 10-6, *A*).

EEG spikes that occur between full-blown seizures are called **interictal spikes.** Similar events can be studied experimentally. These spikes arise from abrupt, long-lasting depolarizations, called **depolarization shifts,** that trigger repetitive action potentials in cortical neurons. These depolarization shifts may reflect several changes in epileptic foci. Such changes include regenerative Ca^{++}-mediated dendritic action potentials in cortical neurons and a reduction in inhibitory interactions in cortical circuits. Electrical field potentials and the release of K^+ and excitatory amino acids from hyperactive neurons may also contribute to the increased cortical excitability.

● **Figure 10-6.** EEG abnormalities in several forms of epilepsy. **A,** EEG during the tonic *(left)* and clonic *(right)* phases of a grand mal seizure. **B,** Spike and wave components of a petit mal seizure. **C,** EEG in temporal lobe epilepsy. **D,** A focal seizure. (Redrawn from Eyzaguirre C, Fidone SJ: Physiology of the Nervous System, 2nd ed. St Louis, Mosby, 1975.)

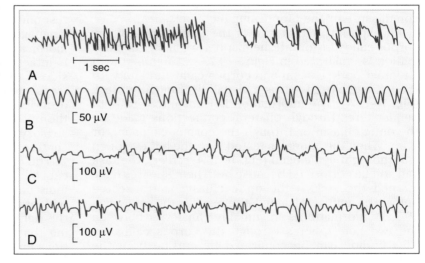

left hemisphere, which may produce deficits in language function **(aphasia),** and (2) by the transient aphasia (inability to speak or write) that results when a short-acting anesthetic is introduced into the left carotid artery. Lesions of the right hemisphere and injection of anesthetic into the right carotid artery do not usually affect language substantially. Differences in the size of an area called the **planum temporale,** which is located in the floor of the lateral fissure, correlate with language dominance. The left planum temporale is usually larger than that of the right hemisphere.

Several areas in the left hemisphere are involved in language. **Wernicke's area** is a large area centered in the posterior part of the superior temporal gyrus behind the auditory cortex. Another important language area, **Broca's area,** is in the posterior part of the inferior frontal gyrus, close to the face representation of the motor cortex. Damage to Wernicke's area results in a **receptive aphasia** in which the person has difficulty understanding spoken and written language; however, speech production remains fluent, if meaningless. Conversely, a lesion in Broca's area causes **expressive aphasia.** Individuals with expressive aphasia have difficulty in speech and in writing, although they can understand language relatively well.

A person with receptive aphasia may not have auditory or visual impairment and one with expressive aphasia may have normal motor control of the muscles responsible for speech or writing. Thus, the terms "sensory aphasia" and "motor aphasia" are misleading. Aphasia does not depend on a deficit of sensation or of motor skill; rather, it is an inability to translate language-encoded sensory information into concepts or to translate concepts into language. However, lesions in the dominant hemisphere may be large enough to result in mixed forms of aphasia, as well as sensory changes or paralysis of some of the muscles used to express language. For example, a lesion of the face representation portion of the motor cortex would result in an inability to manipulate the motor apparatus needed for speaking (vocal cords, tongue, lips) and, consequently, unclear speech because of dysarthria, a mechanical deficit. Such an individual would, however, be able to write if the motor cortex for the upper limb were unaffected.

Interhemispheric Transfer

The two cerebral hemispheres can function somewhat independently, as in the case of language function. However, information must be transferred between the hemispheres to coordinate activity on the two sides of the body. In other words, each hemisphere must know what the other is doing. Much of the information transferred between the two hemispheres is transmitted through the corpus callosum, although some is transmitted through other commissures (e.g., the anterior commissure or the hippocampal commissure).

An experiment that shows the importance of the corpus callosum for interhemispheric transfer of information is illustrated in Figure 10-7, *A*. An animal with an intact optic chiasm and corpus callosum and with the left eye closed learns a visual discrimination task (Fig. 10-7, *A*). The information is transmitted to both hemispheres through bilateral connections made by the optic chiasm or through the corpus callosum, or both. When the animal is tested with the left eye open and the right eye closed (Fig. 10-7, *A, center*), the task can still be performed because both hemispheres have learned the task. If the optic chiasm is transected before the animal is trained, the result is the same (Fig. 10-7, *B*). Information is presumably transferred between the two hemispheres through the corpus callosum. This finding can be confirmed by cutting both the optic chiasm and the corpus callosum before training (Fig. 10-7, *C*). Then the information is not transferred, and each hemisphere must learn the task independently.

A similar experiment has been conducted in human patients who have undergone surgical transection of the corpus callosum to prevent the interhemispheric spread of epilepsy (Fig. 10-8). The optic chiasm remains intact but visual information is directed to one or the other hemisphere by having the subject fix his vision on the central point of the screen. A picture of an object was then flashed to one side of the fixation point so that visual information about the picture reached only the contralateral hemisphere. An opening beneath the screen allowed the patient to manipulate objects that could not be seen. The objects included those shown in the projected pictures. Normal individuals would be able to locate the correct object with either hand. However, patients with a transected corpus callosum could locate the correct object only with the hand ipsilateral to the projected image (contralateral to the hemisphere that received the visual information). The visual information must have had access to the somatosensory and motor areas of the cortex for the hand to explore and recognize the correct object. With the corpus callosum cut, the visual and motor areas are interconnected only on the same side of the brain.

Another test was to ask the patient to verbally identify what object was seen in the picture. The patient would make a correct verbal response to a picture that was projected to the right of the fixation point so that the visual information reached only the left (language dominant) hemisphere. However, the patient could not verbally identify a picture that was presented to the left hemifield so that visual information reached only the right hemisphere.

Similar observations can be made in patients with a transected corpus callosum when different forms of stimuli are used. For example, when such patients are given a verbal command to raise their right arm, they will do so without difficulty. The language centers in the left hemisphere send signals to the ipsilateral motor areas, and these signals produce the movement of the right arm. However, the same patients cannot respond to a command to raise their left arm. The language areas on the left side cannot influence the motor areas on the right unless the corpus callosum is intact. Somatosensory stimuli applied to the right side of the body can be described by patients with a transected corpus callosum, but these patients cannot describe the same stimuli applied to the left side of the body. Information that reaches the right somatosensory areas of the cortex cannot reach the language centers if the corpus callosum has been cut.

The functional capabilities of the two hemispheres can be compared by exploring the performance of individuals with a transected corpus callosum. Such patients solve three-dimensional puzzles better with the right than with the left hemisphere, thus suggesting that the right hemisphere has specialized functions for spatial tasks. Other functions that seem to be more associated with the right than the left hemisphere are facial expression, body language, and speech intonation (Fig. 10-9). The corpus callosum promotes coordination between the two hemispheres. Patients with a transected corpus callosum lack coordination. When they are dressing, for example, one hand may button a shirt while the other tries to unbutton it. Observation of these patients indicates that the two hemispheres can operate quite independently when they are no longer interconnected. However, one hemisphere can express itself with language, whereas the other communicates only nonverbally.

Learning and Memory

Major functions of the higher levels of the nervous system are learning and memory. Learning is a neural

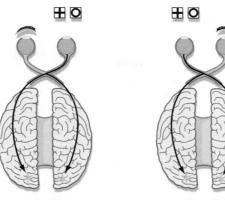

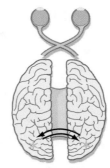

LEARNING
Both hemispheres involved

TESTING
Since both hemispheres involved,
interocular transfer complete

CONCLUSION
Interocular transfer due to intact
optic chiasm and/or
corpus callosum

A

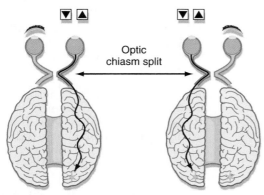

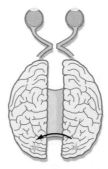

Optic
chiasm split

LEARNING
Right hemisphere trained

TESTING
Left hemisphere knows
problem

CONCLUSION
Learning transferred
via corpus callosum

B

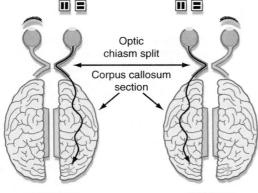

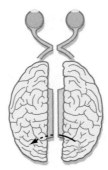

Optic
chiasm split

Corpus callosum
section

LEARNING
Right hemisphere trained

TESTING
Left hemisphere does
not know problem

CONCLUSION
Transfer pathway
was blocked

C

● **Figure 10-7.** Role of the corpus callosum in the interhemispheric transfer of visual information. **A,** Learning involves one eye. Discrimination depends on distinguishing between a cross and a circle. **B,** Discrimination is between triangles oriented with the apex up or down. **C,** Discrimination is between vertical and horizontal bars.

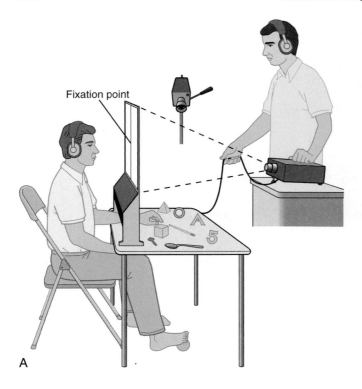

A

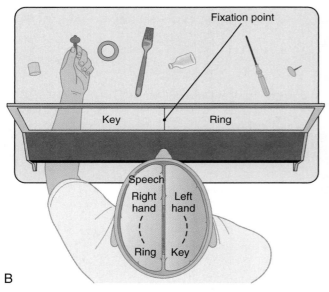

B

● **Figure 10-8.** Tests in a patient with a transected corpus callosum. **A,** The patient fixes on a point on a rear projection screen, and pictures are projected to either side of the fixation point. The hand can palpate objects that correspond to the projected pictures, but these objects cannot be seen. **B,** Response by the left hand to a picture of a key in the left field of view. However, the verbal response is that the patient sees a picture of a ring. (Redrawn from Sperry RW. In Schmitt FO, Worden FG [eds]: The Neurosciences: Third Study Program. Cambridge, MIT Press, 1974.)

> ▶ **IN THE CLINIC**
>
> One of the more striking examples of interhemispheric differences is the phenomenon of "cortical neglect," which is a consequence of a lesion in the parietal cortex of the nondominant, usually right hemisphere. In such cases the patient ignores objects and individuals in his left visual field, draws objects that are incomplete on the left, denies that his left arm and leg are his, and fails to dress the left side of his body. He also denies that he has any such difficulties **(anosognosia).** Although he may respond to touch and pinprick on the left side of his body, he cannot identify objects placed in his left hand. The lesion is adjacent to SI, as well as the visual association cortex, and it suggests that this region plays a special role in the perception of one's body image and immediate extrapersonal space. Similar lesions on the dominant side result only in loss of some higher-order somesthesias, such as agraphesthesia (inability to identify characters drawn on the palm) and astereognosis (inability to identify an object only by touch).

mechanism by which the individual changes behavior as the result of experience. Memory refers to the storage mechanism for what is learned.

The neural circuitry involved in memory and learning in mammals is complex; hence it is difficult to study these mechanisms. Alternative approaches are animal studies, especially in the simpler nervous systems of invertebrates, analysis of the functional consequences of lesions, and anatomic/physiological studies at the cellular and pathway level. For example, by using the marine mollusk *Aplysia* it has been possible to isolate a connection between a single sensory neuron and a motor neuron, which shows aspects of **habituation** (learning not to respond to repetitions of an insignificant stimulus), **sensitization** (increased responsiveness to innocuous stimuli that follow the presentation of a strong or noxious stimulus), and even **associative conditioning** (learning to respond to a previously insignificant event after it has been paired with a significant one). In the case of habituation, the amount of transmitter released in successive responses gradually diminishes. The change involves an alteration in the Ca^{++} current that triggers release of neurotransmitter. The cause of this change is inactivation of presynaptic Ca^{++} channels by repeated action potentials. Long-term habituation can also be produced. In this case the number of synaptic endings and active zones in the remaining terminals decreases.

Long-Term Potentiation

Another model of learning is provided by a synaptic phenomenon called **long-term potentiation (LTP).** LTP has been studied most intensively in slices of the hippocampus in vitro. However, LTP has also been described in the neocortex and in other parts of the nervous system. Repetitive activation of an afferent pathway to the hippocampus or repetitive activation

● **Figure 10-9.** Schematic illustration of the functional specializations of the left and right hemispheres as determined in patients after section of the corpus callosum. (Modified from Siegel A, Sapru HN: Essential Neuroscience, 5th ed. Philadelphia, Lippincott Williams & Wilkins, 2005.)

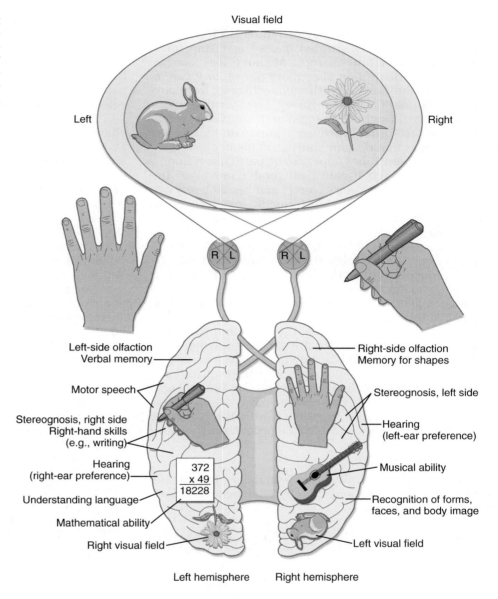

of one of the intrinsic connections increases the responses of pyramidal cells. The increased responses (the LTP) last for hours in vitro (and even days to weeks in vivo). The forms of LTP differ, depending on the particular synaptic system. The mechanism of the enhanced synaptic efficacy seems to involve both presynaptic and postsynaptic events. The neurotransmitters involved in LTP include excitatory amino acids that act on *N*-methyl-D-aspartate (NMDA) receptors, the responses of which are associated with an influx of Ca^{++} into the postsynaptic neuron. Second messenger pathways (including G proteins, Ca^{++}/calmodulin-dependent kinase II, protein kinase G, and protein kinase C) are also involved, and these kinases cause protein phosphorylation and changes in the responsiveness of neurotransmitter receptors. A retrograde messenger, perhaps nitric oxide (or carbon monoxide), may be released from postsynaptic neurons to act on presynaptic endings in such a way that trans-

mitter release is enhanced. Immediate-early genes are also activated during LTP. Hence, changes in gene expression may also be involved.

Another form of synaptic plasticity is **long-term depression** (LTD). LTD has been studied most extensively in the cerebellum, but it also occurs in the hippocampus and in other regions of the central nervous system (CNS). Some of the same factors, such as influx of Ca^{++} and activation of signal transduction mechanism, may account for the induction of LTD, just as for LTP.

Memory

With regard to the stages of memory storage, a distinction between **short-term memory** and **long-term memory** is useful. Recent events appear to be stored in short-term memory by ongoing neural activity because short-term memory persists for only minutes. Short-term memory is used, for instance, to remember a telephone number after calling the operator. Long-term memory can be subdivided into an intermediate form, which can be disrupted, and a long-lasting form, which is difficult to disrupt. Memory loss can be caused by a disruption of memory per se, or it can be a result of interference with the mechanism for recovering information from memory. Long-term memory may involve structural changes in the nervous system because this form of memory can remain intact even after events that disrupt short-term memory.

The temporal lobes appear to be particularly important for memory because bilateral removal of the hippocampal formation severely and permanently disrupts recent memory. Short-term and long-term memories are unaffected, but new long-term memories can no longer be stored. Thus, patients with such deficits remember events before their surgery but fail to recall new events, even with multiple exposure, and must be reintroduced to their therapists repeatedly. This is a loss of declarative memory involving the conscious recall of personal events, words and their meanings, and general history. Such patients, however, can still learn some tasks because they retain procedural memory, the ability to acquire problem-solving, association, and motor skills. If patients are given a complex task to perform (e.g., mirror writing), they will not only improve during the first training session but will also perform better on subsequent days despite their denial of having any experience with the task. The cerebral structures involved in procedural memory are not yet defined.

Neural Plasticity

Damage to the nervous system can induce remodeling of neural pathways and thereby alter behavior. Such remodeling is said to reflect the **plasticity** of the nervous system. The CNS is much more plastic than was once believed. Plasticity is greatest in the developing brain, but some degree of plasticity remains in the adult brain as evidenced by responses to certain manipulations, such as by lesions of the brain, by sensory deprivation, or even by experience.

The capability for developmental plasticity may change for some neural systems at a time referred to as the **critical period.** For example, it is possible to alter some connections formed in the visual pathways during their development by preventing one eye from providing input, but only during an early "critical period" in development. In these visually deprived animals, the visual connections become abnormal (Fig. 10-10), and restoration of normal visual input after this time does not undo the abnormal connections, nor does it restore functional vision from the deprived eye. In addition, similar visual deprivation for a period after several months of age does not result in abnormal connections. The plastic changes seen in such experiments may reflect a competition between fibers for synaptic connections with postsynaptic neurons in the developing nervous system. If a developing neural pathway "loses" in such a competition, the result may be a neurological deficit in the adult.

Phantom limb sensation is an example of neural plasticity in adults. A patient who has suffered the amputation of a limb often perceives sensations on the missing limb when stimulated elsewhere on the body. Functional imaging studies suggest that this is a result of the spread of connections from the surrounding cortical territories into the cortical region that had the amputated limb.

Such remapping can also be seen after surgical amputation of the second and third digits of the hand. Before surgery, each of the digits was represented in discrete and somatotopically organized areas of the postcentral gyrus (S-I). After surgery, the area that represented the amputated digits is now mapped with an enlarged representation of the adjacent digits (Fig. 10-11). Conversely, individuals born with syndactyly (i.e., fusion of two or more digits on the hand) have a single or mostly overlapping representation of these

---

▶ IN THE CLINIC

Two areas important for planning and executing motor tasks are the **parietal cortex** and the **frontal cortex,** the former because it integrates sensory information needed to define the context of a task (see Chapter 7) and the latter because it has neurons that direct all the components for motor execution (see Chapter 9). Mirror neurons have been found in both the **inferior parietal** and the **inferior frontal cortices of macaques.** These cells respond during performance of a specific motor task and also during observation of the same task performed by another animal. Because these mirror cells seem to encode for and respond to very specific and particular tasks, it has been speculated that they may underlie such functions as understanding the intentions of others and empathy, as well as the ability to learn tasks from observation. In humans, EEG activity consistent with the behavior of such mirror neurons has been localized to the **inferior frontal** and **superior parietal lobes.** Autism, which involves an inability to "read" the intentions and emotions of others, has been linked to a lack of mirror neurons by such EEG evidence.

▶ IN THE CLINIC

It was traditional policy to delay corrective surgery for a child born with a congenital cataract until the child was older and more able to cope with the stress of surgery. However, if the correction is deferred until after the "critical period," full recovery of function is unlikely. Similarly, children born with **amblyopia,** a condition characterized by strabismus (cross-eye) because of relative weakness of one of the extraocular muscles, tend to use the unaffected eye in preference. In both cases, early surgery is now common practice so that the cortical circuitry can be correctly sculpted by balanced input from the two eyes.

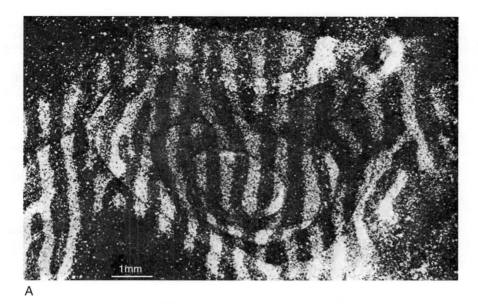

A

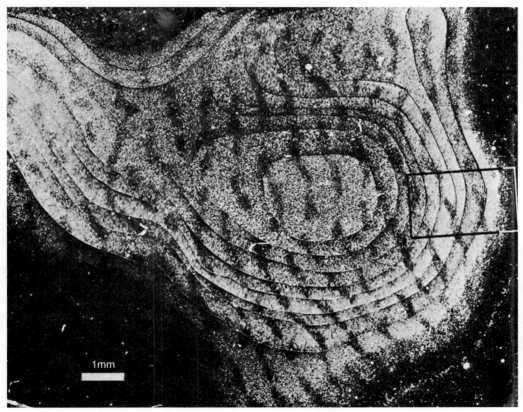

B

● **Figure 10-10.** Plasticity in the visual pathway as a result of sensory deprivation during development. The ocular dominance columns are demonstrated by autoradiography after injection of a radioactive tracer into one eye. The tracer is transported to the lateral geniculate nucleus and then transneurally transported to the striate cortex. The cortex is labeled in bands that alternate with unlabeled bands whose input is from the uninjected eye. **A,** Normal pattern. **B,** Changed pattern in an animal raised with monocular visual deprivation. The injection was made into the nondeprived eye, and the ocular dominance columns for this eye were clearly expanded. In other experiments, it could be shown that the ocular dominance columns for the deprived eye contracted. (**A,** From Hubel DH, Wiesel TN: Proc R Soc Lond B 198:1, 1977; **B,** from LeVay S et al: J Comp Neurol 191:1, 1980.)

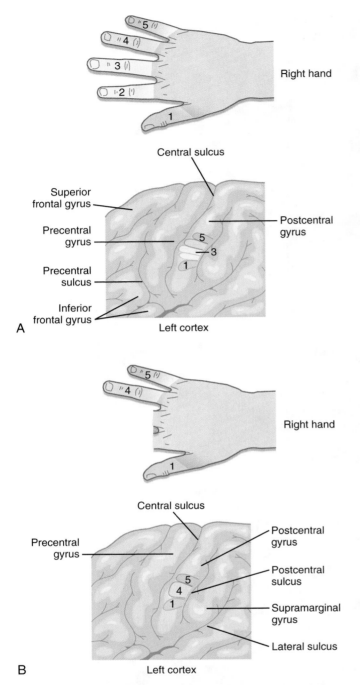

● **Figure 10-11.** Representation of the digit region of the left SI cortex **(A)** and reorganization of this representation **(B)** after amputation of the second and third digits. (From Haines DE [ed]: Fundamental Neuroscience for Basic and Clinical Applications, 3rd ed. Philadelphia, Churchill Livingstone, 2006.)

ing, but the number of cortically recorded receptive fields on the fingertips was likewise increased.

Plastic changes can also occur after injury to the brain in adults. Sprouting of new axons does occur in the damaged CNS. However, the sprouts do not necessarily restore normal function, and many neural pathways do not appear to sprout. Additional knowledge concerning neural plasticity in the adult nervous system is vital if medical therapy is to be improved for many diseases of the nervous system and after neural trauma. Research is currently being conducted to explore the potential of human embryonic stem cells for restoring nervous system function.

■ KEY CONCEPTS

1. The cerebral cortex can be subdivided into lobes based on the pattern of gyri and sulci. Each lobe has distinctive functions, as shown by the effects of lesions or seizures. The left cerebral hemisphere is dominant for language in most individuals. Wernicke's area (in the posterior temporal lobe) is responsible for the understanding of language and Broca's area (in the inferior frontal lobe) for its expression.

2. The cerebral cortex can be subdivided into neocortex, archicortex, and paleocortex. The neocortex typically has six layers, whereas the other types of cortex have fewer layers. The archicortex has three layers, as typified by the hippocampus and dentate gyrus of the hippocampal formation.

3. The neocortex contains a number of cell types, including pyramidal cells, which serve as the output cells, and several kinds of interneurons. The pyramidal cells release an excitatory amino acid neurotransmitter. The inhibitory interneurons are GABAergic. Specific thalamocortical afferent fibers terminate mainly in layer IV of the neocortex; diffuse thalamocortical afferent fibers synapse in layers I and VI. Cortical efferent fibers from layers II and III project to other areas of the cortex; those from layer V project to many subcortical targets, including the spinal cord, brainstem, striatum, and thalamus. Layer VI distributes to the appropriate specific thalamic nucleus.

4. The cortical structure varies in different regions. Agranular cortex is found in the motor areas, whereas granular cortex occurs in the primary sensory receiving areas. Intermediate forms are found elsewhere in the neocortex. Brodmann's area designations reflect these variations in cortical structure and correlate with functionally discrete areas.

5. The EEG varies with the state of the sleep-wake cycle, disease, and other factors. EEG rhythms include alpha, beta, theta, and delta waves. The EEG reflects electrical fields generated by the activity of pyramidal cells. Cortical evoked potentials are stimulus-triggered changes in the EEG and are useful clinical tests of sensory transmission. The

digits in the S-I cortex. After corrective surgery, the independent digits come to have distinctive representations. Even more remarkably, monkeys that were trained on a sensory discrimination task requiring repeated daily use of their fingertips showed cortical differences after training. Not only were the S-I cortical territories of their fingertips larger than before train-

EEG helps in recognition of the various forms of epilepsy. Seizures are associated with depolarization shifts in pyramidal cells. Such shifts are caused by dendritic Ca^{++} spikes and a reduction in inhibitory processing.

6. Sleep can be divided into slow-wave and REM forms. Slow-wave sleep progresses through stages 1 through 4, each with a characteristic EEG pattern. Most dreams occur in REM sleep. Sleep is produced actively by a brainstem mechanism, and its circadian rhythmicity is controlled by the suprachiasmatic nucleus.

7. Information is transferred between the two hemispheres primarily through the corpus callosum. This structure coordinates the two sides of the brain. The right hemisphere is more capable than the left in spatial tasks, facial expression, body language, and speech intonation. The left hemisphere is specialized for the understanding and generation of language, for logic, and for mathematical computation.

8. Learning and memory can be studied on the cellular level, in invertebrates, and in higher animals. Long-term potentiation is mediated by an increased synaptic efficacy that lasts hours to weeks and that involves both presynaptic and postsynaptic changes. Memory includes short-term (minutes), recent, and long-term storage processes and a retrieval mechanism. The hippocampal formation is important for storing declarative memory.

9. Lesion studies and behavioral studies indicate that plasticity occurs in the brain throughout life. However, there appears to be more plasticity early in life, and early "critical periods" are important for the establishment of neural circuitry.

CHAPTER 11

The Autonomic Nervous System and Its Central Control

The main function of the **autonomic nervous system** is to assist the body in maintaining a constant internal environment **(homeostasis).** When internal stimuli signal that regulation of the body's environment is required, the central nervous system (CNS) and its autonomic outflow issue commands that lead to compensatory actions. For example, a sudden increase in systemic blood pressure activates the baroreceptors, which in turn modify the activity of the autonomic nervous system so that the blood pressure is restored toward its previous level (see Chapter 17).

The autonomic nervous system is often regarded as a part of the motor system. However, instead of skeletal muscle, the effectors of the autonomic nervous system are smooth muscle, cardiac muscle, and glands. Because the autonomic nervous system provides motor control of the viscera, it is sometimes called the **visceral motor system.** An older term for this system is the **vegetative nervous system.** This terminology is no longer used because it does not seem appropriate for a system that is important for all levels of activity, including aggressive behavior.

By tradition, the autonomic system is a purely motor system; however, autonomic motor fibers in peripheral nerves are accompanied by visceral afferent fibers that originate from sensory receptors in the viscera. Many of these receptors trigger reflexes, but the activity of some receptors evokes sensory experiences such as pain, hunger, thirst, nausea, and a sense of visceral distention.

The autonomic nervous system also participates in appropriate and coordinated responses to external stimuli. For example, the autonomic nervous system helps regulate pupil size in response to different intensities of ambient light. An extreme example of this regulation is the "fight-or-flight response" that occurs when a threat intensively activates the sympathetic nervous system. Such activation causes a variety of responses. Adrenal hormones are released, the heart rate and blood pressure increase, bronchioles dilate, intestinal motility and secretion are inhibited, glucose metabolism increases, pupils dilate, hairs become erect because of the action of piloerector muscles, cutaneous and splanchnic blood vessels constrict, and blood vessels in skeletal muscle dilate. However, the fight-or-flight response is an uncommon event; it does not represent the usual mode of operation in daily life.

The term autonomic nervous system generally refers to the **sympathetic** and **parasympathetic nervous systems.** In this chapter, the **enteric nervous system** is also included as part of the autonomic nervous system, although it is sometimes considered a separate entity (see also Chapter 32). In addition, because the autonomic nervous system is under CNS control, the central components of the autonomic nervous system are discussed in this chapter. The central components include the hypothalamus and higher levels of the limbic system, which are associated with emotions and with many visceral types of behavior (e.g., feeding, drinking, thermoregulation, reproduction, defense, and aggression) that have survival value.

ORGANIZATION OF THE AUTONOMIC NERVOUS SYSTEM

The primary functional unit of the sympathetic and parasympathetic nervous systems is the two-neuron motor pathway, which consists of a preganglionic neuron, whose cell body is located in the CNS, and a postganglionic neuron, whose cell body is located in one of the autonomic ganglia (Figs. 11-1 and 11-2). The enteric nervous system includes the neurons and nerve fibers in the myenteric and submucosal plexuses, which are located in the wall of the gastrointestinal tract.

The sympathetic preganglionic neurons are located in the thoracic and upper lumbar segments of the spinal cord. For this reason, the sympathetic nervous system is sometimes referred to as the **thoracolumbar division** of the autonomic nervous system. In contrast, the parasympathetic preganglionic neurons are found in the brainstem and in the sacral spinal cord. Hence, this part of the autonomic nervous system is sometimes called the **craniosacral division.** Sympathetic postganglionic neurons are generally found in the paravertebral or prevertebral ganglia. The paravertebral ganglia form two sets of ganglia, one lateral to each side of the vertebral column. Each set of ganglia is linked by longitudinally running axons to form a sympathetic trunk (Figs. 11-1 and 11-2). Prevertebral ganglia are located in the abdominal cavity (Fig.

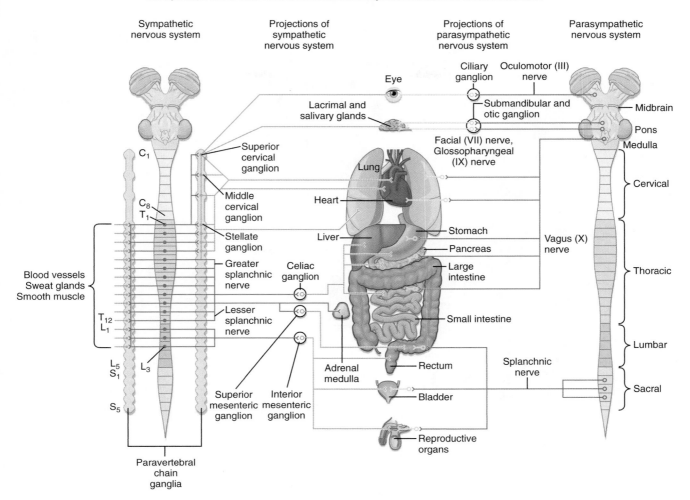

Figure 11-1. Schematic showing the sympathetic and parasympathetic pathways. Sympathetic pathways are shown in red and parasympathetic pathways in blue. Preganglionics are shown in darker shades and postganglionics in lighter shades.

11-1). Thus, paravertebral and prevertebral ganglia are located at some distance from their target organs. In contrast, parasympathetic postganglionic neurons are found in ganglia, which lie near or actually in the walls of the target organs.

Control of the sympathetic and parasympathetic nervous systems of many organs has often been described as antagonistic. This description is not entirely correct. It is more appropriate to consider these two parts of the autonomic control system as working in a coordinated manner—sometimes acting reciprocally and sometimes synergistically—to regulate visceral function. Furthermore, not all visceral structures are innervated by both systems. For example, the smooth muscles and glands in the skin and most of the blood vessels in the body receive sympathetic innervation exclusively; only a small fraction of the blood vessels have parasympathetic innervation. The parasympathetic nervous system does not innervate the body wall, only structures in the head and in the thoracic, abdominal, and pelvic cavities.

The Sympathetic Nervous System

Sympathetic preganglionic neurons are concentrated in the **intermediolateral cell column** (lateral horn) in the thoracic and upper lumbar segments of the spinal cord (Fig. 11-2). Some neurons may also be found in the C8 segment. In addition to the intermediolateral cell column, groups of sympathetic preganglionic neurons are found in other locations, including the lateral funiculus, the intermediate gray matter, and the gray matter dorsal to the central canal.

The axons of preganglionic neurons are often small myelinated nerve fibers known as B fibers (see Table 5-1). However, some are unmyelinated C fibers. They leave the spinal cord in the ventral root and enter the paravertebral ganglion at the same segmental level through a white communicating ramus. White rami are found only from T1 to L2. The preganglionic axon may synapse on postganglionic neurons in this ganglion; may travel rostrally or caudally within the sympathetic trunk and give off collaterals to the ganglia that it passes; or may pass through the ganglion, exit the sympathetic trunk, and enter a splanchnic nerve to

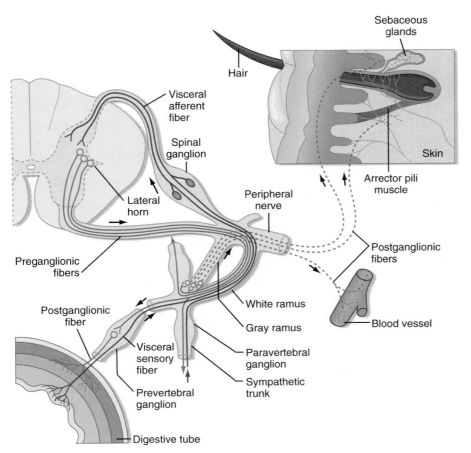

● **Figure 11-2.** Details of the sympathetic pathway at a spinal segment. Autonomic sensory fibers are shown in blue. Sympathetic fibers are in red with preganglionics drawn as solid lines and postganglionics as dashed lines. (Redrawn from Parent A, Carpenter MB: Carpenter's Human Neuroanatomy, 9th ed. p. 295. Philadelphia, Williams & Wilkins, 1996.)

travel to a prevertebral ganglion (Figs. 11-1 and 11-2). A splanchnic nerve is a nerve that innervates the viscera; it contains both visceral afferents and autonomic fibers (sympathetic or parasympathetic).

Postganglionic neurons whose somata lie in paravertebral ganglia generally send their axons through a gray communicating ramus to enter a spinal nerve (Fig. 11-2). Each of the 31 pairs of spinal nerves has a gray ramus. Postganglionic axons are distributed through the peripheral nerves to effectors, such as piloerector muscles, blood vessels, and sweat glands, located in the skin, muscle, and joints. Postganglionic axons are generally unmyelinated (C fibers), although some exceptions exist. The distinction between white and gray rami is a consequence of the relative content of myelinated and unmyelinated axons in these rami.

Preganglionic axons in a splanchnic nerve often travel to a prevertebral ganglion and synapse, or they may pass through the ganglion and an autonomic plexus and end in a more distant ganglion. Some preganglionic axons pass through a splanchnic nerve and end directly on cells of the adrenal medulla, which are equivalent to postganglionic cells.

The sympathetic chain extends from the cervical to the coccygeal levels of the spinal cord. This arrangement serves as a distribution system that enables preganglionic neurons, which are limited to the thoracic and upper lumbar segments, to activate postganglionic neurons that innervate all body segments. However, there are fewer paravertebral ganglia than there are spinal segments because some of the segmental ganglia fuse during development. For example, the superior cervical sympathetic ganglion represents the fused ganglia of C1 through C4, the middle cervical sympathetic ganglion is the fused ganglia of C5 and C6, and the inferior cervical sympathetic ganglion is a combination of the ganglia at C7 and C8. The term **stellate ganglion** refers to fusion of the inferior cervical sympathetic ganglion with the ganglion of T1. The superior cervical sympathetic ganglion provides postganglionic innervation to the head and neck, and the middle cervical and stellate ganglia innervate the heart, lungs, and bronchi.

Generally, the sympathetic preganglionic neurons are distributed to ipsilateral ganglia and thus control autonomic function on the same side of the body. One important exception is that the sympathetic innervation of the intestine and the pelvic viscera is bilateral. As with motor neurons to skeletal muscle, sympathetic preganglionic neurons that control a particular organ are spread over several segments. For example, the sympathetic preganglionic neurons that control sympathetic functions in the head and neck region are distributed in C8 to T5, whereas those that control the adrenal gland are in T4 to T12.

The Parasympathetic Nervous System

The parasympathetic preganglionic neurons are located in several cranial nerve nuclei in the brainstem, as well as in the intermediate region of the S3 and S4 segments of the sacral spinal cord (Fig. 11-1). The cranial nerve nuclei that contain parasympathetic preganglionic neurons are the **Edinger-Westphal nucleus** (cranial nerve III), the **superior** (cranial nerve VII) and **inferior** (cranial nerve IX) **salivatory nuclei,** and the **dorsal motor nucleus** and **nucleus ambiguus** (cranial nerve X). Postganglionic parasympathetic cells are located in cranial ganglia, including the **ciliary ganglion** (preganglionic input is from the Edinger-Westphal nucleus), the **pterygopalatine** and **submandibular ganglia** (input from the superior salivatory nucleus), and the **otic ganglion** (input from the inferior salivatory nucleus). The ciliary ganglion innervates the pupillary sphincter and ciliary muscles in the eye. The pterygopalatine ganglion supplies the lacrimal gland, as well as glands in the nasal and oral pharynx. The submandibular ganglion projects to the submandibular and sublingual salivary glands and to glands in the oral cavity. The otic ganglion innervates the parotid salivary gland and glands in the mouth.

Other parasympathetic postganglionic neurons are located near or in the walls of visceral organs in the thoracic, abdominal, and pelvic cavities. Neurons of the enteric plexus include cells that can also be considered parasympathetic postganglionic neurons. These cells receive input from the vagus or pelvic nerves. The vagus nerves innervate the heart, lungs, bronchi, liver, pancreas, and gastrointestinal tract from the esophagus to the splenic flexure of the colon. The remainder of the colon and rectum, as well as the urinary bladder and reproductive organs, is supplied by sacral parasympathetic preganglionic neurons that travel through the pelvic nerves to postganglionic neurons in the pelvic ganglia.

The parasympathetic preganglionic neurons that project to the viscera of the thorax and part of the abdomen are located in the dorsal motor nucleus of the vagus (see Fig. 4-7 E, F) and the nucleus ambiguus. The dorsal motor nucleus is largely **secretomotor** (it activates glands), whereas the nucleus ambiguus is **visceromotor** (it modifies the activity of cardiac muscle). The dorsal motor nucleus is secretomotor (it activates glands) and visceromotor (it activates the smooth muscle of the gut), whereas the nucleus ambiguus is visceromotor (it modifies the activity of cardiac muscle). Electrical stimulation of the dorsal motor nucleus results in gastric acid secretion, as well as secretion of insulin and glucagon by the pancreas. Although projections to the heart have been described, their function is uncertain. The nucleus ambiguus contains two groups of neurons: (1) a dorsal group **(branchiomotor)** that activates striated muscle in the soft palate, pharynx, larynx, and esophagus and (2) a ventrolateral group that innervates and slows the heart (see also Chapter 18).

Visceral Afferent Fibers

The visceral motor fibers in the autonomic nerves are accompanied by visceral afferent fibers. Most of these afferent fibers supply information that originates from sensory receptors in the viscera. The activity of many of these sensory receptors never reaches the level of consciousness. Instead, these receptors initiate the afferent limb of reflex arcs. Both viscerovisceral and viscerosomatic reflexes are elicited by these afferent fibers. Visceral reflexes operate at a subconscious level, and they are very important for homeostatic regulation and adjustment to external stimuli.

The fast-acting neurotransmitters released by visceral afferent fibers are not well documented, although many of these neurons release an excitatory amino acid transmitter such as glutamate. However, visceral afferent fibers also contain many neuropeptides or combinations of neuropeptides, including angiotensin II, arginine vasopressin, bombesin, calcitonin gene–related peptide, cholecystokinin, galanin, substance P, enkephalin, oxytocin, somatostatin, and vasoactive intestinal polypeptide.

Visceral afferent fibers that mediate sensation include nociceptors that travel in sympathetic nerves, such as the splanchnic nerves. Visceral pain is caused by excessive distention of hollow viscera, contraction against an obstruction, or ischemia. The origin of visceral pain is often difficult to identify because of its diffuse nature and its tendency to be referred to somatic structures (see Chapter 7). Visceral nociceptors in sympathetic nerves reach the spinal cord via the sympathetic chain, white rami, and dorsal roots. The terminals of nociceptive afferent fibers project to the dorsal horn and to the region surrounding the central canal. They activate not only local interneurons, which participate in reflex arcs, but also projection cells, which include spinothalamic tract cells that signal pain to the brain.

A major visceral nociceptive pathway from the pelvis involves a relay in the gray matter of the lumbosacral spinal cord. These neurons send axons into the fasciculus gracilis that terminate in the nucleus gracilis. Thus, the dorsal columns not only contain primary afferents for somatic sensation (their main component) but also second-order neurons of the visceral pain pathway (recall that second-order axons for somatic pain travel in the lateral funiculus as part of the spinothalamic tract). Visceral nociceptive signals are then transmitted to the ventral posterior lateral nucleus of the thalamus and presumably from there to the cerebral cortex. Interruption of this pathway accounts for the beneficial effects of surgically induced lesions of the dorsal column at lower thoracic levels to relieve pain produced by cancer of the pelvic organs.

Other visceral afferent fibers travel in parasympathetic nerves. These fibers are generally involved in reflexes rather than sensation (except for taste afferent fibers; see Chapter 8). For example, the baroreceptor afferent fibers that innervate the carotid sinus are in the glossopharyngeal nerve. They enter the brainstem, pass through the solitary tract, and terminate in the nucleus of the solitary tract (see Fig. 4-7, *D–F*). These neurons connect with interneurons in the brainstem reticular formation. The interneurons, in turn, project to the autonomic preganglionic neurons that control heart rate and blood pressure (see Chapter 18).

The nucleus of the solitary tract receives information from all visceral organs, except those in the pelvis. This nucleus is subdivided into several areas that receive information from specific visceral organs.

The Enteric Nervous System

The enteric nervous system, which is located in the wall of the gastrointestinal tract, contains about 100 million neurons. The enteric nervous system is subdivided into the myenteric plexus, which lies between the longitudinal and circular muscle layers of the gut, and the submucosal plexus, which lies in the submucosa of the gut. The neurons of the myenteric plexus primarily control gastrointestinal motility (see Chapter 26), whereas those in the submucosal plexus primarily regulate body fluid homeostasis (see Chapter 34).

The types of neurons found in the myenteric plexus include not only excitatory and inhibitory motor neurons (which can be considered parasympathetic postganglionic neurons) but also interneurons and primary afferent neurons. Afferent neurons supply mechanoreceptors within the wall of the gastrointestinal tract. These mechanoreceptors form the afferent limb of reflex arcs within the enteric plexus. Local excitatory and inhibitory interneurons process these reflexes, and the output is sent through the motor neurons to smooth muscle cells. Excitatory motor neurons release acetylcholine and substance P; inhibitory motor neurons release dynorphin and vasoactive intestinal polypeptide. The circuitry of the enteric plexus is so extensive that it can coordinate the movements of an intestine that has been completely removed from the body. However, normal function requires innervation by the autonomic preganglionic neurons and regulation by the CNS.

Activity in the enteric nervous system is modulated by the sympathetic nervous system. Sympathetic postganglionic neurons that contain norepinephrine inhibit intestinal motility, those that contain norepinephrine and neuropeptide Y regulate blood flow, and those that contain norepinephrine and somatostatin control intestinal secretion. Feedback is provided by intestinofugal neurons that project back from the myenteric plexus to the sympathetic ganglia.

The submucosal plexus regulates ion and water transport across the intestinal epithelium and glandular secretion. It also communicates with the myenteric plexus to ensure coordination of the functions of the two components of the enteric nervous system. The neurons and neural circuits of the submucosal plexus are not as well understood as those of the myenteric plexus, but many of the neurons contain neuropeptides, and the neural networks are well organized.

AUTONOMIC GANGLIA

The main type of neuron in autonomic ganglia is the postganglionic neuron. These cells receive synaptic connections from preganglionic neurons, and they project to autonomic effector cells. However, many autonomic ganglia also contain interneurons. These interneurons process information within the autonomic ganglia; the enteric plexus can be regarded as an elaborate example of this kind of processing. One type of interneuron found in some autonomic ganglia contains a high concentration of catecholamines. Hence, these interneurons have been called **small, intensely fluorescent (SIF) cells.** SIF cells are believed to be inhibitory.

NEUROTRANSMITTERS

Neurotransmitters in Autonomic Ganglia

The classic neurotransmitter of autonomic ganglia, whether sympathetic or parasympathetic, is acetylcholine. The two classes of acetylcholine receptors in autonomic ganglia are **nicotinic** and **muscarinic receptors,** so named because of their responses to the plant alkaloids **nicotine** and **muscarine.** Nicotinic acetylcholine receptors can be blocked by such agents as **curare** or **hexamethonium,** and muscarinic receptors can be blocked by **atropine.** Nicotinic receptors in autonomic ganglia differ somewhat from those on skeletal muscle cells.

Nicotinic and muscarinic receptors both mediate excitatory postsynaptic potentials (EPSPs), but these potentials have different time courses. Stimulation of preganglionic neurons elicits a fast EPSP, followed by a slow EPSP. The fast EPSP results from activation of nicotinic receptors, which cause ion channels to open. The slow EPSP is mediated by muscarinic receptors (primarily the M_2 receptor—see Chapter 6) that inhibit the **M current,** a current produced by potassium conductance.

Neurons in autonomic ganglia also release neuropeptides that act as neuromodulators. Besides acetylcholine, sympathetic preganglionic neurons may release enkephalin, substance P, luteinizing hormone–releasing hormone, neurotensin, or somatostatin.

Catecholamines such as norepinephrine and dopamine serve as the neurotransmitters of SIF cells in autonomic ganglia.

Neurotransmitters between Postganglionic Neurons and Autonomic Effectors
Sympathetic Postganglionic Neurons

Sympathetic postganglionic neurons typically release norepinephrine, which excites some effector cells but inhibits others. The receptors on target cells may be either α- or β-adrenergic receptors. These receptors are further subdivided into α_1, α_2, β_1, and β_2 receptors. The distribution of these types of receptors and the actions that they mediate when activated by sympathetic postganglionic neurons are listed for various target organs in Table 11-1.

● **Table 11-1.   Responses of Effector Organs to Autonomic Nerve Impulses**

Effector Organs	Receptor Type	Adrenergic Impulses,[1] Responses[2]	Cholinergic Impulses,[1] Responses[2]
Eye			
Radial muscle, iris	α	Contraction (mydriasis) ++	—
Sphincter muscle, iris	α	—	Contraction (miosis) +++
Ciliary muscle	β	Relaxation for far vision +	Contraction for near vision +++
Heart			
Sinoatrial node	β_1	Increase in heart rate ++	Decrease in heart rate; vagal arrest +++
Atria	β_1	Increase in contractility and conduction velocity ++	Decrease in contractility and (usually) increase in conduction velocity ++
Atrioventricular node	β_1	Increase in automaticity and conduction velocity ++	Decrease in conduction velocity; AV block +++
His-Purkinje system	β_1	Increase in automaticity and conduction velocity +++	Little effect
Ventricles	β_1	Increase in contractility, conduction velocity, automaticity, and rate of idioventricular pacemakers +++	Slight decrease in contractility
Arterioles			
Coronary	α, β_2	Constriction +; dilation[3] ++	Dilation +
Skin and mucosa	α	Constriction +++	Dilation[4]
Skeletal muscle	α, β_2	Constriction ++; dilation[3,5] ++	Dilation[6] +
Cerebral	α	Constriction (slight)	Dilation[4]
Pulmonary	α, β_2	Constriction +; dilation[3]	Dilation[4]
Abdominal viscera, renal	α, β_2	Constriction +++; dilation[5] +	—
Salivary glands	α	Constriction +++	Dilation ++
Veins (systemic)	α, β_2	Constriction ++; dilation ++	—
Lung			
Bronchial muscle	β_2	Relaxation +	Contraction ++
Bronchial glands	?	Inhibition (?)	Stimulation +++
Stomach			
Motility and tone	α_2, β_2	Decrease (usually)[7] +	Increase +++
Sphincters	α	Contraction (usually) +	Relaxation (usually) +
Secretion		Inhibition (?)	Stimulation +++
Intestine			
Motility and tone	α_2, β_2	Decrease[7] +	Increase +++
Sphincters	α	Contraction (usually) +	Relaxation (usually) +
Secretion		Inhibition (?)	Stimulation +++
Gallbladder and ducts		Relaxation +	Contraction +
Kidney	β_2	Renin secretion ++	—
Urinary bladder			
Detrusor	β	Relaxation (usually) +	Contraction +++
Trigone and sphincter	α	Contraction +++	Relaxation ++
Ureter			
Motility and tone	α	Increase (usually)	Increase (?)
Uterus	α, β_2	Pregnant: contraction (α); nonpregnant: relaxation (β)	Variable[8]
Sex organs, male	α	Ejaculation +++	Erection +++
Skin			
Pilomotor muscles	α	Contraction ++	
Sweat glands	α	Localized secretion[9] +	Generalized secretion +++
Spleen capsule	α, β_2	Contraction +++; relaxation +	—
Adrenal medulla		—	Secretion of epinephrine and norepinephrine
Liver	α, β_2	Glycogenolysis, gluconeogenesis[10] +++	Glycogen synthesis +
Pancreas			
Acini	α	Decreased secretion +	Secretion ++
Islets (beta cells)	α	Decreased secretion +++	—

● **Table 11-1.** **Responses of Effector Organs to Autonomic Nerve Impulses—cont'd**

Effector Organs	Receptor Type	Adrenergic Impulses,[1] Responses[2]	Cholinergic Impulses,[1] Responses[2]
	β_2	Increased secretion +	—
Fat cells	α, β_1	Lipolysis[10] +++	—
Salivary glands	α	K^+ and water secretion +	K^+ and water secretion +++
	β	Amylase secretion +	—
Lacrimal glands		—	Secretion +++
Nasopharyngeal glands		—	Secretion +++
Pineal gland	β	Melatonin synthesis	—

[1]A long dash (—) signifies no known functional innervation.
[2]Responses are designated + to +++ to provide an approximate indication of the importance of adrenergic and cholinergic nerve activity in control of the various organs and functions listed.
[3]Dilation predominates in situ because of metabolic autoregulatory phenomena.
[4]Cholinergic vasodilation at these sites is of questionable physiological significance.
[5]Over the usual concentration range of physiologically released, circulating epinephrine, a β receptor response (vasodilation) predominates in blood vessels of skeletal muscle and the liver and an α receptor response (vasoconstriction) in blood vessels of other abdominal viscera. The renal and mesenteric vessels also contain specific dopaminergic receptors, activation of which causes dilation, but their physiological significance has not been established.
[6]The sympathetic cholinergic system causes vasodilation in skeletal muscle, but this is not involved in most physiological responses.
[7]It has been proposed that adrenergic fibers terminate at inhibitory β receptors on smooth muscle fibers and at inhibitory α receptors on parasympathetic cholinergic (excitatory) ganglion cells of Auerbach's plexus.
[8]Depends on the stage of the menstrual cycle, the amount of circulating estrogen and progesterone, and other factors.
[9]Palms of the hands and some other sites ("adrenergic sweating").
[10]There is significant variation among species in the type of receptor that mediates certain metabolic responses.
From Goodman LS, Gilman A: The Pharmacological Basis of Therapeutics, 6th ed. New York, Macmillan, 1980.

α_1 Receptors are located postsynaptically, but α_2 receptors may be either presynaptic or postsynaptic. Receptors located presynaptically are generally called **autoreceptors;** they usually inhibit release of transmitter. The effects of agents that excite α_1 or α_2 receptors can be distinguished by using antagonists to block these receptors specifically. For example, prazosin is a selective α_1-adrenergic antagonist, and yohimbine is a selective α_2-adrenergic antagonist. The effects of α_1 receptors are mediated by activation of the inositol triphosphate/diacylglycerol second messenger system (see Chapter 3). In contrast, α_2 receptors decrease the rate of synthesis of cAMP through action on a G protein.

β Receptors are subdivided into β_1 and β_2 receptors on the basis of the ability of antagonists to block them. The proteins that make up the two types of β receptors are similar, with seven membrane-spanning regions connected by intracellular and extracellular domains (see Chapter 3). Agonist drugs that work on β receptors activate a G protein that stimulates adenylyl cyclase to increase the cAMP concentration. This action is terminated by the buildup of guanosine diphosphate.

β Receptors can also be antagonized by the action of α_1 receptors. The number of β receptors can be regulated. If the β receptors are exposed to agonists, they can be desensitized by phosphorylation. In addition, their numbers can be decreased if they become internalized. β Receptors can also increase in number (up-regulation), for example, by denervation. The number of α receptors is likewise regulated.

In addition to releasing norepinephrine, sympathetic postganglionic neurons release neuropeptides such as somatostatin and neuropeptide Y. For example, cells that release both norepinephrine and somatostatin supply the mucosa of the gastrointestinal tract, and cells that release both norepinephrine and neuropeptide Y innervate blood vessels in the gut and the limb. Another chemical mediator in sympathetic postganglionic neurons is ATP.

The endocrine cells of the adrenal medulla are similar in many respects to sympathetic postganglionic neurons (see also Chapter 42). They receive input from sympathetic preganglionic neurons, are excited by acetylcholine, and release catecholamines. However, the cells of the adrenal medulla differ from sympathetic postganglionic neurons in that they release catecholamines into the circulation rather than into a synapse. Moreover, the main catecholamine released is epinephrine, not norepinephrine. In humans, 80% of the catecholamine released by the adrenal medulla is epinephrine and 20% is norepinephrine.

Some sympathetic postganglionic neurons release acetylcholine rather than norepinephrine as their neurotransmitter. For example, sympathetic postganglionic neurons that innervate eccrine sweat glands are cholinergic. The acetylcholine receptors involved are muscarinic, and they are therefore blocked by atropine. Similarly, some blood vessels are innervated by cholinergic sympathetic postganglionic neurons. In addition to releasing acetylcholine, the postganglionic neurons that supply the sweat glands also release neuropeptides, including calcitonin gene–related peptide and vasoactive intestinal polypeptide.

Parasympathetic Postganglionic Neurons

The neurotransmitter released by parasympathetic postganglionic neurons is acetylcholine. The effects of these neurons on various target organs are listed in Table 11-1. Parasympathetic postganglionic actions are mediated by muscarinic receptors. On the basis of binding studies, the action of selective antagonists, and molecular cloning, five types of muscarinic receptors have now been discovered (see Chapter 6). Activation of M_1 receptors enhances the secretion of gastric acid in the stomach. The M_2 receptor is the most abundant receptor type in smooth muscle, including smooth muscle in the intestines, uterus, trachea, and bladder. In addition, it is found in autonomic ganglia and in the heart, where they exert negative chronotropic and inotropic actions (see Chapter 18). M_3 receptors are also found in the smooth muscle of a variety of organs, and although they are less abundant than M_2 receptors, normal contractile patterns appear to require an interaction between the two receptor types. M_4 receptors, like M_2 receptors, are found in autonomic ganglia and thus play a role in synaptic transmission at these sites. M_5 receptors are found in the sphincter muscle of the pupil, the esophagus, and the parotid gland, as well as in cerebral blood vessels.

Muscarinic receptors, like adrenergic receptors, have diverse actions. Some of their effects are mediated by specific second messenger systems. For example, cardiac M_2 muscarinic receptors may act by way of the inositol triphosphate system, and they may also inhibit adenylyl cyclase and thus cAMP synthesis. Muscarinic receptors also open or close ion channels, particularly K^+ or Ca^{++} channels. This action on ion channels is likely to occur through activation of G proteins. A third action of muscarinic receptors is to relax vascular smooth muscle by an effect on endothelial cells, which produce endothelium-derived relaxing factor (EDRF). EDRF is actually nitric oxide, a gas released when arginine is converted to citrulline by nitric oxide synthase (see Chapter 18). Nitric oxide relaxes vascular smooth muscle by stimulating guanyl-

ate cyclase and thereby increasing levels of cGMP, which in turn activates a cGMP-dependent protein kinase (see Chapter 3).

The number of muscarinic receptors is regulated, and exposure to muscarinic agonists decreases the number of receptors by internalization of the receptors.

CENTRAL CONTROL OF AUTONOMIC FUNCTION

The discharges of autonomic preganglionic neurons are controlled by pathways that synapse on autonomic preganglionic neurons. The pathways that influence autonomic activity include spinal cord and brainstem reflex pathways, as well as descending control systems originating at higher levels of the nervous system, such as the hypothalamus.

Examples of Autonomic Control of Particular Organs

The autonomic control of different target organs depends on local reflex circuitry and on signals from parts of the CNS (Table 11-1).

Pupil

The sphincter and dilator muscles of the iris determine the size of the pupil. Activation of sympathetic innervation of the eye dilates the pupil, which occurs during emotional excitement and also in response to painful stimulation. The neurotransmitter at the sympathetic postganglionic synapses is norepinephrine, and it acts at α receptors.

The parasympathetic nervous system exerts an action on pupillary size opposite that of the sympa-

> ### ▶ IN THE CLINIC
>
> **Chagas' disease** is the result of infection by the parasite *Trypanosoma cruzi*. About 18 million people are infected worldwide, and approximately 50,000 die each year as a result of complications from the disease. The most serious forms involve enlargement of the esophagus, colon, and heart. Loss of parasympathetic control is a significant component of the initial stages of the disease; shortly after the initial infection, the parasympathetic neurons innervating the heart, esophagus, and colon are destroyed, which leads to arrhythmias (and potentially sudden death) and aperistalsis. Chronically, cardiomyopathy (malfunction of the heart muscle) that can lead to death occurs in approximately 30% of those infected. Although the pathogenesis of the cardiomyopathy is not fully understood, one leading idea involves autoimmunity. Antibodies against the parasitic antigens have been found to bind to the β-adrenergic and M_2 acetylcholine receptors in the heart. These antibodies not only trigger autoimmune responses that destroy heart muscle but also act as agonists at these receptors and cause inappropriate responses of the cardiovascular system to changing external demands.

> ### ▶ IN THE CLINIC
>
> Sympathetic control of the pupil is sometimes affected by disease. For example, interruption of the sympathetic innervation of the head and neck results in **Horner's syndrome.** This syndrome is characterized by the triad of miosis (abnormal pupillary constriction), ptosis (caused by paralysis of the superior tarsal muscle), and anhidrosis (loss of sweating) on the face. **Enophthalmos** (retraction of the eye into the orbit) also occurs in some animals (rats, cats, and dogs, among others), but in humans no true enophthalmos occurs; however, there is an apparent enophthalmos, an illusion created by partial closure of the eyelid from the ptosis. Horner's syndrome can be produced by a lesion that (1) destroys the sympathetic preganglionic neurons in the upper thoracic spinal cord, (2) interrupts the cervical sympathetic chain, or (3) damages the lower brainstem in the region of the reticular formation, through which pathways descend to the spinal cord to activate sympathetic preganglionic neurons. In the last case there will be a loss of sweating on the side of the body ipsilateral to the lesion.

thetic nervous system. Whereas the sympathetic system elicits pupillary dilation, the parasympathetic system constricts the pupil. The main neurotransmitter at the postganglionic parasympathetic synapse is acetylcholine, which acts on muscarinic receptors. However, neuromodulatory peptides may also be released from some neurons.

Pupil size is reduced by the **pupillary light reflex** and during accommodation for near vision. In the pupillary light reflex, light that strikes the retina is processed by retinal circuits that excite W-type retinal ganglion cells (see Chapter 8). These cells respond to diffuse illumination. The axons of some of the W cells project through the optic nerve and tract to the pretectal area, where they synapse in the olivary pretectal nucleus. This nucleus contains neurons that also respond to diffuse illumination. Activity of neurons of the olivary pretectal nucleus causes pupillary constriction by means of bilateral connections with parasympathetic preganglionic neurons in the Edinger-Westphal nuclei. The reflex results in contraction of the pupillary sphincter muscles in both eyes.

In the **accommodation response,** information from M cells of the retina is transmitted to the striate cortex through the geniculostriate visual pathway (see Chapter 8). The stimulus that triggers accommodation is thought to be a blurred retinal image and disparity of the image between the two eyes. After the information is processed in the visual cortex, signals are transmitted directly or indirectly to the middle temporal cortex, where they activate neurons in a visual area known as MT. MT neurons transmit signals to the midbrain that activate parasympathetic preganglionic neurons in the Edinger-Westphal nuclei bilaterally via their axons in cranial nerve III, which results in pupillary constriction. At the same time signals are transmitted to the ciliary muscle that cause it to contract. This ciliary muscle contraction allows the lens to round up and increase its refractile power.

> ## IN THE CLINIC

The pupillary light reflex is sometimes absent in patients with tertiary (advanced) syphilis, which affects the CNS (i.e., in tabes dorsalis). Although the pupil fails to respond to light, it has a normal accommodation response. This condition is known as the **Argyll Robertson pupil.** The exact mechanism is controversial. One explanation rests on the fact that some optic tract fibers project to the pretectal area in the midbrain. These fibers can be damaged in syphilitic meningitis, possibly by the presence of spirochetes in the subarachnoid space. Note that the pretectal area projects to the Edinger-Westphal nucleus, also in the midbrain, whose cells originate the parasympathetic innervation of the eye, which controls the pupillary sphincter muscle. Although input to the olivary pretectal nucleus is interrupted, the optic tract fibers projecting to the lateral geniculate nucleus are not destroyed, and thus vision is maintained, as is pupillary constriction during accommodation.

Urinary Bladder

The urinary bladder is controlled by reflex pathways in the spinal cord and also by a supraspinal center (Fig. 11-3). The sympathetic innervation originates from preganglionic sympathetic neurons in the upper lumbar segments of the spinal cord. Postganglionic sympathetic axons act to inhibit the smooth muscle **(detrusor muscle)** throughout the body of the bladder, and they also act to excite the smooth muscle of the trigone region and the internal urethral sphincter. The detrusor muscle is tonically inhibited during filling of the bladder, and such inhibition prevents urine from being voided. Inhibition of the detrusor muscle is mediated by the action of norepinephrine on β receptors, whereas excitation of the trigone and internal urethral sphincter is elicited by the action of norepinephrine on α receptors.

The external sphincter of the urethra also helps control voiding. This sphincter is a striated muscle, and it is innervated by motor axons in the pudendal nerves, which are somatic nerves. The motor neurons are located in **Onuf's nucleus,** in the ventral horn of the sacral spinal cord.

The parasympathetic preganglionic neurons that control the bladder are located in the sacral spinal cord (the S2 and S3 or S3 and S4 segments). These cholinergic neurons project through the pelvic nerves and are distributed to ganglia in the pelvic plexus and the bladder wall. Postganglionic parasympathetic neurons in the bladder wall innervate the detrusor muscle, as well as the trigone and sphincter. The parasympathetic activity contracts the detrusor muscle and relaxes the trigone and internal sphincter. These actions result in **micturition,** or urination. Some of the postganglionic neurons are cholinergic and others are purinergic (they release ATP).

Micturition is normally controlled by the **micturition reflex** (see Fig. 11-3). Mechanoreceptors in the bladder wall are excited by both stretch and contraction of the muscles in the bladder wall. Thus, as urine accumulates and distends the bladder, the mechanoreceptors begin to discharge. The pressure in the urinary bladder is low during filling (5 to 10 cm H_2O), but it increases abruptly when micturition begins. Micturition can be triggered either reflexively or voluntarily. In reflex micturition, bladder afferent fibers excite neurons that project to the brainstem and activate the micturition center in the rostral pons **(Barrington's center).** The descending projections also inhibit sympathetic preganglionic neurons that prevent voiding. When a sufficient level of activity occurs in this ascending pathway, micturition is triggered by the micturition center. Commands reach the sacral spinal cord through a reticulospinal pathway. Activity in the sympathetic projection to the bladder is inhibited, and the parasympathetic projections to the bladder are activated. Contraction of muscle in the wall of the bladder causes a vigorous discharge of the mechanoreceptors that supply the bladder wall and thereby further activates the supraspinal loop. The result is complete emptying of the bladder.

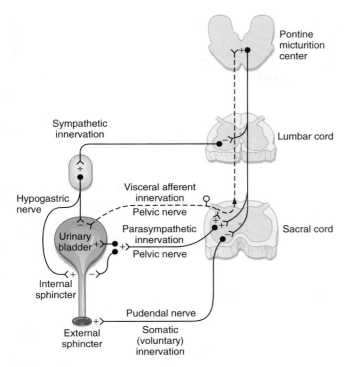

A spinal reflex pathway also exists for micturition. This pathway is operational in newborn infants. However, with maturation, the supraspinal control pathways take on a dominant role in triggering micturition. After spinal cord injury, human adults lose bladder control during the period of spinal shock (urinary incontinence). As the spinal cord recovers from spinal shock, some degree of bladder function is recovered because of enhancement of the spinal cord micturition reflex. However, the bladder has increased muscle tone and fails to empty completely. These circumstances frequently lead to urinary infections.

Autonomic Centers in the Brain

An autonomic center consists of a local network of neurons that respond to input from a particular source and that influence distant neurons by way of long efferent pathways. For example, the micturition center is the autonomic center in the pons that regulates micturition. Many other autonomic centers with diverse functions are also located in the brain. Vasomotor and vasodilator centers are in the medulla, and respiratory centers are in the medulla and pons. Perhaps the greatest concentration of autonomic centers is found in the hypothalamus.

The Hypothalamus

The hypothalamus is part of the diencephalon. Some of the nuclei of the hypothalamus are shown in Figure 11-4. Continuing anteriorly from the hypothalamus are telencephalic structures, the preoptic region and septum. Both the preoptic and septal regions help regulate autonomic function. Important fiber tracts

● **Figure 11-3.** Descending and efferent pathways for reflexes that control the urinary bladder. For clarity, only some of the major involved pathways are shown. (Redrawn from de Groat WC, Booth AM. In Dyck PJ et al (eds): Peripheral Neuropathy, 2nd ed. Philadelphia, WB Saunders, 1984.)

● **Figure 11-4.** Main nuclei of the hypothalamus seen in a view from the third ventricle. Anterior is to the right. (Redrawn from Nauta WJH, Haymaker W: The Hypothalamus. Springfield, IL, Charles C Thomas, 1969.)

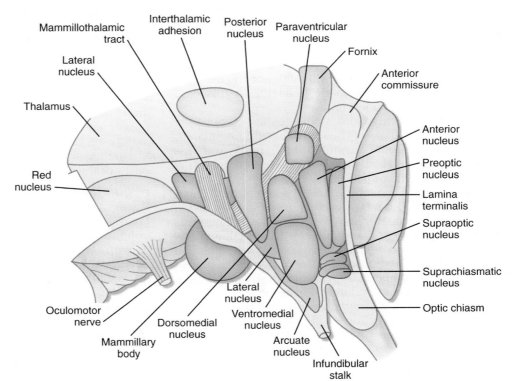

that course through the hypothalamus are the **fornix,** the **medial forebrain bundle,** and the **mammillothalamic tract.** The fornix is used as a landmark to divide the hypothalamus into the medial and lateral hypothalamus.

The hypothalamus has many functions; see Chapter 40 for a discussion of hypothalamic control of endocrine function. Its control of autonomic function is emphasized here.

Temperature Regulation

Homeothermic animals maintain a relatively constant temperature in the face of fluctuating environmental temperatures. When the environmental temperature decreases, the body adjusts by reducing heat loss and by increasing heat production. Conversely, when the temperature rises, the body increases its heat loss and reduces heat production.

Information about the external temperature is provided by thermoreceptors in the skin (and probably other organs such as muscle). Internal temperature is monitored by central thermoreceptive neurons in the anterior hypothalamus. The central thermoreceptors monitor the temperature of blood. The system acts as a servomechanism (a control system that uses negative feedback to operate another system) with a set point at the normal body temperature. Error signals, which represent a deviation from the set point, evoke responses that tend to restore body temperature toward the set point. These responses are mediated by the autonomic, somatic, and endocrine systems.

Cooling causes shivering, which consists of asynchronous muscle contractions that increase heat production. Increases in thyroid gland activity and in sympathetic neural activity tend to increase heat production metabolically. Heat loss is reduced by piloerection and by cutaneous vasoconstriction. Piloerection is effective in animals with fur but not in humans; in the latter, the result is goose bumps. In addition, the hypothalamus, via its widespread connections to cortical regions, will influence the decision to initiate concurrent somatic behavior, in this case possibly putting a jacket on.

Warming the body causes changes in the opposite direction. The activity of the thyroid gland diminishes, which leads to reduced metabolic activity and less heat production. Heat loss is increased by sweating and cutaneous vasodilation.

The hypothalamus serves as the temperature servomechanism. The heat loss responses are organized by the heat loss center, which is composed of neurons in the preoptic region and anterior hypothalamus. As might be expected, lesions here prevent sweating and cutaneous vasodilation, and if the individual is placed in a warm environment, **hyperthermia** will occur. Conversely, electrical stimulation of the heat loss center causes cutaneous vasodilation and inhibits shivering. Heat conservation responses are organized in the posterior hypothalamus by neurons that form a heat production and conservation center. Thus, lesions in the area dorsolateral to the mammillary body interfere with heat production and conservation and can cause

IN THE CLINIC

In fever, the set point for body temperature is elevated. This can be caused by the release of a **pyrogen** by microorganisms. The pyrogen changes the set point, thereby leading to increased heat production by shivering and to heat conservation by cutaneous vasoconstriction.

hypothermia when the subject is in a cold environment. Electrical stimulation in this region of the brain evokes shivering.

Thermoregulatory responses are also produced when the hypothalamus is locally warmed or cooled. These responses reflect the presence of central thermoreceptive neurons in the hypothalamus.

Regulation of Food Intake

Food intake is also regulated by a servomechanism. However, the set point is affected by many factors. Sensory signals that help regulate food intake operate both on a short-term basis to control ingestion and on a long-term basis to control body weight. Glucoreceptors in the hypothalamus sense blood glucose and use this information to control food intake. Their main action occurs when blood glucose levels decrease. Opioid peptides and pancreatic polypeptide stimulate food intake; cholecystokinin inhibits food intake. Insulin and adrenal glucocorticoids also affect food intake (see Chapters 38 and 42).

Lesions of the lateral hypothalamus suppress food intake **(aphagia),** which can cause starvation and death. Electrical excitation of the lateral hypothalamus stimulates eating. These observations suggest that the lateral hypothalamus contains a **feeding center.** Converse effects are produced by manipulation of the ventromedial nucleus of the hypothalamus. A lesion here causes **hyperphagia,** which is an increased food intake that can result in obesity, whereas electrical stimulation of the same region stops the feeding behavior. This area of the hypothalamus is known as the **satiety center.** The feeding and satiety centers operate reciprocally.

Further work is needed to clarify the role of other parts of the nervous system in feeding behavior.

Regulation of Water Intake

Water intake also depends on a servomechanism. Fluid intake is influenced by blood osmolality and volume (Fig. 11-5).

With water deprivation, the extracellular fluid becomes hyperosmotic, which in turn causes the intracellular fluid to become hyperosmotic. The brain contains neurons that serve as osmoreceptors for detection of increases in the osmotic pressure of extracellular fluid (see also Chapter 34). The osmoreceptors appear to be located in the organum vasculosum of the lamina terminalis, which is a circumventricular organ. Circumventricular organs surround the cerebral ventricles and lack a blood-brain barrier. The sub-

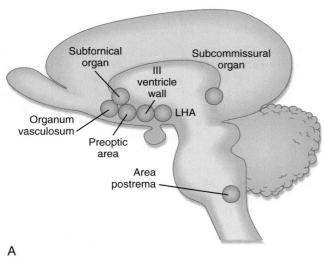

A

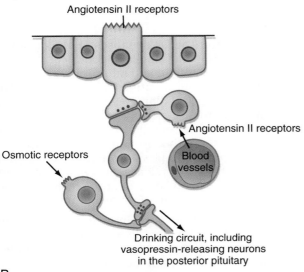

B

● **Figure 11-5.** **A,** Structures thought to play a role in the regulation of water intake in rats. **B,** Neural circuits that signal changes in blood osmolality and volume. (**A,** Redrawn from Shepherd GM: Neurobiology. New York, Oxford University Press, 1983.)

fornical organ and the organum vasculosum are involved in thirst.

Water deprivation also causes a decrease in blood volume, which is sensed by receptors in the low-pressure side of the vasculature, including the right atrium (see also Chapter 17). In addition, decreased blood volume triggers the release of renin by the kidney. Renin breaks down angiotensinogen into angiotensin I, which is then hydrolyzed to angiotensin II (see Chapter 34). This peptide stimulates drinking by an action on angiotensin II receptors in another one of the circumventricular organs, namely, the subfornical organ. Angiotensin II also causes vasoconstriction and release of aldosterone and antidiuretic hormone (ADH).

Insufficient water intake is usually a greater problem than excess water intake. However, when more water is taken in than required, it is easily eliminated by inhibition of the release of ADH from neurons in the supraoptic nucleus at their terminals in the posterior pituitary gland (see Chapter 40). As mentioned previously, signals that inhibit release of ADH include increased blood volume and decreased osmolality of extracellular fluid. Other areas of the hypothalamus, particularly the preoptic region and lateral hypothalamus, help regulate water intake, as do several structures outside the hypothalamus.

Other Autonomic Control Structures

Several regions of the forebrain other than the hypothalamus also play a role in autonomic control. These regions include the central nucleus of the amygdala and the bed nucleus of the stria terminalis, as well as a number of areas of the cerebral cortex. Information reaches these higher autonomic centers from viscera through an ascending system that involves the nucleus of the solitary tract, the parabrachial nucleus, the periaqueductal gray matter, and the hypothalamus. Descending pathways that help control autonomic activity originate in such structures as the paraventricular nucleus of the hypothalamus, the A5 noradrenergic cell group, the rostral ventrolateral medulla, and the raphe nuclei and adjacent structures of the ventromedial medulla.

Neural Influences on the Immune System

Environmental stress can cause immunosuppression, in which the number of helper T cells and the activity of natural killer cells are reduced. Immunosuppression can even be the result of classic conditioning. One mechanism for such an effect involves the release of corticotropin-releasing factor (CRF) from the hypothalamus. CRF causes the release of adrenocorticotropic hormone (ACTH) from the pituitary gland; release of ACTH stimulates the secretion of adrenal corticosteroids, which cause immunosuppression (see Chapter 42). Other mechanisms include direct neural actions on lymphoid tissue. The immune system may also influence neural activity.

Emotional Behavior

The limbic system helps control emotional behavior, in part by an influence on the hypothalamus. The limbic lobe is phylogenetically the oldest part of the cerebral cortex. A circuit that connects the limbic lobe with the hypothalamus (the Papez circuit) regulates emotional behavior. The neural components of this circuit are termed the limbic system (Fig. 11-6, see also Fig. 10-1, _B_).

The Papez circuit indirectly connects many areas of the neocortex to the hypothalamus. Information passes from the cingulate gyrus to the entorhinal cortex and hippocampus and from there via the fornix to the mammillary bodies in the hypothalamus. The mammillothalamic tract then connects the hypothalamus with the anterior thalamic nuclei, which project back to the cingulate gyrus. Other structures included in the limbic system circuitry are the amygdala and the bed nucleus of the stria terminalis.

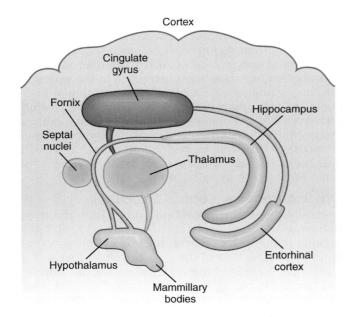

● **Figure 11-6.** The Papez circuit. (From Groves PM, Schlesinger K: Introduction to Biological Psychology, 2nd ed. Dubuque, IA, William C Brown, 1982.)

Bilateral temporal lobe lesions can produce Klüver-Bucy syndrome, which is characterized by loss of the ability to detect and recognize the meaning of objects from visual cues (visual agnosia), a tendency to examine objects orally, attention to irrelevant stimuli, hypersexuality, change in dietary habits, and decreased emotionality. Although this syndrome was originally described following large lesions that included most or all of the temporal lobe, in more recent studies the syndrome has been shown to occur following more selective lesions of the anterior temporal lobe, which highlights the importance of the loss of the amygdala and its role in emotional processing as an underlying factor in the syndrome.

■ KEY CONCEPTS

1. The autonomic nervous system is a motor system that controls smooth muscle, cardiac muscle, and glands. It helps maintain homeostasis and coordinates responses to external stimuli. Its components are the sympathetic, parasympathetic, and enteric nervous systems. Autonomic motor pathways have preganglionic and postganglionic neurons. Preganglionic neurons reside in the CNS, whereas postganglionic neurons lie in peripheral ganglia.

2. Sympathetic preganglionic neurons are located in the thoracolumbar region of the spinal cord, and sympathetic postganglionic neurons are located in paravertebral and prevertebral ganglia. Parasympathetic preganglionic neurons are located in cranial nerve nuclei or in the sacral spinal cord. Parasympathetic postganglionic neurons reside in ganglia located in or near the target organs.

3. Visceral afferent fibers innervate sensory receptors in the viscera. Most function to activate reflexes; for some, activation also leads to conscious sensations.

4. The enteric nervous system includes the myenteric and submucosal plexuses in the wall of the gastrointestinal tract. The myenteric plexus regulates motility, and the submucosal plexus regulates ion and water transport and secretion.

5. Neurotransmitters at the synapses of preganglionic neurons in autonomic ganglia include acetylcholine (acting at both nicotinic and muscarinic receptors) and a number of neuropeptides. Interneurons in the ganglia release catecholamines. Sympathetic postganglionic neurons generally release norepinephrine (acting on adrenergic receptors) as their neurotransmitter, although neuropeptides are also released. Sympathetic postganglionic neurons that supply sweat glands release acetylcholine. Parasympathetic postganglionic neurons release acetylcholine (acting on muscarinic receptors).

6. The pupil is controlled reciprocally by the sympathetic and parasympathetic nervous systems. Sympathetic activity causes pupillary dilation (mydriasis); parasympathetic activity causes pupillary constriction (meiosis).

7. Emptying of the urinary bladder depends on parasympathetic outflow during the micturition reflex. Sympathetic constriction of the internal sphincter of the urethra prevents voiding. The micturition reflex is triggered by stretch receptors, and it is controlled in normal adults by a micturition center in the pons.

8. The hypothalamus contains several centers that control autonomic and other activities, including heat loss, heat production and conservation, feeding and satiety, and fluid intake.

9. The limbic system consists of several cortical and subcortical structures. It controls emotional behavior, in part by activation of the autonomic nervous system.

MUSCLE

James M. Watras

CHAPTER 12

Skeletal Muscle Physiology

Muscle cells are highly specialized cells for the conversion of chemical energy to mechanical energy. Specifically, muscle cells use the energy in ATP to generate force or do work. Because work can take many forms (such as locomotion, pumping blood, or peristalsis), several types of muscle have evolved. The three basic types of muscle are **skeletal muscle, cardiac muscle,** and **smooth muscle.**

Skeletal muscle acts on the skeleton. In limbs, for example, skeletal muscle spans a joint, thereby allowing a lever action. Skeletal muscle is under voluntary control (i.e., controlled by the central nervous system) and plays a key role in numerous activities such as maintenance of posture, locomotion, speech, and respiration. When viewed under the microscope, skeletal muscle exhibits transverse striations (at intervals of 2 to 3 μm) that result from the highly organized arrangement of actin and myosin molecules within the skeletal muscle cells. Thus, skeletal muscle is classified as a **striated muscle.** The heart is composed of cardiac muscle, and although it is also a striated muscle, it is an involuntary muscle (i.e., controlled by an intrinsic pacemaker and modulated by the autonomic nervous system). Smooth muscle (which lacks the striations evident in skeletal and cardiac muscle) is an involuntary muscle typically found lining hollow organs such as the intestine and blood vessels. In all three muscle types, force is generated by the interaction of actin and myosin molecules, a process that requires transient elevation of intracellular [Ca^{++}].

In this chapter attention is directed at the molecular mechanisms underlying contraction of skeletal muscle. Mechanisms for regulating the force of contraction are also addressed. To put this information into perspective, it is important to first examine the basic organization of skeletal muscle.

ORGANIZATION OF SKELETAL MUSCLE

Figure 12-1 illustrates skeletal muscles spanning the elbow joint. The muscles are attached to bone on either side of the joint. The point of attachment closest to the spine is called the **origin,** whereas the point of attachment on the distal region (on the far side of the joint) is called the **insertion.** These points of attachment occur through **tendons** (connective tissue) at the end of the muscle. Note that the point of insertion

is close to the elbow joint, which promotes a broad range of motion. Also note that the joint is spanned by a **flexor** muscle on one side and an **extensor** muscle on the opposite side of the joint. Thus, contraction of the flexor muscle (see the biceps muscle in Fig. 12-1) results in a decrease in the angle of the elbow joint (bringing the forearm closer to the shoulder), whereas contraction of the extensor muscle (see the triceps muscle in Fig. 12-1) results in the reverse motion (extending the arm).

The basic structure of skeletal muscle is shown in Figure 12-2. Each muscle is composed of numerous cells called **muscle fibers.** A connective tissue layer called the **endomysium** surrounds each of these fibers. Individual muscle fibers are then grouped together into **fascicles,** which are surrounded by another connective tissue layer called the **perimysium.** Within the perimysium are the blood vessels and nerves that supply the individual muscle fibers. Finally, fascicles are joined together to form the muscle. The connective tissue sheath that surrounds the muscle is called the **epimysium.** At the ends of the muscle, the connective tissue layers come together to form a tendon, which attaches the muscle to the skeleton. The connective tissue layers are composed mainly of elastin and collagen fibers, and they serve to transmit movement of the actin and myosin molecules to the skeleton to effect movement. The connective tissue layers also contribute to passive tension of muscle and prevent damage to the muscle fibers as a result of overstretching or contraction (or both).

Individual skeletal muscle cells are narrow (≈10 to 80 μm in diameter), but they can be extremely long (up to 25 cm in length). Each skeletal muscle fiber contains bundles of filaments, called **myofibrils,** running along the axis of the cell. The gross striation pattern of the cell results from a repeating pattern in the myofibrils. Specifically, it is the regular arrangement of the thick and thin filaments within these myofibrils coupled with the highly organized alignment of adjacent myofibrils that gives rise to the striated appearance of skeletal muscle. Striations can be observed in intact muscle fibers and in the underlying myofibrils.

A myofibril can be subdivided longitudinally into **sarcomeres** (Fig. 12-3). The sarcomere is demarcated by two dark lines called **Z lines** and represents a repeating contractile unit in skeletal muscle. The average length of a sarcomere is 2 μm. On either side

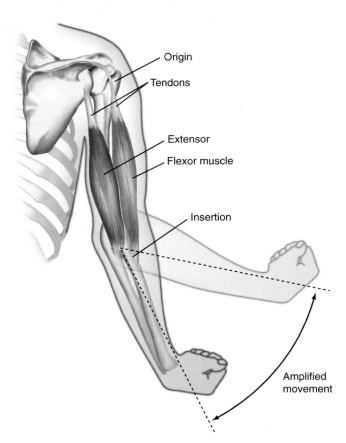

Figure 12-1. Skeletal muscle attaches to the skeleton by way of tendons and typically spans a joint. The proximal and distal points of attachment of the tendon are termed "origin" and "insertion," respectively. Note that the insertion is close to the joint, which allows a broad range of motion. Also note that skeletal muscles span both sides of the joint, which allows both flexion and extension of the forearm.

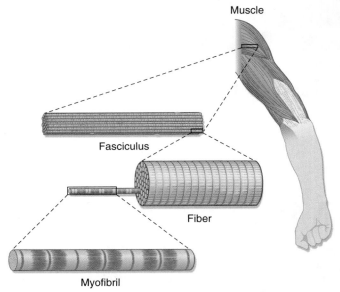

Figure 12-2. Skeletal muscle is composed of bundles of muscle fibers called a fasciculus. A muscle fiber represents an individual muscle cell and contains bundles of myofibrils. The striations are due to the arrangement of thick and thin filaments. See text for details. (Redrawn from Bloom W, Fawcett DW: A Textbook of Histology, 10th ed. Philadelphia, Saunders, 1975.)

of the Z line is a light band (**I band**) that contains thin filaments composed primarily of the protein **actin.** The area between two I bands within a sarcomere is the **A band,** which contains thick filaments composed primarily of the protein **myosin.** The thin actin filaments extend from the Z line toward the center of the sarcomere and overlap a portion of the thick filaments. The dark area at the end of the A band represents this region of overlap between thick and thin filaments. A light area present in the center of the sarcomere is called the **H band.** This area represents the portion of the A band that contains myosin thick filaments, but no thin actin filaments. Thus, thin actin filaments extend from the Z line to the edge of the H band and overlap a portion of the thick filament in the A band. A dark line called the **M line** is evident in the center of the sarcomere and includes proteins that appear to be critical for organization and alignment of the thick filaments in the sarcomere.

As illustrated in Figure 12-3, each myofibril in a muscle fiber is surrounded by **sarcoplasmic reticulum**

(SR). The SR is an intracellular membrane network that plays a critical role in the regulation of intracellular [Ca^{++}]. Invaginations of the sarcolemma, called **T tubules,** pass into the muscle fiber near the ends of the A band (i.e., close to the SR). The SR and the T tubules, however, are distinct membrane systems. The SR is an intracellular network, whereas the T tubules are in contact with the extracellular space. A gap ($\approx$15 nm in width) separates the T tubules from the SR. The portion of the SR nearest the T tubules is called the **terminal cisternae,** and it is the site of Ca^{++} release, which is critical for contraction of skeletal muscle (see later). The longitudinal portions of the SR are continuous with the terminal cisternae and extend along the length of the sarcomere. This portion of the SR contains a high density of Ca^{++} pump protein (i.e., Ca^{++}-ATPase), which is critical for reaccumulation of Ca^{++} in the SR and hence relaxation of the muscle.

The thick and thin filaments are highly organized in the sarcomere of myofibrils (Fig. 12-3). As mentioned, thin actin filaments extend from the Z line toward the center of the sarcomere, whereas thick myosin filaments are centrally located and overlap a portion of the opposing thin actin filaments. The thick and thin filaments are oriented such that in the region of overlap within the sarcomere, each thick myosin filament is surrounded by a hexagonal array of thin actin filaments. It is the Ca^{++}-dependent interaction of the thick myosin and the thin actin filaments that generates the force of contraction after stimulation of the muscle (see later).

The thick myosin filaments are tethered to the Z lines by a cytoskeletal protein called **titin.** Titin is a

● **Figure 12-3.** **A,** Myofibrils are arranged in parallel within a muscle fiber. **B,** Each fibril is surrounded by sarcoplasmic reticulum (SR). Terminal cisternae of the SR are closely associated with T tubules and form a triad at the junction of the I and A bands. The Z lines define the boundary of the sarcomere. The striations are formed by overlap of the contractile proteins. Three bands can be seen, the A band, I band, and H band. An M line is seen in the middle of the H band. **C,** Organization of the proteins within a single sarcomere. The cross-sectional arrangement of the proteins is also illustrated.

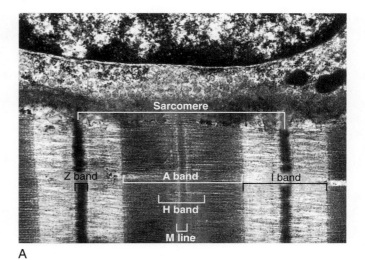

A

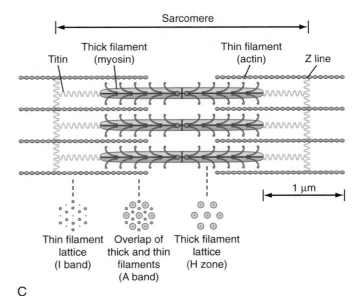

B

C

very large elastic protein (molecular weight in excess of 3000 kDa) that extends from the Z line to the center of the sarcomere and appears to be important for organization and alignment of the thick filaments in the sarcomere. Titin may also serve as a mechanosensor and influence gene expression and protein degradation in a mechanical activity–dependent manner. Some forms of muscular dystrophy have been attributed to defects in titin.

The thin filament is formed by the aggregation of actin molecules (termed **globular actin** or **G-actin**) into a two-stranded helical filament called **F-actin,** or **filamentous actin** (Fig. 12-5). The elongated cytoskeletal protein **nebulin** extends along the length of the thin filament and may participate in regulation of the length of the thin filament. Dimers of the protein **tropomyosin** extend over the entire actin filament and cover myosin binding sites on the actin molecules. Each tropomyosin dimer extends over seven actin molecules, with sequential tropomyosin dimers arranged in a head-to-tail configuration. A **troponin complex** consisting of three subunits **(troponin T, troponin I,** and **troponin C)** is present on each tropomyosin dimer and influences the position of the tropomyosin molecule on the actin filament and hence the ability of tropomyosin to inhibit binding of myosin to the actin filament. Troponin T binds tropomyosin, troponin I facilitates the inhibition of myosin binding to actin by tropomyosin, and troponin C binds Ca^{++}. Binding of Ca^{++} to troponin C promotes the movement of tropomyosin on the actin filament, thereby exposing myosin binding sites and facilitating the interaction of myosin and actin filaments and sarcomere contraction (see later). Additional proteins associated with the thin filament include **tropomodulin, α-actinin,** and **capZ protein.** Tropomodulin is located at the end of the thin filament, toward the center of the sarcomere, and may participate in setting the length of the thin filament. α-Actinin and capZ protein serve to anchor the thin filament to the Z line.

Organization of the thick filament is shown in Figure 12-6. **Myosin** is a large protein (≈480 kDa) that consists of six different polypeptides with one pair of large heavy chains (≈200 kDa) and two pairs of light chains (≈20 kDa). The heavy chains are wound together in an α-helical configuration to form a long rod-like segment, with the N-terminal portion of each heavy chain forming a large globular head. The head region extends away from the thick filament toward the actin thin fila-

● AT THE CELLULAR LEVEL

The muscular dystrophies constitute a group of genetically determined degenerative disorders. **Duchenne's muscular dystrophy** (DMD; described by G.B. Duchenne in 1861) is the most common of the muscular dystrophies and affects 1 in 3500 boys (3 to 5 years of age). Severe muscle wasting occurs, with most patients being wheelchair bound by the age of 12 and many dying of respiratory failure in adulthood (30 to 40 years of age). DMD is an X-linked recessive disease that has been linked to a defect in the dystrophin gene that leads to a deficiency of the dystrophin protein in skeletal muscle, brain, retina, and smooth muscle. **Dystrophin** is a large (427 kDa) protein that is present in low abundance (0.025%) in skeletal muscle. It is localized on the intracellular surface of the sarcolemma in association with several integral membrane glycoproteins (forming a dystrophin-glycoprotein complex). This dystrophin-glycoprotein complex provides a structural link between the subsarcolemmal cytoskeleton of the muscle cell and the extracellular matrix (Fig. 12-4) and appears to stabilize the sarcolemma and hence prevents contraction-induced injury (rupture). The dystrophin-glycoprotein complex may also serve as a scaffold for cell signaling cascades that promote cell survival.

Although defects in the dystrophin-glycoprotein complex are involved in many forms of muscular dystrophy, recent studies have identified some forms of muscular dystrophy that involve other mechanisms. Specifically, a defect in sarcolemma repair (attributed to loss/mutation of the protein dysferlin) appears to underlie at least one form of muscular dystrophy (**limb-girdle muscular dystrophy 2B,** associated with muscle wasting in the pelvic region). Defects in the protein titin (termed titinopathies) have been implicated in other forms of muscular dystrophy (e.g., **limb-girdle muscular dystrophy 2J** and **tibial muscular dystrophy**). The link between titin mutations and muscular dystrophy may reflect a disruption in the ability of titin to bind a signalosome that can inhibit transcription and promote protein degradation. In the latter mechanism, the signalosome has been shown to include a muscle-specific ubiquitin ligase (viz., MuRF2) that can inhibit a transcription factor (viz., serum response factor) by promoting translocation to the cytosol and promote protein degradation (through ubiquitination—see Chapter 1). Mutations in the protease **calpain 3** (resulting in loss of protease activity) have also been implicated in some types of muscular dystrophy (e.g., limb-girdle muscular dystrophy 2A), apparently secondary to apoptosis.

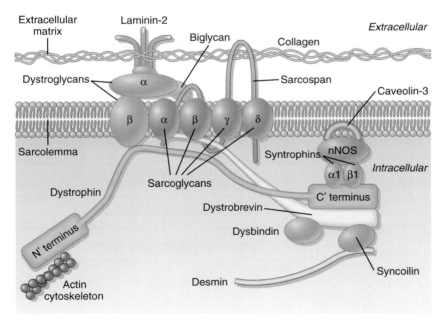

● Figure 12-4. Organization of the dystrophin-glycoprotein complex in skeletal muscle. The dystrophin-glycoprotein complex provides a structural link between the cytoskeleton of the muscle cell and the extracellular matrix, which appears to stabilize the sarcolemma and hence prevents contraction-induced injury (rupture). Duchenne's muscular dystrophy is associated with loss of dystrophin. (Redrawn from Nowak K, and Davies K.E.: EMBO Reports 5:872–876, 2004.)

ment and is the portion of the molecule that can bind to actin. Myosin is also able to hydrolyze ATP, and ATPase activity is located in the globular head as well. The two pairs of light chains are associated with the globular head. One of these pairs of light chains, termed essential light chains, is critical for the ATPase activity of myosin. The other pair of light chains, sometimes called regulatory light chains, may influence the kinetics of myosin and actin binding under certain conditions. Thus, myosin ATPase activity resides in the globular head of myosin and requires the presence of light chains (viz., the "essential" light chains).

Myosin filaments form by a tail-to-tail association of myosin molecules, thereby resulting in a bipolar arrangement of the thick filament. The thick filament then extends on either side of the central bare zone by a head-to-tail association of myosin molecules, thus maintaining the bipolar organization of the thick filament centered on the M line. Such a bipolar arrange-

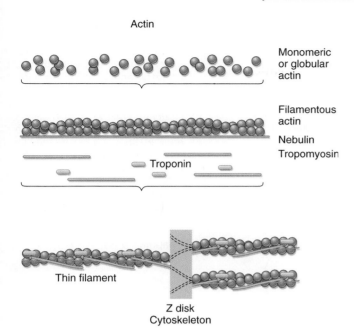

● **Figure 12-5.** Organization of a thin filament. Polymerization of monomeric actin into filamentous actin forms the backbone of the thin filament. The filament contains several other structural/regulatory proteins such as nebulin, tropomyosin, and troponin.

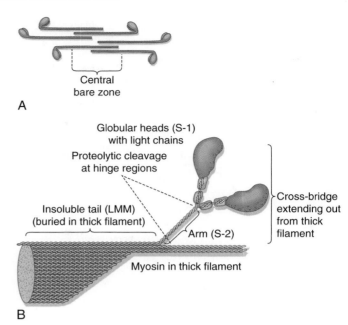

● **Figure 12-6.** Organization of a thick filament. A thick filament is formed by the polymerization of myosin molecules in a tail-to-tail configuration extending from the center of the sarcomere **(A)**. An individual myosin molecule has a tail region and a cross-bridge region. The cross-bridge region is composed of an arm and globular heads **(B)**. The globular heads contain light chains that are important for the function of myosin ATPase activity.

ment is critical for drawing the Z lines together (i.e., shortening the length of the sarcomere) during contraction. The mechanisms controlling this highly organized structure of the myosin thick filament are not clear, although the cytoskeletal protein titin is thought to participate in the formation of a scaffold for organization and alignment of the thick filament in the sarcomere. Additional proteins found in the thick filaments (e.g., **myomesin** and **C protein**) may also participate in the bipolar organization or packing of the thick filament (or both).

CONTROL OF SKELETAL MUSCLE ACTIVITY

Motor Nerves and Motor Units

Skeletal muscle is controlled by the central nervous system. Specifically, each skeletal muscle is innervated by an α **motor neuron.** The cell bodies of α motor neurons are located in the ventral horn of the spinal cord (Fig. 12-7; see also Chapter 9). The motor axons exit via the ventral roots and reach the muscle through mixed peripheral nerves. The motor nerves branch in the muscle, with each branch innervating a single muscle fiber. The specialized cholinergic synapse that forms the **neuromuscular junction** and the neuromuscular transmission process that generates an action potential in the muscle fiber are described in Chapter 6.

A **motor unit** consists of the motor nerve and all the muscle fibers innervated by the nerve. The motor unit is the functional contractile unit because all the muscle cells within a motor unit contract synchronously when the motor nerve fires. The size of motor

units within a muscle varies depending on the function of the muscle. In the rectus muscles of the eye the motor units are small (i.e., only a small number of muscle fibers are innervated by a motor neuron), and thus movement of the eye can be precisely controlled. In contrast, the motor units of the legs are large, which facilitates running. Activation of varying numbers of motor units within a muscle is one way in which the tension developed by a muscle can be controlled (see later).

The neuromuscular junction formed by the α motor neuron is called an **end plate** (see Chapter 6 for details). Acetylcholine released from the α motor neuron at the neuromuscular junction initiates an action potential in the muscle fiber that rapidly spreads along its length. The duration of the action potential in skeletal muscle is less than 5 msec. This contrasts with the duration of the action potential in cardiac muscle, which is approximately 200 msec. The short duration of the skeletal muscle action potential allows very rapid contractions of the fiber and provides yet another mechanism by which the force of contraction can be increased. Increasing tension by repetitive stimulation of the muscle is called tetany (this phenomenon is described in more detail later in this chapter).

Excitation-Contraction Coupling

When an action potential is transmitted along the sarcolemma of the muscle fiber and then down the T tubules, Ca^{++} is released from the terminal cisternae

Input from brain and
higher centers

Spinal cord

Dorsal
root

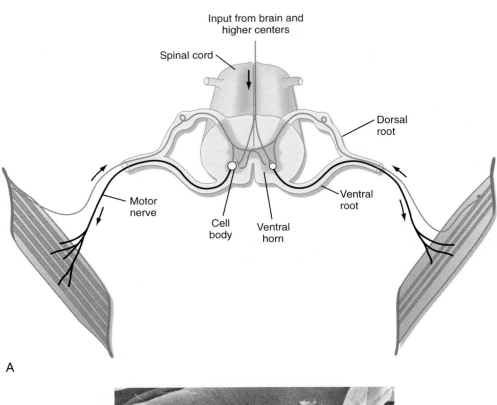

Motor
nerve

Cell
body

Ventral
horn

Ventral
root

A

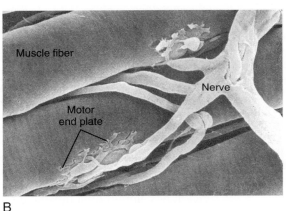

Muscle fiber

Nerve

Motor
end plate

B

● **Figure 12-7.** Skeletal muscle is a voluntary muscle controlled by the central nervous system, with efferent signals (i.e., action potentials) passing through an α motor neuron to muscle fibers. Each motor neuron may innervate many muscle fibers within a muscle, although each muscle fiber is innervated by only one motor neuron **(A). B,** Scanning electron micrograph showing innervation of several muscle fibers by a single motor neuron. (**B,** From Bloom W, Fawcett DW: A Textbook of Physiology, 12th ed. New York, Chapman & Hall, 1994.)

SR into the myoplasm. This release of Ca⁺⁺ from the SR raises intracellular [Ca⁺⁺], which in turn promotes actin-myosin interaction and contraction. The time course for the increase in intracellular [Ca⁺⁺] relative to the action potential and development of force is shown in Figure 12-8. The action potential is extremely short-lived ($\approx$5 msec). The elevation in intracellular [Ca⁺⁺] begins slightly after the action potential and peaks at approximately 20 msec. This increase in intracellular [Ca⁺⁺] initiates a contraction called a twitch.

The mechanism underlying the elevation in intracellular [Ca⁺⁺] involves an interaction between protein in the T tubule and the adjacent terminal cisternae of the SR. As previously described (Fig. 12-3), the T tubule represents an invagination of the sarcolemma that extends into the muscle fiber and forms a close association with two terminal cisternae of the SR. The asso-

ciation of a T tubule with two opposing terminal cisternae is called a **triad.** Although there is a gap ($\approx$15 nm in width) between the T tubule and the terminal cisternae, proteins bridge this gap. Based on their appearance on electron micrographs, these bridging proteins are called **feet** (Fig. 12-9). These feet are the Ca⁺⁺ release channels in the membrane of the terminal cisternae that are responsible for the elevation in intracellular [Ca⁺⁺] in response to the action potential. Because this channel binds the drug **ryanodine,** it is commonly called the **ryanodine receptor (RYR).** RYR is a large protein ($\approx$500 kDa) that exists as a homotetramer. Only a small portion of the RYR molecule is actually embedded in the SR membrane. Most of the RYR molecule appears to be in the myoplasm and spans the gap between the terminal cisternae and the T tubule (Fig. 12-10).

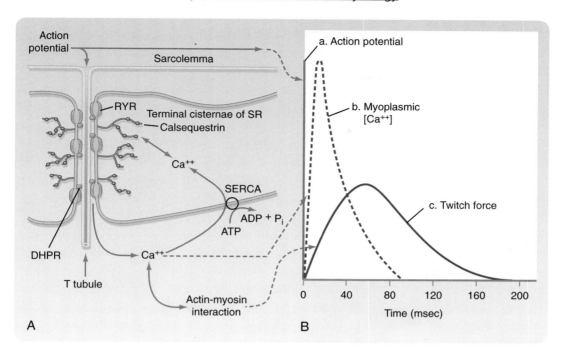

● **Figure 12-8.** Stimulation of a skeletal muscle fiber initiates an action potential in the muscle that travels down the T tubule and induces release of Ca^{++} from the terminal cisternae of the SR **(A).** The rise in intracellular $[Ca^{++}]$ causes a contraction. As Ca^{++} is pumped back into the SR by Ca^{++}-ATPase (SERCA), relaxation occurs. **B,** Time courses of the action potential, myoplasmic Ca^{++} transient, and force of the twitch contraction.

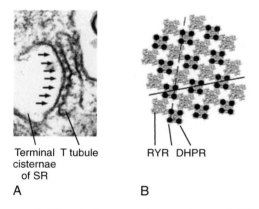

● **Figure 12-9.** **A,** Electron micrograph of a triad illustrating the "feet" between the T tubule and the SR, which are thought to be the ryanodine receptors (RYRs) in the SR. **B,** Each RYR in the SR is associated with four dihydropyridine receptors (DHPRs) in the T tubule. (From Protasi F et al: Biophys J 79:2494, 2000.)

At the T-tubule membrane, the RYR is thought to interact with a protein called the **dihydropyridine receptor (DHPR).** DHPR is an L-type voltage-gated Ca^{++} channel with five subunits. One of these subunits binds the dihydropyridine class of channel blocking drugs and appears to be critical for the ability of the action potential in the T tubule to induce release of Ca^{++} from the SR. However, influx of Ca^{++} into the cell through the DHPR is not needed for the initiation of

Ca^{++} release from the SR. Indeed, skeletal muscle is able to contract in the absence of extracellular Ca^{++} or with a mutated DHPR that does not conduct Ca^{++}. Instead, release of Ca^{++} from the terminal cisternae of the SR is thought to result from a conformational change in the DHPR as the action potential passes down the T tubule, and this conformational change in the DHPR, by means of a protein-protein interaction, opens the RYR and releases Ca^{++} into the myoplasm.

Structural analysis, including the use of freeze-fracture techniques, provides evidence for a close physical association of DHPR and RYR (Fig. 12-9). DHPR in the T-tubule membrane appears to reside directly opposite the four corners of the underlying homotetrameric RYR channel in the SR membrane.

Other proteins that reside near the RYR include **calsequestrin, triadin,** and **junctin** (Fig. 12-10). Calsequestrin is a low-affinity Ca^{++}-binding protein that is present in the lumen of the terminal cisternae. It allows Ca^{++} to be "stored" at high concentration and thereby establishes a favorable concentration gradient that facilitates the efflux of Ca^{++} from the SR into the myoplasm when the RYR opens. Triadin and junctin are in the terminal cisternae membrane and bind both RYR and calsequestrin; they could anchor calsequestrin near the RYR and thereby increase Ca^{++} buffering capacity at the site of Ca^{++} release. **Histidine-rich calcium-binding protein (HRC)** is another low-affinity Ca^{++}-binding protein in the SR lumen, although it is less abundant than calsequestrin. HRC appears to bind triadin in a Ca^{++}-dependent manner, which raises the

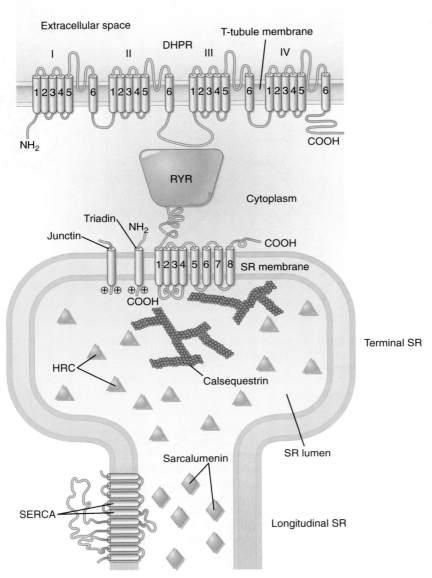

● **Figure 12-10.** Molecular structure and relationships between the dihydropyridine receptor (DHPR) in the T-tubule membrane and the RYR in the SR membrane. Triadin is an associated SR protein that may participate in the interaction of RYR and DHPR. Calsequestrin is a low-affinity Ca++-binding protein that helps accumulate Ca++ in the terminal cisternae. See text for details. (From Rossi AE, Dirksen RT: Muscle Nerve 33:715, 2006.)

● AT THE CELLULAR LEVEL

A variety of mutational studies have been conducted to ascertain the region of the DHPR that is critical for opening of the RYR. One possible site of interaction (depicted in Fig. 12-10) is the myoplasmic loop between transmembrane domains II and III in the α_1 subunit of the DHPR. The voltage-sensing region of the DHPR involved in intramembranous charge movement is thought to reside in the S_4 transmembrane segments of the α_1 subunit. Genetic mutations in the RYR or DHPR, or in both, have been associated with pathological disturbances in myoplasmic [Ca++]. Such disturbances include malignant hyperthermia and central core disease, as described later. These mutations are typically observed in the myoplasmic portion of the RYR, although mutations have also been observed in a myoplasmic loop in the DHPR.

possibility of a role greater than serving simply as a Ca++ buffer.

Relaxation of skeletal muscle occurs as intracellular Ca++ is resequestered by the SR. Uptake of Ca++ into the SR is due to the action of a Ca++ pump (i.e., Ca++-ATPase). This pump is not unique to skeletal muscle and is found in all cells in association with the endoplasmic reticulum. Accordingly, it is named **SERCA**, which stands for **sarcoplasmic endoplasmic reticulum calcium ATPase.** SERCA is the most abundant protein in the SR of skeletal muscle, and it is distributed throughout the longitudinal tubules and the terminal cisternae as well. It transports two molecules of Ca++ into its lumen for each molecule of ATP hydrolyzed.* Thus, the Ca++ transient seen during a twitch contraction (see Fig. 12-8) reflects release of Ca++ from the

*During the transport of Ca++, SERCA exchanges 2 Ca++ ions for 2 H+ ions (i.e., H+ is pumped out of the SR).

terminal cisternae via the RYR and reuptake primarily into the longitudinal portion of the SR by SERCA. The low-affinity Ca^{++}-binding protein **sarcalumenin** is present throughout the longitudinal tubules of the SR and nonjunctional regions of the terminal cisternae and is thought to be involved in the transfer of Ca^{++} from sites of Ca^{++} uptake in the longitudinal tubules to sites of Ca^{++} release in the terminal cisternae. Recent studies suggest that sarcalumenin increases Ca^{++} uptake by SERCA, at least in part by buffering luminal Ca^{++} near the pump.

Actin-Myosin Interaction: Cross-Bridge Formation

As noted, contraction of skeletal muscle requires an increase in intracellular $[Ca^{++}]$. Moreover, the process of contraction is regulated by the thin filament. As shown in Figure 12-11, contractile force (i.e., tension) increases in sigmoidal fashion as intracellular $[Ca^{++}]$ is elevated above 0.1 μM, with half-maximal force occurring at less than 1 μM Ca^{++}. The mechanism by which Ca^{++} promotes this increase in tension is as follows. Ca^{++} released from the SR binds to troponin C. Once bound with Ca^{++}, troponin C facilitates movement of the associated tropomyosin molecule toward the cleft of the actin filament. This movement of tropomyosin

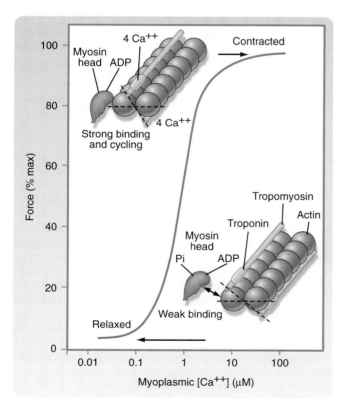

● **Figure 12-11.** The contractile force of skeletal muscle increases in a Ca^{++}-dependent manner as a result of binding of Ca^{++} to troponin C and the subsequent movement of tropomyosin away from myosin binding sites on the underlying actin molecules. See text for details. (Redrawn from Hartshorne DJ. In Lapedes DN, editor: Yearbook of Science and Technology, New York, 1976, McGraw-Hill.)

exposes the myosin binding site on the actin filament and allows a cross-bridge to form and thereby generate tension (see later). Troponin C has four Ca^{++} binding sites. Two of these sites have high affinity for Ca^{++} but also bind Mg^{++} at rest. These sites seem to be involved in controlling and enhancing the interaction between the troponin I and troponin T subunits. The other two

IN THE CLINIC

Genetic diseases causing disturbances in Ca^{++} homeostasis in skeletal muscle include **malignant hyperthermia (MH), central core disease (CCD),** and **Brody's disease (BD).** MH is an autosomal dominant trait that has life-threatening consequences in certain surgical instances. Anesthetics such as halothane or ether and the muscle relaxant succinylcholine can produce uncontrolled release of Ca^{++} from the SR, thereby resulting in skeletal muscle rigidity, tachycardia, hyperventilation, and hyperthermia. This condition is lethal if not treated immediately. There are currently a series of tests (using contractile responses of muscle biopsy specimens) to assess whether a patient has MH. The incidence of MH is approximately 1 in 15,000 children and 1 in 50,000 adults treated with anesthetics. MH is the result of a defect in the SR Ca^{++} release channel (RYR), which becomes activated in the presence of the aforementioned anesthetics and results in the release of Ca^{++} into the myoplasm and hence prolonged muscle contraction (rigidity). The defect in the RYR is not restricted to a single locus. In some cases MH has been linked to a defect in the DHPR of the T tubule.

CCD is a rare autosomal dominant trait that results in muscle weakness, loss of mitochondria in the core of skeletal muscle fibers, and some disintegration of contractile filaments. CCD is often closely associated with MH, so CCD patients are treated as though they are susceptible to MH in surgical situations. It is hypothesized that central cores devoid of mitochondria represent areas of elevated intracellular Ca^{++} secondary to a mutation in the RYR. The loss of mitochondria is thought to occur when they take up the elevated Ca^{++} leading to mitochondrial Ca^{++} overload.

BD is characterized by painless muscle cramping and impaired muscle relaxation during exercise. While running upstairs, for example, muscles may stiffen and temporarily cannot be used. This relaxation abnormality is seen in muscles of the legs, arms, and eyelid, with the response worsened in cold weather. BD can be either autosomal recessive or autosomal dominant and may involve mutations in up to three genes. BD, however, is a rare occurrence (affecting 1 in 10,000,000 births). It appears that BD results from decreased activity of the SERCA1 Ca^{++} pump found in fast-twitch skeletal muscle (see later). The decreased activity of SERCA1 has been associated with mutation in the SERCA1 gene, although there may also be an accessory factor that contributes to the decreased SR Ca^{++} uptake in the fast-twitch skeletal muscle of individuals with BD.

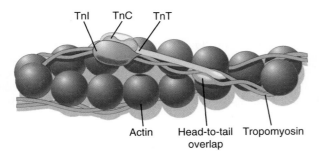

● **Figure 12-12.** Organization of the thin filament showing a double-helical array of tropomyosin on the actin filament, with sequential tropomyosin molecules arranged in a head-to-tail configuration. Such a configuration may promote the interaction of one tropomyosin unit with an adjacent tropomyosin. Also shown is the troponin complex consisting of its three subunits: troponin C (TnC), troponin I (TnI), and troponin T (TnT). See text for details. (From Gordon AM et al: Physiol Rev 80:853, 2000.)

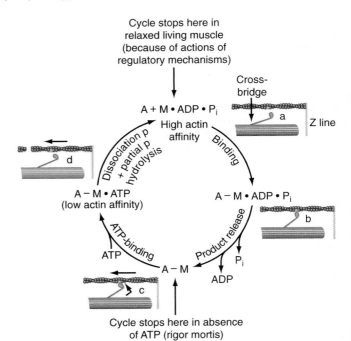

● **Figure 12-13.** Cross-bridge cycle. **State a,** In the relaxed state, ATP is partially hydrolyzed ($M \cdot ADP \cdot P_i$). **State b,** In the presence of elevated myoplasmic Ca^{++}, myosin binds to actin. **State c,** Hydrolysis of ATP is completed and causes a conformational change in the myosin molecule that pulls the actin filament toward the center of the sarcomere. **State d,** A new ATP binds to myosin and causes release of the cross-bridge. Partial hydrolysis of the newly bound ATP recocks the myosin head, which is now ready to bind again and again. If myoplasmic [Ca^{++}] is still elevated, the cycle repeats. If myoplasmic [Ca^{++}] is low, relaxation results.

binding sites have lower affinity and bind Ca^{++} as its concentration rises after release from the SR. Binding of myosin to the actin filaments appears to cause a further shift in tropomyosin. Although a given tropomyosin molecule extends over seven actin molecules, it is hypothesized that the strong binding of myosin to actin results in movement of an adjacent tropomyosin molecule, perhaps exposing myosin binding sites on as many as 14 actin molecules. This ability of one tropomyosin molecule to influence the movement of another may be a consequence of the close proximity of adjacent tropomyosin molecules (Fig. 12-12).

Cross-Bridge Cycling—Sarcomere Shortening

Once myosin and actin have bound, ATP-dependent conformational changes in the myosin molecule result in movement of the actin filaments toward the center of the sarcomere. Such movement shortens the length of the sarcomere and thereby contracts the muscle fiber. The mechanism by which myosin produces force and shortens the sarcomere is thought to involve four basic steps that are collectively termed the cross-bridge cycle (labeled *a* to *d* in Figure 12-13). In the resting state, myosin is thought to have partially hydrolyzed ATP (state *a*). When Ca^{++} is released from the terminal cisternae of the SR, it binds to troponin C, which in turn promotes movement of tropomyosin on the actin filament such that myosin binding sites on actin are exposed. This then allows the "energized" myosin head to bind to the underlying actin (state *b*). Myosin next undergoes a conformational change termed "ratchet action" that pulls the actin filament toward the center of the sarcomere (state *c*). Myosin releases ADP and P_i during the transition to state *c*. Binding of ATP to myosin decreases the affinity of myosin for actin, thereby resulting in the release of myosin from the actin filament (state *d*). Myosin then partially hydrolyzes the ATP, and part of the energy in the ATP is used to recock the head and return to the resting state. If intracellular [Ca^{++}] is still elevated,

myosin will undergo another cross-bridge cycle and produce further contraction of the muscle. The ratchet action of the cross-bridge is capable of moving the thin filament approximately 10 nm. The cycle continues until the SERCA pumps Ca^{++} back into the SR. As [Ca^{++}] falls, Ca^{++} dissociates from troponin C, and the troponin-tropomyosin complex moves and blocks the myosin binding sites on the actin filament. If the supply of ATP is exhausted, as occurs with death, the cycle stops in state "c" with the formation of permanent actin-myosin complexes (i.e., the rigor state). In this state the muscle is rigid and the condition is termed **"rigor mortis."**

As already noted, formation of the thick filaments involves the association of myosin molecules in a tail-to-tail configuration to produce a bipolar orientation (Fig. 12-6). Such a bipolar orientation allows myosin to pull the actin filaments toward the center of the sarcomere during the cross-bridge cycle. The myosin molecules are also oriented in a helical array in the thick filament such that cross-bridges extend toward each of the six thin filaments surrounding the thick filament (Fig. 12-3). These myosin projections/cross-bridges can be seen on electron micrographs of skeletal muscle (Fig. 12-14) and appear to extend perpendicular from the thick filaments at rest. In the

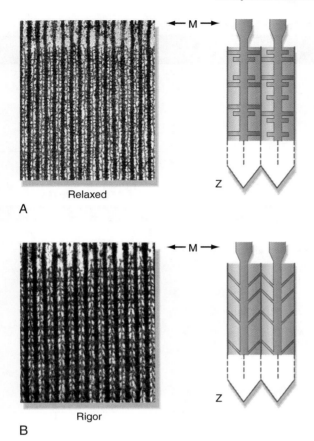

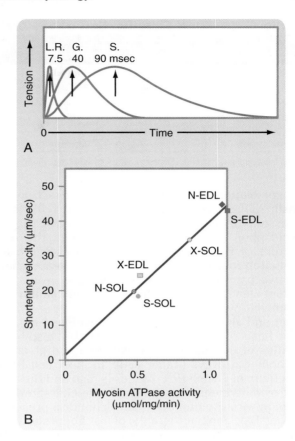

● **Figure 12-14.** Electron micrograph of skeletal muscle in the relaxed and contracted (rigor) states. The direction of the cross-bridges in the contracted state is consistent with a ratchet action of myosin, which pulls actin toward the center of the sarcomere. (Modified from Patton H et al: Textbook of Physiology. Philadelphia, Saunders, 1989.)

● **Figure 12-15.** **A,** Muscles vary in terms of the speed of contraction. G, gastrocnemius of the leg; LR, lateral rectus muscle of the eye; S, soleus muscle of the leg. **B,** The speed of shortening is correlated with myosin ATPase activity. (**A,** From Montcastle V [ed]: Medical Physiology, 12th ed. St. Louis, Mosby, 1974; **B,** from Barany M, Close RI: J Physiol 213:455, 1971.) N-SOL, normal soleus (slow twitch); N-EDL, normal extensor digitorum longus (fast twitch); S-EDL, self-innervated EDL (EDL motor nerve transected and resutured); S-SOL, self-innervated soleus (soleus motor nerve transected and resutured); X-EDL, cross innervated EDL (EDL innervated by soleus motor nerve); X-SOL, cross innervated SOL (soleus innervated by EDL motor nerve).

contracted state, the myosin cross-bridges slant toward the center of the sarcomere, consistent with the ratchet action of the myosin head.

The cross-bridge cycling mechanism just described is called the **sliding filament theory** because the myosin cross-bridge is pulling the actin thin filament toward the center of the sarcomere, thereby resulting in an apparent "sliding" of the thin filament past the thick filament. There is, however, uncertainty about how many myosin molecules contribute to the generation of force and whether both myosin heads in a given myosin molecule are involved. It has been calculated that there may be 600 myosin heads per thick filament, with a stoichiometry of 1 myosin head per 1.8 actin molecules. As a result of steric considerations, it is unlikely that all myosin heads can interact with actin, and calculations suggest that even during maximal force generation, only 20% to 40% of the myosin heads bind to actin.

The conversion of chemical energy (i.e., ATP) to mechanical energy by muscle is highly efficient. In isolated muscle preparations, maximum mechanical efficiency (≈65% efficiency) is obtained at a submaximal force of 30% maximal tension. In humans perform-

ing steady-state ergometer exercise, mechanical efficiencies range from 40% to 57%.

SKELETAL MUSCLE TYPES

Skeletal muscle can be classified as either **fast-twitch** (also called type IIA and type IIB) or **slow-twitch** (also called type I) muscle. As shown in Figure 12-15, the lateral rectus muscle of the eye contracts very quickly, with peak tension attained within 7.5 msec after stimulation. The gastrocnemius muscle of the leg, in contrast, requires 40 msec to develop peak tension. The soleus muscle of the leg requires even longer (≈90 msec) for peak tension to develop. Thus, the soleus muscle is classified as a slow-twitch muscle, whereas the lateral rectus muscle would be classified as a fast-twitch muscle. The gastrocnemius muscle contains a mixture of fast- and slow-twitch fibers and thus exhibits a weighted-average intermediate rate of tension development when the whole muscle is stimulated.

● **Table 12-1. Basic Classification of Skeletal Muscle Fiber Types**

	Type I: Slow Oxidative (Red)	Type IIB: Fast Glycolytic (White)	Type IIA*: Fast Oxidative (Red)
Myosin isoenzyme (ATPase rate)	Slow	Fast	Fast
Sarcoplasmic reticular Ca⁺⁺ pumping capacity	Moderate	High	High
Diameter (diffusion distance)	Moderate	Large	Small
Oxidative capacity: mitochondrial content, capillary density, myoglobin	High	Low	Very high
Glycolytic capacity	Moderate	High	High

*Comparatively infrequent in humans and other primates. In text, the simple designation of type II fiber refers to a fast glycolytic (type IIB) fiber.

A correlation between speed of contraction and myosin ATPase activity is also seen and reflects the expression of different myosin isoforms in the two muscle fiber types (Fig. 12-15). Although the basic structure of the myosin isoforms in fast-twitch and slow-twitch muscles is similar (i.e., two heavy chains with two pairs of light chains), they are products of different genes and thus have different amino acid sequences.

Fast and slow fibers can be distinguished not only on the basis of myosin ATPase activity but also by the activities of enzymes in the oxidative and glycolytic metabolic pathways (Table 12-1). In most fast fibers, the activity of glycolytic enzymes is high and the activity of oxidative enzymes is low. These characteristics correlate with the number of mitochondria present in the fiber. Electron micrographs of fast fibers show only a few mitochondria as compared with the large number seen in slow fibers. Fast fibers also have a much more extensive SR than slow fibers do. Typically, fast fibers and slow fibers are intermixed in most mammalian skeletal muscles.

Because of the dependence of fast fibers on glycolytic metabolism, they fatigue rapidly. Consequently, they are used only occasionally and for brief periods. In contrast, slow fibers meet their metabolic demands by oxidative phosphorylation. As a result, these muscles fatigue more slowly and are therefore used for more sustained activities (e.g., maintenance of posture). Some fast fibers have both high glycolytic and high oxidative capacity. Such fibers, called type IIA, are found in mammals but are uncommon in humans. The fibers that derive their energy primarily from oxidative phosphorylation (i.e., the slow type I fibers and the fast type IIA fibers) contain numerous mitochondria and high levels of the oxygen-binding protein **myoglobin.** Because myoglobin is red, these fibers are sometimes called **"red fibers."** Table 12-2 summarizes some of the differences in the motor units of fast and slow muscles.

In addition to the differences between fast and slow fibers just noted, other muscle proteins are also expressed in a fiber type–specific manner. Such proteins include SERCA, the three troponin subunits, tropomyosin, and C protein. The differential expression of SERCA isoforms (SERCA1 in fast-twitch muscle and SERCA2 in slow-twitch and cardiac muscle) contributes to the differences in the speed of relaxation between fast- and slow-twitch muscle. The activity of SERCA1 is greater than that of SERCA2. Therefore, Ca⁺⁺ reuptake

● **Table 12-2. Properties of Motor Units**

Characteristics	Motor Unit Classification	
	Type I	Type II
Properties of Nerve		
Cell diameter	Small	Large
Conduction velocity	Fast	Very fast
Excitability	High	Low
Properties of Muscle Cells		
Number of fibers	Few	Many
Fiber diameter	Moderate	Large
Force of unit	Low	High
Metabolic profile	Oxidative	Glycolytic
Contraction velocity	Moderate	Fast
Fatigability	Low	High

into the SR occurs more quickly in fast muscles, and as a result, these fibers have a faster relaxation time. The differential expression of troponin and tropomyosin isoforms influences the dependency of contraction on Ca⁺⁺. Slow fibers begin to develop tension at lower [Ca⁺⁺] than fast fibers do. This differential sensitivity to Ca⁺⁺ is related in part to the fact that the troponin C isoform in slow fibers has only a single low-affinity Ca⁺⁺ binding site, whereas the troponin C of fast fibers has two low-affinity binding sites. Changes in the dependence of contraction on Ca⁺⁺, however, are not restricted to differences in the troponin C isoforms. Differences in troponin T and tropomyosin isoforms are also found. Thus, regulation of the dependence of contraction on Ca⁺⁺ is complex and involves contributions from multiple proteins on the thin filament.

The activity pattern of a muscle is a major determinant of whether it adopts a fast-twitch or a slow-twitch phenotype. Thus, it is possible to convert a fast-twitch muscle to a slow-twitch muscle through cross-innervation or chronic electrical stimulation, as discussed later in this chapter. Ca⁺⁺-dependent activation of the phosphatase calcineurin and the transcription factor "nuclear factor from activated T cells" (NFAT) have been implicated in this transition.

MODULATION OF THE FORCE OF CONTRACTION
Recruitment

A simple means of increasing the force of contraction of a muscle is to recruit more muscle fibers. Because all the muscle fibers within a motor unit are activated simultaneously, one recruits more muscle fibers by recruiting more motor units. As already noted, muscle fibers can be classified as fast twitch or slow twitch. The type of fiber is determined by its innervation. Because all fibers in a motor unit are innervated by a single α motor neuron, all fibers within a motor unit are of the same type. Slow-twitch motor units tend to be small (100 to 500 muscle fibers) and are innervated by an α motor neuron that is easily excited. Fast-twitch motor units, by contrast, tend to be large (containing 1000 to 2000 muscle fibers) and are innervated by α motor neurons that are more difficult to excite. Thus, slow-twitch motor units tend to be recruited first. As more and more force is needed, fast-twitch motor units are recruited. The advantage of such a recruitment strategy is that the first muscle fibers recruited are those that have high resistance to fatigue. Moreover, the small size of slow-twitch motor units allows fine motor control at low levels of force. The process of increasing the force of contraction by recruiting additional motor units is termed **spatial summation** because one is "summing" forces from muscle fibers within a larger area of the muscle. This is in contrast to **temporal summation,** which is discussed later.

Tetany

Action potentials in skeletal muscles are quite uniform and lead to the release of a reproducible pulse of Ca^{++} from the SR (Fig. 12-16). A single action potential releases sufficient Ca^{++} to cause a twitch contraction. However, the duration of this contraction is very short because Ca^{++} is very rapidly pumped back into the SR. If the muscle is stimulated a second time before the muscle is fully relaxed, the force of contraction increases (middle panel of Fig. 12-16). Thus, twitch forces are amplified as stimulus frequency increases. At a high level of stimulation, intracellular $[Ca^{++}]$ increases and is maintained throughout the period of stimulation (right panel of Fig. 12-16), and the amount of force developed greatly exceeds that seen during a

twitch. The response is termed tetany. At intermediate stimulus frequency, intracellular $[Ca^{++}]$ returns to baseline just before the next stimulus. However, there is gradual rise in force (middle panel of Fig. 12-16). This phenomenon is termed incomplete tetany. In both cases, the increased frequency of stimulation is said to produce a fusion of twitches.

It is hypothesized that the low force generation during a twitch, as compared with that seen during tetany, is due to the presence of a series elastic component in the muscle. Specifically, when the muscle is stretched a small amount shortly after initiation of the action potential, the muscle generates a twitch force that approximates the maximal tetanic force. This result, coupled with the observation that the size of the intracellular Ca^{++} transient during a twitch contraction is comparable to that seen during tetany, suggests that enough Ca^{++} is released into the myoplasm during a twitch to allow the actin-myosin interactions to produce maximal tension. However, the duration of the intracellular Ca^{++} transient during a twitch is sufficiently short that the contractile elements may not have enough time to fully stretch the series elastic components in the fiber and muscle. As a result, the measured tension is submaximal. Increasing the duration of the intracellular Ca^{++} transient, as occurs with tetany, provides the muscle with sufficient time to completely stretch the series elastic component and thereby results in expression of the full contractile force of the actin-myosin interactions (i.e., maximal tension). Partial stretching of the series elastic component (as might be expected during a single twitch), followed by restimulation of the muscle before complete relaxation, on the other hand, would be expected to yield an intermediate level of tension, similar to that seen with incomplete tetany. The location of the series elastic component in skeletal muscle is not known. One potential source is the myosin molecule itself. In addition, it is likely that there are other sources of the series elastic component, such as the connective tissue and titin.

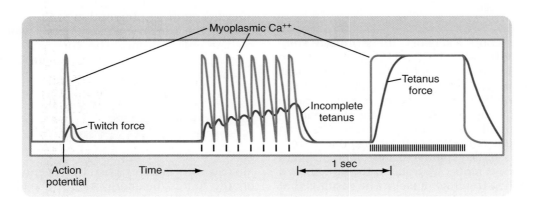

● **Figure 12-16.** Increasing the frequency of electrical stimulation of skeletal muscle results in an increase in the force of contraction. This is attributable to prolongation of the intracellular Ca^{++} transient and is termed tetany. Incomplete tetany results from initiation of another intracellular Ca^{++} transient before the muscle has completely relaxed. Thus, there is a summation of twitch forces. See text for details.

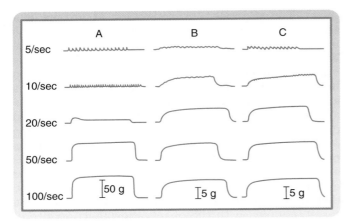

● **Figure 12-17.** Slow-twitch muscles tetanize at a lower stimulation frequency than that required for fast-twitch muscles. **A,** Fast-twitch motor unit in the gastrocnemius muscle. **B,** Slow-twitch motor unit in the gastrocnemius muscle. **C,** Slow-twitch muscle unit in the soleus muscle. The motor units were stimulated at the frequencies indicated on the left. The tension (in grams) generated during concentration is indicated by the vertical arrows. Note the large force generated by the fast-twitch motor unit **(A)**. (From Montcastle V [ed]: Medical Physiology, 12th ed. St. Louis, Mosby, 1974.)

The stimulus frequency needed to produce tetany depends on whether the motor unit consists of slow or fast fibers (Fig. 12-17). Slow fibers can be tetanized at lower frequencies than is the case with fast fibers. The ability of slow-twitch muscle to tetanize at lower stimulation frequencies reflects, at least in part, the longer duration of contraction seen in slow fibers. As also illustrated in Figure 12-17, fast fibers develop a larger maximal force than slow fibers do because fast fibers are larger in diameter than slow fibers and there are more fibers in fast motor units than in slow motor units.

MODULATION OF FORCE BY REFLEX ARCS

Stretch Reflex

Skeletal muscles contain sensory fibers (**muscle spindles**—also called **intrafusal fibers**) that run parallel to the skeletal muscle fibers. The muscle spindles assess the degree of stretch of the muscle, as well as the speed of contraction. In the stretch reflex, rapid stretching of the muscle (e.g., tapping the tendon) lengthens the spindles in the muscle and results in an increased frequency of action potentials in the afferent sensory neurons of the spindle. These afferent fibers in turn excite the α motor neurons in the spinal cord that innervate the stretched muscle. The result is that the reflex arc is a stretch-induced contraction of the muscle that does not require input from high centers in the brain. It should be noted that as the muscle shortens, efferent output to the spindle also occurs, thereby taking the slack out of the spindle and ensuring its ability to respond to stretch at all muscle

lengths. By their action, muscle spindles provide feedback to the muscle in terms of its length and thus help maintain a joint at a given angle.

Golgi Tendon Organ

Golgi tendon organs are located in the tendons of muscles and provide feedback regarding contraction of the muscle. The main component of the tendon organ is an elongated fascicle of collagen bundles that is in series with the muscle fibers and can respond to contractions of individual muscle fibers. A given tendon organ may attach to several fast-twitch or slow-twitch muscle fibers (or both) and sends impulses through Ib afferent nerve fibers in response to muscle contraction. The Ib afferent impulses enter the spinal cord, which can promote inhibition of α motor neurons to the contracting (and synergistic) muscles while promoting excitation of α motor neurons to antagonistic muscles. The inhibitory actions are mediated through interneurons in the cord that release an inhibitory transmitter to the α motor neuron and create an inhibitory postsynaptic potential (IPSP). The Ib afferent impulses are also sent to higher centers (including the motor cortex and cerebellum). It is hypothesized that feedback from the tendon organs in response to muscle contraction may smooth the progression of muscle contraction by limiting the recruitment of additional motor units. Interestingly, the response of the tendon organ is not linearly related to force but rather drops off at higher levels of force, which may facilitate the recruitment of motor units at higher levels of effort.

SKELETAL MUSCLE TONE

The skeletal system supports the body in an erect posture with the expenditure of relatively little energy. Nonetheless, even at rest, muscles normally exhibit some level of contractile activity. Isolated (i.e., denervated) unstimulated muscles are in a relaxed state and are said to be flaccid. However, relaxed muscles in the body are comparatively firm. This firmness, or tone, is caused by low levels of contractile activity in some of the motor units and is driven by reflex arcs from the muscle spindles. Interruption of the reflex arc by sectioning the sensory afferent fibers will abolish this resting muscle tone. The tone in skeletal muscle is distinct from the "tone" in smooth muscle (see Chapter 14).

ENERGY SOURCES DURING CONTRACTION

ATP

Muscle cells convert chemical energy to mechanical energy. ATP is the energy source used for this conversion. The ATP pool in skeletal muscle is small and capable of supporting only a few contractions if not replenished. This pool, however, is continually replenished during contraction, as described later, such that even when the muscle fatigues, ATP stores are only modestly decreased.

Creatine Phosphate

Muscle cells contain creatine phosphate, which is used to convert ADP to ATP and thus replenish the ATP store during muscle contraction. The creatine phosphate store represents the immediate high-energy source for replenishing the ATP supply in skeletal muscle, especially during intense exercise. The enzyme **creatine phosphokinase (CPK)** catalyzes the reaction

$$ADP + Creatine\ phosphate \rightarrow ATP + Creatine$$

Although much of the CPK is present in the myoplasm, a small amount is located in the thick filament (near the M line). The CPK in the thick filament may participate in the rapid resynthesis of ATP near the myosin heads during muscle contraction. The phosphate store created, however, is only about five times the size of the ATP store and thus cannot support prolonged periods of contraction (less than a minute of maximal muscle activity). Skeletal muscle fatigue during intense exercise is associated with depletion of the creatine phosphate store, although as described subsequently, this does not necessarily imply that the fatigue is caused by depletion of the creatine phosphate store. Because the CPK-catalyzed reaction shown above is reversible, the muscle cell replenishes the creatine phosphate pool during recovery from fatigue by using ATP synthesized through oxidative phosphorylation.

Carbohydrates

Muscle cells contain glycogen, which can be metabolized during muscle contraction to provide glucose for oxidative phosphorylation and glycolysis, both of which will generate ATP to replenish the ATP store. Muscle cells can also take up glucose from blood, a process that is stimulated by insulin (see Chapter 38). The cytosolic enzyme phosphorylase releases glucose 1-phosphate residues from glycogen, which are then metabolized by a combination of glycolysis (in the cytosol) and oxidative phosphorylation (in the mitochondria) to yield the equivalent of 37 mol of ATP per mole of glucose 1-phosphate. Blood glucose yields 36 mol of ATP per mole of glucose because 1 ATP is used to phosphorylate glucose at the start of glycolysis. These ATP yields, however, are dependent on an adequate oxygen supply. Under anaerobic conditions, by contrast, metabolism of glycogen and glucose yields only 3 and 2 mol of ATP per mole of glucose 1-phosphate and glucose, respectively (along with 2 mol of lactate). As discussed later, muscle fatigue during prolonged exercise is associated with depletion of glycogen stores in the muscle.

Fatty Acids and Triglycerides

Fatty acids represent an important source of energy for muscle cells during prolonged exercise. Muscle cells contain fatty acids but can also take up fatty acids from blood. In addition, muscle cells can store triglycerides, which can be hydrolyzed when needed to produce fatty acids. The fatty acids are subjected to β oxidation within the mitochondria. For fatty acids to enter the mitochondria, however, they are converted to acyl-carnitine in the cytosol and then transported into the mitochondria, where they are converted to acyl-coenzyme A (CoA). Within the mitochondria, the acyl-CoA is subjected to β oxidation and yields acetyl-CoA, which then enters the citric acid cycle and ultimately produces ATP.

OXYGEN DEBT

If the energy demands of exercise cannot be met by oxidative phosphorylation, an **oxygen debt** is incurred. After completion of exercise, respiration remains above the resting level in order to "repay" this oxygen debt. The extra oxygen consumption during this recovery phase is used to restore metabolite levels (such as creatine phosphate and ATP) and to metabolize the lactate generated by glycolysis. The increased cardiac and respiratory work during recovery also contributes to the increased oxygen consumption seen at this time and explains why more O_2 has to be "repaid" than was "borrowed." Some oxygen debt occurs even with low levels of exercise because slow oxidative motor units consume considerable ATP, derived from creatine phosphate or glycolysis, before oxidative metabolism can increase ATP production to meet steady-state requirements. The oxygen debt is much greater with strenuous exercise, when fast glycolytic motor units are used (Fig. 12-18). The oxygen debt is approximately

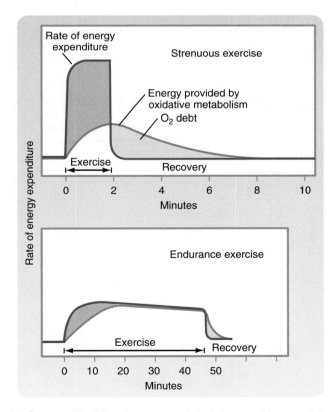

● **Figure 12-18.** An oxygen debt is incurred by exercising muscle when the rate of energy expenditure exceeds the rate of energy production by oxidative metabolism. Both strenuous **(upper panel)** and endurance exercise **(lower panel)** is shown. See text for details.

equal to the energy consumed during exercise minus that supplied by oxidative metabolism (i.e., the dark- and light-colored areas in Fig. 12-18 are roughly equal). As indicated earlier, the additional oxygen used during recovery from exercise represents the energy requirements for restoring normal cellular metabolite levels.

FATIGUE

The ability of muscle to meet energy needs is a major determinant of the duration of the exercise. However, fatigue is not the result of depletion of energy stores. Instead, metabolic byproducts seem to be important factors in the onset of fatigue. Fatigue may potentially occur at any of the points involved in muscle contraction, from the brain to the muscle cells, as well as in the cardiovascular and respiratory systems that maintain energy supplies (i.e., fatty acids and glucose) and O_2 delivery to the exercising muscle.

Several factors have been implicated in **muscle fatigue.** During brief periods of tetany the oxygen supply to the muscle is adequate as long as the circulation is intact. However, the force/stress generated during these brief tetanic periods decays rapidly to a level that can be maintained for long periods (Fig. 12-19). This decay represents the rapid and almost total failure of the fast motor units. The decline in force/stress is paralleled by depletion of glycogen and creatine phosphate stores and accumulation of lactic acid. Importantly, the decline in force/stress occurs when the ATP pool is not greatly reduced, so the muscle fibers do not go into rigor. In contrast, the slow motor units are able to meet the energy demands of

fibers under this condition, and they do not exhibit significant fatigue, even after many hours. Evidently, some factor associated with energy metabolism can inhibit contraction (e.g., in the fast fibers), but this factor has not been clearly identified.

During intense exercise, accumulation of P_i and lactic acid in the myoplasm accounts for muscle fatigue. The accumulation of lactic acid, to levels as high as 15 to 26 mM, decreases myoplasmic pH (from ≈7 to ≈6.2) and inhibits actin-myosin interactions. This decrease in pH reduces the sensitivity of the actin-myosin interaction to Ca^{++} by altering Ca^{++} binding to troponin C and by decreasing the maximum number of actin-myosin interactions. Fast-twitch fibers appear to be slightly more sensitive than slow-twitch muscle fibers to the effects of pH. P_i has also been implicated as an important factor in the development of fatigue during intense exercise inasmuch as phosphate concentrations can increase from around 2 mM at rest to nearly 40 mM in working muscle. Such an elevation in $[P_i]$ can reduce tension by at least the following three different mechanisms: (1) inhibition of Ca^{++} release from the SR, (2) decrease in the sensitivity of contraction to Ca^{++}, and (3) alteration in actin-myosin binding. A number of other factors, including glycogen depletion from a specialized compartment, a localized increase in [ADP], intracellular elevation of $[K^+]$, and generation of oxygen free radicals, have also been implicated in various forms of exercise-induced muscle fatigue. Finally, the central nervous system contributes to fatigue, especially the manner in which fatigue is perceived by the individual (see later).

Regardless of whether the muscle is fatigued as a consequence of high-intensity exercise or prolonged exercise, the myoplasmic ATP level does not decrease substantially. Given the reliance of all cells on the availability of ATP to maintain viability, fatigue has been described as a protective mechanism to minimize the risk of muscle cell injury or death. Consequently, it is likely that skeletal muscle cells have developed redundant systems to ensure that ATP levels do not drop to dangerously low levels and hence risk the viability of the cell.

Most persons tire and cease exercise long before the motor unit fatigues. General physical fatigue may be defined as a homeostatic disturbance produced by work. The basis for the perceived discomfort (or even pain) probably involves many factors. These factors may include a decrease in plasma glucose levels and accumulation of metabolites. Motor system function in the central nervous system is not impaired. Highly motivated and trained athletes can withstand the discomfort of fatigue and will exercise to the point at which some motor unit fatigue occurs. Part of the enhanced performance observed after training involves motivational factors.

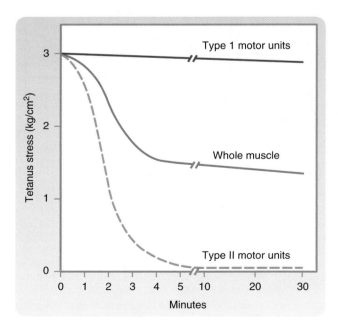

● **Figure 12-19.** A series of brief tetanic stimulations of skeletal muscle result in a rapid decrease in force (tetanic stress; "Whole muscle" in plot) that is attributable to fatigue of fast-twitch (type II) motor units in the muscle. Under these conditions, however, slow-twitch (type I) motor units are fatigue resistant.

GROWTH AND DEVELOPMENT

Skeletal muscle fibers differentiate before they are innervated, and some neuromuscular junctions are formed well after birth. Before innervation, the muscle fibers physiologically resemble slow (type I) cells. **Acetylcholine receptors** are distributed throughout the sarcolemma of these uninnervated cells and are supersensitive to that neurotransmitter. An end plate is formed when the first growing nerve terminal establishes contact with a muscle cell. The cell forms no further association with nerves, and receptors to acetylcholine become concentrated in the end plate membranes. Cells innervated by a small motor neuron form slow (type I) oxidative motor units. Fibers innervated by large motor nerves develop all the characteristics of fast (type II) motor units. Innervation produces major cellular changes, including synthesis of the fast and slow myosin isoforms, which replace embryonic or neonatal variants. Thus, muscle fiber type is determined by the nerves that innervate the fiber.

An increase in muscle strength and size occurs during maturation. As the skeleton grows, the muscle cells lengthen. Lengthening is accomplished by the formation of additional sarcomeres at the ends of the

muscle cells (Fig. 12-20), a process that is reversible. For example, the length of a cell decreases when terminal sarcomeres are eliminated, which can occur when a limb is immobilized with the muscle in a shortened position or when an improperly set fracture leads to a shortened limb segment. Changes in muscle length affect the velocity and extent of shortening but do not influence the amount of force that can be generated by the muscle. The gradual increase in strength and diameter of a muscle during growth is achieved mainly by hypertrophy. Doubling the myofibrillar diameter by adding more sarcomeres in parallel (**hypertrophy,** for example) may double the amount of force generated but has no effect on the maximal velocity of shortening.

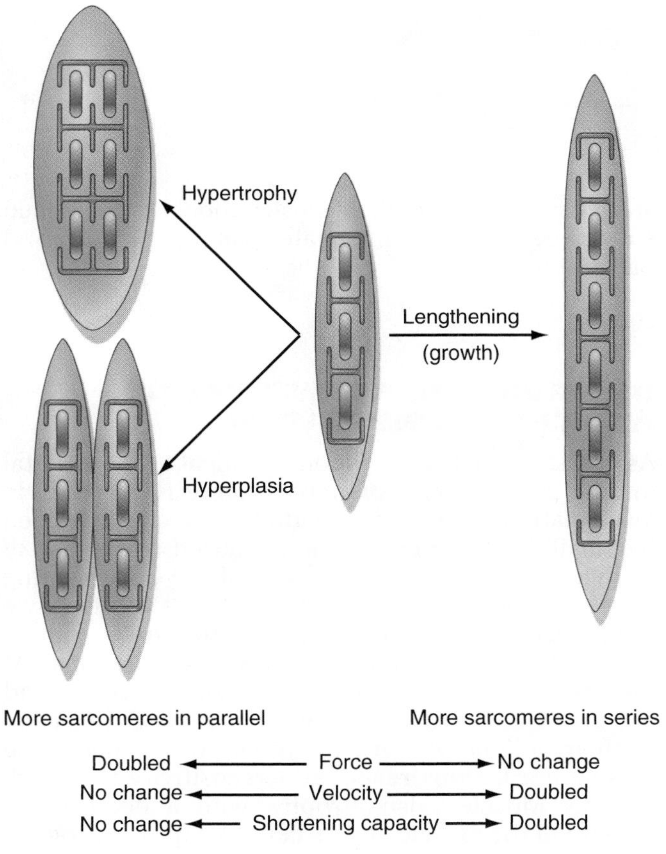

Skeletal muscles have a limited ability to form new fibers (**hyperplasia).** These new fibers result from differentiation of satellite cells that are present in the tissues. However, major cellular destruction leads to replacement by scar tissue.

Muscles must not only be used to maintain normal growth and development but must also experience a load. Muscles immobilized in a cast lose mass. In addition, space flight exposes astronauts to a microgravity environment that mechanically unloads their muscles. Such unloading leads to rapid loss of muscle mass (i.e., **atrophy**) and weakness. Atrophy appears to involve both inhibition of protein synthesis and stimulation of protein degradation.

Muscles that frequently contract to support the body typically have a high number of slow (type I) oxidative motor units. These slow motor units atrophy more rapidly than the fast (type II) motor units during prolonged periods of unloading. This atrophy of slow motor units is associated with a decrease in maximal tetanic force, but an increase in maximal shortening velocity. The increase in velocity is correlated with expression of the fast myosin isoform in these fibers. An important aspect of space medicine is the design of exercise programs that minimize such phenotypic changes during prolonged space flight.

Testosterone is a major factor responsible for the greater muscle mass in males because it has myotrophic action as well as androgenic (masculinization) effects (see Chapter 43). A variety of synthetic molecules, called anabolic steroids, have been designed to enhance muscle growth while minimizing their androgenic action. These drugs are widely used by bodybuilders and athletes in sports in which strength is important. The doses are typically 10- to 50-fold greater than might be prescribed therapeutically for individuals with impaired hormone production. Unfortunately, none of these compounds lack androgenic effects. Hence, at the doses used, they induce serious hormone disturbances, including depressed testosterone production. A major issue is whether these drugs do in fact increase muscle and athletic performance in individuals with normal circulating levels of testosterone. After some 4 decades of use, the scientific facts remain uncertain, and most experimental studies in animals have not documented any significant effects on muscle development. Reports in humans remain

● **Figure 12-20.** Effects of growth on the mechanical output of a muscle cell. Typically, skeletal muscle cell growth involves either lengthening (adding more sarcomeres to the ends of the muscle fibers) or increasing muscle fiber diameter (hypertrophy as a result of the addition of more myofilaments/myofibrils in parallel within the muscle fiber). The formation of new muscle fibers is called hyperplasia, and it is infrequent in skeletal muscle.

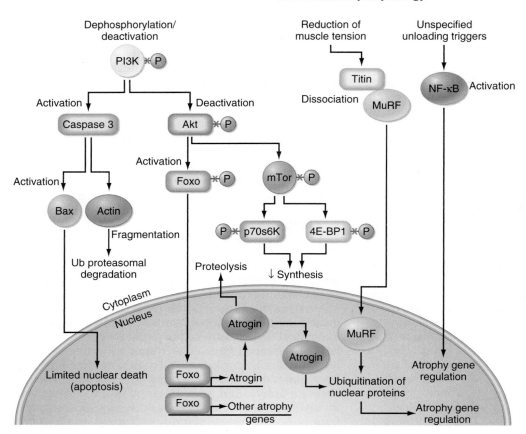

● **Figure 12-21.** Molecular signaling pathways contributing to atrophy of skeletal muscle. A decrease in activity of the PI3K/Akt pathway has been implicated in a variety of muscular atrophies and results in stimulation of proteolysis (through activation of the protease caspase 3 and expression of atrophy genes such as the ubiquitin ligase atrogin), decreased protein synthesis (through activation of an inhibitor of translation, 4E-BP1), and limited nuclear death (apoptosis). Decreased contractile activity also results in release of the ubiquitin ligase MuRF2 from titin and activation of the transcription factor NF-κB, both of which contribute to gene regulation of atrophy. (From Kandarian SC, Jackman RW: Muscle Nerve 33:155-165, 2006.)

● AT THE CELLULAR LEVEL

One factor thought to contribute to the decreased protein synthesis and increased protein degradation during periods of mechanical inactivity is the release of a **ubiquitin ligase (MuRF2)** from titin (Fig. 12-21). Specifically, MuRF2 inhibits transcription by exporting a transcription factor **(serum response factor [SRF])** from the nucleus into the myoplasm. MuRF2 also promotes protein degradation through ubiquitination (see Chapter 1). In addition to the actions of MuRF2, atrophy is also thought to involve inhibition of a **phosphatidylinositol-3-kinase (PI3K)** signaling cascade. Inhibition of PI3K and the serine/threonine kinase Akt appears to contribute to the decrease in protein synthesis by inhibiting eukaryotic translation initiation factor 4E. Decreased activity of PI3K can also stimulate proteolysis through activation of **caspase 3** or through ubiquitination (or both). The increased ubiquitination is thought to result from increased expression of a ubiquitin ligase **(atrogin)** and would complement the increased ubiquitination resulting from release of the ubiquitin ligase MuRF2 from titin, as described earlier.

controversial. Proponents claim increases in strength that provide the edge in world-class performance. Critics argue that these increases are largely placebo effects associated with expectations and motivational factors. The public debate on abuse of anabolic steroids has led to their designation as controlled substances, along with opiates, amphetamines, and barbiturates.

DENERVATION, REINNERVATION, AND CROSS-INNERVATION

As already noted, innervation is critical to the skeletal muscle phenotype. If the motor nerve is cut, muscle fasciculation occurs. **Fasciculation** is characterized by small, irregular contractions caused by release of acetylcholine from the terminals of the degenerating distal portion of the axon. Several days after denervation, muscle fibrillation begins. **Fibrillation** is characterized by spontaneous, repetitive contractions. At this time, the cholinergic receptors have spread out over the entire cell membrane, in effect reverting to their preinnervation embryonic arrangement. The muscle fibrillations reflect supersensitivity to acetylcholine. Muscles also atrophy, with a decrease in the size of the muscle and its cells. Atrophy is progressive in humans, with degeneration of some cells 3 or 4 months after denervation. Most of the muscle fibers are replaced by fat and connective tissue after 1 to 2 years. These changes can be reversed if reinnervation occurs within a few months. Reinnervation is normally achieved by growth of the peripheral stump of motor nerve axons along the old nerve sheath.

Reinnervation of formerly fast (type II) fibers by a small motor axon causes that cell to redifferentiate into a slow (type I) fiber, and vice versa. This suggests that large and small motor nerves differ qualitatively and that the nerves have specific "trophic" effects on the muscle fibers. This "trophic" effect reflects the rate of fiber stimulation. For example, stimulation via electrodes implanted in the muscle can lessen denervation atrophy. More strikingly, chronic low-frequency stimulation of fast motor units causes these units to be converted to slow units. Some conversion toward a typical fast-fiber phenotype can occur when the frequency of contraction in slow units is greatly decreased by reducing the excitatory input. Excitatory input can be reduced by sectioning the appropriate spinal or dorsal root or by severing the tendon, which functionally inactivates peripheral mechanoreceptors.

The frequency of contraction determines fiber development and phenotype through changes in gene expression and protein synthesis. Fibers that undergo frequent contractile activity form many mitochondria and synthesize the slow isoform of myosin. Fibers innervated by large, less excitable axons contract infrequently. Such relatively inactive fibers typically form few mitochondria and have large concentrations of glycolytic enzymes. The fast isoform of myosin is synthesized in such cells.

Intracellular [Ca^{++}] appears to play an important role in expression of the slow myosin isoform. Slow-twitch muscle fibers have a higher resting level of intracellular Ca^{++} than fast-twitch muscle does. In addition, chronic electrical stimulation of fast-twitch muscle is accompanied by a 2.5-fold increase in resting myoplasmic [Ca^{++}] that precedes the increased expression of slow-twitch myosin and decreased expression of fast-twitch myosin. Similarly, chronic elevation of

intracellular Ca^{++} (approximately fivefold) in muscle cells expressing fast-twitch myosin induces a change in gene expression from the fast muscle myosin isoform to the slow myosin isoform within 8 days. An increase in citrate synthetase activity (an indicator of oxidative

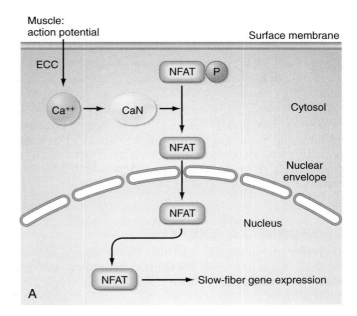

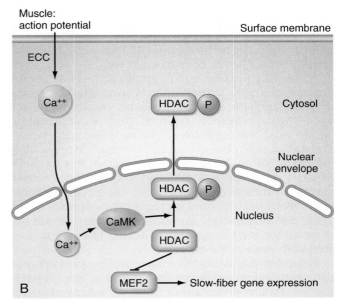

● **Figure 12-22.** Molecular signaling pathways contributing to the transition from fast-twitch muscle to slow-twitch muscle. Chronic electrical stimulation of a fast-twitch muscle in a pattern consistent with a slow-twitch muscle results in development of the slow-twitch muscle phenotype because of dephosphorylation of the transcription factor NFAT by the Ca^{++}-calmodulin–dependent protein phosphatase calcineurin (CaN); this in turn results in nuclear translocation of NFAT and expression of slow-twitch muscle fiber genes **(A).** Activation of the transcription factor MEF2 also appears to contribute to this fiber type transition **(B),** with activation of MEF2 involving Ca^{++}-calmodulin–dependent phosphorylation of an inhibitor (histone deacetylase [HDAC]). (From Liu Y et al: J Muscle Res Cell Motil 26:13-21, 2005.)

● AT THE CELLULAR LEVEL

The transcription factor **nuclear factor from activated T cells (NFAT)** has been implicated in this transition from fast-twitch to slow-twitch muscle (Fig. 12-22, *A*). Specifically, it appears that stimulation of adult fast-twitch muscle cells at a frequency consistent with slow-twitch muscle cells can activate the Ca^{++}-dependent phosphatase calcineurin, which in turn can dephosphorylate NFAT and result in translocation of NFAT from the myoplasm to the nucleus, followed by the transcription of slow-twitch muscle genes (and inhibition of fast-twitch muscle genes). Consistent with this mechanism, expression of constitutively active NFAT in fast-twitch muscle promotes the expression of slow-twitch myosin while inhibiting the expression of fast-twitch myosin. The transcription factor **myocyte enhancing factor 2 (MEF2)** has also been implicated in this transition from fast-twitch to slow-twitch muscle (Fig. 12-22, *B*). Activation of MEF2 is thought to result from Ca^{++}-calmodulin–dependent phosphorylation of an inhibitor of MEF2 (viz., histone deacetylase [HDAC]).

● **Table 12-3.** **Effects of Exercise**

Type of Training	Example	Major Adaptive Response
Learning/coordination skills	Typing	Increased rate and accuracy of motor units (central nervous system)
Endurance (submaximal, sustained efforts)	Marathon running	Increased oxidative capacity in all involved motor units with limited cellular hypertrophy
Strength (brief, maximal efforts)	Weightlifting	Hypertrophy and enhanced glycolytic capacity of the motor units used

capacity) and a decrease in lactate dehydrogenase activity (an indicator of glycolytic capacity) accompany this Ca^{++}-dependent transition from fast-twitch to slow-twitch myosin. These Ca^{++}-dependent changes are reversible by lowering intracellular $[Ca^{++}]$.

RESPONSE TO EXERCISE

Exercise physiologists identify three categories of training regimens and responses: **learning, endurance,** and **strength training** (Table 12-3). Typically, most athletic endeavors involve elements of all three. The learning aspect of training involves motivational factors, as well as neuromuscular coordination. This aspect of training does not involve adaptive changes in the muscle fibers per se. However, motor skills can persist for years without regular training, unlike the responses of muscle cells to exercise.

All healthy persons can maintain some level of continuous muscular activity that is supported by oxidative metabolism. This level can be greatly increased by a regular exercise regimen that is sufficient to induce adaptive responses. The adaptive response of skeletal muscle fibers to endurance exercise is mainly the result of an increase in the oxidative metabolic capacity of the motor units involved. This demand places an increased load on the cardiovascular and respiratory systems and increases the capacity of the heart and respiratory muscles. The latter effects are responsible for the principal health benefits associated with endurance exercise.

Muscle strength can be increased by regular massive efforts that involve most motor units. Such efforts recruit fast glycolytic motor units, as well as slow oxidative motor units. During these efforts, blood supply to the working muscles may be interrupted as tissue pressures rise above intravascular pressure. The reduced blood flow limits the duration of the contraction. Regular maximal-strength exercise, such as weightlifting, induces the synthesis of more myofibrils and hence hypertrophy of the active muscle cells. The increased stress also induces the growth of tendons and bones.

Endurance exercise does not cause fast motor units to become slow, nor does maximal muscular effort produce a shift from slow to fast motor units. Thus, any practical exercise regimen, when superimposed on normal daily activities, probably does not alter muscle fiber phenotype.

DELAYED-ONSET MUSCLE SORENESS

Activities such as hiking or, in particular, downhill running, in which contracting muscles are stretched and lengthened too vigorously, are followed by more pain and stiffness than after comparable exercise that does not involve vigorous muscle stretching and lengthening (e.g., cycling). The resultant dull, aching pain develops slowly and reaches its peak within 24 to 48 hours. The pain is associated with reduced range of motion, stiffness, and weakness of the affected muscles. The prime factors that cause the pain are swelling and inflammation from injury to muscle cells, most commonly near the myotendinous junction. Fast type II motor units are affected more than type I motor units because the maximal force is highest in large cells, where the loads imposed are some 60% greater than the maximal force that the cells can develop. Recovery is slow and depends on regeneration of the injured sarcomeres.

BIOPHYSICAL PROPERTIES OF SKELETAL MUSCLE

The molecular mechanisms of muscle contraction described earlier underlie and are responsible for the biophysical properties of muscle. Historically, these biophysical properties were well described before elucidation of the molecular mechanisms of contraction. They remain important ways of describing muscle function.

Length-Tension Relationship

When muscles contract, they generate force (often measured as tension or stress) and decrease in length. When studying the biophysical properties of muscle, one of these parameters is usually held constant while the other is measured after an experimental maneuver. Accordingly, an **isometric contraction** is one in which muscle length is held constant, and the force generated during the contraction is then measured. An **isotonic contraction** is one in which the force (or tone) is held constant, and the change in length of the muscle is then measured.

When a muscle at rest is stretched, it resists stretch by a force that increases slowly at first and then more rapidly as the extent of stretch increases (Fig. 12-23). This purely passive property is due to the elastic tissue in the muscle. If the muscle is stimulated to contract at these various lengths, a different relationship is obtained. Specifically, contractile force increases as muscle length is increased up to a point (designated L_0 to indicate optimal length). As the muscle is stretched beyond L_0, contractile force decreases. This length-tension curve is consistent with the sliding filament theory. At a very long sarcomere length (3.7 μm), actin filaments no longer overlap with myosin fila-

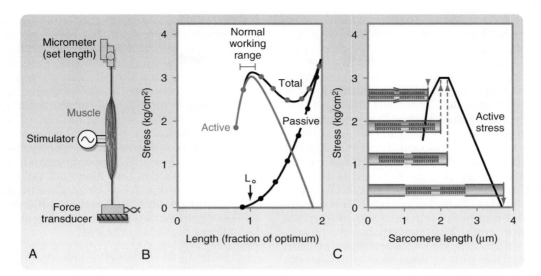

● **Figure 12-23.** Length-tension relationship in skeletal muscle. **A,** Experimental setup in which maximal isometric tetanic tension is measured at various muscle lengths. **B,** How active tension was calculated at various muscle lengths (i.e., by subtracting passive tension from total tension at each muscle length). **C,** Plot of active tension as a function of muscle length, with the predicted overlap of thick and thin filaments at selected points.

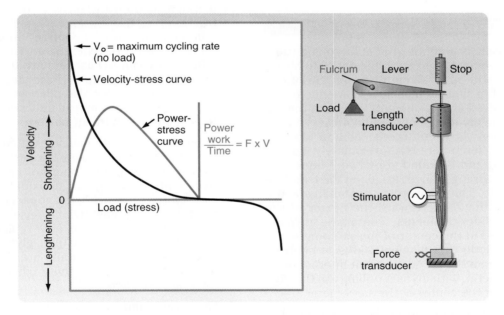

● **Figure 12-24.** Force-velocity relationship of skeletal muscle. The experimental setup is shown on the right. The initial muscle length was kept constant, but the amount of weight that the muscle had to lift during tetanic stimulation varied. Muscle-shortening velocity while lifting these various amounts of weight was measured. See text for details.

ments, so there is no contraction. As muscle length is decreased toward L_0, the amount of overlap increases, and contractile force progressively increases. As sarcomere length decreases below 2 μm, the thin filaments collide in the middle of the sarcomere, and the actin-myosin interaction is disturbed and hence contractile force decreases. Note that for construction of the length-tension curves, muscles were maintained at a given length, and then contractile force was mea-

sured (i.e., isometric contraction). Thus, the length-tension relationship supports the sliding filament theory of muscle contraction described previously.

Force-Velocity Relationship

The velocity at which a muscle shortens is strongly dependent on the amount of force that the muscle must develop (Fig. 12-24). In the absence of any load, the shortening velocity of the muscle is maximal (denoted as V_0). V_0 corresponds to the maximal cycling rate of the cross-bridges (i.e., it is proportional to the maximal rate of energy turnover [ATPase activity] by myosin). Thus, V_0 for fast-twitch muscle is higher than that for slow-twitch muscle. Increasing the load decreases the velocity of muscle shortening until, at maximal load, the muscle cannot lift the load and hence cannot shorten (zero velocity). Further increases in load result in stretching the muscle (negative velocity). The maximal isometric tension (i.e., force at which shortening velocity is zero) is proportional to the number of active cross-bridges between actin and myosin, and it is usually greater for fast-twitch motor units (given the larger diameter of fast-twitch muscle fibers and greater number of muscle fibers in a typical fast-twitch motor unit). The curve labeled "power-stress curve" reflects the rate of work done at each load and shows that the maximal rate of work was done at a submaximal load (viz., when the force of contraction was approximately 30% of the maximal tetanic tension). The latter curve was calculated simply by multiplying the x and y coordinates and then plotting the product as a function of the x coordinate.

■ KEY CONCEPTS

1. Skeletal muscle is composed of numerous muscle cells (muscle fibers) that are typically 10 to 80 μm in diameter and up to 25 cm in length. Striations are apparent in skeletal muscle and are due to the highly organized arrangement of thick and thin filaments in the myofibrils of skeletal muscle fibers. The sarcomere is a contractile unit in skeletal muscle. Each sarcomere is approximately 2 μm in length at rest and is bounded by two Z lines. Sarcomeres are arranged in series along the length of the myofibril. Thin filaments, containing actin, extend from the Z line toward the center of the sarcomere. Thick filaments, containing myosin, are positioned in the center of the sarcomere and overlap the actin thin filaments. Muscle contraction results from the Ca^{++}-dependent interaction of myosin and actin, with myosin pulling the thin filaments toward the center of the sarcomere.

2. Contraction of skeletal muscle is under control of the central nervous system (i.e., voluntary). Motor centers in the brain control the activity of α motor neurons in the ventral horns of the spinal cord. These α motor neurons, in turn, synapse on skeletal muscle fibers. Although each skeletal muscle fiber is innervated by only one motor neuron, a motor neuron innervates several muscle fibers within the muscle. A motor unit refers to all the muscle fibers innervated by a single motor neuron.

3. The motor neuron initiates contraction of skeletal muscle by producing an action potential in the muscle fiber. As the action potential passes down the T tubules of the muscle fiber, dihydropyridine receptors (DHPRs) in the T tubules undergo conformational changes that result in the opening of neighboring SR Ca^{++} channels called ryanodine receptors (RYRs), which then release Ca^{++} to the myoplasm from the SR. The increase in myoplasmic Ca^{++} promotes muscle contraction by exposing myosin binding sites on the actin thin filaments (a process that involves binding of Ca^{++} to troponin C, followed by movement of tropomyosin toward the groove in the thin filament). Myosin cross-bridges then appear to undergo a ratchet action, with the thin filaments pulled toward the center of the sarcomere and contracting the skeletal muscle fiber. Relaxation of the muscle follows as myoplasmic Ca^{++} is resequestered by Ca^{++}-ATPase (SERCA) in the SR.

4. The force of contraction can be increased by activating more motor neurons (i.e., recruiting more muscle fibers) or by increasing the frequency of action potentials in the muscle fiber, which produces tetany. The increased force during tetanic contractions is due to prolonged elevation of intracellular $[Ca^{++}]$.

5. The two basic types of skeletal muscle fibers are distinguished on the basis of their speed of contraction (i.e., fast twitch versus slow twitch). The difference in speed of contraction is attributed to the expression of different myosin isoforms that differ in myosin ATPase activity. In addition to the difference in myosin ATPase activity, fast- and slow-twitch muscles also differ in metabolic activity, fiber diameter, motor unit size, sensitivity to tetany, and recruitment pattern.

6. Typically, slow-twitch muscles are recruited before fast-twitch muscle fibers because of the greater excitability of motor neurons innervating slow-twitch muscles. The high oxidative capacity of slow-twitch muscle fibers supports sustained contractile activity. Fast-twitch muscle fibers, in contrast, tend to be large and typically have low oxidative capacity and high glycolytic capacity. The fast-twitch motor units are thus best suited for short periods of activity when high levels of force are required.

7. Fast-twitch muscle fibers can be converted to slow-twitch muscle fibers (and vice versa), depending on the stimulation pattern. Chronic electrical stimulation of a fast-twitch muscle results in the expression of slow-twitch myosin and decreased expression of fast-twitch myosin, along with an increase in oxidative capacity. The mechanism or mechanisms underlying this change in gene expression are unknown but appear to be secondary to an elevation in resting intracellular $[Ca^{++}]$. The Ca^{++}-dependent phosphatase calcineurin and the transcription factor NFAT have been implicated in this transition from the fast-twitch to the slow-twitch phenotype. Ca^{++}-calmodulin–dependent kinase and the transcription factor MEF2 may also participate in the phenotype transition.

8. Skeletal muscle fibers atrophy after denervation. Muscle fibers depend on the activity of their motor nerves for maintenance of the differentiated phenotype. Reinnervation by axon growth along the original nerve sheath can reverse these changes. Skeletal muscle has a limited capacity to replace cells lost as a result of trauma or disease. Inhibition of the PI3K/Akt signaling pathways appears to contribute to the decreased rate of protein synthesis and increased rate of protein degradation observed during atrophy. The increased protein degradation during atrophy is attributed to increases in both protease activity (e.g., activation of caspase 3) and ubiquitination (through elevated levels of ubiquitin ligases). During disuse-induced atrophy, release of the ubiquitin ligase MuRF2 appears to contribute to decreased transcription and increased protein degradation.

9. Skeletal muscle exhibits considerable phenotypic plasticity. Normal growth is associated with cellular hypertrophy caused by the addition of more myofibrils and more sarcomeres at the ends of the cell to match skeletal growth. Strength training induces cellular hypertrophy, whereas endurance training increases the oxidative capacity of all involved motor units. Training regimens are not able to alter fiber type or the expression of myosin isoforms.

10. Muscle fatigue during exercise is not due to depletion of ATP. The mechanism or mechanisms underlying exercise-induced fatigue are not known, although the accumulation of various metabolic products (lactate, P_i, ADP) has been implicated. Given the importance of preventing depletion of myoplasmic ATP, which would affect the viability of the cell, it is likely that multiple mechanisms may have been developed to induce fatigue and hence lower the rate of ATP hydrolysis before risking injury/death of the skeletal muscle cell.

11. When the energy demands of an exercising muscle cannot be met by oxidative metabolism, an oxygen debt is incurred. Increased breathing during the recovery period after exercise reflects this O_2 debt. The greater the reliance on anaerobic metabolism to meet the energy requirements of muscle contraction, the greater the O_2 debt.

CHAPTER 13

Cardiac Muscle

The function of the heart is to pump blood through the circulatory system, and this is accomplished by the highly organized contraction of cardiac muscle cells. Specifically, the cardiac muscle cells are connected together to form an electrical syncytium, with tight electrical and mechanical connections between adjacent cardiac muscle cells. An action potential initiated in a specialized region of the heart (e.g., the sinoatrial node) is therefore able to pass quickly throughout the heart to facilitate synchronized contraction of the cardiac muscle cells, which is important for the pumping action of the heart. Likewise, refilling of the heart requires synchronized relaxation of the heart, with abnormal relaxation often resulting in pathological conditions.

In this chapter attention is initially directed at the organization of cardiac muscle cells within the heart, including discussion of the tight electrical and mechanical connections. The mechanisms underlying contraction, relaxation, and regulation of the force of contraction of cardiac muscle cells are also addressed. It is noteworthy that although cardiac muscle and skeletal muscle are both striated muscles, there are significant differences in terms of organization, electrical and mechanical coupling, excitation-contraction coupling, and mechanisms to regulate the force of contraction. These differences are also highlighted.

BASIC ORGANIZATION OF CARDIAC MUSCLE CELLS

Cardiac muscle cells are much smaller than skeletal muscle cells. Typically, cardiac muscle cells measure 10 μm in diameter and approximately 100 μm in length. As shown in Figure 13-1, *A*, cardiac cells are connected to each other through **intercalated disks,** which include a combination of mechanical junctions and electrical connections. The mechanical connections, which keep the cells from pulling apart when contracting, include the **fascia adherens** and **desmosomes. Gap junctions** between cardiac muscle cells, on the other hand, provide electrical connections between cells to allow propagation of the action potential throughout the heart. Thus, the arrangement of cardiac muscle cells within the heart is said to form an electrical and mechanical syncytium that allows a single action potential (generated within the sinoatrial node) to pass throughout the heart so that the heart can contract in a synchronous, wave-like fashion. Blood vessels course through the myocardium.

The basic organization of thick and thin filaments in cardiac muscle cells is comparable to that seen in skeletal muscle (see Chapter 12). When viewed by electron microscopy, there are repeating light and dark bands that represent I bands and A bands, respectively (Fig. 13-1, *B*). Thus, cardiac muscle is classified as a striated muscle. The Z line transects the I band and represents the point of attachment of the thin filaments. The region between two adjacent Z lines represents the sarcomere, which is the contractile unit of the muscle cell. The thin filaments are composed of actin, tropomyosin, and troponin and extend into the A band. The A band is composed of thick filaments, along with some overlap of thin filaments. The thick filaments are composed of myosin and extend from the center of the sarcomere toward the Z lines.

Myosin filaments are formed by a tail-to-tail association of myosin molecules in the center of the sarcomere, followed by a head-to-tail association as the thick filament extends toward the Z lines. Thus, the myosin filament is polarized and poised for pulling the actin filaments toward the center of the sarcomere. A cross section of the sarcomere near the end of the A band shows that each thick filament is surrounded by six thin filaments and each thin filament receives cross-bridge attachments from three thick filaments. This complex array of thick and thin filaments is characteristic of both cardiac and skeletal muscle and helps stabilize the filaments during muscle contraction (see Fig. 12-3, *B,* for the hexagonal array of thick and thin filaments in the sarcomere of striated muscle).

There are several proteins that may contribute to the organization of the thick and thin filaments, including meromyosin and C protein (in the center of the sarcomere), which appear to serve as a scaffold for organization of the thick filaments. Similarly, nebulin extends along the length of the actin filament and may serve as a scaffold for the thin filament. α-Actinin anchors the actin filament to the Z line, whereas the protein tropomodulin resides at the end of the actin filament and regulates the length of the thin filament. These proteins are present in both cardiac and skeletal muscle cells.

The thick filaments are tethered to the Z lines by a large elastic protein called **titin.** Although titin was postulated to tether myosin to the Z lines and thus prevent overstretching of the sarcomere, there is evidence indicating that titin may participate in cell signaling (perhaps by acting as a stretch sensor and thus modulating protein synthesis in response to stress). Such signaling by titin has been observed in both

● **Figure 13-1.** **A,** Photomicrograph of cardiac muscle cells (210×). Intercalated disks at either end of a muscle cell are identified in the lower left portion of the micrograph. The intercalated disk physically connects adjacent myocytes and, because of the presence of gap junctions, electrically couples the cells as well so that the muscle functions as an electrical and mechanical syncytium. **B,** Schematic representation of the organization of a sarcomere within a cardiac muscle cell. (**A,** From Telser A: Elsevier's Integrated Histology. St. Louis, Mosby, 2007; **B,** redrawn from Fawcett D, McNutt NS: J Cell Biol 42:1-45, 1969.)

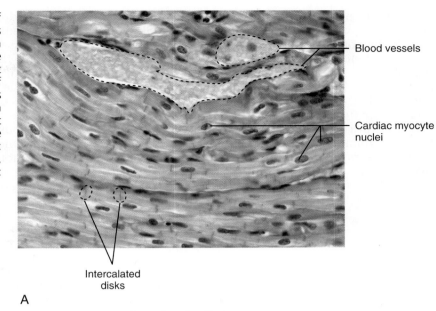

Blood vessels

Cardiac myocyte nuclei

Intercalated disks

A

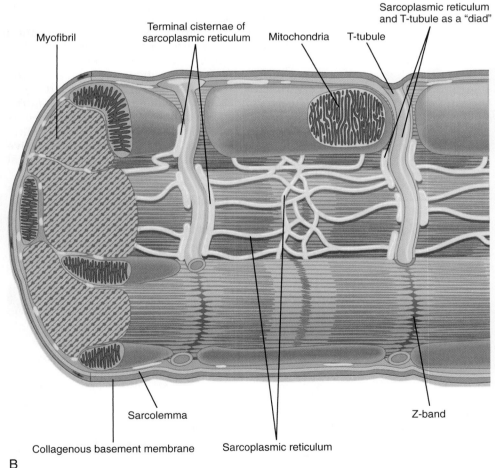

Myofibril

Terminal cisternae of sarcoplasmic reticulum

Mitochondria

T-tubule

Sarcoplasmic reticulum and T-tubule as a "diad"

Sarcolemma

Collagenous basement membrane

Sarcoplasmic reticulum

Z-band

B

cardiac and skeletal muscle cells. Moreover, genetic defects in titin result in atrophy of both cardiac and skeletal muscle cells and may contribute to both cardiac dysfunction and skeletal muscle dystrophies (recently termed **titinopathies**). Titin is also thought to contribute to the ability of cardiac muscle to increase force upon stretch (discussed later).

Although cardiac muscle and skeletal muscle both contain an abundance of connective tissue, there is more connective tissue in the heart. The abundance of connective tissue in the heart helps prevent muscle rupture (as in skeletal muscle), but it also prevents overstretching of the heart. Length-tension analysis of cardiac muscle, for example, shows a dramatic increase in passive tension as cardiac muscle is stretched beyond its resting length (Fig. 13-2). Skeletal muscle, by contrast, tolerates a much greater degree of stretch before passive tension increases to a comparable level. The reason for this difference between cardiac and skeletal muscle is not known, although one possibility is that stretch of skeletal muscle is typically limited by the range of motion of the joint, which in turn is limited by the ligaments/connective tissue surrounding the joint. The heart, on the other hand, appears to rely on the abundance of connective tissue around cardiac muscle cells to prevent over-stretching during periods of increased venous return. During intense exercise, for example, venous return may increase fivefold. However, the heart is capable of pumping this extra volume of blood into the arterial system with only minor changes in the ventricular volume of the heart (i.e., end-diastolic volume increases less than 20%). Although the abundance of connective tissue in the heart limits stretch of the heart during these periods of increased venous return, additional regulatory mechanisms help the heart pump the extra blood that it receives (as discussed later). Conversely, if the heart were to be overstretched, the contractile ability of cardiac muscle cells would be expected to decrease (because of decreased overlap of the thick and thin filaments), thereby resulting in insufficient pumping, increased venous pressure, and perhaps pulmonary edema.

Within cardiac muscle cells, myofibrils are surrounded by the **sarcoplasmic reticulum (SR),** an internal network of membranes (Fig. 13-1, *B*). This is similar to skeletal muscle except that the SR in the heart is less dense and not as well developed. Terminal regions of the SR abut the **T tubule** or lie just below the **sarcolemma** (or both) and play a key role in the elevation of intracellular [Ca^{++}] during an action potential. The mechanism by which an action potential initiates release of Ca^{++} in the heart, however, differs significantly from that in skeletal muscle (as discussed later). The heart contains an abundance of mitochondria, with up to 30% of the volume of the heart being occupied by these organelles. The high density of mitochondria provides the heart with great oxidative capacity, more so than typically seen in skeletal muscle.

The sarcolemma of cardiac muscle also contains invaginations **(T tubules),** comparable to those seen in skeletal muscle. In cardiac muscle, however, T tubules are positioned at the Z lines, whereas in mammalian skeletal muscle, T tubules are positioned at the ends of the I bands. In cardiac muscle there also tends

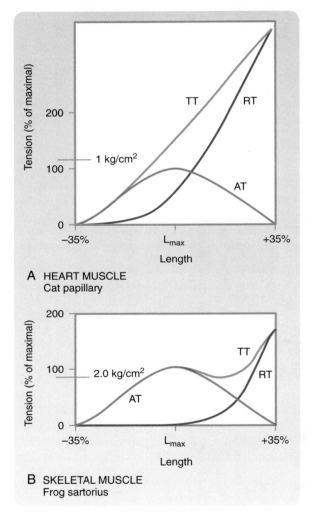

● **Figure 13-2.** Cardiac muscle (panel **A**) has high resistance to stretch when compared with skeletal muscle (panel **B**). When either cardiac or skeletal muscle is stretched, there is an increase in resting tension (RT). If the muscle is then stimulated to contract maximally, it generates more tension (termed total tension—TT). The difference between total tension and resting tension at any given length is the force produced by contraction (e.g., active tension—AT). The bell-shaped dependence of active tension on muscle length is consistent with the sliding filament theory of cardiac and skeletal muscle. It is, however, difficult to stretch cardiac muscle beyond its optimal sarcomere length, as evidenced by the rapid rise in resting tension in the middle of the bell-shaped AT curve.

● AT THE CELLULAR LEVEL

Familial cardiomyopathic hypertrophy (FCH) occurs in approximately 0.2% of the general population but is a leading cause of sudden death in otherwise healthy adults. It has been linked to genetic defects in a variety of proteins in cardiac sarcomeres, including myosin, troponin, tropomyosin, and myosin-binding protein C, a structural protein located in the middle of the A band of the sarcomere. FHC is an autosomal dominant disease, and transgenic studies indicate that expression of only a small amount of the mutated protein can result in development of the cardiomyopathic phenotype. Moreover, mutation of a single amino acid in the myosin molecule is sufficient to produce cardiomyopathic hypertrophy. The pathogenesis of FHC, however, is variable, even within a family with a single gene defect, both in terms of onset and severity, thus suggesting the presence of modifying loci.

to be fewer and less well developed connections between the T tubules and the SR than in skeletal muscle.

CONTROL OF CARDIAC MUSCLE ACTIVITY

Cardiac muscle is an involuntary muscle with an intrinsic pacemaker. The pacemaker represents a specialized cell (located in the **sinoatrial node** of the right atrium) that is able to undergo spontaneous depolarization and generate action potentials. It is important to note that although several cells in the heart are able to depolarize spontaneously, the fastest spontaneous depolarizations occur in cells in the sinoatrial node. Moreover, once a given cell spontaneously depolarizes and fires an action potential, this action potential is then propagated throughout the heart (by specialized conduction pathways and cell-to-cell contact). Thus, depolarization from only one cell is needed to initiate a wave of contraction in the heart (i.e., heartbeat). The mechanism or mechanisms underlying this spontaneous depolarization are discussed in depth in Chapter 16.

As shown in Figure 16-17, once an action potential is initiated in the sinoatrial node, it is propagated between atrial cells via gap junctions, as well as through specialized conduction fibers in the atria. The action potential can pass throughout the atria within approximately 70 msec. For the action potential to reach the ventricles, it must pass through the **atrioventricular node,** after which the action potential passes throughout the ventricle via specialized conduction pathways (**bundle of His** and **Purkinje system**) and gap junctions in the intercalated disks of adjacent cardiac myocytes. The action potential can pass through the entire heart within 220 msec after initiation in the sinoatrial node. Because contraction of a cardiac muscle cell typically lasts 300 msec, this rapid conduction promotes nearly synchronous contraction of heart muscle cells. This is a very different scenario from that of skeletal muscle, where cells are grouped into motor units that are recruited independently as the force of contraction is increased.

Excitation-Contraction Coupling

Blood and extracellular fluids typically contain 1 to 2 mM free Ca^{++}, and it has been known since the days of the physiologist Sidney Ringer (ca. 1882) that the heart requires extracellular Ca^{++} to contract. Thus, an isolated heart typically continues to beat when perfused with a warm ($37°C$), oxygenated, physiological salt solution that contains approximately 2 mM Ca^{++} (e.g., Tyrode's solution), but it stops beating in the absence of extracellular Ca^{++}. This cessation of contractions in Ca^{++}-deficient media is also observed in hearts that are electrically stimulated, thus further demonstrating the importance of extracellular Ca^{++} for contraction of cardiac muscle. This situation is quite different from that of skeletal muscle, which can contract in the total absence of extracellular Ca^{++}.

Examination of the action potential in cardiac muscle reveals a prolonged action potential lasting 150 to 300 msec (Fig. 13-3), which is substantially longer than the action potentials in skeletal muscle ($\approx$5 msec). The long action potential duration in cardiac muscle is due to a slow inward Ca^{++} current

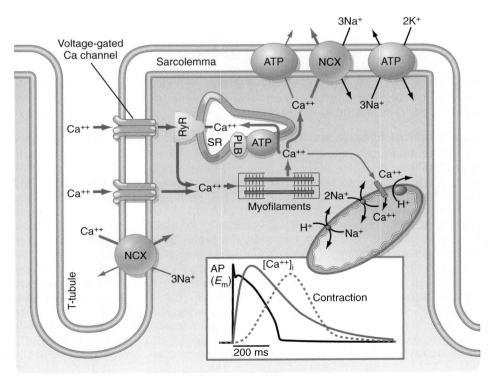

● **Figure 13-3.** Excitation-contraction coupling in the heart requires Ca^{++} influx through L-type Ca^{++} channels in the sarcolemma and T tubules. See text for details. (Redrawn from Bers DM: Nature 415:198-205, 2002.)

through a **voltage-gated L-type Ca^{++} channel** in the sarcolemma. The amount of Ca^{++} coming into the cardiac muscle cell is relatively small and serves as a trigger for release of Ca^{++} from the SR. In the absence of extracellular Ca^{++}, one is still able to initiate an action potential in cardiac muscle, although it is considerably shorter in duration and unable to initiate a contraction. Thus, influx of Ca^{++} during the action potential is critical for triggering release of Ca^{++} from the SR and thus initiating contraction.

The L-type Ca^{++} channel is composed of five subunits (α_1, α_2, β, γ, and δ). The α_1 subunit is also called the **dihydropyridine receptor (DHPR)** because it binds the dihydropyridine class of Ca^{++} channel blocking drugs (e.g., nitrendipine and nimodipine). Although this channel complex is present in both skeletal and cardiac muscle, it serves very different functions in the two muscle types (see later).

In each cardiac muscle sarcomere, terminal regions of the SR abut T tubules and the sarcolemma (Figs. 13-1, *B*, and 13-3). These junctional regions of the SR are enriched in **ryanodine receptors (RYRs;** an SR Ca^{++} release channel). The RYR is a Ca^{++}-gated Ca^{++} channel, so influx of Ca^{++} during an action potential is able to initiate release of Ca^{++} from the SR in cardiac muscle. The amount of Ca^{++} released into the cytosol from the SR is much greater than that entering the cytosol from the sarcolemma, although release of Ca^{++} from the SR does not occur without this entry of "trigger" Ca^{++}. This contrasts with skeletal muscle, where release of Ca^{++} from the SR does not involve entry of Ca^{++} across the sarcolemma but instead results from a voltage-induced conformational change in the DHPR. Thus, excitation-contraction coupling in cardiac muscle is termed **electrochemical coupling** (involving Ca^{++}-induced release of Ca^{++}), whereas excitation-contraction coupling in skeletal muscle is termed **electromechanical coupling** (involving direct interactions between the DHPR in the T tubule and the RYR in the SR). The basis for this difference in Ca^{++} release mechanisms appears to depend on the DHPR isoform because expression of cardiac DHPR in skeletal muscle cells results in a requirement for extracellular Ca^{++} for contraction of these modified skeletal muscle cells.

Contraction Mechanism

As in skeletal muscle, contraction of cardiac muscle is thin filament regulated, with an elevation in intracellular [Ca^{++}] required to promote actin-myosin interaction. At low (<50 nM) intracellular [Ca^{++}], binding of myosin to actin is blocked by tropomyosin. As cytosolic [Ca^{++}] increases during an action potential, however, binding of Ca^{++} to troponin C results in a conformational change in the troponin/tropomyosin complex such that tropomyosin slips into the groove of the actin filament and exposes myosin binding sites on the actin filament. As long as cytosolic [Ca^{++}] remains elevated and hence myosin binding sites are exposed, myosin will bind to actin, undergo a ratchet action, and contract the cardiac muscle cell. Note that because myosin binding sites on actin are blocked at low [Ca^{++}] and exposed during a rise in intracellular

[Ca^{++}], contraction of cardiac muscle is termed "thin filament regulated." This is identical to the situation in skeletal muscle but contrasts with smooth muscle, where contraction is thick filament regulated (see Chapter 14).

During a rise in intracellular [Ca^{++}] and exposure of myosin binding sites on actin, the myosin cross-bridges undergo a series of steps resulting in contraction of the cardiac muscle cell. At rest, the myosin molecules are energized in that they have partially hydrolyzed ATP to "cock the head" and are thus ready to interact with actin. An elevation in intracellular [Ca^{++}] then exposes myosin binding sites on actin and thus allows myosin to bind actin (step 1). The bound myosin subsequently undergoes a power stroke in which the actin filament is pulled toward the center of the sarcomere (step 2). ADP and P$_i$ are released from the myosin head during this step as the energy from ATP is used to contract the muscle. The myosin head moves approximately 70 nm during each ratchet action (cross-bridge cycle). Binding of ATP to myosin decreases the affinity of myosin for actin and thus allows myosin to release from actin (step 3). Myosin then partially hydrolyzes the bound ATP to reenergize ("cock") the head (step 4) and ready the cross-bridge for another cycle. This four-step cycle is identical to that described for skeletal muscle (see Chapter 12).

Cardiac muscle and skeletal muscle differ, however, in the level of intracellular [Ca^{++}] attained after an action potential and hence in the number of actin-myosin interactions. In skeletal muscle, the rise in intracellular [Ca^{++}] and the number of actin-myosin interactions are high after an action potential. In cardiac muscle, the rise in intracellular [Ca^{++}] can be regulated, which affords the heart an important means of modulating the force of contraction without recruiting more muscle cells or undergoing tetany. Recall that in the heart all the muscle cells are activated during a contraction, so recruiting more muscle cells is not an option. Moreover, tetany of cardiac muscle cells would prevent any pumping action and thus be fatal. Consequently, the heart relies on different means of increasing the force of contraction, including varying the amplitude of the intracellular Ca^{++} transient.

Relaxation of Cardiac Muscle

Relaxation of skeletal muscle simply requires reaccumulation of Ca^{++} by the SR through the action of the **SR Ca^{++} pump (SERCA).** Although SERCA plays a key role in the decrease in cytosolic [Ca^{++}] in cardiac muscle, the process is more complex than that in skeletal muscle because some trigger Ca^{++} enters the cardiac muscle cell through the sarcolemmal Ca^{++} channels during each action potential. A mechanism must therefore exist to extrude this trigger Ca^{++}; otherwise, the amount of Ca^{++} in the SR would continuously increase and result in Ca^{++} overload. In particular, some Ca^{++} is extruded from the cardiac muscle cell though the sarcolemmal **3Na$^+$-1Ca^{++} antiporter** and a **sarcolemmal Ca^{++} pump** (Fig. 13-3). Note that extracellular [Ca^{++}] is in the millimolar range, whereas intracellular [Ca^{++}] is submicromolar, so extrusion of Ca^{++} is accomplished against a large chemical gradient. Similarly, [Na$^+$] is considerably higher in the extracellular media than within the cell. The antiporter uses the Na$^+$ gradient across the cell to power the uphill movement of Ca^{++} out of the cell. Because 3 Na$^+$ ions enter the cell in exchange for 1 Ca^{++} ion, the 3Na$^+$-1Ca^{++} antiporter is electrogenic and creates a depolarizing current. The sarcolemmal Ca^{++} pump, on the other hand, uses the energy in ATP to extrude Ca^{++} from the cell. Both extrusion mechanisms and SERCA thus contribute to the relaxation of cardiac muscle by decreasing cytosolic [Ca^{++}].

Although the interaction of actin and myosin requires a relatively small increase in free intracellular [Ca^{++}], the abundance of Ca^{++}-binding proteins in the myoplasm necessitates a much larger increase in total intracellular [Ca^{++}]. The resting intracellular [Ca^{++}] is approximately 50 to 100 nM, with half-maximal force of contraction requiring approximately 600 nM free Ca^{++} (Fig. 13-4). However, because of Ca^{++}-binding proteins such as parvalbumin and troponin C, the total myoplasmic concentration must increase by 70 μM. As already noted, much of this increase in total myoplasmic [Ca^{++}] occurs through release of Ca^{++} from the SR. In a number of species, including rabbits, dogs, cats, guinea pigs, and humans, uptake and release of Ca^{++} by the SR account for approximately 70% of the intracellular Ca^{++} transient. Thus, up to 30% of the rise in intracellular [Ca^{++}] may be attributable to influx of Ca^{++} through voltage-gated Ca^{++} channels in the sarcolemma, with the 3Na$^+$-1Ca^{++} antiporter contributing significantly to Ca^{++} extrusion during relaxation.

The sarcolemmal Ca^{++} pump is in lower abundance than the 3Na$^+$-1Ca^{++} antiporter but has a higher affinity for Ca^{++} and thus may contribute more to the regulation of resting intracellular [Ca^{++}] (Fig. 13-4). The relative contribution of the Ca^{++} extrusion mechanisms, however, varies between species. For example, rat and mouse myocytes rely primarily on Ca^{++} reuptake by the SR (i.e., the SR accounting for 92% of Ca^{++} transport).

REGULATION OF THE FORCE OF CONTRACTION

Intracellular Calcium

Because the heart represents an electrical syncytium, with all of the cardiac muscle cells contracting during a single beat, it is not possible to increase the force of contraction by recruiting more muscle cells. Moreover, tetany of the heart would be lethal because it would defeat the critical pumping action of the heart. The heart has therefore developed alternative strategies to increase the force of contraction. It should be noted that the long action potential found in cardiac muscle, which is due to activation of the voltage-gated L-type Ca^{++} channel, results in a long refractory period, which in turn prevents tetany. Modulation of Ca^{++} influx through L-type Ca^{++} channels during an action potential, however, provides the heart with a mechanism to alter cytosolic [Ca^{++}] and hence the force of contraction.

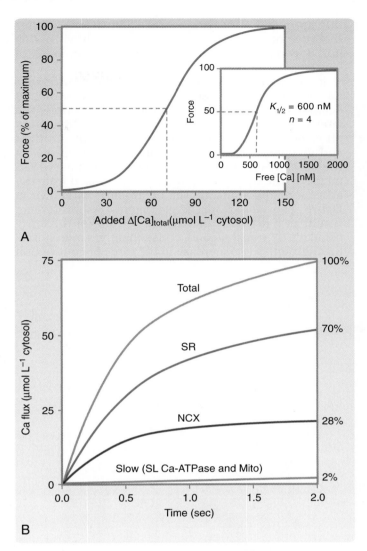

● **Figure 13-4.** Half-maximal force of contraction of cardiac muscles requires a rise in cytosolic free [Ca^{++}] to approximately 600 nM (*inset* to panel **A**). Because of the high Ca^{++} buffering capacity of cytosolic proteins (such as parvalbumin and troponin C), this rise in free Ca^{++} requires an increase in total cytosolic [Ca^{++}] of about 70 μM (panel **A**). Relaxation of the heart occurs by reducing cytosolic free [Ca^{++}], with Ca^{++} sequestration by the SR accounting for the majority of the decrease in cytosolic [Ca^{++}] (≈70%; panel **B**). Some Ca^{++} extrusion occurs through the 3Na$^+$-1Ca^{++} antiporter (≈28%), with very little Ca^{++} extrusion by the sarcolemmal Ca^{++} pump (<2%). NCX, sodium-calcium exchanger. (Redrawn from Bers DM: Nature 415:198-205, 2002.)

A simple means of modulating the force of contraction of cardiac muscle cells in vitro is to vary extracellular [Ca^{++}]. As noted previously, contraction of the heart requires extracellular Ca^{++}. Decreasing extracellular [Ca^{++}] from a normal range of 1 to 2 mM to 0.5 mM, for example, reduces the force of the contraction. This reduction in force of contraction is not associated with a change in the duration of the contraction because the kinetics of Ca^{++} sequestration by the SR and Ca^{++} extrusion has not been modified. Although this approach of varying extracellular [Ca^{++}] to alter the force of contraction is demonstrable in vitro, it is not a common means of modulating the force of cardiac contraction in vivo.

In vivo, an increase in the size of the intracellular Ca^{++} transient and hence the force of contraction occurs in response to sympathetic stimulation (see later and also Chapter 18). Sympathetic stimulation often occurs during periods of excitement or fright and involves activation of β-adrenergic receptors on the heart by norepinephrine (released from nerve terminals in the heart) or epinephrine (released from the adrenal medulla into the bloodstream). As shown in Figure 13-5, the β-adrenergic agonist isoproterenol results in a dramatic increase in the size of the intracellular Ca^{++} transient and, consequently, a more forceful contraction. An increase in the force of contraction

is termed **positive inotropy.** Typically, there is also an increase in the rate of relaxation accompanying this β-adrenergic stimulation that results in a shorter contraction. The increase in the rate of muscle relaxation is termed **positive lusitropy.** The frequency of contractions of the heart also increases with β-adrenergic stimulation and is termed **positive chronotropy.** Thus, β-adrenergic stimulation of the heart produces stronger, briefer, and more frequent contractions.

β-Adrenergic Agonists

The sympathetic nervous system is stimulated when we become excited and is said to prepare the individual for "fight or flight." In the case of the heart, increased levels of the adrenal medullary hormone **epinephrine** or the sympathetic neurotransmitter **norepinephrine** activate β-adrenergic receptors on the cardiac muscle cells, which in turn activates **adenylate cyclase,** increases **cAMP,** and thus promotes cAMP-dependent phosphorylation of numerous proteins in cardiac muscle cells (Fig. 13-6).

Both voltage-gated L-type Ca^{++} channels (responsible for the trigger Ca^{++}) and a protein associated with SERCA, called **phospholamban,** are phosphorylated by cAMP-dependent protein kinase. The combined action of these phosphorylations increases the amount of Ca^{++} in the SR. Specifically, phosphorylation of the sarcolemmal Ca^{++} channel results in more trigger Ca^{++} entering the cell, and phosphorylation of phospholamban increases the activity of SERCA, thereby allowing the SR to accumulate more Ca^{++} before it is extruded by the $3Na^{+}$-$1Ca^{++}$ antiporter and sarcolemmal Ca^{++} pump. The net result is that the SR releases more Ca^{++} into the cytosol during the next action potential, which promotes more actin-myosin interactions and hence greater force of contraction (Fig. 13-6). The increased activity of SERCA after sympathetic stimulation also results in a shortened contraction because of the rapid reaccumulation of Ca^{++} by the SR. This in turn allows the heart to increase its rate of relaxation. An additional consequence of sympathetic stimulation is an increase in heart rate through a direct effect on the pacemaker cells (see Chapter 18).

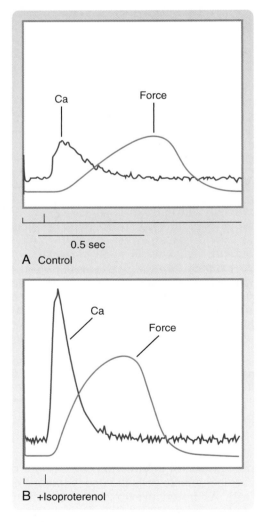

● **Figure 13-5.** Stimulation of β-adrenergic receptors in the heart increases the force of contraction. Electrical stimulation of myocardium results in a transient rise in intracellular [Ca^{++}] and production of force **(A).** Isoproterenol (a β-adrenergic receptor agonist) increases the amplitude of the intracellular Ca^{++} transient and hence the amount of force generated **(B).**

● AT THE CELLULAR LEVEL

The mechanisms underlying the response of the heart to β-adrenergic stimulation is complex and involves cAMP-dependent phosphorylation of several proteins. An **A kinase anchor protein (AKAP)** has been shown to be closely associated with the L-type Ca^{++} channel in the heart, thereby positioning **cAMP-dependent protein kinase** close to the channel and facilitating cAMP-dependent phosphorylation of this channel during sympathetic stimulation. How these cAMP-dependent phosphorylations increase the amplitude of the intracellular Ca^{++} transient and in so doing result in a more forceful, briefer cardiac contraction is discussed in general terms later (see also Chapter 18).

● **Figure 13-6.** Sympathetic stimulation of the heart results in an increase in cytosolic cAMP and hence phosphorylation of several proteins by protein kinase A (PKA). An A kinase anchor protein (AKAP) adjacent to the L-type Ca⁺⁺ channel facilitates phosphorylation of this channel and possibly nearby SR Ca⁺⁺ channels (RyR). Other proteins phosphorylated by PKA include phospholamban (PLB) and troponin I. Muscarinic agonists (e.g., acetylcholine [ACh]), on the other hand, inhibit this sympathetic cascade by inhibiting the production of cAMP by adenylate cyclase (AC). β-AR, β-adrenergic receptor. (Redrawn from Bers DM: Nature 415:198, 2002.)

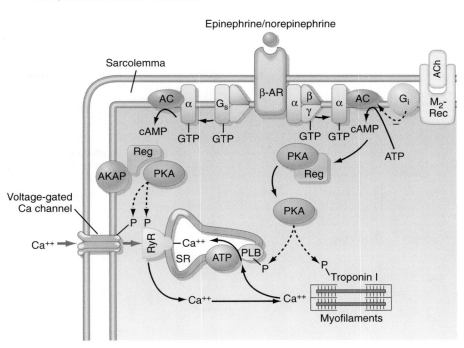

AT THE CELLULAR LEVEL

Mutations in the cardiac ryanodine receptor (RyR2) have been associated with cardiac arrhythmias. Specifically, catecholaminergic polymorphic ventricular tachycardia (CPVT) is an inherited autosomal dominant disease that is typically manifested during childhood as an exercise-induced tachycardia that can progress to arrhythmias during exercise (or stress) and result in sudden death. Approximately 40% of patients with CPVT exhibit a defect in RyR2 that has been associated with increased release of Ca⁺⁺ from the SR. The mutation in RyR2 may involve substitution of a highly conserved amino acid, which differs from malignant hyperthermia, in which splicing errors or deletions within the RYR have been reported. It is hypothesized that during periods of exercise or stress, increased levels of intracellular Ca⁺⁺ (because of the combined effects of β-adrenergic stimulation and increased activity of the mutated RyR2) promote the development of delayed afterdepolarizations (DADs) and hence arrhythmias. Elevation of intracellular [Ca⁺⁺] during diastole is thought to promote the development of DADs through activation of the 3Na⁺-1Ca⁺⁺ antiporter, wherein Ca⁺⁺ extrusion during diastole results in a net inward current sufficient to depolarize the cell to the threshold for an action potential. Treatment of CPVT patients involves antiadrenergic therapy (using β-adrenergic antagonists) or (for unresponsive patients) an implanted defibrillator.

Stretch

Stretching the heart increases the force of contraction both in vivo and in vitro and is an intrinsic mechanism for regulating contractile force. This contrasts with skeletal muscle, which typically exhibits maximal tension at resting length. Stretching of the heart in vivo occurs during times of increased venous return of blood to the heart (e.g., during exercise or when the heart rate is slowed, or both). The **Frank-Starling law of the heart** refers to this ability of the heart to increase its force of contraction when stretched, which occurs at times of increased venous return (Fig. 13-7; also see Chapter 16).

The importance of this mechanism is that it helps the heart pump whatever volume of blood it receives. Thus, when the heart receives a lot of blood, the ventricles are stretched and the force of contraction is increased, thereby ensuring ejection of this extra volume of blood. It should be noted that stretching cardiac muscle also increases passive tension, which helps prevent overstretching of the heart. This passive resistance in the heart is greater than that in skeletal muscle and is attributed to both extracellular matrix (connective tissue) and intracellular elastic proteins **(titin).**

The mechanism underlying this stretch-induced increase in force of contraction appears to involve a change in both sensitivity to Ca⁺⁺ and the level of actin-myosin interactions. The change in the level of actin-myosin interactions is shown in Figure 13-7, *B*. When compared with control cardiac muscle, stretched cardiac muscle exhibits an increased force of contraction at saturating [Ca⁺⁺]. Likewise, shortening cardiac muscle (by precontracting the muscle) results in a less forceful contraction at saturating [Ca⁺⁺] than with either control or stretched cardiac muscle. The mechanism underlying this length-dependent increase in force does not appear to be due to differences in the overlap of thick and thin filaments. Instead, evidence suggests that stretch reduces the space between thick and thin filaments (i.e., interfilament spacing), and this is associated with the ability of more myosin

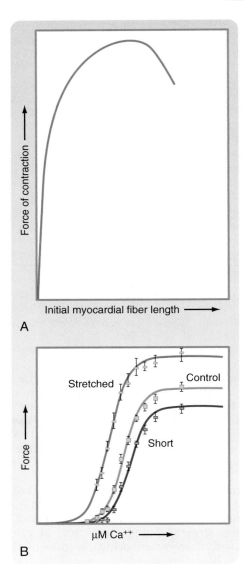

Figure 13-7. Stretching the heart increases the force of contraction **(A).** This is attributable to both an increase in the maximal force of contraction and an increase in the sensitivity of contraction to Ca^{++} **(B)** and reflects an intrinsic regulatory process referred to as the Frank-Starling law of the heart. (**B**, redrawn from Dobesh D, Konhilas J, and de Tombe P: Am J Physiol Heart Circ Physiol 282:1055–1062, 2002.)

molecules to interact with actin (increasing the force at saturating [Ca^{++}]). The intracellular elastic protein titin has been implicated in this length-dependent increase in force because it binds both actin and myosin and might pull the actin and myosin filaments closer together when the muscle/titin is stretched (Fig. 13-8). Consistent with the latter hypothesis, in vitro experiments involving partial proteolysis of titin resulted in attenuation of the length-dependent increase in force.

Stretch also increases sensitivity to Ca^{++} and the level of actin-myosin interactions in cardiac muscle (Fig. 13-7, *B*). Stretched cardiac muscle requires a lower level of Ca^{++} to produce a half-maximal force of contraction than control/unstretched cardiac muscle

does. Moreover, precontracted cardiac muscle requires a higher level of Ca^{++} to produce a half-maximal force of contraction than control/unstretched cardiac muscle does. The mechanism or mechanisms underlying this stretch-induced increase in the sensitivity of cardiac actin-myosin interactions to Ca^{++} are unknown but probably also involve a stretch-induced decrease in spacing between actin and myosin filaments, perhaps involving titin. Interestingly, skeletal muscle does not exhibit this stretch-dependent change in sensitivity to Ca^{++}, although it does contain titin. This difference between muscle types may reflect the expression of different titin isoforms or other proteins (e.g., myosin, troponins, and tropomyosin).

CARDIAC MUSCLE METABOLISM

As in skeletal muscle, myosin uses the energy in ATP to generate force, so the ATP pool, which is small, must be continually replenished. Typically, this replenishment of ATP pools is accomplished by aerobic metabolism, including the oxidation of fats and carbohydrates. During times of ischemia, the **creatine phosphate** pool, which converts ADP to ATP, may decrease. As in skeletal muscle, the creatine phosphate pool is small.

When cardiac muscle is completely deprived of O$_2$ because of occlusion of a coronary vessel (i.e., stopped-flow ischemia), contractions quickly cease (within 30 seconds). This is not due to depletion of either ATP or creatine phosphate because these levels decline more slowly. Even after 10 minutes of stopped-flow ischemia, when creatine phosphate levels are near zero and only 20% of the ATP remains, reperfusion can restore these energy stores, as well as contractile ability. However, prolonging the stopped-flow ischemia for 20 minutes results in further drops in ATP such that reperfusion has considerably less effect with only limited restoration of ATP and creatine phosphate levels or contractile activity.

CARDIAC MUSCLE HYPERTROPHY

Exercise such as endurance running can increase the size of the heart as a result of hypertrophy of individual cardiac muscle cells. Concomitant with this enlarged "athlete's heart" is improved cardiac performance, as assessed by an increase in stroke volume, increased oxygen consumption, and preserved relaxation. Thus, the "athlete's heart" represents an example of "physiological hypertrophy," with beneficial contractile effects.

By contrast, if exposed to chronic pressure overload, the heart may undergo either **concentric left ventricular hypertrophy** or **dilated left ventricular hypertrophy,** with impaired functional consequences. Details regarding the morphological, functional, and mechanistic differences between these various types of hypertrophy can be found elsewhere in this textbook (see Chapter 18).

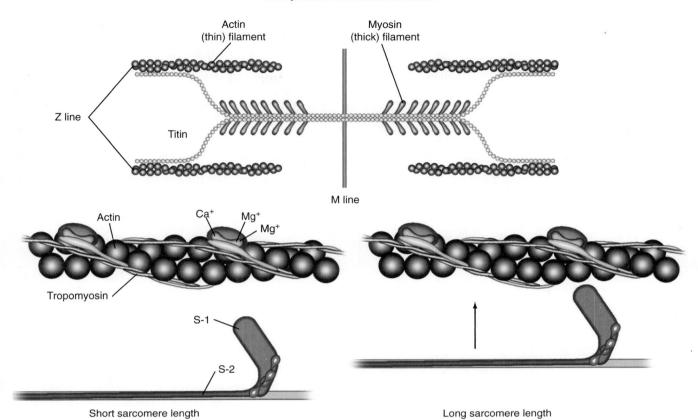

● **Figure 13-8.**   Titin may contribute to the ability of stretch to increase the force of contraction of the heart. Titin binds to both myosin and actin such that stretch of the cardiac muscle may bring the actin filament closer to the myosin head and thus increase the number of myosin heads that interact with actin at a given intracellular [Ca++]. (Redrawn from Moss RL, Fitzsimons DP: Circ Res 90:11-13, 2002.)

Concentric hypertrophy is characterized by thickening of the left ventricular wall and represents a compensatory hypertrophy to the increased load. Dilated hypertrophy is characterized by increased ventricular volume (end-diastolic volume). Both concentric/compensatory left ventricular hypertrophy and dilated left ventricular hypertrophy have been shown to exhibit decreased contractile response to β-adrenergic stimulation, thus limiting the contractile reserve. In dilated left ventricular hypertrophy, normal contractile function, along with the Frank-Starling response, may also be impaired.

The cellular and molecular mechanism or mechanisms underlying the development of cardiac hypertrophy are not clear, although an elevation in intracellular [Ca++] has been implicated.

The link or links between cardiac hypertrophy, decreased cardiac performance, and impaired β-adrenergic response during chronic pressure overload are unclear. Decreased cardiac performance has been attributed to dysregulation of intracellular [Ca++]. Alterations in the level, activity, and phosphorylation status of a variety of proteins, including L-type Ca^{++} channels, phospholamban, SERCA, and RYR, have all been implicated in the Ca++ dysregulation associated with a failing heart (pathological hypertrophy).

● AT THE CELLULAR LEVEL

A modest elevation in intracellular [Ca++] (as a result of increased contractile activity), for example, has been proposed to activate a Ca++-calmodulin–dependent protein phosphatase **(calcineurin)** that can dephosphorylate the transcription factor **NFAT (nuclear factor of activated T cells),** thereby facilitating translocation of NFAT to the nucleus and ultimately promoting protein synthesis and thus hypertrophy (Fig. 13-9). Activation of Ca++-calmodulin–dependent protein kinase has also been implicated in activation of the transcription factor **MEF2** (myocyte enhancer factor 2) by promoting the dissociation (nuclear export) of an inhibitor of MEF2 (viz., **histone deacetylase [HDAC]).**

The impaired β-adrenergic response of cardiac muscle after chronic pressure overload involves, at least in part, a decrease in β-adrenergic receptors because of internalization. Both **phosphatidylinositol-3-kinase (PI3K)** and **β-adrenergic receptor kinase 1** have been implicated in the internalization of β-adrenergic receptors.

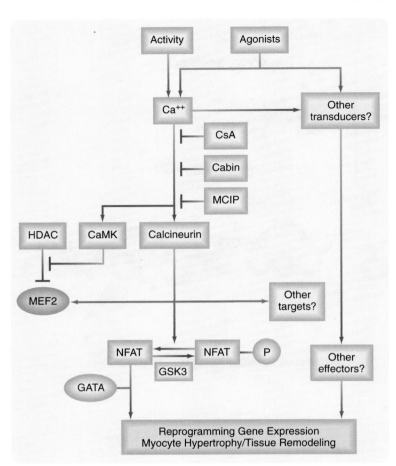

● **Figure 13-9.** Calcium-dependent activation of calcineurin and calmodulin-dependent protein kinase have been implicated in the development of cardiac hypertrophy and involve activation of the transcription factors NFAT, GATA, and MEF2. Cabin, calcineurim binding protein/inhibitor; CaMK, Ca^{++}/calmodulin dependent protein kinase; CsA, cyclosporin; GATA, transcription factor binding to DNA sequence GATA; GSK3, glycogen synthase kinase 3; HDAC, histone deacetylase; MCIP, modulatory calcineurin interacting protein; MEF2, myocyte enhancer factor 2; NFAT, nuclear factor of activated T-cells. (Redrawn from Olson EN, Williams RS: Cell 101:689-692, 2000.)

Finally, there is evidence that cardiac hypertrophy can be dissociated from some functional impairments. Intermittent aortic constrictions, for example, result in decreased β-adrenergic signaling, decreased capillary density, and decreased SERCA2 levels, without evidence of hypertrophy. Activation of PI3K appears to be involved in this response.

■ KEY CONCEPTS

1. Cardiac muscle is an involuntary, striated muscle. Cardiac muscle cells are relatively small (10 μm × 100 μm) and form an electrical syncytium with tight electrical and mechanical connections between adjacent cardiac muscle cells. Action potentials are initiated in the sinoatrial node and spread quickly throughout the heart to allow synchronous contraction, a feature important for the pumping action of the heart.

2. Contraction of cardiac muscle involves the Ca^{++}-dependent interaction of actin and myosin filaments, as in skeletal muscle. However, unlike skeletal muscle, an influx of extracellular Ca^{++} is required. Specifically, the influx of Ca^{++} during an action potential triggers release of Ca^{++} from the SR, which then promotes actin-myosin interaction and contraction.

● AT THE CELLULAR LEVEL

High blood pressure, defects in heart valves, and weakened ventricular walls secondary to myocardial infarction can all lead to heart failure, a leading cause of death. Heart failure may be seen with thickening of the walls of the ventricle or with dilation (i.e., increased volume) of the ventricles.

Studies suggest that dilated cardiomyopathy can be prevented in an animal model by down-regulating a protein called phospholamban. The mechanism underlying this preventive effect of phospholamban down-regulation is thought to involve an increase in SR Ca^{++} uptake activity because phospholamban typically inhibits SERCA. Increased activity of SERCA would facilitate relaxation of the heart as a result of rapid Ca^{++} uptake by the SR. In addition, the force of contraction is increased because more Ca^{++} is available for release. Increased Ca^{++} uptake by the SR may also decrease activation of the Ca^{++}-dependent phosphatases that have been implicated in the development of cardiac hypertrophy.

3. Relaxation of cardiac muscle involves reaccumulation of Ca^{++} by the SR and extrusion of Ca^{++} from the cell via the $3Na^+$-$1Ca^{++}$ antiporter and the sarcolemmal Ca^{++} pump.

4. The force of contraction of cardiac muscle is increased by stretch (Frank-Starling law of the heart) and by sympathetic stimulation. This differs from skeletal muscle, which increases force by recruiting more muscle fibers or by tetany.

5. Hypertrophy of the heart can occur in response to exercise, chronic pressure overload, or genetic mutations. The cardiac hypertrophy resulting from exercise is typically beneficial, with improved cardiac performance, increased oxygen consumption, and normal relaxation. Chronic pressure overload, on the other hand, can result in cardiac hypertrophy that is initially associated with a decreased β-adrenergic response but may progress to dilated cardiac hypertrophy characterized by decreased contractile ability. Genetic mutations resulting in cardiac hypertrophy include familial hypertrophic cardiomyopathy, in which a mutation in a single intracellular protein may alter contractile function and promote a hypertrophic response.

CHAPTER 14

Smooth Muscle

Nonstriated, or smooth, muscle cells are a major component of hollow organs such as the alimentary canal, airways, vasculature, and urogenital tract. Contraction of smooth muscle serves to alter the dimensions of the organ, which may result in either propelling the contents of the organ (as in peristalsis of the intestine) or increasing the resistance to flow (as in vasoconstriction). The basic mechanism underlying contraction of smooth muscle involves an interaction of myosin with actin (as in striated muscle), although there are some important differences. Specifically, contraction of smooth muscle is thick filament regulated and requires an alteration in myosin before it can interact with actin, whereas contraction of striated muscle is thin filament regulated and requires movement of the troponin-tropomyosin complex on the actin filament before myosin can bind to actin. Smooth muscle can contract in response to either electrical or hormonal signals and exhibits the ability to remain contracted for extended periods at low levels of energy consumption, which is important for functions such as maintaining vascular tone and hence blood pressure. An additional feature of smooth muscle (termed "length adaptation") facilitates contraction of smooth muscle over a broad range of lengths, which may be important for emptying a hollow organ at various levels of filling. Thus, regulation of contraction of smooth muscle is complex, sometimes involving multiple intracellular signaling cascades. In the present chapter, effort is made to identify mechanisms underlying this diverse regulation of smooth muscle contraction and, when appropriate, compare these regulatory mechanisms with those observed in striated muscle. Alterations in smooth muscle function/regulation that have been implicated in various pathological conditions are also discussed.

OVERVIEW OF SMOOTH MUSCLE
Types of Smooth Muscle

Smooth muscle has been subdivided into two groups: **single unit** and **multiunit.** In single-unit smooth muscle, the smooth muscle cells are electrically coupled such that electrical stimulation of one cell is followed by stimulation of adjacent smooth muscle cells. This results in a wave of contraction, as in peristalsis. Moreover, this wave of electrical activity, and hence contraction, in single-unit smooth muscle may be initiated by a pacemaker cell (i.e., a smooth muscle cell that exhibits spontaneous depolarization). In con-

trast, multiunit smooth muscle cells are not electrically coupled, so stimulation of one cell does not necessarily result in activation of adjacent smooth muscle cells. Examples of multiunit smooth muscle include the vas deferens of the male genital tract and the iris of the eye. Smooth muscle, however, is even more diverse, with the single-unit and multiunit classifications representing ends of a spectrum. Moreover, the terms single-unit and multiunit represent an oversimplification because most smooth muscles are modulated by a combination of neural elements, with at least some degree of cell-to-cell coupling, and locally produced activators or inhibitors, which also promote a somewhat coordinated response of smooth muscles.

A second consideration when discussing types of smooth muscle is the activity pattern (Fig. 14-1). In some organs, the smooth muscle cells contract rhythmically or intermittently, whereas in other organs, the smooth muscle cells are continuously active and maintain a level of "tone." Smooth muscle exhibiting rhythmic or intermittent activity is termed **phasic smooth muscle** and includes smooth muscles in the walls of the gastrointestinal and urogenital tracts. Such phasic smooth muscle corresponds to the single-unit category described earlier because the smooth muscle cells contract in response to action potentials that propagate from cell to cell. Smooth muscle that is continuously active, on the other hand, is termed **tonic smooth muscle.** Vascular smooth muscle, respiratory smooth muscle, and some sphincters are continuously active. The continuous partial activation of tonic smooth muscle is not associated with action potentials, although it is proportional to membrane potential. Tonic smooth muscle would thus correspond to the multiunit smooth muscle described earlier. Phasic and tonic contractions of smooth muscle result from interactions of actin and myosin filaments, although as discussed later in this chapter, there is a change in cross-bridge cycling kinetics during tonic contraction such that the smooth muscle can maintain force at low energy cost.

STRUCTURE OF SMOOTH MUSCLE CELLS

Smooth muscle cells typically form layers around hollow organs (Fig. 14-2). Blood vessels and airways exhibit a simple tubular structure in which the smooth muscle cells are arranged circumferentially, so contraction reduces the diameter of the tube. This contraction increases resistance to the flow of blood or air but has little effect on the length of the organ. Smooth muscle cell organization is more complex in the gastrointestinal tract. Layers of smooth muscle in both circumferential and longitudinal orientations provide the mechanical action for mixing food and also propelling the luminal contents from the mouth to the anus. Coordination between these layers

depends on a complex system of autonomic nerves linked by plexuses. These plexuses are located between the two muscle layers. The smooth muscle in the walls of saccular structures, such as the urinary bladder or rectum, allows the organ to increase in size with the accumulation of urine or feces. The varied arrangement of cells in the walls of these organs contributes to their ability to reduce internal volume to almost zero during urination or defecation. Smooth muscle cells in hollow organs occur in a spectrum of forms, depending on their function and mechanical loads.

In all hollow organs, the smooth muscle is separated from the contents of the organ by other cellular elements, which may be as simple as vascular endothelium or as complex as the mucosa of the digestive tract. The walls of hollow organs also contain large amounts of connective tissue that bear an increasing share of the wall stress as organ volume increases.

The following sections describe the structural components that enable smooth muscle to set or alter hollow organ volume. These components include contractile and regulatory proteins, force-transmitting systems such as the cytoskeleton, linkages between cells and to the extracellular matrix, and membrane systems that transduce extracellular signals into changes in myoplasmic $[Ca^{++}]$.

Cell-to-Cell Contact

A variety of specialized contact exists between smooth muscle cells. Such contact allows mechanical linkage and communication between the cells (Fig. 14-3). In contrast to skeletal muscle cells, which are normally attached at either end to a tendon, smooth (and cardiac) muscle cells are connected to each other. Because smooth muscle cells are anatomically

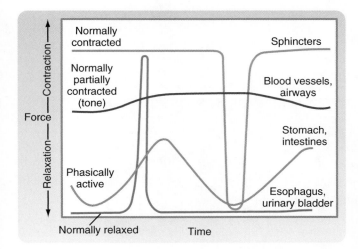

● **Figure 14-1.** Some contractile activity patterns exhibited by smooth muscles. Tonic smooth muscles are normally contracted and generate a variable steady-state force. Examples are sphincters, blood vessels, and airways. Phasic smooth muscles commonly exhibit rhythmic contractions (e.g., peristalsis in the gastrointestinal tract) but may contract intermittently during physiological activities under voluntary control (e.g., voiding of urine and swallowing).

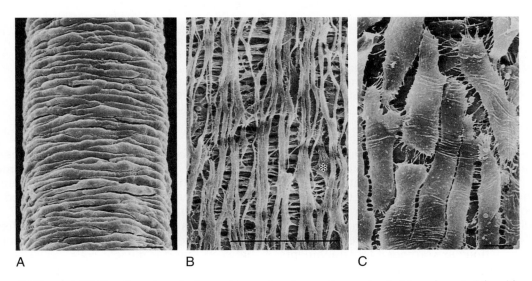

● **Figure 14-2.** Scanning electron micrographs of smooth muscle. **A,** Muscular arteriole with fusiform smooth muscle cells in a circular orientation (*bar,* 20 μm). **B,** Superimposed images of circular *(below)* and longitudinal *(above)* layers of intestinal smooth muscle sandwiching neural components of the myenteric plexus *(asterisk)* (*bar,* 50 mm). **C,** Rectangular smooth muscle cells with thin projections to adjacent cells in a small testicular duct (*bar,* 5 μm). (From Motta PM [ed]: Ultrastructure of Smooth Muscle. Norwell, MA, Kluwer Academic, 1990.)

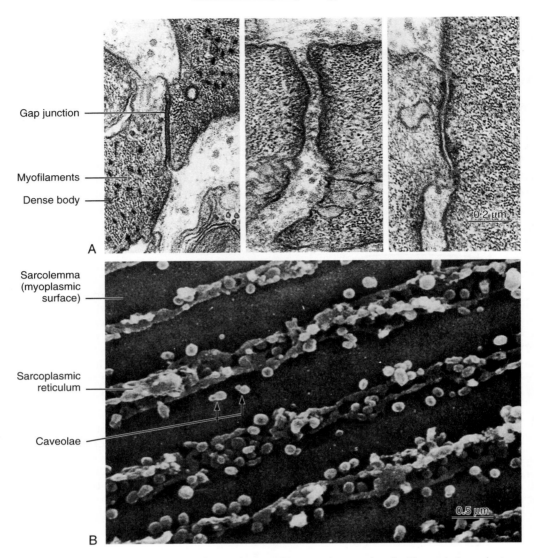

Gap junction

Myofilaments

Dense body

0.2 μm

A

Sarcolemma
(myoplasmic
surface)

Sarcoplasmic
reticulum

Caveolae

0.5 μm

B

● **Figure 14-3.** Junctions and membranes in smooth muscle. **A,** Transmission electron micrograph of junctions between intestinal smooth muscle cells. **B,** Scanning electron micrograph of the inner surface of the sarcolemma of an intestinal smooth muscle cell. Longitudinal rows of caveolae project into the myoplasm *(small, light-colored spheres),* surrounded by darker elements of the tubular sarcoplasmic reticulum. The attachments of thin filaments to the sarcolemma between the rows of membrane elements were removed during preparation of the specimen. (From Motta PM [ed]: Ultrastructure of Smooth Muscle. Norwell, MA, Kluwer Academic, 1990.)

arranged in series, they not only must be mechanically linked but must also be activated simultaneously and to the same degree. This mechanical and functional linkage is crucial to smooth muscle function. If such linkage did not exist, contraction in one region would simply stretch another region without a substantial decrease in radius or increase in pressure. The mechanical connections are provided by attachments to sheaths of connective tissue and by specific junctions between muscle cells.

Several types of junctions are found in smooth muscle (Fig. 14-4). Functional linkage of the cells is provided by **gap junctions.** Gap junctions form low-resistance pathways between cells (see Chapter 2). They also allow chemical communication by diffusion

of low-molecular-weight compounds. In certain tissues, such as the outer longitudinal layer of smooth muscle in the intestine, large numbers of such junctions exist. Action potentials are readily propagated from cell to cell through such tissues.

Adherens junctions (also called dense plaques or attachment plaques) provide mechanical linkage between smooth muscle cells. As depicted in Figure 14-4, the adherens junction appears as thickened regions of opposing cell membranes that are separated by a small gap ($\approx$60 nm) containing dense granular material. Thin filaments extend into the adherens junction to allow the contractile force generated in one smooth muscle cell to be transmitted to adjacent smooth muscle cells.

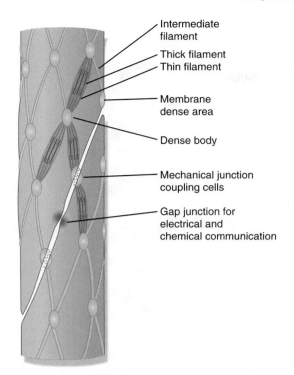

- **Figure 14-4.** Apparent organization of cell-to-cell contacts, cytoskeleton, and myofilaments in smooth muscle cells. Small contractile elements functionally equivalent to a sarcomere underlie the similarities in mechanics between smooth and skeletal muscle. Linkages consisting of specialized junctions or interstitial fibrillar material functionally couple the contractile apparatus of adjacent cells.

Figure 14-3 also shows the presence of **caveolae,** which represent invaginations of the smooth muscle membrane (analogous to T tubules in striated muscle). The **sarcoplasmic reticulum (SR)** extends throughout the smooth muscle cell, although as depicted in Figure 14-3, there are junctional regions of the SR where it abuts regions of the sarcolemma or caveolae, or both. As discussed in a subsequent section, these subsarcolemmal regions of the SR play an important role in the regulation of intracellular [Ca^{++}] and hence smooth muscle tone.

Cells and Membranes

Embryonic smooth muscle cells do not fuse, and each differentiated cell has a single, centrally located nucleus (Fig. 14-5). Though dwarfed by skeletal muscle cells, smooth muscle cells are nevertheless quite large (typically 40 to 600 µm long). These cells are 2 to 10 µm in diameter in the region of the nucleus, and most taper toward their ends. Contracting cells become quite distorted as a result of the force exerted on the cell by attachments to other cells or to the extracellular matrix, and cross sections of these cells are often very irregular.

Smooth muscle cells lack T tubules, the invaginations of the skeletal muscle sarcolemma that provide electrical links to the SR. However, the sarcolemma of smooth muscle has longitudinal rows of tiny sac-like in-pocketings called caveolae (Figs. 14-3 and 14-5).

Caveolae increase the surface-to-volume ratio of the cells and are often closely opposed to the underlying SR. A gap of approximately 15 nm has been observed between the caveolae and the underlying SR, comparable to the gap between the T tubules and terminal SR in skeletal muscle. Moreover, "Ca^{++} sparks" and a variety of Ca^{++}-handling proteins have been observed in the vicinity of caveolae, thus raising the possibility that the caveolae and the underlying SR may contribute to the regulation of intracellular [Ca^{++}] in smooth muscle. The voltage-gated L-type Ca^{++} channel and the 3Na$^+$-1Ca^{++} antiporter, for example, are associated with caveolae. The proteins caveolin and cholesterol are both critical for the formation of caveolae, and it is hypothesized that the caveolae reflect a specialized region of the sarcolemma that may also contain various signaling molecules in addition to the Ca^{++} signaling mentioned earlier.

Smooth muscle also has an intracellular membrane network of SR that serves as an intracellular reservoir for Ca^{++} (Figs. 14-3 and 14-5). Calcium can be released from the SR into the myoplasm when stimulatory neurotransmitters, hormones, or drugs bind to receptors on the sarcolemma. Importantly, intracellular Ca^{++} channels in the SR of smooth muscle include the **ryanodine receptor (RYR),** which is similar to that found in skeletal muscle SR, and the **inositol 1,4,5-trisphosphate (InsP3)**-gated Ca^{++} channel. The RYR is typically activated by a rise in intracellular [Ca^{++}] (i.e., Ca^{++}-induced release of Ca^{++} in response to an influx of Ca^{++} through the sarcolemma). The InsP3-gated Ca^{++} channel is activated by InsP3, which is produced when a hormone or hormones bind to various Ca^{++}-mobilizing receptors on the sarcolemma. Intracellular [Ca^{++}] is lowered through the action of an SR **Ca^{++}-ATPase (SERCA)** and extrusion of Ca^{++} from the cell via a 3Na$^+$-1Ca^{++} antiporter and a sarcolemmal Ca^{++}-ATPase. The amount of SR in smooth muscle cells varies from 2% to 6% of cell volume and approximates that of skeletal muscle. As mentioned earlier, chemical signals such as InsP3 or a localized increase in intracellular [Ca^{++}] (e.g., within the gap between the caveolae and SR) functionally link the sarcolemma and the SR.

Smooth muscle cells contain a prominent rough endoplasmic reticulum and Golgi apparatus, which are located centrally at each end of the nucleus. These structures reflect significant protein synthetic and secretory functions. The scattered mitochondria (Fig. 14-5) are sufficient for oxidative phosphorylation to generate the increased ATP consumed during contraction.

Contractile Apparatus

The thick and thin filaments of smooth muscle cells are about 10,000 times longer than their diameter and are tightly packed. Therefore, the probability of observing an intact filament by electron microscopy is extremely low. In contrast to skeletal muscle, which contains a transverse alignment of thick and thin filaments that results in striations, the contractile filaments in smooth muscle are not in uniform transverse alignment, and thus smooth muscle has no striations.

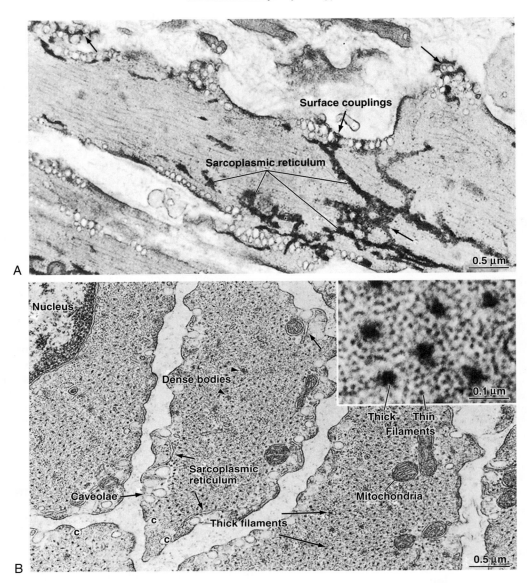

● **Figure 14-5.**   **A,** Longitudinal view of a pulmonary artery smooth muscle cell. The sarcoplasmic reticulum is stained with osmium ferricyanide and appears to form a continuous network throughout the cell consisting of tubules, fenestrated sheets *(long arrows),* and surface couplings at the cell membrane *(short arrows).* **B,** Transverse section of a bundle of venous smooth muscle cells illustrating the regular spacing of thick filaments *(long arrows)* and the relatively large number of surrounding thin (actin) filaments *(inset).* Dense bodies *(arrowheads)* are sites of attachment for the thin actin filaments and equivalent to the Z lines of striated muscles. Elements of sarcoplasmic reticulum *(short arrows)* occur at the periphery of these cells. (From Somlyo AP, Somlyo AV: Smooth muscle structure and function. In Fozzard HA et al [eds]: The Heart and Cardiovascular System, 2nd ed. New York, Raven Press, 1992.)

The lack of striations in smooth muscle does not imply a lack of order. The thick and thin filaments are organized in contractile units that are analogous to sarcomeres.

The thin filaments of smooth muscle have an actin and tropomyosin composition and structure similar to that in skeletal muscle. However, the cellular content of actin and tropomyosin in smooth muscle is about twice that of striated muscle. Smooth muscle lacks troponin and nebulin but contains two proteins not found in striated muscle: **caldesmon** and **calponin.**

The precise roles of these proteins are unknown, but they do not appear to be fundamental to cross-bridge cycling. It has been suggested that calponin may inhibit the binding of unphosphorylated myosin to actin. Most of the myoplasm is filled with thin filaments that are roughly aligned along the long axis of the cell. The myosin content of smooth muscle is only a fourth that of striated muscle. Small groups of three to five thick filaments are aligned and surrounded by many thin filaments. These groups of thick filaments with interdigitating thin filaments are connected to dense bodies or areas (Figs. 14-4 and 14-5) and represent the equivalent of the sarcomere. To maintain alignment of the contractile apparatus along the long axis of the cell, the thick and thin filaments of some smooth muscles do not appear to circumvent the centrally located nucleus but instead may connect to (or near) the nucleus. The contractile apparatus of adjacent cells is mechanically coupled by the links between membrane-dense areas (Fig. 14-4).

Cytoskeleton

The cytoskeleton in smooth muscle cells serves as an attachment point for the thin filaments and permits transmission of force to the ends of the cell. In contrast to skeletal muscle, the contractile apparatus in smooth muscle is not organized into myofibrils, and Z lines are lacking. The functional equivalents of the Z lines in smooth muscle cells are ellipsoidal dense bodies in the myoplasm and dense areas that form bands along the sarcolemma (Figs. 14-3 to 14-5). These structures serve as attachment points for the thin filaments and contain α-actinin, a protein also found in the Z lines of striated muscle. Intermediate filaments with diameters between those of thin filaments (7 nm) and thick filaments (15 nm) are prominent in smooth muscle. These filaments link the dense bodies and areas into a cytoskeletal network (Fig. 14-4). The intermediate filaments consist of protein polymers of **desmin** or **vimentin**.

CONTROL OF SMOOTH MUSCLE ACTIVITY

The contractile activity of smooth muscle can be controlled by numerous factors, including hormones, autonomic nerves, pacemaker activity, and a variety of drugs. Like skeletal or cardiac muscle, contraction of smooth muscle is dependent on Ca^{++}, and the agents just listed induce smooth muscle contraction by increasing intracellular $[Ca^{++}]$. However, in contrast to skeletal or cardiac muscle, action potentials in smooth muscle are highly variable and not always needed to initiate contraction. Moreover, several agents can increase intracellular $[Ca^{++}]$ and hence contract smooth muscle without changing the membrane potential. Figure 14-6 shows various types of action potentials in smooth muscle and the corresponding changes in force. An action potential in smooth muscle can be associated with a slow twitch-like response, and the twitch forces can summate during periods of repetitive action potentials (i.e., similar to tetany in skeletal muscle). Such a pattern of activity is characteristic of single-unit smooth muscle in many viscera.

Periodic oscillations in membrane potential can occur as a result of changes in the activity of Na^+,K^+-ATPase in the sarcolemma. These oscillations in membrane potential can trigger multiple action potentials in the cell. Alternatively, the contractile activity of smooth muscle may not be associated with the generation of action potentials or even a change in membrane potential. In many smooth muscles, the resting membrane potential is sufficiently depolarized (−60 to −40 mV) that a small decrease in membrane potential

can significantly inhibit influx of Ca^{++} through voltage-gated Ca^{++} channels in the sarcolemma. By decreasing Ca^{++} influx, the force developed by smooth muscle decreases. Such a graded response to slight changes in the resting membrane potential is common in multiunit smooth muscles that maintain constant tension (e.g., vascular smooth muscle).

Contraction of smooth muscle in response to an agent that does not produce a change in membrane potential is termed **pharmacomechanical coupling** and typically reflects the ability of the agent to increase the level of the intracellular second messenger InsP3. Other agents result in a decrease in tension, also without a change in membrane potential. These agents typically increase levels of the intracellular second messengers cGMP or cAMP. The molecular mechanisms by which InsP3, cGMP, cAMP, and Ca^{++} alter the contractile force of smooth muscle are presented later.

Phosphorylation of a myosin light chain is required for the interaction of myosin with actin, and although Ca^{++}-dependent phosphorylation plays a key role in this process, the level of myosin phosphorylation (and hence the degree of contraction) is dependent on the relative activities of both **myosin light-chain kinase** (**MLCK,** which promotes phosphorylation) and **myosin phosphatase** (**MP,** which promotes dephosphorylation). Several agonists/hormones increase the level of myosin light-chain phosphorylation by simultaneously activating MLCK through an increase in intracellular $[Ca^{++}]$ and inhibiting MP through a signaling cascade involving the monomeric G protein **RhoA** and its effector **Rho kinase (ROK).** Moreover, hyperactivity of this RhoA/ROK signaling cascade has been implicated in various pathological conditions such as hypertension and vasospasm (discussed later).

INNERVATION OF SMOOTH MUSCLE

Neural regulation of smooth muscle contraction depends on the type of innervation and neurotransmitters released, the proximity of the nerves to the muscle cells, and the type and distribution of the neurotransmitter receptors on the muscle cell membranes (Fig. 14-7). In general, smooth muscle is innervated by the autonomic nervous system. The smooth muscle in arteries is innervated primarily by sympathetic fibers, whereas the smooth muscle in other tissues can have both sympathetic and parasympathetic innervation. In the gastrointestinal tract, smooth muscle is innervated by nerve plexuses that make up the enteric nervous system. The smooth muscle cells of some tissues, such as the uterus, have no innervation.

The neuromuscular junctions and neuromuscular transmission in smooth muscle are functionally comparable to that of skeletal muscle, but structurally less complex. The autonomic nerves that supply smooth muscle have a series of swollen areas, or varicosities, that are spaced at intervals along the axon. These varicosities contain vesicles for the neurotransmitter (Fig. 14-7). The postsynaptic membrane of smooth muscle exhibits little specialization when compared with that of skeletal muscle (see Chapter 6). The syn-

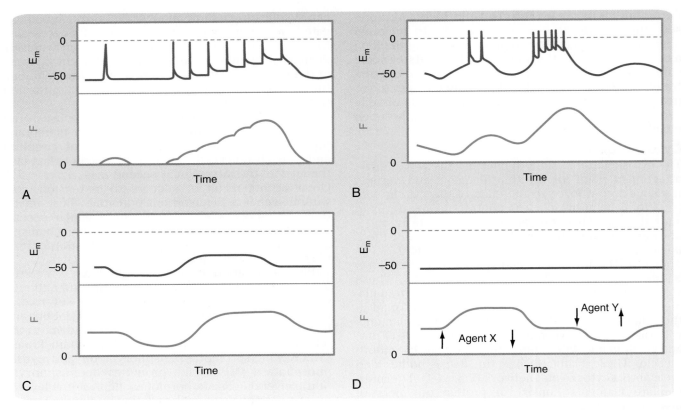

● **Figure 14-6.** Relationships between membrane potential (E_m) and generation of force (F) in different types of smooth muscle. **A,** Action potentials may be generated and lead to a twitch or larger summed mechanical responses. Action potentials are characteristic of single-unit smooth muscles (many viscera). Gap junctions permit the spread of action potentials throughout the tissue. **B,** Rhythmic activity produced by slow waves that trigger action potentials. The contractions are generally associated with a burst of action potentials. Slow oscillations in membrane potential usually reflect the activity of electrogenic pumps in the cell membrane. **C,** Tonic contractile activity may be related to the value of the membrane potential in the absence of action potentials. Graded changes in E_m are common in multiunit smooth muscles (e.g., vascular), where action potentials are not generated and propagated from cell to cell. **D,** Pharmacomechanical coupling; changes in force produced by the addition or removal _(arrows)_ of drugs or hormones that have no significant effect on membrane potential.

aptic cleft is typically about 80 to 120 nm wide but can be as narrow as 6 to 20 nm or even greater than 120 nm. In synapses in which a wide synaptic cleft is found, release of neurotransmitter can affect multiple smooth muscle cells. There are a large number of neurotransmitters that affect smooth muscle activity. A partial listing is provided in Table 14-1.

REGULATION OF CONTRACTION

Contraction of smooth muscle requires the phosphorylation of a myosin light chain. Typically, this phosphorylation occurs in response to a rise in intracellular [Ca^{++}] either after an action potential or in the presence of a hormone/agonist. As depicted in Figure 14-8, a rise in intracellular [Ca^{++}] in smooth muscle results in the binding of 4 Ca^{++} ions to the protein calmodulin, and then the Ca^{++}-calmodulin complex activates MLCK, which phosphorylates the regulatory light chain of myosin. This phosphorylation step is critical for the

> ▶ **IN THE CLINIC**
>
> The enteric nervous system controls many aspects of gastrointestinal function, including motility. Some children are born without enteric nerves in the distal portion of the colon. The absence of nerves is caused by mutant genes that disrupt the signals necessary for the embryonic nerves to migrate to the colon. In these children, normal motility of the colon does not occur and severe constipation results. This condition is called **Hirschsprung's disease.** It can be corrected by surgically removing the portion of the colon that does not contain enteric nerves.

interaction of smooth muscle myosin with actin. In addition to this phosphorylation step in smooth muscle, an ATP molecule is also needed to energize the myosin cross-bridge for the development of force.

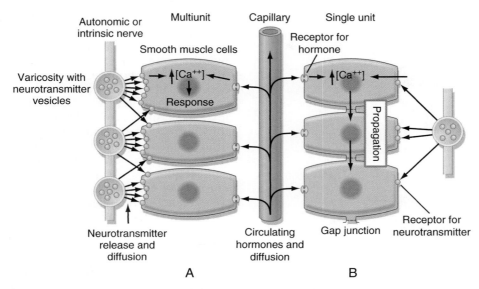

● **Figure 14-7.** Control systems of smooth muscle. Contraction (or inhibition of contraction) of smooth muscles can be initiated by (1) the intrinsic activity of pacemaker cells, (2) neurally released transmitters, or (3) circulating or locally generated hormones or signaling molecules. The combination of a neurotransmitter, hormone, or drug with specific receptors activates contraction by increasing cell Ca^{++}. The response of the cells depends on the concentration of the transmitters or hormones at the cell membrane and the nature of the receptors present. Hormone concentrations depend on diffusion distance, release, reuptake, and catabolism. Consequently, cells lacking close neuromuscular contacts will have a limited response to neural activity unless they are electrically coupled so that depolarization is transmitted from cell to cell. **A,** Multiunit smooth muscles resemble striated muscles in that there is no electrical coupling and neural regulation is important. **B,** Single-unit smooth muscles are like cardiac muscle, and electrical activity is propagated throughout the tissue. Most smooth muscles probably lie between the two ends of the single unit–multiunit spectrum.

● **Table 14-1.**
Modulation of Smooth Muscle Activity by Neurotransmitters, Hormones, and Local Factors

Agonist	Response	Receptor	Second Messenger
Norepinephrine and epinephrine from sympathetic stimulation	Contraction* (predominant) Relaxation[†]	α_1-AR β_2-AR	InsP3 cAMP
Acetylcholine from parasympathetic stimulation	Contraction[‡] (direct) Relaxation[‡] (indirect)	Muscarinic receptor on SMC Muscarinic receptor on EC	
Angiotensin II	Contraction[§]	AT-II receptor	InsP3
Vasopressin	Contraction[§]	Vasopressin receptor	InsP3
Endothelin	Contraction[§]	Endothelin receptor	InsP3
Adenosine	Relaxation[‖]	Adenosine receptor	cAMP

*The predominant effect of sympathetic stimulation is smooth muscle contraction caused by the abundance of α_1-AR relative to β_2-AR in smooth muscle.
[†]Activation of β_2-AR on smooth muscle modulates the degree of smooth muscle contraction during sympathetic stimulation. Therapeutic β_2-AR agonists are important for the relaxation of bronchial smooth muscle during asthmatic attacks.
[‡]Vascular smooth muscles are poorly innervated by the parasympathetic system. During vagal stimulation, however, acetylcholine (ACh) can become elevated in the coronary circulation and result in coronary relaxation (mediated by binding of ACh to endothelial cells). Note that this effect of ACh is indirect because binding of ACh to endothelial cells results in release of the smooth muscle relaxant nitric oxide from the endothelial cells. In regions of the coronary circulation with damaged endothelium, binding of ACh to coronary smooth muscle could promote contraction (vasospasm; direct effect).
[§]A variety of hormones can elevate InsP3 in smooth muscle and thereby result in smooth muscle contraction. Such hormones include angiotensin II, vasopressin, and endothelin, along with the neurotransmitters norepinephrine and acetylcholine. As noted above, however, each hormone/transmitter binds to a specific receptor type.
[‖]During periods of intense muscular activity, adenosine can be released from the working muscle, diffuse to the neighboring vasculature, and promote vasodilation. Thus, adenosine is acting as a local factor to increase blood flow to a specific region (i.e., working muscle).
AR, adrenergic receptor; EC, endothelial cell; InsP3, inositol 1,4,5-trisphosphate; SMC, smooth muscle cell.

Contraction of smooth muscle is thus said to be "thick filament regulated," which contrasts with the "thin filament regulation" of contraction of striated muscle, where binding of Ca^{++} to troponin exposes myosin binding sites on the actin thin filament. The thick filament regulation is attributable to the expression of a distinct myosin isoform in smooth muscle.

The myosin cross-bridge cycle in smooth muscle is similar to that in striated muscle in that after attachment to the actin filament, the cross-bridge undergoes a ratchet action in which the thin filament is pulled toward the center of the thick filament and force is generated. ADP and P_i are released from the myosin head at this time, thereby allowing ATP to bind. ATP

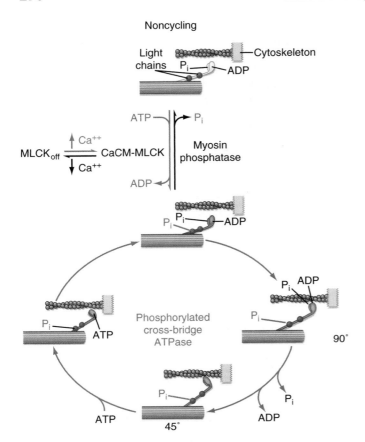

Noncycling

Light chains
Cytoskeleton
P_i
ADP

$ATP \longrightarrow P_i$

$MLCK_{off} \rightleftharpoons CaCM\text{-}MLCK$
$\uparrow Ca^{++}$
$\downarrow Ca^{++}$

Myosin phosphatase

ADP

P_i P_i ADP

P_i ADP $90°$

Phosphorylated cross-bridge ATPase

P_i ATP

P_i

P_i P_i

ATP $45°$ ADP

● **Figure 14-8.** Regulation of smooth muscle myosin interactions with actin by Ca^{++}-stimulated phosphorylation. In the relaxed state, cross-bridges are present as a high-energy myosin-ADP-P_i complex in the presence of ATP. Attachment to actin depends on phosphorylation of the cross-bridge by a Ca^{++}-calmodulin–dependent myosin light-chain kinase (MLCK). Phosphorylated cross-bridges cycle until they are dephosphorylated by myosin phosphatase. Note that cross-bridge phosphorylation at a specific site on a myosin regulatory light chain requires ATP in addition to that used in each cyclic interaction with actin.

ments in the sarcomere of striated muscle. A bipolar arrangement of myosin molecules within the thick filament is thought to allow the myosin cross-bridges to pull the actin filaments toward the center of the thick filament, thus contracting the smooth muscle and hence developing force.

From a structural standpoint, smooth muscle myosin is similar to striated muscle myosin in that they both contain a pair of heavy chains and two pairs of light chains. Despite this similarity, they represent different gene products and thus have different amino acid sequences. As noted, smooth muscle myosin, unlike skeletal muscle myosin, is unable to interact with the actin thin filament unless the regulatory light chain of myosin is phosphorylated. Moreover, the thin filament in smooth muscle lacks troponin, which plays a critical role in the thin filament regulation of contraction in striated muscle (see Chapter 12).

Although intracellular Ca^{++} is required for smooth muscle contraction, the sensitivity of contraction to Ca^{++} is variable. Several hormones/agonists, for example, increase the force of contraction at a given submaximal intracellular $[Ca^{++}]$, thereby resulting in **"Ca^{++} sensitization."** A basic mechanism contributing to Ca^{++} sensitization involves inhibition of MP and a resultant net increase in total myosin light-chain phosphorylation (and hence force) at a given submaximal $[Ca^{++}]$.

decreases the affinity of myosin for actin, which allows the release of myosin from actin. Energy from the newly bound ATP is then used to produce a conformational change in the myosin head (i.e., recocking the head) so that the cross-bridge is ready for another contraction cycle. The cross-bridge cycle continues as long as the myosin cross-bridge remains phosphorylated. Note that although the basic steps of the cross-bridge cycle appear to be the same for striated and smooth muscle, the kinetics of cross-bridge cycling is much slower for smooth muscle.

Cross-bridge cycling continues, with the hydrolysis of 1 ATP molecule per cycle, until myoplasmic $[Ca^{++}]$ falls. With the decrease in $[Ca^{++}]$, MLCK becomes inactive, and the cross-bridges are dephosphorylated by MP (Fig. 14-8).

As indicated in Figure 14-4, the thin filaments in smooth muscle are attached to dense bodies, and the myosin thick filaments appear to reside between two dense bodies and overlap a portion of the thin filaments, much like the overlap of thick and thin fila-

● AT THE CELLULAR LEVEL

Inhibition of MP underlies the phenomenon of Ca^{++} sensitization that occurs in response to activation of the monomeric G protein RhoA signaling cascade (Fig. 14-9). RhoA activates Rho kinase (ROK), which in turn inhibits MP by both direct and indirect mechanisms. Direct inhibition of MP by activated ROK involves ROK phosphorylation of the myosin-binding subunit (MBS) of MP. Indirect inhibition of MP by activated ROK involves phosphorylation of **CPI-17,** an endogenous 17-kDa protein, which then inhibits MP. Hormones/agonists such as catecholamines (acting on α_1-adrenergic receptors), vasopressin, endothelin, angiotensin, and muscarinic agonists increase the sensitivity of smooth muscle contraction to Ca^{++} through activation of RhoA/ROK signaling. ROK can also be activated by arachidonic acid and inhibited by Y-27632, a highly specific inhibitor (Fig. 14-9). Though not shown in Figure 14-9, inactive RhoA is typically located in the cytosol, bound to GDP and an inhibitory protein **(Rho-GDP dissociation inhibitor [GDI]).** Binding of agonist to various G-coupled receptors can activate RhoA by stimulating **guanine nucleotide exchange factor (GEF)** to yield RhoA-GTP, which localizes to the sarcolemma and activates ROK.

Hyperactivity of the RhoA/ROK signaling cascade has been implicated in various pathological conditions such as hypertension and vasospasm. Hyperactivity of RhoA/ROK in the vascular smooth muscle of hypertensive animals, for example, was manifested by increased levels of activated RhoA, up-regulation of ROK, enhancement of agonist-induced Ca^{++} sensitization of contraction, and a greater reduction in blood pressure by ROK inhibitors as compared with normotensive controls. A similar trend was observed in humans in that ROK inhibitors decreased forearm vascular resistance in hypertensive patients to a greater extent than in normotensive controls. ROK inhibitors have also been shown to reverse or prevent experimentally induced cerebral vasospasm and coronary vasospasm, as well as the associated up-regulation of RhoA/ROK and increased myosin light-chain phosphorylation. Hyperactivity of RhoA/ROK has additionally been implicated in bronchial asthma, erectile dysfunction, and preterm labor, as evidenced by the effects of ROK inhibitors. In addition, ROK inhibitors have decreased vascular smooth muscle proliferation and reduced restenosis after balloon angioplasty in rat carotid artery.

Phasic Versus Tonic Contraction

During a phasic contraction, myoplasmic $[Ca^{++}]$, cross-bridge phosphorylation, and force reach a peak and then return to baseline (Fig. 14-10). In contrast, during a tonic contraction, myoplasmic $[Ca^{++}]$ and cross-bridge phosphorylation decline after an initial spike but do not return to baseline levels. During this later phase, force slowly increases and is sustained at a high level (Fig. 14-10). This sustained force is maintained with only 20% to 30% of the cross-bridges phosphorylated, and thus ATP utilization is reduced. The term **"latch state"** refers to this condition of tonic contraction during which force is maintained at low energy expenditure.

The latch state is thought to reflect dephosphorylation of the myosin light chain (Fig. 14-11). When the myosin light chain is phosphorylated, the cross-bridges recycle as long as myoplasmic $[Ca^{++}]$ is elevated. However, if an attached cross-bridge is dephosphorylated by MP, the rate of cross-bridge recycling is decreased because detachment of cross-bridges is slower and the myosin light chain must be rephosphorylated before another cycle can begin. When myoplasmic $[Ca^{++}]$ is high, most of the cross-bridges will be phosphorylated (i.e., the MLCK-to-MP activity ratio is high), and shortening velocities or rates of force development will be relatively high. When myoplasmic $[Ca^{++}]$ falls during tonic contractions, the likelihood that a cross-bridge will be dephosphorylated and spend more time in an attached, force-generating conformation increases. However, a low rate of Ca^{++}-dependent phosphorylation of myosin light chains is essential for contraction. The muscle will relax if $[Ca^{++}]$ falls below that required for binding to calmodulin and activation of MLCK (about 0.1 μM).

Energetics and Metabolism

As already noted, ATP consumption is reduced during the latch state. Under this condition, smooth muscle

Inappropriate contraction of smooth muscle is associated with many pathological situations. One example is sustained vasospasm of a cerebral artery that develops several hours after a subarachnoid hemorrhage. It is thought that free radicals generated as a result of the hemorrhage raise myoplasmic $[Ca^{++}]$ in surrounding arterial smooth muscle cells. The rise in myoplasmic $[Ca^{++}]$ activates MLCK, which leads to cross-bridge phosphorylation and contraction. The vasoconstriction deprives other areas of the brain of oxygen and may lead to permanent injury or death of surrounding neurons. For a few days the cerebral artery remains sensitive to vasoactive agents, and therefore treatment with vasodilators may restore flow. An increase in ROK activity and MP phosphorylation has been observed during cerebral vasospasm. Administration of ROK inhibitors promotes relaxation of the vasospasm and decreases the level of myosin light-chain phosphorylation. The smooth muscle cells cease to respond to the vasodilators after several days, and they lose contractile proteins and secrete extracellular collagen. The lumen of the artery remains constricted as a result of structural and mechanical changes that do not involve active contraction.

uses 300-fold less ATP than would be required by skeletal muscle to generate the same force. Smooth muscle, like skeletal muscle, requires ATP for ion transport to maintain the resting membrane potential, sequester Ca^{++} in the SR, and extrude Ca^{++} from the cell. All these metabolic needs are readily met by oxidative phosphorylation. Fatigue of smooth muscle does not occur unless the cell is deprived of oxygen. However, aerobic glycolysis with lactic acid production normally supports membrane ion pumps even when oxygen is plentiful.

REGULATION OF MYOPLASMIC CALCIUM CONCENTRATION

The mechanisms that couple activation to contraction in smooth muscle involve two Ca^{++} sources: one involving the sarcolemma and the other involving the SR. The sarcolemma regulates Ca^{++} influx and efflux from the extracellular Ca^{++} pool. The SR membranes determine Ca^{++} movement between the myoplasm and the SR pool. Skeletal muscle contraction does not require extracellular Ca^{++} (see Chapter 12). In contrast, extracellular Ca^{++} is important for smooth muscle contraction. Thus, regulation of myoplasmic $[Ca^{++}]$ involves not only the SR but also the sarcolemma (Fig. 14-12). A number of factors can alter the myoplasmic $[Ca^{++}]$ of smooth muscle. This differs from skeletal muscle, in which action potential–induced release of Ca^{++} from the SR fully activates the contractile apparatus.

Sarcoplasmic Reticulum

The role of the smooth muscle SR in regulating myoplasmic $[Ca^{++}]$ is comparable to that of skeletal muscle. Stimulation of the cell opens SR Ca^{++} channels, and

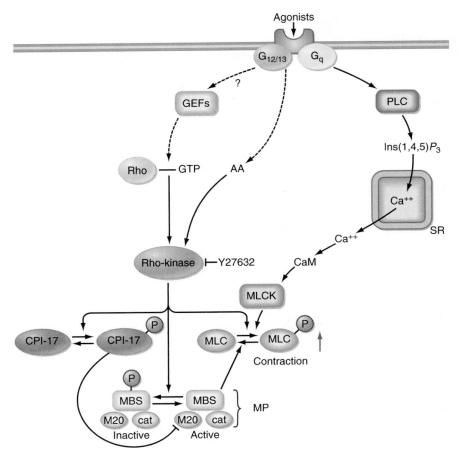

● **Figure 14-9.** RhoA/ROK signaling in smooth muscle. A variety of agonists of G-coupled receptors simultaneously stimulate InsP3 production and activate RhoA/ROK signaling. InsP3 is produced by phospholipase C (PLC)-mediated hydrolysis of PIP2. InsP3 increases intracellular [Ca^{++}] by opening InsP3-gated Ca^{++} channels in the SR, thereby resulting in Ca^{++}-calmodulin–dependent activation of myosin light-chain kinase (MLCK) and subsequent phosphorylation of the myosin regulatory light chain and promotion of actin-myosin interaction (contraction). Activated RhoA (depicted as Rho-GTP) stimulates Rho kinase (ROK), which inhibits myosin phosphatase (MP) by phosphorylating the myosin-binding subunit (MBS) of MP. ROK also inhibits MP indirectly by phosphorylating/activating CPI-17, a 17-kDa inhibitor of MP. The net effect of ROK phosphorylation is a decrease in MP activity, which results in an increased level of myosin light-chain phosphorylation and hence greater force of contraction at a given intracellular [Ca^{++}] (i.e., increased sensitivity of contraction to Ca^{++}). (From Fukata Y, Amano M, and Kaibuchi K: TRENDS in Pharmacol Sci 22:32–39, 2001.)

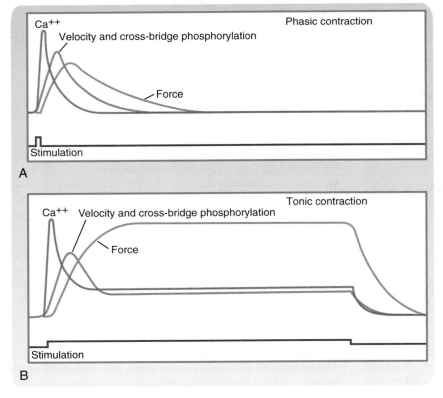

● **Figure 14-10.** Time course of events in cross-bridge activation and contraction in smooth muscle. **A,** A brief period of stimulation is associated with Ca^{++} mobilization, followed by cross-bridge phosphorylation and cycling to produce a brief phasic, twitch-like contraction. **B,** In a sustained tonic contraction produced by prolonged stimulation, the Ca^{++} and phosphorylation levels typically fall from an initial peak. Force is maintained during tonic contractions at a reduced [Ca^{++}] (and hence a low level of myosin light-chain phosphorylation), with lower cross-bridge cycling rates manifested by lower shortening velocities and ATP consumption.

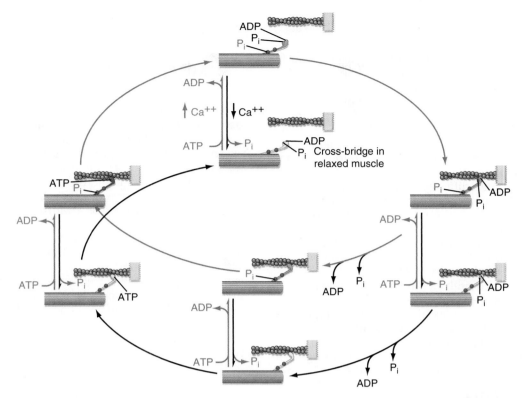

● **Figure 14-11.** Covalent regulation allows eight cross-bridge states in smooth muscle. Phosphorylation by MLCK *(vertical red arrows)* is obligatory for cross-bridge attachment. Phosphorylated cross-bridges cycle comparatively rapidly. Dephosphorylation of a cross-bridge during a cycle by a constitutively active MP *(vertical black arrows)* slows cycling rates and produces the latch state. Calcium regulates cross-bridge cycling by determining phosphorylation rates. Note that ATP is required for both regulation *(vertical arrows)* and cycling *(curved arrows)*.

● **Figure 14-12.** Principal mechanisms determining myoplasmic [Ca++] in smooth muscle. Release of calcium from the SR is a rapid initial event in activation, whereas both the SR and the sarcolemma participate in the subsequent stimulus-dependent regulation of myoplasmic [Ca++]. The sarcolemma integrates many simultaneous excitatory and inhibitory inputs to govern the cellular response. Higher-order regulatory mechanisms can alter the activity of various pumps, exchangers, or enzymes (the *asterisk* designates well-established instances). ATP, process requires ATP hydrolysis; CM, calmodulin; G, guanine nucleotide–binding proteins; IP$_3$, inositol 1,4,5-trisphosphate; MLCK, myosin light-chain kinase; PIP$_2$, phosphatidylinositol bisphosphate; PLC, phospholipase C.

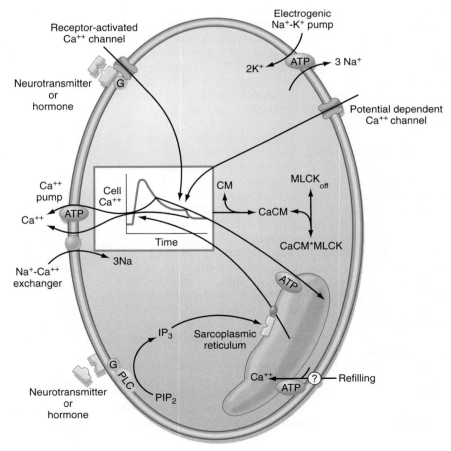

myoplasmic [Ca^{++}] increases rapidly. This release is not linked to voltage sensors, as is the case in skeletal muscle, but to binding of the second messenger InsP3 to receptors in the SR. InsP3 is generated by a stimulus that acts on sarcolemmal receptors that are coupled via a guanine nucleotide–binding protein (G protein) to activate phospholipase C (PLC) (see Chapter 3). PLC hydrolyzes the membrane phospholipid phosphatidylinositol bisphosphate (PIP2) into InsP3 and diacylglycerol. InsP3 then diffuses to the SR and opens the InsP3-gated Ca^{++} channel, thereby resulting in release of Ca^{++} from the SR into the myoplasm. This complex process may permit graded release of Ca^{++} from the SR and also enable many different neurotransmitters and hormones to effect smooth muscle contraction. Calcium is reaccumulated by the SR through the activity of the SERCA, although as indicated later, extrusion of Ca^{++} from the smooth muscle cell also contributes to the reduction in myoplasmic [Ca^{++}]. Refilling of the SR with Ca^{++} not only involves reaccumulation of cytosolic Ca^{++} but also depends on the extracellular [Ca^{++}]. The dependence on extracellular [Ca^{++}] is thought to reflect the operation of a **"store-operated"** Ca^{++} channel present in the sarcolemma at points near underlying SR called **"junctional SR."**

A variety of hormones and neurotransmitters elevate myoplasmic [Ca^{++}] by stimulating InsP3 production. Vascular smooth muscle, for example, is innervated by sympathetic fibers of the autonomic nervous system. These fibers use norepinephrine as a neurotransmitter, which when released binds to α_1-adrenergic receptors on vascular smooth muscle cells and results in G protein–dependent activation of PLC. Activation of PLC results in the production of InsP3, which activates the InsP3-gated Ca^{++} channel in the SR, thereby elevating myoplasmic [Ca^{++}] and causing vasoconstriction. Other agents that promote vasoconstriction by activating the InsP3 cascade include angiotensin II and vasopressin. The development of drugs that block the production of angiotensin II (e.g., angiotensin-converting enzyme [ACE] inhibitors) provides a means of promoting vasodilation that is important for individuals with hypertension or congestive heart failure. As mentioned previously, a variety of agents can produce contraction of smooth muscle without altering membrane potential (i.e., pharmacomechanical coupling). Agonist-induced activation of the InsP3 cascade represents an example of pharmacomechanical coupling. Many of the hormones/agonists that activate PLC through G protein–coupled receptors also promote sarcolemmal Ca^{++} influx and activation of RhoA/ROK. The net effect is a rise in intracellular [Ca^{++}], which activates MLCK, concomitant with a rise in ROK activity, which inhibits MP, both of which act complementarily to promote net myosin light-chain phosphorylation.

In addition to the InsP3 receptor, the SR also contains the Ca^{++}-gated Ca^{++} channel, also called the RYR, which may be activated during periods of Ca^{++} influx through the sarcolemma. Short-lived, spontaneous opening of the RYR resulting in localized elevations in myoplasmic [Ca^{++}] occurs in many cells, including

AT THE CELLULAR LEVEL

Calcium sparks have also been observed to occur in smooth muscle in the presence of an **endothelial-dependent hyperpolarization factor (EDHF)** (Fig. 14-13). Specifically, EDHF appears to be an arachidonic acid metabolite (e.g., **epoxyeicosatrienoic acid [EET]**) that is produced by endothelial cells in response to various stimuli and then released to the underlying vascular smooth muscle. EET has been shown to activate a **transient receptor channel** (e.g., **TRPV4**) in the sarcolemma of smooth muscle that leads to the influx of Ca^{++}, which then opens RYR channels in the SR and results in Ca^{++} sparks. The Ca^{++} sparks in turn activate a large-conductance K$^+$ channel in the sarcolemma (BK$_{Ca}$), and the smooth muscle cell becomes hyperpolarized. Hyperpolarization in turn decreases basal Ca^{++} influx through voltage-gated Ca^{++} channels in the smooth muscle, thereby decreasing intracellular [Ca^{++}] and hence relaxing the smooth muscle, as described earlier.

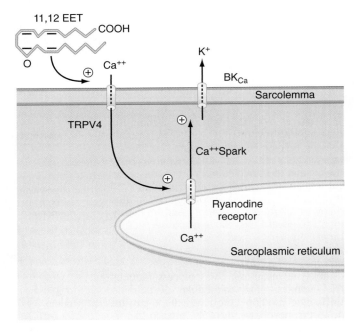

● **Figure 14-13.** An arachidonic acid metabolite (11,12-epoxyeicosatrienoic acid [11,12 EET]) released from endothelial cells can open the transient receptor channel TRPV4 in the underlying smooth muscle to permit the influx of Ca^{++}, which in turn initiates brief openings of the SR ryanodine receptor (Ca^{++} sparks) localized near the sarcolemma. Opening of Ca^{++}-activated K$^+$ channels in the sarcolemma by calcium sparks results in hyperpolarization of the smooth muscle and hence vasodilation. (From Earley S, Heppner T, Nelson M, and Brayden J: Circ Res 97:1270–1279, 2005.)

smooth muscle. When observed with Ca^{++}-sensitive fluorescent dyes, these spontaneous localized elevations in myoplasmic [Ca^{++}] produce brief light flashes and as a result are named **"Ca^{++} sparks."** In smooth muscle, an increase in cAMP has been associated with an increase in the frequency of Ca^{++} sparks, particularly in situations in which the SR is in close proximity to the sarcolemma (i.e., junctional SR, perhaps near caveolae). An increase in the frequency of these sparks hyperpolarizes vascular smooth muscle by activation of a large-conductance Ca^{++}-gated K^+ channel in the sarcolemma. This hyperpolarization then decreases overall myoplasmic $[Ca^{++}]$, and relaxation occurs.

Sarcolemma

Calcium is extruded from the smooth muscle cell by the activity of sarcolemmal Ca^{++}-ATPase and by a $3Na^+$-$1Ca^{++}$ antiporter (i.e., 3 Na^+ ions enter the cell for each Ca^{++} ion extruded). Extrusion of Ca^{++} from the cell competes with sequestration of Ca^{++} in the SR by SERCA and thus reduces the accumulation of Ca^{++} in the SR. It is thought that a decrease in SR $[Ca^{++}]$ results in the release of a **calcium influx factor (CIF)** from the SR, which then activates a **"store-operated"** Ca^{++} channel in the sarcolemma near the junctional SR and allows the SR to completely refill with Ca^{++} from the extracellular fluid. The identity of this CIF and the identity of the store-operated Ca^{++} channel are not yet known. Nevertheless, it is clear that sustained contraction of smooth muscle requires extracellular Ca^{++}. It has been proposed that Ca^{++} refilling may occur in the confined space between the caveolae and peripheral SR of smooth muscle.

In addition to the stimulatory effects of various agents on sarcolemma Ca^{++} channels and InsP3 cascades, there are several inhibitory factors that lower myoplasmic $[Ca^{++}]$ and thereby relax smooth muscle. For example, the dihydropyridine class of Ca^{++} channel blocking drugs decreases the influx of Ca^{++} through sarcolemmal L-type voltage-gated Ca^{++} channels and reduces vasomotor tone. Similarly, drugs that open K^+ channels in the sarcolemma (e.g., hydralazine) promote relaxation (e.g., vasodilation) by hyperpolarizing the membrane potential, which reduces the influx of Ca^{++} through voltage-gated Ca^{++} channels. Conversely, agents that decrease K^+ permeability of the sarcolemma may promote vasoconstriction by inducing membrane depolarization, which then increases influx of Ca^{++} through these same voltage-gated Ca^{++} channels. Smooth muscle also contains receptor-activated Ca^{++} channels. Conductance of these receptor-activated Ca^{++} channels is linked to receptor occupancy.

A variety of drugs and hormones relax smooth muscle by increasing the cellular concentrations of cAMP or cGMP. Nitric oxide (NO) is produced by nerves and vascular endothelial cells, and it relaxes smooth muscle by increasing cGMP. Acetylcholine released from parasympathetic fibers causes vasodilation in some vascular beds as a result of stimulating the production of NO by vascular endothelial cells. The molecular mechanism or mechanisms underlying the cGMP-dependent relaxation of vascular smooth muscle are complex and may involve activation of a myosin light-chain phosphatase, as well as a reduction in intracellular $[Ca^{++}]$, through stimulation of Ca^{++} pumps in the sarcolemma or SR, or both. Similarly, elevation of cAMP in vascular smooth muscle by stimulation of β-adrenergic receptors or activation of adenosine receptors promotes vasodilation through cAMP-dependent phosphorylation. In particular, cAMP-dependent phosphorylation of MLCK has been proposed to attenuate the Ca^{++}-dependent increase in MLCK activity, thereby reducing the ability of MLCK to phosphorylate the regulatory light chain of myosin, although cAMP-dependent relaxation also appears to involve a reduction in intracellular $[Ca^{++}]$. cAMP, for example, has been shown to increase the frequency of Ca^{++} sparks in smooth muscle, which as described earlier, hyperpolarizes the membrane potential by activation of Ca^{++}-gated K^+ channels, thereby reducing the influx of Ca^{++} through voltage-gated Ca^{++} channels. Relaxation of smooth muscle by elevation of cAMP has afforded asthmatics a means of reversing bronchiolar constriction through the use of β$_2$-adrenergic agonists. The local vasodilatory effect of adenosine produced in working muscle during periods of intense exercise has also been attributed, at least in part, to elevated cAMP levels in vascular smooth muscle secondary to adenosine-induced stimulation of purinergic receptors on the sarcolemma of vascular smooth muscle. Adenosine may also activate a sarcolemmal K^+ channel to induce membrane hyperpolarization, which as already noted will decrease the influx of Ca^{++} through voltage-gated Ca^{++} channels and cause vasodilation. Thus, regulation of smooth muscle tone may be under the influence of not only the autonomic nervous system and circulating hormones but also neighboring endothelial cells and skeletal muscle cells via diffusible substances such as NO and adenosine.

DEVELOPMENT AND HYPERTROPHY

During development and growth, the number of smooth muscle cells increases (Fig. 14-14). Smooth muscle tissue mass also increases if an organ is subjected to a sustained increase in mechanical work. This increase in mass is called **compensatory hypertrophy.** A striking example occurs with arterial smooth muscle cells (i.e., in the tunica media of the artery) in hypertensive patients. The increased mechanical load on the muscle cells appears to be the common factor that induces this hypertrophy. Chromosomal replication can result in significant numbers of polyploid muscle cells. The polyploid cells contain multiple sets of the normal number of chromosomes. They synthesize more contractile proteins and thus increase the size of the cell (Fig. 14-14).

The myometrium, which is the smooth muscle component of the uterus, undergoes hypertrophy as parturition (birth) approaches. Hormones play an important role in this response. The smooth muscle is quiescent during pregnancy when the hormone progesterone predominates, and few gap junctions that electrically couple the smooth muscle cells are present. At term, under the dominant influence of estrogen, the myometrium undergoes marked

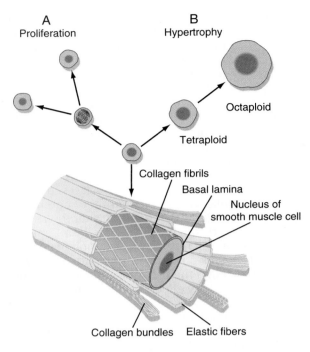

A
Proliferation

B
Hypertrophy

Octaploid

Tetraploid

Collagen fibrils

Basal lamina

Nucleus of
smooth muscle cell

Collagen bundles   Elastic fibers

Protein synthesis and secretion

C

● **Figure 14-14.** Smooth muscle cells carry out many activities. **A,** They retain the capacity to divide during normal growth or in certain pathological responses such as the formation of atherosclerotic plaque. **B,** Cells may also hypertrophy in response to increased loads. Chromosomal replication, not followed by cell division, yields cells with a greater content of contractile proteins. **C,** Smooth muscle cells also synthesize and secrete the constituents of the extracellular matrix.

hypertrophy. Large numbers of gap junctions form just before birth and convert the myometrium to a single-unit tissue to coordinate contraction during parturition.

SYNTHETIC AND SECRETORY FUNCTIONS

The growth and development of tissues that contain smooth muscle are associated with increases in the connective tissue matrix. Smooth muscle cells can synthesize and secrete the materials that make up this matrix, including collagen, elastin, and proteoglycans (Fig. 14-14). The synthetic and secretory capacities are evident when smooth muscle cells are isolated and placed in tissue culture. The cells rapidly lose thick myosin filaments and much of the thin filament lattice, and there is expansion of the rough endoplasmic reticulum and Golgi apparatus. The phenotypically altered cells multiply and lay down connective tissue. This process is reversible, and some degree of redifferentiation with the formation of thick filaments occurs after cell replication ceases. Determinants of the smooth muscle cell phenotype are largely unknown, but hormones and growth factors in blood, as well as mechanical loads on cells, have been implicated in the control of phenotypic modulation.

> ### ► IN THE CLINIC
>
> **Atherosclerosis** is a disease characterized by lesions located in the wall of blood vessels. The lesions are induced by disorders that injure the endothelium, such as hypertension, diabetes, and smoking. Three formed elements (monocytes, T lymphocytes, and platelets) that circulate in the bloodstream act on the damaged vascular endothelium. There, they generate chemotactic factors and mitogens that modify the structure of the surrounding smooth muscle cells. The latter lose most of their thick and thin filaments and develop an extensive rough endoplasmic reticulum and Golgi complex. These cells migrate to the subendothelial space (i.e., the tunica media of the artery), proliferate, and participate in formation of the fatty lesions or the fibrous plaques that characterize atherosclerosis. Inhibition or down-regulation of Rho kinase (ROK) has been shown to promote the regression of atherosclerotic-like lesions in an animal model. The mechanism or mechanisms underlying this beneficial effect of ROK inhibition are unclear but may be related to the regulation of both endothelial permeability and monocyte migration by ROK. That is, hyperactivity of ROK has been implicated in various pathological conditions, including increased transendothelial permeability (perhaps secondary to increased actomyosin activity), whereas inhibition of ROK has been shown to decrease transendothelial migration of monocytes and neutrophils.

> ### ► IN THE CLINIC
>
> Although smooth muscle is involved in physiological adjustments to exercise, sustained changes in the mechanical loading that induce cellular adaptations are usually the result of a pathological condition (e.g., hypertension). A fairly common example in men is **urinary bladder hypertrophy** caused by benign or cancerous enlargement of the prostate gland, which obstructs the bladder outlet. The clinical result is difficulty urinating, distention of the bladder, and impaired emptying. In this situation, the ability of the bladder smooth muscle to contract and develop stress is diminished. The reasons for this remain unexplained, but phenotypic modulation of the smooth muscle cells with altered contractile protein isoform expression and gross anatomic distortion of the bladder wall occurs. Neuromuscular changes also affect myoplasmic Ca^{++} mobilization and cross-bridge phosphorylation. Fortunately, normal structure and function are usually restored after the obstruction is alleviated.

BIOPHYSICAL PROPERTIES OF SMOOTH MUSCLE

Length-Tension Relationship

Smooth muscle contains large amounts of connective tissue composed of **extensible elastin fibrils** and **inextensible collagen fibrils.** Because this extracellular matrix can withstand high distending forces or loads, it is responsible for the passive length-tension curve measured in relaxed tissues. This ability of the matrix also limits organ volume.

When lengths are normalized to the optimal length for the development of force (i.e., L_0), the **length-tension curves** for smooth and skeletal muscle are very similar (Fig. 14-15; see also Chapter 12). However, the length-tension curves of striated and smooth muscle differ quantitatively. For example, smooth muscle cells shorten more than skeletal muscle cells do. In addition, smooth muscle is characteristically only partially activated, and the peak isometric force attained varies with the stimulus. In skeletal muscle, the stimulus (i.e., action potential) always produces a full twitch contraction. Smooth muscle can generate active force comparable to that of skeletal muscle, even though smooth muscle contains only about a fourth as much myosin. This does not imply that the cross-bridges in smooth muscle have greater force-generating capacity. Instead, active cross-bridges in smooth muscle are much more likely to be in the attached, force-generating configuration because of their slow cycling kinetics.

Smooth muscle has the unique ability to shift the length-tension curve, depending on the resting length. Thus, if the smooth muscle is stretched, the length-tension curve will shift to longer lengths over the course of tens of minutes to hours (see Fig. 14-15, *B*). Similarly, if the smooth muscle is allowed to return to a shorter resting length, the length-tension relationship will shift to the left, again over a period of tens of minutes to hours, depending on the stimulation frequency. This unusual property of smooth muscle is termed **"length adaptation."** The molecular basis for this change in the length-tension relationship depending on the resting length of the muscle is thought to involve an alteration in the number of contractile units in series (see Fig. 14-15, *C*).

Force-Velocity Relationship

Smooth and striated muscles both exhibit a hyperbolic dependence of shortening velocity on load. However, contraction velocities are far slower in smooth muscle than in striated muscle. One factor that underlies these slow velocities is that the myosin isoform in smooth muscle cells has low ATPase activity.

Skeletal muscle cells have a **force-velocity curve** in which shortening velocities are determined only by load and the myosin isoform (see Chapter 12). In contrast, both force and shortening velocity, which reflect the number of cycling cross-bridges and their cycling rates, vary in smooth muscle. When activation of smooth muscle is altered, for example, by different frequencies of nerve stimulation or changing hormone

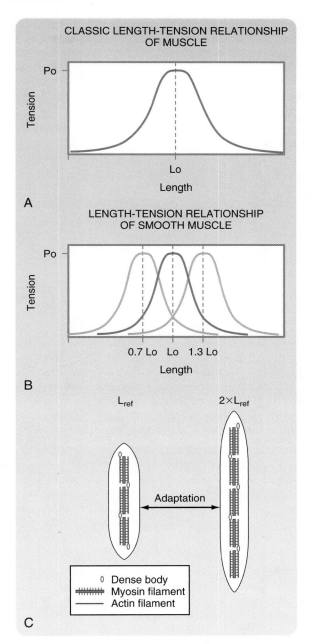

● **Figure 14-15.** Length adaptation of smooth muscle. Both skeletal muscle **(A)** and smooth muscle **(B)** exhibit a bell-shaped length-tension relationship, although the length-tension relationship of smooth muscle can vary. Within a short period after stretching smooth muscle, there is a rightward shift in the length-tension relationship such that maximal force generation occurs at a longer muscle length **(B)**. Likewise, within a brief time after shortening of a smooth muscle, there is a leftward shift in the length-tension relationship **(B)**. The mechanism or mechanisms underlying this length adaptation are hypothesized to reflect a change in the number of contractile units in series **(C)**. (Redrawn from Fust A, and Stephens, N.L.: Can J Physiol Pharmacol 83:865–868, 2005.)

concentrations, a "family" of velocity-stress curves can be derived (Fig. 14-16). This implies that both cross-bridge cycling rates and the number of active cross-bridges in smooth muscle are regulated in some

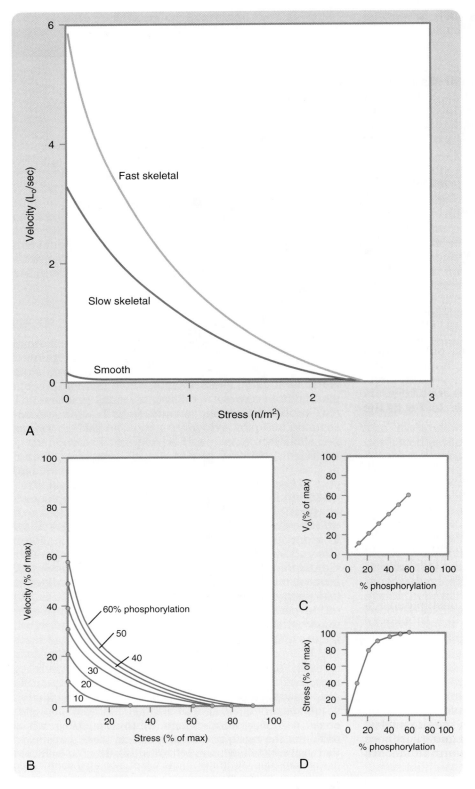

● **Figure 14-16. A,** Force-velocity curves for fast and slow human skeletal muscle cells and smooth muscle. **B,** Smooth muscles have variable force-velocity relationships that are determined by the level of Ca++-stimulated cross-bridge phosphorylation. **C,** Maximal shortening velocities with no load (intercepts on the ordinate in **B**) are directly dependent on cross-bridge phosphorylation by MLCK. **D,** Active force/stress (abscissa intercepts in **B**) rises rapidly with phosphorylation and, near maximal stress, may be generated with only 20% to 30% of the cross-bridges in the phosphorylated state.

way, which is in marked contrast to striated muscle. This difference is conferred by a regulatory system that depends on the phosphorylation of cross-bridges, which in turn depends on myoplasmic [Ca++]. Because myosin light-chain phosphorylation is required for actin-myosin interaction in smooth muscle, a depen-

dence of maximal force on the degree of myosin phosphorylation is expected (i.e., phosphorylation of more myosin molecules results in more actin-myosin interactions and hence more force generated). The variation in maximal shortening velocity as a function of the degree of myosin phosphorylation may reflect dephosphorylation of the myosin light chain while the myosin is still attached to the actin, thus slowing the rate of detachment (i.e., latch state) at low levels of phosphorylation. At higher levels of phosphorylation, the likelihood of latch states would be reduced and the myosin cross-bridges would be released more quickly from actin, thereby yielding a higher shortening velocity at all loads (see Fig. 14-16B).

■ KEY CONCEPTS

1. Smooth muscle cells are linked by a variety of junctions that serve both mechanical and communication roles. These linkages are essential in cells that must contract uniformly.

2. The sarcolemma plays an important role in Ca^{++} exchange between the extracellular fluid and the myoplasm. The sarcolemma of smooth muscle contains numerous caveolae that contribute to the regulation of intracellular [Ca^{++}] and also appear to serve as a scaffold for signaling molecules. The SR contains an intracellular Ca^{++} pool that can be mobilized to transiently increase myoplasmic [Ca^{++}]. Myoplasmic [Ca^{++}] is dependent on extracellular Ca^{++}. Transporters in the sarcolemma that regulate myoplasmic [Ca^{++}] include receptor-mediated Ca^{++} channels, voltage-gated Ca^{++} channels, Ca^{++}-ATPase, and the $3Na^+$-$1Ca^{++}$ antiporter. The SR also regulates myoplasmic [Ca^{++}]. The Ca^{++} channels in the SR open in response to a chemical. Neurotransmitters or hormones that act via receptors in the sarcolemma can activate PLC, followed by generation of the second messenger InsP3. InsP3 then activates InsP3-gated Ca^{++} channels on the SR. Many agonists that activate PLC through G protein–coupled receptors also activate the RhoA/ROK signaling cascade, thereby increasing the sensitivity of smooth muscle contraction to Ca^{++}. Smooth muscle SR also contains Ca^{++}-gated Ca^{++} channels (RYR). Ca^{++} reaccumulates in the SR via SERCA.

3. Smooth muscles contain contractile units that consist of small groups of thick myosin filaments that interdigitate with large numbers of thin filaments attached to Z line equivalents termed dense bodies or membrane-dense areas. No striations are evident. Contraction is caused by a sliding filament–cross-bridge mechanism.

4. Contraction of smooth muscle is dependent on both release of Ca^{++} from the SR and entry of Ca^{++} across the sarcolemma. Smooth muscle lacks tro-ponin. Phosphorylation of cross-bridges by a Ca^{++}-dependent MLCK is necessary for attachment to the thin filament. Dephosphorylation of an attached cross-bridge by MP slows its cycling rates. Higher myoplasmic [Ca^{++}] increases the ratio of MLCK to MP activity, with the result that more of the cross-bridges remain phosphorylated throughout a cycle. This increases shortening velocities.

5. Smooth muscle activity is controlled by nerves (principally autonomic), circulating hormones, locally generated signaling substances, junctions with other smooth muscle cells, and even junctions with other non–smooth muscle cells. A variety of hormones/agonists increase the sensitivity of smooth muscle contraction to Ca^{++} by reducing the activity of MP. Activation of the RhoA/ROK signaling cascade contributes to this inhibition of MP and hence to the increase in sensitivity of smooth muscle contraction to Ca^{++}.

6. The response to sustained or tonic stimulation is a rapid contraction followed by sustained maintenance of force with reduced cross-bridge cycling rates and ATP consumption. This behavior, called the latch state, is advantageous for muscles that may need to withstand continuous external force, such as blood vessels, which must be able to withstand blood pressure. During the latch state, ATP is consumed at less than $\frac{1}{300}$ the rate needed to maintain the same force in skeletal muscle.

7. The length-tension relationships, hyperbolic velocity-load relationships, power output curves, and ability to resist imposed loads are comparable to those of skeletal muscle. Shortening velocities and ATP consumption rates are very low in smooth muscle, in keeping with expression of a myosin isoform with low activity. Uniquely, smooth muscle has the ability to adjust the length-tension relationship when chronically stretched or shortened, a process termed "length adaptation." Smooth muscles also have the unusual ability to alter velocity-stress relationships, which reflects regulation of both the number of active cross-bridges (determining force) and their average cycling rates for a given load (determining velocity).

8. Smooth muscle is also a synthetic and secretory cell with a major role in formation of the extensive extracellular matrix that surrounds and links the cells. Cellular hypertrophy occurs in response to physiological needs, and smooth muscle cells retain the potential to divide.

THE CARDIOVASCULAR SYSTEM

Achilles J. Pappano

CHAPTER 15

Overview of Circulation

The circulatory system transports and distributes essential substances to tissues and removes metabolic byproducts. This system also participates in homeostatic mechanisms such as regulation of body temperature, maintenance of fluid balance, and adjustment of O_2 and nutrient supply under various physiological states. The cardiovascular system that accomplishes these tasks is composed of a pump (the heart), a series of distributing and collecting tubes (blood vessels), and an extensive system of thin vessels (capillaries) that permit rapid exchange between the tissues and vascular channels. Blood vessels throughout the body are filled with a heterogeneous fluid (blood) that is essential for the transport processes performed by the heart and blood vessels. This chapter is a general, functional overview of the heart and blood vessels, whose functions are analyzed in much greater detail in subsequent chapters.

THE HEART

The heart consists of two pumps in series: one pump propels blood through the lungs for exchange of O_2 and CO_2 (the **pulmonary circulation**) and the other pump propels blood to all other tissues of the body (the **systemic circulation**). Flow of blood through the heart is one way (unidirectional). Unidirectional flow through the heart is achieved by the appropriate arrangement of flap valves. Although cardiac output is intermittent, continuous flow to body tissues (periphery) occurs by distention of the aorta and its branches during ventricular contraction **(systole)** and by elastic recoil of the walls of the large arteries with forward propulsion of the blood during ventricular relaxation **(diastole).**

THE CARDIOVASCULAR CIRCUIT

In the normal intact circulation the total volume of blood is constant, and an increase in the volume of blood in one area must be accompanied by a decrease in another. However, the distribution of blood circulating to the different regions of the body is determined by the output of the left ventricle and by the contractile state of the resistance vessels (arterioles) of these

regions. The circulatory system is composed of conduits arranged in series and in parallel (Fig. 15-1). This arrangement, which is discussed in subsequent chapters, has important implications in terms of resistance, flow, and pressure in blood vessels.

Blood entering the right ventricle via the right atrium is pumped through the pulmonary arterial system at a mean pressure about one seventh that in the systemic arteries. The blood then passes through the lung capillaries, where CO_2 in the blood is released and O_2 is taken up. The O_2-rich blood returns via the pulmonary veins to the left atrium, where it is pumped from the ventricle to the periphery, thus completing the cycle.

BLOOD VESSELS

Blood moves rapidly through the aorta and its arterial branches. These branches narrow and their walls become thinner as they approach the periphery. They also change histologically. The aorta is a predominantly elastic structure, but the peripheral arteries become more muscular until at the arterioles, the muscular layer predominates (Fig. 15-2).

In the large arteries, frictional resistance is relatively small and pressures are only slightly less than in the aorta. The small arteries, on the other hand, offer moderate resistance to blood flow. This resistance reaches a maximal level in the arterioles, which are sometimes referred to as the stopcocks of the vascular system. Hence, the pressure drop is greatest across the terminal segment of the small arteries and the arterioles (Fig. 15-3). Adjustment in the degree of contraction of the circular muscle of these small vessels permits regulation of tissue blood flow and aids in the control of arterial blood pressure.

In addition to the reduction in pressure along the arterioles, there is a change from pulsatile to steady blood flow (Fig. 15-3). Pulsatile arterial blood flow, caused by the intermittent ejection of blood from the heart, is damped at the capillary level by a combination of two factors: distensibility of the large arteries and frictional resistance in the small arteries and arterioles.

Many capillaries arise from each arteriole. The total cross-sectional area of the capillary bed is very large despite the fact that the cross-sectional area of each

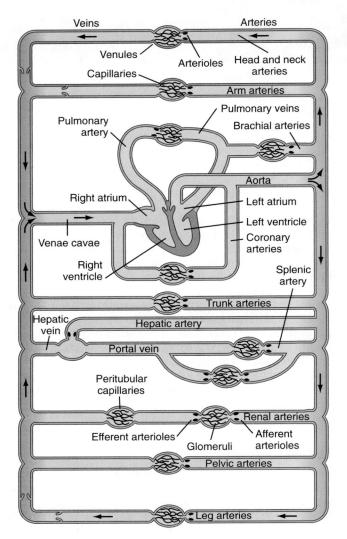

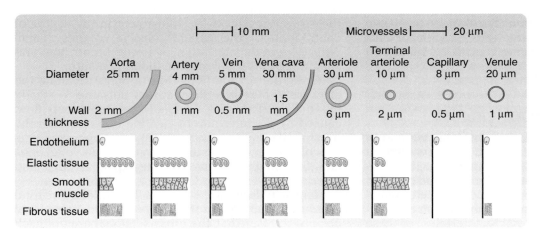

● **Figure 15-1.** Schematic diagram of the parallel and series arrangement of the vessels composing the circulatory system. The capillary beds are represented by thin lines connecting the arteries (on the right) with the veins (on the left). The crescent-shaped thickenings proximal to the capillary beds represent the arterioles (resistance vessels). (Redrawn from Green HD: In Glasser O [ed]: Medical Physics, vol 1. Chicago, Year Book, 1944.)

capillary is less than that of each arteriole. As a result, blood flow velocity becomes quite slow in the capillaries (Fig. 15-3), analogous to the decrease in velocity of flow in the wide regions of a river. Conditions in the capillaries are ideal for the exchange of diffusible substances between blood and tissue because capillaries consist of short tubes with walls that are only one cell thick and flow velocity is low.

On its return to the heart from the capillaries, blood passes through venules and then through veins of increasing size. Pressure within these vessels progressively decreases until the blood reaches the right atrium (Fig. 15-3). Near the heart, the number of veins decreases, the thickness and composition of the vein walls change (Fig. 15-2), the total cross-sectional area of the venous channels diminishes, and the velocity of blood flow increases (Fig. 15-3). Note that the velocity of blood flow and the cross-sectional area at each level of the vasculature are essentially mirror images (Fig. 15-3).

Data from a 20-kg dog (Table 15-1) indicate that between the aorta and the capillaries the number of vessels increases about 3 billion–fold and the total cross-sectional area increases about 500-fold. The volume of blood in the systemic vascular system is greatest in the veins and venules (67%). Only 5% of total blood volume exists in the capillaries, and 11% of total blood volume is found in the aorta, arteries, and arterioles. In contrast, blood volume in the pulmonary vascular bed is about equally divided among the arterial, capillary, and venous vessels. The cross-sectional area of the venae cavae is larger than that of the

▶ IN THE CLINIC

In a patient with hyperthyroidism **(Graves' disease),** basal metabolism is elevated and often associated with arteriolar vasodilation. This reduction in arteriolar resistance diminishes the damping effect on pulsatile arterial pressure and is manifested as pulsatile flow in the capillaries, as observed in the fingernail bed of patients with this ailment.

● **Figure 15-2.** Internal diameter, wall thickness, and relative amounts of the principal components of the vessel walls of the various blood vessels that compose the circulatory system. Cross sections of the vessels are not drawn to scale because of the huge range from aorta and venae cavae to capillary. (Redrawn from Burton AC: Physiol Rev 34:619, 1945.)

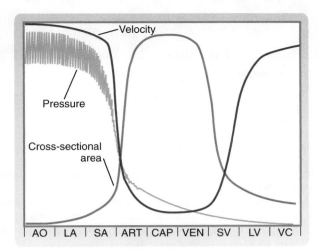

● Figure 15-3. Phasic pressure, velocity of flow, and cross-sectional area of the systemic circulation. The important features are the inverse relationship between velocity and cross-sectional area, the major pressure drop across the small arteries and arterioles, and the maximal cross-sectional area and minimal flow rate in the capillaries. AO, aorta; ART, arterioles; CAP, capillaries; LA, large arteries; LV, large veins; SA, small arteries; SV, small veins; VC, venae cavae; VEN, venules.

● Table 15-1.
Vascular Dimensions in a 20-kg Dog

Vessels	Number	Total Cross-Sectional Area (cm²)	Total Blood Volume (%)
Systemic			
Aorta	1	2.8	
Arteries	40 to 110,000	40	11
Arterioles	2.8×10^6	55	
Capillaries	2.7×10^9	1357	5
Venules	1×10^7	785	
Veins	110 to 660,000	631	67
Venae cavae	2	3.1	
Pulmonary			
Arteries and arterioles	$1\text{-}1.5 \times 10^6$	137	3
Capillaries	2.7×10^9	1357	4
Venules and veins	2×10^6 to 4	210	5
Heart			
Atria	2		5
Ventricles	2		

Data from Milnor WR: Hemodynamics. Baltimore, Williams & Wilkins, 1982.

aorta. Therefore, the velocity of flow is slower in the venae cavae than in the aorta (Fig. 15-3).

■ KEY CONCEPTS

1. The circulatory system consists of a pump (the heart), a series of distributing and collecting tubes (blood vessels), and an extensive system of thin vessels (capillaries) that permit rapid exchange of substances between tissues and blood.

2. Pulsatile pressure is progressively damped by the elasticity of the arterial walls and the frictional resistance of the small arteries and arterioles such that capillary blood flow is essentially nonpulsatile. The greatest resistance to blood flow and hence the greatest pressure drop in the arterial system occurs at the level of the small arteries and arterioles.

3. The velocity of blood flow is inversely related to the cross-sectional area at any point along the vascular system.

CHAPTER 16

Elements of Cardiac Function

ELECTRICAL PROPERTIES OF THE HEART

The cells of the heart, like neurons, are excitable and generate action potentials. These action potentials initiate contraction and thus determine the heart rate. Disorders in electrical activity can induce serious and sometimes lethal disturbances in cardiac rhythm.

In this section the electrical properties of cardiac cells are described. In addition, how these electrical properties account for the **electrocardiogram (ECG)** is considered. The initiation of contraction as a result of the electrical properties of cardiac cells is considered in a later section.

The Cardiac Action Potential

Figure 16-1 illustrates action potentials found in different cardiac cells. Two main types of action potentials occur in the heart and are shown. One type, the fast response, occurs in normal atrial and ventricular myocytes and in the specialized conducting fibers (Purkinje fibers of the heart) and is divided into five phases. The rapid upstroke of the action potential is designated phase 0. The upstroke is followed by a brief period of partial, early repolarization (phase 1) and then by a plateau (phase 2) that persists for about 0.1 to 0.2 second. The membrane then repolarizes (phase 3) until the resting state of polarization (phase 4) is again attained (at point e). Final repolarization (phase 3) develops more slowly than depolarization (phase 0). The other type of action potential, the slow response, occurs in the **sinoatrial (SA) node,** which is the natural pacemaker region of the heart, and in the **atrioventricular (AV) node,** which is the specialized tissue that conducts the cardiac impulse from the atria to the ventricles. The slow-response cells lack the early repolarization phase (phase 1). Other differences between the electrical properties of the fast-response and slow-response cells include the following. The resting membrane potential (phase 4) of the fast-response cells is considerably more negative than that of the slow-response cells. Moreover, the slope of the upstroke (phase 0), the amplitude of the action potential, and the overshoot are greater in the fast-response than in the slow-response cells. The action potential amplitude and the steepness of the upstroke are important determinants of propagation velocity along the myocardial fibers. In slow-response cardiac tissue, the action potential is propagated more slowly and conduction is more likely to be blocked than in fast-response cardiac tissue. Slow conduction and a tendency toward conduction block increase the likelihood of some rhythm disturbances (see the section Reentry).

As noted, the action potential initiates contraction of the myocyte. The relationships between the action potential and contraction of cardiac muscle are shown in Figure 16-2. Rapid depolarization (phase 0) precedes the development of force, and completion of repolarization coincides approximately with peak force. Relaxation of the muscle takes place mainly during phase 4 of the action potential. The duration of contraction usually parallels the duration of the action potential.

The various phases of the cardiac action potential are associated with changes in cell membrane permeability, mainly to Na^+, K^+, and Ca^{++} ions. Changes in cell membrane permeability alter the rate of movement of these ions across the membrane and thereby change the membrane voltage (V_m). These changes in permeability are accomplished by the opening and closing of ion channels that are specific for individual ions (see Chapters 1 and 2).

As with all other cells in the body, the concentration of K^+ inside a cardiac muscle cell ($[K^+]_i$) exceeds the concentration outside the cell ($[K^+]_o$). The reverse concentration gradient exists for Na^+ and Ca^{++}. Estimates of the extracellular and intracellular concentrations of Na^+, K^+, and Ca^{++} and the Nernst equilibrium potentials (see Chapter 1) for these ions are compiled in Table 16-1.

Resting Membrane Voltage

The resting cell membrane has relatively high permeability to K^+; permeability to Na^+ and Ca^{++} is much less. Given the existing chemical gradient for K^+ and V_m, K^+ tends to diffuse from the inside to the outside of the cell. Any flux of K^+ that occurs at the resting membrane potential (i.e., during phase 4) takes place mainly through specific K^+ channels. Several types of K^+ channels exist in cardiac cell membranes. Opening and closing of some of these channels are regulated by V_m, whereas others are controlled by a chemical signal (e.g., the extracellular acetylcholine concentration). The specific K^+ channel through which K^+ passes during phase 4 is a voltage-regulated channel that conducts the **inwardly rectifying K^+ current.** This current is symbolized i_{K1} and is discussed in more detail later. For now, it is necessary only to know how this current is established.

The dependence of V_m on conductance and the intracellular and extracellular concentrations of K^+, Na^+, and other ions is described by the **chord**

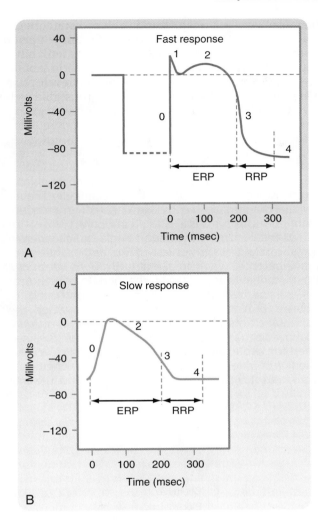

A

B

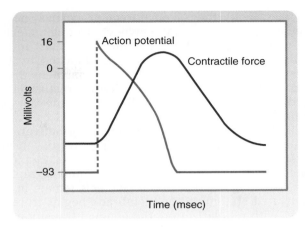

● **Figure 16-2.** Time relationships between the force developed and changes in transmembrane potential in a thin strip of ventricular muscle. (Redrawn from Kavaler F et al: Bull NY Acad Med 41:5925, 1965.)

● **Table 16-1.**
Intracellular and Extracellular Ion Concentrations and Equilibrium Potentials in Cardiac Muscle Cells

Ion	Extracellular Concentrations (mM)	Intracellular Concentrations (mM)*	Equilibrium Potential (mV)
Na⁺	145	10	70
K⁺	4	135	−94
Ca⁺⁺	2	10^{-4}	132

*The intracellular concentrations are estimates of the free concentrations in cytoplasm.
Data from Ten Eick RE et al: Prog Cardiovasc Dis 24:157, 1981.

● **Figure 16-1.** Action potentials of fast-response **(A)** and slow-response **(B)** cardiac fibers. The phases of the action potentials are labeled (see text for details). The effective refractory period (ERP) and the relative refractory period (RRP) are labeled. Note that when compared with fast-response fibers, the resting potential of slow fibers is less negative, the upstroke (phase 0) of the action potential is less steep, the amplitude of the action potential is smaller, phase 1 is absent, and the RRP extends well into phase 4 after the fibers have fully repolarized.

conductance equation (see Chapter 2). In a resting cardiac cell, conductance to K⁺ (g_K) is about 100 times greater than conductance to Na⁺ (g_{Na}). Therefore, V_m is similar to the Nernst equilibrium potential for K⁺. As a result, alterations in extracellular [K⁺] can significantly change V_m, with hypokalemia causing hyperpolarization and hyperkalemia causing depolarization. In contrast, because g_{Na} is so small in the resting cell, changes in [Na⁺]ₒ do not significantly affect V_m.

Fast-Response Action Potentials
Genesis of the Upstroke (Phase 0)
Any stimulus that abruptly depolarizes V_m to a critical value (called the threshold) elicits an action potential. The characteristics of fast-response action potentials are shown in Figure 16-1, *A*. The rapid depolarization (phase 0) is related almost exclusively to the influx of Na⁺ into the myocyte as a result of a sudden increase in g_{Na}. The action potential amplitude (the potential change during phase 0) is dependent on [Na⁺]ₒ. When [Na⁺]ₒ is decreased, the amplitude of the action potential decreases, and when [Na⁺]ₒ is reduced from its normal value of about 140 mEq/L to about 20 mEq/L, the cell is no longer excitable.

When the resting membrane potential, V_m, is suddenly depolarized from −90 mV to the threshold level

---

▶ **IN THE CLINIC**

Fast responses may change to slow responses under certain pathological conditions. For example, in coronary artery disease, a region of cardiac muscle may be deprived of its normal blood supply. As a result, [K⁺] in the interstitial fluid that surrounds the affected muscle cells rises because K⁺ is lost from the inadequately perfused (or ischemic) cells. The action potentials in some of these cells may then be converted from fast to slow responses. Conversion from a fast to a slow response as a result of increasing interstitial [K⁺] is illustrated later in Figure 16-13.

of about −65 mV, the cell membrane properties change dramatically. Na$^+$ enters the myocyte through specific fast **voltage-activated Na$^+$ channels** that exist in the membrane. These channels can be blocked by the puffer fish toxin tetrodotoxin. In addition, many drugs used to treat certain cardiac rhythm disturbances (cardiac arrhythmias) act by blocking these fast Na$^+$ channels.

The Na$^+$ channels open very rapidly or **activate** (in about 0.1 msec), thereby resulting in an abrupt increase in g_{Na}. However, once open, the Na$^+$ channels **inactivate** (time course ≈ 1 to 2 msec), and g_{Na} rapidly decreases (Fig. 16-3). The Na$^+$ channels remain in the inactivated state until the membrane begins to repolarize. With repolarization, the channel transitions to the **closed** state, from which it can then be reopened by another depolarization of V_m to the threshold. These properties of the Na$^+$ channel underlie the basis of the action potential refractory period. When the Na$^+$ channels are in the inactivated state, they cannot be reopened, and another action potential cannot be generated. During this period the cell is said to be in the **effective refractory period.** This prevents a sustained, tetanic contraction of cardiac muscle, which would retard ventricular relaxation and therefore interfere with the normal intermittent pumping action of the heart. As the cell repolarizes (phase 3), the inactivated channels begin to transition to the closed state. During this period, called the **relative refractory period,** another action potential can be generated, but it requires a larger than normal depolarization of V_m. Only when V_m has returned to the resting level (phase 4) are all the Na$^+$ channels closed and thus able to be reactivated by the normal depolarization of V_m.

AT THE CELLULAR LEVEL

Ionic currents through single membrane channels can be measured with the patch clamp technique. The individual channels open and close repeatedly in a random manner. This process is illustrated in Figure 16-4, which shows the current flow through single Na$^+$ channels in a myocardial cell. To the left of the arrow, the membrane potential was clamped at −85 mV. At the arrow, the potential was suddenly changed to −45 mV, at which value it was held for the remainder of the record. Figure 16-4 indicates that immediately after the membrane potential was made less negative, one Na$^+$ channel opened three times in sequence. It remained open for about 2 or 3 msec each time and closed for about 4 or 5 msec between openings. In the open state it allowed 1.5 pA of current to pass. During the first

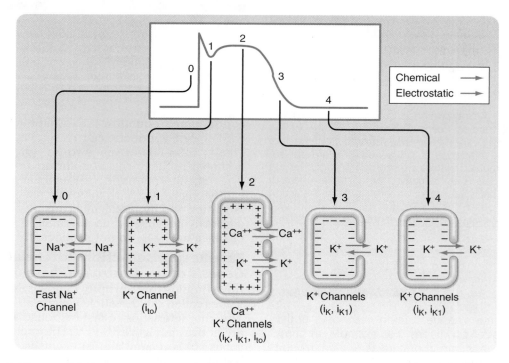

● **Figure 16-3.** Principal ionic currents and channels that generate the various phases of the action potential in a cardiac cell. **Phase 0:** The chemical and electrostatic forces both favor the entry of Na$^+$ into the cell through fast Na$^+$ channels to generate the upstroke. **Phase 1:** The chemical and electrostatic forces both favor the efflux of K$^+$ through i_{to} channels to generate early, partial repolarization. **Phase 2:** During the plateau, the net influx of Ca^{++} through Ca^{++} channels is balanced by the efflux of K$^+$ through i_K, i_{K1}, and i_{to} channels. **Phase 3:** The chemical forces that favor the efflux of K$^+$ through i_K and i_{K1} channels predominate over the electrostatic forces that favor the influx of K$^+$ through these same channels. **Phase 4:** The chemical forces that favor the efflux of K$^+$ through i_K and i_{K1} channels very slightly exceed the electrostatic forces that favor the influx of K$^+$ through these same channels.

● AT THE CELLULAR LEVEL— cont'd

and second openings of this channel, a second channel also opened, but for periods of only 1 msec. During the brief times that both channels were open simultaneously, the total current was 3 pA. After the first channel closed for the third time, both channels remained closed for the rest of the recording, even though the membrane was held constant at −45 mV.

The overall change in ionic conductance of the entire cell membrane at any given time reflects the number of channels that are open at that time. Because the individual channels open and close randomly, the overall membrane conductance represents the statistical probability of the open or closed state of the individual channels. The temporal characteristics of the activation process then represent the time course of the increasing probability that the specific channels will be open rather than the kinetic characteristics of the activation gates in the individual channels. Similarly, the temporal characteristics of inactivation reflect the time course of the decreasing probability that the channels will be open and not the kinetic characteristics of the inactivation gates in the individual channels.

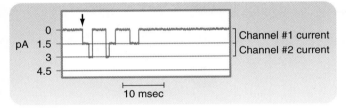

● **Figure 16-4.** Current (in picoamperes) through two individual Na⁺ channels in a cultured heart cell recorded with the patch clamp technique. Membrane voltage was held at −85 mV and then abruptly changed to −45 mV at the arrow and held at this potential for the remainder of the record. (Redrawn from Cachelin AB et al: J Physiol 340:389, 1983.)

Genesis of Early Repolarization (Phase 1)

In many cardiac cells that have a prominent plateau, phase 1 is an early, brief period of limited repolarization. This brief repolarization results in the notch between the end of the upstroke and the beginning of the plateau (Figs. 16-1 and 16-3). Repolarization is brief because of activation of a **transient outward current (i_{to})** carried mainly by K⁺. Activation of K⁺ channels during phase 1 causes a brief efflux of K⁺ from the cell because the cell interior is positively charged and $[K^+]_i$ greatly exceeds $[K^+]_o$ (Fig. 16-3). The cell is briefly and partially repolarized as a result of this transient efflux of K⁺.

The size of the phase 1 notch varies among cardiac cells. It is prominent in myocytes in the epicardial and midmyocardial regions of the left ventricular wall (Fig. 16-5) and in ventricular Purkinje fibers. However, the notch is negligible in myocytes from the endocardial region of the left ventricle (Fig. 16-5) because the density of i_{to} channels is less in these cells. The notch

is also less prominent in the presence of 4-aminopyridine, which blocks the K⁺ channels that carry i_{to}.

Genesis of the Plateau (Phase 2)

During the action potential plateau, Ca⁺⁺ enters myocardial cells through calcium channels (see later) that activate and inactivate much more slowly than the fast Na⁺ channels do. During the flat portion of phase 2 (Figs. 16-1 and 16-3), this influx of Ca⁺⁺ is counterbalanced by the efflux of K⁺. K⁺ exits through channels that conduct mainly the i_{to}, i_K, and i_{K1} currents. The i_{to} current is responsible for phase 1, as described previously, but it is not completely inactivated until after phase 2 has expired. The i_K and i_{K1} currents are described later in this chapter.

Ca⁺⁺ enters the cell via voltage-regulated Ca⁺⁺ channels, which are activated as V_m becomes progressively less negative during the action potential upstroke. Two types of Ca⁺⁺ channels (**L type** and **T type**) have been identified in cardiac tissue. Some of their important characteristics are illustrated in Figure 16-6. L-type channels are so designated because once open they inactivate slowly (Fig. 16-6, lower panel) and provide a "long-lasting" Ca⁺⁺ current. They are the predominant type of Ca⁺⁺ channel in the heart, and they are activated during the action potential upstroke when V_m reaches about −20 mV. L-type channels are blocked by **Ca⁺⁺ channel antagonists** such as verapamil, amlodipine, and diltiazem (Fig. 16-7).

T-type (or "transient") Ca⁺⁺ channels are much less abundant in the heart. They are activated at more negative potentials (about −70 mV) than L-type channels are. They also inactivate more quickly than L-type channels do (Fig. 16-6, upper panel).

Because L-type channels are the most abundant, the following is focused on their function and properties. Opening of Ca⁺⁺ channels results in an increase in Ca⁺⁺ conductance (g_{Ca}) and current (i_{Ca}) soon after the action potential upstroke (Fig. 16-3). Because $[Ca^{++}]_i$ is much less than $[Ca^{++}]_o$ (Table 16-1), the increase in g_{Ca} promotes the influx of Ca⁺⁺ into the cell throughout the plateau. This Ca⁺⁺ influx during the plateau is involved in excitation-contraction coupling, as described later (see also Chapter 13).

Various neurotransmitters and drugs may substantially influence g_{Ca}. The adrenergic neurotransmitter norepinephrine, the β-adrenergic receptor agonist isoproterenol, and various other catecholamines enhance g_{Ca}, whereas the parasympathetic neurotransmitter acetylcholine decreases g_{Ca}. Enhancement of g_{Ca} by catecholamines is the principal mechanism by which they enhance cardiac muscle contractility.

During the plateau (phase 2) of the action potential, the concentration gradient for K⁺ across the cell membrane is virtually the same as it is during phase 4. However, V_m is now positive. Therefore, there is a large gradient that favors efflux of K⁺ from the cell (Fig. 16-3). If g_K were the same during the plateau as it is during phase 4, efflux of K⁺ during phase 2 would greatly exceed the influx of Ca⁺⁺, and a sustained plateau could not be achieved. However, as V_m approaches and then attains positive values near the peak of the action potential upstroke, g_K suddenly

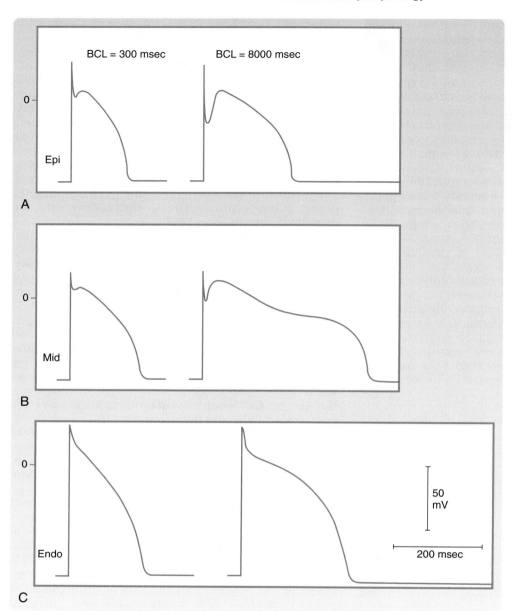

● **Figure 16-5.** Action potentials recorded from the epicardial **(A)**, midmyocardial **(B)**, and endocardial **(C)** regions of the free wall of the canine left ventricle. The preparations were driven at a basic cycle length (BCL) of 300 and 8000 msec. (From Liu D-W et al: Circ Res 72:671, 1993.)

● AT THE CELLULAR LEVEL

To enhance g_{Ca}, catecholamines first bind to β-adrenergic receptors in the cardiac cell membrane. This interaction stimulates the membrane-bound enzyme adenylyl cyclase, which raises the intracellular concentration of cAMP (see also Chapter 3). The rise in the level of cAMP activates cAMP-dependent protein kinase, which in turn promotes phosphorylation of the L-type Ca^{++} channels in the cell membrane and thus augments the influx of Ca^{++} into the cells (Fig. 16-6). Conversely, acetylcholine interacts with muscarinic receptors in the cell membrane to inhibit adenylyl cyclase. In this way, acetylcholine antagonizes the activation of Ca^{++} channels and thereby diminishes g_{Ca}.

▶ IN THE CLINIC

Ca^{++} channel antagonists are substances that block Ca^{++} channels. Examples include the drugs verapamil, amlodipine, and diltiazem. These drugs decrease g_{Ca} and thereby impede the influx of Ca^{++} into myocardial cells. Ca^{++} channel antagonists decrease the duration of the action potential plateau and diminish the strength of the cardiac contraction (Fig. 16-7). Ca^{++} channel antagonists also depress the contraction of vascular smooth muscle and thereby induce generalized vasodilation. This diminished vascular resistance reduces the counterforce (afterload) that opposes the propulsion of blood from the ventricles into the arterial system, as explained in Chapter 17. Hence, vasodilator drugs such as the Ca^{++} channel antagonists are often referred to as afterload-reducing drugs.

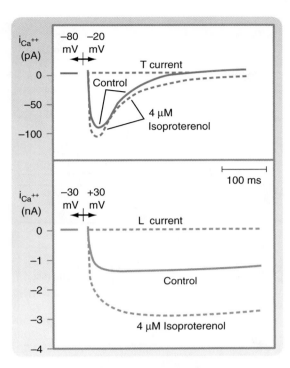

● **Figure 16-6.** Effects of isoproterenol on the Ca⁺⁺ currents conducted by T-type **(upper panel)** and L-type **(lower panel)** Ca⁺⁺ channels in atrial myocytes. **Upper panel,** potential changed from −80 to −20 mV; **lower panel,** potential changed from −30 to +30 mV. (Redrawn from Bean BP: J Gen Physiol 86:1, 1985.)

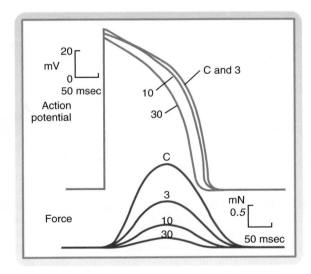

● **Figure 16-7.** Effects of diltiazem, a Ca⁺⁺ channel antagonist, on the action potentials (in millivolts) and isometric contractile forces (in millinewtons) recorded from an isolated papillary muscle. The tracings were recorded under control conditions (C) and in the presence of diltiazem in concentrations of 3, 10, and 30 μmol/L. (Redrawn from Hirth C et al: J Mol Cell Cardiol 15:799, 1983.)

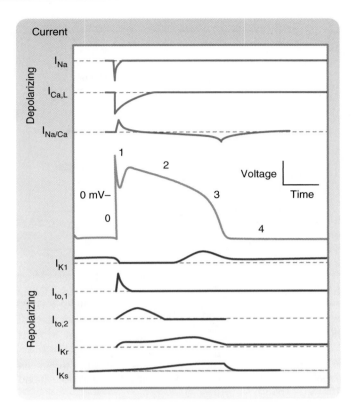

● **Figure 16-8.** Changes in depolarizing **(upper panels)** and repolarizing **(lower panels)** ion currents during the various phases of the action potential in a fast-response cardiac ventricular cell. The inward currents include the fast Na⁺ and L-type Ca⁺⁺ currents. Outward currents are i_{K1}, i_{to}, and the rapid (i_{Kr}) and slow (i_{Ks}) delayed rectifier K⁺ currents. (Redrawn from Tomaselli G, Marbán E: Cardiovasc Res 42:270, 1999.)

decreases (Fig. 16-8). The diminished K⁺ current associated with the reduction in g_K prevents excessive loss of K⁺ from the cell during the plateau.

This reduction in g_K at both positive and low negative values of V_m is called **inward rectification.** Inward rectification is a characteristic of several K⁺ currents, including the i_{K1} current (Fig. 16-9). For these channels, large K⁺ currents flow at negative values of V_m (i.e., g_K is large). However, when V_m is near 0 mV, or positive, as occurs during the plateau (phase 2), little or no K⁺ current flows (i.e., g_K is low). Thus, the substantial g_K that prevails during phase 4 of the cardiac action potential (Fig. 16-8) is largely due to the i_{K1} channels, but current through these channels is greatly diminished during the plateau (Fig. 16-9).

Other K⁺ channels play a role in phase 2 of the action potential. These are characterized as **delayed rectifier (i_k)** channels. These K⁺ channels are closed during phase 4 and are activated very slowly by the potentials that prevail toward the end of phase 0. Hence, activation of these channels tends to increase g_K very gradually during phase 2. These channels play only a minor role during phase 2, but they contribute to the process of final repolarization (phase 3), as described later. Two types of i_k channels exist, depending on their rates of activation. The more slowly

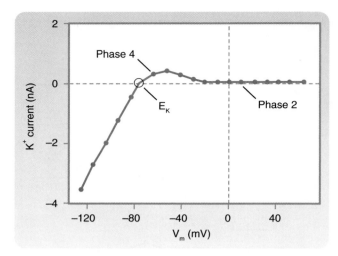

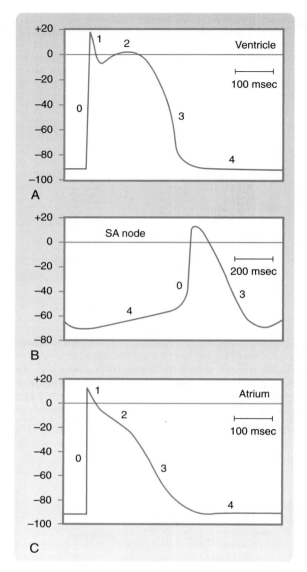

● **Figure 16-9.** Inwardly rectified K⁺ currents recorded from a ventricular myocyte when the potential was changed from a holding potential of −80 mV to various test potentials. Positive values along the vertical axis represent outward currents; negative values represent inward currents. The V_m coordinate of the point *(open circle)* at which the curve intersects the x axis is the reversal potential; it denotes the Nernst equilibrium potential (E_K), at which point the chemical and electrostatic forces are equal. (Redrawn from Giles WR, Imaizumi Y: J Physiol [Lond] <u>405:123, 1988.</u>)

activating channel is designated the **i_{Ks}** channel, whereas the more rapidly activating channel is designated the **i_{Kr}** channel (Fig. 16-8). The duration of the action potential in myocytes in various regions of the ventricular myocardium is determined in part by the relative distributions of these i_{Kr} and i_{Ks} channels.

The action potential plateau persists as long as the efflux of charge carried mainly by K⁺ is balanced by the influx of charge carried mainly by Ca⁺⁺. The effects of altering this balance are demonstrated by the action of the Ca⁺⁺ channel antagonist diltiazem in an isolated papillary muscle preparation (Fig. 16-7). With increasing concentrations of diltiazem, the plateau voltage becomes progressively less positive and the plateau duration diminishes. Conversely, administration of certain K⁺ channel antagonists prolongs the plateau substantially.

Genesis of Final Repolarization (Phase 3)

The process of final repolarization (phase 3) starts at the end of phase 2, when efflux of K⁺ from the cardiac cell begins to exceed influx of Ca⁺⁺. As noted, at least three outward K⁺ currents (i_{to}, i_K, and i_{K1}) contribute to the final repolarization (phase 3) of the cardiac cell (Figs. 16-3 and 16-8).

The transient outward (i_{to}) and the delayed rectifier (i_{Kr}, i_{Ks}) currents help initiate repolarization. These currents are therefore important determinants of the duration of the plateau. For example, the duration of the plateau is substantially less in atrial than in ventricular myocytes (Fig. 16-10) because the magnitude of i_{to} during the plateau is greater in atrial than in ventricular myocytes. As already noted, the duration

● **Figure 16-10.** Typical action potentials (in millivolts) recorded from cells in the ventricle **(A)**, SA node **(B)**, and atrium **(C).** Note that the time calibration in **B** differs from that in **A** and **C.** (From Hoffman BF, Cranefield PF: Electrophysiology of the Heart. New York, McGraw-Hill, 1960.)

of the action potential in ventricular myocytes varies considerably with the location of these myocytes in the ventricular walls (Fig. 16-5). The i_{to} and delayed rectifier (i_K) currents mainly account for these differences. In endocardial myocytes, in which the duration of the action potential is least, the magnitude of i_K is greatest. The converse applies to the midmyocardial myocytes. The magnitude of i_K and the duration of the action potential are intermediate for epicardial myocytes.

The inwardly rectified K⁺ current i_{K1} does not participate in the initiation of repolarization because the conductance of these channels is very small over the range of V_m values that prevail during the plateau. However, the i_{K1} channels contribute substantially to the rate of repolarization once phase 3 has been initiated. As V_m becomes increasingly negative during phase 3, the conductance of the channels that carry the i_{K1} current progressively increases and thereby accelerates repolarization (Fig. 16-3).

Restoration of Ionic Concentrations (Phase 4)

The steady inward leak of Na^+ that enters the cell rapidly during phase 0 and more slowly throughout the cardiac cycle would gradually depolarize the resting membrane voltage were it not for **Na^+,K^+-ATPase,** which is located in the cell membrane (see Chapter 1). Similarly, most of the excess Ca^{++} ions that had entered the cell mainly during phase 2 are eliminated principally by a $3Na^+-1Ca^{++}$ antiporter, which exchanges 3 Na^+ ions for 1 Ca^{++} ion. However, some of the Ca^{++} ions are eliminated by an ATP-driven Ca^{++} pump.

Slow-Response Action Potentials

As described earlier, fast-response action potentials (Fig. 16-1, *A*) consist of four principal components: an upstroke (phase 0), an early partial repolarization (phase 1), a plateau (phase 2), and a final repolarization (phase 3). However, in the slow-response action potential (Fig. 16-1, *B*), the upstroke is much less steep, early repolarization (phase 1) is absent, the plateau is less prolonged and not as flat, and the transition from the plateau to the final repolarization is less distinct.

Blocking fast Na^+ channels with tetrodotoxin in a fast-response fiber can generate slow responses under appropriate conditions. The Purkinje fiber action potential shown in Figure 16-11 clearly exhibits the two response types. In the control tracing (A), the typical fast-response action potential displays a prominent notch as a result of i_{to} that separates the upstroke from the plateau. In action potentials B to E, progressively larger quantities of tetrodotoxin produce a graded blockade of the fast Na^+ channels. The upstroke and notch become progressively less prominent in action potentials B to D. In action potential E, the notch has disappeared and the upstroke is very gradual; this action potential resembles a typical slow response.

Certain cells in the heart, notably those in the SA and AV nodes, exhibit slow-response action potentials. In these cells, depolarization is achieved mainly by influx of Ca^{++} through L-type Ca^{++} channels instead of influx of Na^+ through fast Na^+ channels. Repolarization is accomplished in these fibers by inactivation of the Ca^{++} channels and by the increased K^+ conductance through the i_{K1} and i_K channels (Fig. 16-3).

CONDUCTION IN CARDIAC FIBERS

An action potential traveling along a cardiac muscle fiber is propagated by local circuit currents, much as it is in nerve and skeletal muscle fibers (see Chapter 5). When the wave of depolarization reaches the end of the cell, the impulse is conducted to adjacent cells through gap junctions (see Chapter 2). Impulses pass more readily along the length of the cell (isotropic) than laterally from cell to cell (anisotropic) because gap junctions are preferentially located at the ends of the cell. These channels are rather nonselective in their permeability to ions and have a low electrical resistance that allows ionic current to pass from one cell to another. The electrical resistance of gap junctions is similar to that of cytoplasm. The flow of charge from cell to cell follows the principles of local circuit currents and therefore allows intercellular propagation of the impulse.

Conduction of the Fast Response

The characteristics of conduction differ in fast- and slow-response fibers. In fast-response fibers, fast Na^+ channels are activated when the transmembrane potential of one region of the fiber suddenly changes from a resting value of about -90 mV to the threshold value of about -65 mV. The inward Na^+ current then rapidly depolarizes the cell at that site. This portion of the fiber subsequently becomes part of the depolarized zone, and the border is displaced accordingly. The same process then begins at the new border. This process is repeated again and again, and the border moves continuously down the fiber as a wave of depolarization (Fig. 16-12).

The conduction velocity along the fiber varies directly with the amplitude of the action potential and the rate of change of the potential (dV_m/dt) during phase 0. The amplitude of the action potential equals the potential difference between the fully depolarized and the fully polarized regions of the cell interior. The

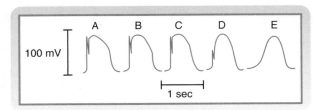

● **Figure 16-11.** Effect of tetrodotoxin, which blocks the fast Na^+ channels, on the action potentials recorded in a Purkinje fiber. The concentration of tetrodotoxin was 0 M in A, 3×10^{-8} M in B, 3×10^{-7} M in C, and 3×10^{-6} M in D and E; E was recorded later than D. (Redrawn from Carmeliet E, Vereecke J: Pflügers Arch 313:300, 1969.)

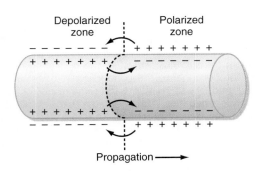

● **Figure 16-12.** The role of local currents in the propagation of a wave of excitation down a cardiac fiber.

magnitude of the local current is proportional to this potential difference (see Chapter 5). Because these local currents shift the potential of the resting zone toward the threshold value, they are local stimuli that depolarize the adjacent resting portion of the fiber to its threshold potential. The greater the potential difference between the depolarized and polarized regions (i.e., the greater the action potential amplitude), the more effective are local stimuli in depolarizing adjacent parts of the membrane and the more rapidly is the wave of depolarization propagated down the fiber.

The rate of change in potential during phase 0 is also an important determinant of conduction velocity. If the active portion of the fiber depolarizes gradually, the local currents between the resting region and the neighboring depolarizing region are small. The resting region adjacent to the active zone is depolarized gradually, and consequently more time is required for each new section of the fiber to reach threshold. This allows some Na^+ channels to inactivate.

The resting membrane potential is also an important determinant of conduction velocity. Changes in the resting membrane potential influence both the amplitude of the action potential and the slope of the upstroke, which in turn alter the conduction velocity (Fig. 16-13). Depolarization of V_m leads to inactivation

of the fast Na^+ channels, which in turn decreases the amplitude of the action potential and the slope of the upstroke, and as a consequence conduction velocity is slowed. In addition to changes in $[K^+]_o$, premature excitation of a cell that has not completely repolarized will also result in a decrease in conduction velocity. This too reflects the fact that when V_m is depolarized, more fast Na^+ channels are inactivated, and thus only a fraction of the Na^+ channels are available to conduct the inward Na^+ current during phase 0.

Conduction of the Slow Response

Local circuits (Fig. 16-12) also propagate the slow response, the conduction characteristics of which differ quantitatively from those of the fast response. The threshold potential is about −40 mV for the slow response, and conduction is much slower than for the

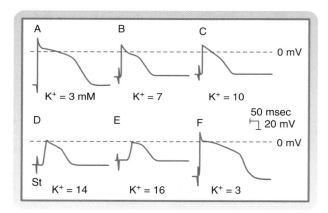

● **Figure 16-13.** Effect of changes in $[K^+]_o$ on the transmembrane action potentials recorded from a Purkinje fiber. The stimulus artifact (St) appears as a biphasic spike to the left of the upstroke of the action potential. The horizontal lines near the peaks of the action potentials denote 0 mV. When $[K^+]_o$ is 3 mM (A and F), the resting V_m is −82 mV and the slope of phase 0 is steep. At the end of phase 0, the overshoot attains a value of 30 mV. Hence, the action potential amplitude is 112 mV. The distance from the stimulus artifact to the beginning of phase 0 is inversely proportional to the conduction velocity. When $[K^+]_o$ is increased gradually to 16 mM (B to E), the resting V_m becomes progressively less negative. At the same time, the amplitudes and durations of the action potentials and the steepness of the upstrokes all diminish. As a consequence, conduction velocity decreases progressively. At $[K^+]_o$ levels of 14 and 16 mM (D and E), the resting V_m attains levels sufficient to inactivate all the fast Na^+ channels and leave the characteristic slow-response action potentials. (From Myerburg RJ, Lazzara R: In Fisch E [ed]: Complex Electrocardiography. Philadelphia, FA Davis, 1973.)

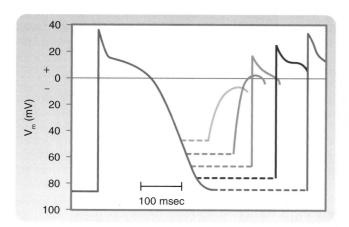

● **Figure 16-14.** Changes in action potential amplitude and upstroke slope as action potentials are initiated at different stages of the relative refractory period of the preceding excitation. (Redrawn from Rosen MR et al: Am Heart J 88:380, 1974.)

fast response. The conduction velocities of the slow response in the SA and AV nodes are about 0.02 to 0.1 m/sec. The fast-response conduction velocities are about 0.3 to 1 m/sec for myocardial cells and 1 to 4 m/sec for the specialized conducting (Purkinje) fibers in the ventricles. Slow responses are more readily blocked than fast responses; that is, conduction ceases before the impulse reaches the end of the myocardial fiber. In addition, fast-response fibers can respond at repetition rates that are much greater than those of slow-response fibers.

CARDIAC EXCITABILITY

Because of the rapid development of artificial pacemakers and other electrical devices for correcting cardiac rhythm disturbances, detailed knowledge of cardiac excitability is essential. The excitability characteristics of various types of cardiac cells differ considerably, depending on whether the action potentials are fast or slow responses.

Fast Response

Once the fast response has been initiated, the depolarized cell is no longer excitable until the cell has partially repolarized (Fig. 16-1, *A*). The interval from the beginning of the action potential until the fiber is able to conduct another action potential is called the effective refractory period. In the fast response, this period extends from the beginning of phase 0 to a point in phase 3 at which repolarization has reached about −50 mV (phase 3 in Fig. 16-1, *A*). At about this value of V_m, many of the fast Na^+ channels have transitioned from the inactivated to the closed state. However, the cardiac fiber is not fully excitable until it has been completely repolarized. Before complete repolarization (i.e., during the relative refractory period), an action potential may be evoked only when the stimulus is stronger than a stimulus that could elicit a response during phase 4.

When a fast response is evoked during the relative refractory period of a previous excitation, its characteristics vary with the membrane potential that exists at the time of stimulation (Fig. 16-14). The later in the relative refractory period that the fiber is stimulated, the greater the increase in the amplitude of the response and the slope of the upstroke because the number of fast Na^+ channels that have recovered from inactivation increases as repolarization proceeds. As a consequence, propagation velocity also increases the later in the relative refractory period that the fiber is stimulated. Once the fiber is fully repolarized, the response is constant no matter what time in phase 4 the stimulus is applied.

Slow Response

In slow-response fibers, the relative refractory period frequently extends well beyond phase 3 (Fig. 16-1, *B*). Even after the cell has completely repolarized, it may be difficult to evoke a propagated response for some time. This characteristic of slow-response fibers is called postrepolarization refractoriness.

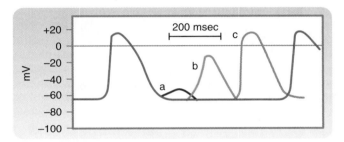

● **Figure 16-15.** Effects of excitation at various times after the initiation of an action potential in a slow-response fiber. In this fiber, excitation very late in phase 3 (or early in phase 4) induces a small, nonpropagated (local) response (a). Later in phase 4, a propagated response (b) can be elicited, but its amplitude is small and the upstroke is not very steep; this response is conducted very slowly. Still later in phase 4, full excitability is regained, and the response (c) displays normal characteristics. (Modified from Singer DH et al: Prog Cardiovasc Dis 24:97, 1981.)

Action potentials evoked early in the relative refractory period are small and the upstrokes are not very steep (Fig. 16-15). The amplitudes and upstroke slopes progressively improve as action potentials are elicited later in the relative refractory period. Recovery of full excitability is much slower than recovery of the fast response. Impulses that arrive early in the relative refractory period are conducted much more slowly than those that arrive late in that period. The long refractory periods also lead to conduction blocks. Even when slow responses recur at low frequency, the fiber may be able to conduct only a fraction of these impulses; for example, in certain conditions only alternate impulses may be propagated (see later).

EFFECTS OF CYCLE LENGTH

Cycle length refers to the time between successive action potentials. Changes in cycle length alter the duration of the action potential in cardiac cells

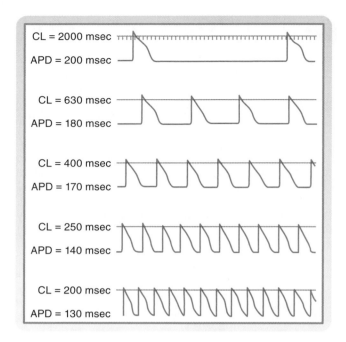

● Figure 16-16. Effect of changes in cycle length (CL) on the action potential duration (APD) of Purkinje fibers. (Modified from Singer D, Ten Eick RE: Am J Cardiol 28:381, 1971.)

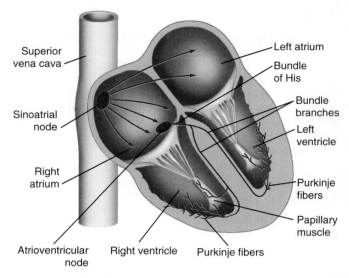

● Figure 16-17. The cardiac conduction system.

(Fig. 16-16; also see Fig. 16-5) and thus change their refractory periods. Consequently, changes in cycle length are often important factors in the initiation or termination of certain arrhythmias (irregular heart rhythms).

The changes in action potential duration produced by stepwise reductions in cycle length from 2000 to 200 msec in a Purkinje fiber are shown in Figure 16-16. Note that as cycle length diminishes, the duration of the action potential decreases. This direct correlation between action potential duration and cycle length is mediated by changes in g_K that involve at least two types of K^+ channels, namely, those that conduct the delayed rectifier K^+ currents i_{Kr} and i_{Ks} and those that conduct the transient outward K^+ current i_{to}.

The i_K current is activated at values of V_m near zero, but the current activates slowly, remains activated for hundreds of milliseconds, and also inactivates very slowly. Consequently, as the basic cycle length diminishes, each action potential tends to occur earlier in the inactivation period of the i_K current initiated by the preceding action potential. Therefore, the shorter the basic cycle length, the greater the outward K^+ current during phase 2 and hence the shorter the action potential duration.

The i_{to} current also influences the relationship between cycle length and action potential duration. The i_{to} current is also activated at near zero potential, and its magnitude varies inversely with cardiac cycle length. Therefore, as cycle length decreases, the consequent increase in the outward K^+ current shortens the plateau.

NATURAL EXCITATION OF THE HEART AND THE ELECTROCARDIOGRAM

Excitation of the heart normally occurs in an ordered fashion, which allows effective pumping of blood. This ordered excitation occurs via the heart's conduction system (Fig. 16-17). The SA node is the pacemaker of the heart and initiates the spread of action potentials throughout the atria. This spread of excitation reaches the AV node, where conduction is slowed such that atrial contraction can occur and the ventricles can be adequately filled. Excitation then spreads rapidly throughout the ventricles via the Purkinje fibers so that the ventricular myocytes contract in a coordinated manner. In the following, the properties of each component of the heart's conduction system are described.

The autonomic nervous system controls various aspects of cardiac function, such as the heart rate and contraction strength. However, cardiac function does not require intact innervation. Indeed, a cardiac transplant patient, whose heart is completely denervated, may still adapt well to stressful situations. The ability of a denervated, transplanted heart to adapt to changing conditions lies in certain intrinsic properties of cardiac tissue, especially its automaticity.

The properties of **automaticity** (the ability to initiate its own beat) and **rhythmicity** (the regularity of pacemaking activity) allow a perfused heart to beat even when it is completely removed from the body. The vertebrate heartbeat is myogenic in origin. If the coronary vasculature of an excised heart is artificially perfused with blood or an oxygenated electrolyte solution, rhythmic cardiac contractions may persist for many hours. At least some cells in the atria and ventricles can initiate beats; such cells reside mainly in nodal tissues or specialized conducting fibers of the heart.

Sinoatrial Node

As noted, the region of the mammalian heart that ordinarily generates impulses at the greatest frequency is the SA node; it is the main cardiac pacemaker. Detailed mapping of the electrical potentials on the surface of the right atrium reveals that two or three sites of automaticity, located 1 or 2 cm from the SA node itself, serve along with the SA node as an atrial pacemaker complex. At times, all these loci initiate impulses simultaneously. At other times, the site of earliest excitation shifts from locus to locus, depending on certain conditions, such as the level of autonomic neural activity.

In humans, the SA node is about 8 mm long and 2 mm thick, and it lies posteriorly in the groove at the junction between the superior vena cava and the right atrium. The sinus node artery runs lengthwise through the center of the node. The SA node contains two principal cell types: (1) small, round cells that have few organelles and myofibrils and (2) slender, elongated cells that are intermediate in appearance between the round and "ordinary" atrial myocardial cells. The round cells are probably the pacemaker cells; the slender, elongated cells probably conduct the impulses within the node and to the nodal margins.

A typical transmembrane action potential recorded from an SA node cell is depicted in Figure 16-10, *B*. When compared with the transmembrane potential recorded from a ventricular myocardial cell (Fig. 16-10, *A*), the resting potential of the SA node cell is usually less negative, the upstroke of the action potential (phase 0) is less steep, the plateau is not sustained, and repolarization (phase 3) is more gradual. These are characteristic attributes of the slow response. As in cells that exhibit the slow response, tetrodotoxin (which blocks the fast Na^+ current) has no influence on the SA nodal action potential because the action potential upstroke is not produced by an inward Na^+ current through fast channels.

The transmembrane potential during phase 4 is much less negative in SA (and AV) nodal automatic cells than in atrial or ventricular myocytes because nodal cells lack the i_{K1} (inward rectifying) type of K^+ channel. Thus, the ratio of g_K to g_{Na} during phase 4 is much less in nodal cells than in myocytes. Hence, during phase 4, V_m deviates much more from the K^+ equilibrium potential (E_K) in nodal cells than it does in myocytes.

The principal feature of a pacemaker cell that distinguishes it from the other cells that we have discussed resides in phase 4. In nonautomatic cells, the potential remains constant during this phase, whereas a pacemaker fiber is characterized by slow diastolic depolarization throughout phase 4. Depolarization proceeds at a steady rate until a threshold is attained, and an action potential is then triggered.

Pacemaker cell frequency may be varied by a change in (1) the rate of depolarization during phase 4, (2) the maximal negativity during phase 4, or (3) the threshold potential (Fig. 16-18). When the rate of slow diastolic depolarization is increased, the threshold

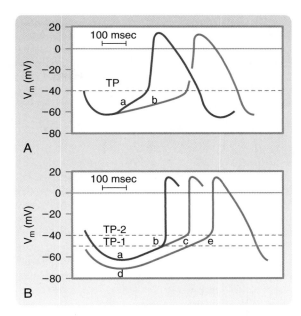

● **Figure 16-18.** Mechanisms involved in the changes in frequency of pacemaker firing. In **A,** a reduction in the slope (from a to b) of slow diastolic depolarization diminishes the firing frequency. In **B,** an increase in the threshold potential (from TP-1 to TP-2) or an increase in the magnitude of the maximum diastolic potential (from a to d) also diminishes the firing frequency. (From Hoffman BF, Cranefield PF: Electrophysiology of the Heart. New York, McGraw-Hill, 1960.)

> ### IN THE CLINIC

Ordinarily, the frequency of pacemaker firing is controlled by the activity of both divisions of the autonomic nervous system. Increased sympathetic nervous activity, through the release of norepinephrine, raises the heart rate principally by increasing the slope of the slow diastolic depolarization. This mechanism of increasing heart rate occurs during physical exertion, anxiety, or certain illnesses such as febrile infectious diseases.

Increased vagal activity, through the release of acetylcholine, diminishes the heart rate by hyperpolarizing the pacemaker cell membrane and reducing the slope of the slow diastolic depolarization. These mechanisms of decreasing the heart rate occur when vagal activity is predominant over sympathetic activity. An extreme example is vasovagal syncope, a brief period of lightheadedness or loss of consciousness caused by an intense burst of vagal activity. This type of syncope is a reflex response to pain or to certain psychological stimuli.

Changes in autonomic neural activity do not usually change the heart rate by altering the threshold level of V_m in the nodal pacemaker cells. However, certain antiarrhythmic drugs, such as quinidine and procainamide, do raise the threshold potential of the automatic cells to less negative values.

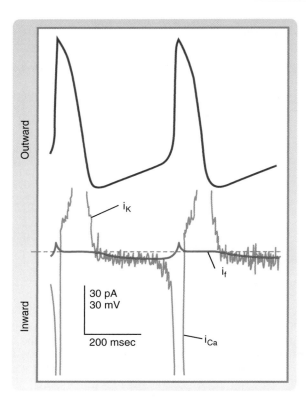

Outward

Inward

i_K

i_f

i_{Ca}

30 pA
30 mV

200 msec

● **Figure 16-19.** The transmembrane potential changes **(top half)** that occur in SA node cells are produced by three principal currents **(bottom half):** (1) the current i_{Ca}; (2) a hyperpolarization-induced inward current, i_f; and (3) an outward K^+ current, i_K. The thin noisy green trace shows net membrane current and the approximate time course of (1) the repolarizing outward K^+ current i_K, (2) the hyperpolarization-induced inward current i_f, and (3) the L-type Ca^{++} current i_{Ca}. The thick bold red line in the current trace indicates the magnitude and direction of estimated I_f. (Redrawn from van Ginneken ACG, Giles W: J Physiol 434:57, 1991.)

● **AT THE CELLULAR LEVEL**

The "f"-current (I_f) in cardiac SA node cells is activated by <u>h</u>yperpolarization and gated by <u>c</u>yclic <u>n</u>ucleotides and is designated HCN. There are four members of the _HCN_ gene family, and such channels are found in central nervous system neurons that generate action potentials repetitively. Transmembrane segment 4 (S_4) has many positively charged amino acids that act as voltage sensors, as also found in voltage-gated Na^+, K^+, and Ca^{++} channels. The dominant channel expressed in heart is derived from the _HCN4_ gene. Mutations in amino acids in S_4 and in the S_4-to-S_5 linker cause marked changes in the voltage dependence of activation such that greater hyperpolarization is needed to open the channel. This effect is like that of acetylcholine, and it has been predicted that the occurrence of such mutations in the human heart could underlie sinus bradycardia and sick sinus syndrome.

diminishes, its opposition to the depolarizing effects of the two inward currents (i_f and i_{Ca}) also gradually decreases. The progressive diastolic depolarization is mediated by the two inward currents i_f and i_{Ca}, which oppose the repolarizing effect of the outward current i_K.

The inward current i_f is activated near the end of repolarization and is carried mainly by Na^+ through specific channels that differ from the fast Na^+ channels. The current was dubbed "funny" because its discoverers had not expected to detect an inward Na^+ current in pacemaker cells at the end of repolarization. This current is activated as the membrane potential becomes hyperpolarized beyond −50 mV. The more negative the membrane potential at this time, the greater the activation of i_f.

The second current responsible for diastolic depolarization is the Ca^{++} current i_{Ca}. This current is activated toward the end of phase 4 as the transmembrane potential reaches a value of about −55 mV (Fig. 16-19). Once the Ca^{++} channels are activated, influx of Ca^{++} into the cell increases. This influx accelerates the rate of diastolic depolarization, which then leads to the action potential upstroke. A decrease in $[Ca^{++}]_o$ (Fig. 16-20) or the addition of Ca^{++} channel antagonists diminishes the amplitude of the action potential and the slope of the slow diastolic depolarization in SA node cells. Recent evidence indicates that additional ion currents, including a sustained (background) inward Na^+ current (i_{Na}), the T-type Ca^{++} current, and the Na/Ca exchange current triggered by spontaneous release of Ca^{++} from the sarcoplasmic reticulum (SR), may also be involved in pacemaking. These observations illustrate the manifold ways to sustain this vital function.*

potential is attained earlier, and the heart rate increases. A rise in the threshold potential delays the onset of phase 0, and the heart rate is reduced. Similarly, when the maximal negative potential is increased, more time is required to reach the threshold potential, when the slope of phase 4 remains unchanged, and the heart rate therefore diminishes.

Ionic Basis of Automaticity

Several ionic currents contribute to the slow diastolic depolarization that characteristically occurs in the automatic cells in the heart. In the pacemaker cells of the SA node, at least three ionic currents mediate the slow diastolic depolarization: (1) an outward K^+ current, i_K; (2) an inward current, i_f, induced by hyperpolarization; and (3) an inward Ca^{++} current, I_{Ca} (Fig. 16-19).

The repetitive firing of the pacemaker cell begins with the delayed rectifier K^+ current i_K. Efflux of K^+ tends to repolarize the cell after the upstroke of the action potential. K^+ continues to move out well beyond the time of maximal repolarization, but its efflux diminishes throughout phase 4 (Fig. 16-19). As the current

---

*The ionic basis for automaticity in the AV node pacemaker cells resembles that in the SA node cells. Similar mechanisms also account for automaticity in ventricular Purkinje fibers, except that the fast Na^+ current rather than i_{Ca} is involved. Also, a voltage- and time-dependent K^+ current rather than the hyperpolarization-induced inward current i_f has been suggested to mediate the slow diastolic depolarization; however, this remains to be clarified.

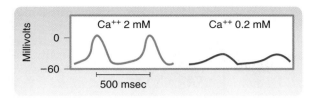

● **Figure 16-20.** Transmembrane action potentials recorded from an SA node pacemaker cell. The concentration of Ca++ in the bath was reduced from 2 to 0.2 mM. (Modified from Kohlhardt M et al: Basic Res Cardiol 71:17, 1976.)

IN THE CLINIC

Regions of the heart other than the SA node may initiate beats in special circumstances. Such sites are called ectopic foci or ectopic pacemakers. Ectopic foci may become pacemakers when (1) their own rhythmicity becomes enhanced, (2) the rhythmicity of the higher-order pacemakers becomes depressed, or (3) all conduction pathways between the ectopic focus and regions with greater rhythmicity become blocked. Ectopic pacemakers may act as a safety mechanism when normal pacemaking centers fail. However, if an ectopic center fires while the normal pacemaking center still functions, the ectopic activity may induce either sporadic rhythm disturbances, such as premature depolarizations, or continuous rhythm disturbances, such as paroxysmal tachycardias (see later section).

The autonomic neurotransmitters affect automaticity by altering membrane ionic currents. The adrenergic transmitters increase all three currents involved in SA nodal automaticity. To increase the slope of diastolic depolarization, the augmentation of i_f and i_{Ca} by adrenergic transmitters must exceed the enhancement of i_K by these same transmitters.

The hyperpolarization induced by acetylcholine released from vagus nerve endings in the heart is achieved by the activation of specific K+ channels, the acetylcholine-regulated K+ channels (K_{ACh}). Acetylcholine also depresses the i_f and i_{Ca} currents. The autonomic neural effects on cardiac cells are described in greater detail in Chapter 18.

When the SA node or other components of the atrial pacemaker complex are excised or destroyed, pacemaker cells in the AV junction generally take over the pacemaker function for the entire heart. After some time, which may vary from minutes to days, automatic cells in the atria usually become dominant again and resume their pacemaker function. Purkinje fibers in the specialized conduction system of the ventricles also display automaticity. Characteristically, these fibers fire at a very slow rate. When the AV junction cannot conduct cardiac impulses from the atria to the ventricles, these idioventricular pacemakers in the Purkinje fiber network initiate the ventricular contractions, but at a frequency of only 30 to 40 beats/min.

IN THE CLINIC

If an ectopic focus in one of the atria suddenly began to fire at a high rate (e.g., 150 impulses/min) in an individual with a normal heart rate of 70 beats/min, the ectopic site would become the pacemaker for the entire heart. If that rapid ectopic focus suddenly stopped firing, the SA node will remain briefly quiescent because of overdrive suppression. The interval from the end of the period of overdrive until the SA node resumes firing is called the sinus node recovery time. In patients with sick sinus syndrome, the sinus node recovery time is prolonged. The consequent period of asystole (absence of a heartbeat) may cause loss of consciousness.

Overdrive Suppression

The automaticity of pacemaker cells diminishes after these cells have been excited at a high frequency. This phenomenon is known as **overdrive suppression.** Because the intrinsic rhythmicity of the SA node is greater than that of the other latent pacemaking sites in the heart, firing of the SA node tends to suppress the automaticity in other loci.

Overdrive suppression results from the activity of membrane Na+,K+-ATPase. A certain amount of Na+ enters the cardiac cell during each depolarization. The more frequently the cell is depolarized, the more Na+ enters the cell per minute. At high excitation frequencies, the activity of Na+,K+-ATPase increases to extrude this larger amount of Na+ from the cell. The activity of Na+,K+-ATPase hyperpolarizes the cell because 3 Na+ ions are extruded by the pump in exchange for 2 K+ ions that enter the cell (see Chapter 1). Therefore, slow diastolic depolarization requires more time to reach the firing threshold. In addition, when the overdrive suddenly ceases, the activity of Na+,K+-ATPase does not slow instantaneously but temporarily remains overactive. This continued extrusion of Na+ opposes the gradual depolarization of the pacemaker cell during phase 4, and it temporarily suppresses the cell's intrinsic automaticity.

Atrial Conduction

From the SA node, the cardiac impulse spreads radially throughout the right atrium (Fig. 16-17) along ordinary atrial myocardial fibers at a conduction velocity of about 1 m/sec. A special pathway, the anterior interatrial myocardial band (or Bachmann's bundle), conducts the SA node impulse directly to the left atrium. The wave of excitation proceeds inferiorly through the right atrium and ultimately reaches the AV node (Fig. 16-17), which is normally the sole entry route of the cardiac impulse to the ventricles.

When compared with the potential recorded from a typical ventricular fiber, the atrial plateau (phase 2) is briefer and less developed, and repolarization (phase 3) is slower (Fig. 16-10). The action potential duration in atrial myocytes is briefer than that in ventricular myocytes because efflux of K+ is greater during

Some people have accessory AV pathways. Because these pathways often serve as a part of a reentry loop (see later), they can be associated with serious cardiac rhythm disturbances. Wolff-Parkinson-White syndrome, a congenital disturbance, is the most common clinical disorder in which a bypass tract of myocardial fibers becomes an accessory pathway between the atria and ventricles. Ordinarily, the syndrome causes no functional abnormality. The disturbance is easily detected on an ECG because a portion of the ventricle is excited via the bypass tract before the remainder of the ventricle is excited via the AV node and His-Purkinje system. This preexcitation can be seen as a bizarre configuration in the ventricular (QRS) complex of the ECG. Occasionally, however, a reentry loop develops in which the atrial impulse travels to the ventricles via one of the two AV pathways (AV node or bypass tract) and then back to the atria through the other of these two pathways. Continuous circling around the loop leads to a very rapid rhythm (supraventricular tachycardia). This rapid rhythm may be incapacitating because it might not allow sufficient time for ventricular filling. Transient block of the AV node by injecting adenosine intravenously or by increasing vagal activity reflexively (by pressing on the neck over the carotid sinus region) usually abolishes the tachycardia and restores a normal sinus rhythm.

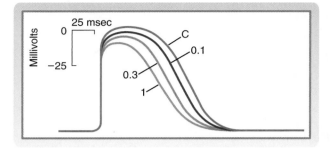

● **Figure 16-21.** Transmembrane potentials recorded from an atrioventricular (AV) node cell under control conditions (C) and in the presence of the Ca^{++} channel antagonist diltiazem at concentrations of 0.1, 0.3, and 1 mmol/L. (Redrawn from Hirth C et al: J Mol Cell Cardiol 15:799, 1983.)

the plateau in atrial myocytes than in ventricular myocytes.

Atrioventricular Conduction

The atrial excitation wave reaches the ventricles via the AV node. In adult humans, this node is approximately 15 mm long, 10 mm wide, and 3 mm thick. The node is situated posteriorly on the right side of the interatrial septum near the ostium of the coronary sinus. The AV node contains the same two cell types as the SA node, but the round cells in the AV node are less abundant and the elongated cells predominate.

The AV node is made up of three functional regions: (1) the AN region, or the transitional zone between the atrium and the remainder of the node; (2) the N region, or the midportion of the AV node; and (3) the NH region, or the zone in which nodal fibers gradually merge with the **bundle of His,** which is the upper portion of the specialized conducting system for the ventricles (Fig. 16-17). Normally, the AV node and the bundle of His are the only pathways along which the cardiac impulse travels from atria to ventricles.

Several features of AV conduction are of physiological and clinical significance. The principal delay in conduction of impulses from the atria to the ventricles occurs in the AN and N regions of the AV node. Conduction velocity is actually less in the N region than in the AN region. However, the path length is substantially greater in the AN than the N region. Conduction

times through the AN and N zones account for the delay between the start of the P wave (the electrical manifestation of atrial excitation) and the QRS complex (the electrical manifestation of ventricular excitation) on an ECG (see later). Functionally, the delay between atrial and ventricular excitation permits optimal ventricular filling during atrial contraction.

In the N region, slow-response action potentials prevail. The resting potential is about −60 mV, the upstroke velocity is low (about 5 V/sec), and the conduction velocity is about 0.05 m/sec.* Tetrodotoxin, which blocks the fast Na$^+$ channels, has virtually no effect on action potentials in this region (or on any other slow-response fibers). Conversely, Ca^{++} channel antagonists decrease the amplitude and duration of the action potentials (Fig. 16-21) and depress AV conduction.

Like other slow-response action potentials, the relative refractory period of cells in the N region extends well beyond the period of complete repolarization; that is, these cells display postrepolarization refractoriness (Fig. 16-15). As the heart rate increases, the time between successive atrial depolarizations is decreased, and conduction through the AV junction slows. Abnormal prolongation of the AV conduction time is called a first-degree AV block (see later). Most of the prolongation of AV conduction induced by a decrease in atrial cycle length takes place in the N region of the AV node.

Impulses tend to be blocked in the AV node at stimulation frequencies that are easily conducted in other regions of the heart. If the atria are depolarized at a high repetition rate, only a fraction (e.g., half) of the atrial impulses might be conducted through the AV junction to the ventricles. The conduction pattern in which only a fraction of the atrial impulses are conducted to the ventricles is called a second-degree AV block (see later). This type of block may protect the ventricles from excessive contraction frequencies,

---

*The shapes of the action potentials in the AN region are intermediate between those in the N region and those in the atria. Similarly, action potentials in the NH region are transitional between those in the N region and those in the bundle of His.

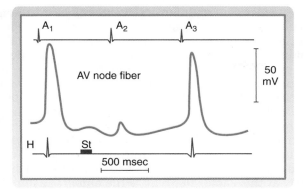

● **Figure 16-22.** Effects of a brief vagal stimulus (St) on the transmembrane potential recorded from an AV nodal fiber. Note that shortly after vagal stimulation, the membrane of the fiber was hyperpolarized. The atrial excitation (A_2) that arrived at the AV node when the cell was hyperpolarized failed to be conducted, as denoted by the absence of a depolarization in the His electrogram (H). The atrial excitations that preceded (A_1) and followed (A_3) excitation A_2 were conducted to the His bundle region. (Redrawn from Mazgalev T et al: Am J Physiol 251:H631, 1986.)

wherein the filling time between contractions might be inadequate.

Retrograde conduction can occur through the AV node. However, the conduction time is significantly longer and the impulse is blocked at lower repetition rates when the impulse is conducted in the retrograde instead of the antegrade direction. Finally the AV node is a common site for reentry (see later).

As in the SA node, the autonomic nervous system regulates AV conduction. Weak vagal activity may simply prolong the AV conduction time. Thus, for any given atrial cycle length, the atrium-to-His (A-H) or atrium-to-ventricle (A-V) conduction time will be prolonged by vagal stimulation. Stronger vagal activity may cause some or all of the impulses arriving from the atria to be blocked in the node. The conduction pattern in which none of the atrial impulses reaches the ventricles is called a third-degree, or complete, AV block (see later). The vagally induced delay or absence of conduction through the AV junction occurs mainly in the N region of the node. This effect of vagal stimulation reflects the action of acetylcholine to hyperpolarize the membrane potential of the conducting fibers in the N region (Fig. 16-22). The greater the hyperpolarization at the time of arrival of the atrial impulse, the more impaired the AV conduction.

Cardiac sympathetic nerves, in contrast, facilitate AV conduction. They decrease the AV conduction time and enhance the rhythmicity of latent pacemakers in the AV junction. The norepinephrine released at the postganglionic sympathetic nerve terminals increases the amplitude and slope of the upstroke of the AV nodal action potentials, principally in the AN and N regions of the node.

Ventricular Conduction

The bundle of His passes subendocardially down the right side of the interventricular septum for about

Conduction of impulses in the right or left bundle branch or in either division of the left bundle branch may be impaired. Conduction blocks may develop in one or more of these conduction pathways as a consequence of coronary artery disease or degenerative processes associated with aging, and they give rise to characteristic ECG patterns. Block of either of the main bundle branches is known as right or left bundle branch block. Block of either division of the left bundle branch is called left anterior or left posterior hemiblock.

1 cm and then divides into the right and left bundle branches (Fig. 16-17). The right bundle branch, a direct continuation of the bundle of His, proceeds down the right side of the interventricular septum. The left bundle branch, which is considerably thicker than the right, arises almost perpendicular from the bundle of His and perforates the interventricular septum. On the subendocardial surface of the left side of the interventricular septum, the left bundle branch splits into a thin anterior division and a thick posterior division.

The right bundle branch and the two divisions of the left bundle branch ultimately subdivide into a complex network of conducting fibers, called Purkinje fibers, that spread out over the subendocardial surfaces of both ventricles.

Purkinje fibers have abundant, linearly arranged sarcomeres, as do myocytes. However, the T tubular system, which is well developed in myocytes, is absent in the Purkinje fibers of many species. Purkinje fibers are the broadest cells in the heart: 70 to 80 μm in diameter, as compared with diameters of 10 to 15 μm for ventricular myocytes. Partly because of the large diameter of the Purkinje fibers, conduction velocity (1 to 4 m/sec) in these fibers exceeds that in any other fiber type within the heart. The increased conduction velocity permits rapid activation of the entire endocardial surface of the ventricles.

The action potentials recorded from Purkinje fibers resemble those of ordinary ventricular myocardial fibers. However, because of the long refractory period of Purkinje fiber action potentials, many premature excitations of the atria are conducted through the AV junction but are then blocked by the Purkinje fibers. Blockade of these atrial excitations prevents premature contraction of the ventricles. This function of protecting the ventricles against the effects of premature atrial depolarization is especially pronounced at slow heart rates because the action potential duration and hence the effective refractory period of the Purkinje fibers vary inversely with the heart rate (Fig. 16-16). At slow heart rates, the effective refractory period of the Purkinje fibers is especially prolonged.* In contrast to Purkinje fibers, the effective refractory period of AV node cells does not change appreciably over the

---

*Similar directional changes in the refractory period also occur in ventricular myocytes in response to changes in rate.

normal range of heart rates and actually increases at very rapid heart rates. Therefore, when the atrium is excited at high repetition rates, it is the AV node that normally protects the ventricles from these excessively high frequencies.

The first portions of the ventricles to be excited by impulses arriving from the AV node are the interventricular septum (except the basal portion) and the papillary muscles. The activation wave spreads into the substance of the septum from both its left and right endocardial surfaces. Early contraction of the septum makes it more rigid and allows it to serve as an anchor point for contraction of the remaining ventricular myocardium. Furthermore, early contraction of the papillary muscles prevents eversion of the AV valves into the atria during ventricular systole.

The endocardial surfaces of both ventricles are activated rapidly, but the wave of excitation spreads from endocardium to epicardium at a slower velocity (about 0.3 to 0.4 m/sec). The epicardial surface of the right ventricle is activated earlier than that of the left ventricle because the right ventricular wall is appreciably thinner than the left. In addition, the apical and central epicardial regions of both ventricles are activated somewhat earlier than their respective basal regions. The last portions of the ventricles to be excited are the posterior basal epicardial regions and a small zone in the basal portion of the interventricular septum.

Reentry

The conditions necessary for reentry are illustrated in Figure 16-23. In each of the four panels a single bundle (S) of cardiac fibers splits into a left (L) and a right (R) branch. A connecting bundle (C) runs between the two branches. Normally the impulse moving down bundle S is conducted along the L and R branches (Fig. 16-23, *A*). As the impulse reaches connecting link C, it enters from both sides and becomes extinguished at the point of collision. The impulse from the left side cannot proceed because the tissue beyond is absolutely refractory; it has just been depolarized from the other direction. The impulse also cannot pass through bundle C from the right for the same reason.

Figure 16-23, *B*, shows that the impulse cannot complete the circuit if an antegrade block exists in the L and R branches of the fiber bundle. Furthermore, if a bidirectional block exists at any point in the loop (e.g., branch R in Fig. 16-23, *C*), the impulse also cannot reenter.

A necessary condition for reentry is that at some point in the loop the impulse can pass in one direction but not in the other. This phenomenon is called unidirectional block. As shown in Figure 16-23, *D*, the impulse may travel down branch L normally but become blocked in the antegrade direction in branch R because of some pathological change in the myocardial cells in that branch. The impulse that was conducted down branch L and through the connecting branch C may then be able to penetrate the depressed region in branch R from the retrograde direction, even though the antegrade impulse had been blocked previously at this same site. Why is the antegrade impulse blocked but not the retrograde impulse? The reason is that the antegrade impulse arrives at the depressed region in branch R earlier than the retrograde impulse does because the path length of the antegrade impulse is very short, whereas the retrograde impulse traverses a much longer path. Therefore, the antegrade impulse may be blocked simply because it arrives at the depressed region during its effective refractory period. If the retrograde impulse is delayed sufficiently, the refractory period may have ended in the affected region, and the impulse can then be conducted back through this region and return to bundle S.

Although unidirectional block is a necessary condition for reentry, it alone cannot cause reentry. For reentry to occur, the effective refractory period of the reentered region must be shorter than the conduction time around the loop. In Figure 16-23, *D*, if the tissue

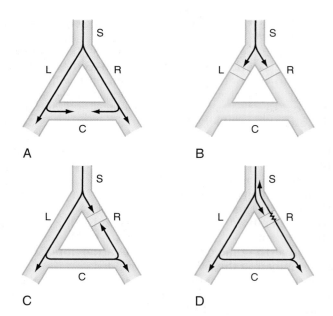

● **Figure 16-23.** The role of unidirectional block in reentry. In **A,** an excitation wave traveling down a single bundle (S) of fibers continues down the left (L) and right (R) branches. The depolarization wave enters the connecting branch (C) from both ends and is extinguished at the zone of collision. In **B,** the wave is blocked in the L and R branches. In **C,** a bidirectional block exists in branch R. In **D,** a unidirectional block exists in branch R. The antegrade impulse is blocked, but the retrograde impulse is conducted through and reenters bundle S.

just beyond the depressed zone in branch R is still refractory from the antegrade depolarization, the retrograde impulse will not be conducted into branch S. Therefore, the conditions that promote reentry are those that prolong the conduction time or shorten the effective refractory period.

The functional characteristics of the various components of the reentry loops responsible for specific cardiac arrhythmias are diverse. Some loops are large and involve entire specialized conduction bundles, whereas others are microscopic. The loop may include myocardial fibers, specialized conducting fibers, nodal cells, and junctional tissues in almost any conceivable arrangement. In addition, the various cardiac cells in the loop may be normal or abnormal.

The propagation velocity along a multicellular cardiac conduction fiber is normally facilitated by the gap junctions that lie between consecutive conducting fibers. Variations in the protein structure of the connexins in the gap junctions can affect the propagation velocity along these fibers. The chemical structure of the specific connexins can vary locally in cardiac tissues and, as a result, can establish local variations in propagation velocity. Such topical variations in velocity might include regions of unidirectional block that induce reentrant rhythm disturbances.

Triggered Activity

Triggered activity is so named because it is always coupled to a preceding action potential. Because reentrant activity is also coupled to a preceding action potential, the arrhythmias induced by triggered activity are usually difficult to distinguish from those induced by reentry. Triggered activity is caused by **afterdepolarizations.** Two types of afterdepolarizations are recognized: **early (EAD)** and **delayed (DAD).** EADs may appear either at the end of the action potential plateau (phase 2) or about midway through repolarization (phase 3), whereas DADs occur near the very end of repolarization or just after full repolarization (phase 4).

Early Afterdepolarizations

EADs are more likely to occur when the prevailing heart rate is slow; a rapid heart rate suppresses EADs (Fig. 16-24). EADs are also more likely to occur in cardiac cells with prolonged action potentials than in cells with shorter action potentials. For example, EADs can be induced more readily in myocytes from the midmyocardial region of the ventricular walls than in

myocytes from the endocardial or epicardial regions because of the longer action potential of midmyocardial myocytes (Fig. 16-5). Certain antiarrhythmic drugs, such as quinidine, prolong the action potential. Consequently, such drugs increase the likelihood that EADs may occur. Hence, antiarrhythmic drugs are also sometimes proarrhythmic.

The direct correlation between a cell's action potential duration and its susceptibility to EADs is probably related to the time required for Ca^{++} channels in the cell membranes to recover from inactivation. When action potentials are sufficiently prolonged, the Ca^{++} channels that were activated at the beginning of the plateau have sufficient time to recover from inactivation and thus may be reactivated before the cell fully repolarizes. This secondary activation could then trigger an EAD.

Delayed Afterdepolarizations

In contrast to EADs, DADs are more likely to occur when the heart rate is high (Fig. 16-25). DADs are associated with elevated $[Ca^{++}]_i$. The amplitudes of DADs are increased by interventions that raise $[Ca^{++}]_i$, such as increasing $[Ca^{++}]_o$ and administering toxic amounts of digitalis glycosides. The elevated levels of intracellular Ca^{++} provoke the oscillatory release of Ca^{++} from the SR. Hence, in myocardial cells, DADs are accompanied by small rhythmic changes in the force developed. The high $[Ca^{++}]_i$ also activates certain membrane channels that permit the passage of Na^+ and K^+. The net flux of these cations constitutes a transient inward

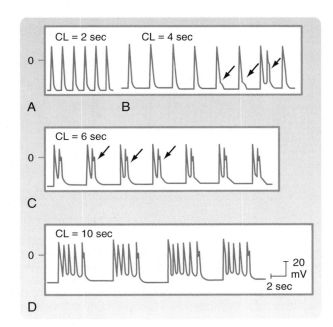

● **Figure 16-24.** Effect of pacing at different cycle lengths (CL) on cesium-induced early afterdepolarizations (EADs) in a Purkinje fiber. **A,** EADs not evident. **B,** EADs first appear *(arrows)*. The third EAD reaches threshold and triggers an action potential *(third arrow)*. **C,** EADs that appear after each driven depolarization trigger an action potential. **D,** Triggered action potentials occur in salvos. (Modified from Damiano BP, Rosen M: Circulation 69:1013, 1984.)

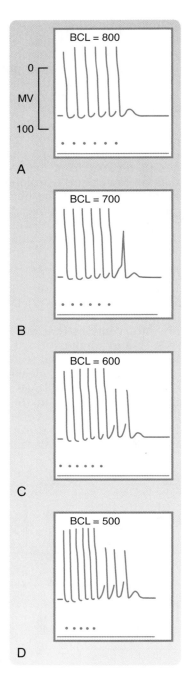

● Figure 16-25. Transmembrane action potentials recorded from Purkinje fibers. Acetylstrophanthidin, a digitalis glycoside, was added to the bath, and sequences of six driven beats (denoted by the *dots*) were produced at a basic cycle length (BCL) of 800 **(A)**, 700 **(B)**, 600 **(C)**, and 500 **(D)** msec. Note that delayed afterpotentials occurred after the driven beats and that these afterpotentials reached threshold after the last driven beat in **B** to **D.** (From Ferrier GR et al: Circ Res 32:600, 1973.)

ELECTROCARDIOGRAPHY

The **ECG** enables physicians to infer the course of the cardiac impulse by recording the variations in electrical potential at various loci on the surface of the body. By analyzing the details of these fluctuations in electrical potential, the physician gains valuable insight into (1) the anatomical orientation of the heart; (2) the relative sizes of its chambers; (3) various disturbances in rhythm and conduction; (4) the extent, location, and progress of ischemic damage to the myocardium; (5) the effects of altered electrolyte concentrations; and (6) the influence of certain drugs (notably digitalis, antiarrhythmic agents, and Ca^{++} channel antagonists). Because electrocardiography is an extensive and complex discipline, only the elementary principles are considered in this section.

Scalar Electrocardiography

In electrocardiography, a lead is the electrical connection from the patient's skin to a recording device **(electrocardiograph)** that measures the electrical activity of the heart. The system of leads used to record routine ECGs is oriented in certain planes of the body. The diverse electrical events that exist in the heart at any moment can be represented by a three-dimensional vector (a quantity with magnitude and direction). A system of recording leads oriented in a given plane detects only the projection of the three-dimensional vector on that plane. The potential difference between two recording electrodes represents the projection of the vector on the line between the two leads. Components of vectors projected on such lines are not vectors but scalar quantities (having magnitude, but not direction). Hence, a recording of changes in the difference in potential between two points on the skin surface over time is called a scalar ECG.

A scalar ECG detects temporal changes in the electrical potential between some point on the surface of the skin and an indifferent electrode or between pairs of points on the skin surface. The cardiac impulse progresses through the heart in a complex three-dimensional pattern. Hence, the precise configuration of the ECG varies from individual to individual, and in any given individual the pattern varies with the anatomic location of the leads. The graphic display of the electrical impulse recorded by an ECG is called a tracing.

In general, a tracing consists of P, QRS, and T waves (Fig. 16-26). The P wave reflects the spread of depolarization through the atria, the QRS wave (or complex) reflects depolarization of the ventricles, and the T wave represents repolarization of the ventricles (repolarization of the atria occurs and is therefore masked during ventricular depolarization). The PR interval (or more precisely, the PQ interval) is a measure of the time from the onset of atrial activation to the onset of ventricular activation; it normally ranges from 0.12 to 0.20 second. A large fraction of this time involves passage of the impulse through the AV conduction system. Pathological prolongations of the PR interval are associated with disturbances in AV conduction. Such disturbances may be produced by

current, i_{ti}, that contributes to the appearance of DADs. The elevated $[Ca^{++}]_i$ may also activate the $3Na^+$-$1Ca^{++}$ antiporter. This electrogenic antiporter, which moves 3 Na^+ ions into the cell for each Ca^{++} ion that it ejects, also creates a net inward cation current that contributes to the appearance of DADs.

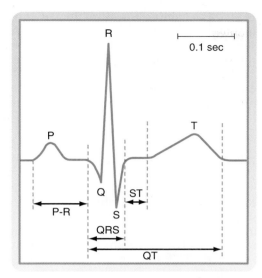

● **Figure 16-26.** Important deflections and intervals of a typical scalar ECG.

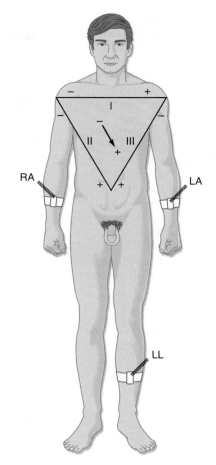

● **Figure 16-27.** Einthoven triangle illustrating the electrocardiographic connections for standard limb leads I, II, and III.

inflammatory, circulatory, pharmacological, or nervous mechanisms.

The configuration and amplitude of the QRS complex vary considerably among individuals. The duration is usually between 0.06 and 0.10 second. An abnormally prolonged QRS complex may indicate a block in the normal conduction pathways through the ventricles (such as a block of the left or right bundle branch). During the ST interval, the entire ventricular myocardium is depolarized. Therefore, the ST segment normally lies on the isoelectric line. Any appreciable deviation of the ST segment from the isoelectric line may indicate ischemic damage to the myocardium. The QT interval, sometimes referred to as the period of "electrical systole" of the ventricles, is closely correlated with the mean action potential duration of the ventricular myocytes. The duration of the QT interval is about 0.4 second, but it varies inversely with the heart rate, mainly because the duration of the myocardial cell action potential varies inversely with the heart rate (Fig. 16-16).

In most leads, the T wave is deflected in the same direction from the isoelectric line as the major component of the QRS complex, although biphasic (that is, oppositely directed) T waves are perfectly normal in certain leads. Deviation of the T wave and QRS complex in the same direction from the isoelectric line indicates that the repolarization process is proceeding in a direction counter to that of the depolarization process. T waves that are abnormal either in direction or in amplitude may indicate myocardial damage, electrolyte disturbances, or cardiac hypertrophy.

Standard Limb Leads

The original ECG lead system was devised by Einthoven about a century ago. In this system, the vector sum of all cardiac electrical activity at any moment is called the **resultant cardiac vector.** This directional electrical force is considered to lie in the center of an equilateral triangle whose apices are located in the left and right shoulders and the pubic region (Fig. 16-27). This triangle, called **Einthoven's triangle,** is oriented in the frontal plane of the body. Hence, only the projection of the resultant cardiac vector on the frontal plane is detected by this system of leads. For convenience, the electrodes are connected to the right and left forearms rather than to the corresponding shoulders because the arms represent simple electrical extensions of leads from the shoulders. Similarly, the leg represents an extension of the lead system from the pubis, and thus the third electrode is generally connected to an ankle (usually the left one).

Certain conventions dictate the manner in which these standard limb leads are connected to the electrocardiograph. Lead I records the potential difference between the left arm (LA) and the right arm (RA). The connections are such that when the potential at LA (V_{LA}) exceeds the potential at RA (V_{RA}), the tracing is deflected upward from the isoelectric line. In Figures 16-27 and 16-28, this arrangement of connections for lead I is designated by a (+) at LA and by a (−) at RA. Lead II records the potential difference between RA and LL (left leg), and the tracing is deflected upward when V_{LL} exceeds V_{RA}. Finally, lead III registers the potential difference between LA and LL, and the tracing is deflected upward when V_{LL} exceeds V_{LA}. These connections were arbitrarily chosen so that the QRS complexes are upright in all three standard limb leads in most normal individuals.

If the frontal projection of a resultant cardiac vector at some moment is represented by an arrow (tail negative, head positive), as in Figure 16-27, the potential difference, $V_{LA} - V_{RA}$, recorded in lead I is represented by the component of the vector projected along the horizontal line between LA and RA, also shown in Figure 16-27. If the vector makes an angle (θ) of 60 degrees with the horizontal line (as in Fig. 16-28, A), the deflection recorded in lead I is upward because the positive arrowhead lies closer to LA than to RA. The deflection in lead II is also upright because the arrowhead lies closer to LL than to RA. The magnitude of the lead II deflection is greater than that in lead I

because in this example the direction of the vector parallels that of lead II; therefore, the magnitude of the projection on lead II exceeds that on lead I. Similarly, in lead III, the deflection is upright and its magnitude equals that in lead I.

If the vector in Figure 16-27, A, is the result of electrical events that occur during the peak of the QRS complex, the orientation of this vector is said to represent the mean electrical axis of the heart in the frontal plane. The positive rotatory direction of this axis is taken to be in the clockwise direction from the horizontal plane (contrary to the usual mathematical convention). In normal individuals, the average mean electrical axis is approximately +60 degrees (as in Fig. 16-28, A). Therefore, QRS complexes are usually upright in all three leads and largest in lead II.

If the mean electrical axis shifts substantially to the right (as in Fig. 16-28, B, where θ = 120 degrees), projections of the QRS complexes on the standard leads change considerably. In this case, the largest upright deflection is in lead III, and the deflection in lead I is inverted because the arrowhead is closer to RA than to LA. Such a shift is termed right axis deviation and occurs with hypertrophy (i.e., increased thickness) of the right ventricle. When the axis shifts to the left, as occurs with hypertrophy of the left ventricle (Fig. 16-28, C, where θ = 0 degrees), the largest upright deflection is in lead I, and the QRS complex in lead III is inverted.

In addition to limb leads I, II, and III, other limb leads that are also oriented in the frontal plane are routinely recorded in patients. These leads are (1) **aVR,** where the right arm is defined as the positive lead and the middle of the heart is defined as the negative lead (i.e., the left arm and ankle leads are connected together); (2) **aVL,** where the left arm is the positive lead and the middle of the heart is defined as the negative lead (i.e., the right arm and ankle leads are connected together); and (3) **aVF,** where the ankle (foot) lead is defined as positive and the middle of the heart is defined as the negative lead (i.e., the two arm leads are connected together). The axes of these leads form angles of +90 degrees for aVF, −30 degrees for aVL, and −150 degrees for aVR (all with respect to the horizontal axis). Finally, leads can be applied to the surface of the chest, so-called **precordial leads,** to determine the

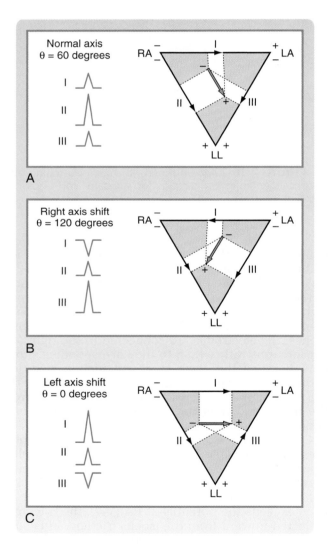

● **Figure 16-28.** Magnitude and direction of the QRS complexes in limb leads I, II, and III when the mean electrical axis (θ) is 60 degrees **(A),** 120 degrees **(B),** and 0 degrees **(C).**

> ### IN THE CLINIC

Changes in the mean electrical axis may occur if the anatomic position of the heart is altered or if the relative mass of the right and left ventricles is abnormal, as it is in certain cardiovascular disturbances. For example, the axis tends to shift toward the left (more horizontal) in short, stocky individuals and toward the right (more vertical) in tall, thin persons. In addition, in left or right ventricular hypertrophy (increased myocardial mass of either ventricle), the axis shifts toward the hypertrophied side.

projections of the cardiac vector on the sagittal and transverse planes of the body. These precordial leads are recorded from six selected points on the anterior and lateral surfaces of the chest in the vicinity of the heart. The leads extend from the right border of the sternum in the fourth intercostal space (V_1) to under the left arm (midaxillary line) in the fifth intercostal space (V_6). Each precordial lead (V_1 to V_6) is defined as a positive lead, whereas the middle of the heart is defined as the negative lead. Detailed analysis of the ECG, as detected by the various lead systems just described, is beyond the scope of this book. Interested students are referred to textbooks on electrocardiography for more information.

ARRHYTHMIAS

Cardiac arrhythmias are disturbances in either impulse initiation or impulse propagation. Disturbances in impulse initiation include those that arise from the SA node and those that originate from various ectopic foci. The principal disturbances in impulse propagation are conduction blocks and reentrant rhythms.

Altered Sinoatrial Rhythms

Mechanisms that vary the firing frequency of cardiac pacemaker cells were described previously. Changes in the firing rate of the SA node are usually produced by the cardiac autonomic nerves. When the firing rate of the SA node is decreased, the heart rate also decreases **(bradycardia).** Conversely, increased SA node firing results in an elevated heart rate **(tachycardia).** Examples of ECGs of sinus tachycardia and sinus bradycardia are shown in Figure 16-29. The P, QRS, and T deflections are all normal, but cardiac cycle duration (the PP interval) is altered. Characteristically, cardiac frequency changes gradually. A rhythmic variation of the PP interval at the respiratory frequency (i.e., a respiratory sinus arrhythmia) is a normal, common occurrence.

Atrioventricular Conduction Blocks

Various physiological, pharmacological, and pathological processes can impede transmission of an impulse through the AV node. The site of block can be localized more precisely by recording the His bundle electrogram (Fig. 16-30). To obtain such tracings, an electrode catheter is introduced into a peripheral vein and threaded centrally into the right side of the heart until the electrode lies in the AV junctional region. When the electrode is properly positioned, a distinct deflection (H in Fig. 16-30) is registered as the cardiac impulse passes through the bundle of His. The time intervals required for propagation from the atrium to the bundle of His (A-H interval) and from the bundle of His to the ventricles (H-V interval) may be measured accurately. Abnormal prolongation of the A-H or H-V interval indicates block above or below the bundle of His, respectively.

● **Figure 16-29.** **A** to **C,** Sinoatrial rhythms.

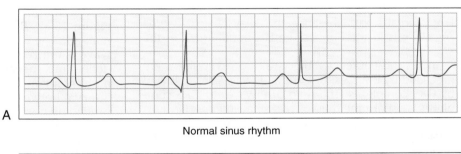

A

Normal sinus rhythm

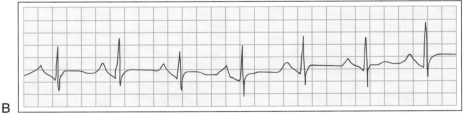

B

Sinus tachycardia

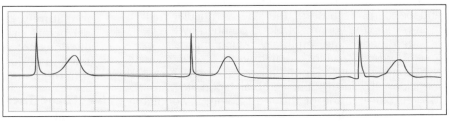

C

Sinus bradycardia

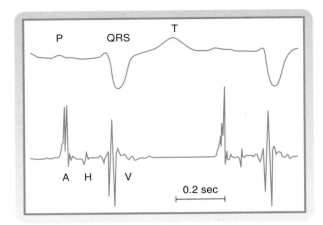

● **Figure 16-30.** His bundle electrogram (**lower tracing,** retouched) and lead II of the scalar electrocardiogram **(upper tracing).** The deflection H, which represents conduction of the impulse over the bundle of His, is clearly visible between the atrial (A) and the ventricular (V) deflections. The conduction time from the atria to the bundle of His is denoted by the A-H interval, and that from the bundle of His to the ventricles, by the H-V interval. (Courtesy of Dr. J. Edelstein.)

> ### IN THE CLINIC
>
> Three degrees of AV block can be distinguished, as shown in Figure 16-31. First-degree AV block is characterized by a prolonged PR interval. In most cases of first-degree block, the A-H interval is prolonged and the H-V interval is normal. Hence, the delay in a first-degree AV block is located above the His bundle (i.e., in the AV node).
>
> In second-degree AV block, all QRS complexes are preceded by P waves, but not all P waves are followed by QRS complexes. The ratio of P waves to QRS complexes is usually the ratio of two small integers (such as 2:1, 3:1, or 3:2). The site of block may be located above or below the His bundle. A block below the bundle is usually more serious than one above the bundle because the former is more likely to evolve into a third-degree block. An artificial pacemaker is frequently implanted when the block is below the bundle.
>
> Third-degree AV block is often referred to as complete heart block because the impulse is completely unable to traverse the AV conduction pathway from atria to ventricles. The most common sites of complete block are distal to the bundle of His. In complete heart block, the atrial and ventricular rhythms are entirely independent. Because of the slow ventricular rhythm that results, the volume of blood pumped by the heart is often inadequate, especially during muscular exercise. Third-degree block is frequently associated with syncope (pronounced lightheadedness), which is caused principally by insufficient cerebral blood flow. Third-degree block is one of the most common conditions that require artificial pacemakers.

Premature Depolarizations

Premature depolarizations occur occasionally in most normal individuals, but they arise more commonly in certain abnormal conditions. Such depolarizations may originate in the atria, AV junction, or ventricles. One type of premature depolarization follows a normally conducted depolarization at a constant time interval (the **coupling interval**). If the normal depolarization is suppressed in some way (e.g., by vagal stimulation), the premature depolarization is also abolished. Such premature depolarizations are called **coupled extrasystoles,** or simply **extrasystoles,** and they generally reflect a reentry phenomenon. A second type of premature depolarization occurs as the result of enhanced automaticity in some ectopic focus. This ectopic center may fire regularly, and a zone of tissue that conducts unidirectionally may protect this center from being depolarized by the normal cardiac impulse. If this premature depolarization occurs at a regular interval or at an integral multiple of that interval, the disturbance is called **parasystole.**

A premature atrial depolarization is shown in Figure 16-32, _A._ With a premature atrial depolarization, the normal interval between beats is shortened. In addition, the configuration of the premature P wave differs from that of the other normal P waves because the course of atrial excitation, which originates at some ectopic focus in the atrium, differs from the normal spread of excitation, which originates at the SA node. The QRS complex of the premature depolarization is generally normal because the ventricular excitation spreads over the usual pathways.

A premature ventricular depolarization is shown in Figure 16-32, _B._ Propagation of the impulse is abnormal, and the configuration of the QRS complex and T wave is entirely different from the normal ventricular deflections because the premature excitation originates at some ectopic focus in the ventricles. The time interval between the premature QRS complex and the preceding normal QRS complex is shortened, whereas the interval after the premature QRS complex and the next normal QRS complex is prolonged. The interval from the QRS complex just before the premature excitation to the QRS complex just after it is virtually equal to the duration of two normal cardiac cycles.

As noted, a compensatory pause usually follows a premature ventricular depolarization. This pause occurs because the ectopic ventricular impulse does not disturb the natural rhythm of the SA node, either because the ectopic ventricular impulse is not conducted retrograde through the AV conduction system or because the SA node had already fired at its natural interval before the ectopic impulse could have reached and depolarized it prematurely. Likewise, the SA nodal impulse generated just before or after the ventricular extrasystole generally does not affect the ventricle because the AV junction and perhaps also the ventricles are still refractory from the premature ventricular excitation.

Ectopic Tachycardias

In contrast to the gradual rate changes that characterize sinus tachycardia, tachycardias that originate from

● **Figure 16-31.** AV blocks. **A,** First-degree block; the PR interval is 0.28 second (normal, <0.20 sec). **B,** Second-degree block (2:1). **C,** Third-degree block; note the dissociation between the P waves and the QRS complexes.

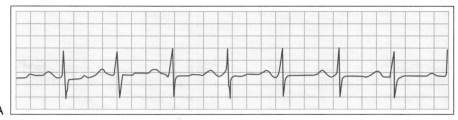

First-degree AV block

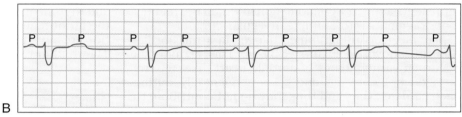

Second-degree AV block (2:1)

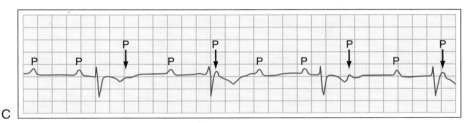

Third-degree AV block

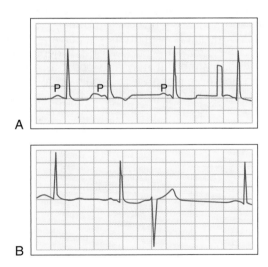

● **Figure 16-32.** Premature atrial depolarization **(A)** and premature ventricular depolarization **(B).** The premature atrial depolarization (the second beat in **A**) is characterized by an inverted P wave and normal QRS complexes and T waves. The interval after the premature depolarization is not much longer than the usual interval between beats. The brief rectangular deflection just before the last depolarization is a standardization signal. The premature ventricular depolarization is characterized by bizarre QRS complexes and T waves and is followed by a compensatory pause.

IN THE CLINIC

Paroxysmal tachycardias that originate either in the atria or in the AV junctional tissues (Fig. 16-33, *A*) are usually indistinguishable, and therefore both are included in the term paroxysmal supraventricular tachycardia. In this tachycardia, the impulse often circles a reentry loop that includes atrial and AV junctional tissue. The QRS complexes are frequently normal because ventricular activation proceeds over the usual pathways.

As its name implies, paroxysmal ventricular tachycardia originates from an ectopic focus in the ventricles. The ECG is characterized by repeated, bizarre QRS complexes that reflect the abnormal intraventricular impulse conduction (Fig. 16-33, *B*). Paroxysmal ventricular tachycardia is much more ominous than supraventricular tachycardia because the former is frequently a precursor of ventricular fibrillation, a lethal arrhythmia described in the next section.

an ectopic focus typically begin and end abruptly. Such ectopic tachycardias are generally called **paroxysmal tachycardias.** Episodes of paroxysmal tachycardia may persist for only a few beats or for many hours or days, and episodes often recur. Paroxysmal tachycardias may result from (1) rapid firing of an ectopic pacemaker, (2) triggered activity secondary to afterpotentials that reach threshold, or (3) an impulse that circles a reentry loop repetitively.

Fibrillation

Under certain conditions, cardiac muscle undergoes an irregular type of contraction that is entirely ineffectual in propelling blood. Such an arrhythmia is termed **fibrillation,** and the disturbance may involve either the atria or the ventricles. Fibrillation probably represents a reentry phenomenon in which the reentry loop fragments into multiple, irregular circuits.

The electrocardiographic changes in atrial fibrillation are shown in Figure 16-34, *A*. This arrhythmia occurs in various types of chronic heart disease. The atria do not contract and relax sequentially during each cardiac cycle, and thus they do not contribute to ventricular filling. Instead, the atria undergo a continuous, uncoordinated rippling motion. P waves do not appear on the ECG, and they are replaced by continuous irregular fluctuations in potential called f waves. The AV node is activated at intervals that may vary considerably from cycle to cycle. Hence, no constant interval occurs between successive QRS complexes or between successive ventricular contractions. Because the strength of ventricular contraction depends on the interval between beats (see Chapter 18), the volume and rhythm of the pulse are irregular. In many patients, the atrial reentry loop and the pattern of AV conduction are more regular than they are in atrial fibrillation. The rhythm is then referred to as atrial flutter.

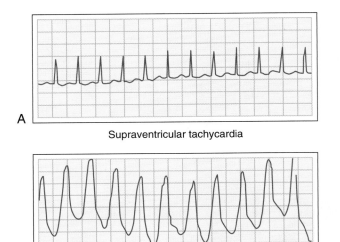

A
Supraventricular tachycardia

B
Ventricular tachycardia

● **Figure 16-33.** **A** and **B,** Paroxysmal tachycardias.

IN THE CLINIC

Atrial fibrillation and flutter are not usually life-threatening; some people with these disturbances can function normally. However, because the atria do not contract and relax rhythmically, blood clots tend to form in the atria. Such clots, if dislodged, may then travel to the pulmonary or systemic vascular beds. Patients with atrial fibrillation or flutter are generally treated with anticoagulant drugs such as dicumarol to prevent the formation of such clots.

Ventricular fibrillation, in contrast, leads to loss of consciousness within a few seconds. The irregular, continuous, uncoordinated twitching of the ventricular muscle fibers pumps no blood. Death ensues unless immediate effective resuscitation is achieved or the rhythm spontaneously reverts to normal, which rarely occurs. Ventricular fibrillation may supervene when the entire ventricle, or some portion of it, is deprived of its normal blood supply. It may also occur as a result of electrocution or in response to certain drugs and anesthetics. On the ECG (Fig. 16-34, *B*), the fluctuations in potential are highly irregular.

● **Figure 16-34.** Atrial and ventricular fibrillation.

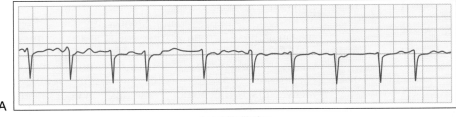

A
Atrial fibrillation

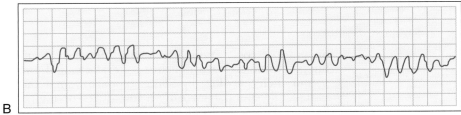

B
Ventricular fibrillation

● AT THE CELLULAR LEVEL

In some individuals the interval between the QRS complex and the T wave is abnormally prolonged, a condition termed long QT syndrome (Fig. 16-35). Several congenital forms of long QT syndrome have been identified in human subjects. Two of the many genes that have been identified as the basis for this syndrome are the *HERG* gene (a K+ channel gene), located on chromosome 7, and the *SCN5A* gene (a Na+ gene), located on chromosome 3. Patients with congenital forms of long QT syndrome may have periodic episodes of syncope (fainting), and about 10% of pediatric subjects with this disorder may die suddenly, without any preceding symptoms. Long QT syndrome may also be acquired inasmuch as a subtle genetic change is not evident until a drug is taken that affects the ion channel involved. Many drugs, including several antiarrhythmic agents, have been identified as causing acquired long QT syndrome.

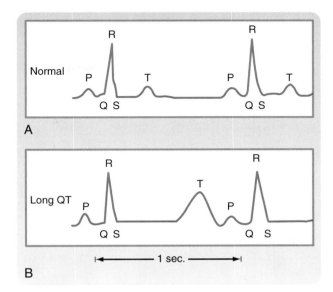

● **Figure 16-35.** Electrocardiograms recorded from a normal subject **(A)** and from a patient with long QT syndrome **(B).**

Ventricular fibrillation is often initiated when a premature impulse arrives during the vulnerable period of the cardiac cycle. This period coincides with the downslope of the T wave of the ECG. During this period the excitability of cardiac cells varies spatially. Some fibers are still in their effective refractory periods, others have almost fully recovered their excitability, and still others are able to conduct impulses, but only at very slow conduction velocities. Consequently, the action potentials are propagated over the chambers in many irregular wavelets that travel along circuitous paths and at various conduction velocities. As a region of cardiac cells becomes excitable again, it is ultimately reentered by one of the wave fronts traveling around the chamber. Hence, the process is self-sustaining.

Atrial fibrillation may be changed to a normal sinus rhythm by drugs that prolong the refractory period. As the cardiac impulse completes the reentry loop, it may then encounter refractory myocardial fibers. When atrial fibrillation does not respond adequately to drugs, electrical defibrillation may be used to correct this condition.

Dramatic therapy is required for ventricular fibrillation. Conversion to a normal sinus rhythm is accomplished by means of a strong electrical current that places the entire myocardium briefly in a refractory state. Techniques have been developed to administer the current safely through the intact chest wall. In successful cases, the SA node again takes over the normal pacemaker function for the entire heart.

▶ IN THE CLINIC

Implantable cardioverter-defibrillator (ICD) devices have recently been developed to prevent death in patients in whom either ventricular fibrillation or paroxysmal ventricular tachycardia has suddenly developed. The former is lethal unless it is treated immediately, and the latter often leads to ventricular fibrillation and sudden death. The ICD device is implanted subcutaneously in the left subclavicular region of the chest wall. Atrial and ventricular leads permit recording of the right atrial and right ventricular electrograms and provide the ability for right atrial or right ventricular pacing, or both. The defibrillation coil in the right atrium permits the application of a strong electrical current to the ventricle and thereby usually terminates the lethal arrhythmia.

task is to consider the relationships between the structure and function of its components.

Relationship of Heart Structure to Function
The Myocardial Cell

Many important morphological and functional differences and similarities exist between myocardial and skeletal muscle cells (see Chapters 12 and 13). Importantly, both are striated as a result of regular arrangement of the contractile proteins actin and myosin, and generation of force and contraction of muscle fiber occur as a result of their interactions (i.e., sliding filament mechanism).

Skeletal muscle and cardiac muscle show similar length-force relationships. This relationship for the heart may be expressed graphically, as in Figure 16-36,

THE CARDIAC PUMP

The great amount of work performed by the heart over an individual's lifetime is impressive. A useful way to understand how the heart accomplishes its important

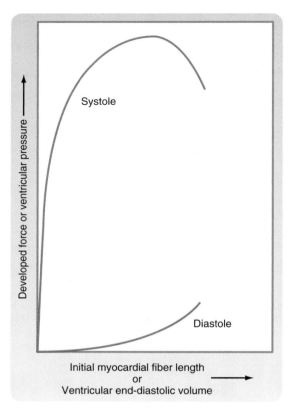

● **Figure 16-36.** Relationship of myocardial resting fiber length (sarcomere length) or end-diastolic volume to the force developed or peak systolic ventricular pressure during ventricular contraction in an intact heart. (Redrawn from Patterson SW et al: J Physiol 48:465, 1914.)

by substituting ventricular systolic pressure for force and end-diastolic ventricular volume for resting myocardial fiber (and hence sarcomere) length. The lower curve in Figure 16-36 represents the increment in pressure produced by each increment in volume when the heart is in diastole. The upper curve represents the peak pressure developed by the ventricle during systole as a function of filling pressure. This curve illustrates the **Frank-Starling relationship** (also called Starling's law of the heart).

The pressure-volume curve during diastole is initially quite flat (compliant), which indicates that large increases in volume can be accommodated with only small increases in pressure. In contrast, the development of systolic pressure is considerable at the lower filling pressures. However, the ventricle becomes much less distensible with greater filling, as evidenced by the sharp rise in the diastolic pressure curve at large intraventricular volumes.

In a normal intact heart, peak force may be attained at a filling pressure of about 12 mm Hg. At this intraventricular diastolic pressure, which is near the upper limit observed in a normal heart, sarcomere length is near its resting length of 2.2 μm. However, the force developed peaks at filling pressures as high as 30 mm Hg. At even higher diastolic pressures

(>50 mm Hg), sarcomere length is not greater than 2.6 μm. This ability of the myocardium to resist stretch at high filling pressures probably resides in the non-contractile constituents of the heart tissue (connective tissue), and it may serve as a safety factor against overloading of the heart in diastole. Usually, ventricular diastolic pressure is about 0 to 7 mm Hg, and the average diastolic sarcomere length is about 2.2 μm. Thus, a normal heart operates on the ascending portion of the Frank-Starling curve depicted in Figure 16-36.

Functional Anatomy
Cardiac Muscle

Cardiac muscle functions as a syncytium; that is, a stimulus applied to any part of the cardiac muscle results in contraction of the entire muscle. Gap junctions with high conductance are present in the intercalated disks between adjacent cells and facilitate conduction of the cardiac impulse from one cell to the next.

Cardiac muscle must contract repetitively for a lifetime, and hence it requires a continuous supply of O_2. Cardiac muscle is therefore very rich in mitochondria. The large number of mitochondria, which have the enzymes necessary for oxidative phosphorylation, permits rapid oxidation of substrates and synthesis of ATP and thus sustains the myocardial energy requirements.

To provide adequate O_2 and substrate for its metabolic machinery, the myocardium is also endowed with a rich capillary supply, about one capillary per fiber. Thus, diffusion distances are short, and O_2, CO_2, substrates, and waste material can move rapidly between the myocardial cell and capillary. The **transverse (T) tubular system** within myocardial cells participates in this exchange of substances between capillary blood and myocardial cells (as described later, the T tubule system also plays a key role in excitation-contraction coupling). The T tubular system is absent or poorly developed in the atrial cells of many mammals.

Excitation-Contraction Coupling

The earliest studies on isolated hearts indicated that optimal concentrations of Na^+, K^+, and Ca^{++} in extracellular fluid are necessary for contraction of cardiac muscle. Without Na^+, the heart is not excitable and will not beat. As already described, the resting membrane potential is independent of the $[Na^+]_o$ gradient across the membrane, but very much dependent on $[K^+]_o$. Decreases or increases in $[K^+]_o$, especially if they are large or occur quickly, can lead to arrhythmias, loss of excitability of the myocardial cells, and even cardiac arrest. Ca^{++} is also essential for cardiac contraction. Removal of Ca^{++} from the extracellular fluid results in decreased contractile force and eventual arrest in diastole. Conversely, an increase in $[Ca^{++}]_o$ enhances contractile force, and very high $[Ca^{++}]_o$ induces cardiac arrest in systole (rigor). The free intracellular $[Ca^{++}]$ is the factor principally responsible for the contractile state of the myocardium.

The process by which the action potential of the cardiac myocyte leads to contraction is termed **excitation-contraction coupling** (see also Chapter 13). Cardiac muscle is excited when a wave of excitation spreads rapidly along the myocardial sarcolemma from cell to cell via gap junctions. Excitation also spreads into the interior of the cells via the T tubules, which invaginate the cardiac fibers at the Z lines. Electrical stimulation at the Z line or the application of Ca^{++} to the Z lines in a skinned (sarcolemma removed) cardiac fiber elicits localized contraction of the adjacent myofibrils. During the plateau (phase 2) of the action potential, permeability of the sarcolemma to Ca^{++} increases. Ca^{++} flows down its electrochemical gradient and enters the cell through Ca^{++} channels in the sarcolemma and in the T tubules.

During the action potential Ca^{++} enters the cell via Ca^{++} channels (e.g., L type). However, the amount of Ca^{++} that enters the cell interior from the extracellular/interstitial fluid is not sufficient to induce contraction of the myofibrils. Instead, it acts as a trigger **(trigger Ca^{++})** to release Ca^{++} from the SR, where the intracellular Ca^{++} is stored (Fig. 16-37). Ca^{++} leaves the SR through Ca^{++} release channels, which are called **ryanodine receptors** because the channel protein,

also called foot protein or junctional processes, binds ryanodine avidly. Cytoplasmic $[Ca^{++}]$ increases from a resting level of about 10^{-7} M to levels of about 10^{-5} M during excitation. This Ca^{++} then binds to the protein troponin C. The Ca^{++}-troponin complex interacts with tropomyosin to unblock active sites between the actin and myosin filaments. This unblocking initiates cross-bridge cycling and hence contraction of the myofibrils.

Mechanisms that raise cytosolic $[Ca^{++}]$ increase the force developed, and those that lower cytosolic $[Ca^{++}]$ decrease the force developed. For example, catecholamines increase the movement of Ca^{++} into the cell by phosphorylation of the sarcolemmal Ca^{++} channels via a cAMP-dependent protein kinase. This in turn releases more Ca^{++} from the SR, and as a result contractile force increases. Increasing $[Ca^{++}]_o$ will increase the amount of Ca^{++} that enters the cell via the Ca^{++} channels and will thereby increase contractile force as just described. Reducing the Na^+ gradient across the sarcolemma will also increase contractile force, an effect mediated by the $3Na^+$-$1Ca^{++}$ antiporter that normally extrudes Ca^{++} from the cell (Fig. 16-37). For example, reducing $[Na^+]_o$ causes less Na^+ to enter the cell in exchange for Ca^{++}, which results in an increase in $[Ca^{++}]_i$ and thus

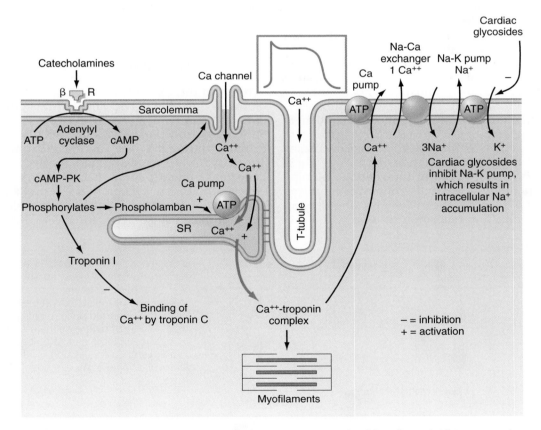

● **Figure 16-37.** Schematic diagram of the movement of calcium in excitation-contraction coupling in cardiac muscle. Influx of Ca^{++} from interstitial fluid during excitation triggers release of Ca^{++} from the sarcoplasmic reticulum (SR). The free cytosolic Ca^{++} activates contraction of the myofilaments (systole). Relaxation (diastole) occurs as a result of uptake of Ca^{++} by the SR, by extrusion of intracellular Ca^{++} by the $3Na^+$-$1Ca^{++}$ antiporter, and to a limited degree by the Ca^{++}-ATPase pump. βR, β-adrenergic receptor; cAMP-PK, cAMP-dependent protein kinase.

contractile force. Raising [Na$^+$]$_i$ will have a similar effect. Indeed, this is the mechanism by which cardiac glycosides increase contractile force. Cardiac glycosides inhibit Na$^+$,K$^+$-ATPase and thereby raise [Na$^+$]$_i$ in the cells. The elevated cytosolic [Na$^+$] reverses the direction of the 3Na$^+$-1Ca^{++} antiporter, and therefore less Ca^{++} is removed from the cell. The increase in [Ca^{++}]$_i$ results in an increase in contractile force. Finally, contractile force is diminished when [Ca^{++}]$_i$ is decreased by a reduction in [Ca^{++}]$_o$, by an increase in the Na$^+$ gradient across the sarcolemma, or by the administration of a Ca^{++} channel antagonist that prevents Ca^{++} from entering the myocardial cell.

At the end of systole, the influx of Ca^{++} stops, and the SR is no longer stimulated to release Ca^{++}. In fact, the SR avidly takes up Ca^{++} by means of a Ca^{++}-ATPase. This SR Ca^{++}-ATPase is similar to but distinct from the Ca^{++}-ATPase found in the sarcolemma. Cytosolic [Ca^{++}] is also reduced during diastole through the action of the 3Na$^+$-1Ca^{++} antiporter in the sarcolemma, as well as by a sarcolemmal Ca^{++}-ATPase (Fig. 16-37).

Cardiac contraction and relaxation are both accelerated by catecholamines. When catecholamines bind to their receptor (β_1-adrenoceptor), adenylyl cyclase is activated, thereby increasing intracellular cAMP levels, which then leads to activation of cAMP-dependent protein kinase A (PKA). PKA has multiple effects in the cell. As already described, it phosphorylates the Ca^{++} channel in the sarcolemma and causes increased entry of Ca^{++} into the cell, thus increasing the force of contraction. In addition, PKA phosphorylates other proteins that facilitate relaxation. One such protein is **phospholamban.** Phospholamban normally inhibits the SR Ca^{++}-ATPase. However, when phosphorylated, the inhibitory action of phospholamban is reduced, and uptake of Ca^{++} into the SR is enhanced. The increased activity of the SR Ca^{++}-ATPase decreases [Ca^{++}]$_i$, thereby causing relaxation. PKA also phosphorylates troponin I, which in turn inhibits binding of Ca^{++} by troponin C. As a result, tropomyosin returns to its position of blocking the myosin binding sites on the actin filaments, and relaxation results.

Myocardial Contractile Machinery and Contractility

Contraction of cardiac muscle is influenced by both **preload** and **afterload** (Fig. 16-38). Preload refers to the force that stretches the relaxed muscle fibers. In the left ventricle, for example, the blood filling and thus stretching the wall during diastole represents the preload. Afterload refers to the force against which the contracting muscle must act. Again from the perspective of the left ventricle, afterload is the pressure in the aorta that must be overcome by the contracting left ventricular muscle to open the aortic valve and eject the blood.

Preload can be increased by greater filling of the left ventricle during diastole (i.e., increasing **end-diastolic volume**). At lower end-diastolic volumes, increments in filling pressure during diastole elicit a greater systolic pressure during the subsequent contraction. Systolic pressure increases until a maximal systolic pressure is reached at the optimal preload (Fig. 16-36). If diastolic filling continues beyond this point, no further increase in the pressure developed will occur. At very high filling pressures, peak pressure development in systole is actually reduced.

At a constant preload, higher systolic pressure can be reached during ventricular contractions by raising the afterload (e.g., increasing aortic pressure by restricting the runoff of arterial blood to the periphery). Incremental increases in afterload produce progressively higher peak systolic pressures. However, if the afterload continues to increase, it becomes so great that the ventricle can no longer generate enough force to open the aortic valve. At this point, ventricular systole is totally isometric (i.e., there is no ejection of blood), and thus no change occurs in ventricular volume during systole. The maximal pressure developed by the left ventricle under these conditions is the maximal isometric force that the ventricle is capable of generating at a given preload. At preloads below the optimal filling volume, an increase in preload can yield greater maximal isometric force (Fig. 16-36).

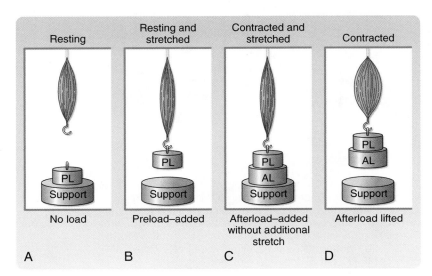

● **Figure 16-38.** Preload and afterload in a papillary muscle. **A,** Resting stage—in the intact heart just before opening of the AV valves. **B,** Preload—in the intact heart at the end of ventricular filling. **C,** Supported preload plus afterload—in the intact heart just before opening of the aortic valve. **D,** Lifting preload plus afterload—in the intact heart, ventricular ejection with a decrease in ventricular volume. AL, afterload; PL, preload; PL + AL, total load.

Resting	Resting and stretched	Contracted and stretched	Contracted
No load	Preload–added	Afterload–added without additional stretch	Afterload lifted
A	B	C	D

In an intact animal, preload and afterload depend on certain characteristics of the vascular system and the behavior of the heart. With respect to the vasculature, the degree of venomotor tone and peripheral resistance influences preload and afterload. With respect to the heart, a change in rate or stroke volume can also alter preload and afterload. Hence, cardiac and vascular factors interact with each other to affect preload and afterload (see Chapter 19).

Contractility defines cardiac performance at a given preload and afterload. Contractility determines the change in peak isometric force (isovolumic pressure) at a given initial fiber length (end-diastolic volume). Contractility can be augmented by certain drugs, such as norepinephrine or digitalis, or by an increase in contraction frequency **(tachycardia).** The increase in contractility **(positive inotropic effect)** produced by these interventions is reflected by incremental increases in the force developed and in the velocity of contraction.

Indices of Contractility

A reasonable index of myocardial contractility can be derived from the contour of ventricular pressure curves (Fig. 16-39). A hypodynamic heart is characterized by an elevated end-diastolic pressure, slowly rising ventricular pressure, and a somewhat reduced ejection phase (curve C, Fig. 16-39). A hyperdynamic heart (curve B, Fig. 16-39) shows reduced end-diastolic pressure, fast-rising ventricular pressure, and a brief ejection phase. The slope of the ascending limb of the ventricular pressure curve indicates the maximal rate

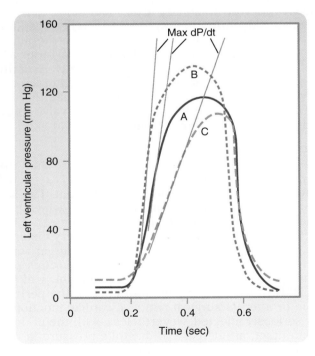

● **Figure 16-39.** Left ventricular pressure curves with tangents drawn to the steepest portions of the ascending limbs to indicate maximal dP/dt values. A, control; B, hyperdynamic heart, as with administration of norepinephrine; C, hypodynamic heart, as in cardiac failure.

of force development by the ventricle. The maximal rate of change in pressure with time, that is, the **maximum dP/dt,** is illustrated by the tangents to the steepest portion of the ascending limbs of the ventricular pressure curves in Figure 16-39. The slope of the ascending limb is maximal during the isovolumic phase of systole (Fig. 16-40). At any given degree of ventricular filling, the slope provides an index of the initial contraction velocity and hence an index of contractility.

Similarly, the contractile state of the myocardium can be obtained from the velocity of blood flow that occurs initially in the ascending aorta during the cardiac cycle (Fig. 16-40). In addition, the **ejection fraction,** which is the ratio of the volume of blood ejected from the left ventricle per beat **(stroke volume)** to the volume of blood in the left ventricle at the end of diastole (end-diastolic volume), is widely used clinically as an index of contractility.

Cardiac Chambers

The atria are thin-walled, low-pressure chambers that function more as large-reservoir conduits of blood for their respective ventricles than as important pumps for the forward propulsion of blood. The ventricles comprise a continuum of muscle fibers originating from the fibrous skeleton at the base of the heart (chiefly around the aortic orifice). These fibers sweep toward the cardiac apex at the epicardial surface. They pass toward the endocardium and gradually undergo an 180-degree change in direction to lie parallel to the epicardial fibers and to form the endocardium and papillary muscles.

At the apex of the heart, the fibers twist and turn inward to form papillary muscles. At the base of the heart and around the valve orifices, these myocardial fibers form a thick, powerful muscle mass that not only decreases the ventricular circumference to implement the ejection of blood but also narrows the AV valve orifices as an aid to closure of the valve. Ventricular ejection is also accomplished by decreasing the longitudinal axis as the heart begins to narrow toward the base. The early contraction of the apical part of the ventricles, coupled with the approximation of the ventricular walls, propels the blood toward the ventricular outflow tracts. The right ventricle, which develops a mean pressure that is about a seventh that developed by the left ventricle, is considerably thinner than the left ventricle.

Cardiac Valves

The cardiac valve leaflets consist of thin flaps of flexible, tough, endothelium-covered fibrous tissue that are firmly attached at the base to the fibrous valve rings. Movement of the valve leaflets is essentially passive, and the orientation of the cardiac valves is responsible for the unidirectional flow of blood through the heart. There are two types of valves in the heart: **atrioventricular** and **semilunar** valves (Figs. 16-41 and 16-42).

Atrioventricular Valves. The tricuspid valve, located between the right atrium and the right

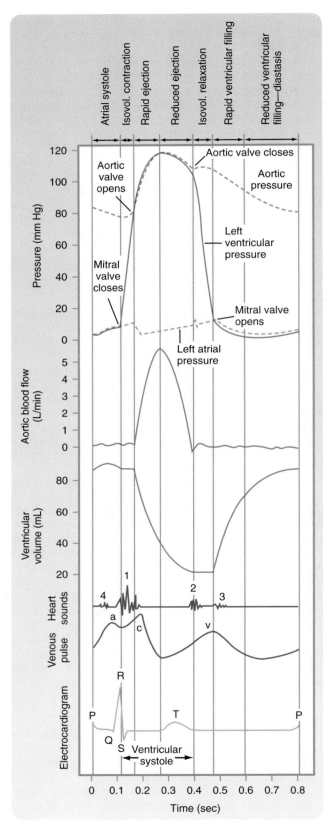

● **Figure 16-40.** Left atrial, aortic, and left ventricular pressure pulses correlated in time with aortic flow, ventricular volume, heart sounds, venous pulse, and the electrocardiogram for a complete cardiac cycle.

ventricle, is made up of three cusps, whereas the mitral valve, which lies between the left atrium and the left ventricle, has two cusps. The total area of the cusps of each AV valve is approximately twice that of the respective AV orifice, so considerable overlap of the leaflets occurs when the valves are in the closed position. Attached to the free edges of these valves are fine, strong ligaments (chordae tendineae) that arise from the powerful papillary muscles of the respective ventricles. These ligaments prevent the valves from becoming everted during ventricular systole.

In a normal heart, the valve leaflets remain relatively close together during ventricular filling. The partial approximation of the valve surfaces during diastole is caused by eddy currents that prevail behind the leaflets and by tension that is exerted by the chordae tendineae and papillary muscles.

Semilunar Valves. The pulmonic and aortic valves are located between the right ventricle and the pulmonary artery and between the left ventricle and the aorta, respectively. These valves consist of three cuplike cusps that are attached to the valve rings (Figs. 16-41 and 16-42). At the end of the reduced ejection phase of ventricular systole, blood flow briefly reverses toward the ventricles. This reversal of blood flow snaps the cusps together and prevents regurgitation of blood into the ventricles. During ventricular systole, the cusps do not lie back against the walls of the pulmonary artery and aorta but instead float in the bloodstream at a point approximately midway between the vessel walls and their closed position. Behind the semilunar valves are small outpocketings (sinuses of Valsalva) of the pulmonary artery and aorta. In these sinuses, eddy currents develop that tend to keep the valve cusps away from the vessel walls. Furthermore, the orifices of the right and left coronary arteries are behind the right and the left cusps, respectively, of the aortic valve. Were it not for the presence of the sinuses of Valsalva and the eddy currents developed therein, the coronary ostia could be blocked by the valve cusps and coronary blood flow would cease.

The Pericardium

The pericardium invests the entire heart and the cardiac portion of the great vessels, and it is reflected onto the cardiac surface as the epicardium. The sac normally contains a small amount of fluid, which provides lubrication for the continuous movement of the enclosed heart. The pericardium is not very distensible, and therefore it strongly resists a large, rapid increase in cardiac size. Hence, the pericardium prevents sudden overdistention of the chambers of the heart. However, in congenital absence of the pericardium or after its surgical removal, cardiac function is not seriously affected. Nevertheless, with the pericardium intact, an increase in diastolic pressure in one ventricle increases the pressure and decreases the compliance of the other ventricle.

Heart Sounds

Four sounds are usually generated by the heart, but only two are ordinarily audible through a stethoscope.

● **Figure 16-41.** Drawing of a heart split perpendicular to the interventricular septum to illustrate the anatomic relationships of the leaflets of the atrioventricular and aortic valves.

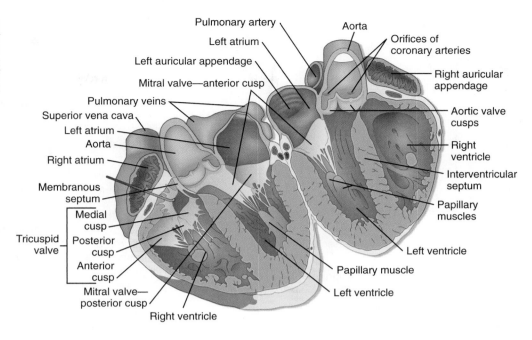

● **Figure 16-42.** Four cardiac valves as viewed from the base of the heart. Note how the leaflets overlap in the closed valves.

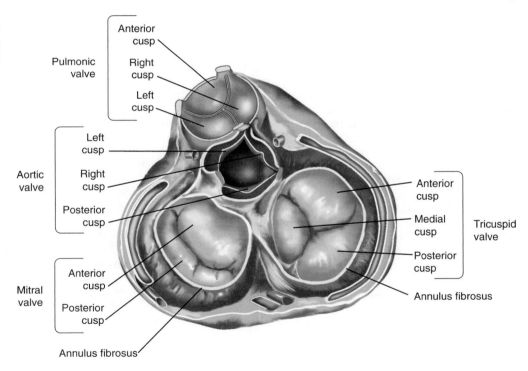

With electronic amplification, the less intense sounds can be detected and recorded graphically as a phonocardiogram. This means of registering faint heart sounds helps delineate the precise timing of the heart sounds relative to other events in the cardiac cycle.

The first heart sound is initiated at the onset of ventricular systole (Fig. 16-43) and reflects closure of the AV valves. It is the loudest and longest of the heart sounds, has a crescendo-decrescendo quality, and is heard best over the apical region of the heart. The tricuspid valve sounds are heard best in the fifth intercostal space just to the left of the sternum; the mitral sounds are heard best in the fifth intercostal space at the cardiac apex.

The second heart sound, which occurs with abrupt closure of the semilunar valves (Fig. 16-43), is composed of higher-frequency vibrations (higher pitch) and is of shorter duration and lower intensity than the first heart sound. The portion of the second sound caused by closure of the pulmonic valve is heard best

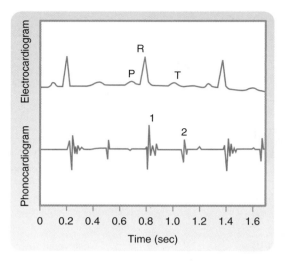

● **Figure 16-43.** Phonocardiogram illustrating the first and second heart sounds and their relationship to the P, R, and T waves of the electrocardiogram.

In overloaded hearts, as in congestive heart failure, when ventricular volume is very large and the ventricular walls are stretched maximally, a third heart sound is often heard. A third heart sound in patients with heart disease is usually a grave sign. When the third and fourth (atrial) sounds are accentuated, as occurs in certain abnormal conditions, triplets of sounds resembling the sound of a galloping horse (called gallop rhythms) may occur.

Mitral insufficiency and mitral stenosis produce, respectively, systolic and diastolic murmurs that are heard best at the cardiac apex. Aortic insufficiency and aortic stenosis, in contrast, produce, respectively, diastolic and systolic murmurs that are heard best in the second intercostal space just to the right of the sternum. The characteristics of the murmurs serve as an important guide in the diagnosis of valvular disease.

in the second thoracic interspace just to the left of the sternum, whereas that caused by closure of the aortic valve is heard best in the same intercostal space but to the right of the sternum. The aortic valve sound is generally louder than the pulmonic, but in cases of pulmonary hypertension the reverse is true. The nature of the second heart sound changes with respiration. During expiration, a single heart sound is heard that reflects simultaneous closing of the pulmonic and aortic valves. However, during inspiration, closure of the pulmonic valve is delayed, mainly as a result of increased blood flow from an inspiration-induced increase in venous return.* With this delayed closure of the pulmonic valve the second heart sound can be resolved into two components; this is termed **physiological splitting** of the second heart sound.

A third heart sound is sometimes heard in children with thin chest walls or in patients with left ventricular failure. It consists of a few low-intensity, low-frequency vibrations heard best in the region of the cardiac apex. The vibrations occur in early diastole and are caused by the abrupt cessation of ventricular distention and by the deceleration of blood entering the ventricles. A fourth, or atrial, sound consists of a few low-frequency oscillations. This sound is occasionally heard in normal individuals. It is caused by the oscillation of blood and cardiac chambers as a result of atrial contraction.

The Cardiac Cycle
Ventricular Systole

Isovolumic Contraction. The phase between the start of ventricular systole and opening of the semilunar valves (when ventricular pressure rises abruptly) is called the isovolumic (literally, "same volume") contraction period. This term is appropriate because ventricular volume remains constant during this brief

period (Fig. 16-40). The onset of isovolumic contraction also coincides with the peak of the R wave on an ECG, initiation of the first heart sound, and the earliest rise in ventricular pressure on the ventricular pressure curve after atrial contraction.

Ejection. Opening of the semilunar valves marks the onset of the ventricular ejection phase, which may be subdivided into an earlier, shorter phase (rapid ejection) and a later, longer phase (reduced ejection). The rapid ejection phase is distinguished from the reduced ejection phase by three characteristics: (1) a sharp rise in ventricular and aortic pressure that terminates at peak ventricular and aortic pressure, (2) an abrupt decrease in ventricular volume, and (3) a pronounced increase in aortic blood flow (Fig. 16-40). The sharp decrease in left atrial pressure seen at the onset of ventricular ejection results from descent of the base of the heart and consequent stretching of the atria. During the reduced ejection period, runoff of blood from the aorta to the peripheral blood vessels exceeds the rate of ventricular output, and therefore aortic pressure declines. Throughout ventricular systole, the blood returning from the peripheral veins to the atria produces a progressive increase in atrial pressure.

Note that during the rapid ejection period, left ventricular pressure slightly exceeds aortic pressure and aortic blood flow accelerates (continues to increase), whereas during the reduced ventricular ejection phase, the reverse holds true. This reversal of the ventricular-aortic pressure gradient in the presence of continuous flow of blood from the left ventricle to the aorta is the result of storage of potential energy in the stretched arterial walls. This stored potential energy decelerates blood flow from the left ventricle into the aorta. The peak of the flow curve coincides with the point at which the left ventricular pressure curve intersects the aortic pressure curve during ejection. Thereafter, flow decelerates (continues to decrease) because the pressure gradient has been reversed.

---

*With inspiration, intrathoracic pressure is reduced (see Chapter 21), which then increases venous blood flow to the right atrium.

Figure 16-40 shows a tracing of a venous pulse curve recorded from a jugular vein. Three waves are apparent. The **a wave** occurs with the rise in pressure caused by atrial contraction. The **c wave** in this tracing is caused by impact of the common carotid artery with the adjacent jugular vein and to some extent by the abrupt closure of the tricuspid valve in early ventricular systole. Finally, the **v wave** reflects the rise in pressure associated with atrial filling. Note that except for the c wave, the venous pulse closely follows the left atrial pressure curve.

At the end of ventricular ejection, a volume of blood approximately equal to that ejected during systole remains in the ventricular cavities. This residual volume is fairly constant in normal hearts. However, residual volume decreases somewhat when the heart rate increases or when peripheral vascular resistance has diminished.

Ventricular Diastole

Isovolumic Relaxation. Closure of the aortic valve produces the characteristic incisura (notch) on the descending limb of the aortic pressure curve, and it also produces the second heart sound (with some vibrations evident on the atrial pressure curve). The incisura marks the end of ventricular systole. The period between closure of the semilunar valves and opening of the AV valves is termed isovolumic relaxation. It is characterized by a precipitous fall in ventricular pressure without a change in ventricular volume.

Rapid Filling Phase. The major portion of ventricular filling occurs immediately after opening of the AV valves. At this point the blood that had returned to the atria during the previous ventricular systole is abruptly released into the relaxing ventricles. This period of ventricular filling is called the rapid filling phase. In Figure 16-40 the onset of the rapid filling phase is indicated by the decrease in left ventricular pressure below left atrial pressure. This pressure reversal opens the mitral valve. The rapid flow of blood from atria to relaxing ventricles produces a transient decrease in atrial and ventricular pressure and a sharp increase in ventricular volume.

Diastasis. The rapid ventricular filling phase is followed by a phase of slow ventricular filling called diastasis. During diastasis, blood returning from the peripheral veins flows into the right ventricle and blood from the lungs flows into the left ventricle. This small, slow addition to ventricular filling is indicated by a gradual rise in atrial, ventricular, and venous pressure and ventricular volume (Fig. 16-40).

Atrial Systole. The onset of atrial systole occurs soon after the beginning of the P wave (atrial depolarization) of the ECG. The transfer of blood from atrium to ventricle achieved by atrial contraction completes the period of ventricular filling. Atrial systole is responsible for the small increases in atrial, ventricular, and venous pressure, as well as ventricular volume (Fig. 16-40). Throughout ventricular diastole, atrial pressure barely exceeds ventricular pressure. This small pressure difference indicates that the pathway through the open AV valves during ventricular filling has low resistance.

Because there are no valves at the junction of the venae cavae and right atrium or the pulmonary veins and left atrium, atrial contraction may force blood in both directions. However, little blood is actually pumped back into the venous tributaries during the brief atrial contraction, mainly because of the inertia of the inflowing blood.

The contribution of atrial contraction to ventricular filling is governed to a great extent by the heart rate and the position of the AV valves. At slow heart rates, filling practically ceases toward the end of diastasis, and atrial contraction contributes little additional filling. During tachycardia, however, diastasis is abbreviated and the atrial contribution can become substantial. Should tachycardia become so great that the rapid filling phase is encroached upon, atrial contraction assumes great importance in rapidly propelling blood into the ventricle during this brief period of the cardiac cycle. If the period of ventricular relaxation is so brief that filling is seriously impaired, even atrial contraction cannot provide adequate ventricular filling. The consequent reduction in cardiac output may result in syncope (fainting).

Pressure-Volume Relationship

The changes in left ventricular pressure and volume throughout the cardiac cycle are summarized in Figure 16-44. Diastolic filling starts at A, when the mitral valve

---

> **IN THE CLINIC**

An increase in myocardial contractility, as produced by catecholamines or by digitalis in a patient with a failing heart, may decrease residual ventricular volume and increase the stroke volume and ejection fraction. In severely hypodynamic and dilated hearts, residual volume can become much greater than stroke volume.

> **IN THE CLINIC**

Atrial contraction is not essential for ventricular filling, as can be observed in patients with atrial fibrillation or complete heart block. In atrial fibrillation, the atrial myofibers contract in a continuous, uncoordinated fashion and therefore cannot pump blood into the ventricles. In complete heart block, the atria and ventricles beat independently of each other. However, ventricular filling may be normal in patients with these two arrhythmias.

In certain disease states, the AV valves may be markedly narrowed (stenotic). Under such conditions, atrial contraction plays a much more important role in ventricular filling than it does in a normal heart.

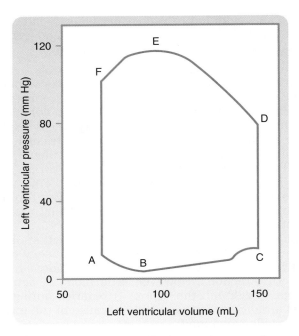

● **Figure 16-44.** Pressure-volume loop of the left ventricle for a single cardiac cycle (ABCDEF).

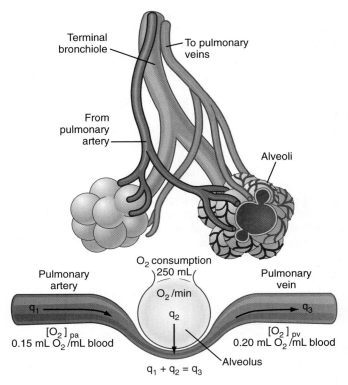

● **Figure 16-45.** Schema illustrating the Fick principle for measuring cardiac output. The change in color from pulmonary artery to pulmonary vein represents the change in color of the blood as venous blood becomes fully oxygenated.

opens, and it terminates at C, when the mitral valve closes. The initial decrease in left ventricular pressure (A to B), despite the rapid inflow of blood from the left atrium, is attributed to progressive ventricular relaxation and distensibility. During the remainder of diastole (B to C), the increase in ventricular pressure reflects ventricular filling and changes in the passive elastic characteristics of the ventricle. Note that only a small increase in pressure accompanies the substantial increase in ventricular volume during diastole (B to C). The small pressure increase reflects the compliance of the left ventricle during diastole. The small increase in pressure just to the left of C is caused by the contribution of atrial contraction to ventricular filling. With isovolumic contraction (C to D), pressure rises steeply, but ventricular volume does not change because the mitral and aortic valves are both closed. At D, the aortic valve opens, and during the first phase of ejection (rapid ejection, D to E), the large reduction in volume is associated with a steady increase in ventricular pressure. This reduction in volume is followed by reduced ejection (E to F) and a small decrease in ventricular pressure. The aortic valve closes at F, and this event is followed by isovolumic relaxation (F to A), which is characterized by a sharp drop in pressure. Ventricular volume does not change during the interval from F to A because the mitral and aortic valves are both closed. The mitral valve opens at A to complete one cardiac cycle.

Measurement of Cardiac Output
The Fick Principle
In 1870 the German physiologist Adolph Fick contrived the first method for measuring cardiac output in intact animals and people. The basis for this method, called

the **Fick principle,** is simply an application of the law of conservation of mass. The principle is derived from the fact that the quantity of O_2 delivered to the pulmonary capillaries via the pulmonary artery, plus the quantity of O_2 that enters the pulmonary capillaries from the alveoli, must equal the quantity of O_2 that is carried away by the pulmonary veins.

The Fick principle is depicted schematically in Figure 16-45. The rate of O_2 delivery to the lungs, q_1, equals the O_2 concentration in pulmonary arterial blood, $[O_2]_{pa}$, times pulmonary arterial blood flow, Q, which equals cardiac output; that is,

● **Equation 16-1**

$$q_1 = Q[O_2]_{pa}$$

Let q_2 be the net rate of O_2 uptake by the pulmonary capillaries from the alveoli. At equilibrium, q_2 equals the O_2 consumption of the body. The rate at which O_2 is carried away by the pulmonary veins, q_3, equals the O_2 concentration in pulmonary venous blood, $[O_2]_{pv}$, times total pulmonary venous flow, which is virtually equal to pulmonary arterial blood flow, Q; that is,

● **Equation 16-2**

$$q_3 = Q[O_2]_{pv}$$

From conservation of mass,

● **Equation 16-3**

$$q_1 + q_2 = q_3$$

Therefore,

● **Equation 16-4**

$$Q[O_2]_{pa} + q_2 = Q[O_2]_{pv}$$

Solving for cardiac output,

● **Equation 16-5**

$$Q = q_2/([O_2]_{pv} - [O_2]_{pa})$$

Equation 16-5 is the statement of the Fick principle.

Determination of cardiac output by this method requires three values: (1) O_2 consumption of the body, (2) the O_2 concentration in pulmonary venous blood ($[O_2]_{pv}$), and (3) the O_2 concentration in pulmonary arterial blood ($[O_2]_{pa}$). O_2 consumption is computed from measurements of the volume and O_2 content of expired air over a given interval. Because the O_2 concentration of peripheral arterial blood is essentially identical to that in the pulmonary veins, $[O_2]_{pv}$ is determined on a sample of peripheral arterial blood withdrawn by needle puncture. The compositions of pulmonary arterial blood and mixed systemic venous blood are virtually identical to one another. Samples for O_2 analysis are obtained from the pulmonary artery or right ventricle through a catheter. A very flexible catheter with a small balloon near the tip can be inserted into a peripheral vein. As the flexible tube is advanced, the flowing blood carries it toward the heart. By following the pressure changes, the physician can advance the catheter tip into the pulmonary artery.

By using the values depicted in Figure 16-45, cardiac output can be calculated as follows. With an O_2 consumption of 250 mL/min, an arterial (pulmonary venous) O_2 content of 0.20 mL O_2/mL blood, and a mixed venous (pulmonary arterial) O_2 content of 0.15 mL O_2/mL blood, cardiac output equals 250/(0.20 − 0.15) = 5000 mL/min.

The Fick principle is also used to estimate the O_2 consumption of organs when blood flow and the O_2 content of arterial and venous blood can be determined. Algebraic rearrangement reveals that O_2 consumption equals blood flow times the arteriovenous O_2 concentration difference. For example, if blood flow through one kidney is 700 mL/min, the arterial O_2 content is 0.20 mL O_2/mL blood, and the renal venous O_2 content is 0.18 mL O_2/mL blood, the rate of O_2 consumption by that kidney must be 700 (0.20 − 0.18) = 14 mL O_2/min.

Cardiac output can be measured noninvasively with Doppler echocardiography. By this method, the velocity of blood in the ascending aorta is measured, and knowing the cross-sectional area of the aorta (also measured by echocardiography) allows the volume of blood ejected in a single beat (i.e., stroke volume) to be determined. Multiplying stroke volume by the heart rate then yields a value for cardiac output in liters per minute.

Cardiac Oxygen Consumption and Work

Consumption of O_2 by the heart depends on the amount and type of activity that the heart performs. Under basal conditions, myocardial O_2 consumption is about 8 to 10 mL/min/100 g of heart. It can increase several-fold during exercise and decrease moderately under such conditions as hypotension and hypothermia. The O_2 content of cardiac venous blood is normally low (about 5 mL/dL), and the myocardium can receive little additional O_2 by further extraction of O_2 from coronary blood. Therefore, increased O_2 demands of the heart must be met mainly by an increase in coronary blood flow (see Chapter 17). In experiments in which the heartbeat is arrested but coronary perfusion is maintained, O_2 consumption falls to 2 mL/min/100 g or less, which is still six to seven times greater than the O_2 consumption of resting skeletal muscle.

Left ventricular work per beat (stroke work) is approximately equal to the product of stroke volume and the mean aortic pressure against which the blood is ejected by the left ventricle. Cardiac work, **W,** may be defined as

● **Equation 16-6**

$$W = \int_{t_1}^{t_2} PdV$$

That is, each small increment in volume that is pumped, **dV,** is multiplied by the associated pressure **P,** and the products **(PdV)** are integrated over the time interval of interest, $t_2 - t_1$, to give total work. Under conditions of steady flow,

● **Equation 16-7**

$$W = PV$$

At resting levels of cardiac output, the kinetic energy component is negligible. However, with high cardiac output, as in strenuous exercise, the kinetic energy component can account for up to 50% of total cardiac work. Simultaneously halving aortic pressure and doubling cardiac output, or vice versa, will result in the same value for cardiac work. However, the O_2 requirements are greater for any given amount of cardiac work when a major proportion of the work is pressure work as opposed to volume work. An increase in cardiac output at a constant aortic pressure (volume work) is accomplished with only a small increase in left ventricular O_2 consumption, whereas increased arterial pressure at constant cardiac output (pressure work) is accompanied by a large increase in myocardial O_2 consumption. Thus, myocardial O_2 consumption may not correlate well with overall cardiac work. The magnitude and duration of left ventricular pressure do correlate with left ventricular O_2 consumption.

The work of the right ventricle is a seventh that of the left ventricle because pulmonary vascular resistance is much less than systemic vascular resistance.

Cardiac Efficiency

The efficiency of the heart may be calculated as the ratio of the work accomplished to the total energy used. If the average O_2 consumption is assumed to be 9 mL/min/100 g for the two ventricles, a 300-g heart will consume 27 mL O_2/min. This value is equivalent to 130 small calories when the respiratory quotient is 0.82. Together, the two ventricles do about 8 kg-m of

> ### ► IN THE CLINIC
>
> The greater energy demand of pressure work than of volume work is clinically important, especially in aortic stenosis. In this condition, left ventricular O_2 consumption is increased, mainly because of the high intraventricular pressure developed during systole. However, coronary perfusion pressure, and hence O_2 supply, is either normal or reduced because of the pressure drop across the narrow orifice of the diseased aortic valve.

work per minute, which is equivalent to 18.7 small calories. Therefore, the gross efficiency of the heart is about 14%.

● **Equation 16-8**

$$18.7/130 \times 100 = 14\%$$

The gross mechanical efficiency of the heart is slightly higher (18%) and is determined by subtracting the O_2 consumption of the nonbeating (asystolic) heart (about 2 mL/min/100 g) from the total cardiac O_2 consumption in the calculation of efficiency. The efficiency of the heart as a pump is relatively low. During physical exercise, efficiency improves because mean blood pressure shows little change, whereas cardiac output and work increase considerably, without a proportional increase in myocardial O_2 consumption. Interestingly, the chemical efficiency of the heart is rather high as indicated by the estimate of 60% for the efficiency of generating ATP from oxidative phosphorylation. The energy expended in cardiac metabolism that does not contribute to the propulsion of blood through the body appears in the form of heat. The energy of flowing blood is also dissipated as heat.

Substrate Utilization

The heart is versatile in its use of substrates, and within certain limits, uptake of a particular substrate is directly proportional to its arterial concentration. The use of one substrate by the heart is also influenced by the presence or absence of other substrates. For example, the addition of lactate to the blood that perfuses a heart metabolizing glucose leads to a reduction in glucose uptake and vice versa. At normal blood concentrations, glucose and lactate are consumed at about equal rates.

In contrast, uptake of pyruvate is very low, as is its arterial concentration. For glucose, the threshold concentration is about 4 mM. Below this blood level, no glucose is taken up by the myocardium. Insulin reduces the glucose threshold and increases the rate of glucose uptake by the heart. A very low threshold exists for cardiac utilization of lactate; insulin does not affect its uptake by the myocardium. Under hypoxic conditions, glucose utilization is facilitated by an increase in the rate of transport across the myocardial cell wall. However, lactate cannot be metabolized by the hypoxic heart and is produced by the heart under anaerobic conditions. Associated with lactate production by the hypoxic heart is the breakdown of cardiac glycogen.

Of the total cardiac O_2 consumption, only 35% to 40% can be accounted for by the oxidation of carbohydrate. Thus, the heart derives the major part of its energy from the oxidation of noncarbohydrate sources, namely, esterified and nonesterified fatty acids, which account for about 60% of the myocardial O_2 consumption in subjects in the postabsorptive state. Various fatty acids have different thresholds for myocardial uptake, but these acids are generally used in direct proportion to their arterial concentration. Ketone bodies, especially acetoacetate, are readily oxidized by the heart, and they contribute a major source of energy in diabetic acidosis. As is true of carbohydrate substrates, use of a specific noncarbohydrate is influenced by the presence of other substrates, whether noncarbohydrate or carbohydrate. Therefore, within certain limits, the heart preferentially uses the substrate that is available in the largest concentration. The contribution to myocardial energy expenditure provided by the oxidation of amino acids is small.

Normally, the heart derives its energy by oxidative phosphorylation, in which each mole of glucose yields 36 mol of ATP. However, during hypoxia, glycolysis takes over, and 2 mol of ATP is provided by each mole of glucose; β oxidation of fatty acids is also curtailed. If hypoxia is prolonged, cellular creatine phosphate and eventually ATP are depleted.

In ischemia, lactic acid accumulates and decreases intracellular pH. This condition inhibits glycolysis, fatty acid use, and protein synthesis, and therefore it results in cellular damage and eventually necrosis of myocardial cells.

■ KEY CONCEPTS

1. The transmembrane action potentials recorded from cardiac myocytes may contain the following five phases:

    Phase 0: The action potential upstroke is initiated when a suprathreshold stimulus rapidly depolarizes the membrane by activating the fast Na^+ channels.
    Phase 1: The notch is an early partial repolarization that is achieved by the efflux of K^+ through transmembrane channels that conduct the transient outward current i_{to}.
    Phase 2: The plateau represents a balance between the influx of Ca^{++} through transmembrane Ca^{++} channels and the efflux of K^+ through several types of K^+ channels.
    Phase 3: Final repolarization is initiated when the efflux of K^+ exceeds the influx of Ca^{++}. The resultant partial repolarization rapidly increases K^+ conductance and restores full repolarization.
    Phase 4: The resting potential of the fully repolarized cell is determined by conductance of the cell membrane to K^+, mainly through i_{K1} channels.

2. Fast-response action potentials are recorded from atrial and ventricular myocardial fibers and from

ventricular specialized conducting (Purkinje) fibers. The action potential is characterized by a large amplitude, a steep upstroke, and a relatively long plateau. The effective refractory period of fast-response fibers begins at the upstroke of the action potential and persists until midway through phase 3. The fiber is relatively refractory during the remainder of phase 3, and it regains full excitability soon after it is fully repolarized (phase 4).

3. Slow-response action potentials are recorded from normal SA and AV nodal cells and from abnormal myocardial cells that have been partially depolarized. The action potential is characterized by a less negative resting potential, a smaller amplitude, a less steep upstroke, and a shorter plateau than is typical of the fast-response action potential. The upstroke in slow-response fibers is produced by the activation of Ca^{++} channels. Slow-response fibers become absolutely refractory at the beginning of the upstroke, and partial excitability may not be regained until very late in phase 3 or until after the fiber is fully repolarized.

4. Normally, the SA node serves as the cardiac pacemaker to initiate the cardiac impulse. This impulse is propagated from the SA node to the atria and ultimately reaches the AV node. After a delay in the AV node, the cardiac impulse is propagated throughout the ventricles. Ectopic foci in the atrium, AV node, or His-Purkinje system may initiate propagated cardiac impulses if the normal pacemaker cells in the SA node are suppressed or if the rhythmicity of the ectopic automatic cells is abnormally enhanced.

5. Under certain abnormal conditions, afterdepolarizations may be triggered by an otherwise normal action potential. EADs arise early in phase 3 of a normal action potential. They are more likely to occur when the basic cycle length of the initiating beats is very long and when the cardiac action potentials are abnormally prolonged. DADs appear late in phase 3 or in phase 4. They are more likely to occur when the basic cycle length of the initiating beats is short and when the cardiac cells are overloaded with Ca^{++}.

6. Reentrant arrhythmias occur when a cardiac impulse traverses a loop of cardiac fibers and reenters previously excited tissue, when the impulse is conducted slowly around the loop, and when the impulse is blocked unidirectionally in some section of the loop.

7. The ECG, which is recorded from the surface of the body, traces the conduction of the cardiac impulse throughout the heart. The ECG may be used to detect and analyze certain cardiac arrhythmias, such as altered sinoatrial rhythms, AV conduction blocks, premature depolarizations, ectopic tachycardias, and atrial and ventricular fibrillation.

8. On excitation, voltage-gated Ca^{++} channels open to admit extracellular Ca^{++} into the cell. The influx of Ca^{++} triggers the release of Ca^{++} from the sarcoplasmic reticulum. The elevated $[Ca^{++}]_i$ elicits contraction of the myofilaments. Relaxation is accomplished via restoration of resting cytosolic $[Ca^{++}]$ by pumping Ca^{++} back into the sarcoplasmic reticulum and exchanging it for extracellular Na^+ across the sarcolemma. Velocity and force of contraction are functions of $[Ca^{++}]_i$. Force and velocity are inversely related, so with no load, velocity is maximal. In an isovolumic contraction, no external shortening occurs.

9. In ventricular contraction, preload is stretch of the fibers by blood during ventricular filling. Afterload is the arterial pressure against which the ventricle ejects the blood. An increase in myocardial fiber length, as occurs with augmented ventricular filling (preload) during diastole, produces a more forceful ventricular contraction. This relationship between fiber length and strength of contraction is known as the Frank-Starling relationship or Starling's law of the heart.

10. Contractility is an expression of cardiac performance at a given preload and afterload. Contractility can be modulated by the autonomic nervous system.

11. Cardiac output can be determined, according to the Fick principle, by measuring the O_2 consumption of the body (q_2) and the oxygen content of arterial ($[O_2]_a$) and mixed venous ($[O_2]_v$) blood. Cardiac output $= q_2/([O_2]_a - [O_2]_v)$. It can also be measured noninvasively by Doppler echocardiography.

12. The myocardium functions only aerobically, and in general it uses substrates in proportion to their arterial concentration.

CHAPTER 17

Properties of the Vasculature

The vasculature consists of a closed system of tubes or vessels that distributes blood from the heart to the tissues and returns blood from the tissues to the heart. It can be divided into three components: the **arterial system,** which takes blood from the heart and distributes it to the tissues; the **venous system,** which returns blood from the tissues to the heart; and the **microcirculation,** which separates the arterial and venous systems and is the site where nutrients and cellular waste products are exchanged between blood and tissues. These components of the vasculature are presented in this chapter. In addition, the properties of blood flow to specific vascular beds and tissues are considered. As an introduction to this material, the physics of blood/fluid flow through the vasculature (i.e., **hemodynamics**) is reviewed.

HEMODYNAMICS

The physics of fluid flow through rigid tubes provides a basis for understanding the flow of blood through blood vessels, even though the blood vessels are not rigid tubules (i.e., they are distensible) and blood is not a simple homogeneous fluid. Knowledge of these physical principles underlies understanding of the interrelationships among velocity of blood flow, blood pressure, and the dimensions of the various components of the systemic circulation.

Velocity of the Bloodstream

Velocity, as relates to fluid movement, is the distance that a particle of fluid travels with respect to time, and it is expressed in units of distance per unit time (e.g., cm/sec). This is in contrast to flow, which is the rate of displacement of a volume of fluid, and it is expressed in units of volume per unit time (e.g., cm^3/sec). In a rigid tube, velocity (v) and flow (Q) are related to one another by the cross-sectional area (A) of the tube:

● Equation 17-1

$$v = Q/A$$

The interrelationships among velocity, flow, and area are shown in Figure 17-1. Because conservation of mass requires that the fluid flowing through a rigid tube be constant, the velocity of the fluid will vary inversely with the cross-sectional area. Thus, fluid flow velocity is greatest in the section of the tube with the smallest cross-sectional area and slowest in the section of the tube with the greatest cross-sectional area.

As shown in Figure 15-3, velocity decreases progressively as blood traverses the arterial system. At the capillaries, velocity decreases to a minimal value. As the blood then passes centrally through the venous system toward the heart, velocity progressively increases again. The relative velocities in the various components of the circulatory system are related only to the respective cross-sectional areas.

Relationship between Velocity and Pressure

The total energy in a hydraulic system consists of three components: pressure, gravity, and velocity. The velocity of blood flow can have an important effect on the pressure within the tube. Consider the effect of velocity on pressure in a tube with different cross-sectional areas (Fig.17-2). An ideal fluid flows in this system, in which the total energy remains constant. The total pressure within the tube equals the lateral (static) pressure plus the dynamic pressure. The gravitational component can be neglected because the tube is horizontal. The total pressures in segments A, B, and C will be equal, provided that the energy loss from viscosity is negligible (viz., this fluid is an "ideal fluid"). The effect of velocity on the dynamic component (P_{dyn}) can be estimated from

● Equation 17-2

$$P_{dyn} = \rho v^2/2$$

where ρ is the density of the fluid (g/cm^3) and v is velocity (cm/sec). The fluid has a density of 1 g/cm^3. In section A, the lateral pressure is 100 mm Hg; note that 1 mm Hg equals 1330 dynes/cm^2. From equation 17-2, $P_{dyn} = 5000$ dynes/cm^2, or 3.8 mm Hg. In the narrow section B of the tube where the velocity is twice as great, $P_{dyn} = 20,000$ dynes/cm^2, or 15 mm Hg. Thus, the lateral pressure in section B will be 15 mm Hg less than the total pressure, whereas the lateral pressure in sections A and C will be only 3.8 mm Hg less. In most arterial locations, the dynamic component will be a negligible fraction of the total pressure. However, at sites of an arterial constriction or obstruction, the high flow velocity is associated with a large kinetic energy, and therefore the dynamic pressure component may increase significantly. Hence, the pressure would be reduced and perfusion of distal segments will be correspondingly decreased. This example helps explain how pressure changes in a vessel that is narrowed by atherosclerosis or spasm of the blood vessel wall. That is, in narrowed sections of a tube, the dynamic component increases significantly because

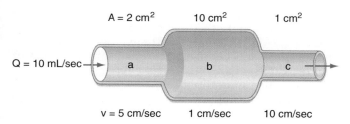

● Figure 17-1. As fluid flows through a tube of variable cross-sectional area, A, the linear velocity, v, varies inversely with the cross-sectional area.

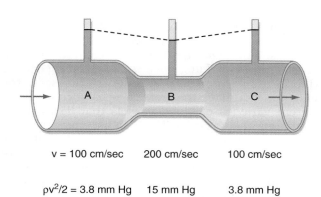

● Figure 17-2. In a narrow section, B, of a tube, the linear velocity, v, and hence the dynamic component of pressure, $\rho v^2/2$, are greater than in the wide sections, A and C, of the same tube. If the total energy is virtually constant throughout the tube (i.e., if the energy loss because of viscosity is negligible), the lateral pressure in the narrow section will be less than the lateral pressure in the wide sections of the tube.

the flow velocity is associated with a large kinetic energy.

Relationship between Pressure and Flow

The most fundamental law that governs the flow of fluids through cylindrical tubes was derived empirically by the French physiologist Poiseuille. He was primarily interested in the physical determinants of blood flow, but he replaced blood with simpler liquids in his measurements of flow through glass capillary tubes. His work was so precise and important that his observations have been designated **Poiseuille's law.**

Poiseuille's Law

Poiseuille's law applies to the steady (i.e., nonpulsatile) laminar flow of newtonian fluids through rigid cylindrical tubes. A newtonian fluid is one whose viscosity remains constant, and laminar flow is the type of motion in which the fluid moves as a series of individual layers, with each layer moving at a velocity different from that of its neighboring layers (Fig. 17-3). In the case of laminar flow through a tube, the fluid consists of a series of infinitesimally thin concentric tubes sliding past one another. Despite the differences between the vascular system (i.e., flow is pulsatile, the vessels are not rigid cylinders, and blood is not a newtonian fluid), Poiseuille's law does provide valu-

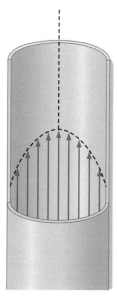

● Figure 17-3. When flow is laminar, all elements of the fluid move in streamlines that are parallel to the axis of the tube; the fluid does not move in a radial or circumferential direction. The layer of fluid in contact with the wall is motionless; the fluid that moves along the central axis of the tube has the maximal velocity.

able insight into the determinants of blood flow through the vascular system.

Poiseuille's law describes the flow of fluids through cylindrical tubes in terms of flow, pressure, the dimensions of the tube, and the viscosity of liquid.

● Equation 17-3

$$Q = \frac{\pi(P_i - P_o)r^4}{8\eta l}$$

where

Q = flow
$P_i - P_o$ = pressure gradient from the inlet (i) of the tube to the outlet (o)
r = radius of the tube
l = length of the tube
η = viscosity of the fluid

As is clear from the equation, flow through the tube will increase as the pressure gradient is increased, and it will decrease as either the viscosity of the fluid or the length of the tube increases. The radius of the tube is a critical factor in determining flow because it is raised to the fourth power. As described later, the radius of a tube is a major determinant of the resistance to flow.

Resistance to Flow

In electrical theory, **Ohm's law** states that the resistance, R, equals the ratio of voltage drop, E, to current flow, I.

● Equation 17-4

$$R = E/I$$

Similarly, in fluid mechanics, hydraulic resistance, R, may be defined as the ratio of the pressure drop, $P_i - P_o$, to flow, Q.

● **Equation 17-5**

$$R = \frac{P_i - P_o}{Q}$$

For the steady, laminar flow of a newtonian fluid through a cylindrical tube, the physical components of hydraulic resistance may be appreciated by rearranging Poiseuille's law to give the hydraulic resistance equation:

● **Equation 17-6**

$$R = \frac{P_i - P_o}{Q} = \frac{8\eta l}{\pi r^4}$$

Thus, when Poiseuille's law applies, the resistance to flow depends only on the dimensions of the tube and the characteristics of the fluid.

The principal determinant of resistance to blood flow through any vessel is the caliber of the vessel because resistance varies inversely as the fourth power of the radius of the tube. In Figure 17-4, the resistance to flow through small blood vessels was measured and the resistance per unit length of vessel (R/l) was plotted against the vessel diameter. As shown, resistance is highest in the capillaries (diameter of 7 μm), and it diminishes as the vessels increase in diameter on the arterial and venous sides of the capillaries. Values of R/l are virtually proportional to

the fourth power of the diameter (or radius) of the larger vessels on both sides of the capillaries.

Changes in vascular resistance occur when the caliber of vessels changes. The most important factor that leads to a change in vessel caliber is contraction of the circular smooth muscle cells in the vessel wall. Changes in internal pressure also alter the caliber of blood vessels and therefore alter the resistance to blood flow through these vessels. Blood vessels are elastic tubes. Hence, the greater the transmural pressure (i.e., the difference between internal and external pressure) across the wall of a vessel, the greater the caliber of the vessel and the less its hydraulic resistance.

It is apparent from Figure 15-3 that the greatest drop in pressure occurs in the very small arteries and arterioles. However, capillaries, which have a mean diameter of about 7 μm, have the greatest resistance to blood flow. Nevertheless, it is the arterioles, not the capillaries, that have the greatest resistance of all the different varieties of blood vessels that lie in series with one another (as in Fig. 15-3). This seeming paradox is related to the relative numbers of parallel capillaries and parallel arterioles. Most simply, there are far more capillaries than arterioles in the systemic circulation, and total resistance across the many capillaries arranged in parallel is much less than total resistance across the fewer arterioles arranged in parallel. In addition, arterioles have a thick coat of circularly arranged smooth muscle fibers that can vary the lumen radius. Even small changes in radius alter resistance greatly, as can be seen from the hydraulic resistance equation (Equation 17-6), wherein R varies inversely with r^4.

Resistances in Series and in Parallel

In the cardiovascular system, the various types of vessels listed along the horizontal axis in Figure 15-3 lie in series with one another. The individual members of each category of vessels are ordinarily arranged in parallel with one another (Fig. 15-1). Thus, capillaries throughout the body are in most instances parallel elements, except for the renal vasculature (in which the peritubular capillaries are in series with the glomerular capillaries) and the splanchnic vasculature (in which the intestinal and hepatic capillaries are aligned in series with each other). The total hydraulic resistance of components arranged in series or in parallel can be derived in the same manner as those for analogous combinations of electrical resistance.

Resistance of Vessels in Series. Three hydraulic resistances, R_1, R_2, and R_3, are arranged in series in the system depicted in Figure 17-5. The pressure drop across the entire system (i.e., the difference between inflow pressure, P_i, and outflow pressure, P_o) consists of the sum of the pressure drops across each of the individual resistances (equation a). In steady state, the flow, Q, through any given cross section must equal the flow through any other cross section. By dividing each component in equation a by Q (equation b), it is evident from the definition of resistance (Equation 17-5) that for resistances in series, the total

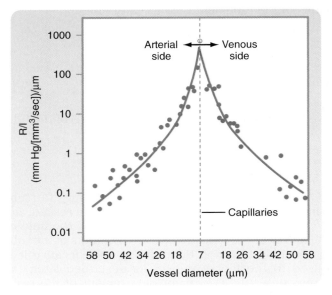

● **Figure 17-4.** Resistance per unit length (R/l) for individual small blood vessels. The capillaries, with a diameter of 7 μm, are denoted by the vertical dashed line. Resistances of the arterioles are plotted to the left and resistances of the venules to the right of the vertical dashed line. For both types of vessels, the resistance per unit length is inversely proportional to the fourth power of the vessel diameter (D). (Redrawn from Lipowsky HH et al: Circ Res 43:738, 1978.)

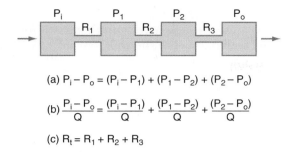

(a) $P_i - P_o = (P_i - P_1) + (P_1 - P_2) + (P_2 - P_o)$

(b) $\dfrac{P_i - P_o}{Q} = \dfrac{(P_i - P_1)}{Q} + \dfrac{(P_1 - P_2)}{Q} + \dfrac{(P_2 - P_o)}{Q}$

(c) $R_t = R_1 + R_2 + R_3$

● **Figure 17-5.** For resistances (R_1, R_2, and R_3) arranged in series, total resistance, R_t, equals the sum of the individual resistances. P, pressure; Q, flow.

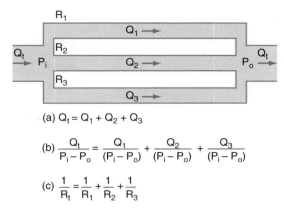

(a) $Q_t = Q_1 + Q_2 + Q_3$

(b) $\dfrac{Q_t}{P_i - P_o} = \dfrac{Q_1}{(P_i - P_o)} + \dfrac{Q_2}{(P_i - P_o)} + \dfrac{Q_3}{(P_i - P_o)}$

(c) $\dfrac{1}{R_t} = \dfrac{1}{R_1} + \dfrac{1}{R_2} + \dfrac{1}{R_3}$

● **Figure 17-6.** For resistances (R_1, R_2, and R_3) arranged in parallel, the reciprocal of the total resistance, R_t, equals the sum of the reciprocals of the individual resistances. P, pressure; Q, flow.

resistance, R_t, of the entire system equals the sum of the individual resistances, that is,

● **Equation 17-7**

$$R_t = R_1 + R_2 + R_3$$

Resistance of Vessels in Parallel. For resistances in parallel, as illustrated in Figure 17-6, inflow and outflow pressure is the same for all tubes. In steady state, the total flow, Q_t, through the system equals the sum of the flows through the individual parallel elements (equation a). Because the pressure gradient ($P_i - P_o$) is identical for all parallel elements, each term in equation a may be divided by that pressure gradient to yield equation b. From the definition of resistance, equation c may be derived. This equation states that for resistances in parallel, the reciprocal of the total resistance, R_t, equals the sum of the reciprocals of the individual resistances, that is,

● **Equation 17-8**

$$1/R_t = (1/R_1) + (1/R_2) + (1/R_3)$$

By considering a few simple illustrations, some of the fundamental properties of parallel hydraulic systems become apparent. For example, if the resistances of the three parallel elements in Figure 17-6 were all equal, then

● **Equation 17-9**

$$R_1 = R_2 = R_3$$

Therefore, from Equation 17-8,

● **Equation 17-10**

$$1/R_t = 3/R_1$$

By equating the reciprocals of these terms,

● **Equation 17-11**

$$R_t = R_1/3$$

Thus, the total resistance is less than the individual resistances. For any parallel arrangement, the total resistance must be less than that of any individual component. For example, consider a system in which a tube with very high resistance is added in parallel to a low-resistance tube. The total resistance of the system must be less than that of the low-resistance component by itself because the high-resistance com-

ponent affords an additional pathway, or conductance, for flow of fluid.

Consider the physiological relationship between the **total peripheral resistance (TPR)** of the entire systemic vascular bed and the resistance of one of its components, such as the renal vasculature. TPR is the ratio of the arteriovenous (AV) pressure difference ($P_a - P_v$) to the flow through the entire systemic vascular bed (i.e., the cardiac output, Q_t). The renal vascular resistance (R_r) would be the ratio of the same AV pressure difference ($P_a - P_v$) to renal blood flow (Q_r).

In an individual with an arterial pressure of 100 mm Hg, a peripheral venous pressure of 0 mm Hg, and a cardiac output of 5000 mL/min, TPR will be 0.02 mm Hg/mL/min, or 0.02 PRU **(peripheral resistance units)**. Normally, blood flow through one kidney would be approximately 600 mL/min. Renal resistance would therefore be 100 mm Hg ÷ 600 mL/min, or 0.17 PRU, which is 8.5 times greater than TPR. An organ such as the kidney, which weighs only about 1% as much as the whole body, has a vascular resistance much greater than that of the entire systemic circulation. Hence, it is not surprising that the resistance to flow would be greater for a component organ, such as the kidney, than for the entire systemic circulation because the systemic circulation has many more alternative pathways for blood to flow than just one kidney.

Laminar and Turbulent Flow

Under certain conditions, fluid flow in a cylindrical tube will be laminar, as illustrated in Figure 17-3. As the fluid moves through the tube, a thin layer of fluid in contact with the tube wall adheres to the wall and hence is motionless. The layer of fluid just central to this external lamina must shear against this motionless layer, and therefore the layer moves slowly, but with a finite velocity. Similarly, the next more central layer moves still more rapidly; the longitudinal velocity profile is that of a paraboloid (Fig. 17-3). The fluid elements in any given lamina remain in that lamina as the fluid moves longitudinally along the tube. The velocity at the center of the stream is maximal and equal to twice the mean velocity of flow across the entire cross section of the tube.

Irregular motions of the fluid elements may develop in the flow of fluid through a tube; such flow is called turbulent. In these conditions, fluid elements do not remain confined to definite laminae, but rapid, radial mixing occurs (Fig. 17-7). Greater pressure is required to force a given flow of fluid through the same tube when the flow is turbulent than when it is laminar. In turbulent flow, the pressure drop is approximately proportional to the square of the flow rate, whereas in laminar flow, the pressure drop is proportional to the first power of the flow rate. Hence, to produce a given flow, a pump such as the heart must do considerably more work if turbulence develops.

Whether turbulent or laminar flow will exist in a tube under given conditions may be predicted on the basis of a dimensionless number called **Reynold's number (N_R).** This number represents the ratio of inertial to viscous forces. For a fluid flowing through a cylindrical tube,

● **Equation 17-12**

$$N_R = \rho D v/\eta$$

where ρ = fluid density, D = tube diameter, v = mean velocity, and η = viscosity. For N_R of 2000 or greater, the flow will usually be laminar; for N_R of 3000 or greater, the flow will be turbulent; and for N_R between 2000 and 3000, the flow will be transitional between laminar and turbulent. Equation 17-12 indicates that high fluid densities, large tube diameters, high flow velocities, and low fluid viscosities predispose to turbulence. In addition to these factors, abrupt variations in tube dimensions or irregularities in the tube walls may produce turbulence.

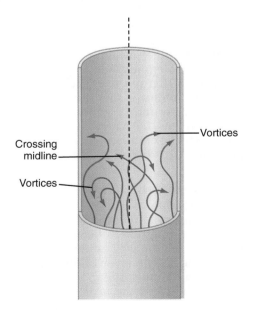

● **Figure 17-7.** In turbulent flow the elements of the fluid move irregularly in axial, radial, and circumferential directions. Vortices frequently develop.

Shear Stress on the Vessel Wall

As blood flows through a vessel, it exerts a force on the vessel wall parallel to the wall. This force is called a shear stress (τ). Shear stress is directly proportional to the flow rate and viscosity of the fluid:

● **Equation 17-13**

$$\tau = \frac{4\eta Q}{\pi r^3}$$

▶ IN THE CLINIC

Turbulence is usually accompanied by audible vibrations. Turbulent flow within the cardiovascular system may be detected with a stethoscope during physical examination. When the turbulence occurs in the heart, the resultant sound is termed a murmur; when it occurs in a vessel, the sound is termed a bruit. In severe anemia, functional cardiac murmurs (murmurs not caused by structural abnormalities) are frequently detectable. The physical basis for such murmurs resides in (1) the reduced viscosity of blood in anemia and (2) the high flow velocities associated with the high cardiac output that usually prevails in anemic patients.

Blood clots, or thrombi, are more likely to develop in turbulent than in laminar flow. A problem with the use of artificial valves in the surgical treatment of valvular heart disease is that thrombi may occur in association with the prosthetic valve. The thrombi may be dislodged and occlude a crucial blood vessel. It is important to design such valves to avert turbulence.

▶ IN THE CLINIC

In certain types of arterial disease, particularly hypertension, the subendothelial layers of vessels tend to degenerate locally, and small regions of the endothelium may lose their normal support. The viscous drag on the arterial wall may cause a tear between a normally supported and an unsupported region of the endothelial lining. Blood may then flow from the vessel lumen through the rift in the lining and dissect between the various layers of the artery. Such a lesion is called a dissecting aneurysm. It occurs most often in the proximal portions of the aorta and is extremely serious. One reason for its predilection for this site is the high velocity of blood flow, with associated large shear rate (du/dy) values at the endothelial wall. Shear stress at the vessel wall also influences many other vascular functions, such as the permeability of the vessel walls to large molecules, the synthetic activity of endothelial cells, the integrity of the formed elements in blood, and blood coagulation. An increase in shear stress on the endothelial wall is also an effective stimulus for the release of nitrous oxide (NO) from vascular endothelial cells; NO is a potent vasodilator (see Microcirculation and Lymphatics).

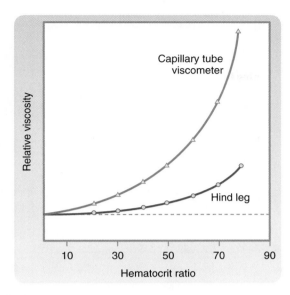

● **Figure 17-8.**   The apparent viscosity of whole blood, relative to that of plasma, increases at a progressively greater rate as the hematocrit ratio increases. For any given hematocrit ratio, the apparent viscosity of blood is less when measured in a biological viscometer (such as the blood vessels) than in a conventional capillary tube viscometer. (Redrawn from Levy MN, Share L: Circ Res 1:247, 1953.)

Rheologic Properties of Blood

The viscosity of a given newtonian fluid at a specified temperature will be constant over a wide range of tube dimensions and flows. However, for a non-newtonian fluid such as blood, viscosity may vary considerably as a function of tube dimensions and flows. Therefore, the term _viscosity_ does not have a unique meaning for blood. The term _apparent viscosity_ is frequently used for the derived value of blood viscosity obtained under the particular conditions of measurement.

Rheologically, blood is a suspension of formed elements, principally erythrocytes, in a relatively homogeneous liquid, the blood plasma. Because blood is a suspension, the apparent viscosity of blood varies as a function of the hematocrit (ratio of the volume of red blood cells to the volume of whole blood). The viscosity of plasma is 1.2 to 1.3 times that of water. The upper curve in Figure 17-8 shows that blood with a normal hematocrit ratio of 45% has an apparent viscosity 2.4 times that of plasma.* In severe anemia, blood viscosity is low. With greater hematocrit ratios, the slope of the curve increases progressively; it is especially steep at the upper range of erythrocyte concentrations.

For any given hematocrit ratio, the apparent viscosity of blood, relative to that of water, depends on the dimensions of the tube used in estimating the viscosity. Figure 17-9 demonstrates that the apparent viscos-

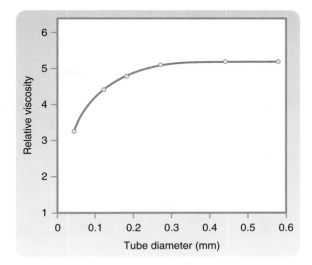

● **Figure 17-9.**   The viscosity of blood relative to that of water increases as a function of tube diameter up to a diameter of about 0.3 mm. (Redrawn from Fåhraeus R, Lindqvist T: Am J Physiol 96:562, 1931.)

ity of blood diminishes progressively as tube diameter decreases below a value of about 0.3 mm. The diameters of the highest-resistance blood vessels, the arterioles, are considerably less than this critical value. This phenomenon therefore reduces the resistance to flow in blood vessels that possess the greatest resistance. The influence of tube diameter on apparent viscosity is explained in part by the actual change in blood composition as it flows through small tubes. The composition of blood changes because the red blood cells tend to accumulate in the faster axial stream, whereas plasma tends to flow in the slower marginal layers. Because the axial portions of the bloodstream contain a greater proportion of red cells and this axial portion will move at greater velocity, the red cells tend to traverse the tube in less time than plasma does. Measurement has shown that red cells do travel faster than plasma through these vascular beds. Furthermore, the hematocrit ratios of the blood contained in the small blood vessels of various tissues are lower than those in blood samples withdrawn from large arteries or veins.

The physical forces responsible for the drift of erythrocytes toward the axial stream and away from the vessel walls when blood is flowing at normal rates are not fully understood. One factor is the great flexibility of red blood cells. At low flow rates, like those in the microcirculation, rigid particles do not migrate toward the central axis of a tube, whereas flexible particles do. The concentration of flexible particles near the tube's central axis is enhanced by increasing the shear rate.

The apparent viscosity of blood diminishes as the flow rate is increased (Fig. 17-10), a phenomenon called shear thinning. The greater the flow, the greater the rate that one lamina of fluid shears against an adjacent lamina. The greater tendency for erythro-

---

*Figure 17-8 also illustrates that the apparent viscosity of blood, when measured in living tissues, is considerably less than the apparent viscosity of the same blood measured in a conventional capillary tube viscometer.

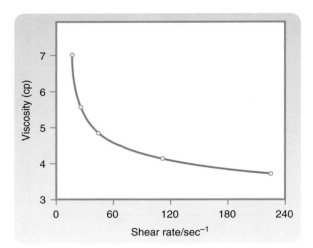

● **Figure 17-10.** Decrease in the viscosity of blood (centipoise) at increasing rates of shear (sec⁻¹). The shear rate refers to the velocity of one layer of fluid relative to that of the adjacent layers and is directionally related to the rate of flow. (Redrawn from Amin TM, Sirs JA: Q J Exp Physiol 70:37, 1985.)

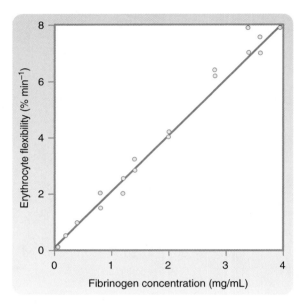

● **Figure 17-11.** Effect of the plasma fibrinogen concentration on the flexibility of human erythrocytes. (Redrawn from Amin TM, Sirs JA: Q J Exp Physiol 70:37, 1985.)

cytes to accumulate in the axial laminae at higher flow rates is partly responsible for this non-newtonian behavior. However, a more important factor is that at very slow flow rates, the suspended cells tend to form aggregates, which increases blood viscosity. As flow is increased, this aggregation decreases, and so also does the apparent viscosity of blood (Fig. 17-10).

The tendency for erythrocytes to aggregate at low flow depends on the concentration of the larger protein molecules in plasma, especially fibrinogen. For this reason, changes in blood viscosity with flow rate are much more pronounced when the concentration of fibrinogen is high. In addition, at low flow rates, leukocytes tend to adhere to the endothelial cells of the microvessels and thereby increase the apparent viscosity of the blood.

The deformability of erythrocytes is also a factor in shear thinning, especially when hematocrit ratios are high. The mean diameter of human red blood cells is about 7 μm, yet they are able to pass through openings with a diameter of only 3 μm. As blood with densely packed erythrocytes flows at progressively greater rates, the erythrocytes become more and more deformed. Such deformation diminishes the apparent viscosity of blood. The flexibility of human erythrocytes is enhanced as the concentration of fibrinogen in plasma increases (Fig. 17-11). If the red blood cells become hardened, as they are in certain spherocytic anemias, shear thinning may diminish.

THE ARTERIAL SYSTEM

Arterial Elasticity

The systemic and pulmonary arterial systems distribute blood to the capillary beds throughout the body. The arterioles are high-resistance vessels of this system that regulate the distribution of flow to the various capillary beds. The aorta, the pulmonary artery, and their major branches have a large amount of elastin in their walls, which makes these vessels highly distensible (i.e., compliant). This distensibility serves to dampen the pulsatile nature of blood flow that results from the heart pumping blood intermittently. When blood is ejected from the ventricles during systole, these vessels distend, and during diastole, they recoil back and propel the blood forward (Fig. 17-12). Thus, the intermittent output of the heart is converted to a steady flow through the capillaries.

The elastic nature of the large arteries also reduces the work of the heart. If these arteries were rigid rather than compliant, the pressure would rise dramatically during systole. This increased pressure would require the ventricles to pump against a large load (i.e., afterload) and thus increase the work of the heart. Instead, as blood is ejected into these vessels, they distend, and the resultant increase in systolic pressure, and thus the work of the heart, is reduced.

Determinants of Arterial Blood Pressure

Arterial blood pressure is routinely measured in patients, and it provides a useful estimate of their

> ◤ **IN THE CLINIC**
>
> As people age, the elastin content of the large arteries is reduced and replaced by collagen. This reduces arterial compliance (Fig. 17-13). Thus, with age, systolic pressure increases, as does the difference between systolic and diastolic blood pressure, called the pulse pressure (see below).

COMPLIANT

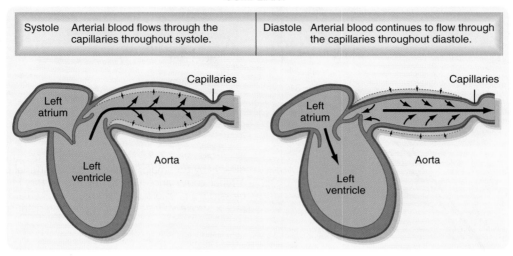

Systole	Arterial blood flows through the capillaries throughout systole.
Diastole	Arterial blood continues to flow through the capillaries throughout diastole.

A When the arteries are normally compliant, a substantial fraction of the stroke volume is stored in the arteries during ventricular systole. The arterial walls are stretched.

B During ventricular diastole the previously stretched arteries recoil. The volume of blood that is displaced by the recoil furnishes continuous capillary flow throughout diastole.

RIGID ARTERIES

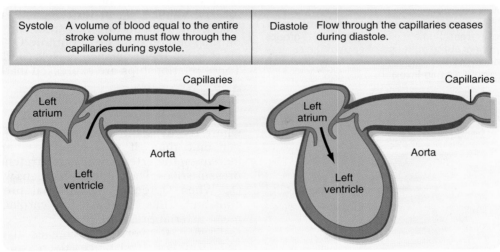

Systole	A volume of blood equal to the entire stroke volume must flow through the capillaries during systole.
Diastole	Flow through the capillaries ceases during diastole.

C When the arteries are rigid, virtually none of the stroke volume can be stored in the arteries.

D Rigid arteries cannot recoil appreciably during diastole.

● **Figure 17-12.** **A** to **D,** When the arteries are normally compliant, blood flows through the capillaries throughout the cardiac cycle. When the arteries are rigid, blood flows through the capillaries during systole, but flow ceases during diastole.

cardiovascular status. Arterial pressure can be defined as **mean arterial pressure,** which is the pressure averaged over time, and as **systolic** (maximal) and **diastolic** (minimal) arterial pressure within the cardiac cycle (Fig. 17-14). The difference between systolic and diastolic pressure is termed **pulse pressure.**

The determinants of arterial blood pressure are arbitrarily divided into "physical" and "physiological" factors (Fig. 17-15). The two physical factors or fluid mechanical characteristics are fluid volume (i.e., blood volume) within the arterial system and the static elastic characteristics (compliance) of the system. The physiological factors are cardiac output (which equals heart rate × stroke volume) and peripheral resistance.

Mean Arterial Pressure
Mean arterial pressure, $\overline{P}_a$, may be estimated from an arterial blood pressure tracing by measuring the area

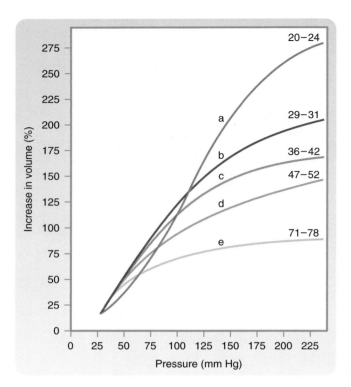

● **Figure 17-13.** Pressure-volume relationships of aortas obtained at autopsy from humans in different age groups (denoted by the numbers at the right end of each of the curves). Note how compliance (ΔV/ΔP) decreases with age. (Redrawn from Hallock P, Benson IC: *J Clin Invest* 16:595, 1937.)

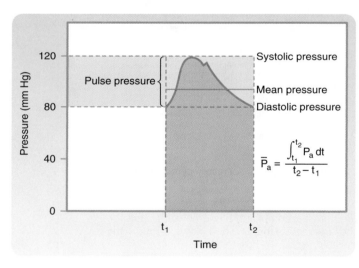

●**Figure 17-14.** Arterial systolic, diastolic, pulse, and mean pressure. Mean arterial pressure ($\overline{P}_a$) represents the area under the arterial pressure curve *(shaded area)* divided by the duration of the cardiac cycle ($t_2 - t_1$).

under the pressure curve and dividing this area by the time interval involved (Fig. 17-14). Alternatively, $\overline{P}_a$ can be satisfactorily approximated from the measured values of systolic (P_s) and diastolic (P_d) pressure by means of the following formula:

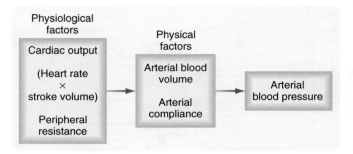

● **Figure 17-15.** Arterial blood pressure is determined directly by two major physical factors: arterial blood volume and arterial compliance. These physical factors in turn are affected by certain physiological factors, namely, cardiac output (heart rate × stroke volume) and peripheral resistance.

● **Equation 17-14**

$$\overline{P}_a = P_d + \frac{P_s - P_d}{3}$$

Consider that mean arterial pressure depends on only two physical factors: mean blood volume in the arterial system and arterial compliance (Fig. 17-16). Arterial volume, V_a, in turn depends on the rate of inflow, Q_h, into the arteries from the heart (cardiac output) and on the rate of outflow, Q_r, from the arteries through the resistance vessels (peripheral runoff). These relationships are expressed mathematically as

● **Equation 17-15**

$$dV_a/dt = Q_h - Q_r$$

where dV_a/dt is the change in arterial blood volume per unit time. If Q_h exceeds Q_r, arterial volume increases, the arterial walls are stretched further, and pressure rises. The converse happens when Q_r exceeds Q_h. When Q_h equals Q_r, arterial pressure remains constant. Thus, increases in cardiac output raise mean arterial pressure, as do increases in peripheral resistance. Conversely, decreases in cardiac output or peripheral resistance decrease mean arterial pressure.

Arterial Pulse Pressure

Arterial pulse pressure is systolic pressure minus diastolic pressure. It is principally a function of just one physiological factor, stroke volume, which determines the change in arterial blood volume (a physical factor) during ventricular systole. This physical factor, plus a second physical factor (arterial compliance), determines the arterial pulse pressure (Fig. 17-16).

Stroke Volume. As described previously, mean arterial pressure depends on cardiac output and peripheral resistance. During the rapid ejection phase of systole, the volume of blood introduced into the arterial system exceeds the volume that exits the system through the arterioles. Arterial pressure and volume therefore rise to a peak pressure, which is systolic pressure. During the remainder of the cardiac cycle (i.e., ventricular diastole), cardiac ejection is

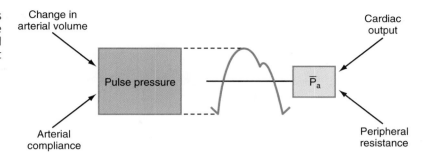

● **Figure 17-16.** The two physical determinants of pulse pressure are arterial compliance (C_a) and the change in arterial volume. The two physiological determinants of mean arterial pressure ($\overline{P}_a$) are cardiac output and total peripheral resistance.

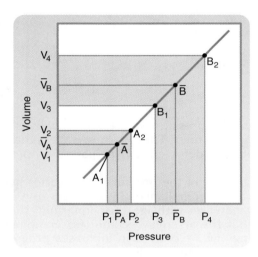

● **Figure 17-17.** Effect of a change in stroke volume on pulse pressure in a system in which arterial compliance remains constant over the prevailing range of pressures and volumes. A larger volume increment [$(V_4 - V_3) > (V_2 - V_1)$] results in a greater mean pressure ($\overline{P}_B > \overline{P}_A$) and a greater pulse pressure [$(P_4 - P_3) > (P_2 - P_1)$].

zero, and peripheral runoff now greatly exceeds cardiac ejection. The resultant decrement in arterial blood volume thus causes pressure to fall to a minimum, which is diastolic pressure. The effect of stroke volume on pulse pressure when arterial compliance is constant is illustrated in Figure 17-17.

Arterial Compliance. Arterial compliance also affects pulse pressure. This relationship is illustrated in Figure 17-18. When cardiac output and TPR are constant, a decrease in arterial compliance results in an increase in pulse pressure. Diminished arterial compliance also imposes a greater workload on the left ventricle (i.e., increased afterload), even if stroke volume, TPR, and mean arterial pressure are equal in the two individuals.

Total Peripheral Resistance and Arterial Diastolic Pressure. As previously discussed, if the heart rate and stroke volume remain constant, an increase in TPR will increase mean arterial pressure. When arterial compliance is constant, an increase in TPR leads to proportional increases in systolic and diastolic pressure such that the pulse pressure is unchanged (Fig. 17-19, *A*). However, arterial compliance is not

Arterial pulse pressure affords valuable clues about a person's stroke volume, provided that arterial compliance is essentially normal. Patients who have severe congestive heart failure or who have suffered a severe hemorrhage are likely to have a very small arterial pulse pressure because their stroke volumes are abnormally small. Conversely, individuals with large stroke volumes, as in aortic valve regurgitation, are likely to have an increased arterial pulse pressure. Similarly, well-trained athletes at rest tend to have large stroke volumes because their heart rates are usually low. The prolonged ventricular filling times in these individuals induce the ventricles to pump a large stroke volume, and hence their pulse pressure is large.

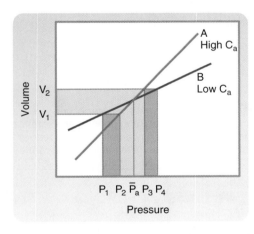

● **Figure 17-18.** For a given volume increment ($V_2 - V_1$), reduced arterial compliance (compliance B < compliance A) results in increased pulse pressure [$(P_4 - P_1) > (P_3 - P_2)$].

linear. As mean arterial pressure increases and the artery is stressed, compliance decreases (Fig. 17-19, *B*). Because of the decrease in arterial compliance with increased arterial pressure, pulse pressure will increase when arterial pressure is elevated.

Peripheral Arterial Pressure Curves

The radial stretch of the ascending aorta brought about by left ventricular ejection initiates a pressure wave that is propagated down the aorta and its

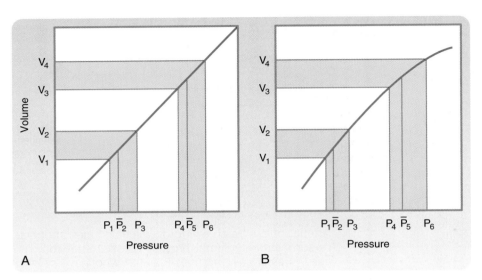

● **Figure 17-19.** Comparison of the effects of a given change in peripheral resistance on pulse pressure when the pressure-volume curve for the arterial system is either rectilinear (A) or curvilinear (B). The increment in arterial volume is the same for both conditions $[(V_4 - V_3) = (V_2 - V_1)]$.

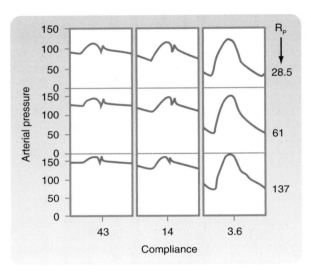

● **Figure 17-20.** Changes in aortic pressure induced by changes in arterial compliance and peripheral resistance (R_p) in an isolated heart preparation. As compliance was reduced from 43 to 14 to 3.6 units, pulse pressure increased significantly. (Modified from Elizinga G, Westerhof N: Circ Res 32:178, 1973.)

▶ **IN THE CLINIC**

In chronic hypertension, a condition characterized by a persistent elevation in TPR, the arterial pressure-volume curve resembles that shown in Figure 17-19, *B*. Because arteries become substantially less compliant when arterial pressure rises, an increase in TPR will elevate systolic pressure more than it will elevate diastolic pressure. Diastolic pressure is elevated in such individuals, but ordinarily not more than 10 to 40 mm Hg above the average normal level of 80 mm Hg. Not uncommonly, however, systolic pressure is elevated by 50 to 100 mm Hg above the average normal level of 120 mm Hg. The combination of increased resistance and diminished arterial compliance is represented in Figure 17-20.

branches. The pressure wave travels much faster than the blood itself does. This pressure wave is the "pulse" that can be detected by palpating a peripheral artery.

The velocity of the pressure wave varies inversely with arterial compliance. In general, transmission velocity increases with age, thus confirming the observation that the arteries become less compliant with advancing age. Velocity also increases progressively as the pulse wave travels from the ascending aorta toward the periphery. This increase in velocity reflects the decrease in vascular compliance in the more distal than in the more proximal portions of the arterial system.

The arterial pressure contour becomes distorted as the wave is transmitted down the arterial system. This distortion in the pressure wave contour is demonstrated in Figure 17-21. These changes in contour are pronounced in young individuals, but they diminish with age. In elderly patients, the pulse wave may be transmitted virtually unchanged from the ascending aorta to the periphery.

Damping of the high-frequency components of the arterial pulse is largely caused by the elastic properties of the arterial walls. Several factors, including wave reflection and resonance, vascular tapering, and pressure-induced changes in transmission velocity, contribute to peaking of the arterial pressure wave.

Blood Pressure Measurement in Humans

In hospital intensive care units, needles or catheters may be introduced into the peripheral arteries of patients to measure arterial blood pressure directly by means of strain gauges. Ordinarily, blood pressure is estimated indirectly by means of a sphygmomanometer.

When blood pressure readings are taken from the arm, systolic pressure may be estimated by palpating the radial artery at the wrist (palpatory method). While pressure in the cuff exceeds the systolic level, no pulse is perceived. As pressure falls just below the systolic level (Fig. 17-22, *A*), a spurt of blood passes

● **Figure 17-21.** Arterial pressure curves recorded from various sites. Aside from the increasing delay in the onset of the initial pressure rise, three major changes occur in the arterial pulse contour as the pressure wave travels distally. First, the systolic portions of the pressure wave become narrowed and elevated. In the figure, the systolic pressure at the level of the knee was 39 mm Hg greater than that recorded in the aortic arch. Second, the high-frequency components of the pulse, such as the incisura (i.e., the notch that appears at the end of ventricular ejection), are damped out and soon disappear. Third, a hump may appear on the diastolic portion of the pressure wave, at a point in the pressure wave just beyond the locus at which the incisura had initially appeared. (From Remington JW, O'Brien LJ: Am J Physiol 218:437, 1970.)

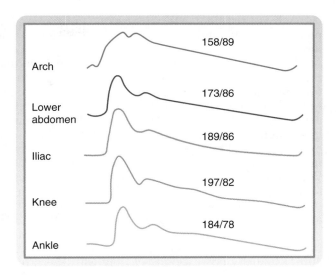

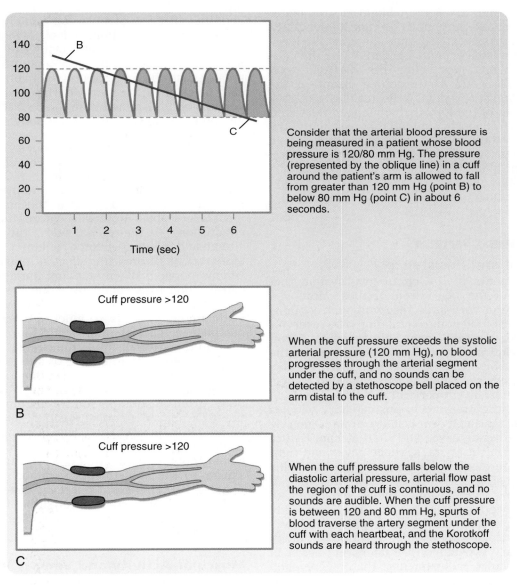

Consider that the arterial blood pressure is being measured in a patient whose blood pressure is 120/80 mm Hg. The pressure (represented by the oblique line) in a cuff around the patient's arm is allowed to fall from greater than 120 mm Hg (point B) to below 80 mm Hg (point C) in about 6 seconds.

When the cuff pressure exceeds the systolic arterial pressure (120 mm Hg), no blood progresses through the arterial segment under the cuff, and no sounds can be detected by a stethoscope bell placed on the arm distal to the cuff.

When the cuff pressure falls below the diastolic arterial pressure, arterial flow past the region of the cuff is continuous, and no sounds are audible. When the cuff pressure is between 120 and 80 mm Hg, spurts of blood traverse the artery segment under the cuff with each heartbeat, and the Korotkoff sounds are heard through the stethoscope.

● **Figure 17-22. A** to **C,** Measurement of arterial blood pressure with a sphygmomanometer.

through the brachial artery under the cuff during the peak of systole, and a slight pulse will be felt at the wrist.

The auscultatory method is a more sensitive and therefore a more precise technique for measuring systolic pressure, and it also permits diastolic pressure to be estimated. The practitioner listens with a stethoscope applied to the skin of the antecubital space over the brachial artery. While the pressure in the cuff exceeds systolic pressure, the brachial artery is occluded and no sounds are heard (Fig. 17-22, *B*). When the inflation pressure falls just below the systolic level (120 mm Hg in Fig. 17-22, *A*), a small spurt of blood escapes the occluding pressure of the cuff, and slight tapping sounds (called Korotkoff sounds) are heard with each heartbeat. The pressure at which the first sound is detected represents systolic pressure. It usually corresponds closely with the directly measured systolic pressure. As the inflation pressure of the cuff continues to fall, more blood escapes under the cuff per beat and the sounds become louder. When the inflation pressure approaches the diastolic level, the Korotkoff sounds become muffled. When the inflation pressure falls just below the diastolic level (80 mm Hg in Fig. 17-22, *A*), the sounds disappear; the pressure reading at this point indicates diastolic pressure. The origin of the Korotkoff sounds is related to the discontinuous spurts of blood that pass under the cuff and meet a static column of blood beyond the cuff; the impact and turbulence generate audible vibrations. Once the inflation pressure is less than diastolic pressure, flow is continuous in the brachial artery, and sounds are no longer heard (Fig. 17-22, *C*).

THE VENOUS SYSTEM

Capacitance and Resistance

Veins are elements of the circulatory system that return blood to the heart from tissues. Moreover, veins constitute a very large reservoir that contains up to 70% of the blood in the circulation. The reservoir function of veins makes them able to adjust blood volume returning to the heart, or preload, so that the needs of the body can be matched when cardiac output is altered (see Chapter 19). This high capacitance is an important property of veins.

The hydrostatic pressure in postcapillary venules is about 20 mm Hg, and it decreases to around 0 mm Hg in the thoracic venae cavae and right atrium. Hydrostatic pressure in the thoracic venae cavae and right atrium is also termed central venous pressure. Veins are very distensible and have very low resistance to blood flow. This low resistance allows movement of blood from peripheral veins to the heart with only small reductions in central venous pressure. Moreover, veins control filtration and absorption by adjusting postcapillary resistance (see later) and assist in the cardiovascular adjustments that accompany changes in body position.

The ability of veins to participate in these various functions depends on their distensibility, or compliance. Venous compliance varies with the position in the body such that veins in the lower limb are less compliant than those at or above the level of the heart. Veins in the lower limbs are also thicker than those in the brain or upper limbs. The compliance of veins, like that of arteries, decreases with age, and the vascular thickening that occurs is accompanied by a reduction in elastin and an increase in collagen content.

Variations in venous return are achieved by adjustments in venomotor tone, respiratory activity (see Chapter 19), and orthostatic stress or gravity.

Gravity

Gravitational forces may profoundly affect cardiac output. For example, soldiers standing at attention for a long time may faint because gravity causes blood to pool in the dependent blood vessels and thereby reduces cardiac output. Warm ambient temperatures interfere with the compensatory vasomotor reactions, and the absence of muscular activity exaggerates these effects. Gravitational effects are amplified in airplane pilots during pullout from dives. The centrifugal force in the footward direction may be several times greater than the force of gravity. Pilots characteristically black out momentarily during the pullout maneuver as blood is drained from the cephalic regions and pooled in the lower parts of the body.

Some explanations that have been advanced to explain the gravitationally induced reduction in cardiac output are inaccurate. For example, it has been argued that when an individual is standing, the force of gravity impedes venous return to the heart from the dependent regions of the body. This statement is incomplete because it ignores the gravitational counterforce on the arterial side of the same vascular circuit, and this counterforce facilitates venous return. Moreover, it ignores the effect of gravity in causing venous pooling. When standing upright, gravity will cause blood to accumulate in the lower extremities and distend both the arteries and veins. Because venous compliance is so much greater than arterial compliance, this distention occurs more on the venous than on the arterial side of the circuit.

The hemodynamic effects of such venous distention (venous pooling) resemble those caused by the hemorrhage of an equivalent volume of blood from the body. When an adult person shifts from a supine position to a relaxed standing position, 300 to 800 mL of blood pools in the legs. This pooling may reduce cardiac output by about 2 L/min. The compensatory adjustments to assumption of a standing position are similar to the adjustments to blood loss (see also Chapter 19). There is a reflex increase in heart rate and cardiac contractility. In addition, both arterioles and veins constrict, with the arterioles being affected to a greater extent than the veins.

Muscular Activity and Venous Valves

When a recumbent person stands but remains at rest, the pressure in the veins rises in the dependent regions of the body (Fig. 17-23). The venous pressure (P_v) in

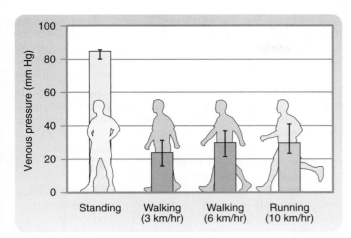

● **Figure 17-23.** Mean pressures (±95% confidence intervals) in the foot veins of 18 human subjects during quiet standing, walking, and running. (From Stick C et al: J Appl Physiol 72:2063, 1992.)

the legs increases gradually and does not reach an equilibrium value until almost 1 minute after standing. The slowness of this rise in P_v is attributable to the venous valves, which permit flow only toward the heart. When a person stands, the valves prevent blood in the veins from falling toward the feet. Hence, the column of venous blood is supported at numerous levels by these valves. Because of these valves, the venous column can be thought of as consisting of many discontinuous segments. However, blood continues to enter the column from many venules and small tributary veins, and the pressure continues to rise. As soon as the pressure in one segment exceeds that in the segment just above it, the intervening valve is forced open. Ultimately, all the valves are open and the column is continuous.

Precise measurement reveals that the final level of P_v in the feet during quiet standing is only slightly greater than that in a static column of blood extending from the right atrium to the feet. This finding indicates that the pressure drop caused by blood flow from the foot veins to the right atrium is very small. This very low resistance justifies considering all the veins as a common venous compliance in the circulatory system model illustrated in Chapter 19.

When an individual who has been standing quietly begins to walk, venous pressure in the legs decreases appreciably (Fig. 17-23). Because of the intermittent venous compression exerted by the contracting leg muscles and because of the operation of the venous valves, blood is forced from the veins toward the heart. Hence, muscular contraction lowers the mean venous pressure in the legs and serves as an auxiliary pump. Furthermore, muscular contraction prevents venous pooling and lowers capillary hydrostatic pressure. In this way, muscular contraction reduces the tendency for edema fluid to collect in the feet during standing.

MICROCIRCULATION AND LYMPHATICS

The circulatory system supplies the tissues with blood in amounts that meet the body's requirements for O_2 and nutrients. The capillaries, whose walls consist of a single layer of endothelial cells, permit rapid exchange of gases, water, and solutes with interstitial fluid. The muscular arterioles, which are the major resistance vessels, regulate regional blood flow to the capillary beds. Venules and veins serve primarily as collecting channels and storage vessels.

The lymphatic system is composed of lymphatic vessels, nodes, and lymphoid tissue. This system collects the fluid and proteins that have escaped from blood and transports them back into the veins for recirculation in blood. In this section we examine in detail the network of the smallest blood vessels of the body, as well as the lymphatic vessels.

Microcirculation

The microcirculation is defined as the circulation of blood through the smallest vessels of the body—arterioles, capillaries, and venules. Arterioles (5 to 100 μm in diameter) have a thick smooth muscle layer, a thin adventitial layer, and an endothelial lining (see Fig. 15-2). Arterioles give rise directly to capillaries (5 to 10 μm in diameter) or in some tissues to metarterioles (10 to 20 μm in diameter), which then give rise to capillaries (Fig. 17-24). Metarterioles can either bypass the capillary bed and connect to venules or directly connect to the capillary bed. Arterioles that give rise directly to capillaries regulate flow through these capillaries by constriction or dilation. The capillaries form an interconnecting network of tubes with an average length of 0.5 to 1 mm.

Functional Properties of Capillaries

In metabolically active organs, such as the heart, skeletal muscle, and glands, capillary density is high. In less active tissues, such as subcutaneous tissue or cartilage, capillary density is low. Capillary diameter also varies. Some capillaries have diameters smaller than those of erythrocytes. Passage through these tiny vessels requires the erythrocytes to become temporarily deformed. Fortunately, normal erythrocytes are quite flexible.

Blood flow in capillaries depends chiefly on the contractile state of arterioles. The average velocity of blood flow in capillaries is approximately 1 mm/sec; however, it can vary from zero to several millimeters per second in the same vessel within a brief period. These changes in capillary blood flow may be random

or rhythmic. The rhythmic oscillatory behavior of capillaries is caused by contraction and relaxation (vasomotion) of the precapillary vessels (i.e., the arterioles and small arteries).

Vasomotion is an intrinsic contractile behavior of vascular smooth muscle and is independent of external input. Changes in transmural pressure (intravascular minus extravascular pressure) also influence the contractile state of precapillary vessels. An increase in transmural pressure, caused either by an increase in venous pressure or by dilation of arterioles, results in contraction of the terminal arterioles. A decrease in transmural pressure causes precapillary vessel relaxation (see Chapter 18). Humoral and possibly neural factors also affect vasomotion. For example, when increased transmural pressure causes the precapillary vessels to contract, the contractile response can be overridden and vasomotion abolished. This effect is accomplished by metabolic (humoral) factors when the O_2 supply becomes too low for the requirements of parenchymal tissue, as occurs in skeletal muscle during exercise.

Although a reduction in transmural pressure relaxes the terminal arterioles, blood flow through the capillaries cannot increase if the reduction in intravascular pressure is caused by severe constriction of the upstream microvessels. Large arterioles and metarterioles also exhibit vasomotion. However, their contraction does not usually completely occlude the lumen of the vessel and arrest blood flow, whereas contraction of the terminal arterioles may arrest blood flow. Thus, the flow rate in capillaries may be altered by contraction and relaxation of small arteries, arterioles, and metarterioles.

Blood flow through the capillaries has been called nutritional flow because it provides for exchange of gases and solutes between blood and tissue. Conversely, blood flow that bypasses the capillaries as it passes from the arterial to the venous side of the circulation has been termed nonnutritional, or shunt, flow (Fig. 17-24). In some areas of the body (e.g., fingertips, ears), true AV shunts exist (see Chapter 18). However, in many tissues, such as muscle, anatomic shunts are lacking. Even in the absence of these shunts, nonnutritional flow can occur. In tissues with metarterioles, nonnutritional flow may be continuous from arteriole to venule during low metabolic activity, when many precapillary vessels are closed. When metabolic activity increases in these tissues, more precapillary vessels open to permit capillary perfusion.

True capillaries lack smooth muscle and are therefore incapable of active constriction. Nevertheless, the endothelial cells that form the capillary wall contain actin and myosin, and they can alter their shape in response to certain chemical stimuli.

Because of their narrow lumens (i.e., small radius), the thin-walled capillaries can withstand high internal pressures without bursting. This property can be explained in terms of the law of Laplace:

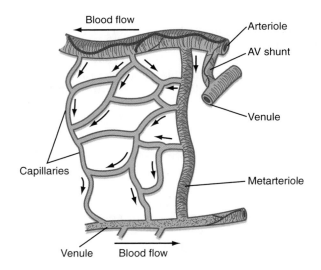

● **Figure 17-24.** Composite schematic drawing of the microcirculation. The circular structures on the arteriole and venule represent smooth muscle fibers, and the branching solid lines represent sympathetic nerve fibers. The arrows indicate the direction of blood flow.

● **Equation 17-16**

$$T = Pr$$

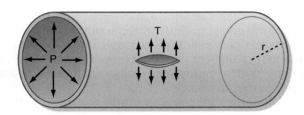

● **Figure 17-25.** Diagram of a small blood vessel to illustrate the law of Laplace: T = Pr, where P = intraluminal pressure, r = radius of the vessel, and T = wall tension as the force per unit length tangential to the vessel wall. Wall tension acts to prevent rupture along a theoretical longitudinal slit in the vessel.

where

T = tension in the vessel wall
P = transmural pressure
r = radius of the vessel

The Laplace equation applies to very thin-walled vessels, such as capillaries. Wall tension opposes the distending force (Pr) that tends to pull apart a theoretical longitudinal slit in the vessel (Fig. 17-25). Transmural pressure in a blood vessel in vivo is essentially equal to intraluminal pressure because extravascular pressure is generally negligible. To calculate wall tension, pressure in mm Hg is converted to dynes per square centimeter according to the equation P = hρg, where h is the height of an Hg column in centimeters, ρ is the density of Hg in g/cm^3, and g is gravitational acceleration in cm/s^2. For a capillary with a pressure of 25 mm Hg and a radius of 5×10^{-4} cm, the pressure (2.5 cm Hg × 13.6 g/cm^3 × 980 cm/sec^2) is 3.33×10^4 dyne/cm. Wall tension is then 16.7 $dyne/cm^2$. For an aorta with a pressure of 100 mm Hg and a radius of 1.5 cm, wall tension is 2×10^5 dyne/cm. Thus, at the pressures normally found in the aorta and capillaries, the wall tension of the aorta is about 12,000 times greater than that of the capillaries. In a person standing quietly, capillary pressure in the feet may reach 100 mm Hg. Even under such conditions, capillary wall tension increases to a value that is still only one three-thousandth of the wall tension in the aorta at the same internal pressure.

The diameter of the resistance vessels (arterioles) is determined by the balance between the contractile force of the vascular smooth muscle and the distending force produced by intraluminal pressure. The greater the contractile activity of the vascular smooth muscle of an arteriole, the smaller its diameter. In small arterioles, contraction can continue to the point at which the vessel is completely occluded. Occlusion is caused by infolding of the endothelium and by trapping of blood cells in the vessel.

With a progressive reduction in intravascular pressure, vessel diameter decreases (as does vessel wall tension—the law of Laplace) and blood flow eventually ceases, although pressure within the arteriole is still greater than tissue pressure. The pressure that causes flow to cease has been called the critical closing pressure, and its mechanism is still controversial. This

critical closing pressure is low when vasomotor activity is reduced by inhibition of sympathetic nerve activity in the vessel and is increased when vasomotor tone is enhanced by activation of the vascular sympathetic nerve fibers.

Vasoactive Role of the Capillary Endothelium

For many years, the endothelium of capillaries was thought to be an inert single layer of cells that served solely as a passive filter to permit the passage of water and small molecules across the blood vessel wall and to retain blood cells and large molecules (proteins) within the vascular compartment. However, the endothelium is now recognized to be an important source of substances that cause contraction or relaxation of vascular smooth muscle.

One of these substances is **prostacyclin (PGI₂)**. PGI₂ can relax vascular smooth muscle via an increase in cAMP (Fig. 17-26). PGI₂ is formed in the endothelium from arachidonic acid, and the process is catalyzed by PGI₂ synthase. The mechanism that triggers synthesis of PGI₂ is not known. However, PGI₂ may be released by an increase in shear stress caused by accelerated blood flow. The primary function of PGI₂ is to inhibit platelet adherence to the endothelium and platelet aggregation and thus prevent intravascular clot formation. PGI₂ also causes relaxation of vascular smooth muscle.

Of far greater importance in endothelium-mediated vascular dilation is the formation and release of **nitric oxide (NO),** a component of endothelium-derived relaxing factor (Fig. 17-26). When endothelial cells are stimulated by acetylcholine or other vasodilator agents (ATP, bradykinin, serotonin, substance P, histamine), NO is released. These agents do not cause vasodilation in blood vessels lacking the endothelium. NO (synthesized from L-arginine) activates guanylyl cyclase in vascular smooth muscle to increase [cGMP], which produces relaxation by decreasing myofilament sensitivity to [Ca⁺⁺]. Release of NO can be stimulated by the shear stress of blood flow on the endothelium.

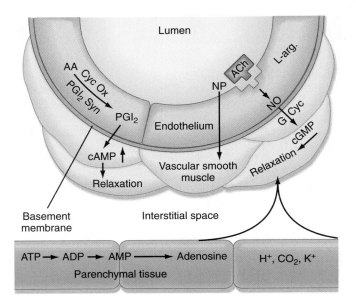

● **Figure 17-26.** Endothelium- and non–endothelium-mediated vasodilation. Prostacyclin (PGI$_2$) is formed from arachidonic acid (AA) by the action of cyclooxygenase (Cyc Ox) and prostacyclin synthase (PGI$_2$ Syn) in the endothelium and elicits relaxation of the adjacent vascular smooth muscle via increases in cAMP. Stimulation of the endothelial cells with acetylcholine (ACh) or other agents (see text) results in the formation and release of an endothelium-derived relaxing factor identified as nitric oxide (NO). NO stimulates guanylyl cyclase (G Cyc) to increase cGMP in the vascular smooth muscle to produce relaxation. The vasodilator agent nitroprusside (NP) acts directly on vascular smooth muscle. Substances such as adenosine, H$^+$, CO$_2$, and K$^+$ can arise in the parenchymal tissue and elicit vasodilation by direct action on vascular smooth muscle.

● AT THE CELLULAR LEVEL

Injury to the endothelium of blood vessels precedes atherosclerosis. The protective effect (antiatherogenic) of the endothelium resides in several properties. Thus, the endothelium regulates adhesion of leukocytes to the vessel wall, suppresses the proliferation of vascular smooth muscle cells, maintains a vessel lining that resists the formation of thrombi, and regulates vascular smooth muscle tone. All these functions involve the action of NO. As indicated previously, production of NO is regulated by many substances and by shear stress acting on the vessel wall.

The drug nitroprusside also increases cGMP by acting directly on vascular smooth muscle; it is not endothelium mediated. Vasodilator agents such as adenosine, H$^+$, CO$_2$, and K$^+$ may be released from parenchymal tissue and act locally on resistance vessels (Fig. 17-26).

Acetylcholine also causes the release of an endothelium-dependent hyperpolarizing factor that underlies the relaxation of adjacent smooth muscle. Although arachidonic acid metabolites have been suggested,

the factor remains unknown. Moreover, how the factor reaches vascular smooth muscle (diffusion through the extracellular space or passage via myoepithelial junctions) is unclear. Nevertheless, there are diverse ways by which endothelial cells communicate with vascular smooth muscle.

The endothelium can also synthesize **endothelin,** a potent vasoconstrictor peptide. Endothelin can affect vascular tone and blood pressure in humans and may be involved in such pathological states as atherosclerosis, pulmonary hypertension, congestive heart failure, and renal failure.

Passive Role of the Capillary Endothelium

Transcapillary Exchange. Solvent and solute move across the capillary endothelial wall by three processes: diffusion, filtration, and pinocytosis. Diffusion is the most important process for transcapillary exchange and pinocytosis is the least important.

DIFFUSION. Under normal conditions, only about 0.06 mL of water per minute moves back and forth across the capillary wall per 100 g of tissue as a result of filtration and absorption. In contrast, 300 mL of water per minute per 100 g of tissue moves across the capillary wall by diffusion, a 5000-fold difference.

When filtration and diffusion are related to blood flow, about 2% of the plasma passing through the capillaries is filtered. In contrast, the diffusion of water is 40 times greater than the rate at which it is brought to the capillaries by blood flow. The transcapillary exchange of solutes is also primarily governed by diffusion. Thus, diffusion is the key factor in providing exchange of gases, substrates, and waste products between capillaries and tissue cells.

The process of diffusion is described by Fick's law (see also Chapter 1):

● **Equation 17-17**

$$J = -DA\frac{\Delta C}{\Delta X}$$

where

J = quantity of a substance moved per unit time
D = free diffusion coefficient for a particular molecule
A = cross-sectional area of the diffusion pathway
$\frac{\Delta C}{\Delta X}$ = concentration gradient of the solute

For diffusion across a capillary wall, Fick's law can also be expressed as

● **Equation 17-18**

$$J = -PS(C_o - C_i)$$

where

P = capillary permeability to the substance
S = capillary surface area
C$_i$ = concentration of the substance inside the capillary
C$_o$ = concentration of the substance outside the capillary

The PS product provides a convenient expression of available capillary surface area because the intrinsic permeability of the capillary is rarely altered much under physiological conditions (capillary permeability may be altered as with a bee sting).

In capillaries, diffusion of lipid-insoluble molecules is restricted to water-filled channels or pores. Movement of solute across the capillary endothelium is complex and involves corrections for attractions between solute and solvent molecules, interactions between solute molecules, pore configuration, and charge on the molecules relative to charge on the endothelial cells. Such solute motion is not simply a matter of random thermal movement of molecules down a concentration gradient. For small molecules, such as water, NaCl, urea, and glucose, the capillary pores offer little restriction to diffusion (i.e., they have a low reflection coefficient—see later). Diffusion of these substances is so rapid that the mean concentration gradient across the capillary endothelium is extremely small. The greater the size of the lipid-insoluble molecules, the more restricted their diffusion through capillaries. Diffusion eventually becomes minimal when the molecular weight of the molecules exceeds about 60,000. With small molecules, the only limitation to net movement across the capillary wall is the rate at which blood flow transports the molecules to the capillary. Transport of these molecules is said to be **flow limited.**

With flow-limited small molecules, the concentration of the molecule in blood reaches equilibrium with its concentration in interstitial fluid at a location near the origin of the capillary from its parent arteriole. Its concentration falls to negligible levels near the arterial end of the capillary (Fig. 17-27, *A*). If the flow is large, the small molecule can still be present at a distant locus downstream in the capillary. A somewhat larger molecule will move farther along the capillary before it reaches an insignificant concentration in blood. Furthermore, the number of still larger molecules that enter the arterial end of the capillary but cannot pass through the capillary pores equals the number that leaves the venous end of the capillary (see Fig. 17-27, *A*).

With large molecules, diffusion across the capillaries becomes the limiting factor **(diffusion limited).** That is, the permeability of a capillary to a large solute molecule limits its transport across the capillary wall. Diffusion of small lipid-insoluble molecules is so rapid that diffusion limits blood-tissue exchange only when distances between capillaries and parenchymal cells are great (e.g., tissue edema or very low capillary density) (Fig. 17-27, *B*).

Movement of lipid-soluble molecules across the capillary wall is not limited to capillary pores (only about 0.02% of the capillary surface) but also occurs directly through the lipid membranes of the entire capillary endothelium. Consequently, lipid-soluble molecules move rapidly between blood and tissue. The degree of lipid solubility (oil-to-water partition coefficient) provides a good index of the ease of transfer of lipid molecules through the capillary endothelium.

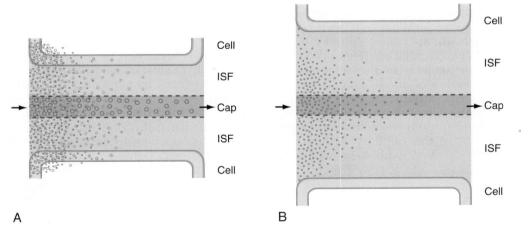

A   B

● **Figure 17-27.** Flow- and diffusion-limited transport from capillaries (Cap) to tissue. **A,** Flow-limited transport. The smallest water-soluble inert tracer particles *(blue dots)* reach negligible concentrations after passing only a short distance down the capillary. Larger particles *(circles)* with similar properties travel farther along the capillary before reaching an insignificant intracapillary concentration. Both substances cross the interstitial fluid (ISF) and reach the parenchymal tissue (Cell). Because of their size, more of the smaller particles are taken up by the tissue cells. The largest particles cannot penetrate the capillary pores and hence do not escape from the capillary lumen except by pinocytotic vesicle transport. An increase in the volume of blood flow or an increase in capillary density increases tissue supply of the diffusible solutes. Note that capillary permeability is greater at the venous end of the capillary (also in the venule, not shown) because of the larger number of pores in this region. **B,** Diffusion-limited transport. When the distance between the capillaries and parenchymal tissue is large as a result of edema or low capillary density, diffusion becomes a limiting factor in the transport of solutes from capillary to tissue, even at high rates of capillary blood flow.

O_2 and CO_2 are both lipid soluble, and they readily pass through endothelial cells. Calculations based on (1) the diffusion coefficient for O_2, (2) capillary density and diffusion distances, (3) blood flow, and (4) tissue O_2 consumption indicate that the O_2 supply of normal tissue at rest and during activity is not limited by diffusion or by the number of open capillaries.

Measurements of the partial pressure of O_2 (PO_2) and O_2 saturation of blood in microvessels indicate that in many tissues, O_2 saturation at the entrance of capillaries has decreased to about 80% as a result of diffusion of O_2 from arterioles and small arteries. Moreover, CO_2 loading and the resulting intravascular shifts in the oxyhemoglobin dissociation curve occur in the precapillary vessels. Hence, in addition to gas exchange at the capillaries, O_2 and CO_2 pass directly between adjacent arterioles and venules and possibly between arteries and veins (countercurrent exchange). This countercurrent exchange represents a diffusional shunt of gas away from the capillaries; this shunt may limit the supply of O_2 to the tissue at low blood flow rates.

CAPILLARY FILTRATION. The permeability of the capillary endothelial membrane is not uniform. Thus, the liver capillaries are quite permeable, and albumin escapes from them at a rate several times greater than that from the less permeable muscle capillaries. Furthermore, permeability is not uniform along the length of the capillary. The venous ends are more permeable than the arterial ends, and permeability is greatest in the venules, a property attributed to the greater number of pores in these regions.

Where does filtration occur? Some water passes through the capillary endothelial cell membranes, but most flows through apertures (pores) in the endothelial walls of the capillaries (Figs. 17-28 and 17-29). The pores in skeletal and cardiac muscle capillaries have diameters of about 4 nm. There are clefts between adjacent endothelial cells in mouse cardiac muscle, and the gap at the narrowest point is about 4 nm. The clefts (pores) are sparse and represent only about 0.02% of the capillary surface area. Pores are absent in cerebral capillaries, where the blood-brain barrier blocks the entry of many small molecules.

In addition to clefts, some of the more porous capillaries (e.g., in the kidney, intestine) contain fenestrations 20 to 100 nm wide, whereas other capillaries (e.g., in the liver) have a discontinuous endothelium (Fig. 17-29). Fenestrations and discontinuous endothelium permit the passage of molecules that are too large to pass through the intercellular clefts of the endothelium.

The direction and magnitude of water movement across the capillary wall can be estimated as the algebraic sum of the hydrostatic and osmotic pressure that exists across the membrane. An increase in intracapillary hydrostatic pressure favors movement of fluid from the vessel interior to the interstitial space, whereas an increase in the concentration of osmotically active particles within vessels favors movement of fluid into the vessels from the interstitial space (Fig. 17-30).

Hydrostatic Forces. Hydrostatic pressure (blood pressure) within capillaries is not constant. Instead, it depends on arterial and venous pressure and on precapillary (arterioles) and postcapillary (venules and small veins) resistance. An increase in arterial or venous pressure elevates capillary hydrostatic pressure, whereas a reduction in arterial or venous pressure has the opposite effect. An increase in arteriolar resistance or closure of arteries reduces capillary pressure, whereas a greater resistance to flow in venules and veins increases capillary pressure.

Hydrostatic pressure is the principal force in capillary filtration. A given change in venous pressure produces a greater effect on capillary hydrostatic pressure than does the same change in arterial pressure. About 80% of an increase in venous pressure is transmitted back to the capillaries.

Capillary hydrostatic pressure (P_c) varies from tissue to tissue. Average values, obtained from direct measurements in human skin, are about 32 mm Hg at the arterial end of capillaries and about 15 mm Hg at the venous end of capillaries at the level of the heart (Fig. 17-30). As discussed previously, when a person stands, hydrostatic pressure increases in the legs and decreases in the head.

Tissue pressure, or more specifically interstitial fluid pressure (P_i) outside the capillaries, opposes capillary filtration. $P_c - P_i$ constitutes the driving force for filtration. Normally, P_i is close to zero, so P_c essentially represents the hydrostatic driving force.

Osmotic Forces. The key factor that restrains fluid loss from capillaries is the osmotic pressure of plasma proteins (such as albumin). This osmotic pressure is called colloid osmotic pressure or oncotic pressure (π_p). The total osmotic pressure of plasma is about 6000 mm Hg (reflecting the presence of electrolytes and other small molecules), whereas oncotic pressure is only about 25 mm Hg. This small oncotic pressure is an important factor in fluid exchange across the capillary because plasma proteins are essentially confined to the intravascular space, whereas electrolytes are virtually equal in concentration on both sides of the capillary endothelium. The relative permeability of solute to water influences the actual magnitude of osmotic pressure. The **reflection coefficient (σ)** is the relative impediment to the passage of a substance through the capillary membrane. The reflection coefficient of water is zero and that of albumin (to which the endothelium is essentially impermeable) is 1. Filterable solutes have reflection coefficients between 0 and 1. In addition, different tissues have different reflection coefficients for the same molecule. Hence, movement of a given solute across the endothelial wall varies with the tissue. True oncotic pressure (π) is defined by the following equation (see also Chapter 1):

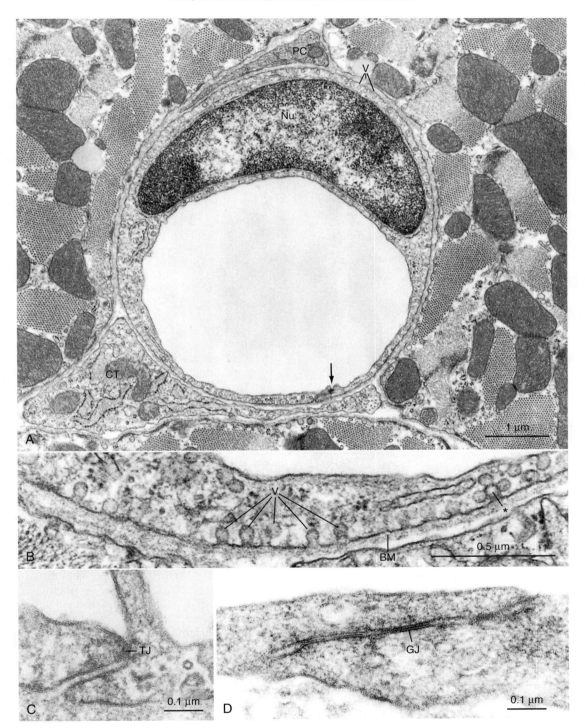

● **Figure 17-28.** **A,** Cross-sectioned capillary in a mouse ventricular wall. The luminal diameter is approximately 4 μm. In this thin section, the capillary wall is formed by a single endothelial cell (Nu, endothelial nucleus), which forms a functional complex *(arrow)* with itself. The thin pericapillary space is occupied by a pericyte (PC) and a connective tissue (CT) cell ("fibroblast"). Note the numerous endothelial vesicles (V). **B,** Detail of the endothelial cell in **A** showing plasmalemmal vesicles (V) attached to the endothelial cell surface. These vesicles are especially prominent in vascular endothelium and are involved in transport of substances across the blood vessel wall. Note the complex alveolar vesicle *(asterisk)*. BM, basement membrane. **C,** Junctional complex in a capillary of a mouse heart. "Tight" junctions (TJ) typically form in these small blood vessels and appear to consist of fusions between apposed endothelial cell surface membranes. **D,** Interendothelial junction in a muscular artery of monkey papillary muscle. Although tight junctions similar to those of capillaries are found in these large blood vessels, extensive junctions that resemble gap junctions in the intercalated disks between myocardial cells often appear in arterial endothelium (example shown at GJ).

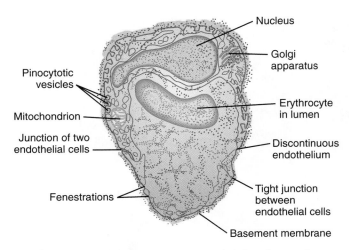

● **Figure 17-29.** Diagrammatic sketch of an electron micrograph of a **composite** capillary in cross section.

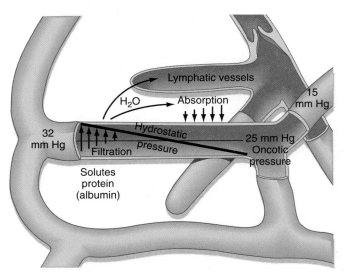

● **Figure 17-30.** Schematic representation of the factors responsible for filtration and absorption across the capillary wall and the formation of lymph.

● **Equation 17-19**

$$\pi = \sigma RT (C_i - C_o)$$

where

σ = reflection coefficient
R = gas constant
T = temperature in degrees Kelvin
C_i and C_o = solute concentration inside and outside the capillary, respectively

Albumin is the most important plasma protein determining oncotic pressure. The average albumin molecule (molecular weight of 69,000) is approximately half the size of the average globulin molecule, and it is present at almost twice the concentration as that of globulins (4.5 versus 2.5 g/dL of plasma). Albumin also exerts a greater osmotic force than can be accounted for solely on the basis of its concentration in plasma. Therefore, it cannot be completely

With prolonged standing, particularly when associated with some elevation of venous pressure in the legs (such as that caused by pregnancy) or with sustained increases in venous pressure (as seen in congestive heart failure), filtration is greatly enhanced, and it exceeds the capacity of the lymphatic system to remove the capillary filtrate from the interstitial space.

The concentration of plasma proteins may also change in different pathological states and thus alter the osmotic force and movement of fluid across the capillary membrane. The plasma protein concentration is increased in dehydration (e.g., water deprivation, prolonged sweating, severe vomiting, diarrhea). In this condition, water moves by osmotic force from the tissues to the vascular compartment. In contrast, the plasma protein concentration is reduced in some renal diseases because of its loss in urine, and edema may occur.

When capillary injury is extensive, as in severe burns, intravascular fluid and plasma protein leak into the interstitial space in the damaged tissues. The protein that escapes from the vessel lumen increases the oncotic pressure of the interstitial fluid. This greater osmotic force outside the capillaries leads to additional fluid loss and possibly to severe dehydration of the patient.

replaced by inert substances of appropriate molecular size, such as dextran. This additional osmotic force becomes disproportionately great at high concentrations of albumin (as in plasma), and this force is weak to absent in dilute solutions of albumin (as in interstitial fluid). The reason for this activity of albumin is its negative charge at normal blood pH. Albumin binds a small number of Cl^- ions, which increases the negative charge and hence the ability to retain more Na^+ inside the capillaries (see Chapter 2). This small increase in the electrolyte concentration of plasma over that of interstitial fluid produced by the negatively charged albumin enhances its osmotic force to that of an ideal solution containing a solute with a molecular weight 37,000. If albumin had a molecular weight of 37,000, it would not be retained by the capillary endothelium because of its small size. Hence, albumin could not function as a counterforce to capillary hydrostatic pressure. If albumin did not exert this enhanced osmotic force, a concentration of about 12 g of albumin/dL of plasma would be required to achieve a plasma oncotic pressure of 25 mm Hg. Such a high albumin concentration would greatly increase blood viscosity and hence would increase resistance to blood flow through the vascular system.

Small amounts of albumin escape from the capillaries and enter the interstitial fluid, where they exert a very small osmotic force (0.1 to 5 mm Hg). This force, π_i, is small because the concentration of albumin in interstitial fluid is low and because at low concentrations, albumin cannot enhance the osmotic force as much as it does at high concentrations.

Balance of Hydrostatic and Osmotic Forces.

The relationship between hydrostatic pressure and oncotic pressure and the role of these forces in regulating fluid passage across the capillary endothelium were expounded by Starling in 1896. This relationship constitutes the Starling hypothesis. It can be expressed by the equation

● **Equation 17-20**

$$Q_f = k[(P_c + \pi_i) - (P_i + \pi_p)]$$

where

Q_f = fluid movement
P_c = capillary hydrostatic pressure
P_i = interstitial fluid hydrostatic pressure
π_p = plasma oncotic pressure
π_i = interstitial fluid oncotic pressure
k = filtration constant for the capillary membrane

Filtration occurs when the algebraic sum is positive; absorption occurs when it is negative.

Traditionally, filtration was considered to occur at the arterial end of the capillary and absorption was considered to occur at its venous end because of the gradient of hydrostatic pressure along the capillary. This scheme is true for an idealized capillary (Fig. 17-30). However, in well-perfused capillaries, arteriolar vasoconstriction can reduce P_c such that absorption is allowed transiently. With continued vasoconstriction, absorption will diminish with time because fluid absorption increases π_i (the interstitial protein concentration rises) and decreases P_i. Direct observations have revealed that many capillaries only filter, whereas others only absorb. In some vascular beds (e.g., the renal glomerulus), hydrostatic pressure in the capillary is high enough to cause filtration along the entire length of the capillary. In other vascular beds (e.g., the intestinal mucosa), the hydrostatic and oncotic forces are such that absorption occurs along the whole capillary.

Capillary pressure depends on several factors, the principal one being the contractile state of the precapillary vessel. Normally, arterial pressure, venous pressure, postcapillary resistance, interstitial fluid hydrostatic and oncotic pressure, and plasma oncotic pressure are relatively constant. A change in precapillary resistance influences fluid movement across the capillary wall. Because water moves so quickly across the capillary endothelium, the hydrostatic and osmotic forces equilibrate along the entire capillary. Hence, in the normal state, filtration and absorption across the capillary wall are well balanced. Only a small percentage (2%) of the plasma that flows through the vascular system is filtered. Of this, about 85% is absorbed in the capillaries and venules. The remainder returns to the vascular system as lymph fluid, along with the albumin that escapes from the capillaries.

In the lungs, mean capillary hydrostatic pressure is only about 8 mm Hg (see Chapter 22). Because plasma oncotic pressure is 25 mm Hg and lung interstitial fluid pressure is approximately 15 mm Hg, the net force slightly favors reabsorption. Despite the predominance of reabsorption, pulmonary lymph is formed.

This lymph consists of fluid that is osmotically withdrawn from the capillaries by the small amount of plasma protein that escapes through the capillary endothelium.

Capillary Filtration Coefficient.

The rate of fluid movement (Q_f) across the capillary membrane depends not only on the algebraic sum of the hydrostatic and osmotic forces across the endothelium (ΔP) but also on the area (A_m) of the capillary wall available for filtration, the distance (Δx) across the capillary wall, the viscosity (η) of the filtrate, and the filtration constant (k) of the membrane. These factors may be expressed by the equation

● **Equation 17-21**

$$Q_r = \frac{kA_m\Delta P}{\eta\Delta X}$$

The dimensions of Q_r are units of flow per unit of pressure gradient across the capillary wall per unit of capillary surface area. This expression, which describes the flow of fluid through the membrane pores, is essentially Poiseuille's law for flow through tubes.

Because the thickness of the capillary wall and the viscosity of the filtrate are relatively constant, they can be included in the filtration constant k. If the area of the capillary membrane is not known, the rate of filtration can be expressed per unit weight of tissue. Hence, the equation can be simplified to

● **Equation 17-22**

$$Q_f = k_t\Delta P$$

where k_t is the capillary filtration coefficient for a given tissue and the units for Q_f are milliliters per minute per 100 g of tissue per mm Hg pressure.

In any given tissue, the filtration coefficient per unit area of capillary surface, and hence capillary permeability, is not changed by various physiological conditions, such as arteriolar dilation and capillary distention, or by such adverse conditions as hypoxia, hypercapnia, or reduced pH. When capillaries are injured (as by toxins or severe burns), significant amounts of fluid and protein leak out of the capillaries into the interstitial space. This increase in capillary permeability is reflected by an increase in the filtration coefficient.

Because capillary permeability is constant under normal conditions, the filtration coefficient can be used to determine the relative number of open capillaries (i.e., the capillary surface area available for filtration in tissue). For example, the increased metabolic activity of contracting skeletal muscle relaxes the precapillary resistance vessels and hence opens more capillaries. This process, called **capillary recruitment**, increases the filtering surface area.

Disturbances in Hydrostatic-Osmotic Balance.

Relatively small changes in arterial pressure may have little effect on filtration. The change in pressure may be countered by adjustments in precapillary resistance vessels (autoregulation; see Chapter 18) so that hydrostatic pressure remains constant in the open capillaries. However, a severe reduction in mean arterial pressure usually evokes arteriolar constriction mediated by the sympathetic nervous system. This response may occur in hemorrhage, and it is often accompanied by a fall in venous pressure. These changes reduce capillary hydrostatic pressure. However, the low blood pressure in hemorrhage causes a decrease in blood flow (and hence in O_2 supply) to the tissue, with the result that vasodilator metabolites accumulate and relax the arterioles. Precapillary vessel relaxation also occurs because of the reduced transmural pressure (autoregulation, see Chapter 18). Consequently, absorption predominates over filtration, and fluid moves from the interstitium into the capillary. These responses to hemorrhage constitute one of the compensatory mechanisms used by the body to restore blood volume (see Chapter 19).

An increase in venous pressure alone, as occurs in the feet when a person stands up, would elevate capillary pressure and enhance filtration. However, the increase in transmural pressure closes precapillary vessels (myogenic mechanism; see Chapter 18), and hence the capillary filtration coefficient actually decreases. This reduction in capillary surface available for filtration prevents large amounts of fluid from leaving the capillaries and entering the interstitial space.

In a normal individual, the filtration coefficient (k_t) for the whole body is about 0.006 mL/min/100 g of tissue/mm Hg. For a 70-kg man, an elevation in venous pressure of 10 mm Hg for 10 minutes would increase filtration from capillaries by 342 mL. Edema does not usually occur because the fluid is returned to the vascular compartment by the lymphatic vessels. When edema develops, it usually appears in the dependent parts of the body, where the hydrostatic pressure is greatest, but its location and magnitude are also determined by the type of tissue. Loose tissues, such as the subcutaneous tissue around the eyes or in the scrotum, are more prone than firm tissues, such as in a muscle, or encapsulated structures, such as in a kidney, to collect larger quantities of interstitial fluid.

PINOCYTOSIS. Some transfer of substances across the capillary wall can occur in tiny pinocytotic vesicles. These vesicles (Figs. 17-28 and 17-29), formed by pinching off of the endothelial cell membrane, can take up substances on one side of the capillary wall, move them across the cell by kinetic energy, and deposit their contents on the other side—a process termed transcytosis. The amount of material transported in this way is very small relative to that moved by diffusion. However, pinocytosis may be responsible for the movement of large (30 nm) lipid-insoluble molecules between blood and interstitial fluid. The number of pinocytotic vesicles in endothelium varies among tissues (muscle > lung > brain), and the number increases from the arterial to the venous end of the capillary.

Lymphatics

The terminal vessels of the lymphatic system consist of a widely distributed, closed-end network of highly permeable lymph capillaries. These lymph capillaries resemble blood capillaries, with two important differences: tight junctions are not present between endothelial cells, and fine filaments anchor lymph vessels to the surrounding connective tissue. With muscular contraction, these fine strands pull on the lymphatic vessels to open spaces between the endothelial cells and permit the entrance of protein and large particles into the lymphatic vessels. The lymph capillaries drain into larger vessels that finally enter the right and left subclavian veins, where they connect with the respective internal jugular veins.

Only cartilage, bone, epithelia, and tissues of the central nervous system lack lymphatic vessels. These vessels return the plasma capillary filtrate to the circulation. This task is accomplished by means of tissue pressure, and it is facilitated by intermittent skeletal muscle activity, lymphatic vessel contractions, and an extensive system of one-way valves. In this respect, lymphatic vessels resemble veins, although the larger lymphatic vessels do have thinner walls than the corresponding veins, and they contain only a small amount of elastic tissue and smooth muscle.

The volume of fluid transported through the lymphatics in 24 hours is about equal to the body's total plasma volume. The lymphatics return about a fourth to half of the circulating plasma proteins to the blood in a day. These vessels are the only means whereby the protein that leaves the vascular compartment can be returned to blood. Net back-diffusion of protein into the capillaries cannot occur against the large protein concentration gradient. If the protein were not removed by the lymph vessels, it would accumulate in interstitial fluid and act as an oncotic force that draws fluid from the blood capillaries and produces edema.

In addition to returning fluid and protein to the vascular bed, the lymphatic system filters the lymph at the lymph nodes and removes foreign particles such as bacteria. The largest lymphatic vessel, the thoracic duct, not only drains the lower extremities but also returns the protein lost through the permeable liver capillaries. Moreover, the thoracic duct carries substances absorbed from the gastrointestinal tract. The principal substance is fat, in the form of chylomicrons.

Lymph flow varies considerably. The flow from resting skeletal muscle is almost nil, and it increases during exercise in proportion to the degree of muscular activity. It is increased by any mechanism that enhances the rate of blood capillary filtration; such mechanisms include increased capillary pressure or permeability and decreased plasma oncotic pressure. When either the volume of interstitial fluid exceeds the drainage capacity of the lymphatics or the lymphatic vessels become blocked, interstitial fluid accumulates and gives rise to clinical edema.

CORONARY CIRCULATION

Functional Anatomy of Coronary Vessels

The right and left coronary arteries arise at the root of the aorta behind the right and left cusps of the aortic valve, respectively. These arteries provide the entire blood supply to the myocardium. The right coronary artery principally supplies the right ventricle and atrium. The left coronary artery, which divides near its origin into the anterior descending and the circumflex branches, mainly supplies the left ventricle and atrium. There is some overlap between the regions supplied by the left and right arteries. In humans, the right coronary artery is dominant (supplying most of the myocardium) in about 50% of individuals. The left coronary artery is dominant in another 20%, and the flow delivered by each main artery is about equal in the remaining 30%. The epicardial distribution of the coronary arteries and veins is illustrated in Figure 17-31.

Coronary arterial blood passes through the capillary beds; most of it returns to the right atrium through the coronary sinus. Some of the coronary venous blood reaches the right atrium via the anterior coronary veins. In addition, vascular communications directly link the myocardial vessels with the cardiac chambers; these communications are the **arteriosinusoidal, arterioluminal,** and **thebesian** vessels. The

● **Figure 17-31.** Anterior and posterior surfaces of the heart illustrating the location and distribution of the principal coronary vessels.

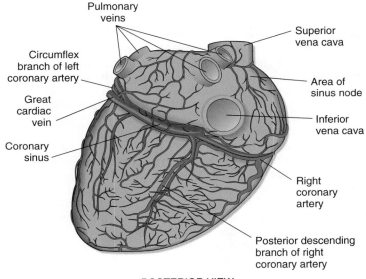

POSTERIOR VIEW

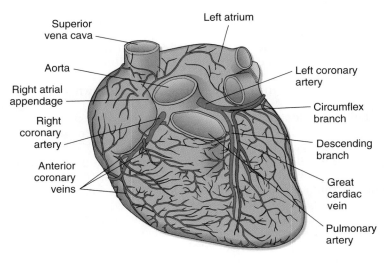

ANTERIOR VIEW

arteriosinusoidal channels consist of small arteries or arterioles that lose their arterial structure as they penetrate the chamber walls, where they divide into irregular, endothelium-lined sinuses. These sinuses anastomose with other sinuses and with capillaries, and they communicate with the cardiac chambers. The arterioluminal vessels are small arteries or arterioles that open directly into the atria and ventricles. The thebesian vessels are small veins that connect capillary beds directly with the cardiac chambers and also communicate with the cardiac veins. All the minute vessels of the myocardium communicate in the form of an extensive plexus of subendocardial vessels. However, the myocardium does not receive significant nutritional blood flow directly from the cardiac chambers.

Factors That Influence Coronary Blood Flow

Physical Factors

The primary factor responsible for perfusion of the myocardium is aortic pressure. Changes in aortic pressure generally evoke parallel directional changes in coronary blood flow. This is caused in part by changes in coronary perfusion pressure. However, the major factor in the regulation of coronary blood flow is a change in arteriolar resistance engendered by changes in the metabolic activity of the heart. When the metabolic activity of the heart increases, coronary resistance decreases; when cardiac metabolism decreases, coronary resistance increases (see Chapter 18).

If a cannulated coronary artery is perfused by blood from a pressure-controlled reservoir, perfusion pressure can be altered without changing aortic pressure and cardiac work. The relationship between initial and steady-state blood flow is shown in the experiment in Figure 17-32. This is an example of autoregulation of blood flow, which is discussed in Chapter 18. Blood pressure is kept within narrow limits by baroreceptor reflex mechanisms. Hence, changes in coronary blood flow are mainly caused by changes in the diameter of coronary resistance vessels in response to the metabolic demands of the heart.

In addition to providing the pressure to move blood through the coronary vessels, the heart also affects its blood supply by the squeezing effect (extravascular compression) of the contracting myocardium on its own blood vessels. The patterns of coronary flow in the left and right coronary arteries are shown in Figure 17-33.

Left ventricular myocardial pressure (pressure within the wall of the left ventricle) is greatest near the endocardium and least near the epicardium. This pressure gradient does not normally impair endocardial blood flow because the greater blood flow to the endocardium during diastole compensates for the greater blood flow to the epicardium during systole. Measurements of coronary blood flow indicate that blood flow to the epicardial and endocardial halves of the left ventricle is approximately equal under normal conditions. Because extravascular compression is greatest at the endocardial surface of the ventricle, the

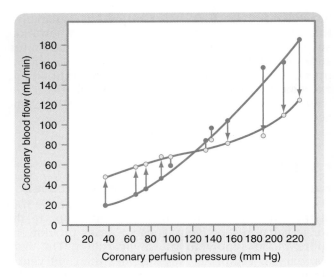

● **Figure 17-32.** Pressure-flow relationships in the coronary vascular bed. At constant aortic pressure, cardiac output, and heart rate, coronary artery perfusion pressure was abruptly increased or decreased from the control level indicated by the point where the two lines cross. The closed circles represent the flows that were obtained immediately after the change in perfusion pressure; the open circles represent the steady-state flows at the new pressures. There is a tendency for flow to return toward the control level (autoregulation of blood flow), and this is most prominent over the intermediate pressure range (about 60 to 180 mm Hg). (From Berne RM, Rubio R: Coronary circulation. In Handbook of Physiology (sect 2): The Cardiovascular System: The Heart, vol 1. Bethesda, MD, American Physiological Society, 1979.)

> ### IN THE CLINIC
>
> The minimal extravascular resistance and absence of left ventricular work during diastole can be used to improve myocardial perfusion in patients with damaged myocardium and low blood pressure. In a method called counterpulsation, an inflatable balloon is inserted into the thoracic aorta through a femoral artery. The balloon is inflated during each ventricular diastole and deflated during each systole. This procedure enhances coronary blood flow during diastole by raising diastolic pressure at a time when coronary extravascular resistance is lowest. Furthermore, it reduces cardiac energy requirements by lowering aortic pressure (afterload) during ventricular ejection.

equality of epicardial and endocardial blood flow indicates that the tone of the endocardial resistance vessels is less than that of the epicardial vessels.

The flow pattern in the right coronary artery is similar to that in the left coronary artery (Fig. 17-33). In contrast to the left ventricle, reversal of blood flow does not occur in the right ventricle in early systole because the thin right ventricle develops a lower pressure during systole. Hence, systolic blood flow

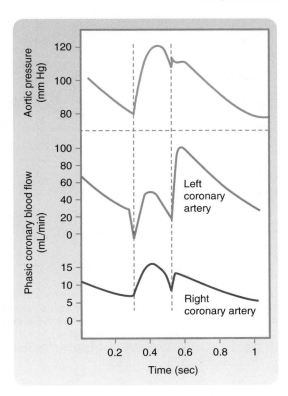

● **Figure 17-33.**   Comparison of phasic coronary blood flow in the left and right coronary arteries. Extravascular compression is so great during early ventricular systole that blood flow in the large coronary arteries supplying the left ventricle is briefly reversed. Maximal left coronary inflow occurs in early diastole, when the ventricles have relaxed and extravascular compression of the coronary vessels is virtually absent. After an initial reversal in early systole, left coronary blood flow follows the aortic pressure until early diastole, when it rises abruptly and then declines slowly as aortic pressure falls during the remainder of diastole.

constitutes a much greater proportion of total coronary inflow than it does in the left coronary artery.

The extent to which extravascular compression restricts coronary inflow can be readily seen when the heart is suddenly arrested in diastole or with the induction of ventricular fibrillation. Figure 17-34, *A,* depicts mean left coronary flow when the vessel was perfused with blood at a constant pressure from a reservoir. When ventricular fibrillation was electrically induced, an immediate and substantial increase in blood flow occurred. A subsequent increase in coronary resistance over a period of many minutes reduced myocardial blood flow to below the level that existed before induction of ventricular fibrillation (Fig. 17-34, *B,* just before stellate ganglion stimulation).

When diastolic pressure in the coronary arteries is abnormally low (such as in severe hypotension, partial coronary artery occlusion, or severe aortic stenosis), the ratio of endocardial to epicardial blood flow falls below a value of 1. This ratio indicates that blood flow to the endocardial regions is more severely impaired than that to the epicardial regions of the ventricle. There is also an increase in the gradient of myocardial lactic acid and myocardial adenosine concentrations from epicardium to endocardium. For this reason, the myocardial damage observed in atherosclerotic heart disease (e.g., after coronary occlusion) is greatest in the inner wall of the left ventricle.

Tachycardia and bradycardia have dual effects on coronary blood flow. A change in heart rate mainly alters diastole. In tachycardia, the proportion of time spent in systole, and consequently the period of restricted inflow, increases. However, this mechanical effect is overridden by the dilation of coronary resistance vessels associated with the increased metabolic activity of the more rapidly beating heart. With bradycardia the opposite occurs; coronary inflow is less restricted (more time in diastole), but so are the metabolic (O_2) requirements of the myocardium.

● **Figure 17-34.**   **A,** Unmasking of the restricting effect of ventricular systole on mean coronary blood flow by induction of ventricular fibrillation during perfusion of the left coronary artery at constant pressure. With the onset of ventricular fibrillation, coronary blood flow increases abruptly because extravascular compression is removed. Flow then gradually returns toward and often falls below the prefibrillation level. This increase in coronary resistance that occurs despite the removal of extravascular compression demonstrates the heart's ability to adjust its blood flow to meet its energy requirements. **B,** Effect of cardiac sympathetic nerve stimulation on coronary blood flow and coronary sinus blood O_2 tension in a fibrillating heart during perfusion of the left coronary artery at constant pressure. (Berne RM: Unpublished observations.)

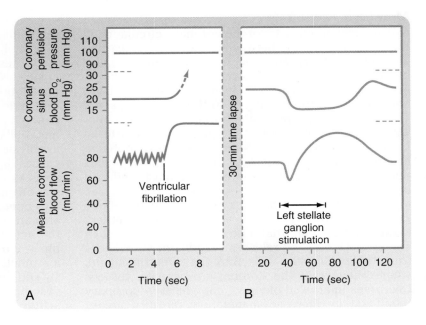

Neural and Neurohumoral Factors

Stimulation of cardiac sympathetic nerves markedly increases coronary blood flow. However, the increase in flow is associated with an increased heart rate and more forceful systole. The stronger contraction and the tachycardia tend to restrict coronary flow. The increase in myocardial metabolic activity, however, tends to dilate coronary resistance vessels. The increase in coronary blood flow evoked by cardiac sympathetic nerve stimulation reflects the sum of these factors. In perfused hearts in which the mechanical effect of extravascular compression is eliminated by cardiac arrest or by ventricular fibrillation, an initial coronary vasoconstriction is often observed. After this initial vasoconstriction, the metabolic effect evokes vasodilation (see Fig. 17-34, *B*).

Furthermore, when β-adrenergic receptor blockade eliminates the positive chronotropic and inotropic effects, activation of the cardiac sympathetic nerves increases coronary resistance. These observations indicate that the primary action of the sympathetic nerve fibers on the coronary resistance vessels is vasoconstriction.

α-Adrenergic receptors (constrictors) and β-adrenergic receptors (dilators) are present on the coronary vessels. Coronary resistance vessels also participate in the baroreceptor and chemoreceptor reflexes, and the sympathetic constrictor tone of the coronary arterioles can be modulated by such reflexes. Nevertheless, coronary resistance is predominantly under local nonneural control.

Vagus nerve stimulation slightly dilates the coronary resistance vessels, and activation of the carotid and aortic chemoreceptors can slightly decrease coronary resistance via the vagus nerves to the heart. Failure of strong vagal stimulation to increase coronary blood flow is not due to lack of muscarinic receptors on the coronary resistance vessels because intracoronary administration of acetylcholine elicits marked vasodilation.

Metabolic Factors

A striking characteristic of the coronary circulation is the close relationship between the level of myocardial metabolic activity and the magnitude of coronary blood flow (Fig. 17-35). This relationship is also found in a denervated heart and in a completely isolated heart, either in the beating or in the fibrillating state. The fibrillating ventricles can fibrillate for many hours when the coronary arteries are perfused with arterial blood from some external source. As already noted, a fibrillating heart uses less O_2 than a pumping heart does, and blood flow to the myocardium is reduced accordingly.

The mechanisms that link the cardiac metabolic rate and coronary blood flow remain unsettled. However, it appears that a decrease in the ratio of O_2 supply to O_2 demand releases vasodilator substances from the myocardial cells into the interstitial fluid, where they relax the coronary resistance vessels. Decreases in arterial blood O_2 content or in coronary blood flow and increases in metabolic rate all decrease

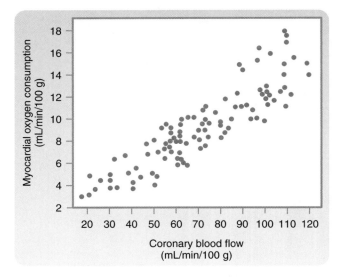

● **Figure 17-35.** Relationship between myocardial O_2 consumption and coronary blood flow during a variety of interventions that increase or decrease the myocardial metabolic rate. (From Berne RM, Rubio R: Coronary circulation. In Handbook of Physiology (sect 2): The Cardiovascular System: The Heart, vol 1. Bethesda, MD, American Physiological Society, 1979.)

the O_2 supply-demand ratio (Fig. 17-36). As a consequence, vasodilator substances are released. These substances dilate the arterioles and thereby adjust the O_2 supply to the O_2 demand. A decrease in O_2 demand diminishes the release of vasodilators and permits greater expression of basal tone.

Numerous metabolites mediate the vasodilation that accompanies increased cardiac work. Accumulation of vasoactive metabolites can also account for the increase in blood flow that results from a brief period of ischemia (i.e., **reactive hyperemia**—see Chapter 18). The duration of the enhanced coronary flow after release of the briefly occluded vessel is, within certain limits, proportional to the duration of the period of occlusion. Among the factors implicated in reactive hyperemia are ATP-sensitive K^+ (K_{ATP}) channels, NO, CO_2, H^+, K^+, hypoxia, and adenosine.

Of these agents, the key factors appear to be adenosine, NO, and opening of the K_{ATP} channels. The contributions of each of these agents and their interaction under basal conditions and during increased myocardial activity are complex. A reduction in oxidative metabolism in vascular smooth muscle reduces ATP synthesis, which in turn opens K_{ATP} channels and causes hyperpolarization. This change in potential reduces entry of Ca^{++} and relaxes coronary vascular smooth muscle to increase flow. A reduction in ATP also opens K_{ATP} channels in cardiac muscle and generates an outward current that reduces the duration of the action potential and limits entry of Ca^{++} during phase 2 of the action potential. This action may serve a protective role during periods of imbalance between O_2 supply and demand. Additionally, the release of vasodilators, such as NO and adenosine, dilates the arterioles and thereby adjusts the O_2 supply to the O_2

● **Figure 17-36.** Imbalance in the O_2 supply–O_2 demand ratio alters coronary blood flow by the rate of release of a vasodilator metabolite from cardiomyocytes. A decrease in the ratio elicits an increase in vasodilator release, whereas an increase in the ratio has the opposite effect.

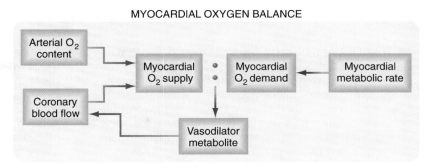

MYOCARDIAL OXYGEN BALANCE

● **Figure 17-37.** Schematic representation of factors that increase (+) or decrease (–) coronary vascular resistance. Intravascular pressure (arterial blood pressure) stretches the vessel wall.

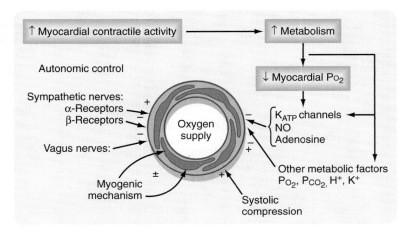

demand. At low concentrations, adenosine appears to activate endothelial K_{ATP} channels and to enhance release of NO. Conversely, at higher concentrations, adenosine acts directly on vascular smooth muscle by activating K_{ATP} channels. Decreased O_2 demand would sustain the ATP level, as well as reduce the amount of vasodilator substances released and permit greater expression of basal tone. If production of all three agents is inhibited, coronary blood flow is reduced, both at rest and during exercise. Furthermore, contractile dysfunction and signs of myocardial ischemia become evident.

According to the adenosine hypothesis, a reduction in myocardial O_2 tension produced by inadequate coronary blood flow, hypoxemia, or increased metabolic activity of the heart leads to release of adenosine from the myocardium. Adenosine enters the interstitial fluid space to reach the coronary resistance vessels and induces vasodilation by activating adenosine receptors. However, it cannot be responsible for the increased coronary flow observed during prolonged enhancement of cardiac metabolic activity because release of adenosine from cardiac muscle is transitory. Little evidence exists that CO_2, H^+, or O_2 play a significant direct role in the regulation of coronary blood flow. Factors that alter coronary vascular resistance are illustrated in Figure 17-37.

Effects of Diminished Coronary Blood Flow

Most of the O_2 in coronary arterial blood is extracted during one passage through the myocardial capillar-

ies. Thus, the supply of O_2 to myocardial cells is flow limited; any substantial reduction in coronary blood flow will curtail O_2 delivery to the myocardium because O_2 extraction is nearly maximal even when blood flow is normal.

A reduction in coronary flow that is neither too prolonged nor too severe to induce myocardial necrosis can still cause substantial (but temporary) dysfunction of the heart. A relatively brief period of severe ischemia followed by reperfusion can result in pronounced mechanical dysfunction (myocardial stunning). However, the heart eventually recovers fully from the dysfunction. Pathophysiologically, the basis for myocardial stunning appears to be a result of intracellular Ca^{++} overload, initiated during the period of ischemia, combined with the generation of OH^- and superoxide free radicals early in the period of reperfusion. These changes impair the responsiveness of myofilaments to Ca^{++}.

Coronary Collateral Circulation and Vasodilators

In the normal human heart, there are virtually no functional intercoronary channels. Abrupt occlusion of a coronary artery or one of its branches leads to ischemic necrosis and eventual fibrosis of the areas of myocardium supplied by the occluded vessel. However, if a coronary artery narrows slowly and progressively over a period of days or weeks, collateral vessels develop and may furnish sufficient blood to the ischemic myocardium to prevent or reduce the extent of necrosis. Collateral vessels may develop between

Myocardial stunning may be evident in patients who have suffered an acute coronary artery occlusion. If the patient is treated sufficiently early by coronary bypass surgery or balloon angioplasty and if adequate blood flow is restored to the ischemic region, the myocardial cells in this region may recover fully. However, for many days or even weeks, the contractility of the myocardium in the affected region may be grossly subnormal.

Prolonged reductions in coronary blood flow (myocardial ischemia) may critically and permanently impair the mechanical and electrical behavior of the heart. Diminished coronary blood flow as a consequence of coronary artery disease (usually coronary atherosclerosis) is one of the most common causes of serious cardiac disease. The ischemia may be global (affects an entire ventricle) or regional (affects some fraction of the ventricle). The impairment in mechanical contraction of the affected myocardium is produced not only by the diminished delivery of O_2 and metabolic substrates but also by the accumulation of potentially harmful substances (e.g., K^+, lactic acid, H^+) in the cardiac tissues. If the reduction in coronary flow to any region of the heart is sufficiently severe and prolonged, necrosis of the affected cardiac cells will result.

The term **myocardial hibernation** is used to describe the phenomenon in which cellular metabolism is down-regulated in cells whose function is impaired by inadequate delivery of O_2 and nutrients. Myocardial hibernation occurs mainly in patients with coronary artery disease, just as myocardial stunning does. The coronary blood flow in these patients is diminished persistently and significantly, and the mechanical function of the heart is impaired. If coronary blood flow is restored to normal by bypass surgery or angioplasty, mechanical function returns to normal.

Numerous surgical attempts have been made to enhance the development of coronary collateral vessels. However, the techniques used do not increase the collateral circulation over and above that produced by coronary artery narrowing alone. When discrete occlusions or severe narrowing occurs in coronary arteries, as in coronary atherosclerosis, the lesions can be bypassed with an artery or a vein graft. Frequently, the narrow segment can be dilated by inserting a balloon-tipped catheter into the diseased vessel via a peripheral artery and then inflating the balloon. Distention of the vessel by balloon inflation (angioplasty) can produce lasting dilation of a narrowed coronary artery (Fig. 17-38), particularly when a drug-eluting stent (the drugs help prevent restenosis) is inserted during angioplasty.

Many drugs are available for use in patients with coronary artery disease to relieve angina pectoris, the chest pain associated with myocardial ischemia. These compounds include organic nitrates/nitrites, Ca^{++} channel antagonists, and β-adrenoceptor antagonists. Organic nitrates and nitrites are metabolized to NO. NO dilates the great veins to reduce venous return (preload), thereby reducing cardiac work (see Chapter 19) and myocardial O_2 requirements. In addition, NO dilates the coronary arteries to increase collateral flow. Importantly, organic nitrates/nitrites do not interfere with coronary autoregulation. Calcium channel antagonists also cause vasodilation; none selectively dilates the coronary vessels. β-Adrenoceptor antagonists reduce the heart rate to indirectly increase coronary flow and oppose the reflex tachycardia seen with organic nitrates/nitrites.

In patients with marked narrowing of a coronary artery, administration of dipyridamole, a vasodilator, can fully dilate normal vessel branches that are parallel to the narrowed segment and thereby reduce the head of pressure to the partially occluded vessel. The reduced pressure to the narrowed vessel will further compromise blood flow to the ischemic myocardium. This phenomenon is known as coronary steal, and it occurs because dipyridamole acts by blocking the cellular uptake and metabolism of endogenous adenosine. Notably, dipyridamole interferes with coronary autoregulation.

branches of occluded and nonoccluded arteries. They originate from preexisting small vessels that undergo proliferative changes of the endothelium and smooth muscle. These changes may occur in response to wall stress and to chemical agents, including vascular endothelial growth factor (VEGF) released by the ischemic tissue.

CUTANEOUS CIRCULATION

The O_2 and nutrient requirements of the skin are relatively small. Unlike other body tissues, the supply of O_2 and nutrients is not the chief factor in the regulation of cutaneous blood flow. The primary function of the cutaneous circulation is to maintain a constant body temperature. Thus, the skin undergoes wide fluctuations in blood flow, depending on whether the body needs to lose or conserve heat. Changes in ambient and internal body temperature activate mechanisms responsible for alterations in skin blood flow.

REGULATION OF SKIN BLOOD FLOW

Neural Factors

The skin contains essentially two types of resistance vessels: arterioles and **arteriovenous anastomoses.** AV anastomoses shunt blood from the arterioles to the venules and venous plexuses; hence, they bypass the capillary bed. Such anastomoses are found in the fingertips, palms of the hands, toes, soles of the feet, ears, nose, and lips. AV anastomoses differ morphologically from arterioles; the anastomoses are either short, straight, or long coiled vessels, about 20 to 40 μm in luminal diameter, and they have thick

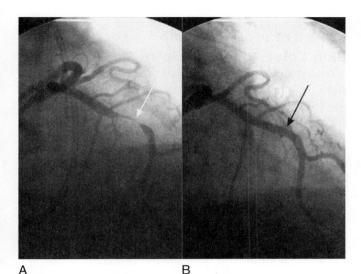

● **Figure 17-38.** **A,** Angiogram (intracoronary radiopaque dye) of a person with marked narrowing of the left anterior descending (LAD) branch of the left coronary artery (white arrow). **B,** The same segment of the coronary artery after angioplasty and insertion of a drug-eluting stent. (Courtesy Dr. Michael Azrin.)

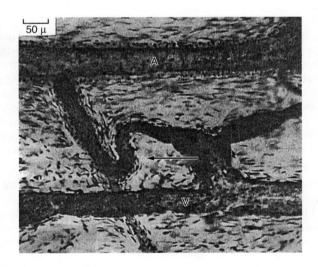

● **Figure 17-39.** AV anastomosis in the ear injected with Berlin blue. A, artery; V, vein; arrow points to an AV anastomosis. The walls of the AV anastomosis in the fingertips are thicker and more cellular. (From Pritchard MML, Daniel PM: J Anat 90:309, 1956.)

IN THE CLINIC

The fingers and toes of some individuals are very sensitive to cold. On exposure to cold, the arterioles to the fingers and toes constrict. The consequent ischemia results in localized blanching of the skin associated with tingling, numbness, and pain. The blanching is followed by cyanosis (a dark blue color of the skin) and later by redness as the arterial spasm subsides. The cause of this condition, called Raynaud's disease, is unknown.

thermore, AV anastomoses are not under metabolic control, and they do not show reactive hyperemia or autoregulation of blood flow. Thus, regulation of blood flow through these anastomotic channels is governed principally by the nervous system in response to reflex activation by temperature receptors or from higher centers of the central nervous system.

Most of the resistance vessels in the skin exhibit some basal tone and are under dual control of the sympathetic nervous system and local regulatory factors. However, neural control predominates. Stimulation of sympathetic nerve fibers induces vasoconstriction, and cutting the sympathetic nerves induces vasodilation. After chronic denervation of the cutaneous blood vessels, the degree of tone that existed before denervation is gradually regained over a period of several weeks. This restoration of tone is accomplished by an enhancement of basal tone. Denervation of the skin vessels results in enhanced sensitivity to catecholamines in circulation (**denervation hypersensitivity**).

Parasympathetic vasodilator nerve fibers do not innervate cutaneous blood vessels. However, stimulation of the sweat glands, which are innervated by sympathetic cholinergic fibers, dilates the skin resistance vessels. Sweat contains an enzyme that lyses a protein (kallidin) in the tissue fluid to produce bradykinin, a polypeptide with potent vasodilator properties. Bradykinin, formed locally, dilates the arterioles and increases blood flow to the skin.

Certain skin vessels, particularly those in the head, neck, shoulders, and upper part of the chest, are regulated by higher centers in the brain. Blushing, in response to embarrassment or anger, and blanching, in response to fear or anxiety, are examples of cerebral inhibition and stimulation, respectively, of the sympathetic nerve fibers to the affected cutaneous regions.

In contrast to AV anastomoses in the skin, the resistance vessels display autoregulation of blood flow and reactive hyperemia. If the arterial inflow to a limb is stopped by inflating a blood pressure cuff briefly, the skin becomes bright red below the point of vascular occlusion when the cuff is subsequently deflated. The increased cutaneous blood flow (reactive hyperemia) is also manifested by distention of the superficial veins in the affected extremity.

muscular walls richly supplied with nerve fibers (Fig. 17-39). These vessels are almost exclusively under sympathetic neural control, and they dilate maximally when their nerve supply is interrupted. Conversely, reflex stimulation of the sympathetic fibers to these vessels may constrict them and obliterate the vascular lumen. Although AV anastomoses do not exhibit basal tone, they are highly sensitive to vasoconstrictor agents such as epinephrine and norepinephrine. Fur-

The Role of Temperature in the Regulation of Skin Blood Flow

The primary function of the skin is to maintain a constant internal environment and protect the body from adverse changes. Ambient temperature is one of the most important external variables with which the body must contend. Exposure to cold elicits a generalized cutaneous vasoconstriction that is especially pronounced in the hands and feet. This response is chiefly mediated by the nervous system. Arrest of the circulation to a hand by a pressure cuff plus immersion of that hand in cold water induces vasoconstriction in the skin of the other extremities that are exposed to room temperature. When the circulation to the chilled hand is not occluded, the reflex generalized vasoconstriction is caused in part by the cooled blood that returns to the general circulation. This returned blood then stimulates the temperature-regulating center in the anterior hypothalamus, which also responds to direct application of cold to evoke cutaneous vasoconstriction.

The skin vessels of the cooled hand also respond directly to cold. Moderate cooling or a brief exposure to severe cold (0°C to 15°C) constricts the resistance and capacitance vessels, including the AV anastomoses. Prolonged exposure to severe cold evokes a secondary vasodilator response. Prompt vasoconstriction and severe pain are elicited by immersion of the hand in ice water. However, this response is soon followed by dilation of the skin vessels, with reddening of the immersed part and alleviation of the pain. With continued immersion of the hand, alternating periods of constriction and dilation occur, but the skin temperature rarely drops as much as it did in response to the initial vasoconstriction. Prolonged severe cold, of course, damages tissue. The rosy faces of people exposed to a cold environment are examples of cold vasodilation. However, blood flow through the skin of the face may be greatly reduced despite the flushed appearance. The red color of the slowly flowing blood is mainly caused by reduced O_2 uptake by the cold skin and the cold-induced shift of the oxyhemoglobin dissociation curve to the left (see Chapter 23).

Direct application of heat to the skin not only dilates the local resistance and capacitance vessels and AV anastomoses but also reflexly dilates blood vessels in other parts of the body. The local effect is independent of the vascular nerve supply, whereas the reflex vasodilation is a combined response to stimulation of the anterior hypothalamus by the returning warmed blood and stimulation of cutaneous heat receptors in the heated regions of the skin.

The close proximity of the major arteries and veins permits countercurrent heat exchange between them. Cold blood that flows in veins from a cooled hand toward the heart takes up heat from adjacent arteries; this warms the venous blood and cools the arterial blood. Heat exchange takes place in the opposite direction when the extremity is exposed to heat. Thus, heat conservation is enhanced during exposure of extremities to cold environments, and heat conservation is minimized during exposure of the extremities to warm environments.

Skin Color: Relationship to Skin Blood Volume, Oxyhemoglobin, and Blood Flow

Skin color is determined mainly by the pigment content. However, the degree of pallor or ruddiness is mainly a function of the amount of blood in the skin, except when the skin is very dark. With little blood in the venous plexus, the skin appears pale, whereas with moderate to large quantities of blood in the venous plexus, the skin displays a color. This color may be red, blue, or some shade between, depending on the degree of oxygenation of the blood. A combination of vasoconstriction and reduced hemoglobin can impart an ashen gray color to the skin. A combination of venous engorgement and reduced hemoglobin content can impart a dark purple hue.

Skin color provides little information about the rate of cutaneous blood flow. Rapid blood flow may be accompanied by pale skin when the AV anastomoses are open, and slow blood flow may be associated with red skin when the skin is exposed to cold.

SKELETAL MUSCLE CIRCULATION

The rate of blood flow in skeletal muscle varies directly with the contractile activity of the tissue and the type of muscle. Blood flow and capillary density in red muscle (slow twitch, high oxidative capacity) are greater than in white muscle (fast twitch, low oxidative capacity). In resting muscle, the precapillary arterioles contract and relax intermittently. Thus, at any given moment, most of the capillary bed is not perfused and total blood flow through quiescent skeletal muscle is low (1.4 to 4.5 mL/min/100 g). During exercise, the resistance vessels relax and muscle blood flow may increase to 15 to 20 times the resting level, depending on the intensity of the exercise.

Regulation of Skeletal Muscle Blood Flow

Neural and local factors regulate muscle circulation. Physical factors such as arterial pressure, tissue pressure, and blood viscosity influence muscle blood flow. However, another physical factor, the squeezing effect of the active skeletal muscle, affects blood flow in the vessels. With intermittent contractions, inflow is restricted, and as previously described, venous outflow is enhanced. The venous valves prevent backflow of blood between contractions and thereby aid in the forward propulsion of blood. With strong sustained contractions, as occurs during exercise, the vascular bed can be compressed to the point where blood flow actually ceases temporarily.

Neural Factors

The resistance vessels of muscle possess a high degree of basal tone; they also display tone in response to continuous low-frequency activity in the sympathetic vasoconstrictor nerve fibers. The basal firing frequency of sympathetic vasoconstrictor fibers is only about 1 to 2 per second, and maximal vasoconstriction occurs at frequencies of about 10 per second.

Vasoconstriction evoked by sympathetic nerve activity is caused by the local release of norepinephrine. Intraarterially injected norepinephrine elicits only vasoconstriction (α-adrenergic receptor). In contrast, low doses of epinephrine produce vasodilation (β-adrenergic receptor), whereas large doses cause vasoconstriction.

Baroreceptor reflexes greatly influence the tonic activity of the sympathetic nerves. An increase in carotid sinus pressure dilates the muscle vascular bed, whereas a decrease in carotid sinus pressure elicits vasoconstriction (Fig. 17-40). When sympathetic constrictor tone is high, the decrease in blood flow evoked by common carotid artery occlusion is small, but the increase in flow after the release of occlusion is large. The vasodilation produced by baroreceptor stimulation is caused by inhibition of sympathetic vasoconstrictor activity.

The resistance vessels in skeletal muscle contribute significantly to maintenance of arterial blood pressure because skeletal muscle constitutes a large fraction of the body's mass and hence the muscle vasculature constitutes the largest vascular bed. Participation of the skeletal muscle vessels in vascular reflexes is important in maintaining normal arterial blood pressure.

A comparison of the sympathetic neural effects on the blood vessels of muscle and skin is summarized in Figure 17-41. Note that the lower the basal tone of the skin vessels, the greater their constrictor response; also note the absence of active cutaneous vasodilation.

Local Factors

In active skeletal muscle, blood flow is regulated by metabolic factors. In resting muscle, neural factors predominate, and they superimpose neurogenic tone on basal tone (Fig. 17-41). Cutting the sympathetic nerves to muscle abolishes the neural component of

vascular tone, and it unmasks the intrinsic basal tone of the blood vessels. The neural and local mechanisms that regulate blood flow oppose each other, and during muscle contraction the local vasodilator mechanism supervenes. However, during exercise, strong sympathetic nerve stimulation slightly attenuates the vasodilation induced by locally released metabolites.

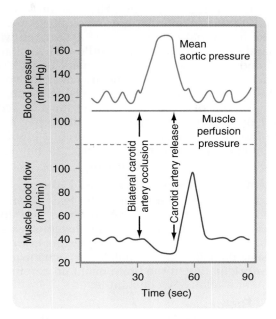

● **Figure 17-40.** Evidence for participation of the muscle vascular bed in vasoconstriction and vasodilation mediated by the carotid sinus baroreceptors after common carotid artery occlusion and release. In this preparation, the sciatic and femoral nerves constituted the only direct connection between the hind leg muscle mass and the rest of the dog. The muscle was perfused by blood at a constant pressure that was completely independent of the animal's arterial pressure. (Redrawn from Jones RD, Berne RM: Am J Physiol 204:461, 1963.)

● **Figure 17-41.** Basal tone and the range of response of resistance vessels in muscle *(dashed lines)* and skin *(shaded area)* to stimulation and section of sympathetic nerves. Peripheral resistance is plotted on a logarithmic scale. (Redrawn from Celander O, Folkow B: Acta Physiol Scand 29:241, 1953.)

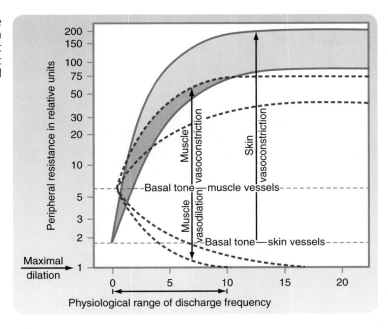

CEREBRAL CIRCULATION

Blood reaches the brain through the internal carotid and vertebral arteries. The vertebral arteries join to form the basilar artery, which in conjunction with branches of the internal carotid arteries, forms the circle of Willis.

A unique feature of the cerebral circulation is that it lies within a rigid structure, the cranium. Because the intracranial contents are incompressible, any increase in arterial inflow must be associated with a comparable increase in venous outflow. The volume of blood and extravascular fluid can vary considerably in most body tissues. In the brain, however, the volume of blood and extravascular fluid is relatively constant; a change in one of these fluid volumes must be accompanied by a reciprocal change in the other. Unlike most other organs, the rate of total cerebral blood flow is maintained within a narrow range; in humans, it averages 55 mL/min/100 g of brain.

Regulation of Cerebral Blood Flow

Of all body tissues, the brain is the least tolerant of ischemia. Interruption of cerebral blood flow for as little as 5 seconds leads to loss of consciousness, and ischemia lasting just a few minutes results in irreversible tissue damage. Local regulatory mechanisms and reflexes originating in the brain maintain cerebral circulation at a relatively constant level.

Neural Factors

The cerebral vessels are innervated by cervical sympathetic nerve fibers that accompany the internal carotid and vertebral arteries into the cranial cavity. The importance of neural regulation of the cerebral circulation is controversial. The sympathetic control of cerebral vessels appears to be weaker than that in other vascular beds, and the contractile state of cerebrovascular smooth muscle appears to depend mainly on local metabolic factors.

Local Factors

Generally, total cerebral blood flow is relatively constant. However, regional blood flow in the brain is associated with regional neural activity. For example, movement of one hand results in increased blood flow only in the hand area of the contralateral sensorimotor and premotor cortex. In addition, talking, reading, and other stimuli to the cerebral cortex are associated with increased blood flow in the appropriate regions of the contralateral cortex (Fig. 17-42). Glucose uptake also corresponds with regional cortical neuronal activity. Thus, when the retina is stimulated by light, uptake of glucose is enhanced in the visual cortex.

The cerebral vessels are very sensitive to CO_2 tension. Increases in arterial blood CO_2 tension (P_{CO_2})

> ### ▶ IN THE CLINIC
>
> Elevated intracranial pressure, as caused by a brain tumor, results in an increase in systemic blood pressure. This response, called Cushing's phenomenon, is apparently evoked by ischemic stimulation of vasomotor regions in the medulla. Cushing's phenomenon helps maintain cerebral blood flow in such conditions as expanding intracranial tumors.

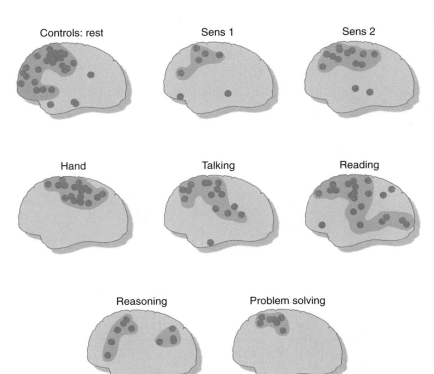

● **Figure 17-42.** Effects of different stimuli on regional blood flow in the contralateral human cerebral cortex. Sens 1, low-intensity electrical stimulation of the hand; Sens 2, high-intensity electrical stimulation of the hand (pain). (Redrawn from Ingvar DH: Brain Res 107:181, 1976.)

elicit marked cerebral vasodilation; inhalation of 7% CO_2 increases cerebral blood flow twofold. Conversely, decreases in P_{CO_2}, as caused by hyperventilation, diminish cerebral blood flow. CO_2 causes these changes by altering perivascular (and probably intracellular vascular smooth muscle) pH, which in turn alters arterial resistance to flow. By independently changing P_{CO_2} and the bicarbonate concentration, pial vessel (vessels of the pia mater) diameter and blood flow were shown to be inversely related to pH, regardless of the level of P_{CO_2}.

CO_2 can diffuse to vascular smooth muscle from brain tissue or from the lumen of the vessels, whereas H^+ in blood is prevented from reaching arteriolar smooth muscle by the blood-brain barrier. Hence, the cerebral vessels dilate when the $[H^+]$ of cerebrospinal fluid is increased, but these vessels dilate only minimally in response to an increase in the $[H^+]$ of arterial blood.

$[K^+]$ also affects cerebral blood flow. Hypoxia, electrical stimulation of the brain, and seizures elicit rapid increases in cerebral blood flow and in perivascular $[K^+]$. The increases in $[K^+]$ are similar in magnitude to those that produce pial arteriolar dilation when K^+ is applied topically to these vessels. However, the increase in $[K^+]$ is not sustained throughout the period of cerebral stimulation. Thus, only the initial increase in cerebral blood flow can be attributed to the release of K^+.

Adenosine affects cerebral blood flow. Adenosine levels in the brain increase in response to ischemia, hypoxemia, hypotension, hypocapnia, electrical stimulation of the brain, and induced seizures. Topically applied adenosine is a potent dilator of the pial arterioles. Any intervention that either reduces the O_2 supply to the brain or increases the O_2 requirements of the brain results in the rapid (within 5 seconds) formation of adenosine in cerebral tissue. Unlike the changes in pH or K^+, the adenosine concentration of the brain increases with initiation of the change in O_2 supply, and it remains elevated throughout the period of O_2 imbalance. The adenosine that is released into cerebrospinal fluid during cerebral ischemia becomes incorporated into adenine nucleotides in cerebral tissue. These local factors—pH, K^+, and adenosine—may all act in concert to adjust cerebral blood flow to the metabolic activity of the brain.

The cerebral circulation displays reactive hyperemia and excellent autoregulation when arterial blood pressure is between 60 and 160 mm Hg. Mean arterial pressures below 60 mm Hg result in reduced cerebral blood flow and then syncope, whereas mean pressures above 160 mm Hg may lead to increased permeability of the blood-brain barrier and consequently to cerebral edema. Hypercapnia or any other potent vasodilator abolishes autoregulation of cerebral blood flow. None of the candidates for metabolic regulation of cerebral blood flow account for this phenomenon. Hence, autoregulation of cerebral blood flow is probably mediated by a myogenic mechanism, but experimental proof is still lacking.

INTESTINAL CIRCULATION

Anatomy

The gastrointestinal tract is supplied by the celiac, superior mesenteric, and inferior mesenteric arteries. The superior mesenteric artery carries more than 10% of the cardiac output. Small mesenteric arteries form an extensive vascular network in the submucosa of the gastrointestinal tract (Fig. 17-43). The arterial branches penetrate the longitudinal and circular muscle layers of the tract, and they give rise to third- and fourth-order arterioles. Some third-order arterioles in the submucosa supply the tips of the villi.

The direction of blood flow in the capillaries and venules in a villus is opposite that in the main arteriole (Fig. 17-43). This arrangement is a countercurrent exchange system. Effective countercurrent exchange also permits diffusion of O_2 from arterioles to venules. At low blood flow rates, a substantial portion of the O_2 may be shunted from arterioles to venules near the base of the villus. This reduces the O_2 supply to the mucosal cells at the tip of the villus. When intestinal blood flow is very low, shunting of O_2 is so great that extensive necrosis of the intestinal villi takes place.

Neural Regulation

Neural control of the mesenteric circulation is almost exclusively sympathetic. Increased sympathetic activity, through α-adrenergic receptors, constricts the mesenteric arterioles and capacitance vessels. These receptors are prepotent in the mesenteric circulation. However, β-adrenergic receptors are also present, so the agonist isoproterenol causes vasodilation.

In response to aggressive behavior or to artificial stimulation of the hypothalamic "defense" area, pronounced vasoconstriction occurs in the mesenteric vascular bed. This vasoconstriction shifts blood flow from the less important intestinal circulation to the more crucial skeletal muscles, heart, and brain.

Autoregulation

Autoregulation of blood flow in the intestinal circulation is not as well developed as in other vascular beds. The principal mechanism responsible for autoregulation is metabolic, although a myogenic mechanism probably also participates (see Chapter 18). The adenosine concentration in mesenteric venous blood rises fourfold after brief arterial occlusion. It also rises during enhanced metabolic activity of the intestinal mucosa, such as during absorption of food. Adenosine, a potent vasodilator in the mesenteric vascular bed, may be the principal metabolic mediator of autoregulation. However, K^+ and altered osmolality may also contribute to autoregulation.

O_2 consumption of the small intestine is more rigorously controlled than blood flow. Experiments have shown that O_2 uptake of the small intestine remains constant when arterial perfusion pressure is varied between 30 and 125 mm Hg.

Functional Hyperemia

Food ingestion increases intestinal blood flow. Secretion of certain gastrointestinal hormones contributes

A

B

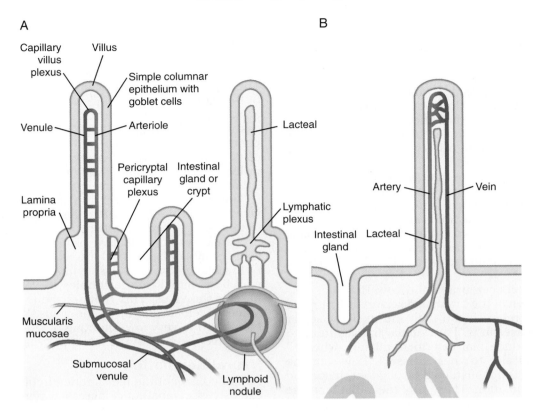

● **Figure 17-43.** Microcirculation pattern of the small intestine. **A,** Capillary plexuses arise from arterioles in the villus and also in the crypt. Blood leaves the crypt via venules that enter the portal circulation. **B,** Lymphatic vessels (lacteals) originate within the villus and eventually form a plexus at the base of the villus. (Redrawn from Kierszenbaum A: Histology and Cell Biology: An Introduction to Pathology. Philadelphia, Mosby, 2002.)

to this hyperemia. Gastrin and cholecystokinin augment intestinal blood flow, and they are secreted when food is ingested. Absorption of food also affects intestinal blood flow. Undigested food has no vasoactive influence, whereas several products of digestion are potent vasodilators. Among the various constituents of chyme, the principal mediators of mesenteric hyperemia are glucose and fatty acids.

HEPATIC CIRCULATION

Anatomy

Blood flow to the liver is normally about 25% of cardiac output. Hepatic blood flow is derived from two sources: the portal vein (about 75%) and the hepatic artery. Because portal venous blood has already passed through the gastrointestinal capillary bed, much of the O_2 of the portal vein blood flow has already been extracted. The hepatic artery delivers the remaining 25% of the blood, which is fully saturated with O_2. Hence, about three fourths of the O_2 used by the liver is derived from hepatic arterial blood.

The small branches of the portal vein and hepatic artery give rise to terminal portal venules and hepatic arterioles (Fig. 17-44). These terminal vessels enter the hepatic acinus (the functional unit of the liver) at its center. Blood flows from these terminal vessels into the sinusoids, which constitute the capillary network of the liver. The sinusoids radiate toward the periphery of the acinus, where they connect with the terminal hepatic venules. Blood from these terminal venules drains into progressively larger branches of the hepatic veins, which are tributaries of the inferior vena cava.

Hemodynamics

Mean blood pressure in the portal vein is about 10 mm Hg, and mean blood pressure in the hepatic artery is about 90 mm Hg. The resistance of the vessels upstream to the hepatic sinusoids is considerably greater than that of the downstream vessels. Consequently, the pressure in the sinusoids is only 2 or 3 mm Hg greater than that in the hepatic veins and inferior vena cava. The ratio of presinusoidal to postsinusoidal resistance in the liver is much greater than it is in almost any other vascular bed. Hence, drugs and other interventions that alter presinusoidal resistance usually affect pressure in the sinusoids and fluid exchange across the sinusoidal wall only slightly. However, changes in hepatic and central venous pressure are transmitted almost quantitatively to the hepatic sinusoids, and they profoundly affect the transsinusoidal exchange of fluids.

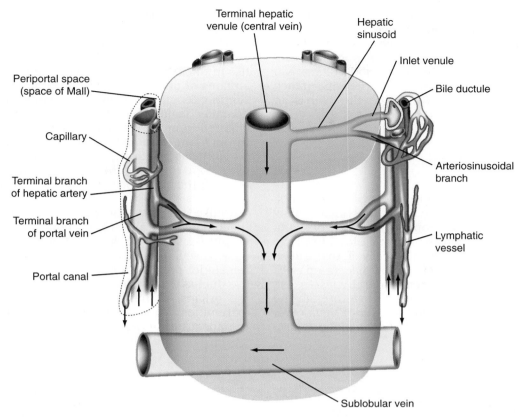

● **Figure 17-44.** Microcirculation of the hepatic acinus. Arrows indicate the direction of blood flow from the terminal portions of the hepatic artery and portal vein to the sinusoids. The mixture of arterial and venous blood flows into the central vein and then passes into the sublobular vein. (Redrawn from Ross MH, Pawling W: Histology: A Text and Atlas: with Correlated Cell and Molecular Biology. Philadelphia, Lippincott Williams & Wilkins, 2006.)

Regulation of Flow

Blood flow in the portal venous and hepatic arterial systems varies reciprocally. When blood flow is curtailed in one system, flow increases in the other but does not fully compensate for the decreased flow in the first system.

The portal venous system does not autoregulate. As portal venous pressure and flow are raised, resistance either remains constant or decreases. The hepatic arterial system does autoregulate, however, and adenosine may be involved in this adjustment of blood flow.

The liver tends to maintain constant O_2 consumption because O_2 extraction from hepatic blood is very efficient. As the rate of O_2 delivery to the liver varies, the liver compensates by an appropriate change in the fraction of O_2 extracted from blood. Such extraction is facilitated by the distance between the presinusoidal vessels at the acinar center and the postsinusoidal vessels at the periphery of the acinus (Fig. 17-44). The substantial distance between these types of vessels prevents countercurrent exchange of O_2, contrary to the countercurrent exchange that occurs in an intestinal villus.

The sympathetic nerves constrict the presinusoidal resistance vessels in the portal venous and hepatic

IN THE CLINIC

When central venous pressure is elevated, as in congestive heart failure, large volumes of plasma water transude from the liver into the peritoneal cavity; this accumulation of fluid in the abdomen is known as **ascites.** Extensive fibrosis of the liver, as in hepatic cirrhosis, markedly increases hepatic vascular resistance and thereby raises pressure substantially in the portal venous system. The consequent increase in capillary hydrostatic pressure through the splanchnic circulation also leads to extensive fluid transudation into the abdominal cavity. The pressure may likewise rise substantially in other veins that anastomose with the portal vein. For example, the esophageal veins may enlarge considerably to form esophageal varices. These varices may rupture and lead to severe, frequently fatal internal bleeding. To prevent these grave problems associated with elevated portal venous pressure in cirrhosis of the liver, an anastomosis (portacaval shunt) is often inserted surgically between the portal vein and inferior vena cava to lower portal venous pressure.

arterial systems. Neural effects on the capacitance vessels are more important, however. The liver contains about 15% of the total blood volume of the body. Under appropriate conditions, as in response to hemorrhage, about half of the hepatic blood volume can be rapidly expelled by constriction of the capacitance vessels (see also Chapter 19). Hence, the liver is an important blood reservoir in humans.

FETAL CIRCULATION

In Utero

Fetal circulation differs from that of postnatal infants. Most importantly, the fetal lungs are functionally inactive, and the fetus depends completely on the placenta for O_2 and nutrients. Oxygenated fetal blood from the placenta passes through the umbilical vein to the liver. Approximately half the flow from the placenta passes through the liver, and the remainder bypasses the liver and reaches the inferior vena cava through the **ductus venosus** (Fig. 17-45). In the inferior vena cava, blood from the ductus venosus joins the blood return-

ing from the lower part of the trunk and the extremities. This combined stream in turn merges with blood from the liver through the hepatic veins.

The streams of blood tend to maintain their identities in the inferior vena cava and are divided into two streams of unequal size by the edge of the interatrial septum (crista dividens). The larger stream, which contains mainly blood from the umbilical vein, is shunted from the inferior vena cava to the left atrium through the **foramen ovale** (Fig. 17-45). The other stream passes into the right atrium, where it merges with blood returning from the upper parts of the body through the superior vena cava and with blood from the myocardium.

Unlike in adults, the ventricles in a fetus operate essentially in parallel. Only a tenth of right ventricular output passes through the lungs because the pulmonary vascular resistance of the fetus is high. The remainder passes from the pulmonary artery through the **ductus arteriosus** to the aorta at a point distal to the origins of the arteries to the head and upper extremities. Blood flows from the pulmonary artery to the aorta because pulmonary vascular resistance is

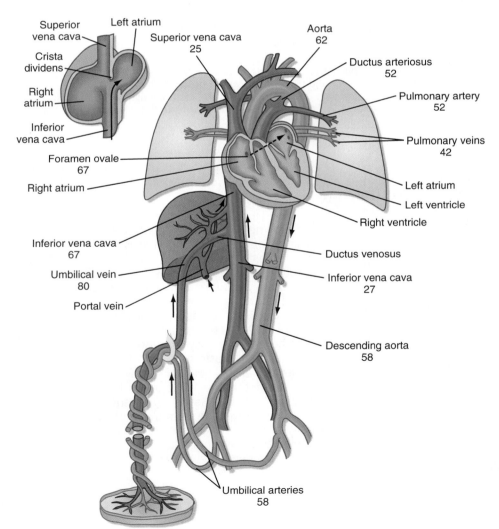

● Figure 17-45. Schematic diagram of the fetal circulation. The numbers represent the percent O_2 saturation of the blood flowing in the indicated blood vessel. Fetal blood that leaves the placenta is 80% saturated, but the saturation of the blood that passes through the foramen ovale is reduced to 67%. This reduction in O_2 saturation is caused by mixing with desaturated blood returning from the lower part of the body and the liver. Addition of the desaturated blood from the lungs reduces the O_2 saturation of left ventricular blood to 62%, which is the level of saturation of the blood reaching the head and upper extremities. The blood in the right ventricle, which is a mixture of desaturated superior vena caval blood, coronary venous blood, and inferior vena caval blood, is only 52% saturated with O_2. When the major portion of this blood traverses the ductus arteriosus and joins that pumped by the left ventricle, the resulting O_2 saturation of the blood traveling to the lower part of the body and back to the placenta is 58%. The inset at upper left illustrates the direction of flow of a major portion of the inferior vena caval blood through the foramen ovale to the left atrium. (Data from Dawes GS et al: J Physiol 126:563, 1954.)

Figure labels:
Superior vena cava
Left atrium
Crista dividens
Right atrium
Inferior vena cava
Superior vena cava 25
Aorta 62
Ductus arteriosus 52
Pulmonary artery 52
Pulmonary veins 42
Foramen ovale 67
Right atrium
Left atrium
Left ventricle
Right ventricle
Inferior vena cava 67
Umbilical vein 80
Portal vein
Ductus venosus
Inferior vena cava 27
Descending aorta 58
Umbilical arteries 58

high and the diameter of the ductus arteriosus is as large as that of the descending aorta.

The large volume of blood that passes through the foramen ovale into the left atrium is joined by blood returning from the lungs, and it is pumped out by the left ventricle into the aorta. Most of the blood in the ascending aorta goes to the head, upper thorax, and arms; the remainder joins blood from the ductus arteriosus and supplies the rest of the body. The amount of blood pumped by the left ventricle is about half that pumped by the right ventricle. The major fraction of the blood that passes down the descending aorta comes from the ductus arteriosus and right ventricle and flows by way of the two umbilical arteries to the placenta.

O_2 saturation of blood occurs at various loci (Fig. 17-45). Thus, the tissues that receive the most highly saturated blood are the liver, heart, and upper parts of the body, including the head.

At the placenta, the chorionic villi dip into the maternal sinuses, and O_2, CO_2, nutrients, and metabolic waste products are exchanged across the membranes. The barrier to exchange prevents equilibration of O_2 between the two circulations at normal rates of blood flow. Therefore, the PO_2 of the fetal blood that leaves the placenta is very low. Were it not for the fact that fetal hemoglobin has a greater affinity for O_2 than adult hemoglobin does, the fetus would not receive an adequate O_2 supply. The fetal oxyhemoglobin dissociation curve is shifted to the left. Therefore, at equal pressures of O_2, fetal blood carries significantly more O_2 than maternal blood does.

In early fetal life, the high glycogen levels that prevail in cardiac myocytes may protect the heart from acute periods of hypoxia. Glycogen levels decrease in late fetal life, and they reach adult levels by term.

Circulatory Changes That Occur at Birth

The umbilical vessels have thick muscular walls that react to trauma, tension, sympathomimetic amines, bradykinin, angiotensin, and changes in PO_2. In animals in which the umbilical cord is not tied, hemorrhage of the newborn is minimized by constriction of these large umbilical vessels in response to the stimuli cited earlier.

Closure of the umbilical vessels increases TPR and the arterial blood pressure of the infant. When blood flow through the umbilical vein ceases, the ductus venosus, a thick-walled vessel with a muscular sphincter, closes. The factor that initiates closure of the ductus venosus is unknown.

Immediately after birth, the asphyxia caused by constriction or clamping of the umbilical vessels, together with cooling of the body, activates the respiratory center of the newborn infant. As the lungs fill with air, pulmonary vascular resistance decreases to about 10% of the value that existed before lung expansion. This change in vascular resistance is not caused by the presence of O_2 in the lungs because the change is just as great if the lungs are filled with N_2. However, filling the lungs with liquid does not reduce pulmonary vascular resistance.

After birth, left atrial pressure is raised above that in the inferior vena cava and right atrium by (1) the decrease in pulmonary resistance, with the consequent large flow of blood through the lungs to the left atrium; (2) the reduction of flow to the right atrium caused by occlusion of the umbilical vein; and (3) the increased resistance to left ventricular output produced by occlusion of the umbilical arteries. Reversal of the pressure gradient across the atria abruptly closes the valve over the foramen ovale, and the septal leaflets fuse over a period of several days.

The decrease in pulmonary vascular resistance causes the pressure in the pulmonary artery to fall to about half its previous level (to about 35 mm Hg). This change in pressure, coupled with a slight increase in aortic pressure, reverses the flow of blood through the ductus arteriosus. However, within several minutes, the large ductus arteriosus begins to constrict. This constriction produces turbulent flow, which is manifested as a murmur in newborn infants. Constriction of the ductus arteriosus is progressive and usually complete within 1 to 2 days after birth. Closure of the ductus arteriosus appears to be initiated by the high PO_2 of the arterial blood passing through it; pulmonary ventilation with O_2 closes the ductus, whereas ventilation with air low in O_2 opens this shunt vessel. Whether O_2 acts directly on the ductus or through the release of a vasoconstrictor substance is not known.

At birth, the walls of the two ventricles are about equal in thickness. In addition, the muscle layer of the pulmonary arterioles is thick; this thickness is partly responsible for the high pulmonary vascular resistance of the fetus. After birth, the thickness of the walls of the right ventricle diminishes, as does the muscle layer of the pulmonary arterioles. In contrast, the left ventricular walls become thicker. These changes progress over a period of weeks after birth.

If a pregnant woman is subjected to hypoxia, the reduced blood PO_2 in the fetus evokes tachycardia and an increase in blood flow through the umbilical vessels. If the hypoxia persists or if flow through the umbilical vessels is impaired, fetal distress occurs and is manifested initially as bradycardia.

The ductus arteriosus occasionally fails to close after birth. In the newborn, this congenital cardiovascular abnormality, called **patent ductus arteriosus,** can sometimes be corrected by the administration of nonsteroidal antiinflammatory agents such as ibuprofen. If this does not result in closure of the ductus or if the child is older, closure must be achieved surgically.

■ KEY CONCEPTS

1. The vascular system is composed of two major subdivisions: the systemic circulation and the pulmonary circulation. These subdivisions are in series with each other and are composed of a number of vessel types (e.g., arteries, arterioles, capillaries) that are aligned in series with one another. In general, the vessels of a given type are arranged in parallel with each other.

2. The mean velocity (v) of blood flow in a given type of vessel is directly proportional to the total blood flow being pumped by the heart, and it is inversely proportional to the cross-sectional area of all the parallel vessels of that type.

3. Poiseuille's law describes blood flow that is steady and laminar in vessels larger than arterioles. However, blood flow is non-newtonian in very small blood vessels (i.e., Poiseuille's law is not applicable).

4. Flow tends to become turbulent when (1) flow velocity is high, (2) fluid viscosity is low, (3) fluid density is great, (4) tube diameter is large, or (5) the wall of the vessel is irregular.

5. Arteries not only conduct blood from the heart to the capillaries but also store some of the ejected blood during each cardiac systole. Hence, blood flow continues through the capillaries during cardiac diastole. Veins return blood to the heart from the capillaries and have a relatively low resistance and high capacitance that serves as a reservoir for blood.

6. The aging process diminishes compliance of the arteries, as well as the veins. The less compliant the arteries, the more work the heart must do to pump a given cardiac output. The less compliant the veins, the less their ability to store blood.

7. Mean arterial pressure varies directly with cardiac output and total peripheral resistance. Arterial pulse pressure varies directly with stroke volume but inversely with arterial compliance.

8. Blood flow through capillaries is chiefly regulated by contraction of arterioles (resistance vessels). The capillary endothelium is the source of NO and PGI_2, which relax vascular smooth muscles.

9. Water and small solutes move between the vascular and interstitial fluid compartments through capillary pores mainly by diffusion, but also by filtration and absorption. Molecules larger than about 60 kDa are essentially confined to the vascular compartment. Lipid-soluble substances, such as CO_2 and O_2, pass directly through the lipid membranes of the capillary; the rate of transfer is directly proportional to their lipid solubility. Large molecules can move across the capillary wall in vesicles by pinocytosis. The vesicles are formed from the lipid membrane of the capillaries.

10. Capillary filtration and absorption are described by the Starling equation:

$$\text{Fluid movement} = k[(P_c + \pi_i) - (P_i + \pi_p)]$$

Filtration occurs when the algebraic sum of these terms is positive; absorption occurs when it is negative.

11. Fluid and protein that have escaped from blood capillaries enter lymphatic capillaries and are transported via the lymphatic system back to the blood vascular compartment.

12. Physical factors that influence coronary blood flow are the viscosity of the blood, frictional resistance of the vessel walls, aortic pressure, and extravascular compression of the vessels within the walls of the left ventricle. Left coronary blood flow is restricted during ventricular systole by extravascular compression, and the flow is greatest during diastole when the intramyocardial vessels are not compressed. Neural regulation of coronary blood flow is much less important than metabolic regulation. Activation of the cardiac sympathetic nerves constricts the coronary resistance vessels. However, the enhanced myocardial metabolism caused by the associated increase in heart rate and contractile force produces vasodilation, which overrides the direct constrictor effect of sympathetic nerve stimulation. Stimulation of the cardiac branches of the vagus nerves slightly dilates the coronary arterioles. A striking parallelism exists between metabolic activity of the heart and coronary blood flow. A decrease in O_2 supply or an increase in O_2 demand apparently releases vasodilators that decrease coronary resistance. Of the known factors (CO_2, O_2, H^+, K^+, adenosine) that can mediate this response, K_{ATP} channels, NO, and adenosine appear to be the most likely candidates, although CO_2, O_2, and H^+ cannot be excluded.

13. Most of the resistance vessels in the skin are under dual control of the sympathetic nervous system and local vasodilator metabolites. The AV anastomoses found in the hands, feet, and face, however, are solely under neural control. The main function of skin blood vessels is to aid in the regulation of body temperature by constricting to conserve heat and by dilating to lose heat. Skin blood vessels dilate directly and reflexly in response to heat, and they constrict directly and reflexly in response to cold.

14. Skeletal muscle blood flow is regulated centrally by the sympathetic nerves and locally by the release of vasodilator metabolites. In subjects at rest, neural regulation of blood flow is paramount, but it yields to metabolic regulation during muscle contractions (such as during exercise).

15. Cerebral blood flow is predominantly regulated by metabolic factors, especially CO_2, K^+, and adenosine. The increased regional cerebral activity

produced by stimuli such as touch, pain, hand motion, talking, reading, reasoning, and problem solving are associated with enhanced blood flow in the activated area of the contralateral cerebral cortex.

16. The microcirculation in intestinal villi constitutes a countercurrent exchange system for O_2. The presence of this countercurrent exchange system places the villi in jeopardy in states of low blood flow. The splanchnic resistance and capacitance vessels are very responsive to changes in sympathetic neural activity.

17. The liver receives about 25% of cardiac output; about three fourths of this output is from the portal vein and about a fourth from the hepatic artery. When flow is diminished in either the portal or hepatic system, flow in the other system usually increases, but not proportionately. The liver tends to maintain constant O_2 consumption, in part because its mechanism for extracting O_2 from blood is so efficient. The liver normally contains about 15% of the total blood volume. It serves as an important blood reservoir for the body.

18. In the fetus, a large percentage of right atrial blood passes through the foramen ovale to the left atrium, and a large percentage of pulmonary arterial blood passes through the ductus arteriosus to the aorta. At birth, the umbilical vessels, ductus venosus, and ductus arteriosus close by contraction of their muscle layers. The reduction in pulmonary vascular resistance caused by lung inflation is the main factor that reverses the pressure gradient between the atria and thereby closes the foramen ovale.

CHAPTER 18

Regulation of the Heart and Vasculature

REGULATION OF HEART RATE AND CONTRACTILITY

Cardiac output is defined as the quantity of blood pumped by the heart each minute. Cardiac output may be varied by changing the **heart rate** or the volume of blood ejected from either ventricle with each heartbeat; this volume is called the **stroke volume.** Mathematically, cardiac output (CO) can be expressed as the product of heart rate (HR) and stroke volume (SV):

● **Equation 18-1**

$$CO = HR \times SV$$

Thus, understanding how cardiac activity is controlled can be gained by considering how the heart rate and stroke volume are regulated. Heart rate is regulated by the activity of the cardiac pacemaker, and stroke volume is directly related to myocardial performance. These two determinants are interdependent because a change in one determinant of cardiac output almost invariably alters the other determinant.

NERVOUS CONTROL OF THE HEART RATE

Although certain local factors, such as temperature changes and stretching of tissue, can affect the heart rate, the autonomic nervous system is the principal means by which the heart rate is controlled.

The average resting heart rate is about 70 beats/min in normal adults, and it is significantly greater in children. During sleep the heart rate decelerates by 10 to 20 beats/min, and during emotional excitement or muscular activity it may accelerate to rates well above 100. In well-trained athletes the resting rate is usually only about 50 beats/min.

Both divisions of the autonomic nervous system tonically influence the cardiac pacemaker, which is normally the sinoatrial (SA) node. The sympathetic system enhances automaticity, whereas the parasympathetic system inhibits it. Changes in heart rate usually involve a reciprocal action of these two divisions of the autonomic nervous system. Thus, the heart rate ordinarily increases with a combined decrease in parasympathetic activity and increase in sympathetic activity; the heart rate decreases with the opposite changes in autonomic neural activity.

Parasympathetic tone usually predominates in healthy, resting individuals. When a resting individual is given atropine, a muscarinic receptor antagonist that blocks parasympathetic effects, the heart rate generally increases substantially. If a resting individual is given propranolol, a β-adrenergic receptor antagonist that blocks sympathetic effects, the heart rate usually decreases only slightly (Fig. 18-1). When both divisions of the autonomic nervous system are blocked, the heart rate of young adults averages about 100 beats/min. The rate that prevails after complete autonomic blockade is called the **intrinsic heart rate.**

Parasympathetic Pathways

The cardiac parasympathetic fibers originate in the medulla oblongata, in cells that lie in the dorsal motor nucleus of the vagus or in the nucleus ambiguus (see Chapter 11). The precise location of the parasympathetic fibers varies among species. In humans, centrifugal vagal fibers pass inferiorly through the neck near the common carotid arteries and then through the mediastinum to synapse with postganglionic vagal cells. These cells are located either on the epicardial surface or within the walls of the heart. Most of the vagal ganglion cells are located in epicardial fat pads near the SA and atrioventicular (AV) nodes.

The right and left vagi are distributed to different cardiac structures. The right vagus nerve affects the SA node predominantly; stimulation of this nerve slows SA nodal firing and can even stop the firing for several seconds. The left vagus nerve mainly inhibits AV conduction tissue to produce various degrees of AV block (see Chapter 16). However, the distribution of the efferent vagal fibers is overlapping such that left vagal stimulation also depresses the SA node and right vagal stimulation impedes AV conduction.

The SA and AV nodes are rich in cholinesterase, an enzyme that rapidly hydrolyzes the neurotransmitter acetylcholine (ACh). The effects of a given vagal stimulus decay very quickly (Fig. 18-2, *A*) when vagal stimulation is discontinued because ACh is rapidly destroyed. In addition, vagal effects on SA and AV nodal function have a very short latency ($\approx$50 to 100 msec) because the ACh released quickly activates special ACh-regulated K$^+$ channels (K_{ACh}) in the cardiac cells. These channels open quickly because the muscarinic receptor is coupled directly to the K_{ACh} channel by a guanine nucleotide–binding protein (G_i). These two features of the vagus nerves—brief latency and rapid decay of the response—permit them to exert beat-by-beat control of SA and AV nodal function.

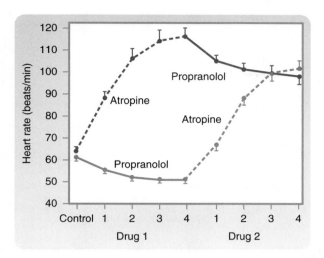

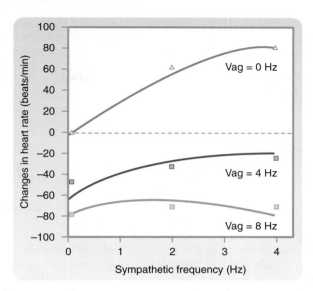

● **Figure 18-1.** Effects of four equal doses of atropine (muscarinic receptor antagonist that blocks parasympathetic effects) and propranolol (β-adrenergic receptor antagonist that blocks sympathetic effects) on the heart rate of 10 healthy young men. In half of the trials, atropine was given first *(top curve);* in the other half, propranolol was given first *(bottom curve).* (Redrawn from Katona PG et al: J Appl Physiol 52:1652, 1982.)

● **Figure 18-3.** Changes in heart rate when the vagus and cardiac sympathetic nerves are stimulated simultaneously. The sympathetic nerves are stimulated at 0, 2, and 4 Hz and the vagus nerves at 0, 4, and 8 Hz. (Modified from Levy MN, Zieske H: J Appl Physiol 27:465, 1969.)

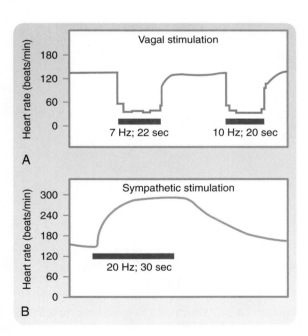

● **Figure 18-2.** Changes in heart rate evoked by stimulation *(horizontal bars)* of the vagus **(A)** and sympathetic nerves **(B).** (Modified from Warner HR, Cox A: J Appl Physiol 17:349, 1962.)

Parasympathetic influences usually predominate over sympathetic effects at the SA node, as shown in Figure 18-3. When the frequency of sympathetic stimulation increases from 0 to 4 Hz, the heart rate increases by about 80 beats/min in the absence of vagal stimulation (Vag = 0 Hz). However, when the vagi are stimulated at 8 Hz, increasing the sympathetic stimulation

frequency from 0 to 4 Hz has only a negligible influence on heart rate.

Sympathetic Pathways

The cardiac sympathetic fibers originate in the intermediolateral columns of the upper five or six thoracic and lower one or two cervical segments of the spinal cord (see Chapter 11). These fibers emerge from the spinal column through the white communicating branches and enter the paravertebral chains of ganglia. The preganglionic and postganglionic neurons synapse mainly in the stellate or middle cervical ganglia, depending on the species. In the mediastinum, the postganglionic and preganglionic parasympathetic fibers join to form a complicated plexus of mixed efferent nerves to the heart.

The postganglionic cardiac sympathetic fibers in this plexus approach the base of the heart along the adventitial surface of the great vessels. From the base of the heart, these fibers are distributed to the various chambers as an extensive epicardial plexus. They then penetrate the myocardium, usually accompanying the coronary vessels.

In contrast to abrupt termination of the response after vagal activity, the effects of sympathetic stimulation decay gradually after stimulation is stopped (Fig. 18-2, *B*). Nerve terminals take up to 70% of the norepinephrine released during sympathetic stimulation; much of the remainder is carried away by the bloodstream. These processes are slow. Furthermore, the facilitatory effects of sympathetic stimulation on the heart attain steady-state values much more slowly than do the inhibitory effects of vagal stimulation. The onset of the cardiac response to sympathetic stimulation begins slowly for two main reasons. First, norepinephrine appears to be released slowly from the sympathetic nerve terminals. Second, the cardiac effects of the neurally released norepinephrine are mediated mainly by a relatively slow second messenger system involving cAMP (see Chapter 3). Hence, sympathetic activity alters the heart rate and AV conduction much more slowly than vagal activity does. Although vagal activity can exert beat-by-beat control of cardiac function, sympathetic activity cannot.

Control by Higher Centers

Stimulation of various brain regions can have significant effects on cardiac rate, rhythm, and contractility (see Chapter 11). In the cerebral cortex, centers that regulate cardiac function are located in the anterior half of the brain, principally in the frontal lobe, the orbital cortex, the motor and premotor cortex, the anterior portion of the temporal lobe, the insula, and the cingulate gyrus. Stimulation of the midline, ventral, and medial nuclei of the thalamus elicits tachycardia. Stimulation of the posterior and posterolateral regions of the hypothalamus can also change the heart rate. Stimuli applied to the H2 fields of Forel in the diencephalon evoke various cardiovascular responses, including tachycardia; these changes resemble those observed during muscular exercise. Undoubtedly, the cortical and diencephalic centers initiate the cardiac reactions that occur during excitement, anxiety, and other emotional states. The hypothalamic centers also initiate the cardiac response to alterations in environmental temperature. Experimentally induced temperature changes in the preoptic anterior hypothalamus alter the heart rate and peripheral resistance.

Stimulation of the parahypoglossal area of the medulla reciprocally activates cardiac sympathetic pathways and inhibits cardiac parasympathetic pathways. In certain dorsal regions of the medulla, distinct cardiac accelerator (increase the heart rate) and augmentor (increase cardiac contractility) sites have been detected in animals with transected vagi. The accelerator regions are more abundant on the right side, whereas the augmentor sites are more prevalent on the left. A similar distribution also exists in the hypothalamus. Therefore, the sympathetic fibers mainly descend ipsilaterally through the brainstem.

Baroreceptor Reflex

Sudden changes in arterial blood pressure initiate a reflex that evokes an inverse change in heart rate (Fig. 18-4). Baroreceptors located in the aortic arch and carotid sinuses are responsible for this reflex. The inverse relationship between heart rate and arterial blood pressure is generally most pronounced over an intermediate range of arterial blood pressure. Below this intermediate range, the heart rate maintains a constant, high value; above this pressure range, the heart rate maintains a constant, low value.

The effects of these changes in carotid sinus pressure on activity in the cardiac autonomic nerves are presented in Figure 18-5, which shows that over an intermediate range of carotid sinus pressure (100 to 180 mm Hg), reciprocal changes are evoked in efferent vagal and sympathetic neural activity. Below this range

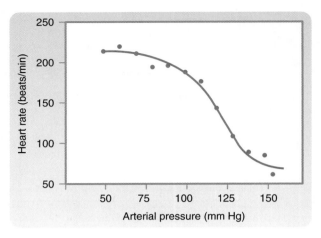

● **Figure 18-4.** Heart rate as a function of mean arterial pressure.

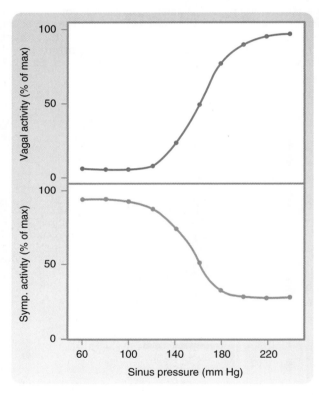

● **Figure 18-5.** Effects of changes in pressure in isolated carotid sinuses on neural activity in cardiac vagal and sympathetic efferent nerve fibers. (Adapted from Kollai M, Koizumi K: Pflügers Arch 413:365, 1989.)

of carotid sinus pressure, sympathetic activity is intense and vagal activity is virtually absent. Conversely, above the intermediate range of carotid sinus pressure, vagal activity is intense and sympathetic activity is minimal.

Bainbridge Reflex, Atrial Receptors, and Atrial Natriuretic Peptide

In 1915, Bainbridge reported that infusing blood or saline into dogs accelerated their heart rate. This

● Figure 18-6. Intravenous infusions of blood or electrolyte solutions tend to increase the heart rate via the Bainbridge reflex and to decrease the heart rate via the baroreceptor reflex. The actual change in heart rate induced by such infusions is the result of these two opposing effects.

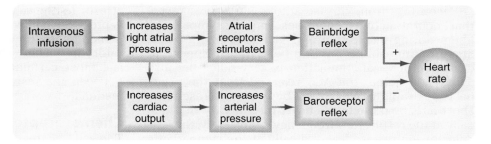

increase did not seem to be tied to arterial blood pressure because the heart rate rose regardless of whether arterial blood pressure did or did not change. However, Bainbridge also noted that the heart rate increased whenever central venous pressure rose sufficiently to distend the right side of the heart. Bilateral transection of the vagi abolished this response. This is termed the **Bainbridge reflex.**

Many investigators have confirmed Bainbridge's observations and have noted that the magnitude and direction of the response depend on the prevailing heart rate. When the heart rate is slow, intravenous infusions usually accelerate the heart. At more rapid heart rates, however, infusions ordinarily slow the heart. What accounts for these different responses? Increases in blood volume not only evoke the so-called Bainbridge reflex but also activate other reflexes (notably the baroreceptor reflex). These other reflexes tend to elicit opposite changes in heart rate. Therefore, changes in heart rate evoked by an alteration in blood volume are the result of these antagonistic reflex effects (Fig. 18-6). Evidently, the Bainbridge reflex predominates over the baroreceptor reflex when blood volume rises, but the baroreceptor reflex prevails over the Bainbridge reflex when blood volume diminishes.

Both atria have receptors that are affected by changes in blood volume and that influence the heart rate. These receptors are located principally in the venoatrial junctions: in the right atrium at its junctions with the venae cavae and in the left atrium at its junctions with the pulmonary veins. Distention of these atrial receptors sends afferent impulses to the brainstem in the vagi. The efferent impulses are carried from the brainstem to the SA node by fibers from both autonomic divisions.

The cardiac response to these changes in autonomic neural activity is highly selective. Even when the reflex increase in heart rate is large, changes in ventricular contractility are generally negligible. Furthermore, the neurally induced increase in heart rate is not usually accompanied by an increase in sympathetic activity in the peripheral arterioles.

Stimulation of the atrial receptors increases not only the heart rate but also urine volume. Reduced activity in the renal sympathetic nerve fibers may partially account for this diuresis. However, the principal mechanism appears to be a neurally mediated reduction in **vasopressin (antidiuretic hormone)** secretion by the posterior pituitary gland (see Chapters 34 and 40). Stretch of the atrial walls also releases **atrial natri-**

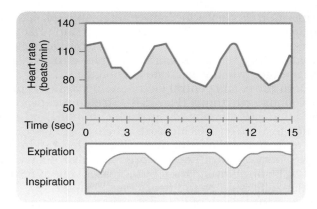

● Figure 18-7. Respiratory sinus arrhythmia. Note that the heart rate increases during inspiration and decreases during expiration (Modified from Warner MR et al. Am J Physiol 251: H1134, 1986).

> ### ▶ IN THE CLINIC
>
> In congestive heart failure, NaCl and water are retained, mainly because stimulation by the renin-angiotensin system increases the release of aldosterone from the adrenal cortex. The plasma level of ANP is also increased in congestive heart failure. By enhancing the renal excretion of NaCl and water, this peptide gradually reduces fluid retention and the consequent elevations in central venous pressure and cardiac preload.

uretic peptide (ANP) from the atria.* ANP, a 28–amino acid peptide, exerts potent diuretic and natriuretic effects on the kidneys (see also Chapter 34) and vasodilator effects on the resistance and capacitance vessels. Thus, ANP is an important regulator of blood volume and blood pressure.

Respiratory Sinus Arrhythmia

Rhythmic variations in heart rate, occurring at the frequency of respiration, are detectable in most individuals and tend to be more pronounced in children. The heart rate typically accelerates during inspiration and decelerates during expiration (Fig. 18-7).

---

*The myocytes of the ventricles secrete a related peptide in response to stretch. This peptide, termed **brain natriuretic peptide (BNP)** because of its initial discovery in the central nervous system, has actions similar to those of ANP (see Chapter 34).

Recordings from cardiac autonomic nerves reveal that neural activity increases in the sympathetic fibers during inspiration and increases in the vagal fibers during expiration. The heart rate response to cessation of vagal stimulation is very quick because as already noted, the ACh released from the vagus nerves is rapidly hydrolyzed by cholinesterase. This short latency permits the heart rate to vary rhythmically at the respiratory frequency. Conversely, the norepinephrine released periodically at the sympathetic endings is removed very slowly. Therefore, the rhythmic variations in sympathetic activity that accompany inspiration do not induce any appreciable oscillatory changes in heart rate. Thus, respiratory sinus arrhythmia is almost entirely brought about by changes in vagal activity. In fact, respiratory sinus arrhythmia is exaggerated when vagal tone is enhanced.

Both reflex and central factors help initiate respiratory sinus arrhythmia (Fig. 18-8). Stretch receptors in the lungs are stimulated during inspiration, and this action leads to a reflex increase in heart rate. The afferent and efferent limbs of this reflex are located in the vagus nerves. Intrathoracic pressure also decreases during inspiration and thereby increases venous return to the right side of the heart (see Chapter 19). The consequent stretch of the right atrium elicits the Bainbridge reflex. After the time delay required for the increased venous return to reach the left side of the heart, left ventricular output increases and raises arterial blood pressure. This rise in blood pressure in turn reduces the heart rate through the baroreceptor reflex.

Central factors are also responsible for respiratory cardiac arrhythmia. The respiratory center in the medulla directly influences the cardiac autonomic centers (Fig. 18-8). In heart-lung bypass experiments, the chest is open, the lungs are collapsed, venous return is diverted to a pump-oxygenator, and arterial blood pressure is maintained at a constant level. In such experiments, rhythmic movement of the rib cage attests to the activity of the medullary respiratory centers. Such movement of the rib cage is often accompanied by rhythmic changes in heart rate at the respiratory frequency. This respiratory cardiac arrhythmia is almost certainly induced by a direct interaction between the respiratory and cardiac centers in the medulla.

Chemoreceptor Reflex

The cardiac response to peripheral chemoreceptor stimulation illustrates the complex interactions that may ensue when one stimulus excites two organ systems simultaneously. In intact animals, stimulation of the carotid chemoreceptors consistently increases ventilatory rate and depth (see Chapter 24), but ordinarily it changes the heart rate only slightly. The magnitude of the ventilatory response determines whether the heart rate increases or decreases as a result of carotid chemoreceptor stimulation. Mild chemoreceptor-induced stimulation of respiration decreases the heart rate moderately; more pronounced stimulation increases the heart rate only slightly. If the pulmonary response to chemoreceptor stimulation is blocked, the heart rate response may be greatly exaggerated, as described later.

The cardiac response to peripheral chemoreceptor stimulation is the result of primary and secondary reflex mechanisms (Fig. 18-9). The principal effect of the primary reflex stimulation is to excite the medullary vagal center and thereby decrease the heart rate. The respiratory system mediates secondary reflex effects. The respiratory stimulation by arterial chemoreceptors tends to inhibit the medullary vagal center. This inhibition varies with the level of concomitant stimulation of respiration; small increases in respiration inhibit the vagal center slightly, whereas large increases in ventilation inhibit the vagal center more profoundly.

An example of the primary inhibitory influence is shown in Figure 18-10. In this example, the lungs are

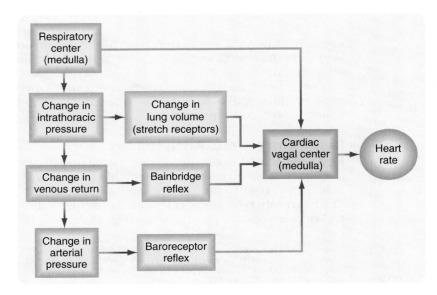

● **Figure 18-8.** Respiratory sinus arrhythmia is generated by a direct interaction between the respiratory and cardiac centers in the medulla, as well as by reflexes that originate from stretch receptors in the lungs, stretch receptors in the right atrium (the Bainbridge reflex), and baroreceptors in the carotid sinuses and aortic arch.

Figure 18-9. The primary effect of stimulation of peripheral chemoreceptors on the heart rate is to excite the cardiac vagal center in the medulla and thus to decrease the heart rate. Peripheral chemoreceptor stimulation also excites the respiratory center in the medulla. This effect produces hypocapnia and increases lung inflation, both of which secondarily inhibit the medullary vagal center. Thus, these secondary influences attenuate the primary reflex effect of peripheral chemoreceptor stimulation on heart rate.

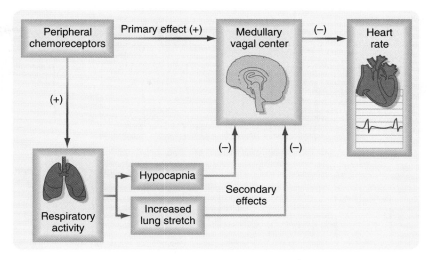

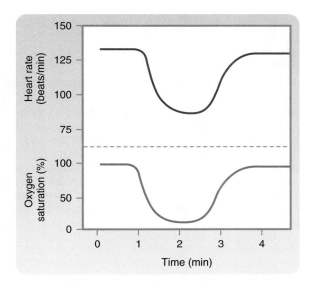

Figure 18-10. Changes in heart rate with carotid chemoreceptor stimulation during total heart bypass. The lungs remain deflated and respiratory gas exchange is accomplished by an artificial oxygenator. The lower tracing represents the oxygen saturation of the blood perfusing the carotid chemoreceptors. The blood perfusing the remainder of the body, including the myocardium, is fully saturated with oxygen. (Modified from Levy MN et al: Circ Res 18:67, 1966.)

completely collapsed and blood oxygenation is accomplished with an artificial oxygenator. When the carotid chemoreceptors are stimulated, an intense bradycardia and some degree of AV block ensue. Such effects are mediated primarily by efferent vagal fibers.

The pulmonary hyperventilation that is ordinarily evoked by carotid chemoreceptor stimulation influences the heart rate secondarily, both by initiating more pronounced pulmonary inflation reflexes and by producing hypocapnia (Fig. 18-9). Both influences tend to depress the primary cardiac response to chemoreceptor stimulation and thereby accelerate the heart. Hence, when pulmonary hyperventilation is not prevented, the primary and secondary effects neutralize

▶ IN THE CLINIC

The electrocardiogram in Figure 18-11 was recorded from a quadriplegic patient who could not breathe spontaneously and required tracheal intubation and artificial respiration. When the tracheal catheter was briefly disconnected (near the beginning of the top strip in the figure) to permit nursing care, profound bradycardia quickly developed. The patient's heart rate was 65 beats/min just before the tracheal catheter was disconnected. In less than 10 seconds after cessation of artificial respiration, his heart rate dropped to about 20 beats/min. This bradycardia could be prevented by blocking the effects of efferent vagal activity with atropine, and its onset could be delayed considerably by hyperventilating the patient before disconnecting the tracheal catheter.

each other, and carotid chemoreceptor stimulation affects the heart rate only moderately.

Ventricular Receptor Reflexes

Sensory receptors located near the endocardial surfaces of the ventricles initiate reflex effects similar to those elicited by the arterial baroreceptors. Excitation of these endocardial receptors diminishes the heart rate and peripheral resistance. Other sensory receptors have been identified in the epicardial regions of the ventricles. Although all these ventricular receptors are excited by various mechanical and chemical stimuli, their exact physiological functions remain unclear.

REGULATION OF MYOCARDIAL PERFORMANCE

Intrinsic Regulation of Myocardial Performance

As noted previously, the heart can initiate its own beat in the absence of any nervous or hormonal control.

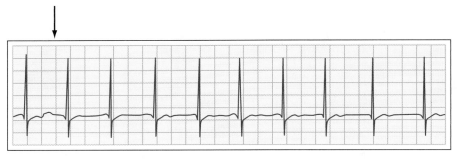

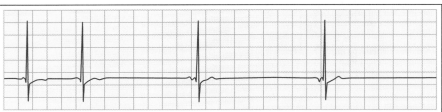

● Figure 18-11. Electrocardiogram of a 30-year-old quadriplegic man who could not breathe spontaneously and required tracheal intubation and artificial respiration. The two strips are continuous. (Modified from Berk JL, Levy MN: Eur Surg Res 9:75, 1977.)

▶ IN THE CLINIC

Ventricular receptors have been implicated in the initiation of **vasovagal syncope,** a feeling of lightheadedness or brief loss of consciousness that may be triggered by psychological or orthostatic stress. The ventricular receptors are believed to be stimulated by reduced ventricular filling volume combined with vigorous ventricular contraction. In a person standing quietly, ventricular filling is diminished because blood tends to pool in the veins in the abdomen and legs, as explained in Chapter 17. Consequently, the reduction in cardiac output and arterial blood pressure leads to a generalized increase in sympathetic neural activity via the baroreceptor reflex (Fig. 18-5). The enhanced sympathetic activity to the heart evokes a vigorous ventricular contraction that thereby stimulates the ventricular receptors. Excitation of the ventricular receptors is believed to initiate the autonomic neural changes that evoke vasovagal syncope, namely, a combination of a profound, vagally mediated bradycardia and generalized arteriolar vasodilation mediated by a reduction in sympathetic neural activity.

▶ IN THE CLINIC

The heart is partially or completely denervated in various clinical situations: (1) a surgically transplanted heart is totally denervated, although the intrinsic, postganglionic parasympathetic fibers persist; (2) atropine blocks vagal effects on the heart, and propranolol blocks sympathetic β-adrenergic influences; (3) certain drugs, such as reserpine, deplete cardiac norepinephrine stores and thereby restrict or abolish sympathetic control; and (4) in chronic congestive heart failure, cardiac norepinephrine stores are often severely diminished, and any sympathetic influences are attenuated.

The myocardium can also adapt to changing hemodynamic conditions by means of mechanisms that are intrinsic to cardiac muscle itself. For example, racing greyhounds with denervated hearts perform almost as well as those with intact innervation. Their maximal running speed decreases by only 5% after complete cardiac denervation. In these dogs, the threefold to fourfold increase in cardiac output during a race is achieved principally by an increase in stroke volume. Normally, the increase in cardiac output with exercise is accompanied by a proportionate increase in heart rate; stroke volume does not change much (see Chapter 19). This adaptation in the denervated heart is not achieved entirely by intrinsic mechanisms; cir-

culating catecholamines undoubtedly contribute. For example, if β-adrenergic receptor antagonists are given to greyhounds with denervated hearts, their racing performance is severely impaired.

Two principal intrinsic mechanisms, namely, the **Frank-Starling mechanism** and **rate-induced regulation,** enable the myocardium to adapt to changes in hemodynamic conditions. The Frank-Starling mechanism **(Starling's law of the heart)** is invoked in response to changes in the resting length of myocardial fibers. Rate-induced regulation is evoked by changes in the frequency of the heartbeat.

Frank-Starling Mechanism

About a century ago, the German physiologist Otto Frank and the English physiologist Ernest Starling independently studied the response of isolated hearts to changes in preload and afterload (see Chapter 16). When ventricular filling pressure (preload) is increased, ventricular volume increases progressively and after several beats attains a constant, larger volume. At equilibrium, the volume of blood ejected by the ventricles (stroke volume) with each heartbeat increases to equal the greater quantity of venous return to the right atrium.

The increased ventricular volume facilitates ventricular contraction and enables the ventricles to pump a greater stroke volume. This increase in ventricular volume is associated with an increase in length of the individual ventricular cardiac fibers. The increase in fiber length alters cardiac performance mainly by altering the number of myofilament cross-bridges that interact (see Chapter 16). More recent evidence indicates that the principal mechanism involves a stretch-induced change in the sensitivity of cardiac myofilaments to Ca^{++} (see Chapter 16). An optimal fiber length exists, however. Excessively high filling pressures that overstretch the myocardial fibers may depress rather than enhance the pumping capacity of the ventricles.

Starling also showed that isolated heart preparations could adapt to changes in the counterforce to the ventricular ejection of blood during systole (i.e., afterload). As the left ventricle contracts, it does not eject blood into the aorta until the ventricle has developed a pressure that just exceeds the prevailing aortic pressure (see Chapter 16). The aortic pressure during ventricular ejection essentially constitutes the left ventricular afterload. In Starling's experiments, arterial pressure was controlled by a hydraulic device in the tubing that led from the ascending aorta to the right atrial blood reservoir. Venous return to the right atrium was held constant by maintaining the hydrostatic level of the blood reservoir. As Starling raised arterial pressure to a new, constant level, the left ventricle responded at first to the increased afterload by pumping a diminished stroke volume. Because venous return was held constant, the diminution in stroke volume was accompanied by a rise in ventricular diastolic volume, as well as by an increase in the length of the myocardial fibers. This change in end-diastolic fiber length finally enabled the ventricle to pump a normal stroke volume against the greater peripheral resistance. Again, a change in the number of cross-bridges between the thick and thin filaments probably contributes to this adaptation, but the major factor appears to be a stretch-induced change in the sensitivity of the contractile proteins to Ca^{++}.

Cardiac adaptation to alterations in heart rate also involves changes in ventricular volume. During bradycardia, for example, the increased duration of diastole permits greater ventricular filling. The consequent increase in myocardial fiber length increases stroke volume. Therefore, the reduction in heart rate may be fully compensated by the increase in stroke volume, and cardiac output may therefore remain constant.

When cardiac compensation involves ventricular dilation, one must consider how the increased size of the ventricle affects the generation of intraventricular pressure. According to the Laplace relationship (see Chapter 17), if the ventricle enlarges, the force required by each myocardial fiber to generate a given intraventricular systolic pressure must be appreciably greater than that developed by the fibers in a ventricle of normal size. Thus, more energy is required for a dilated heart to perform a given amount of external work than for a normal-sized heart. Hence, computation of after-load on contracting myocardial fibers in the walls of the ventricles must consider ventricular dimensions along with intraventricular (and aortic) pressure.

The relatively rigid pericardium that encloses the heart determines the pressure-volume relationship at high levels of pressure and volume. The pericardium limits heart volume even under normal conditions, when an individual is at rest and the heart rate is slow. In patients with **chronic congestive heart failure,** the sustained cardiac dilation and hypertrophy may stretch the pericardium considerably. In such patients, the pericardial limitation of cardiac filling is exerted at pressures and volumes entirely different from those in normal individuals.

To assess changes in ventricular performance, the Frank-Starling mechanism is often represented by a family of **ventricular function curves.** To construct a control ventricular function curve, for example, blood volume is altered over a range of values, and stroke work (i.e., stroke volume × mean arterial pressure) and end-diastolic ventricular pressure are measured at each step. Similar observations are then made during the desired experimental intervention. For example, the ventricular function curve obtained during infusion of norepinephrine lies above and to the left of the control ventricular function curve (Fig. 18-12). Clearly, for a given level of left ventricular end-diastolic pressure (an index of preload), the left ventricle performs more work during the norepinephrine infusion than

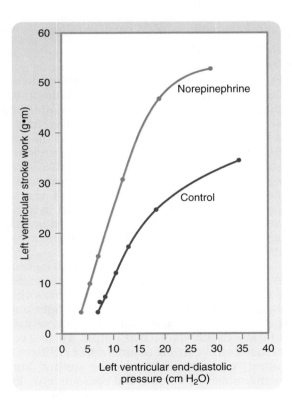

● **Figure 18-12.** A constant infusion of norepinephrine shifts the ventricular function curve to the left. This shift signifies an enhancement in ventricular contractility. (Redrawn from Sarnoff SJ et al: Circ Res 8:1108, 1960.)

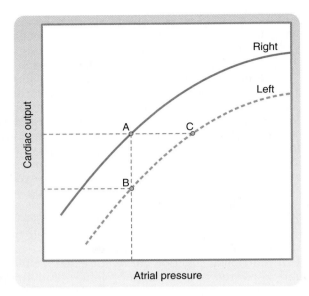

● **Figure 18-13.** Relationships between the output of the right and left ventricles and mean pressure in the right and left atria, respectively. At any given level of cardiac output, mean left atrial pressure (e.g., point C) exceeds mean right atrial pressure (point A).

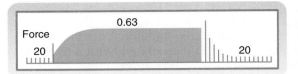

● **Figure 18-14.** Changes in development of force in an isolated papillary muscle from a cat as the interval between contractions is varied from 20 seconds to 0.63 second and then back to 20 seconds. (Redrawn from Koch-Weser J, Blinks JR: *Pharmacol Rev* 15:601, 1963.)

IN THE CLINIC

The greater left than right atrial pressure accounts for the observation that in individuals with congenital atrial septal defects in which the two atria communicate with each other via a patent foramen ovale, the direction of shunt flow is usually from left to right.

during control conditions. Hence, the upward and leftward shift of the ventricular function curve signifies improved ventricular contractility. Conversely, a shift downward and to the right indicates impaired contractility and a tendency toward **cardiac failure.**

Balance between Right and Left Ventricular Output

The Frank-Starling mechanism is well suited to match cardiac output to venous return. Any sudden, excessive output by one ventricle soon causes an increase in venous return to the second ventricle. The consequent increase in diastolic fiber length in the second ventricle augments the output of that ventricle to correspond to the output of its mate. In this way, the Frank-Starling mechanism maintains a precise balance between the output of the right and left ventricles. Because the two ventricles are arranged in series in a closed circuit, any small, but maintained imbalance in output of the two ventricles would otherwise be catastrophic.

The curves that relate cardiac output to mean atrial pressure for the two ventricles do not coincide; the curve for the left ventricle usually lies below that for the right ventricle (Fig. 18-13). At equal right and left atrial pressure (points A and B), right ventricular output exceeds left ventricular output. Hence, venous return to the left ventricle (a function of right ventricular output) exceeds left ventricular output, and left ventricular diastolic volume and pressure rise. By the Frank-Starling mechanism, left ventricular output therefore increases (from B toward C). Only when the output of both ventricles is identical (points A and C) is equilibrium reached. Under such conditions, however, left atrial pressure (C) exceeds right atrial

pressure (A). This is precisely the relationship that ordinarily prevails.

Rate-Induced Regulation

Myocardial performance is also regulated by changes in the frequency at which the myocardial fibers contract. The effects of changes in contraction frequency on the force developed in an isometrically contracting papillary muscle are shown in Figure 18-14. Initially, the cardiac muscle strip is stimulated to contract once every 20 seconds. When the muscle is suddenly made to contract once every 0.63 second, the force developed increases progressively over the next several beats. At the new steady state, the force developed is more than five times as great as at the larger contraction interval. A return to the larger interval (20 seconds) has the opposite influence on the development of force.

The rise in the force developed when the contraction interval is decreased is caused by a gradual increase in $[Ca^{++}]_i$. Two mechanisms contribute to the rise in $[Ca^{++}]$: an increase in the number of depolarizations per minute and an increase in the inward Ca^{++} current per depolarization.

In the first mechanism, Ca^{++} enters the myocardial cell during each action potential plateau (see Chapter 16). As the interval between beats is diminished, the number of plateaus per minute increases. Although the duration of each action potential (and of each plateau) decreases as the interval between beats is reduced, the overriding effect of the increased number of plateaus per minute on the influx of Ca^{++} prevails, and $[Ca^{++}]_i$ increases.

In the second mechanism, as the interval between beats is suddenly diminished, the inward Ca^{++} current (i_{Ca}) progressively increases with each successive beat until a new steady state is attained at the new basic cycle length. In an isolated ventricular myocyte, influx of Ca^{++} into the myocyte increases on successive depolarizations (Fig. 18-15). Both the increased magnitude and the slowed inactivation of i_{Ca} result in greater Ca^{++} influx into the myocyte during the later depolarizations than during the first depolarization. This greater Ca^{++} influx strengthens contraction.

Transient changes in the intervals between beats also profoundly affect the strength of contraction. When the left ventricle contracts prematurely (Fig. 18-16, beat A), the premature contraction (extrasystole) itself is weak, whereas contraction B (postextrasystolic contraction) after the compensatory pause is very strong. In the intact circulatory system, this response depends partly on the Frank-Starling mechanism. Inadequate time for ventricular filling just before the premature beat results in the weak premature contraction. Subsequently, the exaggerated degree of filling associated with the long compensatory pause (Fig. 18-16, beat B) contributes to the vigorous postextrasystolic contraction.

The weakness of the premature beat is directly related to its degree of prematurity. Thus, the earlier the premature beat, the weaker its force of contraction. The curve that relates strength of contraction of a premature beat to the coupling interval is called a **mechanical restitution curve.** Figure 18-17 shows the restitution curve obtained by varying the coupling intervals of test beats in an isolated ventricular muscle preparation.

Restitution of the force of contraction depends on the time course of the intracellular circulation of Ca^{++} in cardiac myocytes during contraction and relaxation. During relaxation, the Ca^{++} that dissociates from the contractile proteins is taken up by the sarcoplasmic reticulum for subsequent release. However, there is a lag of about 500 to 800 msec before this Ca^{++} is available for release from the sarcoplasmic reticulum in response to the next depolarization. Thus, the strength of the premature beat is reduced because the time during the preceding relaxation is insufficient to allow much of the Ca^{++} taken up by the sarcoplasmic reticulum to become available for release during the

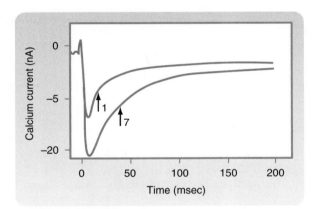

● **Figure 18-15.** Calcium currents induced in a myocyte during the first and seventh depolarizations in a consecutive sequence of depolarizations. The arrows indicate the half-times of inactivation. Note that during the seventh depolarization, the maximal inward Ca^{++} current and the half-time of inactivation were greater than the respective values for the first depolarization. (Modified from Lee KS: Proc Natl Acad Sci U S A 84:3941, 1987.)

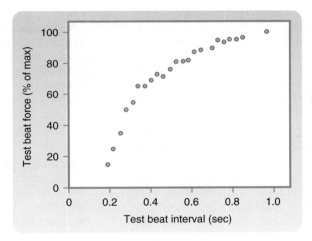

● **Figure 18-17.** Force generated during premature contractions in an isolated ventricular muscle preparation. The muscle was stimulated to contract once per second. Periodically, the muscle was stimulated prematurely. The scale along the x axis denotes the time between the driven and the premature beat. The y axis denotes the ratio of the contractile force of the premature beat to that of the driven beat. (Modified from Seed WA, Walker JM: Cardiovasc Res 22:303, 1988.)

● **Figure 18-16.** In an isovolumic left ventricle preparation, a premature ventricular systole (beat A) is typically weak, whereas the postextrasystolic contraction (beat B) is characteristically strong, and the enhanced contractility may diminish over a few beats (e.g., contraction C). (From Levy MN: Unpublished tracing.)

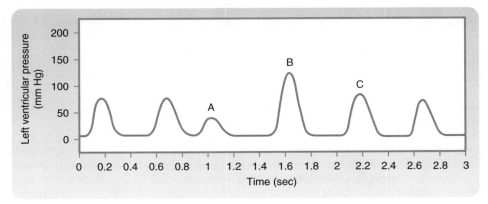

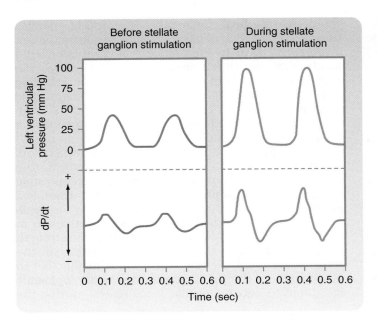

● **Figure 18-18.** In an isovolumic left ventricle preparation, stimulation of cardiac sympathetic nerves evokes a substantial rise in peak left ventricular pressure and in the maximal rates of rise and fall in intraventricular pressure (dP/dt). (From Levy MN: Unpublished tracing.)

premature beat. Conversely, the postextrasystolic beat is considerably stronger than normal because more Ca++ is released from the sarcoplasmic reticulum as a result of the relatively large amount of Ca++ taken up by it during the time that had elapsed from the end of the last regular beat until the beginning of the postextrasystolic beat.

Extrinsic Regulation of Myocardial Performance

Although a completely isolated heart can adapt well to changes in preload and afterload, various extrinsic factors also influence the heart in an individual. Often, these extrinsic regulatory mechanisms may overwhelm the intrinsic mechanisms. The extrinsic regulatory factors may be subdivided into nervous and chemical components.

Nervous Control

Sympathetic Influences. Sympathetic nervous activity enhances atrial and ventricular contractility. The alterations in ventricular contraction evoked by electrical stimulation of the left stellate ganglion in an isovolumic left ventricle preparation are shown in Figure 18-18. Note that the duration of systole is reduced and the rate of ventricular relaxation is increased during the early phases of diastole; both these effects assist ventricular filling. For any given cardiac cycle length, the abbreviated systole allows more time for diastole and hence for ventricular filling.

Sympathetic nervous activity also enhances myocardial performance by altering intracellular Ca++ dynamics (see Chapter 16). Neurally released norepinephrine or circulating catecholamines interact with β-adrenergic receptors on the cardiac cell membranes (Fig. 18-19). This interaction activates adenylyl cyclase, which raises intracellular levels of cAMP (see Chapter 3). Consequently, protein kinases that promote the phosphorylation of various proteins are activated

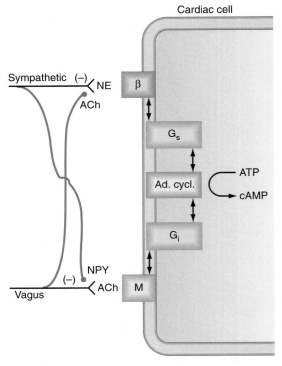

● **Figure 18-19.** Interneuronal and intracellular mechanisms responsible for interactions between the sympathetic and parasympathetic systems in the neural control of cardiac function. ACh, acetycholine; Ad cycl, adenylyl cyclase; β, β-adrenergic receptor; Gs and Gi, stimulatory and inhibitory G proteins; M, muscarinic receptor; NE, norepinephrine; NPY, neuropeptide Y. (From Levy MN: In Kulbertus HE, Franck G [eds]: Neurocardiology. Mt. Kisco, NY, Futura, 1988.)

within the myocardial cells. Phosphorylation of phospholamban facilitates reuptake of Ca++ by the sarcoplasmic reticulum, and phosphorylation of troponin I reduces the sensitivity of contractile proteins to Ca++. These effects facilitate relaxation and reduce end-

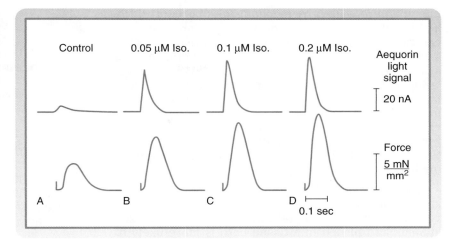

● **Figure 18-20.** Effects of various concentrations of isoproterenol (Iso) on the aequorin light signal (in nA) and contractile force (in mN/mm²) in a rat ventricular muscle injected with aequorin. The aequorin light signal reflects the instantaneous changes in intracellular [Ca⁺⁺]. (Modified from Kurihara S, Konishi M: Pflügers Arch 409:427, 1987.)

diastolic pressure (see Chapter 19). Phosphorylation of specific sarcolemmal proteins also activates Ca⁺⁺ channels in the membranes of myocardial cells.

Activation of Ca⁺⁺ channels increases the influx of Ca⁺⁺ during the action potential plateau, and more Ca⁺⁺ is released from the sarcoplasmic reticulum in response to each cardiac excitation. The contractile strength of the heart is thereby increased. Figure 18-20 shows the correlation between the contractile force in a thin strip of ventricular muscle and the free [Ca⁺⁺] (indicated by the aequorin light signal) in the myoplasm as the concentration of isoproterenol (a β-adrenergic agonist) is increased.

The overall effect of increased cardiac sympathetic activity in intact animals can best be appreciated in terms of families of ventricular function curves. When the frequency of electrical stimulation applied to the left stellate ganglion increases, the ventricular function curves shift progressively to the left. The changes parallel those produced by infusions of norepinephrine (Fig. 18-12). Hence, for any given left ventricular end-diastolic pressure, the ventricle can perform more work as sympathetic nervous activity is increased.

Parasympathetic Influences. The vagus nerves inhibit the cardiac pacemaker, atrial myocardium, and AV conduction tissue. The vagus nerves also depress the ventricular myocardium, but the effects are less pronounced than in the atria. In isovolumic left ventricle preparations, vagal stimulation decreases peak left ventricular pressure, the maximal rate of pressure development (dP/dt), and the maximal rate of pressure decline during diastole (Fig. 18-21). In pumping heart preparations, the ventricular function curve shifts to the right during vagal stimulation.

At least two mechanisms underlie the vagal effects on ventricular myocardium. First, the ACh released from vagus nerve endings can interact with muscarinic receptors in the cardiac cell membrane (Fig. 18-19). This interaction inhibits adenylyl cyclase, which consequently diminishes [cAMP]ᵢ and thus decreases the cAMP-dependent increase in contractility. Second, the ACh released from vagal endings can also inhibit the release of norepinephrine from neighboring sym-

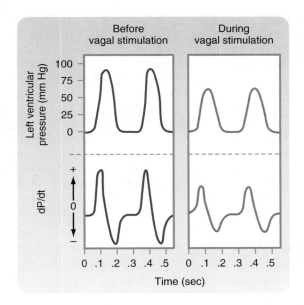

● **Figure 18-21.** In an isovolumic left ventricle preparation, when the ventricle is paced at a constant frequency, vagal stimulation decreases peak left ventricular pressure and diminishes the maximal rates of rise and fall in pressure (dP/dt). (From Levy MN: Unpublished tracing.)

pathetic nerve endings (Fig. 18-19). Thus, vagal activity can decrease ventricular contractility partly by antagonizing any stimulatory effects that concomitant sympathetic activity may be exerting on ventricular contractility. Similarly, sympathetic nerves release norepinephrine and certain neuropeptides, including neuropeptide Y (NPY). NPY inhibits the release of ACh from neighboring vagal fibers (Fig. 18-19).

Chemical Control

Adrenomedullary Hormones. The adrenal medulla is essentially a component of the autonomic nervous system (see Chapters 11 and 42). The principal hormone secreted by the adrenal medulla is epinephrine; some norepinephrine is also released. The rate of secretion of these catecholamines by the adrenal medulla is regulated by mechanisms that control the activity of the sympathetic nervous system. Thus, concentrations of catecholamines in blood rise under the same conditions that activate the sympathetic nervous system. However, the cardiovascular effects of circulating catecholamines are probably minimal under normal conditions. Moreover, the pronounced changes in myocardial contractility seen with exercise, for example, are mediated mainly by the norepinephrine released from cardiac sympathetic nerve fibers rather than by the catecholamines released from the adrenal medulla.

Adrenocortical Hormones. How adrenocortical steroids influence myocardial contractility is controversial. Cardiac muscle taken from adrenalectomized animals and placed in a tissue bath is more likely to fatigue in response to stimulation than is cardiac muscle obtained from normal animals. In some species, however, adrenocortical hormones enhance contractility. In addition, the glucocorticoid hydrocortisone potentiates the cardiotonic effects of catecholamines. This potentiation is mediated in part by the ability of adrenocortical steroids to inhibit the extraneuronal catecholamine uptake mechanisms.

Thyroid Hormones. Thyroid hormones enhance myocardial contractility. Rates of ATP hydrolysis and Ca^{++} uptake by the sarcoplasmic reticulum are increased in experimental hyperthyroidism; the opposite effects occur in hypothyroidism. Thyroid hormones increase cardiac protein synthesis, and this response leads to cardiac hypertrophy. These hormones also affect the composition of myosin isoen-

> ## ◥ IN THE CLINIC
>
> Cardiovascular problems are common in adrenocortical insufficiency (Addison's disease). Blood volume tends to fall, which may lead to severe hypotension and cardiovascular collapse, the so-called addisonian crisis (see Chapter 42).

> ## ● AT THE CELLULAR LEVEL
>
> Thyroid hormone exerts its cardiac actions by two paths, genomic and nongenomic. The genomic route involves interaction of thyroxine (T_3) with nuclear receptors that regulate the transcription of T_3-responsive genes. In hyperthyroidism, there is increased mRNA for cardiac myocyte proteins involved in regulating $[Ca^{++}]_i$ (SERCA, ryanodine channel) and contractile proteins (myosin heavy chain, actin, troponin I). Consequently, the rates of contraction and relaxation increase as ATP hydrolysis and O_2 consumption do. There is less efficient use of ATP and greater fractional loss of heat in the hyperthyroid state. If untreated, severe hyperthyroidism can result in heart failure.

> ## ◥ IN THE CLINIC
>
> Cardiac activity is depressed in patients with inadequate thyroid function (hypothyroidism). The converse is true in patients with overactive thyroid glands (hyperthyroidism). Characteristically, hyperthyroid patients exhibit tachycardia, high cardiac output, and arrhythmias such as atrial fibrillation. In hyperthyroid subjects, sympathetic neural activity may be increased, or the sensitivity of the heart to such activity may be enhanced. Studies have shown that thyroid hormone increases the density of β-adrenergic receptors in cardiac tissue (see also Chapter 41). In experimental animals, the cardiovascular manifestations of hyperthyroidism may be simulated by the administration of excess thyroxine.

zymes in cardiac muscle. By increasing isoenzymes with the greatest ATPase activity, thyroid hormones enhance myocardial contractility.

The cardiovascular changes in thyroid dysfunction also depend on indirect mechanisms. Thyroid hyperactivity increases the body's metabolic rate, which in turn results in arteriolar vasodilation. The consequent reduction in total peripheral resistance increases cardiac output, as explained in Chapter 19.

Insulin. Insulin has a positive inotropic effect on the heart. The effect of insulin is evident even when hypoglycemia is prevented by glucose infusions and when β-adrenergic receptors are blocked. Indeed, the positive inotropic effect of insulin is potentiated by β-adrenergic receptor antagonists. The enhanced contractility cannot be explained satisfactorily by the concomitant augmentation of glucose transport into myocardial cells.

Glucagon. Glucagon has potent positive inotropic and chronotropic effects on the heart. This endogenous hormone is probably not important in normal regulation of the cardiovascular system, but it has been used clinically to enhance cardiac performance. The effects of glucagon on the heart and certain metabolic effects are similar to those of catecholamines. Both glucagon and catecholamines activate adenylyl cyclase to increase myocardial levels of cAMP. The catecholamines activate adenylyl cyclase by interacting with β-adrenergic receptors, but glucagon activates this enzyme by a different mechanism. Nevertheless, the rise in cAMP increases influx of Ca^{++} through Ca^{++} channels in the sarcolemma and facilitates release and reuptake of Ca^{++} by the sarcoplasmic reticulum, just as catecholamines do.

Anterior Pituitary Hormones. The cardiovascular derangements in hypopituitarism are related principally to the associated deficiencies in adrenocortical and thyroid function. Growth hormone affects the myocardium, at least in combination with thyroxine. In hypophysectomized animals, growth hormone alone has little effect on the depressed heart, whereas thyroxine by itself restores adequate cardiac performance under basal conditions. However, when blood volume or peripheral resistance is increased, thyroxine alone does not restore adequate cardiac function, but the combination of growth hormone and thyroxine does reestablish normal cardiac performance. In certain animal models of heart failure, administration of growth hormone alone increases cardiac output and myocardial contractility.

Blood Gases

Changes in cardiac performance as a result of stimulation of central and peripheral chemoreceptors have been described. These effects usually predominate. However, direct effects of O_2 and CO_2 on the myocardium do occur.

Oxygen. Hypoxia has a biphasic effect on myocardial performance. Mild hypoxia stimulates performance, but more severe hypoxia depresses performance because oxidative metabolism is limited.

Carbon Dioxide and Acidosis. An increase in P_{CO_2} ($\downarrow$pH) has a direct depressant effect on the heart. This effect is mediated by changes in intracellular pH.

A reduction in intracellular pH, induced by an increase in P_{CO_2}, diminishes the amount of Ca^{++} released from the sarcoplasmic reticulum in response to excitation. The diminished pH also decreases the sensitivity of the myofilaments to Ca^{++}. Increases in intracellular pH have the opposite effect; that is, they enhance sensitivity to Ca^{++}.

REGULATION OF THE PERIPHERAL CIRCULATION

The peripheral circulation is essentially under dual control: centrally through the nervous system and locally by conditions in tissues surrounding the blood vessels. The relative importance of these two control mechanisms varies in different tissues (see Chapter 17).

The arterioles are involved in regulating the rate of blood flow throughout the body. These vessels offer the greatest resistance to the flow of blood pumped to the tissues by the heart, and thus these vessels are important in the maintenance of arterial blood pressure. The walls of these resistance vessels are composed in large part of smooth muscle fibers that allow the diameter of the vessel lumen to vary. When this smooth muscle contracts strongly, the endothelial lining folds inward and completely obliterates the vessel lumen. When the smooth muscle is completely relaxed, the vessel lumen is maximally dilated. Some resistance vessels are closed at any given time. In addition, the smooth muscle in these vessels is partially contracted (which accounts for the tone of these vessels). If all the resistance vessels in the body dilated simultaneously, arterial blood pressure would fall precipitously.

Vascular smooth muscle controls total peripheral resistance, arterial and venous tone, and the distribution of blood flow throughout the body. The properties of vascular smooth muscle are discussed in Chapter

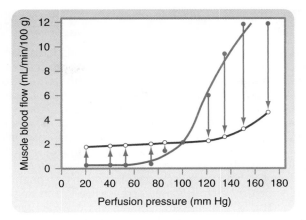

● **Figure 18-22.** Pressure-flow relationship in the skeletal muscle vascular bed. Closed circles represent the flows obtained immediately after abrupt changes in perfusion pressure from the control level (point where lines cross). Open circles represent the steady-state flows obtained at the new perfusion pressure. (Redrawn from Jones RD, Berne RM: Circ Res 14:126, 1964.)

14. In the following sections, intrinsic and extrinsic control of vascular smooth muscle tone, and thus perfusion of peripheral tissues, is reviewed.

Intrinsic or Local Control of Peripheral Blood Flow
Autoregulation and Myogenic Regulation

In certain tissues, blood flow is adjusted to the existing metabolic activity of the tissue. Furthermore, when tissue metabolism is steady, changes in perfusion pressure (arterial blood pressure) evoke changes in vascular resistance that tend to maintain a constant blood flow. This mechanism, which is illustrated graphically in Figure 18-22, is commonly referred to as **autoregulation of blood flow.** When pressure is abruptly increased or decreased from a control pressure of 100 mm Hg, flow increases or decreases, respectively. However, even with pressure maintained at its new level, blood flow returns toward the control level within 30 to 60 seconds. Over the pressure range of 20 to 120 mm Hg, the steady-state flow is relatively constant. Calculation of hydraulic resistance (pressure/flow) across the vascular bed during steady-state conditions shows that the resistance vessels constrict with an elevation in perfusion pressure but dilate with a reduction in perfusion pressure. This response to perfusion pressure is independent of the endothelium because it is identical in intact vessels and in vessels that have been stripped of their endothelium. According to the myogenic mechanism, vascular smooth muscle contracts in response to an increase in the pressure difference across the wall of a blood vessel (transmural pressure), and it relaxes in response to a decrease in transmural pressure. The signaling mechanisms that allow distention of a vessel to elicit contraction are unknown. However, because stretch of vascular smooth muscle has been shown to raise $[Ca^{++}]_i$, an increase in transmural pressure is believed to activate membrane Ca^{++} channels.

⬤ AT THE CELLULAR LEVEL

Transient receptor potential (TRP) channels have been implicated in the myogenic mechanism. These channels are mammalian homologues of a *Drosophila melanogaster* gene that when mutated, allows only a transient response to a sustained light stimulus. The pressure-induced vasoconstrictive response of an artery (myogenic response) appears to have the following signal path: pressure → increased phospholipase C activity → synthesis of diacylglycerol → activation of TRP channel → smooth muscle depolarization and opening of L-type Ca^{++} channels that increase $[Ca^{++}]_i$ and muscle tone. This is a means to regulate vascular resistance. Other TRP channel types have been proposed to participate in chronic hypoxic pulmonary hypertension and in the vasoconstriction caused by the α-adrenergic agonist norepinephrine.

In normal subjects, blood pressure is maintained at a fairly constant level via the baroreceptor reflex. Hence, the myogenic mechanism may play little role in regulating blood flow to tissues under normal conditions. However, when a person changes from a lying to a standing position, transmural pressure rises in the lower extremities, and the precapillary vessels constrict in response to this imposed stretch.

Endothelium-Mediated Regulation

As described in Chapter 17, the endothelium lining the vasculature produces a number of substances that can relax (e.g., nitric oxide) or contract (e.g., angiotensin II and endothelin) vascular smooth muscle. Thus, the endothelium can play an important role in regulating blood flow to specific vascular beds.

Metabolic Regulation

The metabolic activity of a tissue governs blood flow in that tissue. Any intervention that results in an inadequate O_2 supply prompts the formation of vasodilator metabolites that are released from the tissue and act locally to dilate the resistance vessels. When the metabolic rate of the tissue increases or O_2 delivery to the tissue decreases, more vasodilator substances are released (see Chapter 17).

Candidate Vasodilator Substances. Many substances have been proposed as mediators of metabolic vasodilation. Some of the earliest vasodilators suggested were lactic acid, CO_2, and H^+. However, the decrease in vascular resistance caused by supernormal concentrations of these vasodilators is much less than the dilation seen when metabolic activity is increased physiologically.

Alterations in Po_2 can change the contractile state of vascular smooth muscle. An increase in Po_2 elicits contraction; a decrease elicits relaxation. However, measurements of Po_2 in resistance vessels indicate that over a wide range of Po_2 values (11 to 343 mm Hg), Po_2 and arteriolar diameter are not well correlated. Hence, the observed changes in arteriolar diameter are more compatible with the release of a vasodilator metabolite from the tissue than with a direct effect of Po_2 on vascular smooth muscle.

Potassium ions, inorganic phosphate ions, and interstitial fluid osmolarity can also induce vasodilation. Both K^+ and phosphate are released and osmolarity is increased during skeletal muscle contraction. Therefore, these factors may contribute to active hyperemia (increased blood flow caused by enhanced tissue activity). However, significant increases in the phosphate concentration and in osmolarity are not always observed during muscle contraction, and they may increase blood flow only transiently. Therefore, they probably do not mediate the vasodilation observed during muscular activity. Potassium is released at the onset of skeletal muscle contraction or with an increase in cardiac muscle activity. Hence, release of K^+ could underlie the initial decrease in vascular resistance observed in response to physical exercise or to increased cardiac work. However, release of K^+ is not sustained, yet continued arteriolar dilation persists throughout the period of enhanced muscle activity. Furthermore, reoxygenated venous blood obtained from active cardiac and skeletal muscles does not elicit vasodilation when the blood is infused into a test vascular bed. It is unlikely that oxygenation of venous blood alters its K^+ or phosphate content or its osmolarity and thereby neutralizes its vasodilator effect. Therefore, some agent other than K^+ must mediate the vasodilation associated with metabolic activity of the tissue.

Adenosine, which contributes to the regulation of coronary blood flow, may also participate in control of the resistance vessels in skeletal muscle. In addition, some prostaglandins may be important vasodilator mediators in certain vascular beds. Thus, many candidates have been proposed as mediators of metabolic vasodilation, and the relative contribution of each remains to be determined.

Basal Vessel Tone. Metabolic control of vascular resistance by the release of a vasodilator substance requires the existence of a basal vessel tone. Tonic activity in vascular smooth muscle is readily demonstrable, but in contrast to tone in skeletal muscle, the tone in vascular smooth muscle is independent of the nervous system. Thus, some metabolic factor must be responsible for maintaining this tone. The following factors may be involved: (1) the myogenic response to the stretch imposed by blood pressure, (2) the high Po_2 of arterial blood, or (3) the presence of Ca^{++}.

Reactive Hyperemia. If arterial inflow to a vascular bed is stopped temporarily, blood flow on release of the occlusion immediately exceeds the flow that prevailed before occlusion, and the flow gradually returns to the control level. This increase in blood flow is called reactive hyperemia. This type of experiment provides evidence for the existence of a local metabolic factor that regulates tissue blood flow.

In the experiment shown in Figure 18-23, blood flow to the leg was stopped by clamping the femoral artery for 15, 30, and 60 seconds. Release of the 60-second

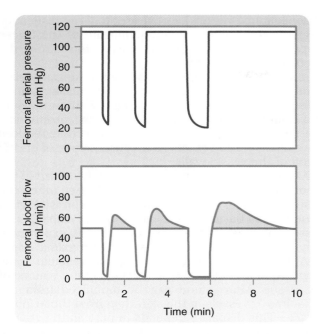

● **Figure 18-23.** Reactive hyperemia in the hind limb of the leg after 15-, 30-, and 60-second occlusion of the femoral artery. (From Berne RM: Unpublished observations.)

▶ **IN THE CLINIC**

Disease of the arterial walls can lead to obstruction of the arteries, and symptoms, called intermittent claudication, appear when the arterial disease occurs in the legs. The symptoms consist of leg pain when the subject walks or climbs stairs, and the pain is relieved by rest. The disease is called thromboangiitis obliterans, and it appears most frequently in men who are smokers. With minimal walking, the resistance vessels become maximally dilated by local release of metabolites; when the O_2 demand of the muscles increases with more rapid walking, blood flow cannot increase sufficiently to meet the muscle needs for O_2, and pain caused by muscle ischemia results.

occlusion resulted in a peak blood flow that was 70% greater than the control flow, and the flow returned to the control level within 110 seconds.

Within limits, peak flow and particularly the duration of reactive hyperemia are proportional to the duration of the occlusion (Fig. 18-23). If the extremity is exercised during the occlusion period, reactive hyperemia is increased. These observations and the close relationship that exists between metabolic activity and blood flow in an unoccluded limb are consistent with a metabolic mechanism in the local regulation of tissue blood flow.

Coordination of Arterial and Arteriolar Dilation.
When the vascular smooth muscle of arterioles relaxes in response to vasodilator metabolites whose release is caused by a decrease in the ratio of O_2 supply to O_2 demand of the tissue, resistance may diminish concomitantly in the small upstream arteries that feed these arterioles. The result is a blood flow greater than that produced by arteriolar dilation alone. There are two possible mechanisms for this coordination of arterial and arteriolar dilation. First, the vasodilation in the microvessels may be propagated, and when dilation is initiated in the arterioles, it can propagate along the vessels from the arterioles back to the small arteries. Second, the metabolite-mediated dilation of the arterioles accelerates blood flow in the feeder arteries. This greater blood flow velocity increases the shear stress on the arterial endothelium, which in turn can induce vasodilation by release of nitric oxide.

Extrinsic Control of Peripheral Blood Flow
Sympathetic Neural Vasoconstriction

Several regions in the cerebral medulla influence cardiovascular activity. Stimulation of the dorsal lateral medulla (pressor region) evokes vasoconstriction, cardiac acceleration, and enhanced myocardial contractility. Stimulation of cerebral centers caudal and ventromedial to the pressor region decreases arterial blood pressure. This depressor area exerts its effect by direct inhibition of spinal regions and by inhibition of the medullary pressor region. These areas are not true anatomic centers in which a discrete group of cells is discernible, but they constitute "physiological" centers.

The cerebrospinal vasoconstrictor regions are tonically active. Reflexes or humoral stimuli that enhance this activity increase the frequency of impulses that reach the terminal neural branches to the vessels. A constrictor neurohumor (norepinephrine) is released at the terminals to elicit a constrictive α-adrenergic effect on the resistance vessels. Inhibition of the vasoconstrictor areas diminishes the impulse frequency in the efferent nerve fibers, and vasodilation results. Thus, neural regulation of the peripheral circulation is achieved mainly by altering the impulse frequency in the sympathetic nerves to the blood vessels. Surgical section of the sympathetic nerves to an extremity abolishes sympathetic vascular tone and thereby increases blood flow to that limb. With time, vascular tone is regained by an increase in basal (intrinsic) tone.

Both the pressor and depressor regions may undergo rhythmic changes in tonic activity that are manifested as oscillations in arterial pressure. Some rhythmic changes **(Traube-Hering waves)** occur at the frequency of respiration and are caused by a cyclic fluctuation in sympathetic impulses to the resistance vessels. Other fluctuations in sympathetic activity **(Mayer waves)** occur at a frequency lower than that of respiration.

Sympathetic Constrictor Influence on Resistance and Capacitance Vessels

Vasoconstrictor fibers of the sympathetic nervous system supply the arteries, arterioles, and veins; the neural influence on larger vessels is much less than it is on arterioles and small arteries. Capacitance vessels (veins) respond more to sympathetic nerve stimulation than resistance vessels do; the capacitance vessels are maximally constricted at a lower stimulation frequency than the resistance vessels are. However, capacitance vessels lack β-adrenergic receptors, and they do respond less to vasodilator metabolites. Norepinephrine is the neurotransmitter released at the sympathetic nerve terminals in blood vessel. Factors such as circulating hormones and particularly locally released substances mediate the release of norepinephrine from the nerve terminals.

The response of the resistance and capacitance vessels to stimulation of sympathetic fibers is illustrated in Figure 18-24. When arterial pressure is held constant, stimulation of sympathetic fibers reduces blood flow (constriction of resistance vessels) and decreases the blood volume of the tissue (constriction

of capacitance vessels). Constriction of the resistance vessels established a new equilibrium of the forces responsible for filtration and absorption across the capillary wall (see Chapter 17).

In addition to active changes (contraction and relaxation of vascular smooth muscle) in vessel caliber, passive changes are also caused by alterations in intraluminal pressure. An increase in intraluminal pressure distends the vessels, and a decrease reduces the caliber of the vessels as a consequence of elastic recoil of the vessel walls.

At basal vascular tone, approximately a third of the blood volume of a tissue can be mobilized when the sympathetic nerves are stimulated at physiological frequencies. Basal tone is very low in capacitance vessels; if these vessels are denervated experimentally, the increases in volume evoked by maximal doses of ACh are small. Therefore, at basal vascular tone, blood volume is close to the maximal blood volume of the tissue. More blood can be mobilized from the capacitance vessels in the skin than from those in the muscle. This disparity depends in part on the greater sensitivity of the skin vessels to sympathetic stimulation, but also in part because basal tone is lower in skin vessels than in muscle vessels. Therefore, in the absence of a neural influence, skin capacitance vessels contain more blood than muscle capacitance vessels do.

Physiological stimuli mobilize blood from capacitance vessels. For example, during physical exercise, activation of sympathetic nerve fibers constricts the peripheral veins and hence augments cardiac filling pressure. In arterial hypotension (as in hemorrhage), the capacitance vessels constrict and thereby correct the decreased central venous pressure associated with blood loss.

Parasympathetic Neural Influence

The efferent fibers of the cranial division of the parasympathetic nervous system innervate the blood vessels of the head and some of the viscera, whereas fibers of the sacral division innervate blood vessels of the genitalia, bladder, and large bowel. Skeletal muscle and skin do not receive parasympathetic innervation. The effect of cholinergic fibers on total vascular resistance is small because only a small proportion of the

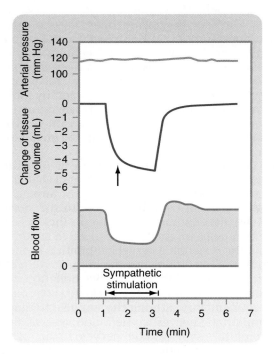

● **Figure 18-24.** Effect of sympathetic nerve stimulation (2 Hz) on blood flow and tissue volume of the lower limb. The arrow denotes the change in slope of the tissue volume curve at the point where the decrease in volume caused by emptying of capacitance vessels ceases and loss of extravascular fluid becomes evident. The abrupt decrease in tissue volume is caused by movement of blood out of the capacitance vessels and out of the lower limb. The late, slow progressive decline in volume (to the right of the *arrow*) was caused by extravascular fluid moving into the capillaries and hence away from the tissue. The loss of tissue fluid results from the lowered capillary hydrostatic pressure secondary to constriction of the resistance vessels. (From Mellander S: Acta Physiol Scand Suppl 50[176]:1, 1960.)

> ### IN THE CLINIC
>
> In hemorrhagic shock, the resistance vessels constrict and thereby assist in the maintenance of normal arterial blood pressure. With arterial hypotension, the enhanced arteriolar constriction also leads to a small mobilization of blood from the tissue by virtue of recoil of the postarteriolar vessels when intraluminal pressure is reduced. Furthermore, extravascular fluid is mobilized because of greater fluid absorption into the capillaries in response to the lowered capillary hydrostatic pressure (see also Chapter 19).

resistance vessels of the body receive parasympathetic fibers.

Stimulation of the parasympathetic fibers to the salivary glands induces marked vasodilation. A vasodilator polypeptide, bradykinin, formed locally from the action of an enzyme on a plasma protein substrate in the glandular lymphatics mediates this vasodilation. Bradykinin is formed in other exocrine glands, such as the lacrimal and sweat glands. Its presence in sweat may be partly responsible for the dilation of cutaneous blood vessels.

Humoral Factors

Epinephrine and norepinephrine exert a powerful effect on peripheral blood vessels. In skeletal muscle, low concentrations of epinephrine dilate resistance vessels (β-adrenergic effect), but high concentrations produce constriction (α-adrenergic effect). In all vascular beds the primary effect of norepinephrine is vasoconstriction. When stimulated, the adrenal gland can release epinephrine and norepinephrine into the systemic circulation. However, under physiological conditions, the effect of catecholamine release from the adrenal medulla is less important than norepinephrine release from sympathetic nerve endings.

Vascular Reflexes

Areas of the cerebral medulla that mediate sympathetic and vagal effects are under the influence of neural impulses that originate in the baroreceptors, chemoreceptors, hypothalamus, cerebral cortex, and skin. These areas of the medulla are also affected by changes in the blood concentrations of CO_2 and O_2.

Arterial Baroreceptors. The baroreceptors (or pressoreceptors) are stretch receptors located in the carotid sinuses and in the aortic arch (Figs. 18-25 and 18-26). The carotid sinuses are the slightly widened areas at the origins of the internal carotid arteries. Impulses that arise in the carotid sinus travel up the carotid sinus nerve (nerve of Hering) to the glossopharyngeal nerve (cranial nerve IX) and, via the latter, to the nucleus of the tractus solitarius (NTS) in the medulla. The NTS is the site of the central projections of the chemoreceptors and baroreceptors. Stimulation of the NTS inhibits sympathetic nerve outflow to the peripheral blood vessels (depressor effect), whereas lesions of the NTS produce vasoconstriction (pressor effect). Impulses that arise in the aortic arch baroreceptors reach the NTS via afferent fibers in the vagus nerves.

Baroreceptor nerve terminals in the walls of the carotid sinus and aortic arch respond to the vascular stretch and deformation induced by changes in arterial blood pressure. The frequency of firing of these nerves is enhanced by an increase in arterial blood pressure and diminished by a reduction in arterial blood pressure. An increase in impulse frequency, as occurs with a rise in arterial pressure, inhibits the cerebral vasoconstrictor regions and results in peripheral vasodilation and lowering of arterial blood pressure. Bradycardia brought about by activation of the cardiac branches of the vagus nerves contributes to this lowering of blood pressure.

The carotid sinus baroreceptors are more sensitive than those in the aortic arch. Changes in carotid sinus pressure evoke greater changes in systemic arterial pressure and peripheral resistance than do equivalent changes in aortic arch pressure.

The receptors in the carotid sinus walls respond more to pulsatile pressure than to constant pressure.

● **Figure 18-25.** Diagrammatic representation of the carotid sinus and carotid body and their innervation. (Redrawn from Adams WE: The Comparative Morphology of the Carotid Body and Carotid Sinus. Springfield, IL, Charles C Thomas, 1958.)

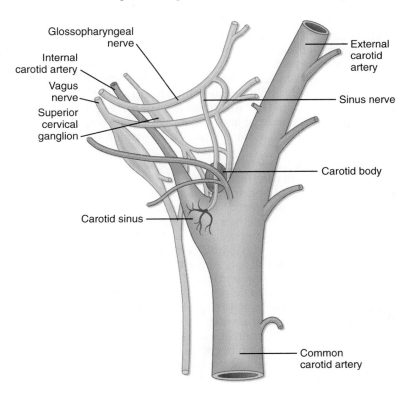

Glossopharyngeal nerve

Internal carotid artery

Vagus nerve

Superior cervical ganglion

External carotid artery

Sinus nerve

Carotid body

Carotid sinus

Common carotid artery

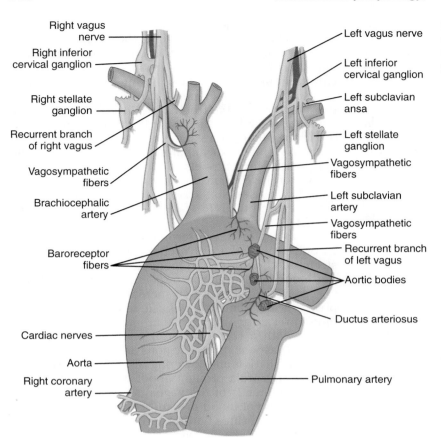

Right vagus nerve
Right inferior cervical ganglion
Right stellate ganglion
Recurrent branch of right vagus
Vagosympathetic fibers
Brachiocephalic artery
Baroreceptor fibers
Cardiac nerves
Aorta
Right coronary artery

Left vagus nerve
Left inferior cervical ganglion
Left subclavian ansa
Left stellate ganglion
Vagosympathetic fibers
Left subclavian artery
Vagosympathetic fibers
Recurrent branch of left vagus
Aortic bodies
Ductus arteriosus
Pulmonary artery

● **Figure 18-26.** Anterior view of the aortic arch showing the innervation of the aortic bodies and baroreceptors. (Modified from Nonidez JF: *Anat Rec* 69:299, 1937.)

This is illustrated in Figure 18-27, which shows that at normal levels of mean arterial blood pressure (about 100 mm Hg), a barrage of impulses from a single fiber of the sinus nerve is initiated in early systole by the pressure rise; only a few spikes occurred during late systole and early diastole. At lower arterial pressure, these phasic changes are even more evident, but the overall discharge frequency is reduced. The blood pressure threshold for evoking sinus nerve impulses is about 50 mm Hg; maximal sustained firing is reached at around 200 mm Hg. Because the baroreceptors adapt, their response at any mean arterial pressure level is greater to a large than to a small pulse pressure.

The increases in resistance that occur in response to reduced pressure in the carotid sinus vary from one peripheral vascular bed to another. These variations allow blood flow to be redistributed. The resistance changes elicited by altering carotid sinus pressure are greatest in the femoral vessels, less in the renal vessels, and least in the mesenteric and celiac vessels.

In addition, the sensitivity of the carotid sinus reflex can be altered. Local application of norepinephrine or stimulation of sympathetic nerve fibers to the carotid sinuses enhances the sensitivity of its receptors such that a given increase in intrasinus pressure produces a greater depressor response. Baroreceptor sensitivity decreases in hypertension because the carotid sinuses become stiffer as a result of the high intraarterial pressure. Consequently, a given increase in carotid sinus

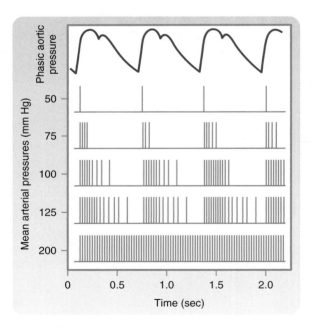

● **Figure 18-27.** Relationship of phasic aortic blood pressure in the firing of a single afferent nerve fiber from the carotid sinus at different levels of mean arterial pressure.

pressure elicits a smaller decrease in systemic arterial pressure than it does at a normal level of blood pressure. Thus, the set point of the baroreceptors is raised in hypertension such that the threshold is increased and the pressure receptors are less sensitive to changes in transmural pressure. As would be expected, denervation of the carotid sinus can produce temporary and, in some instances, prolonged hypertension.

The arterial baroreceptors play a key role in short-term adjustments in blood pressure in response to relatively abrupt changes in blood volume, cardiac output, or peripheral resistance (as in exercise). However, long-term control of blood pressure—over a period of days or weeks—is determined by the fluid balance of the individual, namely, the balance between fluid intake and fluid output. By far the single most important organ in the control of body fluid volume, and hence blood pressure, is the kidney (see also Chapter 34).

Cardiopulmonary Baroreceptors. Cardiopulmonary receptors are located in the atria, ventricles, and pulmonary vessels. These baroreceptors are innervated by vagal and sympathetic afferent nerves. Cardiopulmonary reflexes are tonically active and can alter peripheral resistance in response to changes in intracardiac, venous, or pulmonary vascular pressure.

The atria contain two types of cardiopulmonary baroreceptors: those activated by the tension developed during atrial systole (A receptors) and those activated by stretch of the atria during atrial diastole (B receptors). Stimulation of these atrial receptors sends impulses up vagal fibers to the vagal center in the medulla. Consequently, sympathetic activity is decreased to the kidney and increased to the sinus node. These changes in sympathetic activity increase renal blood flow, urine flow, and heart rate.

Activation of the cardiopulmonary receptors can also initiate a reflex that lowers arterial blood pressure by inhibiting the vasoconstrictor center in the cerebral medulla. Stimulation of the cardiopulmonary receptors inhibits release of angiotensin, aldosterone, and vasopressin (antidiuretic hormone); interruption of the reflex pathway has the opposite effects.

The role that activation of these baroreceptors plays in the regulation of blood volume is apparent in the body's responses to hemorrhage. The reduction in blood volume (hypovolemia) enhances sympathetic

vasoconstriction in the kidney and increases the secretion of renin, angiotensin, aldosterone, and antidiuretic hormone (see also Chapter 19). The renal vasoconstriction (primarily afferent arterioles) reduces glomerular filtration and increases release of renin from the kidney. Renin acts on a plasma substrate to yield angiotensin II, which releases aldosterone from the adrenal cortex. The enhanced release of antidiuretic hormone decreases renal water excretion, and the release of aldosterone decreases renal NaCl excretion. The kidneys retain salt and water, and hence blood volume increases. Angiotensin II (formed from angiotensin I by angiotensin-converting enzyme) also raises systemic arteriolar tone.

Peripheral Chemoreceptors. These chemoreceptors consist of small, highly vascular bodies in the region of the aortic arch (aortic bodies, Fig. 18-26) and just medial to the carotid sinuses (carotid bodies, Fig. 18-25). These vascular bodies are sensitive to changes in the P_{O_2}, P_{CO_2}, and pH of blood. Although they primarily regulate respiration, they also influence the vasomotor regions. A reduction in arterial blood P_{O_2} stimulates the chemoreceptors. The increased activity in afferent nerve fibers from the carotid and aortic bodies stimulates the vasoconstrictor regions and thereby increases the tone of resistance and capacitance vessels.

The chemoreceptors are also stimulated by increased arterial blood P_{CO_2} and by reduced pH. However, the reflex effect is small in comparison to the direct effects of hypercapnia (high P_{CO_2}) and acidosis on the vasomotor regions in the medulla. When hypoxia and hypercapnia occur simultaneously, the effects of the chemoreceptors are greater than the sum of the effects of each of the two stimuli when they act alone.

Chemoreceptors are also located in the heart. These cardiac chemoreceptors are activated by ischemia of cardiac muscle, and they transmit the precordial pain (angina pectoris) associated with an inadequate blood supply to the myocardium.

Hypothalamus. Optimal function of the cardiovascular reflexes requires integrity of the pontine and hypothalamic structures. Furthermore, these structures are responsible for behavioral and emotional control of the cardiovascular system (see also Chapter 11). Stimulation of the anterior hypothalamus produces a fall in blood pressure and bradycardia, whereas stimulation of the posterolateral region of the hypothalamus increases blood pressure and the heart rate. The hypothalamus also contains a temperature-regulating center that affects blood vessels in the skin. Stimulation by the application of cold to the skin or by cooling of the blood perfusing the hypothalamus results in constriction of the skin vessels and heat conservation, whereas warm stimuli to the skin result in cutaneous vasodilation and enhanced heat loss.

Cerebrum. The cerebral cortex also affects blood flow distribution in the body. Stimulation of the motor and premotor areas affects blood pressure; usually, a

> **IN THE CLINIC**
>
> In some individuals, the carotid sinus is abnormally sensitive to external pressure. Hence, tight collars or other forms of external pressure over the region of the carotid sinus may elicit marked hypotension and fainting. Such hypersensitivity is known as the carotid sinus syndrome.

pressor response occurs. However, vasodilation and depressor responses may be evoked, as in blushing or fainting, in response to an emotional stimulus.

Skin and Viscera. Painful stimuli can elicit either pressor or depressor responses, depending on the magnitude and location of the stimulus. Distention of the viscera often evokes a depressor response, whereas painful stimuli to the body surface generally evoke a pressor response.

Pulmonary Reflexes. Inflation of the lungs initiates a reflex that induces systemic vasodilation and a decrease in arterial blood pressure. Conversely, collapse of the lungs evokes systemic vasoconstriction. Afferent fibers that mediate this reflex are in the vagus nerves and possibly also in the sympathetic nerves. Stimulation of these fibers by stretch of the lungs inhibits the vasomotor areas. The magnitude of the depressor response to lung inflation is directly related to the degree of inflation and to the existing level of vasoconstrictor tone (see also Chapter 22).

Central Chemoreceptors. Increases in P_{CO_2} stimulate chemosensitive regions of the medulla (the central chemoreceptors), and they elicit vasoconstriction and increased peripheral resistance. A reduction in P_{CO_2} below normal levels (in response to hyperventilation) decreases tonic activity in these areas in the medulla and thereby decreases peripheral resistance. The chemosensitive regions are also affected by changes in pH. Lowering of blood pH stimulates and a rise in blood pH inhibits these cerebral areas. These effects of changes in P_{CO_2} and blood pH may operate through changes in cerebrospinal fluid pH, as may also the respiratory center.

P_{O_2} has little direct effect on the medullary vasomotor region. The primary effect of hypoxia is mediated by reflexes via the carotid and aortic chemoreceptors. A moderate reduction in P_{O_2} stimulates the vasomotor region, but a severe reduction depresses vasomotor activity in the same manner by which other areas of the brain are depressed by very low O_2 tension.

Balance between Extrinsic and Intrinsic Factors in Regulation of Peripheral Blood Flow

Dual control of peripheral vessels by intrinsic and extrinsic mechanisms evokes a number of important vascular adjustments. Such regulatory mechanisms enable the body to direct blood flow to areas where it is most needed and away from areas that have fewer requirements. In some tissues, the effects of the extrinsic and intrinsic mechanisms are fixed; in other tissues, the ratio is changeable and depends on the state of activity of that tissue.

In the brain and heart, which are vital structures with limited tolerance for a reduced blood supply, intrinsic flow-regulating mechanisms are dominant. For instance, massive discharge of the vasoconstrictor region via the sympathetic nerves, which might occur in severe, acute hemorrhage, has negligible effects on the cerebral and cardiac resistance vessels, whereas the cutaneous, renal, and splanchnic blood vessels become greatly constricted (see also Chapter 19).

In the skin, extrinsic vascular control is dominant. The cutaneous vessels not only participate strongly in a general vasoconstrictor discharge but also respond selectively via hypothalamic pathways to subserve the heat loss and heat conservation functions required for regulation of body temperature. However, intrinsic control can be elicited by local temperature changes that modify or override the central influence on resistance and capacitance vessels (see also Chapter 17).

In skeletal muscle, the extrinsic and intrinsic mechanisms interact. In resting skeletal muscle, neural control (vasoconstrictor tone) is dominant, as can be demonstrated by the large increase in blood flow that occurs immediately after section of the sympathetic nerves to the tissue. After the onset of exercise, the intrinsic flow-regulating mechanism assumes control, and vasodilation occurs in the active muscles because of the local increase in metabolites. Vasoconstriction occurs in the inactive tissues as a manifestation of the general sympathetic discharge. However, constrictor impulses that reach the resistance vessels of the active muscles are overridden by the local metabolic effect. Operation of this dual control mechanism thus provides increased blood flow where it is required and shunts it away from relatively inactive areas (see also Chapter 17). Similar effects may be achieved in response to an increase in P_{CO_2}. Normally, the hyperventilation associated with exercise keeps P_{CO_2} at normal levels. However, if P_{CO_2} is increased, generalized vasoconstriction would occur because CO_2 stimulates the medullary vasoconstrictor region. In active muscles, where $[CO_2]$ would be highest, the smooth muscle of the arterioles would relax in response to the local P_{CO_2}. Factors that affect and are affected by the vasomotor region are summarized in Figure 18-28.

▶ IN THE CLINIC

Cerebral ischemia, which may occur because of excessive pressure exerted by an expanding intracranial tumor, results in a marked increase in peripheral vasoconstriction. The stimulation is probably caused by local accumulation of CO_2 and a reduction in O_2 and possibly by excitation of intracranial baroreceptors. With prolonged, severe ischemia, central depression eventually supervenes, and blood pressure falls.

■ KEY CONCEPTS

1. Cardiac function is regulated by a number of intrinsic and extrinsic mechanisms. The principal intrinsic mechanisms that regulate myocardial contraction are the Frank-Starling mechanism and rate-induced regulation.

2. The heart rate is regulated mainly by the autonomic nervous system. Sympathetic nervous activity increases the heart rate, whereas para-

● **Figure 18-28.** Schematic diagram illustrating neural input and output of the vasomotor region (VR). IX, glossopharyngeal nerve; X, vagus nerve.

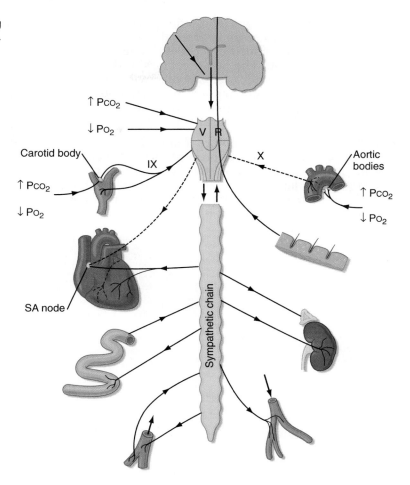

sympathetic (vagal) activity decreases the heart rate. When both systems are active, the vagal effects usually dominate. The autonomic nervous system regulates myocardial performance mainly by varying the Ca^{++} conductance of the cell membrane via the adenylyl cyclase system.

3. The following reflexes regulate the heart rate: the baroreceptor, chemoreceptor, pulmonary inflation, atrial receptor (Bainbridge), and ventricular receptor reflexes.

4. Certain hormones, such as epinephrine, adrenocortical steroids, thyroid hormones, insulin, glucagon, and anterior pituitary hormones, regulate myocardial performance. Changes in the arterial blood concentrations of O_2, CO_2, and H^+ directly alter cardiac function and indirectly alter it via the chemoreceptors.

5. The arterioles (resistance vessels) mainly regulate blood flow through their downstream capillaries. Smooth muscle, which makes up most of the walls of arterioles, contracts and relaxes in response to neural and humoral stimuli. Neural regulation of blood flow is almost completely accomplished by the sympathetic nervous system. Sympathetic nerves to blood vessels are tonically active; inhibition of the vasoconstrictor center in the medulla

reduces peripheral vascular resistance. Stimulation of the sympathetic nerves constricts the resistance and capacitance (veins) vessels. Parasympathetic fibers innervate the head, viscera, and genitalia; they do not innervate the skin and muscle.

6. Autoregulation of blood flow occurs in most tissues. This process is characterized by a constant blood flow in the face of a change in perfusion pressure. Autoregulation is mediated by a myogenic mechanism whereby an increase in transmural pressure elicits a contraction of vascular smooth muscle and a decrease in transmural pressure elicits a relaxation.

7. The striking parallelism between tissue blood flow and tissue O_2 consumption indicates that blood flow is regulated largely by a metabolic mechanism. A decrease in the O_2 supply–to–O_2 demand ratio of a tissue releases vasodilator metabolites that dilate arterioles and thereby enhance the O_2 supply.

8. The baroreceptors in the internal carotid arteries and aorta are tonically active and regulate blood pressure on a moment-to-moment basis. An increase in arterial pressure stretches these receptors to initiate a reflex that inhibits the medullary

vasoconstrictor center and induces vasodilation. Conversely, a decrease in arterial pressure disinhibits the vasoconstrictor center and induces vasoconstriction. The baroreceptors in the internal carotid arteries predominate over those in the aorta, and they respond more vigorously to changes in pressure (stretch) than they do to elevated or reduced nonpulsatile pressure.

9. Peripheral chemoreceptors (carotid and aortic bodies) and central chemoreceptors in the medulla oblongata are stimulated by a decrease in blood P_{O_2} and by an increase in blood P_{CO_2}. Stimulation of these chemoreceptors increases the rate and depth of respiration, but it also produces peripheral vasoconstriction. Cardiopulmonary baroreceptors are also present in the cardiac chambers and large pulmonary vessels. They have less influence on blood pressure but participate in regulation of blood volume.

10. Peripheral resistance and hence blood pressure are affected by stimuli that arise in the skin, viscera, lungs, and brain. The combined effect of neural and local metabolic factors distributes blood to active tissues and diverts it from inactive tissues. In vital structures, such as in the heart and brain and in contracting skeletal muscle, the metabolic factors predominate.

CHAPTER 19

Integrated Control of the Cardiovascular System

REGULATION OF CARDIAC OUTPUT AND BLOOD PRESSURE

Four factors control cardiac output: heart rate, myocardial contractility, preload, and afterload (Fig. 19-1). Heart rate and myocardial contractility are strictly cardiac factors, although they are controlled by various neural and humoral mechanisms. Preload and afterload are factors that are mutually dependent on function of the heart and the vasculature and are important determinants of cardiac output. Preload and afterload are themselves determined by cardiac output and by certain vascular characteristics. Preload and afterload will be called coupling factors because they constitute a functional coupling between the heart and blood vessels. To understand regulation of cardiac output, the nature of the coupling between the heart and the vascular system must be appreciated.

In this chapter, two kinds of graphs are used to analyze interactions between the cardiac and vascular components of the circulatory system. The first curve is called the **cardiac function curve.** It is an expression of the well-known **Frank-Starling relationship** and it illustrates the dependence of cardiac output on preload (i.e., central venous, or right atrial, pressure). The cardiac function curve is a characteristic of the heart itself and is usually studied in hearts completely isolated from the rest of the circulation. This curve has already been discussed in detail in Chapters 16 and 17. We use this curve later in this chapter in association with the other characteristic curve to analyze interactions between the heart and the vasculature.

The second curve, called the **vascular function curve,** defines the dependence of central venous pressure on cardiac output. This relationship depends only on certain vascular system characteristics, namely, peripheral vascular resistance, arterial and venous compliance, and blood volume. The vascular function curve is entirely independent of the characteristics of the heart. Because of this independence, it can be derived experimentally even if a mechanical pump replaces the heart.

VASCULAR FUNCTION CURVE

The vascular function curve defines the changes in central venous pressure that are caused by changes in cardiac output. In this curve, central venous pressure is the dependent variable (or response), and cardiac output is the independent variable (or stimulus). These variables are opposite those of the cardiac function curve, in which central venous pressure (or preload) is the independent variable and cardiac output is the dependent variable.

The simplified model of the circulation shown in Figure 19-2 helps explain how cardiac output determines the level of central venous pressure. In this model, all essential components of the cardiovascular system have been lumped into four basic elements. The right and left sides of the heart, as well as the pulmonary vascular bed, constitute a **pump-oxygenator,** much like an artificial heart-lung machine used to perfuse the body during open-heart surgery. The high-resistance microcirculation is designated the **peripheral resistance.** Finally, the compliance of the system is subdivided into **arterial compliance (C_a)** and **venous compliance (C_v).** As defined in Chapter 17, the compliance (C) of a blood vessel is the change in volume (ΔV) that is accommodated in that vessel per unit change in transmural pressure (ΔP); that is,

● **Equation 19-1**

$$C = \Delta V/\Delta P$$

Venous compliance is about 20 times greater than arterial compliance. In our example, the ratio of C_v to C_a is set at 19:1 to simplify calculations.*

To show how a change in cardiac output causes an inverse change in central venous pressure, our hypothetical model will have certain characteristics that mimic those of an average adult person (Fig. 19-2, *A*). The flow (Q_h) generated by the heart (i.e., cardiac output) will be 5 L/min; mean arterial pressure, P_a, will be 102 mm Hg; and central venous pressure, P_v, will be 2 mm Hg. Peripheral resistance, R, is the ratio of the arteriovenous pressure difference ($P_a - P_v$) to flow (Q_r) through the resistance vessels; this ratio will equal 20 mm Hg/L/min.

An arteriovenous pressure difference of 100 mm Hg is sufficient to force a flow (Q_r) of 5 L/min through a peripheral resistance of 20 mm Hg/L/min (Fig. 19-2, *A*).

---

*Thus, if it were necessary to add x mL of blood to the arterial system to produce a 1–mm Hg increase in arterial pressure, 19x mL of blood would need to be added to the venous system to raise venous pressure by the same amount.

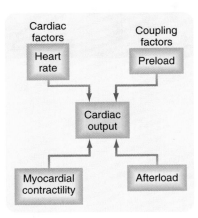

● **Figure 19-1.** The four factors that determine cardiac output.

Under equilibrium conditions, this flow (Q_r) is precisely equal to the flow (Q_h) pumped by the heart. From heartbeat to heartbeat, the volume (V_a) of blood in the arteries and the volume (V_v) of blood in the veins remain constant because the volume of blood transferred from the veins to the arteries by the heart equals the volume of blood that flows from the arteries through the resistance vessels and into the veins.

Effects of Cardiac Arrest on Arterial and Venous Pressure

Figure 19-2, *B,* shows the circulation at the very beginning of an episode of cardiac arrest; that is, $Q_h = 0$. In the instant immediately after arrest of the heart, the volume of blood in the arteries (V_a) and veins (V_v) has not had time to change appreciably. Because arterial pressure and venous pressure depend on V_a and V_v, respectively, these pressures are identical to the respective pressures in Figure 19-2, *A* (i.e., $P_a = 102$ and $P_v = 2$). This arteriovenous pressure gradient of 100 mm Hg forces a flow (Q_r) of 5 L/min through the peripheral resistance of 20 mm Hg/L/min. Thus, although cardiac output (Q_h) now equals 0 L/min, flow through the microcirculation equals 5 L/min because the potential energy stored in the arteries by the preceding pumping action of the heart causes blood to be transferred from arteries to veins. This transfer occurs initially at the control rate, even though the heart can no longer transfer blood from the veins to the arteries.

As the heart continues in arrest, blood flow through the resistance vessels causes the blood volume in the arteries to decrease progressively and the blood volume in the veins to increase progressively at the same absolute rate. Because the arteries and veins are elastic structures, arterial pressure falls gradually and the venous pressure rises gradually. This process continues until arterial and venous pressures become equal (Fig. 19-2, *C*). Once this condition is reached, flow (Q_r) from the arteries to the veins through the resistance vessels is zero, as is Q_h.

When the effects of cardiac arrest reach this equilibrium state (Fig. 19-2, *C*), the pressure attained in the arteries and veins depends on the relative compliance of these vessels. If arterial compliance (C_a) and venous compliance (C_v) are equal, the decline in P_a would equal the rise in P_v because the decrease in arterial volume would equal the increase in venous volume (principle of conservation of mass). Both P_a and P_v would attain the average of their combined values in Figure 19-2, *A;* that is, $P_a = P_v = (102 + 2)/2 = 52$ mm Hg. However, C_a and C_v in a living subject are not equal. Veins are much more compliant than arteries; the compliance ratio (C_v/C_a) is approximately 19, the ratio that we have assumed for the model. When the effects of cardiac arrest reach equilibrium in an intact subject, the pressure in the arteries and veins is much less than the average value of 52 mm Hg that occurs when C_a and C_v are equal. Hence, transfer of blood from arteries to veins at equilibrium induces a fall in arterial pressure 19 times greater than the concomitant rise in venous pressure. As Figure 19-2, *C,* shows, P_v would increase by 5 mm Hg (to 7 mm Hg), whereas P_a would fall by $19 \times 5 = 95$ mm Hg (to 7 mm Hg). This equilibrium pressure, which prevails in the absence of flow, is referred to as either **mean circulatory pressure** or **static pressure.** The pressure in the static system reflects the total blood volume in the system and the overall compliance of the system.

The example of cardiac arrest aids our understanding of the vascular function curve. One can now begin to assemble a vascular function curve (Fig. 19-3). The independent variable (plotted along the x axis) is cardiac output, and the dependent variable (plotted along the y axis) is central venous pressure. Two important points on this curve can be derived from the example in Figure 19-2. One point (A in Fig. 19-3) represents the control state; that is, when cardiac output is 5 L/min, P_v is 2 mm Hg (as depicted in Fig. 19-2, *A*). Then, when the heart is arrested (cardiac output = 0), P_v becomes 7 mm Hg at equilibrium (Fig. 19-2, *C*); this pressure is the mean circulatory pressure (P_{mc} in Fig. 19-3).

The inverse relationship between P_v and cardiac output simply denotes that when cardiac output is suddenly decreased, the rate at which blood flows from arteries to veins through the capillaries is temporarily greater than the rate at which the heart pumps blood from the veins back into the arteries. During that transient period, a net volume of blood is transferred from arteries to veins; hence, P_a falls and P_v rises.

Now let us suddenly increase cardiac output. This example will illustrate how a third point (B in Fig. 19-3) on the vascular function curve is derived. Consider that the arrested heart is suddenly restarted and immediately begins pumping blood from the veins into the arteries at a rate of 1 L/min (Fig. 19-2, *D*). When the heart first begins to beat, the arteriovenous pressure gradient is zero, and no blood is transferred from the arteries through the capillaries and into the veins. Thus, when beating resumes, blood is depleted from the veins at the rate of 1 L/min, and arterial blood volume is repleted from venous blood volume at that same absolute rate. Hence, P_v begins to fall and P_a

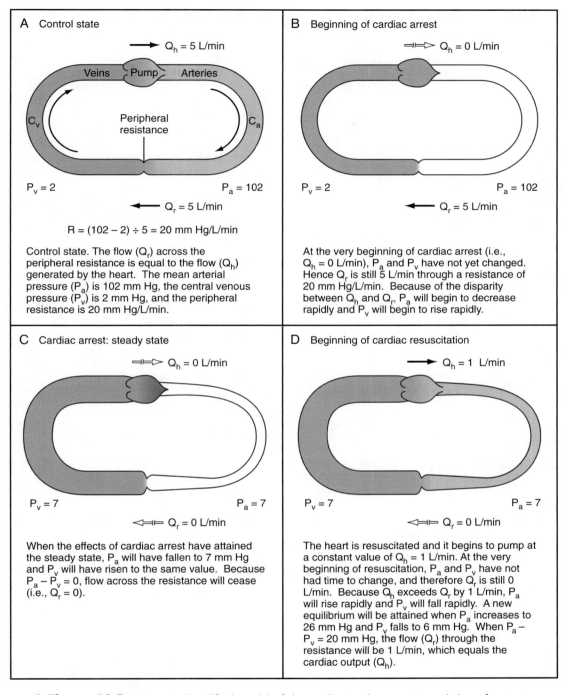

A   Control state

$Q_h = 5$ L/min

Veins | Pump | Arteries

C_v C_a

Peripheral resistance

$P_v = 2$ $P_a = 102$

$Q_r = 5$ L/min

$$R = (102 - 2) \div 5 = 20 \text{ mm Hg/L/min}$$

Control state. The flow (Q_r) across the peripheral resistance is equal to the flow (Q_h) generated by the heart. The mean arterial pressure (P_a) is 102 mm Hg, the central venous pressure (P_v) is 2 mm Hg, and the peripheral resistance is 20 mm Hg/L/min.

B   Beginning of cardiac arrest

$Q_h = 0$ L/min

$P_v = 2$ $P_a = 102$

$Q_r = 5$ L/min

At the very beginning of cardiac arrest (i.e., $Q_h = 0$ L/min), P_a and P_v have not yet changed. Hence Q_r is still 5 L/min through a resistance of 20 mm Hg/L/min. Because of the disparity between Q_h and Q_r, P_a will begin to decrease rapidly and P_v will begin to rise rapidly.

C   Cardiac arrest: steady state

$Q_h = 0$ L/min

$P_v = 7$ $P_a = 7$

$Q_r = 0$ L/min

When the effects of cardiac arrest have attained the steady state, P_a will have fallen to 7 mm Hg and P_v will have risen to the same value. Because $P_a - P_v = 0$, flow across the resistance will cease (i.e., $Q_r = 0$).

D   Beginning of cardiac resuscitation

$Q_h = 1$ L/min

$P_v = 7$ $P_a = 7$

$Q_r = 0$ L/min

The heart is resuscitated and it begins to pump at a constant value of $Q_h = 1$ L/min. At the very beginning of resuscitation, P_a and P_v have not had time to change, and therefore Q_r is still 0 L/min. Because Q_h exceeds Q_r by 1 L/min, P_a will rise rapidly and P_v will fall rapidly. A new equilibrium will be attained when P_a increases to 26 mm Hg and P_v falls to 6 mm Hg. When $P_a - P_v = 20$ mm Hg, the flow (Q_r) through the resistance will be 1 L/min, which equals the cardiac output (Q_h).

● **Figure 19-2.   A** to **D,** Simplified model of the cardiovascular system consisting of a pump, arterial compliance (C_a), peripheral resistance, and venous compliance (C_v).

begins to rise. Because of the difference in arterial and venous compliance, P_a will rise at a rate 19 times faster than the rate at which P_v will fall.

The resultant arteriovenous pressure gradient causes blood to flow through the peripheral resistance. If the heart maintains a constant output of 1 L/min, P_a will continue to rise and P_v will continue to fall until the pressure gradient becomes 20 mm Hg. This gradient will force a flow of 1 L/min through a resistance of 20 mm Hg/L/min. This gradient will be

achieved by a 19–mm Hg rise (to 26 mm Hg) in P_a and a 1–mm Hg fall (to 6 mm Hg) in P_v. This equilibrium value of $P_v = 6$ mm Hg for a cardiac output of 1 L/min also appears on the vascular function curve of Figure 19-3 (point B). The 1–mm Hg reduction in P_v reflects a net transfer of blood from the venous to the arterial side of the circuit.

The reduction in P_v that can be evoked by a sudden increase in cardiac output is limited. At some critical maximal value of cardiac output, sufficient fluid will be transferred from the venous to the arterial side of the circuit for P_v to fall below ambient pressure. In a system of very distensible vessels, such as the venous system, the vessels will be collapsed by the greater external pressure (see Chapter 17). This venous collapse impedes venous return to the heart. Hence, it limits the maximal value of cardiac output to 7 L/min in this example (Fig. 19-3), regardless of the capabilities of the pump.

Factors That Influence the Vascular Function Curve
Dependence of Venous Pressure on Cardiac Output
Experimental and clinical observations have shown that changes in cardiac output do indeed evoke the alterations in P_a and P_v that have been predicted by our simplified model.

Blood Volume
The vascular function curve is affected by variations in total blood volume. During circulatory standstill (zero cardiac output), mean circulatory pressure depends only on total vascular compliance and blood volume. For a given vascular compliance, mean circulatory pressure is increased when blood volume is expanded **(hypervolemia)** and is decreased when blood volume is diminished **(hypovolemia).** This rela-

IN THE CLINIC

Cardiac output may decrease abruptly when a major coronary artery suddenly becomes occluded in a human patient. The **acute heart failure** that occurs as a result of **myocardial infarction** (death of myocardial tissue) is usually accompanied by a fall in arterial blood pressure and a rise in central venous pressure.

tionship is illustrated by the y axis intercepts in Figure 19-4, where mean circulatory pressure is 5 mm Hg after hemorrhage and 9 mm Hg after transfusion, as compared with a value of 7 mm Hg at normal blood volume **(normovolemia or euvolemia).**

From Figure 19-4 it is also apparent that the cardiac output at which $P_v = 0$ varies directly with blood volume. Therefore, the maximal value of cardiac output becomes progressively more limited as the total blood volume is reduced. However, the central venous pressure at which the veins collapse (illustrated by the sharp change in slope of the vascular function curve) is not significantly altered by changes in blood volume. This pressure depends only on the ambient pressure surrounding the central veins. Ambient pressure is the pleural pressure in the thorax (see Chapter 21).

Venomotor Tone
The effects of changes in venomotor tone on the vascular function curve closely resemble those for changes in blood volume. In Figure 19-4, for example, the transfusion curve could also represent increased venomotor tone, whereas the hemorrhage curve could represent decreased tone. During circulatory standstill, for a given blood volume the pressure within the vascular system will rise as smooth muscle tension exerted within the vascular walls increases (these contractile changes in arteriolar and venous smooth muscle are under nervous and humoral control). The fraction of the blood volume located within the arterioles is very small, whereas the blood volume in the veins is large (see Table 15-1). Thus, changes in peripheral resistance (arteriolar tone) have no significant effect on mean circulatory pressure, but changes in venous tone can alter mean circulatory pressure appreciably. Hence, mean circulatory pressure rises

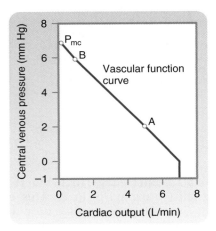

●**Figure 19-3.** Changes in central venous pressure produced by changes in cardiac output. The mean circulatory pressure (or static pressure), P_{mc}, is the equilibrium pressure throughout the cardiovascular system when cardiac output is 0. Points B and A represent the values of venous pressure at a cardiac output of 1 and 5 L/min, respectively.

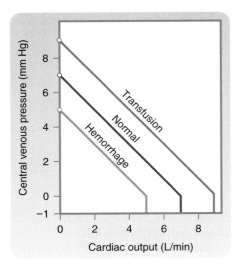

●**Figure 19-4.** Effects of increased blood volume (transfusion curve) and decreased blood volume (hemorrhage curve) on the vascular function curve. Similar shifts in the vascular function curve can be produced by increases and decreases, respectively, in venomotor tone.

with increased venomotor tone and falls with diminished venomotor tone.

Experimentally, the mean circulatory pressure attained about 1 minute after abrupt circulatory standstill is usually substantially above 7 mm Hg, even when blood volume is normal. This high pressure level is attributable to the generalized venoconstriction that is caused by cerebral ischemia, activation of chemoreceptors, and reduced excitation of baroreceptors. If resuscitation fails, this reflex response subsides as central nervous activity ceases, and mean circulatory pressure usually falls to a value close to 7 mm Hg.

Blood Reservoirs

Venoconstriction is considerably greater in certain regions of the body than in others. In effect, vascular beds that undergo significant venoconstriction constitute blood reservoirs. The skin's vascular bed is one of the major blood reservoirs in humans. Blood loss evokes profound subcutaneous venoconstriction, which gives rise to the characteristically pale appearance of the skin in response to hemorrhage. Diversion of blood away from the skin frees several hundred milliliters of blood that can be perfused through more vital regions of the body. The vascular beds of the liver, lungs, and spleen are also important blood reservoirs. In humans, however, the volume changes in the spleen are considerably less extensive (see also Exercise and Hemorrhage).

Peripheral Resistance

The changes in the vascular function curve induced by alterations in arteriolar tone are shown in Figure 19-5. The amount of blood in the arterioles is small—they contain only about 3% of total blood volume (see Chapter 15). Changes in the contractile state of arterioles do not significantly alter mean circulatory pressure. Thus, vascular function curves that represent different peripheral resistances converge at a common point on the abscissa.

P_v varies inversely with **total peripheral resistance (TPR)** when all other factors remain constant. Physiologically, the relationship between P_v and TPR can be explained as follows: if cardiac output is held constant, a sudden increase in TPR causes a progressively greater volume of blood to be retained in the arterial system. Blood volume in the arterial system continues to increase until P_a rises sufficiently to force a flow of blood equal to cardiac output through the resistance vessels. If total blood volume does not change, this increase in arterial blood volume is accompanied by an equivalent decrease in venous blood volume. Hence, an increase in TPR diminishes P_v proportionately. This relationship between TPR and P_v, together with the inability of peripheral resistance to affect mean circulatory pressure, accounts for the clockwise rotation of the vascular function curves in response to increased arteriolar constriction (see Fig. 19-5). Similarly, arteriolar dilation produces a counterclockwise rotation from the same vertical axis intercept. A higher maximal level of cardiac output is attainable when the arterioles are dilated than when they are constricted (Fig. 19-5).

Interrelationships between Cardiac Output and Venous Return

Cardiac output and venous return are tightly linked. Except for small, transient disparities, the heart cannot pump any more blood than is delivered to it through the venous system. Similarly, because the circulatory system is a closed circuit, venous return to the heart must equal cardiac output over any appreciable time interval. The flow around the entire closed circuit depends on the capability of the pump, the characteristics of the circuit, and the total fluid volume of the system.

Thus, cardiac output and venous return are simply two terms for the flow around this closed circuit. Cardiac output is the volume of blood being pumped by the heart per unit time. Venous return is the volume of blood returning to the heart per unit time. At equilibrium, these two flows are equal. In the following section we apply certain techniques of circuit analysis to gain some insight into the control of flow around the circuit.

RELATING THE CARDIAC FUNCTION CURVE TO THE VASCULAR FUNCTION CURVE

Coupling between the Heart and the Vasculature

In accordance with Starling's law of the heart, cardiac output depends closely on right atrial (or central venous) pressure. Furthermore, right atrial pressure is approximately equal to right ventricular end-diastolic pressure because the normal tricuspid valve acts as a low-resistance junction between the right atrium and ventricle. Graphs of cardiac output as a function of central venous pressure (P_v) are called **cardiac function curves;** extrinsic regulatory influences may be expressed as shifts in such curves.

A typical cardiac function curve is plotted on the same coordinates as a normal vascular function curve in Figure 19-6. The cardiac function curve is plotted

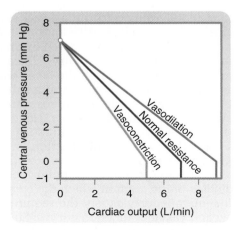

● **Figure 19-5.** Effects of arteriolar dilation and constriction on the vascular function curve.

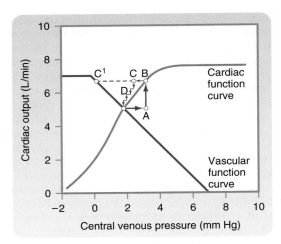

● **Figure 19-6.** Typical vascular and cardiac function curves plotted on the same coordinate axes. Note that to plot both curves on the same graph, the x and y axes for the vascular function curves had to be reversed; compare the assignment of axes with that in Figures 19-3, 19-4, and 19-5. The coordinates of the equilibrium point, at the intersection of the cardiac and vascular function curves, represent the stable values of cardiac output and central venous pressure at which the system tends to operate. Any perturbation (e.g., a sudden increase in venous pressure to point A) institutes a sequence of changes in cardiac output and venous pressure that restore these variables to their equilibrium values.

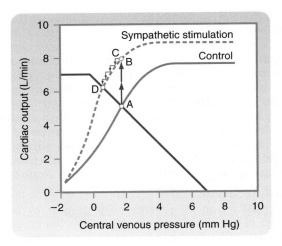

● **Figure 19-7.** Enhancement of myocardial contractility, as by cardiac sympathetic nerve stimulation, causes the equilibrium values of cardiac output and central venous pressure (P_v) to shift from the intersection (point A) of the control vascular and cardiac function curves (continuous curve) to the intersection (point D) of the same vascular function curve with the cardiac function curve *(dashed curve)* that represents the response to sympathetic stimulation.

according to the usual convention; that is, the independent variable (P_v) is plotted along the abscissa, and the dependent variable (cardiac output) is plotted along the ordinate. From the Frank-Starling mechanism, the cardiac function curve reveals that a rise in P_v increases cardiac output.

Conversely, the vascular function curve describes an inverse relationship between cardiac output and P_v; that is, a rise in cardiac output diminishes P_v. P_v is the dependent variable (or response) and cardiac output is the independent variable (or stimulus) for the vascular function curve. Therefore, to plot a vascular function curve in the conventional manner, P_v should be scaled along the y axis and cardiac output along the x axis.

To plot the cardiac and vascular function curves on the same set of axes requires a modification of the plotting convention for one of these curves. We arbitrarily violate the convention for the vascular function curve. Note that the vascular function curve in Figure 19-6 is intended to reflect how P_v (scaled along the x axis) varies in response to a change in cardiac output (scaled along the y axis).

When the cardiovascular system is represented by a given pair of cardiac and vascular function curves, the intersection of these two curves defines the **equilibrium point** of that system. The coordinates of this equilibrium point represent the values of cardiac output and P_v at which the system tends to operate. Only transient deviations from such values of cardiac output and P_v are possible, as long as the given cardiac and vascular function curves accurately describe the system.

The tendency to operate about this equilibrium point may best be illustrated by examining the response to a sudden change. Consider the changes caused by a sudden rise in P_v from the equilibrium point to point A in Figure 19-6. This change in P_v might be caused by the rapid injection, during ventricular diastole, of a given volume of blood on the venous side of the circuit and simultaneous withdrawal of an equal volume from the arterial side of the circuit. Thus, although P_v rises, total blood volume remains constant.

As defined by the cardiac function curve, this elevated P_v would increase cardiac output (from A to B) during the next ventricular systole. The increased cardiac output would then transfer a net quantity of blood from the venous to the arterial side of the circuit, with a consequent reduction in P_v. In one heartbeat the reduction in P_v would be small (from B to C) because the heart would transfer only a fraction of the total venous blood volume to the arterial side. As a result of this reduction in P_v, cardiac output during the very next beat diminishes (from C to D) by an amount dictated by the cardiac function curve. Because D is still above the intersection point, the heart will pump blood from the veins to the arteries at a rate greater than that at which blood will flow across the peripheral resistance from arteries to veins. Hence, P_v will continue to fall. This process will continue in diminishing steps until the point of intersection is reached. Only one specific combination of cardiac output and venous pressure—the equilibrium point, denoted by the coordinates of the point at which the curves intersect—will simultaneously satisfy the requirements of the cardiac and vascular function curves. Stable operation of the system at the equilibrium point (A, in Fig. 19-6) indicates that cardiac output equals venous return.

Myocardial Contractility

Combinations of cardiac and vascular function curves also help explain the effects of alterations in ventricular contractility on cardiac output and P_v. In Figure 19-7, the lower cardiac function curve represents the control state, whereas the upper curve reflects the influence of increased myocardial contractility. This pair of curves is analogous to the "family" of ventricular function curves shown in Figure 18-12. The enhanced ventricular contractility represented by the upper curve in Figure 19-7 can be produced by electrical stimulation of the cardiac sympathetic nerves. When the effects of such neural stimulation are restricted to the heart, the vascular function curve is unaffected. Therefore, only one vascular function curve is needed for this hypothetical intervention (Fig. 19-7).

During the control state of the model, the equilibrium values for cardiac output and P_v are designated by point A in Figure 19-7. Cardiac sympathetic nerve stimulation abruptly raises cardiac output to point B because of the enhanced myocardial contractility. However, this high cardiac output increases the net transfer of blood from the venous to the arterial side of the circuit, and consequently, P_v subsequently begins to fall (to point C). The reduction in P_v then leads to a small decrease in cardiac output. However, cardiac output is still sufficiently high to effect the net transfer of blood from the venous to the arterial side of the circuit. Thus, P_v and cardiac output both continue to fall gradually until a new equilibrium point (D) is reached. This equilibrium point is located at the intersection of the vascular function curve and the new cardiac function curve. Point D lies above and to the left of the control equilibrium point (A) and indicates that sympathetic stimulation can evoke greater cardiac output despite the lower level of P_v.

The biological response to enhancement of myocardial contractility is mimicked by the hypothetical change predicted by our model. As depicted in Figure 19-8, sympathetic nerves innervating the heart are stimulated during the time denoted by the two arrows. During neural stimulation, cardiac output (aortic flow) rose quickly to a peak value and then fell gradually to a steady-state value significantly greater than the control level. The increased aortic flow was accompanied by reductions in right and left atrial pressure (P_{RA} and P_{LA}).

Blood Volume

Changes in blood volume do not directly affect myocardial contractility, but they do influence the vascular function curve in the manner shown in Figure 19-4. Thus, to understand how changes in blood volume affect cardiac output and P_v, the appropriate cardiac function curve is plotted along with the vascular function curves that represent the control and experimental states (Fig. 19-9).

When blood volume is increased by a blood transfusion, the equilibrium point (B), which denotes the values of cardiac output and P_v after transfusion, lies above and to the right of the control equilibrium point

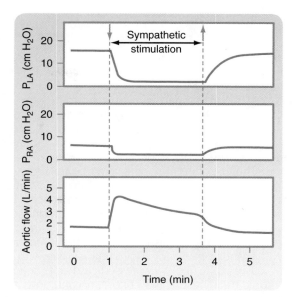

● **Figure 19-8.** During electrical stimulation of the cardiac sympathetic nerve fibers, aortic blood flow (cardiac output) increased while pressure in the left atrium (P_{LA}) and right atrium (P_{RA}) diminished. These data conform to the conclusions derived from Figure 19-7, in which the equilibrium values of cardiac output and venous pressure are observed to shift from point A to point D (i.e., cardiac output increased, but central venous pressure decreased) during cardiac sympathetic nerve stimulation. (Redrawn from Sarnoff SJ et al: Circ Res 8:1108, 1960.)

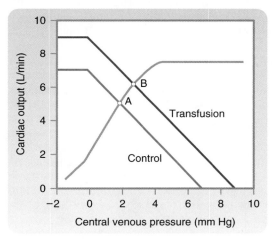

● **Figure 19-9.** After a blood transfusion, the vascular function curve is shifted to the right. Therefore, cardiac output and venous pressure are both increased, as denoted by translocation of the equilibrium point from A to B.

(A). Thus, transfusion increases both cardiac output and P_v. Hemorrhage causes the opposite effect. Mechanistically, the change in ventricular filling pressure (central venous pressure) evoked by a given change in blood volume alters cardiac output by changing the sensitivity of the contractile proteins to the prevailing concentration of intracellular Ca^{++} (see Chapters 17

▶ IN THE CLINIC

Heart failure is a general term that applies to conditions in which the pumping capability of the heart is impaired to the extent that the tissues of the body are not adequately perfused. In heart failure, myocardial contractility is impaired. Heart failure may be acute or chronic. Consequently, in a graph of cardiac and vascular function curves, the cardiac function curve is shifted downward and to the right, as depicted in Figure 19-10.

Acute heart failure may be caused by toxic concentrations of drugs or by certain pathological conditions such as coronary artery occlusion. In acute heart failure, blood volume does not change immediately. In Figure 19-10, therefore, the equilibrium point shifts from the intersection (A) of the normal curves to the intersection (B or C) of the normal vascular function curve with one of the curves that depict depressed cardiac function.

Chronic heart failure may occur in conditions such as essential hypertension or ischemic heart disease. In chronic heart failure, both the cardiac function and vascular function curves shift. The vascular function curve shifts because of an increase in blood volume caused in part by fluid retention by the kidneys. The fluid retention is related to the concomitant reduction in glomerular filtration rate and the decreased renal excretion of NaCl and water (see also Chapter 34). The resultant hypervolemia is reflected by a rightward shift of the vascular function curve, as shown in Figure 19-10. Hence, with moderate degrees of heart failure, P_v is elevated, but cardiac output may be normal (D). With more severe degrees of heart failure, P_v is still greater, but cardiac output is subnormal (E).

and 18). For reasons explained earlier, pure increases or decreases in venomotor tone elicit responses that are like those evoked by increases or decreases, respectively, in total blood volume.

Peripheral Resistance

Analysis of the effects of changes in peripheral resistance on cardiac output and P_v is complex because both the cardiac and vascular function curves shift. When peripheral resistance increases (Fig. 19-11), the vascular function curve is rotated counterclockwise, but it converges on the same P_v axis intercept as the control curve does. Note that vasoconstriction causes a counterclockwise rotation of the vascular function curve in Figure 19-11 but a clockwise rotation in Figure 19-5. The direction of rotation differs because the axes for the vascular function curves were reversed in these two figures, as explained earlier. The cardiac function curve in Figure 19-11 is also shifted downward because at any given P_v, the heart is able to pump less blood against the greater cardiac afterload imposed by the increased peripheral resistance. Because both curves in Figure 19-11 are displaced downward, the new equilibrium point, B, falls below the control point, A; that is, an increase in peripheral resistance diminishes cardiac output.

Whether point B falls directly below point A or lies slightly to the right or left of it depends on the magnitude of the shift in each curve. For example, if a given increase in peripheral resistance shifts the vascular function curve more than it does the cardiac function curve, equilibrium point B will fall below and to the left of A; that is, both cardiac output and P_v will diminish. Conversely, if the cardiac function curve is displaced more than the vascular function curve, point B falls below and to the right of point A; that is, cardiac output decreases, but P_v rises.

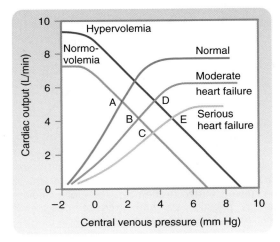

● **Figure 19-10.** Moderate or severe heart failure shifts the cardiac function curves downward and to the right. Before changes in blood volume, cardiac output decreases and central venous pressure rises (from control equilibrium point A to point B or point C). After the increase in blood volume that usually occurs in heart failure, the vascular function curve is shifted to the right. Hence, central venous pressure may be elevated with no reduction in cardiac output (point D) or (in severe heart failure) with some reduction in cardiac output (point E).

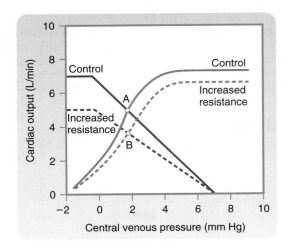

● **Figure 19-11.** An increase in peripheral resistance shifts the cardiac and vascular function curves downward. At equilibrium, cardiac output is less (B) when peripheral resistance is high than when it is normal (A).

A MORE COMPLETE THEORETICAL MODEL: THE TWO-PUMP SYSTEM

The preceding discussion shows that the interrelationships between cardiac output and central venous pressure are complex, even in an oversimplified circulation model that includes only one pump and just the systemic circulation. In reality, the cardiovascular system includes the systemic and pulmonary circulations and two pumps: the left and right ventricles. Thus, the interrelationships among ventricular output, arterial pressure, and atrial pressure are much more complex.

Figure 19-12 shows a more complete, but still oversimplified cardiovascular system model that has two pumps in series (the left and right ventricles) and two vascular beds in series (the systemic and pulmonary vasculature). The series arrangement requires that the flow pumped by the two ventricles be virtually equal to each other over any substantial period; otherwise, all the blood would ultimately accumulate in one or the other of the vascular systems. Because the cardiac function curves for the two ventricles differ substantially, the filling (atrial) pressures for the two ventricles must differ appropriately to ensure equal stroke volumes (see Fig. 18-13).

> ### ▶ IN THE CLINIC
>
> Any change in contractility that affects the two ventricles differently alters the distribution of blood volume in the two vascular systems. If a coronary artery to the left ventricle becomes occluded, left ventricular contractility will be impaired and **acute left ventricular failure** will ensue. In the instant after occlusion, left atrial pressure will not change and the left ventricle will begin to pump a diminished flow. If the right ventricle is not affected by the acute coronary artery occlusion, the right ventricle will initially continue to pump the normal flow. The disparate right and left ventricular output will result in a progressive increase in left atrial pressure and a progressive decrease in right atrial pressure. Therefore, left ventricular output will increase toward the normal value and right ventricular output will fall below the normal value. This process will continue until the output of the two ventricles again becomes equal. At this new equilibrium, the output of the two ventricles will be subnormal. The elevated left atrial pressure will be accompanied by an equally elevated pulmonary venous pressure, which can have serious clinical consequences. The high pulmonary venous pressure can increase lung stiffness and lead to respiratory distress by increasing the mechanical work of pulmonary ventilation (see Chapter 22). Furthermore, the high pulmonary venous pressure will elevate the hydrostatic pressure in the pulmonary capillaries and may lead to the transudation of fluid from the pulmonary capillaries to the pulmonary interstitium or into the alveoli **(pulmonary edema),** which may be lethal.

Two basic principles to remember about ventricular function are that (1) the left ventricle pumps blood through the systemic vasculature, and (2) the right ventricle pumps blood through the pulmonary vasculature. However, these principles do not necessarily imply that both ventricles are essential to perfuse the systemic and pulmonary vascular beds adequately. To better understand the relationships between the two ventricles and the two vascular beds, let us examine right ventricular function in more detail.

In the circulatory system model shown in Figure 19-12, consider the hemodynamic consequences that would occur if the right ventricle suddenly ceased its pump function but instead served merely as a passive, low-resistance conduit between the systemic veins and the pulmonary arteries. Under these conditions, the only functional pump would be the left ventricle, which would then be required to pump blood through both the systemic and pulmonary resistances (for our purposes, consider the resistance to the flow of blood through the inactive right ventricle to be negligible).

Normally, pulmonary vascular resistance is about 10% as great as systemic vascular resistance. Because the two resistances are in series with one another, total resistance would be 10% greater than systemic resistance alone (see Chapter 17). In a normal cardiovascular system, a 10% increase in systemic vascular resistance would increase mean arterial pressure (and hence left ventricular afterload) by approximately 10%. This increase would not drastically affect left ventricular function. Under certain conditions, however, this increase in mean arterial pressure could significantly alter the function of the cardiovascular system. If the 10% increase in total resistance is achieved by adding a small resistance (i.e., pulmonary vascular resistance) to that of the much larger systemic resistance and if the pulmonary vascular resistance is separated from the systemic resistance by a large compliance (the combined systemic venous and

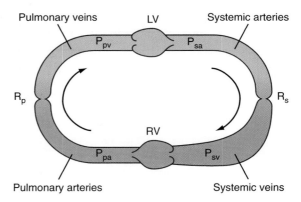

● **Figure 19-12.** Simplified cardiovascular system model that consists of the left (LV) and right (RV) ventricles, systemic (R_s) and pulmonary (R_p) vascular resistance, systemic arterial and venous compliance, and pulmonary arterial and venous compliance. P_{sa} and P_{sv} are the pressures in the systemic arteries and veins, respectively; P_{pa} and P_{pv} are the pressures in the pulmonary arteries and veins, respectively.

pulmonary arterial compliance), the 10% increase in total resistance could drastically impair operation of the cardiovascular system.

The simulated effects of inactivating the pumping action of the right ventricle in a hydraulic analogue of the circulatory system are shown in Figure 19-13. In the model, the right and left ventricles generate cardiac outputs that vary directly with their respective filling pressures. Under control conditions (when the right ventricle is functioning normally), the output of the left and right ventricles is equal (5 L/min). The right ventricular pumping action causes the pressure in the pulmonary artery (not shown) to exceed the pressure in the pulmonary veins (P_{pv}) by an amount that will force fluid through the pulmonary vascular resistance at a rate of 5 L/min.

When the right ventricle ceases pumping (arrow 1), the systemic venous and pulmonary arterial systems, along with the right ventricle itself, become a common passive conduit with a large compliance. When the right ventricle ceases to transfer blood actively from

the pulmonary veins to the pulmonary arteries, pulmonary arterial pressure (P_{pa}) decreases rapidly (not shown) and systemic venous pressure (P_{sv}) rises rapidly to a common value (about 5 mm Hg). At this low pressure, however, fluid flows from the pulmonary arteries to the pulmonary veins at a greatly reduced rate. At the start of right ventricular arrest, the left ventricle is pumping fluid from the pulmonary veins to the systemic arteries at the control rate of 5 L/min, which greatly exceeds the rate at which blood returns to the pulmonary veins once the right ventricle ceases to operate. Hence, pulmonary venous pressure (P_{pv}) drops sharply. Because pulmonary venous pressure is the preload for the left ventricle, left ventricular (cardiac) output drops abruptly as well and attains a steady-state value of about 2.5 L/min. This effect in turn leads to a rapid reduction in systemic arterial pressure (P_{sa}). In short, stoppage of right ventricular pumping markedly curtails cardiac output, systemic arterial pressure, and pulmonary venous pressure and raises systemic venous pressure moderately (Fig. 19-13).

Most of the hemodynamic problems induced by inactivation of the right ventricle can be reversed by increasing the fluid (blood) volume of the system (arrow 2, Fig. 19-13). If fluid is added until pulmonary venous pressure (left ventricular preload) is raised to its control value, cardiac output and systemic arterial pressure are restored almost to normal, but systemic venous pressure is abnormally elevated. If left ventricular function is normal, adding a normal left ventricular preload will evoke a normal left ventricular output. The 10% increase in peripheral resistance caused by adding the pulmonary vascular resistance to that of the systemic vascular resistance does not impose a serious burden on left ventricular pumping capacity.

When the right ventricle is inoperative, however, pulmonary blood flow will not be normal unless the usual pulmonary arteriovenous pressure gradient (about 10 to 15 mm Hg) prevails. Hence, systemic venous pressure (P_{sv}) must exceed pulmonary venous pressure (P_{pv}) by this amount. Maintenance of high systemic venous pressure may lead to the accumulation of tissue fluid (edema) in dependent regions of the body, a characteristic finding in patients with right ventricular heart failure.

With these findings in mind, one may characterize the principal function of the right ventricle as follows. From the viewpoint of providing sufficient flow of blood to all tissues in the body, the left ventricle alone can carry out this function. Operation of the two ventricles in series is not essential to provide adequate blood flow to the tissues. The crucial function of the right ventricle is to prevent the rise in systemic venous (and pulmonary arterial) pressure that would be required to force the normal cardiac output through the pulmonary vascular resistance. A normal right ventricle, by preventing an abnormal rise in systemic venous pressure, prevents the development of extensive edema in dependent regions of the body.

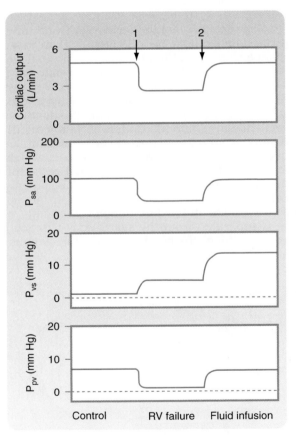

● **Figure 19-13.** Changes in cardiac output, systemic arterial pressure (P_{sa}), systemic venous pressure (P_{sv}), and pulmonary venous pressure (P_{pv}) evoked by simulated right ventricular (RV) failure and by simulated infusion of fluid in the circulatory model shown in Figure 19-12. At arrow 1, the pumping action of the right ventricle was discontinued (simulated RV failure), and the right ventricle served only as a low-resistance conduit. At arrow 2, the fluid volume in the system was expanded, and the right ventricle continued to serve only as a conduit. (Modified from Furey SA et al: Am Heart J 107:404, 1984).

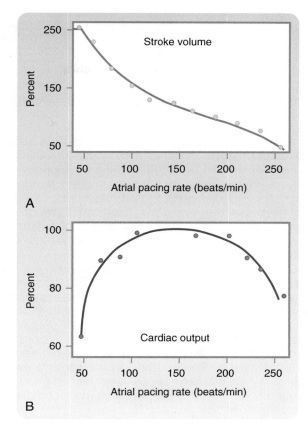

IN THE CLINIC

Clinically, **right ventricular heart failure** may be caused by occlusive disease predominantly of the coronary vessels to the right ventricle. These vessels are affected much less commonly than the vessels to the left ventricle. The major hemodynamic effects of acute right heart failure are pronounced reductions in cardiac output and arterial blood pressure, and the principal treatment is infusion of blood or plasma. Bypass of the right ventricle (by anastomosing the right atrium to the pulmonary artery) may be performed surgically in patients with certain **congenital cardiac defects,** such as severe narrowing of the tricuspid valve or maldevelopment of the right ventricle. The effects of acute right heart failure or right ventricular bypass are directionally similar to those predicted above by analysis of the model shown in Figure 19-13.

● **Figure 19-14.** Changes in stroke volume **(A)** and cardiac output **(B)** induced by changing the rate of atrial pacing. (Redrawn from Kumada M et al: Jpn J Physiol 17:538, 1967.)

ROLE OF THE HEART RATE IN CONTROL OF CARDIAC OUTPUT

Cardiac output is the product of stroke volume and heart rate. Analysis of the control of cardiac output has thus far been restricted to the control of stroke volume, and the role of heart rate has not been considered. Analysis of the effect of a change in heart rate on cardiac output is complex because a change in heart rate alters the other three factors (preload, afterload, and contractility) that determine stroke volume (Fig. 19-1). An increase in heart rate, for example, shortens the duration of diastole. Hence, ventricular filling is diminished; that is, preload is reduced. If an increase in heart rate altered cardiac output, arterial pressure would change; that is, afterload would be altered. Finally, a rise in heart rate would increase the net influx of Ca^{++} per minute into myocardial cells (see also Chapter 16), and this influx would enhance myocardial contractility.

The effects of changes in heart rate on cardiac output have been studied extensively, and the results are similar to those shown in Figure 19-14. As atrial pacing frequency is gradually increased, stroke volume progressively diminishes (Fig. 19-14, _A_). The decrease in stroke volume is caused by the reduced time for ventricular filling. The change in stroke volume is not inversely proportional to the change in heart rate because the direction of the change in cardiac output (Q_h) is markedly influenced by the actual level of the heart rate (Fig. 19-14, _B_). For example, as pacing frequency is increased from 50 to 100 beats/min, the increase in heart rate augments Q_h. Because $Q_h = SV \times HR$, the decrease in stroke volume (SV) over this frequency range must be proportionately less than the increase in heart rate (HR).

Over the frequency range from about 100 to 200 beats/min, however, Q_h is not affected significantly by changes in pacing frequency (Fig. 19-14, _B_). Hence, as pacing frequency is increased, the decrease in stroke volume must be approximately equal to the increase

in heart rate. In addition, generalized vascular autoregulation tends to keep tissue blood flow constant (see also Chapter 17). This adaptation leads to changes in preload and afterload that also keep Q_h nearly constant.

Finally, at excessively high pacing frequencies (above 200 beats/min, Fig. 19-14), further increases in heart rate decrease Q_h. Therefore, the induced decrease in stroke volume must have exceeded the increase in heart rate at this high range of pacing frequencies. At such high pacing frequencies, the ventricular filling time is so severely restricted that compensation is inadequate and cardiac output decreases sharply. Although the relationship of Q_h to heart rate is characteristically that of an inverted U in the general population, the relationship varies quantitatively among subjects and among physiological states.

Strong correlations between heart rate and cardiac output must be interpreted cautiously. In exercising subjects, for example, cardiac output and heart rate usually increase proportionately, and stroke volume may remain constant or increase only slightly (see Exercise). The temptation is great to conclude that the increase in cardiac output during exercise must be caused solely by the observed increase in heart rate. However, Figure 19-14 shows that over a wide range

◢ IN THE CLINIC

The characteristic relationship between cardiac output and heart rate explains the urgent need for treatment of patients who have excessively slow or excessively fast heart rates. Profound **bradycardia** (slow rate) may occur as a result of a very slow sinus rhythm in patients with **sick sinus syndrome** or as a result of a slow idioventricular rhythm in patients with **complete atrioventricular block.** In either rhythm disturbance, the capacity of the ventricles to fill during a prolonged diastole is limited (often by the noncompliant pericardium). Hence, cardiac output usually decreases substantially because the very slow heart rate cannot be counterbalanced by a sufficiently large stroke volume. Consequently, these bradycardias often require the installation of an artificial pacemaker.

Excessively high heart rates in patients with **supraventricular** or **ventricular tachycardias** frequently require emergency treatment because these patients have cardiac output that may be critically low. In such patients, the filling time is so restricted at very high heart rates that even small additional reductions in filling time cause disproportionately severe reductions in filling volume. Slowing the tachycardia to a more normal rhythm can generally be accomplished pharmacologically, but electrical cardioversion may be required in emergencies (see Chapter 16).

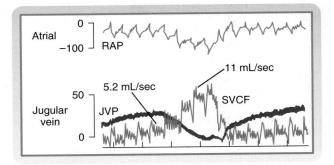

● **Figure 19-15.** During a normal inspiration, intrathoracic, right atrial (RAP), and jugular venous (JVP) pressure decrease, and flow in the superior vena cava (SVCF) increases (from 5.2 to 11 mL/sec). All pressures are in mm H_2O. Femoral arterial pressure (not shown) did not change substantially during the normal inspiration.

of heart rates, a change in heart rate may have little influence on cardiac output. The principal increase in cardiac output during exercise must therefore be attributed to other factors. Such ancillary factors include the pronounced reduction in peripheral vascular resistance because of the vasodilation in the active skeletal muscles and the increased contractility of cardiac muscle associated with the generalized increase in sympathetic neural activity. Nevertheless, the increase in heart rate is still an important factor. Abundant data show that if the heart rate cannot increase normally during exercise, the augmentation in cardiac output and the capacity for exercise are severely limited. Because stroke volume changes only slightly during exercise, the increase in heart rate may play an important permissive role in augmenting cardiac output during physical exercise.

ANCILLARY FACTORS THAT AFFECT THE VENOUS SYSTEM AND CARDIAC OUTPUT

In earlier sections of this chapter, the interrelationships between central venous pressure and cardiac output were simplified by restricting the discussion to the effects evoked by individual variables. However, because the cardiovascular system is regulated by so many feedback control loops, its responses are rarely simple. A change in blood volume, for example, not only affects cardiac output directly by the Frank-Star-

ling mechanism but also triggers reflexes that alter other aspects of cardiac function (such as the heart rate, atrioventricular conduction, and myocardial contractility) and other characteristics of the vascular system (such as peripheral resistance and venomotor tone). Several other factors, especially gravity (see Chapter 17) and respiration, also regulate cardiac output.

Circulatory Effects of Respiratory Activity

The normal, periodic activity of the respiratory muscles causes rhythmic variations in vena caval flow (Fig. 19-15). During respiration, the reduction in intrathoracic pressure is transmitted to the lumens of the thoracic blood vessels. The reduction in central venous pressure during inspiration increases the pressure gradient between extrathoracic and intrathoracic veins. The consequent acceleration in venous return to the right atrium is shown in Figure 19-15 as an increase in superior vena caval blood flow from 5.2 mL/sec during expiration to 11 mL/sec during inspiration.

The exaggerated reduction in intrathoracic pressure achieved by a strong inspiratory effort against a closed glottis (called **Müller's maneuver**) does not increase venous return proportionately. The extrathoracic veins collapse near their entry into the chest when their internal pressures fall below the ambient level. As the veins collapse, flow into the chest momentarily stops (see Chapter 17). The cessation of flow raises pressure upstream and forces the collapsed segment to open again.

During normal expiration, flow into the central veins decelerates. However, the mean rate of venous return during normal respiration exceeds the flow during a brief period of **apnea** (cessation of respiration). Hence, normal inspiration apparently facilitates venous return more than normal expiration impedes it. In part, this facilitation of venous return is implemented by the valves in the veins of the extremities. These valves prevent any reversal of flow during expiration. Thus, the respiratory muscles and venous valves constitute an auxiliary pump for venous return.

The dramatic increase in intrathoracic pressure induced by coughing constitutes an auxiliary pumping mechanism for the blood despite its concurrent tendency to impede venous return. Because patients undergoing certain diagnostic procedures, such as coronary angiography or electrophysiological testing of cardiac function, are at increased risk for ventricular fibrillation, they are trained to cough rhythmically on command during such procedures. If ventricular fibrillation does occur, each cough can generate substantial increases in arterial blood pressure, and enough cerebral blood flow may be promoted to sustain consciousness. The cough raises intravascular pressure equally in the intrathoracic arteries and veins. Blood is propelled through the extrathoracic tissues because the increased pressure is transmitted to the extrathoracic arteries, but not to the extrathoracic veins because the venous valves prevent backflow from the intrathoracic to the extrathoracic veins.

In most forms of artificial respiration (mouth-to-mouth resuscitation, mechanical respiration), lung inflation is achieved by applying endotracheal pressure above atmospheric pressure, and expiration occurs by passive recoil of the thoracic cage (see Chapter 21). Thus, lung inflation is accompanied by an appreciable rise in intrathoracic pressure. Vena caval flow decreases sharply during the phase of positive pressure lung inflation when the endotracheal pressure progressively rises. When negative endotracheal pressure is used to facilitate deflation, vena caval flow accelerates more than when the lungs are allowed to deflate passively.

Sustained expiratory efforts increase intrathoracic pressure and thus impede venous return. Straining against a closed glottis (termed **Valsalva's maneuver**) regularly occurs during coughing, defecation, and heavy lifting. Intrathoracic pressures in excess of 100 mm Hg have been recorded in trumpet players, and pressures higher than 400 mm Hg have been observed during paroxysms of coughing. Such increases in pressure are transmitted directly to the lumens of the intrathoracic arteries. After coughing stops, arterial blood pressure may fall precipitously because of the preceding impediment to venous return.

INTERPLAY OF CENTRAL AND PERIPHERAL FACTORS IN CONTROL OF THE CIRCULATION

The primary function of the circulatory system is to deliver the nutrients needed for tissue metabolism and growth and to remove the products of metabolism. Previously, we examined the contributions of the components of the cardiovascular system to maintain adequate tissue perfusion under different physiological conditions. In this section, we explore the interrelationships among the various components of the circulatory system. The autonomic nervous system and the baroreceptors and chemoreceptors play key roles in regulating the cardiovascular system. Control of fluid balance by the kidneys, with maintenance of a constant blood volume, is also very important.

In any well-regulated system, one way to evaluate the extent and sensitivity of its regulatory mechanisms is to disturb the system and to observe how it restores the preexisting steady state. Two such disturbances, physical exercise and hemorrhage, are used in the following sections to illustrate operation of the various regulatory factors.

Exercise

The cardiovascular adjustments that occur during exercise consist of a combination of neural and local (chemical) factors. Neural factors include (1) central command, (2) reflexes that originate in the contracting muscle, and (3) the baroreceptor reflex.

Central command is the cerebrocortical activation of the sympathetic nervous system that produces cardiac acceleration, increased myocardial contractile force, and peripheral vasoconstriction. Reflexes are activated intramuscularly by stimulation of mechanoreceptors (by stretch, tension) and chemoreceptors (by metabolic products) in response to muscle contraction. Impulses from these receptors travel centrally via small myelinated (group III) and unmyelinated (group IV) afferent nerve fibers. Group IV unmyelinated fibers may represent the muscle chemoreceptors, as no morphological chemoreceptor has been identified. The central connections of this reflex are unknown, but the efferent limb consists of sympathetic nerve fibers to the heart and peripheral blood vessels. The baroreceptor reflex is described in Chapter 18, and local factors that influence skeletal muscle blood flow (metabolic vasodilators) are described in Chapter 17. Vascular chemoreceptors are important in regulation of the cardiovascular system during exercise. Evidence for this assertion comes from the observations that the pH, P_{CO_2}, and P_{O_2} of arterial blood remain normal during exercise and that the vascular chemoreceptors are located on the arterial side of the circulatory system.

Mild to Moderate Exercise

In humans or trained animals, anticipation of physical activity inhibits vagal nerve impulses to the heart and increases sympathetic discharge. The result is an increase in heart rate and myocardial contractility. The tachycardia and enhanced contractility increase cardiac output.

Peripheral Resistance. When cardiac stimulation occurs, the sympathetic nervous system also changes vascular resistance in the periphery. Sympathetic-mediated vasoconstriction increases vascular resistance and thereby diverts blood away from the skin, kidneys, splanchnic regions, and inactive muscle (Fig. 19-16). This increased vascular resistance persists throughout the period of exercise.

Cardiac output and blood flow to active muscles increase with progressive increases in the intensity of exercise. Blood flow to the myocardium increases, whereas flow to the brain is unchanged. Skin blood flow initially decreases during exercise, and then it increases as body temperature rises with increments in the duration and intensity of exercise. Skin blood flow finally decreases when the skin vessels constrict as total body O_2 consumption nears its maximal value (Fig. 19-16).

The major circulatory adjustment to prolonged exercise occurs in the vasculature of the active muscles. Local formation of vasoactive metabolites dilates the resistance vessels markedly. This dilation progresses with increases in the intensity of exercise. Potassium is one of the vasodilator substances released by the contracting muscle, and this ion may be partly responsible for the initial decrease in vascular resistance in the active muscles. Other contributing factors may be the release of adenosine and a decrease in tissue pH during sustained exercise. The local accumulation of metabolites relaxes the terminal arterioles, and blood flow through the muscle may increase 15- to 20-fold above the resting level. This metabolic vasodilation of the precapillary vessels in active muscles occurs very soon after the onset of exercise. The decrease in TPR enables the heart to pump more blood at a lesser load, and it pumps more

efficiently than if TPR were unchanged (see Chapters 17 and 18).

Marked changes in the capillary circulation also occur during exercise. At rest, only a small percentage of the capillaries are perfused, whereas in actively contracting muscle, all or nearly all of the capillaries contain flowing blood **(capillary recruitment).** The surface area available for exchange of gases, water, and solutes is increased many times. Furthermore, hydrostatic pressure in the capillaries is increased because of relaxation of the resistance vessels. Hence, water and solutes move into the muscle tissue. Tissue pressure rises and remains elevated during exercise as fluid continues to move out of the capillaries; this tissue fluid is carried away by the lymphatics. Lymph flow is increased as a result of the rise in capillary hydrostatic pressure and the massaging effect of the contracting muscles on the valve-containing lymphatic vessels (see Chapter 17).

Contracting muscle avidly extracts O_2 from the perfusing blood and thereby increases the arteriovenous O_2 difference (Fig. 19-17). This release of O_2 from blood is facilitated by the shift in the oxyhemoglobin dissociation curve during exercise. During exercise, the

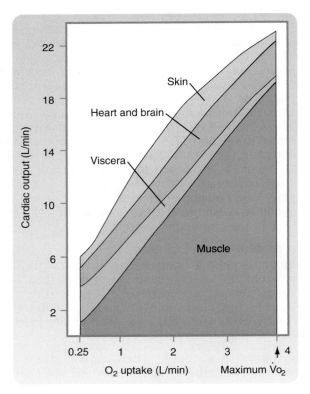

● **Figure 19-16.** Approximate distribution of cardiac output at rest and at different levels of exercise up to the maximal O_2 consumption (($\dot{V}O_2$max) in a normal young man. (Redrawn from Ruch HP, Patton TC: Physiology and Biophysics, 12th ed. Philadelphia, Saunders, 1974.)

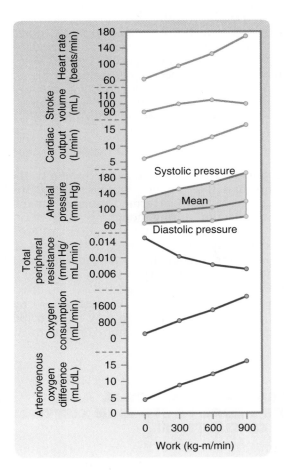

● **Figure 19-17.** Effect of different levels of exercise on several cardiovascular variables. (Data from Carlsten A, Grimby G: The Circulatory Response to Muscular Exercise in Man. Springfield, IL, Charles C Thomas, 1966.)

high concentration of CO_2 and the formation of lactic acid reduce tissue pH. This decrease in pH plus the increase in temperature in the contracting muscle shifts the oxyhemoglobin dissociation curve to the right (see Chapter 23). Therefore, at any given P_{O_2}, less O_2 is held by the hemoglobin in the red cells, and consequently more O_2 is available for the tissues. Oxygen consumption may increase as much as 60-fold, with only a 15-fold increase in muscle blood flow. Muscle myoglobin may serve as a limited O_2 store during exercise, and it can release the attached O_2 at very low partial pressures. However, myoglobin can also facilitate O_2 transport from capillaries to mitochondria by serving as an O_2 carrier.

Cardiac Output. Because the enhanced sympathetic drive and the reduced parasympathetic inhibition of the sinoatrial node continue during exercise, tachycardia persists. If the workload is moderate and constant, the heart rate will reach a certain level and remain there throughout the period of exercise. However, if the workload increases, the heart rate increases concomitantly until a plateau of about 180 beats/min is reached during strenuous exercise. In contrast to the large increase in heart rate, the increase in stroke volume is only about 10% to 35%, the larger values occurring in trained individuals (Fig. 19-17). In well-trained distance runners, whose cardiac output can reach six to seven times the resting level, stroke volume attains about twice the resting value.

Thus, the increase in cardiac output observed during exercise is correlated principally with an increase in heart rate. If the baroreceptors are denervated, the cardiac output and heart rate responses to exercise are small in comparison to those in individuals with normally innervated baroreceptors. However, with total cardiac denervation, exercise still increases cardiac output as much as it does in normal individuals. This increase in cardiac output is achieved chiefly by means of an elevated stroke volume. However, if a β-adrenergic receptor antagonist is given to dogs with denervated hearts, exercise performance is impaired. The β-adrenergic receptor antagonist prevents the cardiac acceleration and enhanced contractility caused by increased amounts of circulating catecholamines. Therefore, the increase in cardiac output necessary for maximal exercise performance is limited.

Venous Return. In addition to the contribution made by sympathetically mediated constriction of the capacitance vessels in both exercising and nonexercising parts of the body, venous return is aided by the auxiliary pumping action of the working skeletal muscles and the muscles of respiration (see also Chapters 21 and 24). The intermittently contracting muscles compress the veins that course through them. Because the venous valves are oriented toward the heart, the contracting muscle pumps blood back toward the right atrium (see Chapter 17). In exercise, the flow of venous blood to the heart is also aided by the deeper

● **Figure 19-18.** Cardiovascular adjustments in exercise. C, vasoconstrictor activity; D, vasodilator activity; IX, glossopharyngeal nerve; VR, vasomotor region; X, vagus nerve; +, increased activity; –, decreased activity.

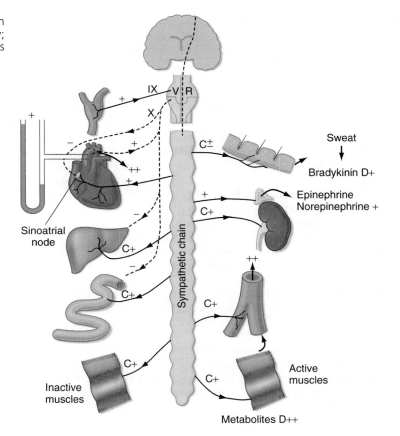

and more frequent respirations that increase the pressure gradient between the abdominal and thoracic veins (intrathoracic pressure becomes more negative during exercise).

In humans, blood reservoirs do not contribute much to the circulating blood volume. In fact, blood volume is usually reduced slightly during exercise, as evidenced by a rise in the hematocrit ratio. This decrease in blood volume is caused by water loss externally through sweating and enhanced ventilation and by fluid movement into the contracting muscle. However, fluid loss is counteracted in several ways. Fluid loss from the vascular compartment into the contracting muscles eventually reaches a plateau as interstitial fluid pressure rises and opposes the increased hydrostatic pressure in capillaries of the active muscle. Fluid loss is partially offset by movement of fluid from the splanchnic regions and inactive muscle into the bloodstream. This influx of fluid results from (1) a decrease in hydrostatic pressure in the capillaries of these tissues and (2) an increase in plasma osmolarity because of movement of osmotically active molecules into blood from the contracting muscle. Reduced urine formation by the kidneys also helps conserve body water.

The large volume of venous blood returning to the heart is so effectively pumped through the lungs and out into the aorta that central venous pressure remains essentially constant. Thus, the Frank-Starling mechanism of a greater initial fiber length does not account for the greater stroke volume in moderate exercise. X-ray films of individuals at rest and during exercise reveal a decrease in heart size during exercise. However, during maximal or near-maximal exercise, right atrial pressure and end-diastolic ventricular volume do increase, and the Frank-Starling mechanism contributes to the enhanced stroke volume in very vigorous exercise.

Arterial Pressure. If the exercise involves a large proportion of the body musculature, such as in running or swimming, the reduction in total vascular resistance can be considerable. Nevertheless, arterial pressure starts to rise with the onset of exercise, and the increase in blood pressure roughly parallels the severity of the exercise performed (Fig. 19-17). Therefore, the increase in cardiac output is proportionally greater than the decrease in TPR. The vasoconstriction produced in the inactive tissues by the sympathetic nervous system (and to some extent by the release of catecholamines from the adrenal medulla) is important for maintenance of normal or increased blood pressure. Sympathectomy or drug-induced block of the adrenergic sympathetic nerve fibers decreases arterial pressure (hypotension) during exercise.

Sympathetic neural activity also elicits vasoconstriction in active skeletal muscle when additional muscles are recruited. In experiments in which one leg is working at maximal levels and then the other leg starts to work, blood flow decreases in the first working leg. Furthermore, blood levels of norepinephrine rise significantly during exercise, and most of the norepi-

nephrine is released from sympathetic nerves to the active muscles.

As body temperature rises during exercise, the skin vessels dilate in response to thermal stimulation of the heat-regulating center in the hypothalamus, and TPR decreases further. This reduction in TPR would reduce blood pressure were it not for the increased cardiac output and the constriction of arterioles in the renal, splanchnic, and other tissues.

In general, mean arterial pressure rises during exercise as a result of the increase in cardiac output. However, the effect of enhanced cardiac output is offset by an overall decrease in TPR, and therefore mean blood pressure increases only slightly. Vasoconstriction in the inactive vascular beds helps maintain normal arterial blood pressure for adequate perfusion of the active tissues. The actual mean arterial pressure attained during exercise thus represents a balance between cardiac output and TPR (see Chapter 17). Systolic pressure usually increases more than diastolic pressure, which results in an increase in pulse pressure (Fig. 19-17). The larger pulse pressure is primarily attributable to a greater stroke volume, but also to more rapid ejection of blood by the left ventricle and diminished peripheral runoff during the brief ventricular ejection period (see also Chapter 17).

Severe Exercise

During exhaustive exercise, the compensatory mechanisms begin to fail. The heart rate attains a maximal level of about 180 beats/min, and stroke volume reaches a plateau. The heart rate may then decrease and result in a fall in blood pressure. The subject also frequently becomes dehydrated. Sympathetic vasoconstrictor activity supersedes the vasodilator influence on vessels of the skin such that the rate of heat loss is decreased. Body temperature is normally elevated in exercise. A reduction in heat loss through cutaneous vasoconstriction can lead to very high body temperatures and to acute distress during severe exercise. Tissue pH and blood pH decrease as a result of increased lactic acid and CO_2 production. The reduced pH may be a key factor that determines the maximal amount of exercise that a given individual can tolerate. Muscle pain, a subjective feeling of exhaustion, and loss of the will to continue determine exercise tolerance. A summary of the neural and local effects of exercise on the cardiovascular system is diagrammed in Figure 19-18.

Postexercise Recovery

When exercise stops, the heart rate and cardiac output quickly decrease—the sympathetic drive to the heart is essentially removed. In contrast, TPR remains low for some time after the exercise is stopped, presumably because vasodilator metabolites have accumulated in the muscles during the exercise period. As a result of the reduced cardiac output and persistence of vasodilation in the muscles, arterial pressure falls, often below preexercise levels, for brief periods. Blood pressure is then stabilized at normal levels by the baroreceptor reflexes.

Limits of Exercise Performance

The two main factors that limit skeletal muscle performance in humans are the rate of O_2 utilization by the muscles and the O_2 supply to the muscles. However, O_2 use by muscle is probably not a critical factor. During exercise, maximal O_2 consumption ($\dot{V}O_2$max) by a large percentage of the body's muscle mass is unchanged or increases only slightly when additional muscles are activated. In fact, during exercise of a large muscle mass, as in vigorous bicycling, the addition of bilateral arm exercise without change in the cycling effort produces only a small increase in cardiac output and $\dot{V}O_2$max. However, the additional arm exercise decreases blood flow to the legs. This centrally mediated (baroreceptor reflex) vasoconstriction during maximal cardiac output prevents the fall in blood pressure that would otherwise be caused by metabolically induced vasodilation in the active muscle. If muscle O_2 use were a significant limiting factor, recruitment of more contracting muscles would entail the use of much more O_2 to meet the enhanced O_2 requirements.

Limitation of the O_2 supply could be caused by inadequate oxygenation of blood in the lungs or limitation of the supply of O_2-laden blood to the muscles. Failure to oxygenate blood fully by the lungs can be excluded because even with the most strenuous exercise at sea level, arterial blood is fully saturated with O_2. Therefore, O_2 delivery to the active muscles (or blood flow because the arterial blood O_2 content is normal) appears to be the limiting factor in muscle performance. This limitation could be caused by the inability to increase cardiac output beyond a critical level. In turn, this inability is caused by a limitation in stroke volume because the heart rate reaches maximal levels before $\dot{V}O_2$max is reached. Hence, the major factor that limits muscle performance is the pumping capacity of the heart.

Physical Training and Conditioning

The response of the cardiovascular system to regular exercise is to increase its capacity to deliver O_2 to the active muscles and improve the ability of the muscle to use O_2. $\dot{V}O_2$max varies with the level of physical conditioning. Training progressively increases $\dot{V}O_2$max, which reaches a plateau at the highest level of conditioning. Highly trained athletes have a lower resting heart rate, a greater stroke volume, and lower peripheral resistance than they had before training or after deconditioning. The low resting heart rate is caused by a higher vagal tone and a lower sympathetic tone. During exercise, the maximal heart rate of a trained individual is the same as that in an untrained person, but it is attained at a higher level of exercise.

A trained person also exhibits low vascular resistance in the muscles. If an individual exercises one leg regularly over an extended period and does not exercise the other leg, vascular resistance is lower and $\dot{V}O_2$max is higher in the "trained" leg than in the "untrained" leg. Physical conditioning is also associated with greater extraction of O_2 from the blood (greater arteriovenous O_2 difference) by the muscles.

> ### ▶ IN THE CLINIC
>
> Endurance training, such as running or swimming, increases left ventricular volume without increasing left ventricular wall thickness. In contrast, strength exercises, such as weightlifting, increase left ventricular wall thickness (hypertrophy) with little effect on ventricular volume. However, this increase in wall thickness is small relative to that observed in chronic hypertension, in which afterload is persistently elevated because of high peripheral resistance.

With long-term training, capillary density in skeletal muscle increases. Also, an increase in the number of arterioles may account for the decrease in muscle vascular resistance. The number of mitochondria increases, as do the oxidative enzymes in mitochondria. In addition, levels of ATPase activity, myoglobin, and enzymes involved in lipid metabolism increase in response to physical conditioning.

Hemorrhage

The cardiovascular system is the principal system affected in an individual who has lost a large quantity of blood. Arterial systolic, diastolic, and pulse pressures decrease, and the arterial pulse is rapid and feeble. The cutaneous veins collapse, and they fill slowly when compressed centrally. The skin is pale, moist, and slightly cyanotic. Respiration is rapid, but the depth of respiration may be shallow or deep.

Course of Arterial Blood Pressure Changes

Cardiac output decreases as a result of blood loss. The amount of blood removed when donating blood ($\approx 10\%$) is well tolerated, and there is little change in mean arterial blood pressure. This is not the case when greater amounts are lost from the circulation. The changes in mean arterial pressure evoked by acute hemorrhage are illustrated in Figure 19-19. If sufficient blood is rapidly withdrawn to decrease mean arterial pressure to 50 mm Hg, the pressure then tends to rise spontaneously toward the control level over the next 20 or 30 minutes. In some individuals (curve A, Fig. 19-19), this trend continues and normal pressure is regained within a few hours. In others (curve B, Fig. 19-19), the pressure rises initially after the cessation of hemorrhage. The pressure then begins to decline, and it continues to fall at an accelerating rate until death ensues. This progressive deterioration in cardiovascular function is termed hemorrhagic shock. At some time after the hemorrhage, the deterioration in the cardiovascular system becomes irreversible. A lethal outcome can be prevented only temporarily by any known therapy, including massive transfusions of donor blood.

Compensatory Mechanisms

The changes in arterial pressure immediately after acute blood loss (Fig. 19-19) indicate that certain compensatory mechanisms must be operative. Any mechanism that raises arterial blood pressure toward normal in response to a reduction in pressure is designated a negative-feedback mechanism. This mechanism is termed negative because the direction of the secondary change in pressure is opposite the direction of the initiating change after the acute blood loss. The following negative-feedback responses are evoked: (1) baroreceptor reflexes, (2) chemoreceptor reflexes, (3) cerebral ischemia responses, (4) reabsorption of tissue fluids, (5) release of endogenous vasoconstrictor substances, and (6) renal conservation of salt and water.

Baroreceptor Reflexes. The reductions in mean arterial pressure and pulse pressure during hemorrhage decrease stimulation of the baroreceptors in the carotid sinuses and aortic arch (see Chapter 18). Several cardiovascular responses are thus evoked, all of which tend to restore the normal level of arterial pressure. Such responses include reduction of vagal tone and enhancement of sympathetic tone, increased heart rate, and enhanced myocardial contractility.

The increased sympathetic tone also produces generalized venoconstriction, which has the same hemodynamic consequences as transfusion of blood (Fig. 19-9). Sympathetic activation constricts certain blood reservoirs. This vasoconstriction acts as an autotransfusion of blood into the circulation. In humans, the cutaneous, pulmonary, and hepatic branches of the vasculature constitute the principal blood reservoirs.

Generalized arteriolar constriction is a prominent response to the reduced baroreceptor stimulation during hemorrhage. The reflex increase in peripheral resistance minimizes the fall in arterial pressure caused by the reduction in cardiac output. Figure 19-20 shows the effect of an 8% blood loss on mean aortic pressure. When both vagi were cut to eliminate the influence of the aortic arch baroreceptors and only the carotid sinus baroreceptors were operative (Fig. 19-20, *A*), this hemorrhage decreased mean aortic pressure by 14%. This pressure change did not differ significantly from the decline in pressure (12%) evoked by the same hemorrhage before vagotomy (not shown). When the carotid sinuses were denervated and the aortic baroreceptor reflexes were intact, the 8% blood loss decreased mean aortic pressure by 38% (see Fig. 19-20, *B*). Hence, the carotid sinus baroreceptors were more effective than the aortic baroreceptors in attenuating the fall in pressure. The aortic baroreceptor reflex must also have been operative, however, because when both sets of afferent baroreceptor pathways were interrupted (see Fig. 19-20, *C*), an 8% blood loss reduced arterial pressure by 48%.

Arteriolar constriction is widespread during hemorrhage but it is by no means uniform. Vasoconstriction is most pronounced in the cutaneous, skeletal muscle, and splanchnic vascular beds, and it is slight or absent in the cerebral and coronary circulations in response to hemorrhage. In many instances, cerebral and coronary vascular resistance is diminished. The reduced cardiac output is redistributed to favor flow through the brain and the heart.

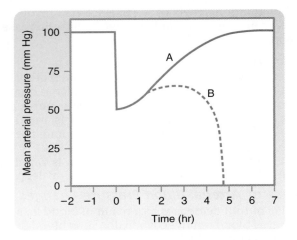

● **Figure 19-19.** Changes in mean arterial pressure after rapid hemorrhage. At time zero, blood is rapidly removed, thereby reducing the mean arterial pressure to 50 mm Hg. After a period in which the pressure returns toward the control level, some individuals continue to improve until the control pressure is attained *(curve A).* However, in other individuals, the pressure will begin to decline until death ensues *(curve B).*

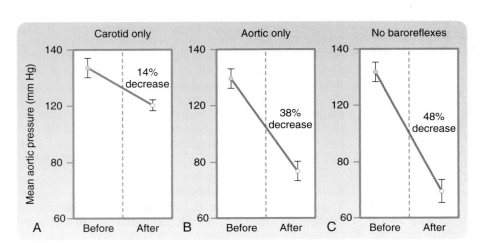

A   B   C

● **Figure 19-20.** Changes in mean aortic pressure in response to an 8% blood loss in three groups of individuals. **A,** The carotid sinus baroreceptors were intact and the aortic reflexes were interrupted. **B,** The aortic reflexes were intact and the carotid sinus reflexes were interrupted. **C,** All sinoaortic reflexes were abrogated. (Data from Shepherd JT: Circulation 50:418, 1974; derived from the data of Edis AJ: Am J Physiol 221:1352, 1971.)

In the early stages of mild to moderate hemorrhage, renal resistance changes only slightly. The tendency for increased sympathetic activity to constrict the renal vessels is counteracted by autoregulatory mechanisms (see Chapters 18 and 32). With more prolonged and severe hemorrhage, however, renal vasoconstriction becomes intense.

The severe renal and splanchnic vasoconstriction during hemorrhage favors the heart and brain. However, if such constriction persists too long, it may be detrimental. Frequently, patients survive the acute hypotensive period of a prolonged, severe hemorrhage, only to die several days later from the kidney failure that results from renal ischemia. Intestinal ischemia may also have dire effects. For example, intestinal bleeding and extensive sloughing of the mucosa can occur after only a few hours of hemorrhagic hypotension. Furthermore, the diminished splanchnic flow swells the centrilobular cells in the liver (i.e., those cells closest to the central vein). The resulting obstruction of the hepatic sinusoids raises portal venous pressure, and this response intensifies intestinal blood loss.

Chemoreceptor Reflexes. Reductions in arterial pressure below about 60 mm Hg do not evoke any additional responses through the baroreceptor reflexes because this pressure level constitutes the threshold for stimulation (see Chapter 18). However, low arterial pressure may stimulate peripheral chemoreceptors because inadequate local blood flow leads to hypoxia in the chemoreceptor tissue. Chemoreceptor excitation may then enhance the already existent peripheral vasoconstriction evoked by the baroreceptor reflexes. In addition, respiratory stimulation assists venous return by the auxiliary pumping mechanism described earlier (see also Chapter 24).

Cerebral Ischemia. When arterial pressure falls below about 40 mm Hg as a consequence of blood loss, the resulting cerebral ischemia activates the sympathoadrenal system. The sympathetic nervous discharge is several times greater than the maximal neural activity that occurs when the baroreceptors cease to be stimulated. The vasoconstriction and increase in myocardial contractility may be pronounced. With more severe degrees of cerebral ischemia, however, the vagal centers also become activated. The resulting bradycardia aggravates the hypotension that initiated the cerebral ischemia

Reabsorption of Tissue Fluids. The arterial hypotension, arteriolar constriction, and reduced venous pressure during hemorrhagic hypotension lower hydrostatic pressure in the capillaries. The balance of these forces promotes the net reabsorption of interstitial fluid into the vascular compartment (see Chapter 17). The rapidity of this response is displayed in Figure 19-21. When 45% of the estimated blood volume was removed over a 30-minute period, mean arterial blood pressure declined rapidly and then was largely restored to near the control level. Plasma colloid osmotic pressure declined markedly during the bleed-

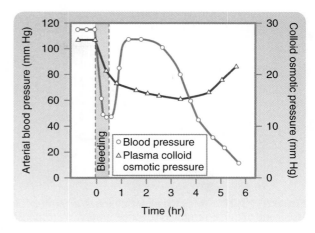

● **Figure 19-21.** Changes in arterial blood pressure and plasma colloid osmotic pressure in response to withdrawal of 45% of the estimated blood volume over a 30-minute period, beginning at time zero. (Redrawn from Zweifach BW: Anesthesiology 41:157, 1974.)

ing and continued to decrease more gradually for several hours. The reduction in colloid osmotic pressure reflects dilution of the blood by tissue fluids that contain little protein.

Considerable quantities of fluid may thus be drawn into the circulation during hemorrhage. About 0.25 mL of fluid per minute per kilogram of body weight may be reabsorbed by the capillaries. Thus, approximately 1 L of fluid per hour might be autoinfused from the interstitial spaces into the circulatory system of an average individual after acute blood loss.

Substantial quantities of fluid may shift slowly from the intracellular to the extracellular space. This fluid exchange is probably mediated by secretion of cortisol from the adrenal cortex in response to hemorrhage. Cortisol appears to be essential for the full restoration of plasma volume after hemorrhage.

Endogenous Vasoconstrictors. The catecholamines epinephrine and norepinephrine are released from the adrenal medulla in response to the same stimuli that evoke widespread sympathetic nervous discharge (see Chapter 42). Blood levels of catecholamines are high during and after hemorrhage. When blood loss is such that arterial pressure is reduced to 40 mm Hg, the level of catecholamines increases as much as 50-fold. Epinephrine comes almost exclusively from the adrenal medulla, whereas norepinephrine is derived from both the adrenal medulla and peripheral sympathetic nerve endings. These humoral substances reinforce the effects of the sympathetic nervous activity listed previously.

Vasopressin (antidiuretic hormone), a potent vasoconstrictor, is secreted by the posterior pituitary gland in response to hemorrhage (see Chapters 34 and 40). The plasma concentration of vasopressin rises progressively as arterial blood pressure diminishes (Fig. 19-22). The receptors responsible for the augmented release of vasopressin are the aortic arch and

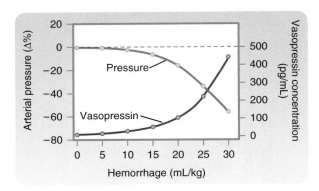

● **Figure 19-22.** Mean percent changes in arterial blood pressure and plasma vasopressin concentration in response to blood loss. (Redrawn from Shen YT et al: Circ Res 68:1422, 1991.)

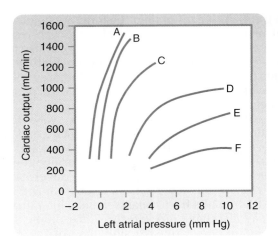

● **Figure 19-23.** Ventricular function curve for the left ventricle during the course of hemorrhagic shock. Curve A represents the control function curve; curve B, 117 minutes; curve C, 247 minutes; curve D, 280 minutes; curve E, 295 minutes; and curve F, 310 minutes after the initial hemorrhage. (Redrawn from Crowell JW, Guyton AC: Am J Physiol 203:248, 1962.)

carotid sinus baroreceptors (high pressure) and stretch receptors in the left atrium (low pressure).

The diminished renal perfusion during hemorrhagic hypotension leads to the secretion of renin from the juxtaglomerular apparatus (see Chapter 34). This enzyme acts on a plasma protein, angiotensinogen, to form the decapeptide angiotensin I, which in turn is cleaved to the active octapeptide angiotensin II by <u>a</u>ngiotensin-<u>c</u>onverting <u>e</u>nzyme (ACE); angiotensin II is a very powerful vasoconstrictor.

Renal Conservation of Salt and Water. Fluid and electrolytes are conserved by the kidneys during hemorrhage in response to various stimuli, including the increased secretion of vasopressin noted previously (Fig. 19-22) and increased renal sympathetic nerve activity, which enhances NaCl reabsorption by the nephron (decreased excretion). The lower arterial pressure decreases the glomerular filtration rate, which also curtails the excretion of water and electrolytes. In addition, the elevated levels of angiotensin II, as described earlier, stimulate the release of aldosterone from the adrenal cortex. Aldosterone, in turn, stimulates reabsorption of NaCl by the nephrons. Thus, NaCl and water excretion is decreased (see also Chapter 34).

Decompensatory Mechanisms

In contrast to negative-feedback mechanisms, hemorrhage also evokes latent positive-feedback mechanisms. These mechanisms exaggerate any primary change initiated by the blood loss. Specifically, positive-feedback mechanisms aggravate the hypotension induced by blood loss and tend to initiate "vicious" cycles, which may lead to death.

Whether a positive-feedback mechanism will lead to a vicious cycle depends on the gain of that mechanism. Gain is the ratio of the secondary change evoked by a given mechanism to the initiating change itself. A gain greater than 1 induces a vicious cycle; a gain less than 1 does not. Consider a positive-feedback mechanism with a gain of 2. If mean arterial pressure were to decrease by 10 mm Hg, a positive-feedback mechanism with a gain of 2 would then evoke a secondary

reduction in pressure of 20 mm Hg, which in turn would cause a further decrease of 40 mm Hg. Thus, each change would induce a subsequent one that is twice as great. Hence, mean arterial pressure would decline at an ever-increasing rate until death occurred. This process is depicted in curve B in Figure 19-19.

Conversely, a positive-feedback mechanism with a gain of 0.5 also exaggerates any change in mean arterial pressure, but the change would not necessarily lead to death. If arterial pressure suddenly decreased by 10 mm Hg, a positive-feedback mechanism would initiate a secondary, additional fall of 5 mm Hg. This decrease, in turn, would provoke a further decrease of 2.5 mm Hg. The process would continue in ever-diminishing steps until arterial pressure approached an equilibrium value.

Some of the more important positive-feedback mechanisms that are evident during hemorrhage include (1) cardiac failure, (2) acidosis, (3) central nervous system depression, (4) aberrations in blood clotting, and (5) depression of the mononuclear phagocytic system (MPS).*

Cardiac Failure. The role of cardiac failure in the progression of shock during hemorrhage is controversial. All investigators agree that the heart fails terminally, but opinions differ about the importance of cardiac failure during earlier stages of hemorrhagic hypotension. Shifts to the right in ventricular function curves (Fig. 19-23) provide evidence of a progressive

---

*The MPS (previously called the reticuloendothelial system) consists of macrophages that are distributed throughout the body. They are derived from bone marrow and exist for a short period in circulating blood as monocytes. They then migrate into tissues, where they phagocytose foreign material and present antigens to lymphocytes to initiate the adaptive immune response. Cells of the MPS include the Kupffer cells of the liver, alveolar macrophages, microglia, and Langerhans cells.

depression in myocardial contractility during hemorrhage.

The hypotension induced by hemorrhage reduces coronary blood flow and therefore depresses ventricular function. The consequent reduction in cardiac output further reduces arterial pressure, a classic example of a positive-feedback mechanism. Furthermore, reduced blood flow to peripheral tissues leads to an accumulation of vasodilator metabolites that decrease peripheral resistance and therefore aggravate the fall in arterial pressure.

Acidosis. The inadequate blood flow during hemorrhage affects the metabolism of all cells. The decreased O_2 delivery to cells accelerates tissue production of lactic acid and other acid metabolites. Moreover, impaired kidney function prevents adequate excretion of the excess H^+, and generalized metabolic acidosis ensues. The resulting depressant effect of acidosis on the heart further reduces tissue perfusion and thus aggravates the metabolic acidosis. Acidosis also reduces the reactivity of the heart and resistance vessels to neurally released and circulating catecholamines and thereby intensifies the hypotension.

Central Nervous System Depression. The hypotension in shock reduces cerebral blood flow. Moderate degrees of cerebral ischemia induce pronounced sympathetic nervous stimulation of the heart, arterioles, and veins, as noted earlier. In severe hypotension, however, the cardiovascular centers in the brainstem eventually become depressed because of inadequate cerebral blood flow. The resulting loss of sympathetic tone then reduces cardiac output and peripheral resistance. The consequent reduction in mean arterial pressure intensifies the inadequate cerebral perfusion.

Endogenous opioids, such as enkephalins and β-endorphin, may be released into the brain substance and into the circulation in response to the same stresses that provoke circulatory shock. Opioids are stored, along with catecholamines, in secretory granules in the adrenal medulla and in sympathetic nerve terminals, and they are released together in response to stress. Similar stimuli release β-endorphin and adrenocorticotropic hormone from the anterior pituitary gland. Opioids depress the brainstem centers that mediate some of the compensatory autonomic adaptations to blood loss, endotoxemia, and other shock-provoking stress. Conversely, the opioid antagonist naloxone improves cardiovascular function and survival in various forms of shock.

Aberrations in Blood Clotting. The alterations in blood clotting after hemorrhage are typically biphasic. An initial phase of hypercoagulability is followed by a secondary phase of hypocoagulability and fibrinolysis. In the initial phase, platelets and leukocytes adhere to the vascular endothelium, and intravascular clots, or thrombi, develop within a few minutes of the onset of severe hemorrhage. Coagulation may be extensive throughout the small blood vessels.

The initial phase is further enhanced by the release of thromboxane A_2 from various ischemic tissues.

Thromboxane A_2 aggregates platelets. As more platelets aggregate, more thromboxane A_2 is released and more platelets are trapped. This form of positive feedback intensifies and prolongs the clotting tendency. The mortality from certain standard shock-provoking procedures has been reduced considerably by the administration of anticoagulants such as heparin.

Mononuclear Phagocytic System. During the course of hemorrhagic hypotension, MPS function becomes depressed. The phagocytic activity of the MPS is modulated by an opsonic protein. The opsonic activity in plasma diminishes during shock, and this change may account in part for the depression in MPS function. As a result, antibacterial and antitoxin defense mechanisms are impaired. Endotoxins from the normal bacterial flora of the intestine constantly enter the circulation. Ordinarily, they are inactivated by the MPS, principally in the liver. When the MPS is depressed, these endotoxins invade the general circulation. Endotoxins produce profound, generalized vasodilation, mainly by inducing the synthesis of an isoform of nitric oxide synthase in the smooth muscle of blood vessels throughout the body. The profound vasodilation aggravates the hemodynamic changes caused by blood loss.

In addition to their role in inactivating endotoxin, macrophages release many of the mediators associated with shock. These mediators include acid hydrolases, neutral proteases, oxygen free radicals, certain coagulation factors, and the following arachidonic acid derivatives: prostaglandins, thromboxanes, and leukotrienes. Macrophages also release certain monokines that modulate temperature regulation, intermediary metabolism, hormone secretion, and the immune system.

Interactions of Positive- and Negative-Feedback Mechanisms

Hemorrhage provokes a multitude of circulatory and metabolic derangements. Some of these changes are compensatory and others are decompensatory. Some of these feedback mechanisms possess high gain and others possess low gain. Furthermore, the gain of any specific mechanism varies with the severity of the hemorrhage. For example, with only a slight loss of blood, mean arterial pressure is maintained within the normal range and the gain of the baroreceptor reflexes is high. With greater losses of blood, when mean arterial pressure is below 60 mm Hg (i.e., below the threshold for the baroreceptors), further reductions in pressure have no additional influence through the baroreceptor reflexes. Hence, below this critical pressure, the baroreceptor reflex gain is zero or near zero.

Generally, with minor degrees of blood loss, the gains of negative-feedback mechanisms are high, whereas those of positive-feedback mechanisms are low. The opposite is true with more severe hemorrhage. The gains of the various mechanisms add algebraically. Therefore, whether a vicious cycle develops depends on whether the sum of the positive and negative gains exceeds 1. Total gains in excess of 1 are of course more likely with severe losses of blood. Therefore, to avert a vicious cycle, serious hemorrhages must be treated quickly and intensively, preferably by whole blood transfusion, before the process becomes irreversible.

■ KEY CONCEPTS

1. Two important relationships between cardiac output (Q_h) and central venous pressure (P_v) prevail in the cardiovascular system. With respect to the heart, Q_h varies directly with P_v (or preload) over a very wide range of P_v. This relationship is represented by the cardiac function curve, and it expresses the Frank-Starling mechanism. In the vascular system, P_v varies inversely with Q_h. This relationship is represented by the vascular function curve, and it reflects the fact that as Q_h increases, a greater fraction of the total blood volume resides in the arteries and a smaller volume resides in the veins.

2. The principal cardiac mechanisms that govern cardiac output are the changes in numbers of myocardial cross-bridges that interact and in the affinity of the contractile proteins for Ca^{++}. The principal factors that govern the vascular function curve are arterial and venous compliance, peripheral vascular resistance, and total blood volume.

3. The equilibrium values of Q_h and P_v that prevail under a given set of conditions are determined by the intersection of the cardiac and vascular function curves. At very low and very high heart rates, the heart is unable to pump an adequate Q_h. At very low heart rates, the increase in filling during diastole cannot compensate for the small number of cardiac contractions per minute. At very high heart rates, the large number of contractions per minute cannot compensate for the inadequate filling time.

4. Gravity influences Q_h because the veins are so compliant, and substantial quantities of blood tend to pool in the veins of dependent portions of the body. Respiration changes the pressure gradient between the intrathoracic and extrathoracic veins. Hence, respiration serves as an auxiliary pump, which may affect the mean level of Q_h and induce rhythmic changes in stroke volume during the various phases of the respiratory cycle.

5. In anticipation of exercise, vagus nerve impulses to the heart are inhibited and the sympathetic nervous system is activated by central command. The result is an increase in heart rate, myocardial contractile force, and regional vascular resistance. In addition, vascular resistance increases in the skin, kidneys, splanchnic regions, and inactive muscles and decreases markedly in the active muscles. The overall effect is a pronounced reduction in total peripheral resistance, which along with the auxiliary pumping action of the contracting skeletal muscles, greatly increases venous return. The increase in heart rate and myocardial contractility, both induced by the activation of cardiac sympathetic nerves, enables the heart to transfer blood to the pulmonary and systemic circulations, thereby increasing cardiac output. Stroke volume increases only slightly. O_2 consumption and blood O_2 extraction increase, and systolic pressure and mean blood pressure increase slightly. As body temperature rises during exercise, the skin blood vessels dilate. However, when the heart rate becomes maximal during severe exercise, the skin vessels constrict. This increases the effective blood volume but causes greater increases in body temperature and a feeling of exhaustion. The limiting factor in exercise performance is delivery of blood to the active muscles.

6. Acute blood loss induces tachycardia, hypotension, generalized arteriolar constriction, and generalized venoconstriction. Acute blood loss invokes a number of negative-feedback (compensatory) mechanisms, such as baroreceptor and chemoreceptor reflexes, responses to moderate cerebral ischemia, reabsorption of tissue fluids, release of endogenous vasoconstrictors, and renal conservation of water and electrolytes. Acute blood loss also invokes a number of positive-feedback (decompensatory) mechanisms, such as cardiac failure, acidosis, central nervous system depression, aberrations in blood coagulation, and depression of the mononuclear phagocytic system. The outcome of acute blood loss depends on the sum of gains of the positive- and negative-feedback mechanisms and on the interactions between these mechanisms.

THE RESPIRATORY SYSTEM

Michelle M. Cloutier and Roger S. Thrall

CHAPTER 20

Structure and Function of the Respiratory System

The primary function of the lung is gas exchange, which consists of movement of O_2 into the body and removal of CO_2. The lung also plays a role in host defense by functioning as a primary barrier between the outside world and the inside of the body. Finally, the lung is a metabolic organ that synthesizes and metabolizes numerous compounds. This chapter provides an overview of lung anatomy (i.e., upper and lower airways, muscles, innervation), growth and development of the normal and aging lung, and the fluids lining various anatomic sites, with special emphasis on unique features relative to the lung. Metabolic features of the lung are discussed in Chapter 25.

LUNG ANATOMY

The lungs are contained in a space with a volume of approximately 4 L, but they have a surface area for gas exchange that is the size of a tennis court ($\sim$85 m^2). This large surface area is composed of myriads of independently functioning respiratory units. Unlike the heart but similar to the kidneys, the lungs demonstrate functional unity; that is, each unit is structurally identical and functions just like every other unit. Because the divisions of the lung and the sites of disease are designated by their anatomic locations (right upper lobe, left lower lobe, etc.), it is essential to understand pulmonary anatomy in order to clinically relate respiratory physiology and pathophysiology. In adults, the lung weighs approximately 1 kg, with lung tissue accounting for 60% of the weight and blood the remainder. **Alveolar spaces** are responsible for most of the lung's volume; these spaces are divided by tissue known collectively as the **interstitium.** The interstitium is composed primarily of lung collagen fibers and is a potential space for fluid and cells to accumulate.

Upper Airways—Nose, Sinuses, Larynx

The respiratory system begins at the nose and ends in the most distal **alveolus.** Thus, the **nasal cavity,** the **posterior pharynx,** the **glottis** and **vocal cords,** the **trachea,** and all divisions of the **tracheobronchial tree** are included in the respiratory system. The **upper airway** consists of all structures from the nose to the vocal cords, including sinuses and the larynx, whereas the **lower airway** consists of the trachea, airways, and alveoli. The major function of the upper airways is to "condition" inspired air so that by the time it reaches the trachea, it is at body temperature and fully humidified. The nose also functions to filter, entrap, and clear particles larger than 10 μm in size. Finally, the nose provides the sense of smell. Neuronal endings in the roof of the nose above the **superior turbinate** carry impulses through the **cribriform plate** to the **olfactory bulb.** The volume of the nose in an adult is approximately 20 mL, but its surface area is greatly increased by the **nasal turbinates,** which are a series of three continuous ribbons of tissue that protrude into the nasal cavity (Fig. 20-1). In humans, the volume of air entering the **nares** each day is on the order of 10,000 to 15,000 L. Resistance to airflow in the nose during quiet breathing accounts for approximately 50% of the total resistance of the respiratory system, which is about 8 cm H_2O/L/sec. Nasal resistance increases with viral infections and with increased airflow, such as during exercise. When nasal resistance becomes too high, mouth breathing begins.

The interior of the nose is lined by respiratory epithelium interspersed with surface secretory cells. These secretory cells produce important immunoglobulins, inflammatory mediators, and interferons, which are the first line in host defense. The paranasal **sinuses,** including the **frontal sinuses,** the **maxillary sinus,** the **sphenoid sinus,** and the **ethmoid sinus,** are lined by ciliated epithelium, and they nearly surround the nasal passages. The cilia facilitate the flow of mucus from the upper airways and clear the main nasal passages approximately every 15 minutes. The sinuses have two major functions—they lighten the skull, which makes upright posture easier, and they offer resonance to the voice. They may also protect the brain during frontal trauma. The fluid covering their surface is continually being propelled into the nose. In some sinuses (e.g., the **maxillary sinus**), the opening **(ostium)** is at the upper edge, which makes them particularly susceptible to retention of mucus. The ostia are readily obstructed in the presence of nasal edema, and retention of secretions and secondary infection **(sinusitis)** can result.

The major structures of the larynx include the **epiglottis, arytenoids,** and **vocal cords** (Fig. 20-1). With some infections, these structures can become **edematous** (swollen) and contribute significantly to airflow

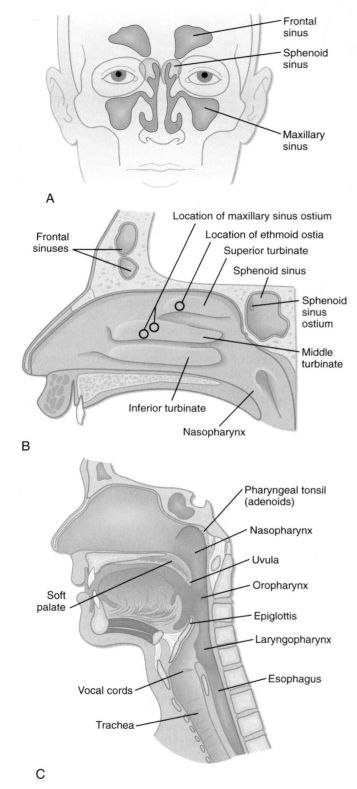

A

B

C

● **Figure 20-1.** Anterior and lateral view drawings of the head and neck illustrating upper airway anatomy. **A,** Anterior view of the paranasal sinuses. **B,** Lateral view of the nasal passage structures demonstrating the superior, middle, and inferior turbinates and sinus ostia. **C,** Lateral midsagittal section of the head and neck showing the three divisions of the pharynx and surrounding upper airway structures.

resistance. The epiglottis and arytenoids "hood" or cover the vocal cords during swallowing. Thus, under normal circumstances, the epiglottis and arytenoids function to prevent aspiration of food and liquid into the lower respiratory tract. The act of swallowing food after **mastication** (chewing) usually occurs within 2 seconds, and it is closely synchronized with muscle reflexes that coordinate opening and closing of the airway. Hence, air is allowed to enter the lower airways and food and liquids are kept out. Patients with some neuromuscular diseases have altered muscle reflexes and can lose this coordinated swallowing mechanism. Thus, they may become susceptible to aspiration of food and liquid, which poses a risk for **pneumonia.**

Lower Airways—Trachea, Bronchi, Bronchioles, Respiratory Unit

The right lung, located in the right **hemithorax,** is divided into three lobes **(upper, middle,** and **lower)** by two interlobular fissures (oblique, horizontal), whereas the left lung, located in the left hemithorax, is divided into two lobes **(upper, including the lingula,** and **lower)** by an **oblique fissure** (Fig. 20-2). Both the right and left lungs are covered by a thin membrane called the **visceral pleura** and are encased by another membrane called the **parietal pleura.** The interface of these two pleuras allows for smooth gliding of the lung as it expands in the chest and produces a potential space. Air can enter between the visceral and parietal pleuras because of either trauma, surgery, or rupture of a group of alveoli creating a **pneumothorax.** Fluid can also enter this space and create a **pleural effusion** or, in the case of severe infection, **empyema.**

The **trachea** bifurcates (branches) into two main stem bronchi (Fig. 20-3). These main stem bronchi then divide (like the branches of a tree) into lobar bronchi (one for each lobe), which in turn divide into segmental bronchi (Figs. 20-3 and 20-4) and into smaller and smaller branches **(bronchioles)** until reaching the **alveolus** (Fig. 20-5). The region of the lung supplied by a segmental bronchus is the functional anatomic unit of the lung. Bronchi and bronchioles differ not only in size but also by the presence of cartilage, the type of epithelium, and their blood supply (Table 20-1). The airways continue to divide in a dichotomous or asymmetric branching pattern until they form terminal bronchioles that are distinguished by being the smallest airways without alveoli. Each branching of the respiratory bronchioles results in decreased diameter; however, the total surface area for that generation increases in size and number until the respiratory bronchiole terminates in an opening to a group of alveoli (Fig. 20-5).

The region of the lung supplied by a segmental bronchus is called a **bronchopulmonary segment** and is the functional **anatomic** unit of the lung. Because of its structure, segments of the lung that have become irreversibly diseased can easily be surgically removed. The basic **physiological** unit of the lung is the respiratory or gas-exchanging unit **(respiratory unit),** which consists of the respiratory bronchioles, the alveolar ducts, and the alveoli (Figs. 20-4 and 20-5). Bronchi

● **Figure 20-2.** Topography of the lung demonstrating the lobes, segments, and fissures. The fissures (or chasms) demarcate the lobes in each lung. Numbers refer to specific bronchopulmonary segments, as presented in Figure 20-3. SVC, superior vena cava.

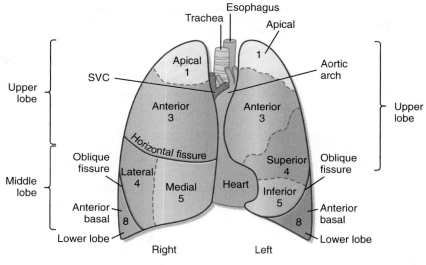

ANTERIOR VIEW

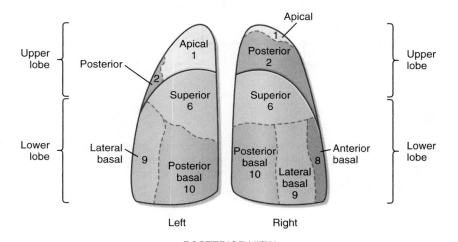

POSTERIOR VIEW

● **Figure 20-3.** Bronchopulmonary segments, anterior view: 1, apical; 2, posterior; 3, anterior; 4, lateral (superior); 5, medial (inferior); 6, superior; 7, medial basal; 8, anterior basal; 9, lateral basal; 10, posterior basal. The numbers are the same as in Figure 20-2.

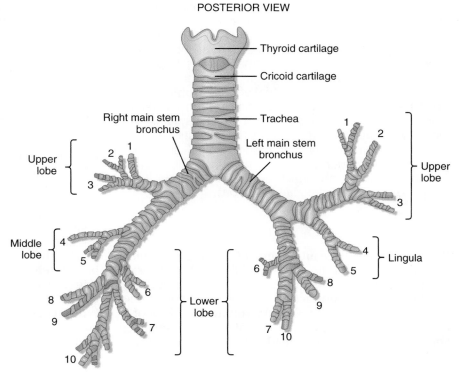

● **Table 20-1.** **Anatomic Characteristics of Bronchi and Bronchioles**

	Cartilage	Diameter (mm)	Epithelium	Blood Supply	Alveoli	Volume (mL)
Bronchi	Yes	>1	Pseudostratified Columnar	Bronchial	No	—
Terminal bronchioles	No	<1	Cuboidal	Bronchial	No	>150
Respiratory bronchioles	No	<1	Cuboidal	Pulmonary	Yes	2500

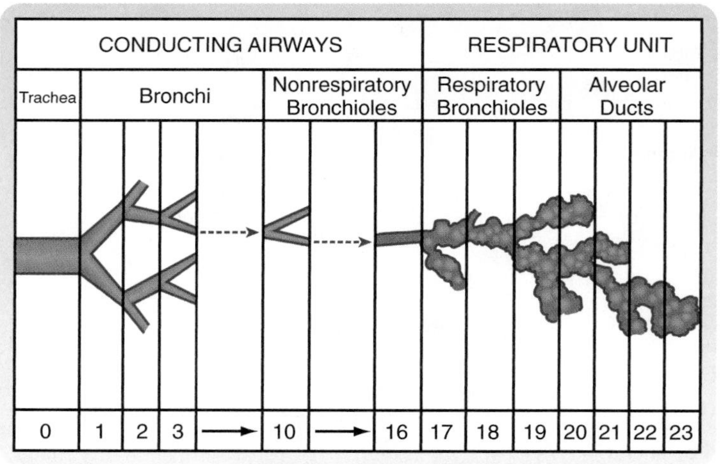

CONDUCTING AIRWAYS			RESPIRATORY UNIT	
Trachea	Bronchi	Nonrespiratory Bronchioles	Respiratory Bronchioles	Alveolar Ducts

| 0 | 1 | 2 | 3 | → | 10 | → | 16 | 17 | 18 | 19 | 20 | 21 | 22 | 23 |

● **Figure 20-4.** Conducting airways and alveolar units of the lung. The relative size of the alveolar unit is greatly enlarged. Numbers at the bottom indicate the approximate number of generations from trachea to alveoli, which may vary from as few as 10 to as many as 23. (From Weibel ER: Morphometry of the Human Lung. Heidelberg, Germany, Springer-Verlag, 1963.)

▶ **IN THE CLINIC**

The conducting airways are involved in several major pulmonary diseases collectively referred to as **chronic obstructive pulmonary disease (COPD),** including asthma, bronchiolitis, chronic bronchitis, and cystic fibrosis. Obstruction of airflow through the airways is commonly caused by increased mucus, airway inflammation, and smooth muscle constriction. **Asthma** involves both large and small airways and is characterized by inflammation, predominantly mediated by lymphocytes and eosinophils, in the airways and reversible airway smooth muscle constriction (bronchospasm). **Bronchiolitis** is a disease of the small airways. It usually occurs in young infants and is caused by viruses, most commonly **respiratory syncytial virus. Chronic bronchitis,** a disease of smokers, is associated with a marked increase in mucus-secreting cells in the airways and an increase in mucus production. **Cystic fibrosis** is a genetically inherited disease that adversely affects chloride channels in exocrine glands. In the lung this results in obstruction via abnormal mucus accumulation and leads to recurrent pulmonary infections.

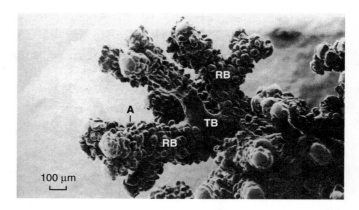

100 μm

● **Figure 20-5.** The airway from the terminal bronchiole to the alveolus. A, alveolus; RB, respiratory bronchiole; TB, terminal bronchiole. Note the absence of alveoli in the terminal bronchiole.

that contain cartilage and nonrespiratory bronchioles (i.e., lacking alveoli) in which cartilage is absent serve to move gas from the airways to the alveoli and are referred to as the **conducting airways.** This area of the lung is approximately 150 mL in volume (or ≈30% of a normal breath), does not participate in gas exchange, and forms the **anatomic dead space.** The respiratory

bronchioles with alveoli and the area from the terminal or nonrespiratory bronchioles to the alveoli are where all gas exchange occurs. This region is only approximately 5 mm long, but it is the single largest volume of the lung at approximately 2500 mL and has a surface area of 70 m² when the lung and chest wall are at the resting volume (Table 20-1).

The alveoli are polygonal in shape and about 250 μm in diameter. An adult has around 5 × 10⁸ alveoli (Fig. 20-6), which are composed of type I and type II epithelial cells. Under normal conditions **type I** and **type II** cells exist in a 1:1 ratio. The type I cell occupies 96% to 98% of the surface area of the alveolus, and it is the primary site for gas exchange. The thin cyto-

● **Figure 20-6.** Alveoli. The terminal respiratory unit consists of the alveoli (A) and the alveolar ducts (AD) arising from a respiratory bronchiole (RB). Each unit is roughly spherical, as suggested by the dashed outline. Pulmonary venous vessels (PV) are peripherally located. TB identifies a terminal bronchiole. PA identifies a pulmonary artery. **Figure insert,** Type I and II alveolar cells. A large fraction of the alveolar wall consists of capillaries (C) and their contents. The alveolar walls are folded and the alveoli (A) are collapsed because this section is from a human lung surgical specimen that was excised and immediately immersed in fixative. This procedure also accounts for the red blood cells in the alveolar air spaces. M, alveolar macrophage; I, type I cell; II, type II cell.

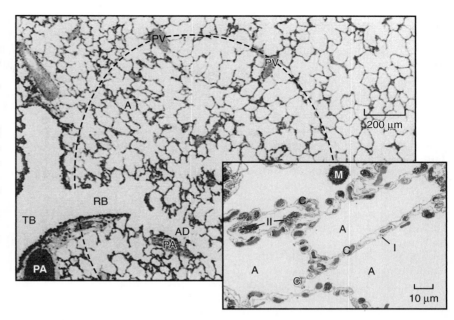

plasm of type I cells is ideal for optimal gas diffusion. In addition, the basement membrane of type I cells and the capillary endothelium are fused, which minimizes the distance for gas diffusion and thereby facilitates gas exchange. The type II epithelial cell is small and cuboidal and is usually found in the "corners" of the alveolus, where it occupies 2% to 4% of its surface area. Type II cells synthesize **pulmonary surfactant,** which reduces surface tension in the alveolar fluid and is responsible for regeneration of the alveolar structure subsequent to injury.

Gas exchange occurs in the alveoli through a dense meshlike network of capillaries and alveoli called the **alveolar-capillary network.** The barrier between gas in the alveoli and the red blood cell is only 1 to 2 μm in thickness and consists of type I alveolar epithelial cells, capillary endothelial cells, and their respective basement membranes. O_2 and CO_2 passively diffuse across this barrier into plasma and red blood cells. Red blood cells pass through the network in less than 1 second, which is sufficient time for CO_2 and O_2 gas exchange.

In response to injury and type I cell death, the type II cell replicates and differentiates into type I cells to restore normal alveolar architecture. This repair process is an example of phylogeny recapitulating ontogeny because during embryonic development the epithelium of the alveolus is entirely composed of type II cells and only very late in gestation do type II cells differentiate into type I cells and form the "normal" alveolar epithelium for optimal gas exchange.

Lung Interstitium

The lung interstitial space or interstitium is composed of connective tissue, smooth muscle, lymphatics, capillaries, and a variety of other cells. Under normal conditions the interstitial space is very small and at times cannot be discerned by light microscopy, especially in alveolar compartments. However, in pathological conditions it can become enlarged with the influx of inflammatory cells and edema fluid, which can interfere with gas exchange in the alveoli.

Fibroblasts are prominent cells in the interstitium of the lung. They synthesize and secrete collagen and elastin, which are the extracellular proteins that play a major role in matrix formation and in the physiology of the lung. **Collagen** is the major structural component of the lung that limits lung distensibility. **Elastin** is the major contributor to elastic recoil of the lung. **Cartilage** is a tough, resilient connective tissue that supports the conducting airways of the lung and encircles about 80% of the trachea. The amount of cartilage decreases down the respiratory system and disappears at the level of the bronchioles. In addition to cartilage, the airway epithelium rests on spiral bands of smooth muscle, which can dilate or constrict in response to chemical, irritant, or mechanical stimulation. **Kultschitzky cells,** neuroendocrine cells, are found in clumps throughout the tracheobronchial tree and secrete biogenic amines, including dopamine and 5-hydroxytryptamine (serotonin). These cells are more numerous in a fetus than in an adult, and they appear to be the cells of origin for a rare bronchial tumor called bronchial carcinoid.

BLOOD SUPPLY TO THE LUNG— PULMONARY AND BRONCHIAL CIRCULATIONS

The lung has two separate blood supplies. The **pulmonary circulation** brings deoxygenated blood from the right ventricle to the gas-exchanging units for removal of CO_2 and oxygenation before blood is returned to the left atrium for distribution to the rest of the body. The

bronchial circulation arises from the aorta and provides nourishment to the lung parenchyma. The circulation to the lung is unique in its duality and ability to accommodate large volumes of blood at low pressure.

Pulmonary Circulation

The pulmonary capillary bed is the largest vascular bed in the body. It covers a surface area of 70 to 80 m², which is nearly as large as the alveolar surface area. The network of capillaries is so dense that it might be considered to be a sheet of blood interrupted by small vertical supporting posts (Fig. 20-7). The capillary volume in the lung at rest is approximately 70 mL. During exercise, this volume increases and approaches 200 mL. This increase occurs, in part, through the recruitment of closed or compressed capillary segments as increased cardiac output raises pulmonary vascular pressure. In addition, open capillaries can enlarge as their internal pressure rises. This occurs when the lungs fill with blood, as it does in left heart failure, which is associated with elevated left atrial pressure. The pulmonary veins return blood to the left atrium through supernumerary conventional branches. Because of their larger numbers and thinner walls, the pulmonary veins provide a large reservoir for blood, and they can either increase or decrease their capacitance to provide constant left ventricular output in the face of variable pulmonary arterial flow. Pulmonary arteries and veins with diameters larger than 50 μm contain smooth muscle. These vessels actively regulate their diameter and thus alter resistance to blood flow.

Bronchial Circulation

The bronchial arteries, usually three in number, provide a source of oxygenated, systemic blood to the lungs. These arteries accompany the bronchial tree and divide with it (Fig. 20-8). They nourish the walls of the bronchi, bronchioles, blood vessels, and nerves, and they perfuse the lymph nodes and most of the visceral pleura. Approximately a third of the blood returns to the right atrium through the bronchial veins, whereas the remainder drains into the left atrium via pulmonary veins. In the presence of diseases such as cystic fibrosis, the bronchial arteries,

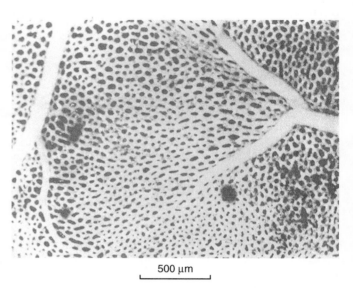

500 μm

● **Figure 20-7.** View of an alveolar wall showing the dense network of capillaries. A small artery and vein can also be seen. The individual capillary segments are so short that the blood forms an almost continuous sheet. (From Maloney JE, Castle BL: Respir Physiol 7:150, 1969.)

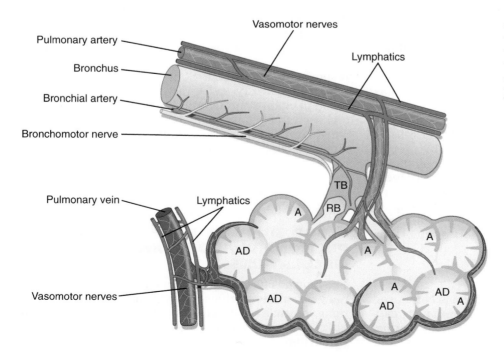

● **Figure 20-8.** Anatomic relationship between the pulmonary artery, the bronchial artery, the airways, and the lymphatics. A, alveoli; AD, alveolar ducts; RB, respiratory bronchioles; TB, terminal bronchioles.

which normally receive only 1% to 2% of cardiac output, increase in size (hypertrophy) and receive as much as 10% to 20% of cardiac output. The erosion of inflamed tissue into these vessels secondary to bacterial infection is responsible for the **hemoptysis** (coughing up blood) that occurs in this disease.

INNERVATION

Breathing is automatic and under control of the central nervous system (CNS). The peripheral nervous system (PNS) includes both sensory and motor components. The PNS conveys and integrates signals from the environment to the CNS. Sensory and motor neurons of the PNS transmit signals from the periphery to the CNS. Somatic motor neurons innervate skeletal muscles, and autonomic neurons innervate smooth muscle, cardiac muscle, and glands. The lung is innervated by the autonomic nervous system of the PNS, which is under CNS control (Fig. 20-9). There are four distinct components of the autonomic nervous system: **parasympathetic** (constriction), **sympathetic** (relaxation), **nonadrenergic noncholinergic inhibitory** (relax-

ation), and **nonadrenergic noncholinergic stimulatory** (constriction).

Stimulation of the parasympathetic system leads to airway constriction, blood vessel dilation, and increased glandular secretion. Stimulation of the sympathetic system causes airway relaxation, blood vessel constriction, and inhibition of glandular secretion (Fig. 20-10). The functional unit of the autonomic nervous system is composed of preganglionic and postganglionic neurons in the CNS and postganglionic neurons in the ganglia of the specific organ. As with most organ systems, the CNS and PNS work in cohort to maintain homeostasis. There is no voluntary motor innervation in the lung, nor are there pain fibers. Pain fibers are found only in the pleura.

The parasympathetic innervation of the lung originates from the medulla in the brainstem (cranial nerve X, the **vagus**). Preganglionic fibers from the vagal nuclei descend in the vagus nerve to ganglia adjacent to airways and blood vessels in the lung. Postganglionic fibers from the ganglia then complete the network by innervating smooth muscle cells, blood vessels, and bronchial epithelial cells (including goblet cells and submucosal glands). The anatomic locations of

● **Figure 20-9.**   Innervation of the lungs. The autonomic innervation (motor and sensory) of the lung and the somatic (motor) nerve supply to the intercostal muscles and diaphragm are depicted.

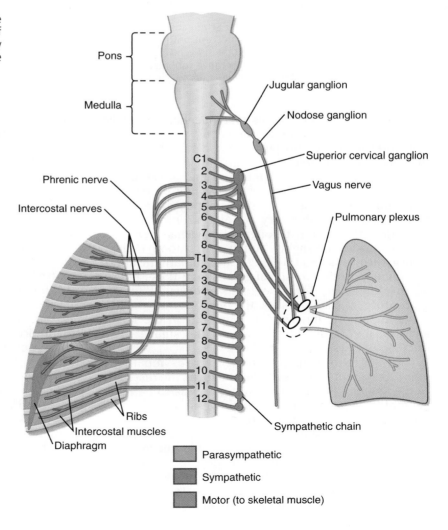

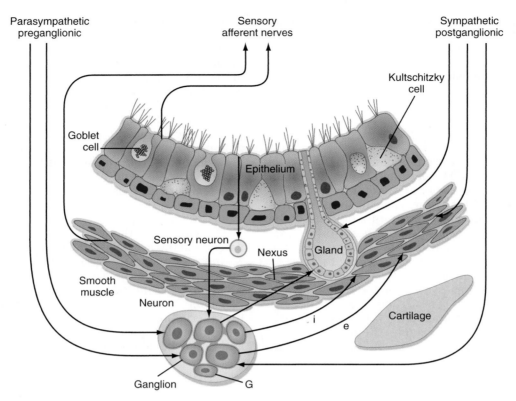

● **Figure 20-10.** Schematic summary of the innervation of the airways. Parasympathetic, preganglionic fibers descend into the vagus and terminate in the ganglia. The ganglia contain excitatory neurons that are cholinergic and inhibitory neurons that are nonadrenergic. Other neurons with an integrative function are probably also present. Glial cells (G) are present in the ganglia. Postganglionic fibers to the smooth muscle are excitatory (e) or inhibitory (i).

the parasympathetic nervous system enhance specific organ responses without influencing other organs. Both preganglionic and postganglionic fibers contain excitatory (cholinergic) and inhibitory (nonadrenergic) motor neurons. **Acetylcholine** and **substance P** are neurotransmitters of excitatory motor neurons; **dynorphin** and **vasoactive intestinal peptide** are neurotransmitters of inhibitory motor neurons. Parasympathetic stimulation through the vagus nerve is responsible for the slightly constricted smooth muscle tone in the normal resting lung. Parasympathetic fibers also innervate the bronchial glands, and these fibers, when stimulated, increase the synthesis of mucus glycoprotein, which raises the viscosity of mucus. Parasympathetic innervation is greater in the larger airways, and it diminishes toward the smaller conducting airways in the periphery.

Whereas the response of the parasympathetic nervous system is very specific and local, the response of the sympathetic nervous system tends to be more general. Mucous glands and blood vessels are heavily innervated by the sympathetic nervous system; however, airway smooth muscle is not. Neurotransmitters of the adrenergic nerves include **norepinephrine** and dopamine, although dopamine has no influence on the lung. Stimulation of the sympathetic nerves in mucous glands increases water secretion. This upsets the balanced response of increased water

and increased viscosity between the sympathetic and parasympathetic pathways. Adrenergic fibers, though present in some animal species, are absent in humans. In addition to the sympathetic and parasympathetic systems, afferent nerve endings are present in the epithelium and in smooth muscle cells.

Central Control of Respiration

Breathing is an automatic, rhythmic, and centrally regulated process with voluntary control. The CNS and, in particular, the **brainstem** function as the main control center for respiration (Fig. 20-11). Regulation of respiration requires (1) generation and maintenance of a respiratory rhythm; (2) modulation of this rhythm by sensory feedback loops and reflexes that allow adaptation to various conditions while minimizing energy costs; and (3) recruitment of respiratory muscles that can contract appropriately for gas exchange.

The **central pattern generator (CPG)** is composed of several groups of cells in the brainstem that have the property of a pacemaker. The CPG integrates peripheral input from stretch receptors in the lung and O_2 receptors in the carotid body with central input from the **hypothalamus** and **amygdala.** This input may be excitatory or inhibitory. In addition, because phrenic nerve output is absent between inspiratory efforts, an inspiratory on-off switch appears to operate

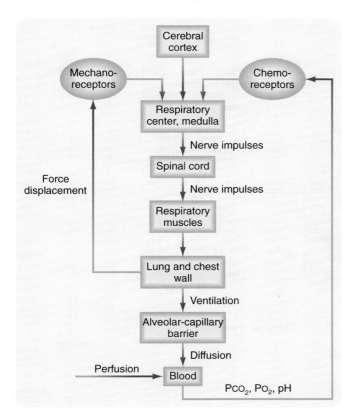

● **Figure 20-11.** Block diagram of the respiratory control system.

in the system, and this switch inhibits the CPG during exhalation. Control of respiration is described in greater detail in Chapter 24.

MUSCLES OF RESPIRATION— DIAPHRAGM, EXTERNAL INTERCOSTALS, SCALENE

The major muscles of respiration include the **diaphragm,** the **external intercostals,** and the **scalene,** which are all skeletal muscles. Skeletal muscles provide the driving force for ventilation; the force of contraction increases when they are stretched and decreases when they shorten. The force of contraction of respiratory muscles increases at larger lung volumes.

The process of respiration or gas exchange begins with the act of inspiration, which is initiated by contraction of the **diaphragm.** On contraction, the diaphragm protrudes into the abdominal cavity and moves the abdomen outward to create negative pressure inside the chest. The opening of the **glottis** in the upper airway creates a portal that connects the outside world to the respiratory system. Because gases flow from higher to lower pressure, air moves into the lungs from the outside, much like the way a vacuum cleaner sucks air into the canister. Lung volume increases at inspiration and oxygen (O_2) is taken into

the lung, whereas during exhalation the diaphragm relaxes, pressure inside the chest increases, and carbon dioxide (CO_2) and other gases flow passively out of the lungs.

The diaphragm is the major muscle of respiration and it divides the thoracic cavity from the abdominal cavity (Fig. 20-12). Contraction of the diaphragm forces the abdominal contents downward and forward. This increases the vertical dimension of the chest cavity and creates a pressure difference between the thorax and abdomen. In adults, the diaphragm can generate airway pressures of up to 150 to 200 cm H_2O during maximal inspiratory effort. During quiet breathing (tidal breathing), the diaphragm moves approximately 1 cm; however, during deep-breathing maneuvers (vital capacity), the diaphragm can move as much as 10 cm. The diaphragm is innervated by the right and left phrenic nerves, which have their origins at the third to fifth cervical segments of the spinal cord (C3 to C5).

The other important muscles of inspiration are the external intercostal muscles, which pull the ribs upward and forward during inspiration (Fig. 20-10). This causes an increase in both the lateral and antero-posterior diameter of the thorax. Innervation of the external intercostal muscles originates from **intercostal nerves** that arise from the same level of the spinal cord. Paralysis of these muscles has no significant effect on respiration because respiration is primarily dependent on the diaphragm. This is why individuals with low spinal cord injuries can breathe on their own. It is only when the injury is above C3 that individuals are completely dependent on a ventilator.

Accessory muscles of inspiration (the scalene muscles, which elevate the **sternocleidomastoid;** the **alae nasi,** which cause nasal flaring; and small muscles in the neck and head) do not contract during normal breathing. However, they do contract vigorously during exercise, and when airway obstruction is significant, they actively pull up on the rib cage. During normal breathing they anchor the sternum and upper ribs. Because the upper airway must remain patent during inspiration, the pharyngeal wall muscles **(genioglossus** and **arytenoid)** are also considered to be muscles of inspiration. All of the rib cage muscles are voluntary muscles that are supplied by intercostal arteries and veins and innervated by motor and sensory intercostal nerves.

Exhalation during normal breathing is passive, but it becomes active during exercise and hyperventilation. The most important muscles of exhalation are those of the abdominal wall **(rectus abdominis, internal** and **external oblique,** and **transversus abdominis)** and the **internal intercostal muscles,** which oppose the external intercostal muscles (i.e., they pull the ribs downward and inward). The inspiratory muscles do the work of breathing. During normal breathing, work is low and the inspiratory muscles have significant reserve. Respiratory muscles can be trained to do more work, but there is a finite limit to the work that they can perform. Respiratory muscle weakness can impair movement of the chest wall, and

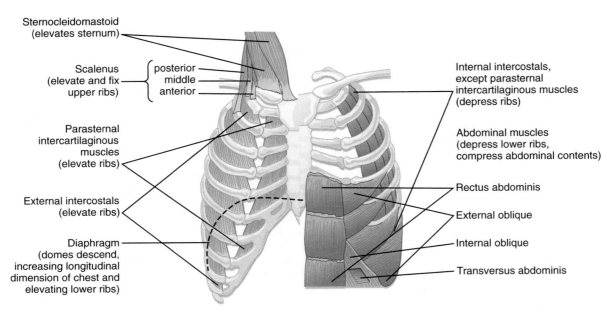

Sternocleidomastoid (elevates sternum)

Scalenus (elevate and fix upper ribs) { posterior / middle / anterior

Parasternal intercartilaginous muscles (elevate ribs)

External intercostals (elevate ribs)

Diaphragm (domes descend, increasing longitudinal dimension of chest and elevating lower ribs)

Internal intercostals, except parasternal intercartilaginous muscles (depress ribs)

Abdominal muscles (depress lower ribs, compress abdominal contents)

Rectus abdominis

External oblique

Internal oblique

Transversus abdominis

A   **Muscles of inspiration**   **Muscles of expiration**

B   Diaphragm muscle

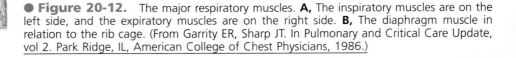

● **Figure 20-12.** The major respiratory muscles. **A,** The inspiratory muscles are on the left side, and the expiratory muscles are on the right side. **B,** The diaphragm muscle in relation to the rib cage. (From Garrity ER, Sharp JT. In Pulmonary and Critical Care Update, vol 2. Park Ridge, IL, American College of Chest Physicians, 1986.)

respiratory muscle fatigue is a major factor in the development of respiratory failure.

FLUIDS LINE THE LUNG EPITHELIUM AND PLAY IMPORTANT PHYSIOLOGICAL ROLES

The respiratory system is lined with three very different and highly significant fluids: **periciliary fluid, mucus,** and **surfactant.** Periciliary fluid and mucus are components of the mucociliary clearance system and line the epithelium of the conducting airways from the trachea to the terminal bronchioles. Together they form the basis for the **mucociliary clearance system,** which aids in the removal of particulates (e.g., bacteria, viruses, toxins) from the lung and will be discussed further in Chapter 25. Surfactant lines the epithelium of the alveolus and provides an "antistick" function

that decreases surface tension in the alveolus. The cells involved in mucociliary clearance and the production of mucus and surfactant are described next.

Cells of the Mucociliary Clearance System

The respiratory tract to the level of the bronchioles is lined by a **pseudostratified, ciliated columnar epithelium** (Fig. 20-10). These cells maintain the level of periciliary fluid, a 5-μm layer of water and electrolytes in which cilia and the mucociliary transport system function. The depth of the periciliary fluid is maintained by the movement of various ions, mainly chloride secretion and sodium absorption, across the epithelium. Mucus and inhaled particles are removed from the airways by the rhythmic beating of the cilia on the top of the pseudostratified, columnar epithelium. Each epithelial cell contains about 250 cilia.

IN THE CLINIC

Because respiratory muscles provide the driving force for ventilation, diseases that affect the mechanical properties of the lung affect the muscles of respiration. For example, in chronic obstructive pulmonary disease (COPD), the work of breathing is increased secondary to airflow obstruction. Exhalation is no longer passive but requires active, expiratory muscle contraction. In addition, total lung capacity (TLC) is increased. The greater TLC forces the diaphragm downward, shortens the muscle fibers, and decreases the radius of curvature. As a result, the function and efficiency of the diaphragm are decreased. Respiratory muscles can fatigue just as other skeletal muscles do when the workload increases. Respiratory muscles can also weaken in patients with neuromuscular diseases (e.g., **Guillain-Barré syndrome, myasthenia gravis**). In these diseases, sufficient respiratory muscle weakness can impair movement of the chest wall and result in respiratory failure even though the mechanical properties of the lung and chest wall are normal.

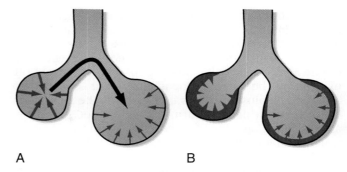

A   B

● **Figure 20-13.** Surface forces in a sphere attempt to reduce the area of the surface and generate pressure within the sphere. By Laplace's law, the pressure generated is inversely proportional to the radius of the sphere. **A,** Surface forces in the smaller sphere generate higher pressure *(heavier arrows)* than those in the larger sphere *(lighter arrows)*. As a result, air moves from the small sphere (higher pressure) to the larger sphere (lower pressure; *black arrow*). This causes the small sphere to collapse and the large sphere to become overdistended. **B,** Surfactant *(shaded layer)* lowers surface tension and lowers it more in the smaller sphere than in the larger sphere. The net result is that the pressure in the small and larger spheres is similar and the spheres are stabilized.

Cells Regulating Mucus Production

Goblet or **surface secretory cells** are interspersed among the epithelial cells in a ratio of approximately one goblet cell to five ciliated cells. They produce mucus in the airways and increase in number in response to chronic cigarette smoke (and environmental pollutants) and thus contribute to the increased mucus and airway obstruction observed in smokers.

Submucosal tracheobronchial glands are present wherever there is cartilage in the tracheobronchial tree. These glands empty to the surface epithelium through a ciliated duct, and they are lined by mucus-secreting **mucous** and **serous** cells (Fig. 20-10). Submucosal tracheobronchial glands increase in number and size in chronic bronchitis, and they extend down to the level of the bronchioles in pulmonary disease.

In normal individuals, **Clara cells** are found at the level of the bronchioles, where the goblet cells and submucosal glands have disappeared. Although their function is controversial, they contain granules with nonmucinous material and may have a secretory function. In addition, they may play a role in epithelial regeneration after injury.

Surfactant and Surface Tension

The alveoli are lined with a predominantly lipid-based substance called **surfactant** that reduces surface tension. Surface tension is a force caused by water molecules at the air-liquid interface that tends to minimize surface area, thereby making it more difficult to inflate the lung. The effect of surface tension on lung inflation is illustrated by comparing the volume-pressure curves of a saline-filled versus an air-filled lung. Higher pressure is required to fully inflate the lung with air than with saline because of the higher surface tension forces in air-filled versus saline-filled lungs.

Surface tension is a measure of the attractive force of the surface molecules per unit length of material to which they are attached. The units of surface tension are those of a force applied per unit length. For a sphere (such as an alveolus), the relationship between the pressure within the sphere (P_s) and the tension in the wall is described by the law of Laplace:

● **Equation 20-1**

$$P_s = \frac{2T}{r}$$

where T is the wall tension (dynes/cm) and r is the radius of the sphere.

In the absence of surfactant, the surface tension at the air-liquid interface would remain constant and the transmural (transalveolar) pressure needed to keep it at that volume would be greater at lower lung (alveolar) volumes (Fig. 20-13, *A*). Thus, greater transmural pressure would be required to produce a given increase in alveolar volume at lower lung volumes than at higher lung volumes. Surfactant stabilizes the inflation of alveoli because it allows the surface tension to increase as the alveoli become larger (Fig. 20-13, *B*). As a result, the transmural pressure required to keep an alveolus inflated increases as lung volume (and transpulmonary pressure) increases, and it decreases as lung volume decreases. The unique feature of surfactant is that although it decreases the surface tension of alveoli overall, the surfactant can change its surface tension at different lung volumes. Specifically, in the presence of surfactant there is an increase in surface tension at high lung volume and a decrease at low lung volume. The result is that the lung can maintain alveoli at many different volumes. Otherwise, small alveoli would empty into large alveoli.

In addition to surfactant, another mechanism, namely, interdependence, contributes to stability of the alveoli. Alveoli, except for those on the pleural surface, are surrounded by other alveoli. The tendency of one alveolus to collapse is opposed by the traction exerted by the surrounding alveoli. Thus, collapse of a single alveolus stretches and distorts the surrounding alveoli, which in turn are connected to other alveoli. Small openings **(pores of Kohn)** in the alveolar walls connect adjacent alveoli, whereas the **canals of Lambert** connect the terminal airways to adjacent alveoli. The pores of Kohn and the canals of Lambert provide collateral ventilation and prevent alveolar collapse **(atelectasis).**

Composition and Function of Surfactant

Pulmonary surfactant is a complex mixture of phospholipids, neutral lipids, fatty acids, and proteins. Surfactant is 85% to 90% lipids, predominantly phospholipids, and 10% to 15% proteins. The major phospholipid is phosphatidylcholine, approximately 75% of which is present as **dipalmitoyl phosphatidylcholine** (DPPC). DPPC is the major surface-active component in surfactant, and it decreases surface tension. The second most abundant phospholipid is phosphatidylglycerol (PG), which accounts for 1% to 10% of total surfactant. These lipids are important in formation of the monolayer on the alveolar-air interface, and PG is important in the spreading of surfactant over a large surface area. Surfactant is secreted by type II cells and thus must spread over the entire surface area of the alveolus. This is accomplished with the aid of surfactant components such as PG, which have spreading properties. Cholesterol and cholesterol esters account for the majority of the neutral lipids; their precise functional role is not yet fully understood, but they may aid in stabilizing the lipid structure.

Four specific surfactant proteins **(SP-A, SP-B, SP-C, SP-D)** make up 2% to 5% of the weight of surfactant. The most studied is SP-A, which is expressed in alveolar type II cells and in Clara cells in the lung. SP-A is involved in the regulation of surfactant turnover, in immune regulation within the lung, and in the formation of tubular myelin. Tubular myelin is the term used to describe a precursor stage of surfactant as it is initially secreted from the type II cell and has not yet spread. Two hydrophobic surfactant-specific proteins are SP-B and SP-C. SP-B may be involved in tubular myelin formation and the surface activity (i.e., surface tension, spreading ability) of surfactant, and it may increase the intermolecular and intramolecular order of the phospholipid bilayer. SP-C may be involved in the spreading ability and surface tension activity of surfactant. The function of SP-D is unknown at this time.

Secretion of surfactant into the airway occurs via exocytosis of the lamellar body by constitutive and regulated mechanisms. Numerous agents, including β-adrenergic agonists, activators of protein kinase C, leukotrienes, and purinergic agonists, stimulate the exocytosis of surfactant. The major routes of clearance of pulmonary surfactant within the lung are reuptake by type II cells, absorption into the lymphatics, and clearance by alveolar macrophages. In summary, pulmonary surfactant serves several physiological roles, including (1) reducing the work of breathing by decreasing surface tension forces; (2) preventing collapse and sticking of alveoli on expiration; and (3) stabilizing alveoli, especially those that tend to deflate at low surface tension.

> ### ▶ IN THE CLINIC
>
> In 1959, Avery and Mead discovered that the lungs of premature infants who died of hyaline membrane disease (HMD) were deficient in surfactant. HMD, also known as infant respiratory distress syndrome (RDS), is characterized by progressive atelectasis and respiratory failure in premature infants. It is a major cause of morbidity and mortality in the neonatal period. The major surfactant deficiency in premature infants is lack of PG. In general, as the level of PG increases in amniotic fluid, the mortality rate decreases. Research in this field has culminated in successful attempts to treat HMD in premature infants with surfactant replacement therapy. Today, surfactant replacement therapy is standard care for premature infants.

THE LYMPHATIC SYSTEM

Host defense and removal of lymph fluid from the lung are the major functions of the lymphatic network in the lung. Interstitial fluid enters lymphatic vessels via lymphatic capillaries. The lymphatic fluid drains to larger lymphatic vessels, and it eventually returns to the blood by way of large veins. Changes in tissue pressure and contractions of the lymphatic vessels drive the interstitial fluid into the lymphatic capillaries. The lymphatic capillaries are highly specialized to allow the transfer of fluid from the interstitial spaces into the lymphatic capillaries. Although the lymphatic capillaries are somewhat similar to blood capillaries, they have several distinct features that aid in fluid movement and clearance: (1) there are no tight junctions between endothelial cells, (2) fine filaments anchor the lymph vessels to adjacent connective tissue such that with each muscle contraction the endothelial junctions open to allow fluid movement, and (3) valves enhance lymph flow in one direction. Chapter 25 will provide additional details about the lymphatic system and the immune functions of the lungs.

LUNG DEVELOPMENT, GROWTH, AND AGING

The epithelium of the lung arises as a pouch from the primitive foregut at approximately 22 to 26 days after fertilization of the ovum. This single lung bud branches into primitive right and left lungs. Over the next 2 to 3 weeks, further branching occurs to create the irregular dichotomous branching pattern. Reid has described "three laws of lung development": (1) the bronchial tree has developed by week 16 of intrauterine life; (2) alveoli develop after birth, the number of alveoli increases until the age of 8 years, and the size of alveoli increases until growth of the chest wall is completed at adulthood; and (3) preacinar vessels (arteries and veins) parallel the development of the airways, whereas intraacinar vessels parallel that of the alveoli. Thus, intrauterine events that occur before 16 weeks of gestation will affect the number of airways. A condition known as **congenital diaphragmatic hernia** is an example of a congenital lung disease. It occurs at 6 to 8 weeks of gestation and is due to failure of the pleuroperitoneal canal to close and separate the chest and abdominal cavities; it results in a decreased number of alveoli.

Growth of the lungs is similar and relatively proportional to growth in body length and stature. The rate of development is fastest in the neonatal and adolescent (≈11 years of age) periods, with girls maturing earlier than boys. Although the growth rate slows after adolescence, the body and lungs increase in size steadily until adulthood. Improvement in lung function occurs at all stages of growth development; however, once optimal size has been attained in early adulthood (20 to 25 years of age), lung function starts to decline with age. The decrease in lung function with age, estimated at less than 1% per year, appears to begin earlier and proceed faster in individuals who smoke or are exposed to toxic environmental factors. The major physiological insufficiencies caused by aging involve ventilatory capacity and ventilatory responses, especially during exercise, and they result in a mismatch of abnormal ventilation with normal perfusion. In addition, gas diffusion decreases with age, most likely as a result of a decrease in alveolar surface area. Age-related decreases in lung function and altered morphology parallel biochemical observations of increased elastin within the lung, which could explain some of the functional abnormalities.

■ KEY CONCEPTS

1. The lung demonstrates anatomic and physiological unity; that is, each unit (bronchopulmonary segment) is structurally identical and it functions just like every other unit.

2. The circulation to the lung is unique in its dual circulation and ability to accommodate large volumes of blood at low pressure. The pulmonary circulation brings deoxygenated blood from the right ventricle to the gas-exchanging units. The bronchial circulation arises from the aorta and provides nourishment to the lung parenchyma.

3. Inspiration is the active phase of breathing; the muscles of the chest wall, mainly the diaphragm, contract and move down into the abdomen, thereby resulting in negative pressure inside the chest. Gas then flows from higher to lower pressure.

4. The surface tension–reducing and antistick properties of surfactant diminish the work of breathing and help stabilize alveoli.

5. The respiratory center is located in the medulla in the brainstem and regulates respiration with input from sensory feedback loops and reflexes in the lung and chest wall and from chemoreceptors that respond to changes in O_2 and CO_2.

CHAPTER 21

Mechanical Properties of the Lung and Chest Wall: Static and Dynamic

Lung mechanics is the study of the mechanical properties of the lung and the chest wall (which includes the rib cage, diaphragm, abdominal cavity, and anterior abdominal muscles). The primary function of the lung is gas exchange. To achieve this primary function, air must be moved in and out of the lung. The mechanical properties of the lung and chest wall determine the ease or difficulty of this air movement. An understanding of lung mechanics is important to comprehend both how the lung works normally and how the lung works in the presence of disease because almost all lung diseases affect the mechanical properties of the lung. In addition, death from lung disease is almost always due to an inability to overcome the altered mechanical properties of the lung or chest wall, or both. Lung mechanics includes static mechanics (the mechanical properties of a lung whose volume is not changing with time) and dynamic mechanics (properties of a lung whose volume is changing with time). Both are described in this chapter.

STATIC LUNG MECHANICS

Lung Volumes

Clinical evaluation of lung function and the study of static lung mechanics begin with the measurement of lung volumes (Fig. 21-1) and the factors that determine these volumes. All lung volumes are subdivisions of **total lung capacity (TLC),** the total volume of air that can be contained in the lung. Lung volumes are reported in liters either as volumes or as capacities. A capacity is composed of two or more volumes. Many lung volumes are measured with a **spirometer.** The patient is asked to first breathe normally into the spirometer, and the volume of air (the **tidal volume [V_T]**) that is moved with each quiet breath is measured. The subject then inhales maximally and exhales forcefully and completely, and the volume of that exhaled air is measured. The total volume of exhaled air, from a maximal inspiration to a maximal exhalation, is the **vital capacity (VC). Residual volume (RV)** is the air remaining in the lung after a complete exhalation. TLC is the sum of VC and RV; it is the total volume of air contained in the lungs, and it includes the volume of air that can be moved (VC) and the volume of air that is always present (trapped) in the lung (RV). **Func-**

tional residual capacity (FRC) is the volume of air in the lung at the end of exhalation during quiet breathing and is also called the resting volume of the lung. FRC is composed of RV and the **expiratory reserve volume (ERV;** the volume of air that can be exhaled from FRC to RV).

The ratio of RV to TLC **(RV/TLC ratio)** is used to distinguish different types of pulmonary disease. In normal individuals, this ratio is usually less than 0.25. Thus, in a healthy individual, approximately 25% of the total volume of air in the lung is trapped. An elevated RV/TLC ratio, secondary to an increase in RV out of proportion to any increase in TLC, is seen in diseases associated with airway obstruction, known as **obstructive pulmonary diseases.** An elevated RV/TLC ratio can also be caused by a decrease in TLC, which occurs in individuals with **restrictive lung diseases.** Measurement of these lung volumes is described later.

Determinants of Lung Volume

What determines the volume of air in the lung at TLC or at RV? The answer lies in the properties of the lung parenchyma and in the interaction between the lungs and the chest wall. The lungs and chest wall always move together in healthy individuals. The lung contains elastic fibers that stretch when stress is applied, thereby resulting in an increase in lung volume, and that recoil passively when this stress is released, thereby resulting in a decrease in lung volume. The elastic recoil of the lung parenchyma is very high. In the absence of external forces (such as the force generated by the chest wall), the lung will become almost airless (10% of TLC). Similarly, chest wall volume can increase when the respiratory muscles are stretched and decrease when respiratory muscle length is shortened. In the absence of the lung parenchyma, the volume of the chest wall is approximately 60% of TLC.

Lung volumes are determined by the balance between the lung's elastic properties and the properties of the muscles of the chest wall. The maximum volume of air contained within the lung and the chest wall (i.e., TLC) is controlled by the muscles of inspiration. With increasing lung volume, the chest wall muscles lengthen progressively. As these muscles lengthen, their ability to generate force decreases. TLC occurs when the inspiratory chest wall muscles

● **Figure 21-1.** The various lung volumes and capacities. ERV, expiratory reserve volume; FRC, functional residual capacity; FVC, forced vital capacity; IC, inspiratory capacity; IRV, inspiratory reserve volume; RV, residual volume; TLC, total lung capacity; VC, vital capacity; V_T, tidal volume.

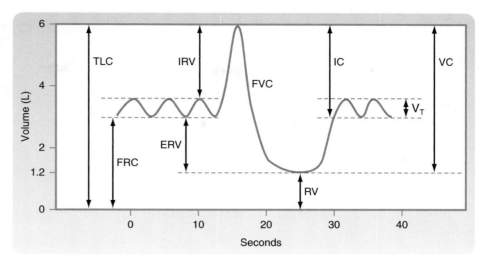

are unable to generate the additional force needed to further distend the lung and chest wall. Similarly, the minimal volume of air in the lung (i.e., RV) is controlled by the expiratory muscle force. Decreasing lung volume results in shortening of the expiratory muscles, which in turn results in a decrease in muscle force. The decrease in lung volume is also associated with an increase in the outward recoil pressure of the chest wall. RV occurs when expiratory muscle force is insufficient to further reduce chest wall volume.

FRC, or the volume of the lung at the end of a normal exhalation, is determined by the balance between the elastic recoil pressure generated by the lung parenchyma to become smaller (inward recoil) and the pressure generated by the chest wall to become larger (outward recoil). When the chest wall muscles are weak, FRC decreases (lung elastic recoil > chest wall muscle force). In the presence of airway obstruction, FRC increases because of premature airway closure, which traps air in the lung.

Measurement of Lung Volumes

RV and TLC can be measured in two ways: by helium dilution and by body plethysmography. Both are used clinically and provide valuable information about lung function and lung disease. The helium dilution technique is the older and simpler method, but it is often less accurate than body plethysmography, which requires sophisticated and expensive equipment.

In normal individuals, the FRC measured by helium dilution and the FRC measured by plethysmography are the same. This is not true in individuals with lung disease. The FRC measured by helium dilution measures the volume of gas in the lung that communicates with the airways, whereas the FRC measured by plethysmography measures the total volume of gas in the lung at the end of a normal exhalation. If a significant amount of gas is trapped in the lung (because of premature airway closure), the FRC determined by plethysmography will be considerably greater than that measured by helium dilution.

> **IN THE CLINIC**

In the helium dilution technique, a known concentration of an inert gas (such as helium) is added to a box of known volume. The box is then connected to a volume that is unknown (the lung volume to be measured). After adequate time for distribution of the inert gas, the new concentration of the inert gas is measured. The change in concentration of the inert gas is then used to determine the new volume in which the inert gas has been distributed (Fig. 21-2). Specifically,

$$C_1 \times V_1 = C_2 (V_1 + V_2)$$

Measurement of lung volumes with a body plethysmograph (body box) uses Boyle's gas law, which states that pressure multiplied by volume is constant (at a constant temperature). The subject sits in an airtight box (Fig. 21-3) and breathes through a mouthpiece that is connected to a flow sensor (pneumotach). The subject then makes panting respiratory effort against a closed mouthpiece. During the expiratory phase of the maneuver, the gas in the lung becomes compressed, lung volume decreases, and the pressure inside the box falls because the gas volume in the box increases. By knowing the volume of the box and measuring the change in pressure of the box at the mouth, the change in volume of the lung can be calculated. Thus,

$$P_1 \times V = P_2 (V - \Delta V)$$

where P_1 and P_2 are mouth pressures and V is FRC.

Lung Compliance

Lung compliance (C_L) is a measure of the elastic properties of the lung. It is a measure of how easily the lung is distended. Lung compliance is defined as the change in lung volume resulting from a 1–cm H_2O change in the distending pressure of the lung. The units of

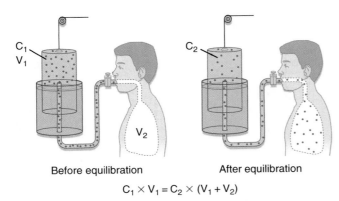

Figure 21-2. Measurement of lung volume by helium dilution.

$$C_1 \times V_1 = C_2 \times (V_1 + V_2)$$

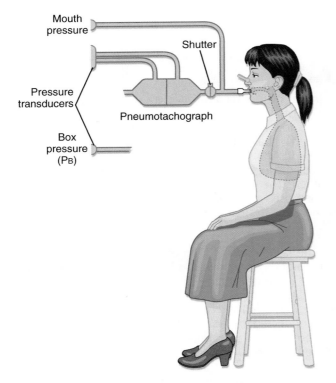

Figure 21-3. The body plethysmograph.

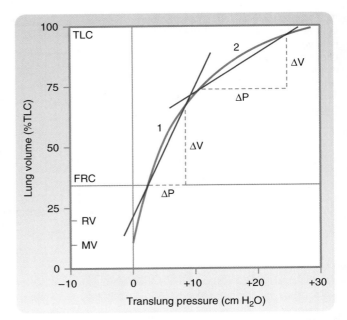

Figure 21-4. Deflation pressure-volume (PV) curve. Because of hysteresis caused by surfactant, the deflation PV curve is used for measurements. Compliance at any point along this curve is the change in volume per change in pressure. From the curve it can be seen that lung compliance varies with lung volume. Compare the compliance at 1 versus 2. By convention, lung compliance is the change in pressure in going from FRC to FRC +1 L.

compliance are mL (or L)/cm H_2O. High lung compliance refers to a lung that is readily distended. Low lung compliance, or a "stiff" lung, is a lung that is not easily distended. The compliance of the lung is thus

● Equation 21-1

$$C_L = \frac{\Delta V}{\Delta P}$$

where ΔV is the change in volume and ΔP is the change in pressure. Graphically, lung compliance is the slope of the line between any two points on the deflation limb of the pressure-volume loop (Fig. 21-4). The compliance of a normal human lung is about 0.2 L/cm H_2O, but it varies with lung volume. Note that the lung is

less distensible at high lung volumes. For this reason, compliance is corrected for the lung volume at which it is measured (specific compliance) (Fig. 21-5). Changes in lung compliance are associated with certain types of lung disease (e.g., restrictive lung diseases) and are of great clinical importance. Compliance measurements are not often performed for clinical purposes, however, because they require placement of an esophageal balloon. The esophageal balloon, which is connected to a pressure transducer, is an excellent surrogate marker for pleural pressure. The change in pleural pressure (P_{pl}) is measured as a function of the change in lung volume; that is, $C_L = \Delta V / \Delta P_{pl}$.

The compliance of the lung is affected by several respiratory disorders. In emphysema, an obstructive lung disease usually of smokers associated with destruction of the alveolar septa and pulmonary capillary bed, the lung is more compliant; that is, for every 1–cm H_2O increase in pressure, the increase in volume is greater than in a normal lung (Fig. 21-6). In contrast, in pulmonary fibrosis, a restrictive lung disease associated with increased collagen fiber deposition in the interstitial space, the lung is noncompliant; that is, for every 1–cm H_2O change in pressure, the change in volume is less.

Lung–Chest Wall Interactions

The lung and chest wall move together as a unit in healthy people. Separating these structures is the **pleural space,** which is best thought of as a potential

● **Figure 21-5.** Relationship between compliance and lung volume. Imagine a lung in which a 5–cm H_2O change in pressure results in a 1-L change in volume. If half of the lung is removed, the compliance will decrease, but when corrected for volume of the lung, there is no change (specific compliance). Even when the lung is reduced by 90%, the specific compliance is unchanged.

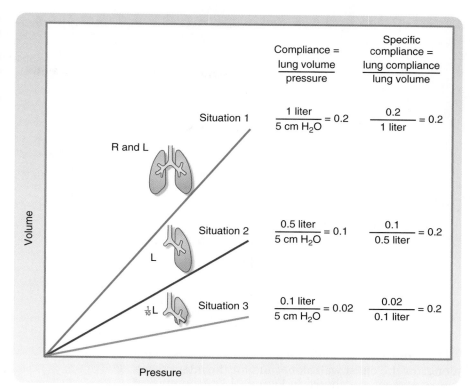

● **Equation 21-2**

$$P_L = P_A - P_{pl}$$

The lung requires positive transpulmonary pressure to increase its volume, and lung volume increases with increasing transpulmonary pressure (Fig. 21-6). The lung assumes its smallest size when transpulmonary pressure is zero. The lung, however, is not totally devoid of air when transpulmonary pressure is zero because of the surface tension–lowering properties of surfactant (see Chapter 20).

The **transmural pressure across the chest wall** (P_w) is the difference between pleural pressure and the pressure surrounding the chest wall (P_b), which is the barometric pressure or body surface pressure. That is,

● **Equation 21-3**

$$P_w = P_{pl} - P_b$$

During inspiration, the chest wall expands to a larger volume. Because pleural pressure is negative relative to atmospheric pressure during quiet breathing, the transmural pressure across the chest wall is negative.

The pressure across the respiratory system (P_{rs}) is the sum of the pressure across the lung and the pressure across the chest wall. That is,

● **Equation 21-4**

$$P_{rs} = P_L + P_w$$
$$= (P_A - P_{pl}) + (P_{pl} - P_b)$$
$$= P_A - P_b$$

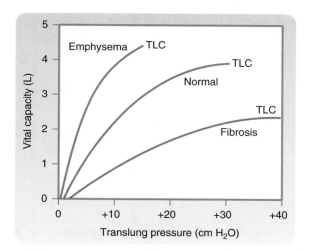

● **Figure 21-6.** Fibrosis/emphysema pressure-volume curve.

space. Because the lung and chest wall move together, changes in their respective volumes are equal. An understanding of the pressures that surround the lung and chest wall and result in changes in lung volume is essential to comprehend how the lungs work. The pressure changes across the lung and across the chest wall are defined as transmural pressure. For the lung, this transmural pressure is called the **transpulmonary** (or translung) **pressure** (P_L), and it is defined as the pressure difference between the air spaces (alveolar pressure [P_A]) and the pressure surrounding the lung (pleural pressure]P_{pl}]). That is,

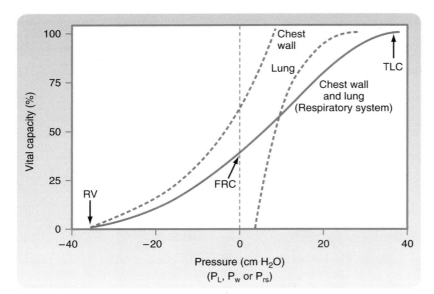

The pressure-volume relationships for the lung alone, for the chest wall alone, and for the intact respiratory system are shown in Figure 21-7. A number of important observations can be made by examining the pressure-volume curves of the lung, chest wall, and respiratory system. Note that the transmural pressure across the respiratory system at FRC is zero. At TLC, both lung pressure and chest wall pressure are positive, and they both require positive transmural distending pressure. The resting volume of the chest wall is the volume at which the transmural pressure for the chest wall is zero, and it is approximately 60% of TLC. At volumes greater than 60% of TLC, the chest wall is recoiling inward and positive transmural pressure is needed, whereas at volumes below 60% of TLC, the chest wall tends to recoil outward.

The transmural pressure for the lung alone flattens at pressures greater than 20 cm H_2O because the elastic limits of the lung have been reached. Thus, further increases in transmural pressure produce no change in volume and compliance is low. Further distention is limited by the connective tissue (collagen, elastin) of the lung. If further pressure is applied, the alveoli near the lung surface can rupture and air can escape into the pleural space. This is called **pneumothorax.**

The relationship between pleural, alveolar, and elastic recoil pressure is shown in Figure 21-8. Alveolar pressure is the sum of the pleural pressure and elastic recoil pressure of the lung.

$$P_A = P_{el} + P_{pl}$$

Because $P_L = P_A - P_{pl}$,

● **Equation 21-5**

$$P_L = (P_{el} + P_{pl}) - P_{pl}$$

Thus,

$$P_L = P_{el}$$

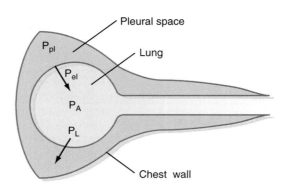

● **Figure 21-8.** Relationship between transpulmonary pressure (P_L) and the pleural (P_{pl}), alveolar (P_A), and elastic recoil (P_{el}) pressures of the lung. Alveolar pressure is the sum of pleural pressure and elastic recoil pressure. Transpulmonary pressure is the difference between pleural pressure and alveolar pressure.

In general, P_L is the pressure distending the lung, whereas P_{el} is the pressure tending to collapse the lung.

Pressure-Volume Relationships

Air flows into and out of the airways from areas of higher pressure to areas of lower pressure. In the absence of a pressure gradient, there is no airflow. **Minute ventilation** is the volume of gas that is moved per unit of time. It is equal to the volume of gas moved with each breath times the number of breaths per minute:

● **Equation 21-6**

$$\dot{V}_E = V_T \times f$$

where $\dot{V}_E$ is minute ventilation in mL or L/min, V_T is tidal volume in mL or L, and f is the frequency or number of breaths per minute.

▶ IN THE CLINIC

To understand the relationship between changes in pressure and changes in volume, it is helpful to examine the pressure changes during inspiration and exhalation (Fig. 21-9). In normal individuals during tidal volume breathing, alveolar pressure decreases at the start of inspiration. This decrease in alveolar pressure is usually small (1 to 3 cm H_2O). It is much larger in individuals with airway obstruction because of the larger pressure drop that occurs across obstructed airways.

Pressure within the pleural space (pleural pressure) also falls during inspiration. This decrease equals the lung elastic recoil, which increases as the lung inflates. Pressure drops along the airways as gas flows from atmospheric pressure (zero) to the pressure in the alveolus (negative relative to atmospheric pressure). Airflow stops when alveolar pressure and atmospheric pressure become equal.

On exhalation, the diaphragm moves higher into the chest, pleural pressure increases (i.e., becomes less negative), alveolar pressure becomes positive, the glottis opens, and gas again flows from a higher (alveolus) to a lower (atmospheric) pressure. In the alveolus, the driving force for exhalation is the sum of the elastic recoil of the lung and pleural pressure.

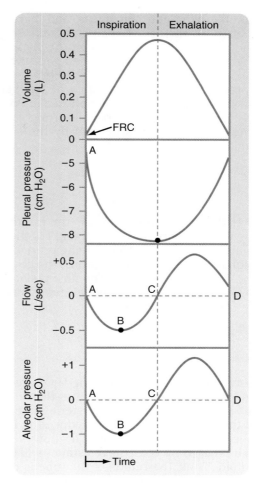

● **Figure 21-9.** Changes in alveolar and pleural pressure during a tidal volume breath. Inspiration is to the left of the vertical dotted line and exhalation is to the right. Positive (relative to atmosphere) pressures are above the horizontal dotted line and negative pressures are below. See text for details. At points of no airflow (points A and C), alveolar pressure is zero.

Before inspiration begins, the pleural pressure in normal individuals is approximately –5 cm H_2O. Thus, the pressure in the pleural space is negative relative to atmospheric pressure (by convention, atmospheric pressure is considered to be 0). This negative pressure is created by the inward elastic recoil pressure of the lung, and it acts to pull the lung away from the chest wall. Just before inspiration begins, alveolar pressure is zero because with no gas flow, there is no pressure drop along the airways. With the onset of inspiration, the muscles of the diaphragm and chest wall shorten, which causes a downward movement of the diaphragm and outward and upward movement of the rib cage. Alveolar pressure falls below zero, and when the glottis opens, gas moves into the airways.

Note that at the resting volume of the lung (FRC), the elastic recoil of the lung acts to decrease lung volume, but this inward recoil is offset by the outward recoil of the chest wall, which acts to increase lung volume. At FRC, these forces are equal and opposite, and the muscles are relaxed. When the chest is opened, as during thoracic surgery, the lung recoils until transpulmonary pressure is zero and the chest wall increases in size. The lungs do not, however, become airless but retain approximately 10% of their TLC.

DYNAMIC LUNG MECHANICS

In this section we examine the principles that control air movement into and out of the lung. Dynamics is

that aspect of mechanics that studies physical systems in motion.

Airflow in Airways

Air flows through the airways when there is a pressure difference at the two ends of the airway. During inspiration, the diaphragm contracts, pleural pressure becomes more negative (relative to atmospheric pressure), and gas flows into the lung (from the higher to the lower pressure). Gas exchange to meet the changing metabolic needs of the body depends on the speed at which fresh gas is brought to the alveoli and the rapidity with which the metabolic products of respiration (i.e., CO_2) are removed. Two major factors determine the speed at which gas flows into the airways for a given pressure change: the pattern of gas flow and the resistance to airflow by the airways. We examine each of these factors here.

There are two major patterns of gas flow in the airways—laminar and turbulent flow. Laminar flow is parallel to the airway walls and is present at low flow rates. As the flow rate increases and particularly as the airways divide, the flow stream becomes unsteady and small eddies occur. At higher flow rates, the flow stream is disorganized and turbulence occurs.

The pressure-flow characteristics of laminar flow were first described by the French physician Poiseuille and apply both to liquids and to air. In straight circular tubes, the flow rate ($\dot{V}$), is defined by the following equation:

● **Equation 21-7**

$$\dot{V} = \frac{P\pi r^4}{8\eta l}$$

where P is the driving pressure, r is the radius of the tube, η is the viscosity of the fluid, and l is the length of the tube. It can be seen that driving pressure (P) is proportional to the flow rate ($\dot{V}$); thus, the greater the pressure, the greater the flow. The flow resistance, R, across a set of tubes is defined as the change in driving pressure (ΔP) divided by the flow rate, or

● **Equation 21-8**

$$R = \frac{\Delta P}{\dot{V}} = \frac{8\eta l}{\pi r^4}$$

The units of resistance are cm $H_2O/L \cdot sec$. This equation for laminar flow demonstrates that the radius of the tube is the most important determinant of resistance. If the radius of the tube is reduced in half, the resistance will increase 16-fold. If, however, tube length is increased twofold, the resistance will increase only twofold. Thus, the radius of the tube is the principal determinant of resistance. Stated another way, resistance is inversely proportional to the fourth power of the radius, and it is directly proportional to the length of the tube and to the viscosity of the gas.

In turbulent flow, gas movement occurs both parallel and perpendicular to the axis of the tube. Pressure is proportional to the flow rate squared. The viscosity of the gas increases with increasing gas density, and therefore the pressure drop increases for a given flow. Overall, gas velocity is blunted because energy is consumed in the process of generating eddies and chaotic movement. As a consequence, higher driving pressure is needed to support a given turbulent flow than to support a given laminar flow.

Whether flow through a tube is laminar or turbulent depends on the Reynolds number. The Reynolds number (R_e) is a dimensionless value that expresses the ratio of two dimensionally equivalent terms (kinematic/viscosity).

● **Equation 21-9**

$$R_e = \frac{2rvd}{\eta}$$

where d is the fluid density, v is the average velocity, r is the radius, and η is the viscosity. In straight tubes, turbulence occurs when the Reynolds number is greater than 2000. From this relationship it can be seen that turbulence is most likely to occur when the average velocity of the gas flow is high and the radius is large. In contrast, a low-density gas, such as helium, is less likely to cause turbulent flow.

Although these relationships apply well to smooth cylindrical tubes, application of these principles to a complicated system of tubes, such as the conducting airways, is difficult. As a result, much of the flow in the airways demonstrates characteristics of both laminar and turbulent flow. During quiet breathing, gas flow at the mouth is approximately 1 L/sec. Gas velocities of 150 cm/sec will occur in an adult with a tracheal diameter of 3 cm. Because air has a density of 0.0012 g/mL and a viscosity of 1.83×10^{-4} g/cm/sec, the Reynolds number is greater than 2000. Hence, turbulent flow occurs in the trachea, even during quiet breathing.

Turbulence is also promoted by the glottis and vocal cords, which produce some irregularity and obstruction in the airways. As gas flows distally, the total cross-sectional area increases dramatically, and gas velocities decrease significantly. As a result, gas flow becomes more laminar in the smaller airways, even during maximal ventilation. Overall, the gas flow in the larger airways (nose, mouth, glottis, and bronchi) is turbulent, whereas the gas flow in the smaller airways is laminar. Breath sounds heard with a stethoscope reflect turbulent airflow. Laminar flow is silent.

Airway Resistance

Airflow resistance is the second major factor that determines rates of airflow in the airways. Airflow resistance in the airways (R_{aw}) differs in airways of different size. In moving from the trachea toward the alveolus, individual airways become smaller while the number of airway branches increases dramatically. R_{aw} is equal to the sum of the resistance of each of these airways (i.e., $R_{aw} = R_{large} + R_{medium} + R_{small}$). From Poiseuille's equation, one might conclude that the major site of airway resistance is in the smallest airways. In fact, however, the major site of resistance along the bronchial tree is the large bronchi. The smallest airways contribute very little to the overall total resistance of the bronchial tree (Fig. 21-10). The reason for this is twofold. First, airflow velocity decreases substantially as the effective cross-sectional area increases (i.e., flow becomes laminar). Second and most important, the airway generations exist in parallel rather than in series. The resistance of airways in parallel is the inverse of the sum of the individual resistances; therefore, the overall resistance of the small airways is very small. As an example, assume that each of three tubes has a resistance of 3 cm H_2O. If the tubes are in series, the total resistance (R_{tot}) is the sum of the individual resistances:

● **Equation 21-10**

$$R_{tot} = R_1 + R_2 + R_3 = 3 + 3 + 3 = 9 \text{ cm } H_2O/L \cdot sec$$

If the tubes are in parallel (as they are in small airways), the total resistance is the sum of the inverse of the individual resistances:

● **Equation 21-11**

$$1/R_{tot} = 1/R_1 + 1/R_2 + 1/R_3 = 1/3 + 1/3 + 1/3$$

$$R_{tot} = 1 \text{ cm } H_2O/L \cdot sec$$

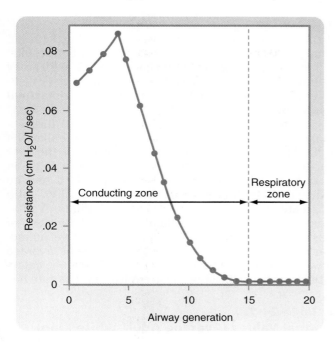

● **Figure 21-10.** Airway resistance as a function of the airway generation. In a normal lung, most of the resistance to airflow occurs in the first eight airway generations.

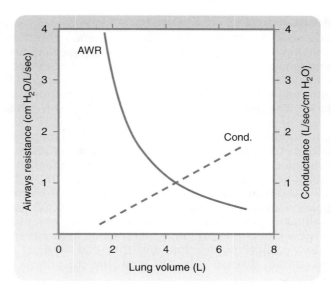

● **Figure 21-11.** Airway resistance (AWR) and conductance (Cond.) as a function of lung volume.

This relationship is in marked contrast to the pulmonary blood vessels, in which most of the resistance is located in the small vessels. Thus, as airway diameter decreases, the resistance offered by each individual airway increases, but the large increase in the number of parallel pathways reduces the resistance at each generation of branching. During normal breathing, approximately 80% of the resistance to airflow at FRC occurs in airways with diameters greater than 2 mm. Because the small airways contribute so little to total lung resistance, measurement of airway resistance is a poor test for detecting small-airway obstruction.

Factors That Contribute to Airway Resistance

In healthy individuals, airway resistance is approximately 1 cm $H_2O/L \cdot sec$. One of the most important factors affecting resistance is lung volume. Increasing lung volume increases the caliber of the airways. As a result, resistance to airflow decreases with increasing lung volume, and it increases with decreasing lung volume. If the reciprocal of resistance (i.e., conductance) is plotted against lung volume, the relationship between lung volume and conductance is linear (Fig. 21-11). Factors that increase airway resistance include airway mucus, edema, and contraction of bronchial smooth muscle, all of which decrease the caliber of the airways.

The density and viscosity of the inspired gas also affect airway resistance. When scuba diving, gas density rises and results in an increase in airway resistance; this increase can cause problems for individuals with asthma and obstructive pulmonary disease.

Breathing a low-density gas such as an oxygen-helium mixture results in a decrease in airway resistance and has been exploited in the treatment of **status asthmaticus,** a condition associated with increased airway resistance because of a combination of bronchospasm, airway inflammation, and mucus.

Neurohumoral Regulation of Airway Resistance

In addition to the effects of disease, airway resistance is regulated by various neural and humoral agents. Stimulation of efferent vagal fibers, either directly or reflexively, increases airway resistance and decreases anatomic dead space secondary to airway constriction (recall that the vagus nerve innervates airway smooth muscle). In contrast, stimulation of the sympathetic nerves and release of the postganglionic neurotransmitter norepinephrine inhibit airway constriction. Reflex stimulation of the vagus nerve by the inhalation of smoke, dust, cold air, or other irritants can also result in airway constriction and coughing. Agents such as histamine, acetylcholine, thromboxane A_2, prostaglandin F_2, and leukotrienes (LTB_4, LTC_4, and LTD_4) are released by resident (e.g., mast cells and airway epithelial cells) and recruited (e.g., neutrophils and eosinophils) airway cells in response to various triggers, such as allergens and viral infections. These agents act directly on airway smooth muscle to cause constriction and an increase in airway resistance. Inhalation of methacholine, a derivative of acetylcholine, is used to diagnose airway hyperresponsiveness, which is one of the cardinal features of asthma. Although everyone is capable of responding to methacholine, airway obstruction develops in patients with asthma at much lower concentrations of inhaled methacholine.

Measurement of Expiratory Flow

Measurement of expiratory flow rates and expiratory volumes is an important clinical tool for evaluating and monitoring respiratory diseases. Commonly used clinical tests have the patient inhale maximally to TLC and then exhale as rapidly and completely as possible to RV. The test results are displayed either as a **spirogram** or as a **flow-volume curve/loop**. Results from individuals with suspected lung disease are compared with results predicted from normal healthy volunteers. Predicted or normal values vary with age, gender, ethnicity, height, and to a lesser extent, weight (Table 21-1). Abnormalities in values indicate abnormal pulmonary function and can be used to predict abnormalities in gas exchange. These values can detect the presence of abnormal lung function long before respiratory symptoms develop, and they can be used to determine disease severity and the response to therapy.

IN THE CLINIC

In a methacholine challenge test, spirometry measurements are made after the patient inhales increasing concentrations of methacholine. The test is stopped when FEV_1 falls by 20% or more or when a maximum concentration (25 mg/mL) of methacholine has been inhaled. The concentration of methacholine that produces a 20% decrease in FEV_1 is called the PC (provocation concentration) 20. The lower the PC20, the more sensitive is an individual to methacholine. Most individuals with asthma have a PC20 less than 8 mg/mL of methacholine.

The Spirogram

A spirogram displays the volume of gas exhaled against time (Fig. 21-12, *A*) and provides four major test results: (1) **forced vital capacity (FVC)**, (2) **forced expiratory volume in 1 second (FEV_1)**, (3) the **ratio of FEV_1 to FVC (FEV_1/FVC)**, and (4) the **average midmaximal expiratory flow (FEF_{25-75})**.

The total volume of air that is exhaled during a maximal forced exhalation from TLC to RV is called the FVC. The volume of air that is exhaled in the first second during the maneuver is called the FEV_1. In normal individuals, 75% to 80% of the FVC can be exhaled in the first second. Thus, the FEV_1/FVC ratio is greater than 75% to 80% in normal adults. A ratio less than 75% suggests difficulty exhaling because of obstruction and is a hallmark of obstructive pulmonary disease. One expiratory flow rate—the average flow rate over the middle section of VC—can be calculated from the spirogram. This expiratory flow rate has

● **Table 21-1.**

Normal Values (Average Adult White Man)

Lung Volumes	
Functional residual capacity (FRC)	2.4 L
Total lung capacity (TLC)	6 L
Tidal volume (V_T)	0.5 L
Breathing frequency (f)	12/min
Mechanics	
Pleural pressure (P_{pl}), mean	−5 cm H_2O
Chest wall compliance (C_w) at FRC	0.2 L/cm H_2O
Lung compliance (C_L) at FRC	0.2 L/cm H_2O
Airway resistance (R_{aw})	2.0 cm H_2O/L/sec

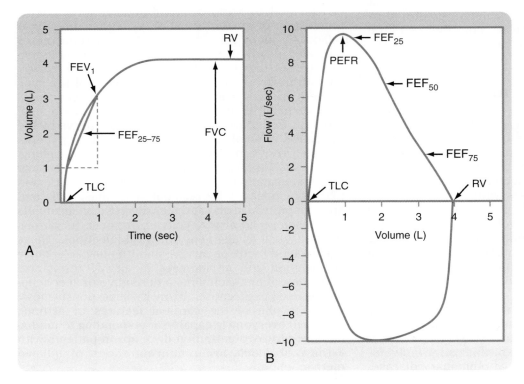

● **Figure 21-12.** The clinical spirogram **(A)** and flow-volume loop **(B).** The subject takes a maximal inspiration and then exhales as rapidly, as forcibly, and as maximally as possible. The volume exhaled is plotted as a function of time. In the spirogram that is reported in clinical settings, exhaled volume increases from the bottom of the trace to the top **(A).** This is in contrast to the physiologist's view of the same maneuver (see Fig. 21-1), in which the exhaled volume increases from the top to the bottom of the trace. Note the locations of TLC and RV on both tracings.

several names, including **MMEF (midmaximal expiratory flow)** and FEF_{25-75} (forced expiratory flow from 25% to 75% of VC). Although it can be calculated from the spirogram, today's spirometers automatically calculate FEF_{25-75}.

Flow-Volume Loop

A newer way of measuring lung function clinically is the flow-volume curve or loop. A flow-volume curve or loop is created by displaying the instantaneous flow rate during a forced maneuver as a function of the volume of gas. This instantaneous flow rate can be displayed both during exhalation (expiratory flow-volume curve) and during inspiration (inspiratory flow-volume curve) (Fig. 21-12, *B*). Expiratory flow rates are displayed above the horizontal line and inspiratory flow rates below the horizontal line. The flow-volume loop yields data for three main pulmonary function tests: (1) the FVC; (2) the greatest flow rate achieved during the expiratory maneuver, called the **peak expiratory flow rate (PEFR),** and (3) expiratory flow rates. When the expiratory flow-volume curve is divided into quarters, the instantaneous flow rate at which 50% of the VC remains to be exhaled is called the FEF_{50} (also known as the $\dot{V}_{max50}$), the instantaneous flow rate at which 75% of the VC has been exhaled is called the FEF_{75} ($\dot{V}_{max75}$), and the instantaneous flow rate at which 25% of the VC has been exhaled is called the FEF_{25} ($\dot{V}_{max25}$).

Determinants of Maximal Flow

The shape of the flow-volume loop reveals important information about normal lung physiology that can be altered by disease. Inspection of the flow-volume loop reveals that the maximum inspiratory flow is the same or slightly greater than the maximum expiratory flow. Three factors are responsible for the maximum inspiratory flow. First, the force that is generated by the inspiratory muscles decreases as lung volume increases above RV. Second, the recoil pressure of the lung increases as the lung volume increases above RV. This opposes the force generated by the inspiratory muscles and reduces maximum inspiratory flow. However, airway resistance decreases with increasing lung volume as the airway caliber increases. The combination of inspiratory muscle force, recoil of the lung, and changes in airway resistance causes maximal inspiratory flow to occur about halfway between TLC and RV.

During exhalation, maximal flow occurs early (in the first 20%) in the maneuver, and flow rates decrease progressively toward RV. Even with increasing effort, maximal flow decreases as RV is approached. This is known as "expiratory flow limitation" and can be demonstrated by asking an individual to perform three forced expiratory maneuvers with increasing effort. Figure 21-13 shows the results of these three maneuvers. As effort increases, peak expiratory flow increases. However, the flow rates at lower lung volumes converge; this indicates that with modest effort, maximal expiratory flow is achieved. No amount of effort will increase the flow rates as lung volume

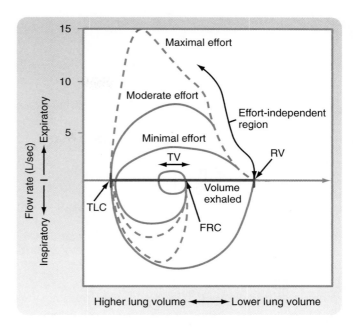

● **Figure 21-13.** Isovolume curves. Three superimposed expiratory flow maneuvers are made with increasing effort. Note that peak inspiratory and expiratory flow rates are dependent on effort, whereas expiratory flow rates later in expiration are independent of effort.

decreases. For this reason, expiratory flow rates at lower lung volumes are said to be "effort independent" and "flow limited" because maximal flow is achieved with modest effort and no amount of additional effort can increase the flow rate beyond this limit. In contrast, events early in the expiratory maneuver are said to be "effort dependent"; that is, increasing effort generates increasing flow rates. In general, the first 20% of the flow in the expiratory flow-volume loop is effort dependent.

Flow Limitation and the Equal Pressure Point

Why is expiratory flow limited? Factors that limit expiratory flow are important because many lung diseases affect these factors and thus affect the volume and speed with which air is moved into and out of the lung. Flow limitation occurs when the airways, which are intrinsically floppy, distensible tubes, become compressed. The airways become compressed when the pressure outside the airway exceeds the pressure inside the airway. How and when this occurs is important to understand lung disease. Figure 21-14 shows the events that occur during expiratory flow limitation at two different lung volumes. The collective airways and alveoli are surrounded by the pleural space and the chest wall. The airways are shown as tapered tubes because the total or collective airway cross-sectional area decreases from the alveoli to the trachea. At the start of exhalation, but before any gas flow occurs, the pressure inside the alveolus (P_A) is

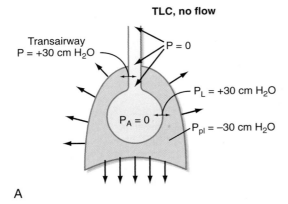

TLC, no flow

Transairway
P = +30 cm H_2O

P = 0

P_L = +30 cm H_2O

P_A = 0

P_{pl} = –30 cm H_2O

A

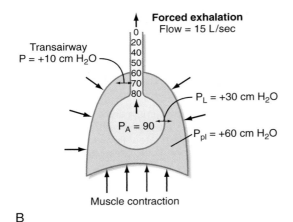

Forced exhalation
Flow = 15 L/sec

Transairway
P = +10 cm H_2O

0
20
40
50
60
70
80

P_L = +30 cm H_2O

P_A = 90

P_{pl} = +60 cm H_2O

Muscle contraction

B

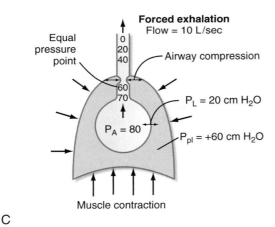

Forced exhalation
Flow = 10 L/sec

Equal
pressure
point

0
20
40

Airway compression

60
70

P_L = 20 cm H_2O

P_A = 80

P_{pl} = +60 cm H_2O

Muscle contraction

C

● **Figure 21-14.** Flow limitation. **A,** End inspiration, before the start of exhalation. **B,** At the start of a forced exhalation. **C,** Expiratory flow limitation later in a forced exhalation. Expiratory flow limitation occurs at locations where airway diameter is narrowed as a result of negative transmural pressure. See text for further explanation.

zero (no airflow), and pleural pressure (in this example) is –30 cm H_2O. Transpulmonary pressure is thus +30 cm H_2O ($P_L = P_A – P_{pl}$). Because there is no flow, the pressure inside the airways is zero and the pressure across the airways (P_{ta}, transairway pressure) is +30 cm H_2O [$P_{ta} = P_{airway} – P_{pl} = 0 – (–30$ cm $H_2O)$]. This positive transpulmonary and transairway pressure holds the alveoli and airways open.

When exhalation begins and the expiratory muscles contract, pleural pressure rises to +60 cm H_2O (in this example). Alveolar pressure also rises, in part because of the increase in pleural pressure (+60 cm H_2O) and in part because of the elastic recoil pressure of the lung at that lung volume (which in this case is 30 cm H_2O). Alveolar pressure is the sum of pleural pressure and elastic recoil pressure (i.e., $P_A = P_{el} + P_{pl} = 30$ cm $H_2O + 60$ cm $H_2O = 90$ cm H_2O in this example). This is the driving pressure for expiratory gas flow. Because alveolar pressure exceeds atmospheric pressure, gas begins to flow from the alveolus to the mouth when the glottis opens. As gas flows out of the alveoli, the transmural pressure across the airways decreases (i.e., the pressure head for expiratory gas flow dissipates). This occurs for two reasons: first, there is a resistive pressure drop caused by the frictional pressure loss associated with flow (expiratory airflow resistance), and second, as the cross-sectional area of the airways decreases toward the trachea, gas velocity increases. This acceleration of gas flow further decreases the pressure.

Thus, as air moves out of the lung, the driving pressure for expiratory gas flow decreases. In addition, the mechanical tethering that holds the airways open at high lung volumes diminishes as lung volume decreases. There is a point between the alveoli and the mouth at which the pressure inside the airways equals the pressure that surrounds the airways. This point is called the **equal pressure point.** Airways toward the mouth become compressed because the pressure outside is greater than the pressure inside **(dynamic airway compression).** As a consequence, the transairway pressure now becomes negative [$P_{ta} = P_{aw} – P_{pl} = 58 – (+60) = –2$ cm H_2O just beyond the equal pressure point]. No amount of effort will increase the flow further because the higher pleural pressure tends to collapse the airway at the equal pressure point, just as it also tends to increase the gradient for expiratory gas flow. Under these conditions, airflow is independent of the total driving pressure. Hence, the expiratory flow is effort independent and flow limited. It is also why airway resistance is greater during exhalation than during inspiration. In the absence of lung disease, the equal pressure point occurs in airways that contain cartilage, and thus they resist collapse. The equal pressure point, however, is not static. As lung volume decreases and as elastic recoil pressure decreases, the equal pressure point moves closer to the alveoli.

What happens in individuals with lung disease? Imagine an individual with airway obstruction secondary to a combination of mucus accumulation and airway inflammation. At the start of exhalation, the driving pressure for expiratory gas flow is the same as in a normal individual; that is, the driving pressure is the sum of the elastic recoil pressure and pleural pressure. As exhalation proceeds, however, the resistive drop in pressure is greater than in the normal individual because of the greater decrease in airway radius secondary to the accumulation of mucus and the inflammation. As a result, the equal pressure point now occurs in small airways that are devoid of cartilage. These airways collapse. This collapse is known as **premature airway closure.** Premature airway closure results in a less than maximal exhalation that is known as air trapping and produces an increase in lung volume. The increase in lung volume initially helps offset the increase in airway resistance caused by the accumulation of mucus and inflammation because it results in an increase in airway caliber and elastic recoil. As the disease progresses, however, inflammation and accumulation of mucus increase further, there is a greater increase in expiratory resistance, and maximal expiratory flow rates decrease.

Individuals with premature airway closure frequently have **crackles,** also sometimes called **rales,** a popping sound usually heard during inspiration on auscultation. These crackles are due to the opening of airways during inspiration that closed (i.e., were compressed) during the previous exhalation. Crackles can be due to mucus accumulation, airway inflammation, fluid in the airways, or any mechanism responsible for airway narrowing or compression. They are also heard in individuals with emphysema, in which there is a decrease in lung elastic recoil. In fact, acute and chronic lung diseases can change the expiratory flow-volume relationship by changes in (1) static lung recoil pressure, (2) airway resistance and the distribution of resistance along the airways, (3) loss of mechanical tethering of intraparenchymal airways, (4) changes in the stiffness or mechanical properties of the airways, and (5) differences in the severity of the aforementioned changes in various lung regions.

Dynamic Compliance

One additional measurement of dynamic lung mechanics should be mentioned before leaving this subject, and this is the measurement of dynamic compliance. A dynamic pressure-volume curve can be created by having an individual breathe over a normal lung volume range (usually from FRC to FRC +1 L). The mean dynamic compliance of the lung (dyn C_L) is calculated as the slope of the line that joins the end-inspiratory and end-expiratory points of no flow (Fig. 21-15).

Dynamic compliance is always less than static compliance, and it increases during exercise. This is because during tidal volume breathing, a small change in alveolar surface area is insufficient to bring additional surfactant molecules to the surface and thus the lung is less compliant. During exercise, the opposite occurs; there are large changes in tidal volume and more surfactant material is incorporated into the air-liquid interface. Therefore, the lung is more compliant.

Sighing and yawning increase dynamic compliance by increasing tidal volume and restoring the normal surfactant layer. Both these respiratory activities are important for maintaining normal lung compliance. In contrast to the lung, the dynamic compliance of the chest wall is not significantly different from its static compliance.

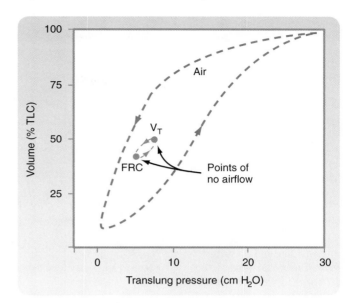

● **Figure 21-15.** Inflation-deflation pressure-volume curve. The direction of inspiration and exhalation is shown by the arrows. The difference between the inflation and deflation pressure-volume curves is due to the variation in surface tension with changes in lung volume. Note the slope of the line joining points of no airflow. This slope is less steep than the slope from the deflation pressure-volume curve at the same lung volume.

WORK OF BREATHING

Breathing requires the use of respiratory muscles (diaphragm, intercostals, etc.), which expends energy. Work is required to overcome the inherent mechanical properties of the lung (i.e., elastic and flow-resistive forces) and to move both the lungs and the chest wall. This work is known as the **work of breathing.** Changes in the mechanical properties of the lung or chest wall (or both) in the presence of disease result in an increase in the work of breathing. Respiratory muscles can perform increased work over long periods. However, like other skeletal muscles, they can fatigue and respiratory failure may ensue. Respiratory muscle fatigue is the most common cause of **respiratory failure,** a process in which gas exchange is inadequate to meet the metabolic needs of the body. In the respiratory system, the work of breathing is calculated by multiplying the change in volume by the pressure exerted across the respiratory system. That is,

Work of breathing (W) = Pressure (P)
× Change in volume (ΔV)

Although methods are not available to measure the total amount of work involved in breathing, one can estimate the mechanical work by measuring the volume and pressure changes during a respiratory cycle. Analysis of pressure-volume curves can be used to illustrate these points (Fig. 21-16). In Figure 21-16, A represents a respiratory cycle of a normal lung. The static inflation-deflation curve is represented by line ABC. The total mechanical workload is represented by the trapezoidal area OAECD. Breakdown of the

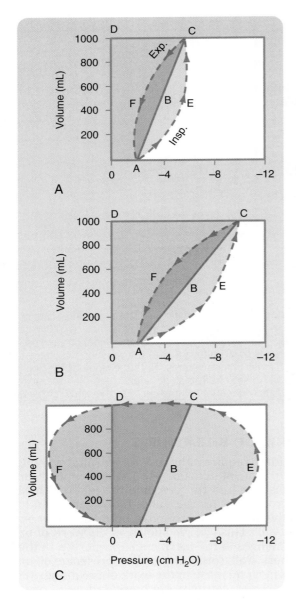

● **Figure 21-16.** Mechanical work done during a respiratory cycle in a normal lung **(A)**, a lung with reduced compliance **(B)**, and a lung with increased airway resistance **(C)**.

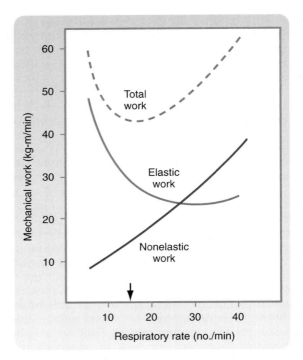

● **Figure 21-17.** Effect of the respiratory rate on the elastic, nonelastic, and total mechanical work of breathing at a given level of alveolar ventilation. Subjects tend to adopt the respiratory rate at which the total work of breathing is minimal *(arrow)*.

trapezoidal areas of Figure 21-16, *A,* enables one to appreciate the individual aspects of the mechanical workload, which include the following:

OABCD: work necessary to overcome elastic resistance

AECF: work necessary to overcome nonelastic resistance

AECB: work necessary to overcome nonelastic resistance during inspiration

ABCF: work necessary to overcome nonelastic resistance during exhalation (represents stored elastic energy from inspiration)

In restrictive lung diseases, such as pulmonary fibrosis, lung compliance is decreased and the pres-

sure-volume curve is shifted to the right. This results in a significant increase in the work of breathing (Fig. 21-16, *B*), as indicated by the increase in the trapezoidal area of OAECD. In obstructive lung diseases, such as asthma or chronic bronchitis, airway resistance is elevated (Fig. 21-16, *C*), and greater negative pleural pressure is needed to maintain normal inspiratory flow rates. In addition to the increase in total inspiratory work (OAECD), individuals with obstructive lung disease have an increase in positive pleural pressure during exhalation because of the increase in resistance and the increased expiratory workload, which is visualized as area DFO. The stored elastic energy, represented by area ABCF of Figure 21-16, *A*, is not sufficient, and additional energy is needed for exhalation. With time or disease progression, these respiratory muscles can fatigue and result in respiratory failure. The work of breathing is also increased when deeper breaths are taken (an increase in tidal volume requires more elastic work to overcome) and when the respiratory rate increases (an increase in minute ventilation requires more flow resistance force to overcome) (Fig. 21-17). Normal individuals and individuals with lung disease adopt respiratory patterns that minimize the work of breathing. For this reason, individuals with pulmonary fibrosis (increased elastic work) breathe more shallowly and rapidly, and those with obstructive lung disease (normal elastic work) breathe more slowly and deeply.

► IN THE CLINIC

Chronic obstructive pulmonary disease (COPD) is a general term that includes diseases such as emphysema and chronic bronchitis. COPD most commonly occurs in individuals who smoke, in whom pathologic changes in the lung consistent with both emphysema and chronic bronchitis can coexist. For individuals with COPD in whom emphysema is a major component, the elastic tissue in the alveolar and capillary walls is progressively destroyed, which results in increased lung compliance and decreased elastic recoil. The decrease in elastic recoil results in movement of the equal pressure point toward the alveolus and premature airway closure. This produces air trapping and increases in RV, FRC, and TLC. Airway resistance is also increased. These increases in lung volumes increase the work of breathing by stretching the respiratory muscles and decreasing their efficiency.

In chronic bronchitis, accumulation of mucus and airway inflammation cause the equal pressure point to move toward the alveolus, which leads to premature airway closure and increases in RV, FRC, and TLC. Airway resistance and the work of breathing are increased, but lung compliance is normal.

In restrictive lung diseases such as pulmonary fibrosis, lung compliance is decreased. Lung volumes are decreased but flow rates are reasonably normal. The changes in pulmonary function values in obstructive and restrictive pulmonary diseases are shown in Table 21-2.

In the third trimester of pregnancy, the enlarged uterus increases intraabdominal pressure and restricts movement of the diaphragm. The FRC, as a result, decreases. This change in lung volume results in decreased lung compliance and increased airway resistance in otherwise healthy women.

● **Table 21-2.**

Patterns of Abnormalities in Pulmonary Function Test Results

Pulmonary Function Measurement	Obstructive Pulmonary Disease	Restrictive Pulmonary Disease
FVC (L)	Decrease	Decrease
FEV_1 (L)	Decrease	Decrease
FEV_1/FVC	Decrease	Normal
FEF_{25-75} (L/sec)	Decrease	Normal to increased
PEFR (L/sec)	Decrease	Normal
FEF_{50} (L/sec)	Decrease	Normal
FEF_{75} (L/sec)	Decrease	Normal
Slope of FV curve	Decrease	Normal to increased

■ KEY CONCEPTS

1. Lung volumes are determined by the balance between the lung's elastic recoil properties and the properties of the muscles of the chest wall. Positive transpulmonary pressure is needed to increase lung volume. The pressure across the respiratory system is zero at points of no airflow (end inspiration and end exhalation). At FRC, the pressure difference across the respiratory system is zero, and lung elastic recoil pressure, which operates to decrease lung volume, and the pressure generated by the chest wall to become larger are equal and opposite.

2. Lung compliance is a measure of the elastic properties of the lung. Loss of elastic recoil is seen in patients with emphysema and is associated with an increase in lung compliance, whereas in diseases associated with pulmonary fibrosis, lung compliance is decreased.

3. Resistance to airflow is the change in pressure per unit of flow. Airway resistance varies with the inverse of the fourth power of the radius and is higher in turbulent than in laminar flow. The major site of airway resistance is the first eight airway generations. Airway resistance decreases with increases in lung volume and with decreases in gas density.

4. The equal pressure point is the point at which the pressure inside and surrounding the airway is the same. The location of the equal pressure point is dynamic. Specifically, as lung volume and elastic recoil decrease, the equal pressure point moves toward the alveolus in normal individuals. In individuals with chronic obstructive pulmonary disease (COPD), the equal pressure point at any lung volume is closer to the alveolus.

5. Pulmonary function tests (spirometry, flow-volume loop, body plethysmography) can detect abnormalities in lung function before individuals become symptomatic. Test results are compared with results obtained in normal individuals and vary with gender, ethnicity, age, and height. COPD is characterized by increases in lung volumes and airway resistance and by decreases in expiratory flow rates. Emphysema, a specific type of COPD, is further characterized by increased lung compliance. Restrictive lung diseases are characterized by decreases in lung volume, normal expiratory flow rates and resistance, and a marked decrease in lung compliance.

CHAPTER 22

Ventilation (V̇), Perfusion (Q̇), and V̇/Q̇ Relationships

Ventilation and pulmonary blood flow (perfusion) are important components of gas exchange in the lung. However, the major determinant of normal gas exchange and thus the level of PO_2 and PCO_2 in blood is the relationship between ventilation and perfusion. This relationship is called the V̇/Q̇ ratio.

VENTILATION

Ventilation is the process by which air moves in and out of the lung. As previously described, minute (or total) ventilation (V̇$_E$) is the volume of air that enters or leaves the lung per minute and it is described by

● **Equation 22-1**

$$\dot{V}_E = f \times TV$$

where f is the frequency or number of breaths per minute and TV, also known as V_T, is the tidal volume, or volume of air inspired (or exhaled) per breath. Tidal volume varies with age, gender, body position, and metabolic activity. In an average-sized adult at rest, tidal volume is 500 mL. In children, it is 3 to 5 mL/kg.

ALVEOLAR VENTILATION
Composition of Air

Inspiration brings ambient air to the alveoli, where O_2 is taken up and CO_2 is excreted. Alveolar ventilation thus begins with ambient air. Ambient air is a gas mixture composed of N_2 and O_2, with minute quantities of CO_2, argon, and inert gases. The composition of a gas mixture can be described in terms of either gas fractions or the corresponding partial pressure. Because ambient air is a gas, it obeys the gas laws.

When these gas laws are applied to ambient air, two important principles arise. The first is that when the components are viewed in terms of gas fractions (F), the sum of the individual gas fractions must equal one.

● **Equation 22-2**

$$1.0 = F_{N_2} + F_{O_2} + F_{argon} \text{ and other gases}$$

It follows, then, that the sum of the **partial pressures** (in mm Hg) or the **tensions** (in torr) of a gas must be equal to the total pressure. Thus, at sea level, where atmospheric pressure is 760 mm Hg, the partial

pressures of the gases in air (also known as barometric pressure (P_b)) are

● **Equation 22-3**

$$P_b = P_{N_2} + P_{O_2} + P_{argon} \text{ and other gases}$$
$$760 \text{ mm Hg} = P_{N_2} + P_{O_2} + P_{argon} \text{ and other gases}$$

The second important principle is that the partial pressure of a gas (P_{gas}) is equal to the fraction of that gas in the gas mixture (F_{gas}) times the total or ambient (barometric) pressure.

● **Equation 22-4**

$$P_{gas} = F_{gas} \times P_b$$

Ambient air is composed of approximately 21% O_2 and 79% N_2. Therefore, the partial pressure of O_2 in ambient air (PO_2) is

● **Equation 22-5**

$$P_{O_2} = F_{O_2} \times P_b$$
$$P_{O_2} = 0.21 \times 760 \text{ mm Hg}$$
$$= 159 \text{ mm Hg or } 159 \text{ torr}$$

This is the O_2 tension (i.e., the partial pressure of O_2) of ambient air at the mouth at the start of inspiration. The O_2 tension at the mouth can be altered in one of two ways—by changing the fraction of O_2 or by changing barometric (atmospheric) pressure. Thus, ambient O_2 tension can be increased through the administration of supplemental O_2 and is decreased at high altitude.

As inspiration begins, the ambient air is brought into the airways, where it becomes warmed to body

● Table 22-1.

Total and Partial Pressures of Respiratory Gases in Ideal Alveolar Gas and Blood at Sea Level (760 mm Hg)

	Ambient Air (Dry)	Moist Tracheal Air	Alveolar Gas (R = 0.8)	Systemic Arterial Blood	Mixed Venous Blood
P_{O_2}	159	150	102	90	40
P_{CO_2}	0	0	40	40	46
P_{H_2O}, 37°C	0	47	47	47	47
P_{N_2}	601	563	571*	571	571
P_{TOTAL}	760	760	760	760	704†

*P_{N_2} is increased in alveolar gas by 1% because R is less than 1 normally.
†P_{TOTAL} is less in venous than in arterial blood because P_{O_2} has decreased more than P_{CO_2} has increased.

temperature and humidified. Inspired gases become saturated with water vapor, which exerts a partial pressure and dilutes the total pressure of the other gases. Water vapor pressure at body temperature is 47 mm Hg. To calculate the partial pressure of a gas in a humidified mixture, the water vapor partial pressure must be subtracted from the total barometric pressure. Thus, in the conducting airways the partial pressure of O_2 is

● Equation 22-6

$$P_{trachea O_2} = (P_b - P_{H_2O}) \times F_{O_2}$$
$$= (760 - 47 \text{ mm Hg}) \times 0.21$$
$$= 150 \text{ mm Hg}$$

and the partial pressure of N_2 is

● Equation 22-7

$$P_{trachea N_2} = (760 - 47 \text{ mm Hg}) \times 0.79$$
$$= 563 \text{ mm Hg}$$

Note that the total pressure has remained 760 mm Hg (150 + 563 + 47 mm Hg). Water vapor pressure, however, has reduced the partial pressures of O_2 and N_2. The conducting airways do not participate in gas exchange. Therefore, the partial pressures of O_2, N_2, and water vapor remain unchanged in the airways until the gas reaches the alveolus.

Alveolar Gas Composition

When the inspired gas reaches the alveolus, O_2 is transported across the alveolar membrane, and CO_2 moves from the capillary bed into the alveolus. The process by which this occurs is described in Chapter 23. At the end of inspiration and with the glottis open, the total pressure in the alveolus is atmospheric; thus, the partial pressures of the gases in the alveolus must equal the total pressure, which in this case is atmospheric. The composition of the gas mixture, however, is changed and can be described as

● Equation 22-8

$$1.0 = F_{O_2} + F_{N_2} + F_{H_2O} + F_{CO_2} + F_{argon} \text{ and other gases}$$

N_2 and argon are inert gases, and therefore the fraction of these gases in the alveolus does not change over time. The fraction of water vapor also does not change because the gas is already fully saturated with water vapor and is at body temperature by the time that it reaches the trachea. As a consequence of gas exchange, the fraction of O_2 in the alveolus decreases

and the fraction of CO_2 in the alveolus increases. Because of changes in the fractions of O_2 and CO_2, the partial pressure exerted by these gases also changes. The partial pressure of O_2 in the alveolus (P_{AO_2}) is given by the **alveolar gas equation,** which is also called the **ideal alveolar oxygen equation:**

● Equation 22-9

$$P_{AO_2} = P_{IO_2} - \frac{P_{ACO_2}}{R}$$

$$= (P_b - P_{H_2O}) \times F_{IO_2} - \frac{P_{ACO_2}}{R}$$

where P_{IO_2} is the inspired partial pressure of O_2, which is equal to the fraction (F) of inspired O_2 (F_{IO_2}) times barometric pressure (P_b) minus water vapor pressure (P_{H_2O}). P_{ACO_2} is the CO_2 tension of alveolar gas, and R is the respiratory exchange ratio or **respiratory quotient.** The respiratory quotient is the ratio of CO_2 excreted ($\dot{V}_{CO_2}$) to the O_2 taken up ($\dot{V}_{O_2}$) by the lungs. This quotient is the amount of CO_2 produced relative to the amount of O_2 consumed by metabolism and is dependent on caloric intake. The respiratory quotient varies between 0.7 and 1.0 and is 0.7 in states of exclusive fatty acid metabolism and 1.0 in states of exclusive carbohydrate metabolism. Under normal dietary conditions, the respiratory quotient is assumed to be 0.8. Thus, the quantity of O_2 taken up exceeds the quantity of CO_2 that is released in the alveoli.

The partial pressures of O_2, CO_2, and N_2 from ambient air to the alveolus are shown in Table 22-1.

The fraction of CO_2 in the alveolus is a function of the rate of CO_2 production by the cells during metabolism and the rate at which the CO_2 is eliminated from the alveolus. This process of elimination of CO_2 is known as **alveolar ventilation.** The relationship between CO_2 production and alveolar ventilation is defined by the **alveolar carbon dioxide equation,**

● Equation 22-10

$$\dot{V}_{CO_2} = \dot{V}_A \times F_{ACO_2}$$

where $\dot{V}_{CO_2}$ is the rate of CO_2 production by the body, $\dot{V}_A$ is alveolar ventilation, and F_{ACO_2} is the fraction of CO_2 in dry alveolar gas. This relationship demonstrates that the rate of elimination of CO_2 from the alveolus is related to alveolar ventilation and to the fraction of CO_2 in the alveolus. Alveolar P_{ACO_2} is defined by the following:

● **Equation 22-11**

$$P_{ACO_2} = F_{ACO_2} \times (P_b - P_{H_2O})$$

Hence, we can substitute in the previous equation and demonstrate the following relationship:

● **Equation 22-12**

$$P_{ACO_2} = \dot{V}_{CO_2} \times \frac{P_b - P_{H_2O}}{\dot{V}_A}$$

This equation demonstrates several important relationships. First, there is an inverse relationship between the partial pressure of CO_2 in the alveolus (P_{ACO_2}) and alveolar ventilation ($\dot{V}_A$), irrespective of the exhaled CO_2. Specifically, if ventilation is doubled, P_{ACO_2} will decrease by 50%. Conversely, if ventilation is decreased by half, the partial pressure of CO_2 in the alveolus will double. Second, at a constant alveolar ventilation ($\dot{V}_A$), doubling of the metabolic production of CO_2 ($\dot{V}_{CO_2}$) will double the partial pressure of CO_2 in the alveolus. The relationship between alveolar ventilation and alveolar P_{CO_2} is shown in Figure 22-1.

Arterial Gas Composition

In normal individuals, arterial P_{CO_2} is tightly regulated and maintained at about 40 mm Hg. Increases or decreases in arterial P_{CO_2}, particularly when associated with changes in arterial pH, have profound effects on cell function, including enzyme and transport protein activity. Specialized chemoreceptors monitor P_{CO_2} in arterial blood and in the brainstem (Chapter 24), and minute ventilation varies in accordance with the level of P_{CO_2}.

An increase in arterial P_{CO_2} results in **respiratory acidosis** (pH <7.35), whereas a decrease in arterial P_{CO_2} results in **respiratory alkalosis** (pH >7.45). **Hypercapnia** is defined as an elevation in arterial P_{CO_2}, and it is secondary to inadequate alveolar ventilation (hypoventilation) relative to CO_2 production. Conversely, hyperventilation occurs when alveolar ventilation exceeds CO_2 production, and it decreases arterial P_{CO_2} **(hypocapnia).**

Distribution of Ventilation

Ventilation is not uniformly distributed in the lung, in large part because of the effects of gravity. In the upright position, alveoli near the apex of the lung are more expanded than alveoli at the base. Gravity pulls the lung downward and away from the chest wall. As a result, pleural pressure is less at the apex than at the base of the lung, and static translung pressure ($P_L = P_A - P_{pl}$) is increased; this results in an increase in alveolar volume at the apex. Because of the difference in alveolar volume at the apex and at the base of the lung (Fig. 22-2), alveoli at the lung base are located along the steep portion of the pressure-volume curve, and they receive more of the ventilation (i.e., they have greater compliance). In contrast, the alveoli at the apex are closer to the top of the pressure-volume curve. They have lower compliance and thus receive

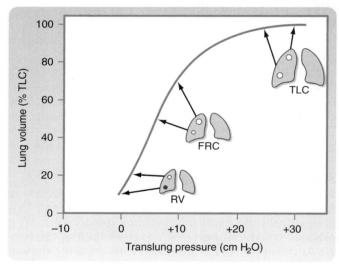

● **Figure 22-2.** Regional distribution of lung volume, including alveolar size and location on the pressure-volume curve of the lung at different lung volumes. Because of suspension of the lung in the upright position, the pleural pressure (P_{pl}) and translung pressure (P_L) of units at the apex will be greater than those at the base. These lung units will be larger at any lung volume than units at the base. The effect is greatest at residual volume (RV), is less at functional residual capacity (FRC), and disappears at total lung capacity (TLC). Note also that because of their location on the pressure-volume curve, inspired air will be differentially distributed to these lung units; the lung units at the apex are less compliant and will receive a smaller proportion of the inspired air than the lung units at the base, which are more compliant (i.e., reside at a steeper part of the pressure-volume curve).

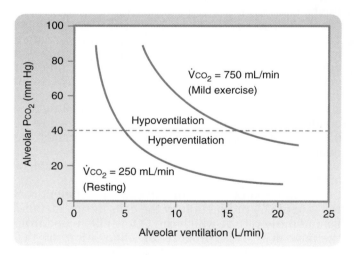

● **Figure 22-1.** Alveolar P_{CO_2} as a function of alveolar ventilation in the lung. Each line corresponds to a given metabolic rate associated with a constant production of CO_2 ($\dot{V}_{CO_2}$ isometabolic line). Normally, alveolar ventilation is controlled to maintain an alveolar P_{CO_2} of about 40 torr. Thus, at rest, when $\dot{V}_{CO_2}$ is approximately 250 mL/min, alveolar ventilation of 5 L/min will result in an alveolar P_{CO_2} of 40 mm Hg. A 50% decrease in ventilation at rest (i.e., from 5 to 2.5 L/min) results in doubling of alveolar P_{CO_2}. During exercise, CO_2 production is increased ($\dot{V}_{CO_2} = 750$ mL/min), and to maintain a normal P_{CO_2}, ventilation must increase (in this case to 15 L/min). Again, however, a 50% reduction in ventilation (15 to 7.5 L/min) will result in doubling of P_{CO_2}.

proportionately less of the tidal volume. The effect of gravity is less pronounced when one is supine rather than upright, and it is less when one is supine rather than prone. This is because the diaphragm is pushed cephalad when one is supine, and it affects the size of all of the alveoli.

In addition to gravitational effects on the distribution of ventilation, ventilation in the terminal respiratory units is not uniform. This is caused by variable airway resistance (R) or compliance (C), and it may be described quantitatively by the **time constant** (τ):

● **Equation 22-12**

$$\tau = R \times C$$

Alveolar units with long time constants fill and empty slowly. Thus, an alveolar unit with increased airway resistance or increased compliance will take longer to fill and longer to empty. In normal adults, the respiratory rate is about 12 breaths per minute, the inspiratory time is about 2 seconds, and the expiratory time is about 3 seconds. In normal individuals this time is sufficient to approach equilibrium (Fig. 22-3). In the presence of increased resistance or increased compliance, however, equilibrium is not reached.

Single-Breath Nitrogen Test

The single-breath N_2 test can be used to assess the uniformity of ventilation. The subject takes a single maximal inspiration of 100% O_2. During the subsequent exhalation, [N_2] in the exhaled air is measured. Air (100% O_2, 0% N_2) initially exits from the conducting airways; then [N_2] begins to rise as alveolar emptying occurs. Finally, there is a plateau [N_2] as only the alveoli that contain N_2 empty (Fig. 22-4).

DEAD SPACE

With each breath, air fills the conducting airways and the alveoli. Dead space ventilation is ventilation to airways that do not participate in gas exchange. There are two types of dead space, anatomic dead space and physiological dead space. **Anatomic dead space** (V_D) is composed of the volume of gas that fills the conducting airways. Thus,

● **Equation 22-13**

$$V_T = V_D + V_A$$

where V refers to volume and the subscripts T, D, and A refer to tidal, dead space, and alveolar. A "dot" above V denotes a volume per unit of time (n). Thus,

● **Equation 22-14**

$$V_T \times n = (V_D \times n) + (V_A \times n)$$

or

● **Equation 22-15**

$$\dot{V}_E = \dot{V}_D + \dot{V}_A$$

where $\dot{V}_E$ is the exhaled minute volume, $\dot{V}_D$ is the dead space per minute, and $\dot{V}_A$ is alveolar ventilation per minute.

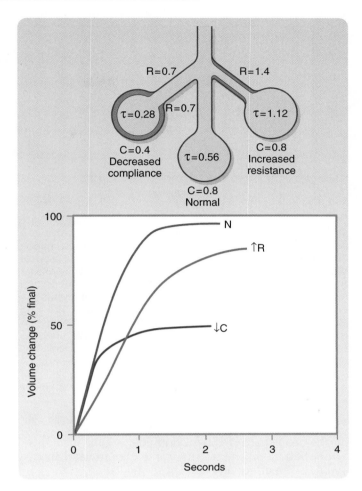

● **Figure 22-3.** Examples of local regulation of ventilation as a result of variation in the resistance (R) or compliance (C) of individual lung units. In the upper schema are shown the individual resistance and compliance of three different lung units. In the lower graph are shown the volume of these three lung units as a function of time. In the upper schema, the normal lung has a time constant (τ) of 0.56 second. This unit reaches 97% of final equilibrium in 2 seconds, the normal inspiratory time, as shown in the lower graph. The unit at the right has a twofold increase in resistance; hence its time constant is doubled. That unit fills more slowly and reaches only 80% equilibrium during a normal breath *(graph)*. The unit is underventilated. The unit on the left has reduced compliance (stiff), which acts to reduce its time constant. This unit fills faster than the normal unit but receives only half the ventilation of a normal unit.

In a healthy adult, the volume of gas contained in the conducting airways at functional residual capacity (FRC) is approximately 100 to 200 mL, as compared with the 3 L of gas in the entire lung. The ratio of the volume of the conducting airways (dead space) to tidal volume describes the fraction of each breath that is wasted in "filling" the conducting airways. This volume is related to tidal volume (V_T) and to minute ventilation ($\dot{V}_E$) in the following way:

● **Equation 22-16**

$$\dot{V}_D = \frac{V_D}{V_T} \times \dot{V}_E$$

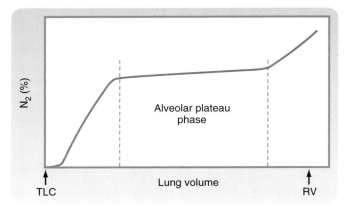

● **Figure 22-4.** The single-breath N_2 washout curve is a simple useful pulmonary function test of the regional distribution of ventilation. It clearly shows that not all lung units have equal $\dot{V}/\dot{Q}$. The well-ventilated units (short time constant) empty faster than less well ventilated units (long time constant). The portion of the curve up to the first vertical dashed line represents the washout of dead space air mixed with alveolar gas. The long alveolar plateau rises slowly (<2%) if the distribution of ventilation is relatively uniform, as shown here. The final phase, after the second vertical line, shows very late, slowly emptying alveoli. This phase is accentuated with age.

IN THE CLINIC

If the dead space is 150 mL and tidal volume increases from 500 to 600 mL for the same minute ventilation, what is the effect on dead space ventilation?

$$V_T = 500 \text{ mL}$$

$$V = \frac{150 \text{mL}}{500 \text{mL}} \times \dot{V}$$

$$= 0.30 \times \dot{V}_E$$

$$V_D = \frac{150 \text{mL}}{600 \text{mL}} \times \dot{V}_E$$

$$= 0.25 \times \dot{V}_E$$

As tidal volume increases, dead space ventilation decreases for the same minute ventilation.

Dead space ventilation (V_D) thus varies inversely with tidal volume (V_T). The larger the tidal volume, the smaller the dead space ventilation. Normally, V_D/V_T is 20% to 30% of minute ventilation.

Physiological Dead Space Ventilation

The second type of dead space is physiological dead space. Alveoli that are perfused but not ventilated are often found in diseased lungs. The **total** volume of gas in each breath that does not participate in gas exchange is called the **physiological dead space ventilation.** This volume includes the anatomic dead space and the dead space secondary to the ventilated but not perfused alveoli. The physiological dead space is always at least as large as the anatomic dead space, and in the presence of disease it may be considerably larger.

IN THE CLINIC

Dead space in the lungs can be determined by measuring P_{CO_2} in alveolar gas and in mixed expired gas. Exhaled gas is collected in a bag over a period of time, and arterial P_{CO_2} (which is the same as alveolar P_{CO_2}) and the P_{CO_2} in the collection bag (P_{ECO_2}) are measured. CO_2 in mixed expired gas is diluted relative to that in alveolar gas, and the extent of the dilution is a function of the wasted ventilation. Dead space volume as a function of tidal volume (V_D/V_T) is described by the following equation:

$$\frac{V_D}{V_T} = 1 - \frac{P_{ECO_2}}{P_{ACO_2}}$$

This is called the Bohr dead space equation, named after the physiologist Christian Bohr.

Dead space ventilation can also be measured by Fowler's method. The patient takes a single breath of 100% O_2 and then exhales into a tube that continuously measures the N_2 concentration in the exhaled gas. As the patient exhales, the anatomic dead space empties first. This volume contains 100% O_2 and 0% N_2 because it has not participated in any gas exchange. As the alveoli begin to empty, O_2 partial pressure falls and N_2 partial pressure begins to rise. Finally, the partial pressure of N_2 is almost uniform, and it represents alveolar gas almost entirely. This phase of expired air exhalation is called the alveolar plateau. The volume with initially 0% N_2 plus half of the rising N_2 volume is equal to the anatomic dead space.

Fowler's and Bohr's methods do not measure exactly the same thing. Fowler's method measures the volume of the conducting airways down to the level at which the inspired gas is rapidly diluted with gas already in the lung. Thus, Fowler's method measures anatomic dead space. In contrast, Bohr's method measures the volume of the lung that does not eliminate CO_2. Thus, Bohr's method measures physiological dead space.

PERFUSION

Perfusion is the process by which deoxygenated blood passes through the lung and becomes reoxygenated.

The Pulmonary Circulation

The pulmonary circulation begins with the right atrium. Deoxygenated blood from the right atrium enters the right ventricle via the tricuspid valve, and it is then pumped under low pressure (9 to 24 mm Hg) into the pulmonary artery through the pulmonic valve. The pulmonary artery (pulmonary trunk), which is about 3 cm in diameter, branches quickly (5 cm from the right ventricle) into the right and left main pulmonary arteries, which supply blood to the right and left lungs, respectively. **The arteries of the pulmonary circulation are the only arteries in the body that carry deoxygenated blood.** The deoxygenated blood in the pulmonary arteries passes through a progressively smaller series of branching vessels (vessel diameters: arteries, >500 μm; arterioles, 10 to 200 μm; capillaries, <10 μm) that end in a complex meshlike network of capillaries (see Chapter 20, Fig. 20-7). The sequential branching pattern of the pulmonary arteries follows the pattern of airway branching. The functions of the pulmonary circulatory system are to (1) reoxygenate the blood and dispense with CO_2, (2) aid in fluid balance in the lung, and (3) distribute metabolic products to and from the lung. Oxygenation of red blood cells occurs in the capillaries that surround the alveoli, where the pulmonary capillary bed and the alveoli come together in the alveolar wall in a unique configuration for optimal gas exchange (Fig. 22-5). Gas exchange occurs through this alveolar-capillary network.

The total blood volume of the pulmonary circulation is about 500 mL, which is about 10% of the circulating blood volume. Approximately 75 mL of blood is present in the alveolar-capillary network of healthy adults at any one time. During exercise, this blood volume increases to 150 to 200 mL because of the recruitment of new capillaries secondary to an increase in pressure and flow. This recruitment of new capillaries is a unique feature of the lung, and it allows for compensation and adjustments to stress, as in the case of exercise. The oxygenated blood leaves the alveolus through a network of small pulmonary venules (15 to 500 μm in diameter) and veins. These small vessels quickly coalesce to form larger pulmonary veins (>500 μm in diameter) through which the oxygenated blood returns to the left atrium of the heart. In contrast to arteries, arterioles, and capillaries, which closely follow the branching patterns of the airways, venules and veins run quite distant from the airways.

Structural Features of the Pulmonary and Bronchial Circulation
Structure of the Pulmonary Circulation
The arteries of the pulmonary circulation are thin walled, with minimal smooth muscle. They are seven times more compliant than systemic vessels, and they are easily distensible. This highly compliant state of the pulmonary arterial vessels requires lower pressure for blood flow through the pulmonary circulation than do the more muscular, noncompliant arterial walls of the systemic circulation. The vessels in the pulmonary circulation, under normal circumstances, are in a dilated state and have larger diameters than do similar arteries in the systemic system. All these factors contribute to a very compliant, low-resistance circulatory system, which aids in the flow of blood through the pulmonary circulation via the relatively weak pumping action of the right ventricle. This low-resistance, low-work system also explains why the right ventricle is less muscular than the left ventricle. The pressure gradient differential for the pulmonary circulation from the pulmonary artery to the left

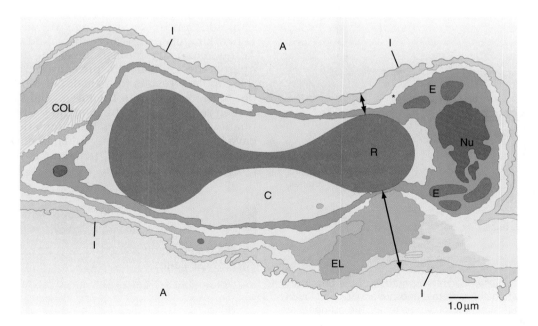

● **Figure 22-5.**   Cross section of an alveolar wall showing the path for diffusion of O_2 and CO_2. The thin side of the alveolar wall barrier *(short double arrow)* consists of type I epithelium (I), interstitium (*) formed by the fused basal laminae of the epithelial and endothelial cells, capillary endothelium (E), plasma in the alveolar capillary (C), and finally the cytoplasm of the red blood cell (R). The thick side of the gas exchange barrier *(long double arrow)* has an accumulation of elastin (EL), collagen (COL), and matrix that jointly separate the alveolar epithelium from the alveolar capillary endothelium. As long as the red blood cells are flowing, O_2 and CO_2 diffusion probably occurs across both sides of the air-blood barrier. A, alveolus; Nu, nucleus of the capillary endothelial cell.

atrium is only 6 mm Hg (14 mm Hg in the pulmonary artery minus 8 mm Hg in the left atrium) (Fig. 22-6). This pressure gradient differential is almost 15 times less than the pressure gradient differential of 87 mm Hg present in the systemic circulation (90 mm Hg in the aorta minus 3 mm Hg in the right atrium).

Structures of the Extraalveolar and Alveolar Vessels and the Pulmonary Microcirculation

Though not well defined anatomically, vessels in the pulmonary circulation can be divided into three categories (extraalveolar, alveolar, and microcirculation) based on differences in their physiological properties. The extraalveolar vessels (arteries, arterioles, veins, and venules) are larger than their systemic counterparts. They are not influenced by alveolar pressure changes, but they are affected by intrapleural and interstitial pressure changes. Thus, the caliber of extraalveolar vessels is affected by lung volume and by lung elastin. At high lung volumes, the decrease in pleural pressure increases the caliber of extraalveolar

vessels, whereas at low lung volumes, an increase in pleural pressure decreases vessel caliber. In contrast, alveolar capillaries reside within the interalveolar septa, and they are very sensitive to changes in alveolar pressure but not to changes in pleural or interstitial pressure. Positive pressure ventilation increases alveolar pressure and compresses these capillaries and thus blocks blood flow. This effect is discussed later in this chapter. Finally, the pulmonary microcirculation refers to the small vessels that participate in liquid and solute exchange in maintenance of fluid balance in the lung.

Structure of the Alveolar-Capillary Network

The sequential branching of the pulmonary arteries culminates in a dense meshlike network of capillaries that surround alveoli. This alveolar-capillary network is composed of thin epithelial cells of the alveolus and endothelial cells of the vessels and their supportive matrix and has an alveolar surface area of about 70 m^2 (about the size of a tennis court). The structural matrix and the tissue components of this alveolar-capillary network provide the only barrier between gas in the airway and blood in the capillary. The cells of this barrier, which is 1 to 2 µm thick, include type I alveolar epithelial cells, capillary endothelial cells, and their respective basement membranes, which are back to back. Surrounded mostly by air, this alveolar-capillary network creates an ideal environment for gas exchange. Red blood cells pass through the capillary component of this network in single file in less than 1 second, which is sufficient time for CO_2 and O_2 gas exchange.

In addition to gas exchange, the alveolar-capillary network regulates the amount of fluid within the lung. At the pulmonary capillary level, the balance between hydrostatic and oncotic pressure across the wall of the capillary results in a small net movement of fluid out of the vessels into the interstitial space. The fluid is then removed from the lung interstitium by the lymphatic system and enters the circulation via the vena cava in the area of the lung hilus. In normal adults, an average of 30 mL of fluid per hour is returned to the circulation via this route.

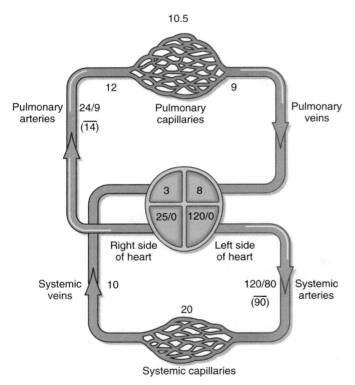

● **Figure 22-6.** Schematic representation of the phasic and mean pressures within the systemic and pulmonary circulations in a normal, resting human adult lying supine. The numbers are millimeters of mercury (mm Hg) for easy comparison. The driving pressure in the systemic circuit is $P_{ao} - P_{ra} = 90 - 3 = 87$ mm Hg, whereas the driving pressure in the pulmonary circuit is $P_{pa} - P_{la} = 14 - 8 = 6$ mm Hg. Cardiac output must be the same in both circuits in the steady state because they are in series. The resistance to flow through the lungs is less than 10% that of the rest of the body. Note that the pressure in the left heart chambers is higher than that in the right side of the heart. Any congenital openings between the right and left sides of the heart favor left-to-right flow.

Starling's equation is used to calculate fluid movement across capillaries:

$$\text{Flux (flow in mL/min)} = K_{fc}\,[(P_{IV} - P_{is}) - \sigma_d\,(\pi_{IV} - \pi_{is})]$$

where

K_{fc} = capillary filtration coefficient of the total number of perfused capillaries
P_{IV} = intravascular hydrostatic pressure
P_{is} = interstitial hydrostatic pressure
σ_d = reflection coefficient (reflects the permeability of the membrane to protein)
π_{IV} = intravascular colloid osmotic pressure
π_{is} = interstitial colloid osmotic pressure

Starling's equation illustrates the forces that create the net flux of fluid out of the pulmonary capillaries (Fig. 22-7). Type I and II alveolar epithelial cells establish a tight barrier that restricts fluid from entering the air space. This barrier is very important because any fluid in the air space will interfere with gas diffusion. The alveolar-capillary network is also very fragile and susceptible to various injurious agents. Type I cells are very disposed to injury, perhaps because of their thin, elongated shape and large surface area. In interstitial lung diseases, type I cells die, thereby leaving a denuded alveolar epithelium with increased permeability that allows increased fluid movement into the air spaces and thus results in impaired gas exchange. Injury to type I cells also results in proliferation of the cuboidal-shaped type II epithelial cells and differentiation into type I cells, which restores the normal lung architecture and permeability.

The Bronchial Circulation

The bronchial circulation is a separate circulatory system in the lung that provides systemic arterial blood to the trachea, upper airways, surface secretory cells, glands, nerves, visceral pleural surface, lymph nodes, pulmonary arteries, and pulmonary veins. The bronchial circulation perfuses the upper respiratory tract; it does not reach the terminal or respiratory bronchioles or the alveolus. Venous blood from the capillaries of the bronchial circulation flows to the heart through either true bronchial veins or bronchopulmonary veins. True bronchial veins are present in the region of the lung hilus, and blood flows into the azygos, hemiazygos, or intercostal veins before entering the right atrium. The bronchopulmonary veins are formed through a network of tributaries from the bronchial and pulmonary circulatory vessels that anastomose and form vessels with an admixture of blood from both circulatory systems. Blood from these anastomosed vessels returns to the left atrium through pulmonary veins. About two thirds of the total bronchial circulation is returned to the heart via the pulmonary veins and this anastomosis route. The bronchial circulation receives only about 1% of total cardiac output as compared with almost 100% for the pulmonary circulation.

PULMONARY VASCULAR RESISTANCE

Blood flow in the pulmonary circulations is pulsatile and influenced by pulmonary vascular resistance (PVR), gravity, alveolar pressure, and the arterial-to-venous pressure gradient. PVR is the change in pressure from the pulmonary artery (P_{PA}) to the left atrium (P_{LA}) divided by the flow (Q_T), which is cardiac output.

● **Equation 22-17**

$$PVR = \frac{P_{PA} - P_{LA}}{Q_T}$$

Under normal circumstances,

● **Equation 22-18**

$$PVR = \frac{14\,mm\,Hg - 8\,mm\,Hg}{6\,L/min} = 1.0\,mm\,Hg/L/min$$

This resistance is about 10 times less than that in the systemic circulation. The pulmonary circulation has two unique features, noted previously, that allow increased blood flow on demand without an increase in pressure. First, with increased demand, such as during exertion or exercise, pulmonary vessels that are normally closed are recruited. Second, the blood vessels in the pulmonary circulation are highly distensible and increase their diameter with only a minimal increase in pulmonary arterial pressure.

Lung volume affects PVR through its influence on alveolar capillaries (Fig. 22-8). At end inspiration, the air-filled alveoli compress the alveolar capillaries and increase PVR. In contrast to the capillary beds in the systemic circulation, the capillary bed in the lung accounts for about 40% of PVR. The larger extraalveolar vessels increase in diameter at end inspiration because of radial traction and elastic recoil, and their PVR is lower at higher lung volume. During exhalation, the deflated alveoli apply the least resistance to the alveolar capillaries and their PVR is diminished, whereas the higher pleural pressure during exhalation increases the PVR of extraalveolar vessels. As a result of these opposite effects of lung volume on PVR, total PVR in the lung is lowest at FRC.

DISTRIBUTION OF PULMONARY BLOOD FLOW

Because the pulmonary circulation is a low-pressure/low-resistance system, it is influenced by gravity much

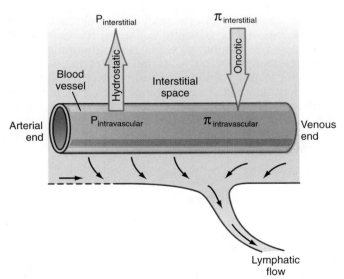

PULMONARY CAPILLARY FLUID BALANCE

● **Figure 22-7.** Factors influencing lung fluid balance. Starling's equation summarizes the balance of forces favoring fluid flux into or out of the pulmonary vessels. Normally there is a net flux of fluid out of the vessels into the interstitium, which is drained from the interstitial space by the lymphatic system.

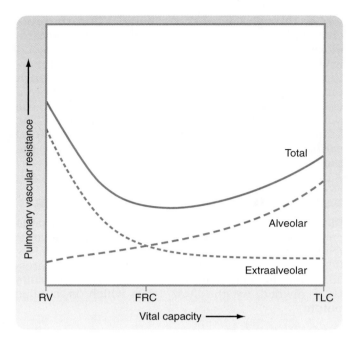

● **Figure 22-8.** Schematic representation of the effects of changes in vital capacity on total pulmonary vascular resistance and the contributions to the total afforded by alveolar and extraalveolar vessels. During inflation from residual volume (RV) to total lung capacity (TLC), resistance to blood flow through alveolar vessels increases, whereas resistance through extraalveolar vessels decreases. Thus, changes in total pulmonary vascular resistance form a U-shaped curve during lung inflation, with the nadir at FRC.

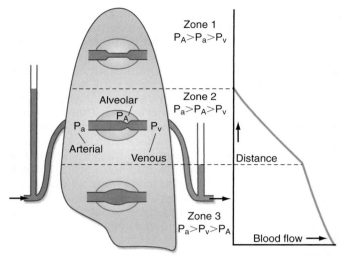

● **Figure 22-9.** Model to explain the uneven distribution of blood flow in the lung based on the pressures affecting the capillaries. (From West JB et al: J Appl Physiol 19:713, 1964.)

more dramatically than the systemic circulation is. This gravitational effect contributes to an uneven distribution of blood flow in the lung. In normal upright subjects at rest, blood flow increases from the apex of the lung to the base of the lung, where it is greatest. Similarly, in a supine individual, blood flow is less in the uppermost (anterior) regions and greater in the lower (posterior) regions. Under conditions of stress, such as exercise, the difference in blood flow in the apex and base of the lung in upright subjects becomes less, mainly because of the increase in arterial pressure.

On leaving the pulmonary artery, blood must travel against gravity to the apex of the lung in upright subjects. For every 1-cm increase in height above the heart, there is a corresponding decrease in hydrostatic pressure equal to 0.74 mm Hg. Thus, the pressure in a pulmonary artery segment that is 10 cm above the heart will be 7.4 mm Hg less than the pressure in a segment at the level of the heart. Conversely, a pulmonary artery segment 5 cm below the heart will have a 3.7–mm Hg increase in pulmonary arterial pressure. This effect of gravity on blood flow affects arteries and veins equally and results in wide variations in arterial and venous pressure from the apex to the base of the lung. These variations will influence both flow and ventilation-perfusion relationships.

In addition to the pulmonary arterial pressure (P_a) to pulmonary venous pressure (P_v) gradients, differences in pulmonary alveolar pressure (P_A) also influence blood flow in the lung. Classically, the lung has been divided into three functional zones (Fig. 22-9). Zone 1 represents the lung apex, where P_a is so low that it can be exceeded by P_A. The capillaries collapse because of the greater external P_A, and blood flow ceases. Under normal conditions this zone does not exist; however, this state could be reached during positive pressure mechanical ventilation or if P_a decreased sufficiently (such as might occur with a marked decrease in blood volume). In zone 2, or the upper third of the lung, P_a is greater than P_A, which is also greater than P_v. Because P_A is greater than P_v, the greater external P_A partially collapses the capillaries and causes a "damming" effect. This phenomenon is often referred to as the "waterfall" effect. In zone 3, P_a is greater than P_v, which is greater than P_A, and blood flows in this area in accordance with the pressure gradients. Thus, pulmonary blood flow is greater in the base of the lung because the increased transmural pressure distends the vessels and lowers the resistance.

ACTIVE REGULATION OF BLOOD FLOW

Blood flow in the lung is regulated primarily by the passive mechanisms described previously. There are, however, several active mechanisms that regulate blood flow. Although the smooth muscle around pulmonary vessels is much thinner than that around systemic vessels, it is sufficient to affect vessel caliber and thus PVR. O_2 levels have a major impact on blood flow. **Hypoxic vasoconstriction** occurs in small arterial vessels in response to decreased alveolar P_{O_2}. The response is local, and it may be a protective response by shifting blood flow from hypoxic areas to well-perfused areas in an effort to enhance gas exchange. Isolated, local hypoxia does not alter PVR; approximately 20% of the vessels need to be hypoxic before a change in PVR can be measured. Low inspired O_2 levels as a result of exposure to high altitude will have a greater effect on PVR because all vessels are affected. High levels of inspired O_2 can dilate pulmonary vessels and decrease PVR. Other factors and some hormones (Table 22-2) can influence vessel caliber, but their effects are usually local, short-lived, and important only in pathological conditions.

VENTILATION-PERFUSION RELATIONSHIPS

Both ventilation (V̇) and lung perfusion (Q̇) are essential elements in normal lung function, but they are insufficient to ensure normal gas exchange. The ventilation-perfusion ratio (also referred to as the V̇/Q̇ ratio) is defined as the ratio of ventilation to blood flow. This ratio can be defined for a single alveolus, for a group of alveoli, or for the entire lung. At the level of a single alveolus, the ratio is defined as alveolar ventilation ($\dot{V}_A$) divided by capillary flow. At the level of the lung, the ratio is defined as total alveolar ventilation divided by cardiac output. In normal individuals, alveolar ventilation is about 4.0 L/min, whereas pulmonary blood flow is about 5.0 L/min. Thus, in a normal lung the overall ventilation-perfusion ratio is about 0.8, but the range of V̇/Q̇ ratios varies widely in different lung units. When ventilation exceeds perfusion, the ventilation-perfusion ratio is greater than one (V̇/Q̇ >1), and

when perfusion exceeds ventilation, the ventilation-perfusion ratio is less than 1 (V̇/Q̇ <1). Mismatching of pulmonary blood flow and ventilation results in impaired O_2 and CO_2 transfer. In individuals with cardiopulmonary disease, mismatching of pulmonary blood flow and alveolar ventilation is the most frequent cause of systemic arterial **hypoxemia** (reduced blood PO_2).

A normal ventilation-perfusion ratio does not mean that ventilation and perfusion to that lung unit are normal; it simply means that the relationship between ventilation and perfusion is normal. For example, in lobar pneumonia, ventilation to the affected lobe is decreased. If perfusion to this area remains unchanged, perfusion would exceed ventilation; that is, the ventilation-perfusion ratio would be less than 1 (V̇/Q̇ <1). However, the decreased ventilation to this area produces hypoxic vasoconstriction in the pulmonary capillary bed supplying this lobe. This results in a decrease in perfusion to the affected area and a more "normal" ventilation-perfusion ratio. Nonetheless, neither the ventilation nor the perfusion to this area is normal (both are decreased), but the relationship between the two approaches the normal range.

Regional Differences in Ventilation-Perfusion Ratios

The ventilation-perfusion ratio varies in different areas of the lung. In an upright subject, ventilation increases more slowly than blood flow from the apex of the lung to the base. Hence, the V̇/Q̇ ratio at the apex of the lung is much greater than 1, whereas the V̇/Q̇ ratio at the base of the lung is much less than 1. The relationship between ventilation and perfusion from the apex to the base of the lung is shown in Figure 22-10.

Alveolar-Arterial PO_2 Difference

Alveolar CO_2 and arterial CO_2 are equal. The same is not true for alveolar and arterial O_2. Even in normal individuals, alveolar O_2 is slightly greater than arterial O_2. The difference between alveolar O_2 (PAO_2) and arterial PO_2 (PaO_2) is called the alveolar-arterial PO_2 difference ($AaDO_2$). An increased in $AaDO_2$ is a hallmark of abnormal O_2 exchange. This small difference is not caused by "imperfect" gas exchange, but by the small number of veins that bypass the lung and empty directly into the arterial circulation. The thebesian vessels of the left ventricular myocardium drain directly into the left ventricle (rather than into the coronary sinus in the right atrium), and some bronchial and mediastinal veins drain into the pulmonary veins. This results in venous admixture and a decrease in arterial PO_2. (This is an example of an anatomic shunt; see later.) Approximately 2% to 3% of cardiac output is **shunted** in this way.

Clinically, the effectiveness of gas exchange is determined by measuring O_2 and CO_2 in arterial blood. Alveolar PO_2 is calculated from the alveolar air equation. The difference, then, between the calculated alveolar PO_2 and the measured arterial PO_2 is $AaDO_2$. In normal individuals breathing room air, $AaDO_2$ is less than 15 mm Hg. The mean value rises approximately

● Table 22-2.
Factors and Hormones That Regulate Pulmonary Blood Flow

Pulmonary Vasoconstrictors
Low PAO_2
Thromboxane A_2
α-Adrenergic catecholamines
Angiotensin
Leukotrienes
Neuropeptides
Serotonin
Endothelin
Histamine
Prostaglandins
High CO_2
Pulmonary Vasodilators
High PAO_2
Prostacyclin
Nitric oxide
Acetylcholine
Bradykinin
Dopamine
β-Adrenergic catecholamines

Ventilation-Perfusion Relationships

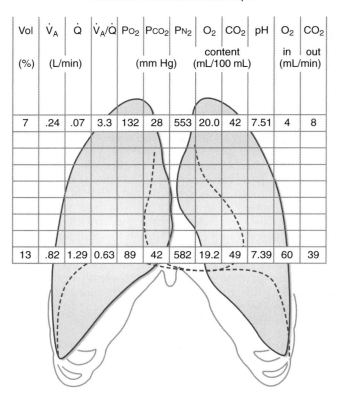

Vol	$\dot{V}_A$	$\dot{Q}$	$\dot{V}_A/\dot{Q}$	PO_2	PCO_2	PN_2	O_2	CO_2	pH	O_2	CO_2
							content			in	out
(%)	(L/min)			(mm Hg)			(mL/100 mL)			(mL/min)	
7	.24	.07	3.3	132	28	553	20.0	42	7.51	4	8
13	.82	1.29	0.63	89	42	582	19.2	49	7.39	60	39

● **Figure 22-10.** Regional differences in gas exchange in a normal lung. Only the apical and basal values are shown for clarity.

3 mm Hg per decade of life. Hence, an $AaDO_2$ less than 25 mm Hg is considered to be the upper limit of normal.

Abnormalities in arterial PO_2 can occur in the presence or absence of an abnormal $AaDO_2$. Hence, the relationship between PaO_2 and $AaDO_2$ is useful in determining the cause of an abnormal PaO_2 and in predicting the response to therapy (particularly to

● **Table 22-3. Causes of Hypoxemia**

Cause	Arterial PO_2	$AaDO_2$	Arterial PO_2 Response to 100% O_2
Anatomic shunt	Decreased	Increased	No significant change
Decreased FIO_2	Decreased	Normal	Increased
Physiological shunt	Decreased	Increased	Decreased
Low ventilation-perfusion ratio	Decreased	Increased	Increased
Diffusion abnormality	Decreased	Increased	Increased
Hypoventilation	Decreased	Normal	Increased

supplemental O_2 administration). Causes of a reduction in arterial PO_2 (arterial hypoxemia) and their effect on $AaDO_2$ are shown in Table 22-3. Each of these causes is discussed in greater detail later.

ARTERIAL BLOOD GAS ABNORMALITIES

Arterial hypoxemia is defined as an arterial PO_2 less than 80 mm Hg in an adult who is breathing room air at sea level. **Hypoxia** occurs when there is insufficient O_2 to carry out normal metabolic functions; hypoxia often occurs when arterial PO_2 is less than 60 mm Hg. **Hypercapnia** is defined as an increase in arterial PCO_2 above the normal range (40 ± 2 mm Hg), and **hypocapnia** is an abnormally low arterial PCO_2 (usually less than 35 mm Hg).

VENTILATION-PERFUSION IN A SINGLE ALVEOLUS

Anatomic Shunt

A useful way to examine the relationship between ventilation and perfusion is the two–lung unit model (Fig. 22-11). Two alveoli are ventilated, each of which is supplied by blood from the heart. When ventilation is uniform, half the inspired gas goes to each alveolus, and when perfusion is uniform, half the cardiac output goes to each alveolus. In this normal unit, the ventilation-perfusion ratio in each of the alveoli is the same and is equal to 1. The alveoli are perfused by mixed venous blood that is deoxygenated and contains increased arterial PCO_2. Alveolar O_2 is higher than mixed venous O_2, and this provides a gradient for movement of O_2 into blood. In contrast, mixed venous CO_2 is greater than alveolar CO_2, and this provides a gradient for movement of CO_2 into the alveolus. Note that in this ideal model, alveolar-arterial O_2 values do not differ.

An anatomic shunt occurs when mixed venous blood bypasses the gas exchange unit and goes directly into arterial blood (Fig. 22-12). Alveolar ventilation, the distribution of alveolar gas, and the composition of alveolar gas are normal, but the distribution of cardiac output is changed. Some of the cardiac output goes through the pulmonary capillary bed that

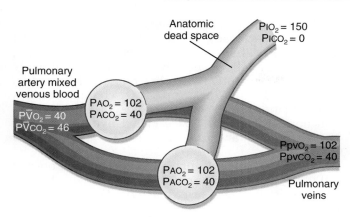

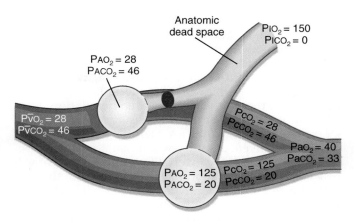

● **Figure 22-11.** Simplified lung model showing two normal parallel lung units. Both units receive equal quantities of fresh air and blood flow for their size. The blood and alveolar gas partial pressures, P, are normal values in a resting person.

● **Figure 22-13.** Schema of a physiological shunt (venous admixture). Notice the marked decrease in arterial P_{O_2} in comparison to P_{CO_2}. The $A a D_{O_2}$ is 85 mm Hg.

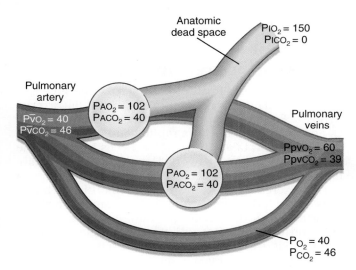

● **Figure 22-12.** Right-to-left shunt. Alveolar ventilation is normal, but a portion of the cardiac output bypasses the lung and mixes with oxygenated blood. PaO_2 will vary depending on the size of the shunt.

supplies the gas exchange units, whereas the rest of it bypasses the gas exchange units and goes directly into arterial blood. The blood that bypasses the gas exchange unit is "shunted," and because the blood is deoxygenated, the model is called a **right-to-left shunt.** Most anatomic shunts occur within the heart, and they occur when deoxygenated blood from the right atrium or ventricle crosses the septum and mixes with blood from the left atrium or ventricle. The effect of this right-to-left shunt is to mix deoxygenated blood with oxygenated blood, and it results in varying degrees of arterial hypoxemia.

An important feature of an anatomic shunt is that the response to giving the individual 100% O_2 to breathe is blunted. The blood that bypasses the gas-exchanging units is never exposed to the enriched O_2, and thus it continues to be deoxygenated. The P_{O_2} in the blood that is not being shunted increases and mixes with the

deoxygenated blood. Thus, the degree of persistent hypoxemia in response to 100% O_2 varies with the extent of the shunted blood. Normally, the hemoglobin in the blood that perfuses the ventilated alveoli is almost fully saturated. Therefore, most of the added O_2 is in the form of dissolved O_2 (see Chapter 24).

The arterial P_{CO_2} in an anatomic shunt is not usually increased even though the shunted blood has an elevated level of CO_2. The reason for this is that the central chemoreceptors respond to any elevation in CO_2 with an increase in ventilation and reduce arterial P_{CO_2} to the normal range. If the hypoxemia is severe, the increased respiratory drive secondary to the hypoxemia increases the ventilation and can decrease arterial P_{CO_2} to below the normal range.

Physiological Shunt

A physiological shunt (also known as venous admixture) can develop when ventilation to lung units is absent in the presence of continuing perfusion (Fig. 22-13). In the two–lung unit model, all of the ventilation now goes to the other lung unit, whereas perfusion is equally distributed between both lung units. The lung unit without ventilation but with perfusion has a $\dot{V}/\dot{Q}$ ratio of 0. The blood perfusing this unit is mixed venous blood; because there is no ventilation, no gas is exchanged in the unit, and the blood leaving this unit continues to be mixed venous blood. The effect of a physiological shunt on oxygenation is similar to the effect of an anatomic shunt; that is, deoxygenated blood bypasses a gas-exchanging unit and admixes with arterial blood. Clinically, **atelectasis** (which is obstruction to ventilation of a gas-exchanging unit with subsequent loss of volume) is an example of a lung region with a $\dot{V}/\dot{Q}$ of 0. Causes of atelectasis include mucous plugs, airway edema, foreign bodies, and tumors in the airway.

VENTILATION-PERFUSION MISMATCHING: LOW $\dot{V}/\dot{Q}$

Mismatching between ventilation and perfusion is the most frequent cause of arterial hypoxemia in patients with respiratory disorders. In the most common example, the composition of mixed venous blood, total blood flow (cardiac output), and the distribution of blood flow are normal. However, when alveolar ventilation is distributed unevenly between the two gas exchange units (Fig. 22-14) and blood flow is equally distributed, the unit with decreased ventilation has a $\dot{V}/\dot{Q}$ ratio of less than 1, whereas the unit with the increased ventilation has a $\dot{V}/\dot{Q}$ of greater than 1. This causes the alveolar and end-capillary gas compositions to vary. Both the arterial O_2 and CO_2 content will be abnormal in the blood that has come from the unit with the decreased ventilation ($\dot{V}/\dot{Q}$ <<<1). The unit with the increased ventilation ($\dot{V}/\dot{Q}$ >1) will have a lower CO_2 and a higher O_2 content because it is being overventilated. The actual arterial Po_2 and Pco_2 will vary, depending on the relative contribution of each of these units to arterial blood. The alveolar-arterial O_2 gradient ($AaDo_2$) will be increased because the relative overventilation of one unit does not fully compensate (either by adding extra O_2 or by removing extra CO_2) for underventilation of the other unit. The failure to compensate is greater for O_2 than for CO_2 because of the flatness of the upper part of the oxyhemoglobin dissociation curve as opposed to the slope of the CO_2 dissociation curve (see Chapter 23). In other words, increased ventilation will increase alveolar Po_2, but it adds little extra O_2 content to the blood because hemoglobin is close to being 100% saturated in the overventilated areas. This is not the case for CO_2, where the steeper slope of the CO_2 curve results in removal of more CO_2 when ventilation increases. Thus, because CO_2 moves by diffusion, as long as a CO_2 gradient is maintained, CO_2 diffusion will occur.

ALVEOLAR HYPOVENTILATION

Alveolar O_2 is determined by a balance between the rate of O_2 uptake and the rate of O_2 replenishment by ventilation. O_2 uptake depends on blood flow through the lung and the metabolic demands of the tissues. If ventilation decreases, alveolar Po_2 will decrease and arterial Po_2 will subsequently decrease. In addition, alveolar ventilation and alveolar CO_2 are directly related. When ventilation is halved, the alveolar CO_2 content and thus the arterial CO_2 content doubles (see Equation 22-8). Ventilation insufficient to maintain normal levels of CO_2 is called **hypoventilation.** Hypoventilation always decreases PaO_2 and increases $PaCO_2$.

One of the hallmarks of hypoventilation is a normal $AaDo_2$. Hypoventilation reduces alveolar O_2, which in turn results in a decrease in arterial O_2. Because gas exchange is normal, the difference between alveolar and arterial O_2 remains normal. Hypoventilation is seen in individuals with diseases associated with muscle weakness and in association with drugs that reduce the respiratory drive. In the presence of hypoventilation, however, areas of atelectasis develop rapidly; atelectasis creates regions with $\dot{V}/\dot{Q}$ ratios of 0, and the $AaDo_2$ then rises.

DIFFUSION ABNORMALITIES

Abnormalities in diffusion of O_2 across the alveolar-capillary barrier could potentially result in arterial hypoxia. Equilibration between alveolar and capillary O_2 and CO_2 content occurs rapidly and in a fraction of the time that it takes for red blood cells to transit the pulmonary capillary network. Hence, diffusion equilibrium almost always occurs in normal subjects, even during exercise, when the transit time of red blood cells through the lung increases significantly. An alveolar-arterial Po_2 difference attributable to incomplete diffusion **(diffusion disequilibrium)** has been observed in normal individuals only during exercise at high altitude (≥10,000 feet). Even in individuals with abnormal diffusion capacity, diffusion disequilibrium at rest is unusual but is possible during exercise and at altitude. **Alveolar capillary block,** or thickening of the air-blood barrier, is an uncommon cause of hypoxemia. Even with a thickened alveolar wall there is sufficient time for gas diffusion unless the red blood cell transit time is increased.

MECHANISMS OF HYPERCAPNIA

Two major mechanisms account for the development of **hypercapnia** (elevated Pco_2): hypoventilation and wasted ventilation. As noted previously, alveolar ventilation and alveolar CO_2 are inversely related. When ventilation is halved, alveolar CO_2 and arterial CO_2 double. Hypoventilation always decreases PaO_2 and increases $PaCO_2$ and thereby results in a hypoxemia that responds to an enriched source of O_2. Wasted or dead space ventilation occurs when pulmonary blood flow is interrupted in the presence of normal ventilation. This occurs most often because of a pulmonary embolus that obstructs blood flow. The embolus halts blood flow to pulmonary areas with normal ventilation

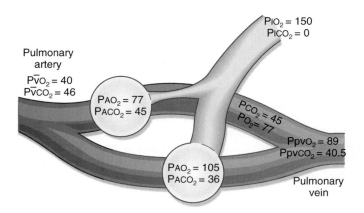

● **Figure 22-14.** Effects of ventilation-perfusion mismatching on gas exchange. The decrease in ventilation to the one lung unit could be due to mucus obstruction, airway edema, bronchospasm, a foreign body, or a tumor.

($\dot{V}/\dot{Q} = \infty$). In this situation the ventilation is wasted because it fails to oxygenate any of the mixed venous blood. The ventilation to the perfused regions of the lung is less than ideal (i.e., there is relative "hypoventilation" to this area because it now receives all the pulmonary blood flow with "normal" ventilation). If compensation does not occur, $PaCO_2$ would increase and PaO_2 would decrease. Compensation after a pulmonary embolus, however, begins almost immediately; local bronchoconstriction occurs and the distribution of ventilation shifts to the areas being perfused. As a result, changes in arterial CO_2 and O_2 content are minimized.

EFFECT OF 100% OXYGEN ON ARTERIAL BLOOD GAS ABNORMALITIES

One of the ways that a right-to-left shunt can be distinguished from other causes of hypoxemia is by having the individual breathe 100% O_2 through a nonrebreathing facemask for approximately 15 minutes. When the subject breathes 100% O_2, all of the N_2 in the alveolus is replaced by O_2. Thus, alveolar O_2, from the alveolar air equation, is

● **Equation 22-19**

$$PaO_2 = 1.0\ (P_b - PH_2O) - PaCO_2/0.8$$
$$= 1.0\ (760 - 47) - 40/0.8$$
$$= 663\ mm\ Hg$$

In a normal lung the alveolar O_2 content rapidly increases, and it provides the gradient for transfer of O_2 into capillary blood. This is associated with a marked increase in arterial O_2 content (Table 22-3). Similarly, over the 15-minute period of breathing enriched O_2, even areas with very low $\dot{V}/\dot{Q}$ ratios will develop high alveolar O_2 pressure as the N_2 is replaced by O_2. In the presence of normal perfusion to these areas, there is a gradient for gas exchange, and the end-capillary blood is highly enriched in O_2. In contrast, in the presence of a right-to-left shunt, oxygenation is not corrected because mixed venous blood continues to flow through the shunt and mix with blood that has perfused normal units. The poorly oxygenated blood from the shunt lowers the arterial O_2 content and maintains the $AaDO_2$. An elevated alveolar-arterial O_2 difference during a properly conducted study with 100% O_2 signifies the presence of a right-to-left shunt; the magnitude of the difference can be used to quantify the proportion of the cardiac output that is being shunted.

EFFECT OF CHANGING CARDIAC OUTPUT

Change in cardiac output is the only nonrespiratory factor that affects gas exchange. Decreasing cardiac output diminishes the O_2 content and increases the CO_2 content of mixed venous blood. Increasing the

cardiac output has the opposite effect. This change in O_2 and CO_2 content will have little effect on arterial O_2 and CO_2 levels in individuals with normal lungs, unless cardiac output is extremely low. In the presence of lung disease secondary to ventilation-perfusion mismatching or in the presence of an anatomic shunt, the composition of mixed venous blood will have a significant effect on the arterial levels of O_2 and CO_2. For any level of $\dot{V}/\dot{Q}$ abnormality, a decrease in cardiac output is associated with an increasingly abnormal PaO_2.

REGIONAL DIFFERENCES

We have already discussed regional differences in ventilation and perfusion and the relationship between ventilation and perfusion. We have also discussed the effects of various physiological abnormalities (e.g., shunt, $\dot{V}/\dot{Q}$ mismatch, and hypoventilation) on arterial O_2 and CO_2 levels. Before leaving this topic, however, it should be noted that because the $\dot{V}/\dot{Q}$ ratio varies in different regions of the lung, the end-capillary blood coming from these regions will have different O_2 and CO_2 levels. These differences are shown in Figure 22-10, and they demonstrate the complexity of the lung. First, recall that the volume of the lung at the apex is less than the volume at the base. As previously described, ventilation and perfusion are less at the apex than at the base, but the differences in perfusion are greater than the differences in ventilation. Thus, the $\dot{V}/\dot{Q}$ ratio is high at the apex and low at the base. This difference in ventilation-perfusion ratios is associated with a difference in alveolar O_2 and CO_2 content between the apex and the base. The alveolar O_2 content is higher and the alveolar CO_2 content is lower in the apex than in the base. This results in differences in end-capillary contents for these gases. End-capillary PO_2 is lower, and consequently the O_2 content is lower in end-capillary blood at the lung base than at the apex. In addition, there is significant variation in blood pH in the end capillaries in these regions because of the variation in CO_2 content. During exercise, blood flow to the apex increases and becomes more uniform in the lung; as a result, the difference between the content of gases in the apex and in the base of the lung diminishes with exercise.

■ KEY CONCEPTS

1. The sum of the partial pressures of a gas is equal to the total pressure. The partial pressure of a gas (P_{gas}) is equal to the fraction of the gas in the gas mixture (F_{gas}) times the total pressure (P_{tot}). The conducting airways do not participate in gas exchange. Therefore, the partial pressures of O_2, N_2, and water vapor in humidified air remain unchanged in the airways until the gas reaches the alveolus. The partial pressure of O_2 in the alveolus is given by the alveolar air equation. This equation is used to calculate $AaDO_2$, the most useful measurement of abnormal arterial O_2.

2. The relationship between CO_2 production and alveolar ventilation is defined by the alveolar CO_2 equation. There is an inverse relationship between the partial pressure of CO_2 in the alveolus ($Paco_2$) and alveolar ventilation (V_A), irrespective of the exhaled quantity of CO_2. In normal individuals, alveolar $Paco_2$ is tightly regulated to remain constant at around 40 mm Hg.

3. The volume of air in the conducting airways is called the anatomic dead space. Dead space ventilation (V_D) varies inversely with tidal volume (V_T). The total volume of gas in each breath that does not participate in gas exchange is called the physiological dead space ventilation. It includes the anatomic dead space and the dead space secondary to ventilated, but not perfused alveoli.

4. The pulmonary circulation is a low-pressure, low-resistance system. The arteries of the pulmonary circulation are thin walled, and they have minimal smooth muscle. The pulmonary vessels are seven times more compliant than the systemic vessels. Recruitment of new capillaries is a unique feature of the lung and allows for adjustments in stress, as in the case of exercise. Pulmonary vascular resistance is the change in pressure from the pulmonary artery (P_{PA}) to the left atrium (P_{LA}) divided by cardiac output (Q_T). This resistance is about 10 times less than in the systemic circulation.

5. There are regional differences in ventilation and perfusion that are due in large part to the effects of gravity. The ventilation-perfusion ratio (also referred to as the $\dot{V}/\dot{Q}$ ratio) is defined as the ratio of ventilation to blood flow. In a normal lung, the overall ventilation-perfusion ratio is about 0.8. When ventilation exceeds perfusion, the ventilation-perfusion ratio is greater than 1 ($\dot{V}/\dot{Q} > 1$), and when perfusion exceeds ventilation, the ventilation-perfusion ratio is less than 1 ($\dot{V}/\dot{Q} < 1$). The $\dot{V}/\dot{Q}$ ratio at the top of the lung is high (increased ventilation relative to very little blood flow), whereas the $\dot{V}/\dot{Q}$ ratio at the bottom of the lung is very low. In normal individuals breathing room air, the $AaDo_2$ is less than 15 mm Hg.

6. There are five mechanisms of arterial hypoxemia: anatomic shunt, physiological shunt, $\dot{V}/\dot{Q}$ mismatching, diffusion abnormalities, and hypoventilation. There are two mechanisms of hypercapnia: increase in dead space and hypoventilation. A change in cardiac output is the only nonrespiratory factor that affects gas exchange.

CHAPTER 23

Oxygen and Carbon Dioxide Transport

The respiratory and circulatory systems function together to transport sufficient oxygen (O_2) from the lungs to the tissues to sustain normal cellular activity and to transport carbon dioxide (CO_2) from the tissues to the lungs for expiration. CO_2, a product of active cellular glucose metabolism, is transported from the tissues via systemic veins to the lungs, where it is expired (Fig. 23-1). To enhance uptake and transport of these gases between the lungs and tissues, specialized mechanisms (e.g., O_2-hemoglobin binding and HCO_3^- transport of CO_2) have evolved that enable O_2 uptake and CO_2 expiration to occur simultaneously. Moreover, these specialized mechanisms facilitate uptake of O_2 and expiration of CO_2. To gain an understanding of the mechanisms involved in the transport of these gases, one must consider gas diffusion properties, as well as transport and delivery mechanisms.

GAS DIFFUSION

Gas movement throughout the respiratory system occurs predominantly via diffusion. The respiratory and circulatory systems contain several unique anatomic and physiological features to facilitate gas diffusion: (1) large surface areas for gas exchange (alveolar to capillary and capillary to tissue membrane barriers) with short distances to travel, (2) substantial partial pressure gradient differences, and (3) gases with advantageous diffusion properties. Transport and delivery of O_2 from the lungs to the tissue and vice versa for CO_2 are dependent on basic gas diffusion laws.

Gases in the Lung Diffuse from Regions of Higher to Lower Partial Pressure

The process of gas diffusion is passive and similar whether diffusion occurs in a gaseous or liquid state. The rate of diffusion of a gas through a liquid is described by **Graham's law,** which states that the rate is directly proportional to the solubility coefficient of the gas and inversely proportional to the square root of its molecular weight. Calculation of the diffusion properties for O_2 and CO_2 reveals that CO_2 diffuses approximately 20 times faster than O_2 does. Rates of O_2 diffusion from the lungs into blood and from blood into tissue, and vice versa for CO_2, are predicted by **Fick's law** of gas diffusion (Fig. 23-2). Fick's law states that the diffusion of a gas ($\dot{V}_{gas}$) across a sheet of tissue is directly related to the surface area (A) of the tissue, the diffusion constant (D) of the specific gas, and the partial pressure difference ($P_1 - P_2$) of the gas on each side of the tissue and is inversely related to tissue thickness (T). That is,

● **Equation 23-1**

$$\dot{V}_{gas} = A \times D \times \frac{P_1 - P_2}{T}$$

The ratio $A \cdot D/T$ represents the conductance of a gas from the alveolus to blood. The diffusing capacity of the lung (D_L) is its conductance ($A \cdot D/T$) when considered for the entire lung; thus, applying Fick's equation, D_L can be calculated as follows:

● **Equation 23-2**

$$\dot{V} = A \cdot D \frac{\Delta(P_1 - P_2)}{T}$$
$$\dot{V} = D_L(P_1 - P_2)$$
$$D_L = \frac{\dot{V}}{P_1 - P_2}$$

Fick's law of diffusion could be used to assess the diffusion properties of O_2 in the lung, except that ΔP (alveolar – capillary P_{O_2}) cannot be determined because capillary P_{O_2} cannot be measured. This limitation can be overcome by using carbon monoxide (CO) rather than O_2. Because CO has low solubility in the capillary membrane, the rate of CO equilibrium across the capillary is slow and the partial pressure of CO in capillary blood remains close to zero. This is in contrast to the high solubility of CO in blood. Thus, the only limitation for diffusion of CO is the alveolar-capillary membrane, which makes CO a useful gas for calculating D_L. The capillary partial pressure (P_2 above) is essentially zero for CO, and therefore D_L can be measured from $\dot{V}_{CO}$ and the average partial pressure of CO in the alveolus. That is,

● **Equation 23-3**

$$\dot{V}_{co} = D_L(P_1 - P_2)$$
$$D_{LCO} = \frac{\dot{V}_{co}}{P_1 - P_2} = \frac{\dot{V}_{co}}{P_{ACO}}$$

Assessment of D_{LCO} has become a classic measurement of the diffusion barrier of the alveolar-capillary membrane. It is useful in the differential diagnosis of certain restrictive and obstructive lung diseases, such as interstitial pulmonary fibrosis and emphysema.

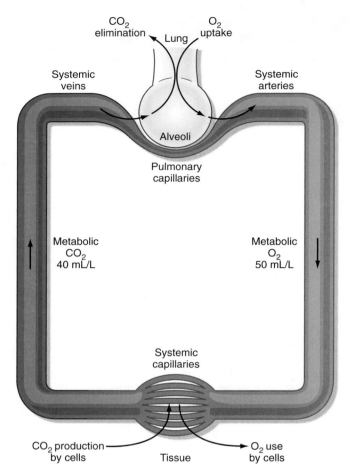

● **Figure 23-1.** Oxygen and CO_2 transport in arterial and venous blood. Oxygen in arterial blood is transferred from arterial capillaries to tissues. The flow rates for O_2 and CO_2 are shown for 1 L of blood. The ratio of CO_2 production to O_2 consumption is the respiratory exchange ratio, R, which at rest is approximately 0.80.

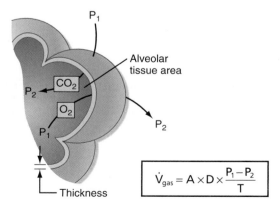

$$\dot{V}_{gas} = A \times D \times \frac{P_1 - P_2}{T}$$

● **Figure 23-2.** Fick's law states that diffusion of a gas across a sheet of tissue is directly related to the surface area of the tissue, the diffusion constant of the specific gas, the partial pressure difference of the gas on each side of the tissue and is inversely related to tissue thickness.

A patient with interstitial pulmonary fibrosis (a restrictive lung disease) inhales a single breath of 0.3% CO from residual volume to total lung capacity. He holds his breath for 10 seconds and then exhales. After discarding the exhaled gas from the dead space, a representative sample of alveolar gas from late in exhalation is obtained. The average alveolar CO pressure is 0.1 mm Hg, and 0.25 mL of CO has been taken up. The diffusion capacity for CO in this patient is

$$D_{LCO} = \frac{V_{CO}}{P_{ACO}} = 0.25\,mL / 10\,sec \times \frac{60\,sec/min}{0.1\,mmHg}$$

$$= 15\,mL/min/mmHg$$

The normal range for D_{LCO} is 20 to 30 mL/min/ mm Hg. Patients with interstitial pulmonary fibrosis have an initial alveolar inflammatory response with subsequent scar formation within the interstitial space. The inflammation and scar tissue thicken the interstitial space and thus make it more difficult for gas diffusion to occur, which results in decreased D_{LCO}. This is a classic characteristic of certain types of restrictive lung disease; gas readily enters the alveolus but is inhibited in its ability to diffuse into blood.

Oxygen and Carbon Dioxide Exchange in the Lung Is Perfusion Limited

Different gases have different solubility factors. Gases that are insoluble in blood (i.e., anesthetic gases, nitrous oxide and ether) do not chemically combine with proteins in blood and equilibrate rapidly between alveolar gas and blood. The equilibration occurs in less time than the 0.75 second that the red blood cell spends in the capillary bed (capillary transit time). The diffusion of insoluble gases between alveolar gas and blood is considered **perfusion limited** because the partial pressure of gas in the blood leaving the capillary has reached equilibrium with alveolar gas and is limited only by the amount of blood perfusing the alveolus. In contrast, a **diffusion limited** gas, such as CO, has low solubility in the alveolar-capillary membrane but high solubility in blood because of its high affinity for **hemoglobin** (Hgb). These features prevent the equilibration of CO between alveolar gas and blood during the red blood cell transit time.

The high affinity of CO for Hgb enables large amounts of CO to be taken up in blood with little or no appreciable increase in its partial pressure. Gases that are chemically bound to Hgb do not exert a partial pressure in blood. Like CO, both CO_2 and O_2 have relatively low solubility in the alveolar-capillary membrane but high solubility in blood because of their ability to bind to Hgb. However, their rate of equilibration is sufficiently rapid for complete equilibration to occur during the transit time of the red blood cell within the capillary. Equilibration for O_2 and CO_2 usually occurs within 0.25 second. Thus, O_2 and CO_2 transfer is normally perfusion limited. The partial pressure of a dif-

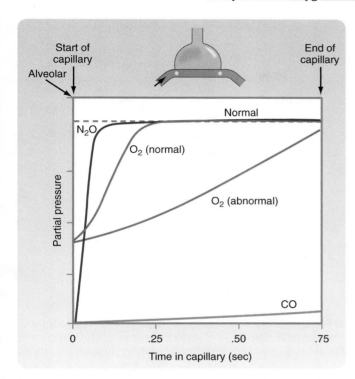

● **Figure 23-3.** Uptake of nitrous oxide (N_2O), CO, and O_2 in blood relative to their partial pressures and the transit time of the red blood cell in the capillary. For gases that are perfusion limited (N_2O and O_2), their partial pressures have equilibrated with alveolar pressure before exiting the capillary. In contrast, the partial pressure of CO, a gas that is diffusion limited, does not reach equilibrium with alveolar pressure. O_2 uptake in rare conditions can become diffusion limited.

fusion limited gas (i.e., CO) does not reach equilibrium with the alveolar pressure over the time that it spends in the capillary (Fig. 23-3). Although CO_2 has a greater rate of diffusion in blood than O_2 does, it has a lower membrane-blood solubility ratio and consequently takes approximately the same amount of time to reach equilibration in blood.

Diffusion limitation for O_2 and CO_2 would occur if red blood cells spent less than 0.25 second in the capillary bed. Occasionally, this can be seen in very fit athletes during vigorous exercise and in healthy subjects who exercise at high altitude.

OXYGEN TRANSPORT

Oxygen is carried in blood in two forms: dissolved O_2 and O_2 bound to Hgb. The dissolved form is measured clinically in an arterial blood gas sample as PaO_2. Only a small percentage of O_2 in blood is in the dissolved form, and its contribution to O_2 transport under normal conditions is almost negligible. However, dissolved O_2 can become a significant factor in conditions of severe hypoxemia. Binding of O_2 to Hgb to form **oxyhemoglobin** within red blood cells is the primary transport mechanism of O_2. Hgb not bound to O_2 is referred to

as deoxyhemoglobin or reduced Hgb. The O_2-carrying capacity of blood is enhanced about 65 times by its ability to bind to Hgb.

Hemoglobin

Hgb is the major transport molecule for O_2. The Hgb molecule is a protein with two major components: four nonprotein heme groups each containing iron in the reduced ferrous (Fe^{+++}) form, which is the site of O_2 binding, and a globin portion consisting of four polypeptide chains. Normal adults have two α-globin chains and two β-globin chains (HgbA), whereas children younger than 1 year have fetal Hgb (HgbF) consisting of two α chains and two γ chains. This difference in the structure of HgbF increases its affinity for O_2 and aids in the transport of O_2 across the placenta. In addition, HgbF is not inhibited by 2,3-diphosphoglycerate (2,3-DPG), a product of glycolysis, thus further enhancing O_2 uptake.

Binding of O_2 to Hgb alters the ability of Hgb to absorb light. This effect of O_2 on Hgb is responsible for the change in color between oxygenated arterial blood (bright red) and deoxygenated venous blood (dark-red bluish). Binding and dissociation of O_2 with Hgb occur in milliseconds, thus facilitating O_2 transport because red blood cells spend 0.75 second in the capillaries. There are approximately 280 million Hgb molecules per red blood cell, which provides an efficient mechanism to transport O_2. Myoglobin, a protein similar in structure and function to Hgb, has only one subunit of the Hgb molecule. It aids in the transfer of O_2 from blood to muscle cells and in the storage of O_2, which is especially critical in O_2-deprived conditions.

Abnormalities of the Hgb molecule occur with mutations in the amino acid sequence (i.e., sickle cell disease) or in the spatial arrangement of the globin polypeptide chains and result in abnormal function. Compounds such as CO, nitrites (nitric oxide [NO]), and cyanides can oxidize the iron molecule in the heme group and change it from the reduced ferrous state to the ferric state (Fe^{++++}), which reduce the ability of O_2 to bind to Hgb.

The Oxyhemoglobin Dissociation Curve

In the alveoli the majority of O_2 in plasma quickly diffuses into red blood cells and chemically binds to Hgb. This process is reversible such that Hgb gives up its O_2 to the tissue. The oxyhemoglobin dissociation curve illustrates the relationship between PO_2 in blood and the number of O_2 molecules bound to Hgb (Fig. 23-4). The **S** shape of the curve demonstrates the dependence of Hgb saturation on PO_2, especially at partial pressures lower than 60 mm Hg. The clinical significance of the flat portion of the oxyhemoglobin dissociation curve (>60 mm Hg) is that a drop in PO_2 over a wide range of partial pressures (100 to 60 mm Hg) has only minimal effect on Hgb saturation, which remains at 90% to 100%, a level sufficient for normal O_2 transport and delivery. The clinical significance of the steep portion (<60 mm Hg) of the curve is that a large amount of O_2 is released from Hgb with only a small change in PO_2, which facilitates the release and diffusion of O_2

IN THE CLINIC

In an inherited homozygous condition known as sickle cell disease, individuals have an amino acid substitution (valine for glutamic acid) on the β chain of the Hgb molecule. This creates a sickle cell Hgb (HgbS), which when not bound to oxygen (deoxyhemoglobin or desaturated Hgb), can transform into a gelatinous material that distorts the normal biconcave shape of the red blood cell to a crescent or "sickle" form. This change in shape increases the tendency of the red blood cell to form thrombi or clots that obstruct small vessels and creates a clinical condition known as "acute sickle cell episode." The symptoms of such an episode vary depending on the site of the obstruction (i.e., stroke, pulmonary infarction) but are commonly associated with intense pain. The spleen is a common site of infarction, and the ensuing tissue damage compromises the immune capabilities of individuals and renders them susceptible to recurrent infections. In the homozygous form this is a life-shortening condition; however, in the heterozygous form, individuals are resistant to malaria. Thus, there is a survival advantage to a heterozygous individual in regions of the world where malaria is prevalent, which may explain why the sickle cell mutation has been preserved through evolution. The increased affinity of HgbF for O_2 renders advantages to individuals with sickle cell disease in that the cells do not desaturate as much when O_2 is released from Hgb to the tissue and thus are less likely to sickle. Sickle cell disease is most prevalent in individuals of African American descent but is also observed in Hispanic, Turkish, Asian, and other ethnic groups.

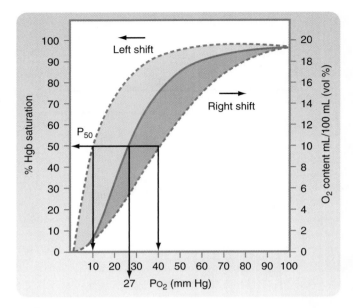

● **Figure 23-4.** Oxyhemoglobin dissociation curve showing the relationship between the partial pressure of O_2 in blood and the percentage of Hgb binding sites that are occupied by oxygen molecules (percent saturation). Adult hemoglobin (HgbA) is about 50% saturated at a P_{O_2} of 27 mm Hg, 90% saturated at 60 mm Hg, and about 98% saturated at 100 mm Hg. The P_{50} is the partial pressure at which Hgb is 50% saturated with O_2. When the O_2 dissociation curve shifts to the right, P_{50} increases. When the curve shifts to the left, P_{50} decreases.

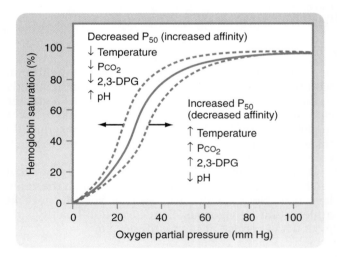

● **Figure 23-5.** Factors that shift the oxyhemoglobin dissociation curve.

into tissue. The point on the curve where 50% of Hgb is saturated with O_2 is called the P_{50}, and it is 27 mm Hg in normal adults (Fig. 23-4).

Physiological Factors That Shift the Oxyhemoglobin Dissociation Curve

The oxyhemoglobin dissociation curve can be shifted in numerous clinical conditions either to the right or to the left (Fig. 23-5). The curve is shifted to the right when the affinity of Hgb for O_2 decreases, which enhances O_2 dissociation. This results in decreased Hgb binding to O_2 at a given P_{O_2}, thus increasing the P_{50}. When the affinity of Hgb for O_2 increases, the curve is shifted to the left, which reduces the P_{50}. In this state, O_2 dissociation and delivery to tissue are inhibited. Shifts to the right or left of the dissociation curve have little effect when they occur at O_2 partial pressures within the normal range (80 to 100 mm Hg). However, at O_2 partial pressures below 60 mm Hg (steep part of the curve), shifts in the oxyhemoglobin dissociation curve can dramatically influence O_2 transport.

pH and CO_2

Changes in blood pH shift the oxyhemoglobin dissociation curve. An increase in CO_2 production by tissue

and release into blood results in the generation of hydrogen ions (H^+) and a decrease in pH. This shifts the dissociation curve to the right, which has a beneficial effect by aiding in the release of O_2 from Hgb for diffusion into tissues. The shift to the right in the dissociation curve is due to the decrease in pH and to a direct effect of CO_2 on Hgb. This effect of CO_2 on the affinity of Hgb for O_2 is known as the **Bohr effect,** and it serves to enhance O_2 uptake in the lungs and delivery of O_2 to tissues. Conversely, as blood passes through the lungs, CO_2 is exhaled, thereby resulting in an increase in pH, which causes a shift to the left in the oxyhemoglobin dissociation curve. Increased body temperature, such as during exercise, shifts the oxyhemoglobin dissociation curve to the right and enables more O_2 to be released to tissues where it is needed because the demand increases. During cold weather, a decrease in body temperature, especially in the extremities (lips, fingers, toes, and ears), shifts the O_2 dissociation curve to the left (higher Hgb affinity). In this instance PaO_2 may be normal, but release of O_2 in these extremities is not facilitated. That is why these anatomic areas display a bluish coloration with exposure to cold.

2,3-Diphosphoglycerate

Mature red blood cells do not have mitochondria, and therefore they respire via anaerobic glycolysis. Large quantities of a metabolic intermediary, 2,3-DPG, are formed in the red blood cell during glycolysis, and the affinity of Hgb for O_2 decreases as 2,3-DPG levels increase. Thus, the oxyhemoglobin dissociation curve shifts to the right. Although the binding sites of 2,3-DPG and O_2 differ on the Hgb molecule, binding of 2,3-DPG creates an allosteric effect that inhibits the binding of O_2. Conditions that increase 2,3-DPG include hypoxia, decreased Hgb, and increased pH. Decreased levels of 2,3-DPG are observed in stored blood samples and thus may present a problem to transfusion recipients because of the greater affinity of Hgb for O_2, which inhibits the unloading of O_2 to tissues.

Fetal Hemoglobin

As discussed previously, fetal Hgb has a greater affinity for O_2 than adult Hgb does. Fetal Hgb thus shifts the oxyhemoglobin dissociation curve to the left.

Carbon Monoxide

Carbon monoxide (CO) binds to the heme group of the Hgb molecule at the same site as O_2 and forms **carboxyhemoglobin** (HgbCO). A major difference between the ability of CO versus CO_2 to bind to Hgb is illustrated by comparing the oxyhemoglobin and carboxyhemoglobin dissociation curves. The affinity of CO for Hgb is about 200 times greater than it is for O_2 (Fig. 23-6). Thus, small amounts of CO can greatly influence the binding of O_2 to Hgb. In the presence of CO, the affinity of Hgb for O_2 is enhanced. This shifts the dissociation curve to the left, which further prevents the unloading and delivery of O_2 to tissues. As the PCO of blood approaches 1.0 mm Hg, all of the Hgb binding sites are occupied by CO, and Hgb is unable to bind to O_2. This situation is not compatible with life and is the cause of death in individuals with CO poisoning. In healthy individuals, HgbCO occupies about 1% to 2% of the Hgb binding sites; however, in cigarette smokers and in individuals who reside in high-density urban traffic areas, occupation of Hgb binding sites can be increased to 10%. Levels above 5% to 7% are considered hazardous. Treatment of individuals with high levels of CO, such as after inhaling car exhaust or

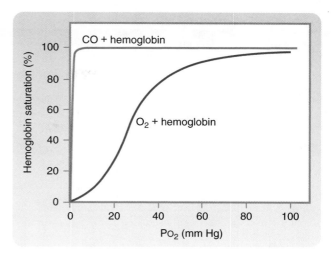

● **Figure 23-6.** Oxyhemoglobin and carboxyhemoglobin dissociation curves.

inhaling smoke from a burning building, consists of administering high concentrations of O_2 to displace CO from Hgb. Increasing the ambient pressure above atmospheric pressure, through the use of a barometric chamber, substantially increases the O_2 tension, which promotes the dissociation of CO from Hgb. Another gas, NO, has great affinity (200,000 times greater than O_2) for Hgb, and it binds irreversibly to Hgb at the same site as O_2 does. Endothelial cells synthesize NO, which has vasodilation properties. Thus, NO is used therapeutically as an inhalant in patients with pulmonary hypertension to reduce pressure. Although NO poisoning is not common, one should be cautious when administering NO therapy for long periods. Hgb-bound CO and NO is referred to as methemoglobin. Under normal conditions, about 1% to 2% of Hgb is bound to CO and NO.

Oxygen Saturation, Content, and Delivery

Each Hgb molecule can bind up to four O_2 atoms, and each gram of Hgb can bind up to 1.34 mL of O_2. The term **O_2 saturation** (SO_2) refers to the amount of O_2 bound to Hgb relative to the maximal amount of O_2 (100% O_2 capacity) that can bind Hgb. At 100% O_2 capacity, the heme groups of the Hgb molecules are fully saturated with O_2, and at 75% SO_2, three of the four heme groups are occupied. Binding of O_2 to each heme group increases the affinity of the Hgb molecule to bind additional O_2. The O_2 content in blood is the sum of the O_2 bound to Hgb and the dissolved O_2. Oxygen content is decreased in the presence of increased CO_2 and CO and in individuals with anemia (Fig. 23-7).

Oxygen delivery from the lungs to tissues is dependent on several factors, including cardiac output, the Hgb content of blood, and the ability of the lung to oxygenate the blood. Not all of the O_2 carried in blood is unloaded at the tissue level. The actual O_2 extracted from blood by the tissue is the difference between the arterial O_2 content and the venous O_2 content times

● **Table 23-1. Tissue Hypoxia**

Type of Hypoxia	Cause	PaO₂	CaO₂	Amount of O₂ Delivered	Amount of O₂ Used
Hypoxic	Pulmonary disease with ↓ PaO₂ ↓ V̇/Q̇ ratio	Low	Low	Low	Normal
Circulatory	Vascular disease Arteriovenous shunt	Normal	Normal	Low	Normal
Anemic	CO poisoning Anemia	Normal	Low	Normal	Normal
Histotoxic	Cyanide poisoning Sodium azide	Normal	Normal	Normal	Low

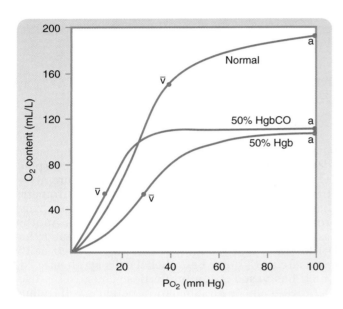

● **Figure 23-7.** A comparison of O₂ content curves under three conditions shows why HgbCO dramatically reduces the O₂ transport system. Fifty percent HgbCO represents binding of half the circulating Hgb with CO. The 50% Hgb and 50% HgbCO curves show the same decreased O₂ content in arterial blood. However, CO has a profound effect in lowering venous Po₂. The arterial (a) and mixed venous (v̄) points of constant cardiac output are indicated.

cardiac output. Under normal conditions, Hgb leaves the tissue 75% saturated with O₂, and only about 25% is actually used by tissues. Hypothermia, relaxation of skeletal muscles, and an increase in cardiac output reduce O₂ consumption. Conversely, a decrease in cardiac output, anemia, hyperthermia, and exercise increase O₂ consumption.

Tissue hypoxia refers to a condition in which insufficient O₂ is available to cells to maintain adequate aerobic metabolism. Thus, anaerobic metabolism is stimulated and results in the generation of increased levels of lactate and H⁺ and the subsequent formation of lactic acid. The net result can lead to a significant decrease in blood pH. In cases of severe hypoxia, the extremities, toes, and fingertips may appear blue-gray **(cyanotic)** because of lack of O₂ and increased deoxyhemoglobin. There are four major types of tissue hypoxia (Table 23-1) that can occur via different mech-

anisms, the most common being **hypoxic hypoxia.** Hypoxic hypoxia is caused by a variety of lung diseases (e.g., chronic obstructive pulmonary disease, pulmonary fibrosis, neuromuscular diseases) that result in decreased Pao₂ or Cao₂, or both, with a subsequent decrease in the delivery of O₂ to tissues. **Circulatory (stagnate) hypoxia** is caused by reduced blood flow to an organ and is usually due to a vascular disease or an arteriovenous shunt. **Anemic hypoxia** is caused by an inability of blood to carry sufficient O₂ because of either low Hgb (anemia) or an inability of Hgb to carry O₂ (as in the case of CO poisoning). **Histotoxic hypoxia** is often caused by poisons (i.e., cyanide, sodium azide, and some pesticides) that block the electron transport system in mitochondria and prevent the utilization of O₂ by the cell.

Erythropoiesis

Tissue oxygenation depends on the concentration of Hgb and thus on the number of red blood cells available in the circulation. Red blood cell production **(erythropoiesis)** in the bone marrow is controlled by the hormone **erythropoietin,** which is synthesized in the kidney by cortical interstitial cells. Although Hgb levels are normally very stable, decreased O₂ delivery, low Hgb concentration, and low PaO₂ stimulate the secretion of erythropoietin. This increases the production of red blood cells. Chronic renal disease damages the cortical interstitial cells and thereby suppresses their ability to synthesize erythropoietin. This causes anemia, along with decreased Hgb because of the lack of erythropoietin. Erythropoietin replacement therapy effectively increases red blood cell production.

CO₂ TRANSPORT
Glucose Metabolism and CO₂ Production

CO₂ is produced at a rate of approximately 200 mL/min under healthy conditions, and typically, 80 molecules of CO₂ will be expired by the lung for every 100 molecules of O₂ that enter the capillary bed. The ratio of expired CO₂ to O₂ uptake is referred to as the **respiratory exchange ratio** and, under normal conditions, is 0.8 (80 CO₂ to 100 O₂). This ratio is similar at the tissue to blood compartment, where it is referred to as the **respiratory quotient.**

The body has enhanced storage capabilities for CO₂ as compared with O₂, and hence PaO₂ is much more sensitive to changes in ventilation than Pa_{CO_2} is. Whereas Pa_{O_2} is dependent on several factors, in addition to alveolar ventilation, arterial Pa_{CO_2} is solely dependent on alveolar ventilation and CO_2 production. There is an inverse relationship between alveolar ventilation and Pa_{CO_2}.

Bicarbonate and CO_2 Transport

In blood CO_2 is transported in red blood cells primarily as bicarbonate (HCO_3^-), but also as dissolved CO_2 and as carbamino protein complexes (i.e., CO_2 binds to plasma proteins and to Hgb) (Fig. 23-8). Once CO_2 diffuses through the tissue and enters plasma, it quickly dissolves. The reaction of CO_2 with H_2O to form carbonic acid (H_2CO_3) provides the major pathway for the generation of HCO_3^- in red blood cells (Equation 23-4):

● **Equation 23-4**

$$CO_2 + H_2O \leftrightarrow H_2CO_3 \leftrightarrow H^+ + HCO_3^-$$

This reaction normally proceeds quite slowly; however, it is catalyzed within red blood cells by the enzyme **carbonic anhydrase.** The HCO_3^- diffuses out of the red blood cell in exchange for Cl^-, the **chloride shift,** which helps the cell maintain its osmotic equilibrium.

The chemical reaction just described and in Figure 23-8 is reversible and can be shifted to the right to generate more HCO_3^- in response to more CO_2 entering the blood from tissues, or it can be shifted to the left as CO_2 is exhaled in the lungs, thereby reducing HCO_3^-. The free H^+ is quickly buffered within the red blood cell by binding to Hgb. Buffering of H^+ ion is critical to keep the reaction moving toward the synthesis of HCO_3^-; high levels of free H^+ (low pH) will shift the reaction to the left.

REGULATION OF H^+ ION CONCENTRATION AND ACID-BASE BALANCE

The H^+ ion concentration (pH) has a dramatic effect on many metabolic processes within cells, and regulation of pH is essential for normal homeostasis. In the

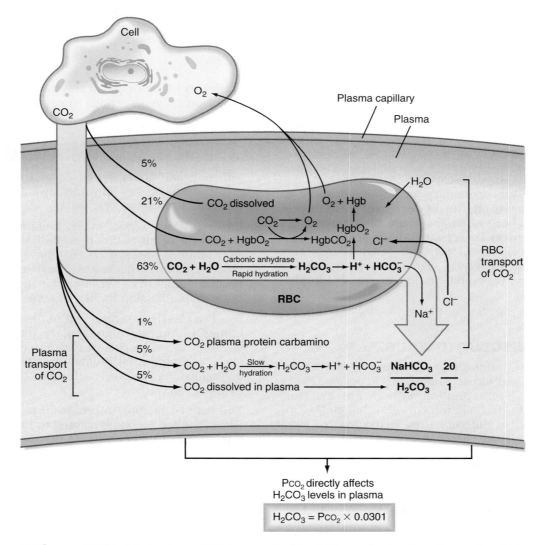

● **Figure 23-8.** Mechanisms of CO_2 transport in blood. The predominant mechanism by which CO_2 is transported from tissue cells to the lung is in the form of HCO_3^-. RBC, red blood cell.

clinical setting, blood pH is measured to assess the concentration of H^+. The normal pH range for adults is 7.35 to 7.45 and is maintained by the lung, kidney, and chemical buffer systems (see Chapter 36). In the respiratory system, conversion of CO_2 to HCO_3^-, as illustrated below, provides a major mechanism to buffer and regulate the H^+ concentration (pH):

● **Equation 23-5**

$$CO_2 + H_2O \leftrightarrow H_2CO_3 \leftrightarrow H^+ + HCO_3^-$$
$$\updownarrow$$
$$H^+ + Hgb \leftrightarrow H \times Hgb$$

As PA_{CO_2} changes, so does the concentration of HCO_3^- and H_2CO_3, as well as Pa_{CO_2}.

The **Henderson-Hasselbalch** equation is used to calculate how changes in CO_2 and HCO_3^- affect pH.

● **Equation 23-6**

$$pH = pK' + \frac{\log[HCO_3^-]}{\alpha P_{CO_2}}$$

or

● **Equation 23-7**

$$pH = 6.1 + \frac{\log[HCO_3^-]}{0.03 P_{CO_2}}$$

In these equations the amount of CO_2 is determined from the partial pressure of CO_2 (P_{CO_2}) and its solubility (α) in solution. For plasma at 37°C, α has a value of 0.03. Also, pK' is the negative logarithm of the overall dissociation constant for the reaction and has a value of 6.1 for plasma at 37°C.

Acute hyperventilation secondary to exercise or anxiety reduces P_{CO_2}, thereby increasing pH (respiratory alkalosis). Conversely, if P_{CO_2} increases because of hypoventilation secondary to an overdose of a respiratory depressant, the pH decreases (respiratory acidosis). Acid-base imbalances are also caused by metabolic disorders such as metabolic acidosis (e.g., lactic acidosis, ketoacidosis, and renal failure; see Chapter 36) and metabolic alkalosis (e.g., hypokalemia, hypochloremia, vomiting, high doses of steroids; see Chapter 36).

THE CO₂ DISSOCIATION CURVE

In contrast to O_2, the dissociation curve for CO_2 in blood is linear and directly related to P_{CO_2} (Fig. 23-9). The degree of Hgb saturation with O_2 has a major effect on the CO_2 dissociation curve. Although O_2 and CO_2 bind to Hgb at different sites, deoxygenated Hgb has greater affinity for CO_2 than oxygenated Hgb does. Thus, deoxygenated blood (venous blood) freely takes up and transports more CO_2 than oxygenated arterial blood does. The deoxygenated Hgb more readily forms carbamino compounds and also more readily binds free H^+ ions released during the formation of HCO_3^-. The effect of changes in oxyhemoglobin saturation on the relationship of CO_2 content to P_{CO_2} is referred to as the **Haldane effect** and is reversed in the lung when O_2 is transported from the alveoli to red blood cells.

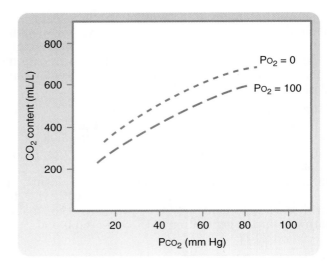

● **Figure 23-9.** Blood CO_2 equilibrium curves (arterial and venous). Venous blood can transport more CO_2 than arterial blood can at any given P_{CO_2}. When compared with the $HgbO_2$ equilibrium curve, the CO_2 curves are essentially straight lines between a P_{CO_2} of 20 and 80 mm Hg.

This effect is illustrated by a shift to the left in the CO_2 dissociation curve in venous blood as compared with arterial blood.

■ KEY CONCEPTS

1. Diffusion and transport of O_2 and CO_2 are determined by basic gas diffusion laws and depend on differential pressure gradients.

2. Gases (nitrous oxide, ether, helium) that have a rapid rate of air-to-blood equilibration are perfusion limited. Gases (CO) that have a slow air-to-blood equilibration rate are diffusion limited. Under normal conditions, O_2 transport is perfusion limited but can be diffusion limited in some situations.

3. D_{LCO} is a classic measurement of the diffusion capabilities of the alveolar-capillary membrane. It is useful in the diagnosis of restrictive lung diseases such as interstitial pulmonary fibrosis and in distinguishing between chronic bronchitis and emphysema.

4. The major transport mechanism of O_2 in blood is within the red blood cell bound to Hgb, and for CO_2 it is within red blood cells in the form of HCO_3^-.

5. Tissue hypoxia occurs when insufficient amounts of O_2 are supplied to the tissue to conduct normal levels of aerobic metabolism.

6. The reversible reaction of CO_2 with H_2O to form H_2CO_3 with its subsequent dissociation to HCO_3^- and H^+ is catalyzed by the enzyme carbonic anhydrase within red blood cells and is the major pathway for generation of HCO_3^-.

7. The CO_2 dissociation curve from blood is linear and directly related to PCO_2. PCO_2 is solely dependent on alveolar ventilation and CO_2 production.

8. The O_2 dissociation curve is **S** shaped. In the plateau area (above 60 mm Hg), increasing or decreasing PO_2 has only a minimal effect on Hgb saturation from 100 to 90%. This ensures adequate Hgb saturation over a large range of PO_2 values.

9. The CO_2-to-HCO_3^- pathway plays a critical role in the regulation of H^+ ions and in maintaining acid-base balance in the body.

CHAPTER 24

Control of Respiration

We breathe without thinking, and we can willingly modify our breathing pattern and even hold our breath. Control of ventilation, which is discussed in this chapter, includes the generation and regulation of rhythmic breathing by the respiratory center in the brainstem and its modification by the input of information from higher brain centers and from systemic receptors. The goal of breathing, from a mechanical perspective, is to minimize work and, from a physiological perspective, to maintain blood gases and, specifically, to regulate arterial P_{CO_2}. Another goal of breathing is to maintain acid-base balance in the brain by regulating arterial P_{CO_2}. Automatic respiration begins at birth. In utero, the placenta, not the lung, is the organ of gas exchange in the fetus. Its microvilli interdigitate with the maternal uterine circulation, and O_2 transport and CO_2 removal from the fetus occur by passive diffusion across the maternal circulation.

VENTILATORY CONTROL: AN OVERVIEW

There are four major sites of ventilatory control: (1) the **respiratory control center,** (2) **central chemoreceptors,** (3) **peripheral chemoreceptors,** and (4) **pulmonary mechanoreceptors/sensory nerves.** The respiratory control center is located in the medulla oblongata of the brainstem and is composed of multiple nuclei that generate and modify the basic ventilatory rhythm. The center consists of two main parts: (1) a ventilatory pattern generator, which sets the rhythmic pattern, and (2) an integrator, which controls generation of the pattern, processes input from higher brain centers and chemoreceptors, and controls the rate and amplitude of the ventilatory pattern. Input to the integrator arises from higher brain centers, including the cerebral cortex, hypothalamus, amygdala, limbic system, and cerebellum.

Central chemoreceptors are located in the central nervous system just below the ventrolateral surface of the medulla. These central chemoreceptors detect changes in the P_{CO_2} and pH of interstitial fluid in the brainstem, and they modulate ventilation. Peripheral chemoreceptors are located on specialized cells in the aortic arch **(aortic bodies)** and at the bifurcation of the internal and external carotid arteries **(carotid bodies)** in the neck. These peripheral chemoreceptors sense the P_{O_2}, P_{CO_2}, and pH of arterial blood, and they feed information back to the integrator nuclei in the medulla through the vagus nerves and carotid sinus

nerves, which are branches of the glossopharyngeal nerves. Pulmonary mechanoreceptors and sensory nerve stimulation, in response to lung inflation or to stimulation by irritants or release of local mediators in the airways, modify the ventilatory pattern.

The collective output of the respiratory control center to motor neurons located in the anterior horn of the spinal column controls the muscles of respiration, and this output determines the automatic rhythmic pattern of respiration. Motor neurons located in the cervical region of the spinal column control the activity of the diaphragm through the **phrenic nerves,** whereas other motor neurons located in the thoracic region of the spine control the intercostal muscles and the accessory muscles of respiration.

In contrast to automatic respiration, voluntary respiration bypasses the respiratory control center in the medulla. The neural activity controlling voluntary respiration originates in the motor cortex, and signaling passes directly to motor neurons in the spine through the **corticospinal tracts.** The motor neurons to the respiratory muscles act as the final site of integration of the voluntary (corticospinal tract) and automatic (ventrolateral tracts) control of ventilation. Voluntary control of these muscles competes with automatic influences at the level of the spinal motor neurons, and this competition can be demonstrated by breath holding. At the start of the breath hold, voluntary control dominates the spinal motor neurons. However, as the breath hold continues, the automatic ventilatory control eventually overpowers the voluntary effort and limits the duration of the breath hold. Motor neurons also innervate muscles of the upper airway. These neurons are located within the medulla near the respiratory control center. They innervate muscles in the upper airways through the cranial nerves. When activated, they dilate the pharynx and large airways at the initiation of inspiration.

RESPONSE TO CO₂

Ventilation is regulated by P_{CO_2}, P_{O_2}, and pH in arterial blood. Arterial P_{CO_2} is the most important of these regulators. Both the rate and depth of breathing are controlled to maintain Pa_{CO_2} close to 40 mm Hg. In a normal awake individual, there is a linear rise in ventilation as arterial P_{CO_2} reaches and exceeds 40 mm Hg (Fig. 24-1). Changes in Pa_{CO_2} are sensed by central and peripheral chemoreceptors, and they transmit this information to the medullary respiratory centers. The respiratory

● **Figure 24-1.** Relationship between Paco₂ and alveolar ventilation in awake normal states, during sleep, after narcotic ingestion and deep anesthesia, and in the presence of metabolic acidosis. Both the slopes of the response (sensitivity) and the position of the response curves (threshold, the point at which the curve crosses the x axis) are changed, thus indicating differences in ventilatory responses and response thresholds.

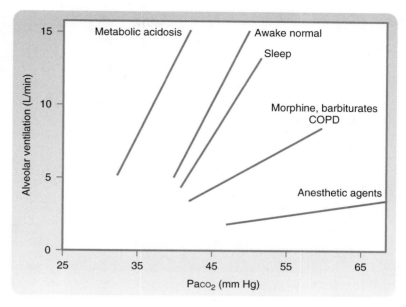

CONTROL OF VENTILATION: THE DETAILS

The Respiratory Control Center

control center then regulates minute ventilation and thereby maintains arterial PCO_2 within the normal range. In the presence of a normal PAO_2, ventilation increases by about 3 L/min for each millimeter rise in $PaCO_2$. The response to an increase in $PACO_2$ is further increased in the presence of a low PaO_2 (Fig. 24-2). With a low PaO_2, ventilation is greater for any given $PACO_2$, and the increase in ventilation for a given increment in $PACO_2$ is enhanced (the slope is greater).

The slope of the minute ventilation response as a function of the inspired CO_2 is termed the ventilatory response to CO_2 and is a test of CO_2 sensitivity. It is important to recognize that this relationship is amplified by low O_2 (Fig. 24-2, *B*). The enhanced responsiveness to low O_2 occurs because different mechanisms are responsible for sensing PO_2 and PCO_2 in the peripheral chemoreceptors. Thus, the presence of both hypercapnia and hypoxemia (often called asphyxia when both changes are present) has an additive effect on chemoreceptor output and on the resulting ventilatory stimulation.

The ventilatory drive or response to changes in PCO_2 can be reduced by hyperventilation and by drugs, such as morphine, barbiturates, and anesthetic agents, that depress the respiratory center and decrease the ventilatory response to both CO_2 and O_2 (Fig. 24-1). In these instances, the stimulus is inadequate to stimulate the motor neurons that innervate the muscles of respiration. It is also depressed during sleep.

In addition, the ventilatory response to changes in PCO_2 is reduced if the work of breathing is increased, which can occur in individuals with chronic obstructive pulmonary disease (COPD) (Fig. 24-1). This effect occurs primarily because the neural output of the respiratory center is less effective in promoting ventilation as a result of the mechanical limitation to ventilation.

When the brain is transected experimentally between the medulla and the pons, periodic breathing is maintained, thus demonstrating that the inherent rhythmicity of breathing originates in the medulla. Although no single group of neurons in the medulla has been found to be the breathing "pacemaker," two distinct nuclei within the medulla are involved in generation of the respiratory pattern (Fig. 24-3). One nucleus is the **dorsal respiratory group** (DRG), which is composed of cells in the **nucleus tractus solitarius** located in the dorsomedial region of the medulla. Cells in the DRG receive afferent input from the 9th and 10th cranial nerves, which originate from airways and the lung and are thought to constitute the initial intracranial processing station for this afferent input. The second group of medullary cells is the **ventral respiratory group** (VRG), located in the ventrolateral region of the medulla. The VRG is composed of three cell groups: the **rostral nucleus retrofacialis,** the **caudal nucleus retroambiguus,** and the **nucleus paraambiguus.** The VRG contains both inspiratory and expiratory neurons. The nucleus retrofacialis and the caudally located cells of the nucleus retroambiguus are active during exhalation, whereas the rostrally located cells of the nucleus retroambiguus are active during inspiration. The nucleus paraambiguus has inspiratory and expiratory neurons that travel in the vagus nerve to the laryngeal and pharyngeal muscles. Discharges from cells in these areas excite some cells and inhibit other cells.

At the level of the respiratory control center, inspiration and exhalation involve three phases—one inspiratory and two expiratory (Fig. 24-4). Inspiration begins with an abrupt increase in discharge from cells

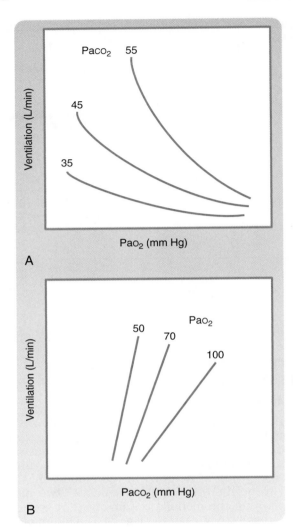

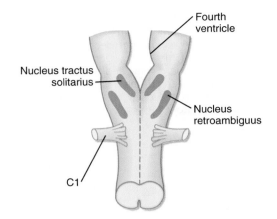

● **Figure 24-3.** The respiratory control center is located in the medulla (the most primitive portion of the brain). The neurons are mainly in two areas called the nucleus tractus solitarius and the nucleus retroambiguus.

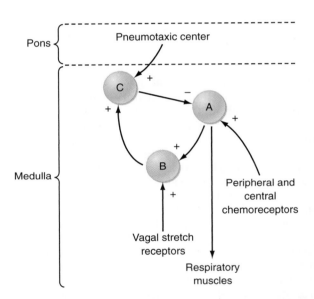

● **Figure 24-2.** The effects of hypoxia **(A)** and hypercapnia **(B)** on ventilation as the other respiratory gas partial pressure is varied. **A,** At a given Pa_{CO_2}, ventilation increases more and more as Pa_{O_2} decreases. When Pa_{CO_2} is allowed to decrease (the normal condition) during hypoxia, there is little stimulation of breathing until P_{O_2} falls below 60 mm Hg. The hypoxic response is mediated through the carotid body chemoreceptors. **B,** The sensitivity of the ventilatory response to CO_2 is enhanced by hypoxia.

● **Figure 24-4.** The basic wiring diagram of the brainstem ventilatory controller. The signs of the main output *(arrows)* of the neuron pools indicate whether the output is excitatory (+) or inhibitory (−). Pool A provides tonic inspiratory stimuli to the muscles of breathing. Pool B is stimulated by pool A and provides additional stimulation to the muscles of breathing, and pool B stimulates pool C. Other brain centers feed into pool C (inspiratory cutoff switch), which sends inhibitory impulses to pool A. Afferent information (feedback) from various sensors acts at different locations: chemoreceptors act on pool A and intrapulmonary sensory fibers act via the vagus nerves on pool B. A pneumotaxic center in the anterior pons receives input from the cerebral cortex, and it modulates the pool C group.

in the nucleus tractus solitarius, the nucleus retroambiguus, and the nucleus paraambiguus, followed by a steady ramplike increase in firing rate throughout inspiration. This leads to progressive contraction of the respiratory muscles during automatic breathing. At the end of inspiration, an off-switch event results in a marked decrease in neuron firing, at which point exhalation begins. At the start of exhalation (phase I of expiration), a paradoxical increase in inspiratory neuron firing slows the expiratory phase down by increasing inspiratory muscle tone and expiratory neuron firing. This inspiratory neuron firing decreases and stops during phase II of exhalation. Although many different neurons in the DRG and VRG are involved in ventilation, each cell type appears to have

a specific function. For example, the **Hering-Breuer reflex** is an inspiratory inhibitory reflex that arises from afferent stretch receptors located in the smooth muscles of the airways. Increasing lung inflation stimulates these stretch receptors and results in early exhalation by stimulating the neurons associated with the off-switch phase of inspiratory muscle control. Thus,

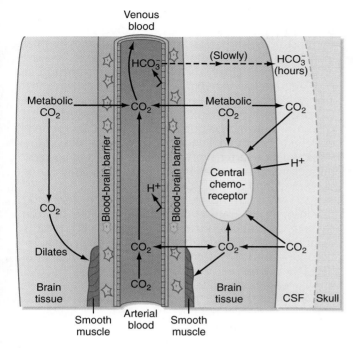

● **Figure 24-5.** CO_2 and the blood-brain barrier. Arterial CO_2 crosses the blood-brain barrier and rapidly equilibrates with CSF CO_2. H^+ and HCO_3^- ions cross the barrier slowly. Arterial CO_2 combines with metabolic CO_2 to dilate the smooth muscle. When compared with arterial blood, the pH of CSF is lower and the PCO_2 is higher, with little protein buffering.

● **Table 24-1.**

Normal Values for the Composition of Cerebrospinal Fluid and Arterial Blood

	CSF	Arterial
pH	7.33	7.40
PCO_2 (mm Hg)	44	40
HCO_3^- (mEq/L)	22	24

● **AT THE CELLULAR LEVEL**

The **Henderson-Hasselbalch equation** relates the pH of CSF to $[HCO_3^-]$:

$$pH = pK + \log \frac{[HCO_3]}{\alpha \cdot P_{CO_2}}$$

where α is the solubility coefficient (0.03 mmol/L/mm Hg) and pK is the negative logarithm of the dissociation constant for carbonic acid (6.1). The Henderson-Hasselbalch equation demonstrates that an increase in CSF PCO_2 will decrease the pH of CSF at any given $[HCO_3^-]$. The decrease in pH will stimulate the central chemoreceptors and thereby increase ventilation. Thus, CO_2 in blood regulates ventilation by its effect on the pH of CSF. The resulting hyperventilation reduces the PCO_2 in the blood, and therefore in CSF, and returns the pH of CSF toward a normal value. Furthermore, cerebral vasodilation accompanies an increase in arterial PCO_2, and this enhances the diffusion of CO_2 into CSF. By contrast, an increase in CSF $[HCO_3^-]$ will increase the pH of CSF at any given PCO_2.

rhythmic breathing depends on a continuous (tonic) inspiratory drive from the DRG and an intermittent (phasic) expiratory drive from the cerebrum, thalamus, cranial nerves, and ascending sensory tracts in the spinal cord.

Central Chemoreceptors

A chemoreceptor is a receptor that responds to a change in the chemical composition of blood or other fluid around it. Central chemoreceptors are specialized cells on the ventrolateral surface of the medulla. Chemoreceptors are sensitive to the pH of the surrounding extracellular fluid. Because this extracellular fluid is in contact with cerebrospinal fluid (CSF), changes in the pH of CSF affect ventilation by acting on these chemoreceptors

CSF is an ultrafiltrate of plasma that is secreted continuously by the **choroid plexus** and is reabsorbed by the arachnoid villi. Because it is in contact with the extracellular fluid in the brain, the composition of CSF is influenced by the metabolic activity of the cells in the surrounding area and the composition of the blood. Although the origin of CSF is plasma, the composition of CSF is not the same as that of plasma because the **blood-brain barrier** exists between the two sites (Fig. 24-5). The blood-brain barrier is composed of endothelial cells, smooth muscle, and the **pial** and **arachnoid membranes,** and it regulates the movement of ions between blood and CSF. In addition, the choroid plexus also determines the ionic composition of CSF by trans-

porting ions into and out of CSF. The blood-brain barrier is relatively impermeable to H^+ and HCO_3^- ions, but it is very permeable to CO_2. Thus, the PCO_2 in CSF parallels the arterial PCO_2 tension. CO_2 is also produced by cells of the brain as a product of metabolism. As a consequence, the PCO_2 in CSF is usually a few mm Hg higher than that in arterial blood, so the pH is slightly more acidic (7.33) than in plasma (Table 24-1).

Changes in arterial PCO_2, by altering pH, activate homeostatic mechanisms that return the pH back toward normal. The blood-brain barrier regulates the pH of CSF by adjusting the ionic composition and $[HCO_3^-]$ of CSF. These changes in CSF $[HCO_3^-]$, however, occur slowly, over a period of several hours, whereas changes in CSF PCO_2 can occur within minutes. Thus, compensation for changes in the pH of CSF requires hours to fully develop.

Peripheral Chemoreceptors

The **carotid** and **aortic bodies** are peripheral chemoreceptors that respond to changes in arterial PO_2 (not the O_2 content), PCO_2, and pH, and they transmit afferent information to the central respiratory control center. The peripheral chemoreceptors are the only chemoreceptors that respond to changes in PO_2. The peripheral chemoreceptors are also responsible for approximately 40% of the ventilatory response to CO_2. These chemoreceptors are small, highly vascularized structures. They consist of type I **(glomus)** cells that are rich in mitochondria and endoplasmic reticulum. They also have several types of cytoplasmic granules (synaptic vesicles) that contain various neurotransmitters, including dopamine, acetylcholine, norepinephrine, and neuropeptides. Afferent nerve fibers synapse with type I cells, and they transmit information to the brainstem through the carotid sinus nerve (carotid body) and vagus nerve (aortic body). Type I cells are the cells primarily responsible for sensing PO_2, PCO_2, and pH. In response to even small decreases in arterial PO_2 there is an increase in chemoreceptor discharge, which enhances respiration. The response is robust when arterial PO_2 decreases below 75 mm Hg. Thus, ventilation is regulated by changes in arterial and CSF pH via effects on peripheral and central chemoreceptors (Fig. 24-6).

IN THE CLINIC

Imagine flying from New York City to Denver. The barometric pressure in New York is about 760 mm Hg, whereas in the mountains surrounding Denver, Colorado, it is 600 mm Hg. At sea level, the PO_2 in arterial blood is approximately 95 mm Hg (using the alveolar air equation [see Chapter 22], $PAO_2 = [(760 - 47) \times 0.21] - [40/0.8] = 100$ mm Hg. If the alveolar-arterial PO_2 difference [$AaDO_2$] is 5 mm Hg, $PaO_2 = 100 - 5 = 95$ mm Hg). In the CSF, pH would be about 7.33, PCO_2 would be 44 mm Hg (arterial PCO_2 + CO_2 produced by metabolism of brain cells), and HCO_3^- would be approximately 22 mEq/L.

There is an abrupt decrease in PIO_2 when you arrive in the mountains ($PIO_2 = [600 - 47] \times 0.21 = 116$ mm Hg), and alveolar and arterial O_2 decrease ($PAO_2 = 116 - [40/0.8] = 66$ mm Hg; $PaO_2 = 61$ mm Hg, assuming no change in $AaDO_2$). This decrease in arterial O_2 stimulates the peripheral chemoreceptors and thereby increases ventilation. The increase in ventilation decreases arterial PCO_2 and elevates arterial pH. The result of this increase in ventilation is to minimize the hypoxemia by increasing PAO_2. (For example, assume that $PACO_2$ decreases to 30 mm Hg. Then, $PAO_2 = [(600 - 47) \times 0.21] - [30/0.8] = 78$ mm Hg, a 12–mm Hg increase in PAO_2.)

The decrease in arterial PCO_2 also decreases the PCO_2 of CSF. Because [HCO_3^-] is unchanged, the pH of CSF increases. This increase in the pH of CSF attenuates the rate of discharge of the central chemoreceptors and decreases their contribution to the ventilatory drive. Over the next 12 to 36 hours, [HCO_3^-] in CSF decreases as acid-base transporter proteins in the blood-brain barrier reduce [HCO_3^-]. Consequently, the pH of CSF returns toward normal. Central chemoreceptor discharge increases and minute ventilation is further increased. At the same time that [HCO_3^-] in CSF decreases, HCO_3^- is gradually excreted from plasma by the kidneys. This results in a gradual return of arterial

pH toward normal. Peripheral chemoreceptor stimulation increases further as arterial pH becomes normal (peripheral chemoreceptors are inhibited by the elevated arterial pH). Finally, within 36 hours of arriving at high altitude, minute ventilation increases significantly. This delayed response is greater than the immediate effect of the hypoxemia on ventilation. This further increase in ventilation is due to both central and peripheral chemoreceptor stimulation. Thus, by the end of the weekend, both arterial pH and CSF pH are approaching normal; minute ventilation is increased, arterial PO_2 is decreased, and arterial PCO_2 is decreased.

You now return home. When you land in New York, the inspired PO_2 returns to normal, and the hypoxic stimulus to ventilation is removed. Arterial PO_2 returns to normal and the peripheral chemoreceptor stimulation to ventilation decreases. This increases arterial [CO_2] toward normal, which in turn increases CSF [CO_2]. This increase is associated with a decrease in the pH of CSF as [HCO_3^-] in CSF is now reduced and ventilation is augmented. Over the next 12 to 36 hours, acid-base transporters in the blood-brain barrier transport HCO_3^- back into CSF, and the pH of CSF gradually returns toward normal. Similarly, the pH of blood decreases as arterial PCO_2 rises because arterial [HCO_3^-] decreases. This stimulates the peripheral chemoreceptors, and minute ventilation remains augmented. Over the next 12 to 36 hours, the kidney increases blood [HCO_3^-] (see Chapter 36), arterial pH returns to normal, and minute ventilation returns to normal.

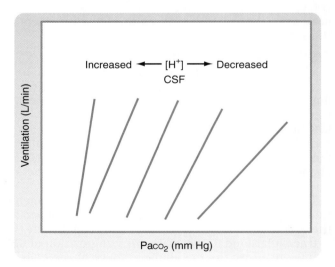

● **Figure 24-6.** The ventilatory response to PCO_2 is affected by the [H^+] of CSF and brainstem interstitial fluid. During chronic metabolic acidosis (e.g., diabetic ketoacidosis), the [H^+] of CSF is increased and the ventilatory response to inspired PCO_2 is increased (steeper slope). Conversely, during chronic metabolic alkalosis (a relatively uncommon condition), the [H^+] of CSF is decreased and the ventilatory response to inspired PCO_2 is decreased (reduced slope). The positions of the response lines are also shifted, thus indicating altered thresholds.

● **Table 24-2.** **Reflexes and Sensory Nerves in the Respiratory Tract**

Reflex	Stimuli	End-Organ Location	Receptor Type
Hering-Breuer inflation reflex Hering-Breuer deflation reflex Bronchodilation Tachycardia Hyperpnea	Lung inflation	Airway smooth muscle cells	Myelinated, vagal, slowly adapting receptor
Cough Mucus secretion Bronchoconstriction Hering-Breuer deflation reflex	Lung hyperinflation Exogenous and endogenous agents Histamine Prostaglandin	Among airway epithelial cells	Myelinated, vagal, rapidly adapting receptors (irritant receptors)
Apnea, followed by tachypnea Bronchoconstriction Bradycardia Hypotension Mucus secretion	Large hyperinflation Exogenous and endogenous agents Capsaicin Phenyl diguanide Histamine Bradykinin Serotonin Prostaglandins	Pulmonary interstitial space Close to the pulmonary circulation Close to the bronchial circulation	Unmyelinated, vagal, C fiber endings (J receptors)

Pulmonary Mechanoreceptors
Chest Wall and Lung Reflexes

Several reflexes that arise from the chest wall and lungs affect ventilation and ventilatory patterns (Table 24-2). The **Hering-Breuer inspiratory-inhibitory reflex** is stimulated by increases in lung volume, especially those associated with an increase in both ventilatory rate and tidal volume. This stretch reflex is mediated by vagal fibers, and when elicited, it results in cessation of inspiration by stimulating the off-switch neurons in the medulla. This reflex is inactive during quiet breathing and appears to be most important in newborns. Stimulation of nasal or facial receptors with cold water initiates the **diving reflex.** When this reflex is elicited, **apnea,** or cessation of breathing, and bradycardia occur. This reflex protects individuals from aspirating water in the initial stages of drowning. Activation of receptors in the nose is responsible for the sneeze reflex.

The **aspiration** or **sniff reflex** can be elicited by stimulation of mechanical receptors in the nasopharynx and pharynx. This is a strong, short-duration inspiratory effort that brings material from the nasopharynx to the pharynx, where it can be swallowed or expectorated. The mechanical receptors responsible for the sniff reflex are also important in swallowing by inhibiting respiration and causing laryngeal closure. Only newborn infants can breathe and swallow simultaneously, which allows more rapid ingestion of nutrients.

The larynx contains both superficial and deep receptors. Activation of the superficial receptors results in apnea, cough, and expiratory movements that protect the lower respiratory tract from aspirating foreign material. The deep receptors are located in the skeletal muscles of the larynx, and they control muscle fiber activation, as in other skeletal muscles.

Sensory Receptors and Reflexes

There are three major types of sensory receptors located in the tracheobronchial tree that respond to a variety of different stimuli and result in changes in the lung's mechanical properties, alterations in the respiratory pattern, and the development of respiratory symptoms. Inhaled dust, noxious gases, or cigarette smoke stimulates **irritant receptors** in the trachea and large airways that transmit information through myelinated vagal afferent fibers. Stimulation of these receptors results in an increase in airway resistance, reflex apnea, and coughing. These receptors are also known as **rapidly adapting pulmonary stretch receptors. Slowly adapting pulmonary stretch receptors** respond to mechanical stimulation, and they are activated by lung inflation. They also transmit information through myelinated, vagal afferent fibers. The increased lung volume in people with obstructive pulmonary disease stimulates these pulmonary stretch receptors and delays the onset of the next inspiratory effort. This explains the long, slow expiratory effort in these individuals, and it is essential to minimize dynamic, expiratory airway compression. Finally, specialized sensory receptors occur in the lung parenchyma and respond to chemical or mechanical stimulation in the lung interstitium. These receptors are called **juxtaalveolar or J receptors.** They transmit their afferent input through unmyelinated, vagal C fibers. They may be responsible for the sensation of **dyspnea** (abnormal shortness of breath) and the rapid, shallow ventilatory patterns that occur in interstitial lung edema and some inflammatory lung states.

Somatic receptors are also located in the intercostal muscles, rib joints, accessory muscles of respiration, and tendons, and they respond to changes in the length and tension of the respiratory muscles. Although they do not directly control respiration, they do provide information about lung volume and play a role in terminating inspiration. They are especially important in individuals with increased airway resistance and decreased pulmonary compliance because they can augment muscle force within the same breath. Somatic receptors also help minimize the chest wall distortion during inspiration in newborns, who have very compliant rib cages.

EXERCISE

The ability to exercise depends on the capacity of the cardiac and respiratory systems to increase delivery of O_2 to tissues and remove CO_2 from the body. Ventilation increases immediately when exercise begins, and this increase in minute ventilation closely matches the increase in O_2 consumption and CO_2 production that accompanies exercise (Fig. 24-7). Ventilation is linearly related to both CO_2 production and O_2 consumption at low to moderate levels (Fig. 24-7). During maximal exercise, a fit individual can achieve an O_2 consumption of 4 L/min with a minute volume of 120 L/min, which is almost 15 times the resting level.

Exercise is remarkable because of the lack of significant changes in blood gases. Except at maximal exertion, changes in arterial PCO_2 and PO_2 are minimal during exercise. Arterial pH remains within normal values during moderate exercise. During heavy exercise, arterial pH begins to fall as lactic acid is liberated from muscles during anaerobic metabolism. This decrease in arterial pH stimulates ventilation that is out of proportion to the level of exercise. The level of exercise at which sustained metabolic (lactic) acidosis begins is called the **anaerobic threshold** (Fig. 24-7).

ABNORMALITIES IN THE CONTROL OF BREATHING

Changes in the ventilatory pattern can occur for both primary and secondary reasons. During sleep, approximately a third of normal individuals have brief epi-

The clinical history of individuals with **Obstructive Sleep Apnea** (OSA) is very similar among patients. A spouse usually reports that the individual snores. The snoring becomes louder and louder and then stops while the individual continues to make vigorous respiratory efforts (Fig. 24-8). The individual then awakens, falls back to sleep, and continues the same process repetitively throughout the night. Individuals with OSA awaken when the arterial hypoxemia and hypercapnia stimulate both peripheral and central chemoreceptors. Respiration is restored briefly before the next apneic event occurs. Individuals with OSA can have hundreds of these events each night that interrupt sleep.

Complications of OSA include sleep deprivation, polycythemia, right-sided cardiac failure (cor pulmonale), and pulmonary hypertension secondary to the recurrent, hypoxic events. OSA is common in individuals with obesity and in those with excessive compliance of the hypopharynx, upper airway edema, and structural abnormalities of the upper airway.

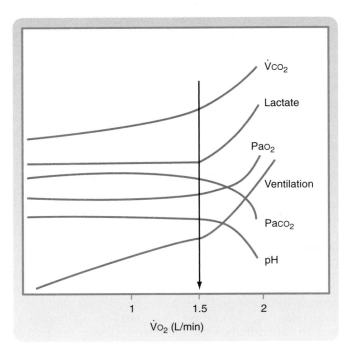

Figure 24-7. Oxygen consumption ($\dot{V}O_2$) as a function of the metabolic changes that occur during exercise. The anaerobic threshold *(arrow)* is the point at which the illustrated variables change and is due to lactic acidosis.

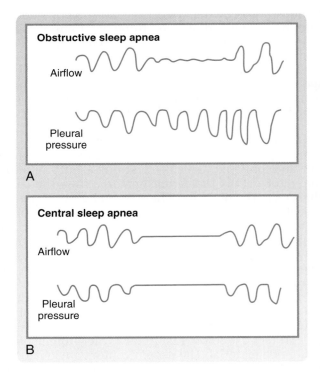

Figure 24-8. The two main types of sleep apnea. **A,** In obstructive sleep apnea, the pleural pressure oscillations increase as CO_2 rises. This indicates that resistance to airflow is very high as a result of upper airway obstruction. **B,** Central sleep apnea is characterized by no attempt to breathe, as demonstrated by no oscillations in pleural pressure.

sodes of apnea or hypoventilation that have no significant effects on arterial PO_2 or PCO_2. The apnea usually lasts less than 10 seconds, and it occurs in the lighter stages of slow-wave and rapid eye movement (REM) sleep. In **sleep apnea** syndromes, the duration of apnea is abnormally prolonged, and it changes arterial PO_2 and PCO_2. There are two major categories of sleep apnea (Fig. 24-8). The first is **obstructive sleep apnea** (OSA). OSA is the most common of the sleep apnea syndromes, and it occurs when the upper airway (generally the hypopharynx) closes during inspiration. Although the process is similar to what happens during snoring, it is more severe, obstructs the airway, and causes cessation of airflow.

The second sleep apnea syndrome is called **central sleep apnea.** This variant of apnea occurs when the ventilatory drive to the respiratory motor neurons decreases. Individuals with central sleep apnea have repeated episodes of apnea every night, during which they make no respiratory effort (Fig. 24-8). The degree of hypercapnia and hypoxemia in individuals with central sleep apnea is less than that in individuals with OSA, but the same complications (polycythemia, etc.) can occur when central sleep apnea is recurrent and severe.

Cheyne-Stokes ventilation is another abnormality of ventilatory control that is characterized by varying tidal volume and ventilatory frequency (Fig. 24-9). After a period of apnea, tidal volume and respiratory frequency increase progressively over several breaths, and then they progressively decrease until apnea occurs. This irregular breathing pattern is seen in some individuals with central nervous system dis-

eases, head trauma, and increased intracranial pressure. It is also present on occasion in normal individuals during sleep at high altitude. The mechanism of Cheyne-Stokes respiration is not known. In some individuals it appears to be due to slow blood flow in the

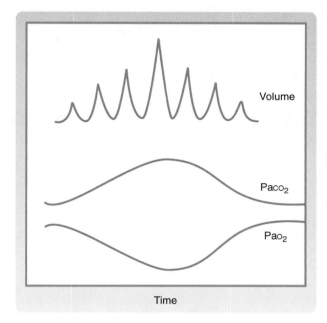

● **Figure 24-9.** In Cheyne-Stokes breathing, tidal volume and consequently arterial blood gases wax and wane. Generally, Cheyne-Stokes breathing is a sign of vasomotor instability, particularly low cardiac output.

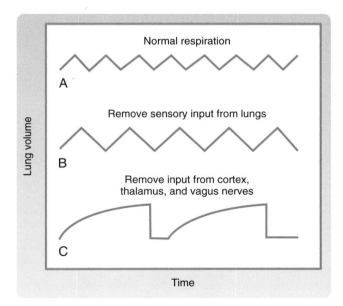

● **Figure 24-10.** Some patterns of breathing. **A,** Normal breathing at about 15 breaths/min. **B,** The effect of removing sensory input from various lung receptors (mainly stretch) is to lengthen each breathing cycle and increase tidal volume so that alveolar ventilation is not significantly affected. **C,** When input from the cerebral cortex and thalamus is also eliminated together with vagal blockade, the result is prolonged inspiratory activity broken after several seconds by brief expirations (apneusis).

> ### ▶ IN THE CLINIC
>
> **Central alveolar hypoventilation** (CAH), also known as Ondine's curse, is a rare disease in which voluntary breathing is intact but abnormalities in automaticity exist. It is the most severe of the central sleep apnea syndromes. As a result, people with CAH can breathe as long as they do not fall asleep. For these individuals, mechanical ventilation or, more recently, bilateral diaphragmatic pacing (similar to a cardiac pacemaker) can be lifesaving.

> ### ▶ IN THE CLINIC
>
> **Sudden infant death syndrome** (SIDS) is the most common cause of death in infants in the first year of life outside the perinatal period. Although the cause of SIDS is not known, abnormalities in ventilatory control, particularly in CO_2 responsiveness, have been implicated. Placing infants on their back to sleep (reducing the potential for CO_2 rebreathing) has dramatically decreased (but not eliminated) the death rate from this syndrome.

brain associated with periods of overshooting and undershooting ventilatory effort in response to changes in P_{CO_2}.

Apneustic breathing is another abnormal breathing pattern that is characterized by sustained periods of inspiration separated by brief periods of exhalation (Fig. 24-10, *C*). The mechanism of this ventilatory pattern appears to be a loss of inspiratory-inhibitory activities resulting in the augmented inspiratory drive. The pattern sometimes occurs in individuals with central nervous system injury.

■ KEY CONCEPTS

1. Ventilatory control is composed of the respiratory control center, central chemoreceptors, peripheral chemoreceptors, and pulmonary mechanoreceptors/sensory nerves. Arterial P_{CO_2} is the major factor that influences ventilation.

2. The respiratory control center is composed of the dorsal respiratory group and the ventral respiratory group. Rhythmic breathing depends on a continuous (tonic) inspiratory drive from the dorsal respiratory group and on intermittent (phasic) expiratory input from the cerebrum, thalamus, cranial nerves, and ascending spinal cord sensory tracts. The peripheral and central chemoreceptors respond to changes in P_{CO_2} and pH. The peripheral chemoreceptors (carotid and aortic bodies) are the only chemoreceptors that respond to changes in P_{O_2}.

3. Acute hypoxia and chronic hypoxia affect breathing differently because the slow adjustments in CSF $[H^+]$ in chronic hypoxia alter sensitivity to CO_2.

4. Irritant receptors protect the lower respiratory tract from particles, chemical vapors, and physical factors, primarily by inducing cough. C fiber J receptors in the terminal respiratory units are stimulated by distortion of the alveolar walls (by lung congestion or edema).

5. The two most important clinical abnormalities of breathing are obstructive and central sleep apnea.

CHAPTER 25

Nonrespiratory Functions of the Lung

Although gas exchange is the primary function of the lung, the lung is also a major defense organ that protects the inside of the body from the outside world, and it is an important organ for metabolism. To cope with the inhalation of ubiquitous foreign substances, the respiratory system and, in particular, the conducting airways have developed unique structural features (e.g., the mucociliary clearance system), as well as specialized adaptive and innate immune response mechanisms. In addition, because the lung receives the total cardiac output, it is uniquely positioned to act as a metabolic regulator of venous blood before its entry into the systemic circulation. This chapter provides insight into mucociliary clearance and the immune defense systems of the lung, as well as describes the metabolic capabilities of the lung.

MUCOCILIARY CLEARANCE SYSTEM

The mucociliary clearance system protects the lower respiratory system by trapping and removing inhaled pathogenic viruses and bacteria, in addition to nontoxic and toxic particulates (e.g., pollen, ash, mineral dust, mold spores, and organic particles), from the lungs. These particulates are inhaled with each breath and must be removed from the lungs. The three major components of the mucociliary clearance system are two fluid layers referred to as the sol **(periciliary fluid)** and gel **(mucus layer)** phases and the **cilia,** which are positioned on the surface of the airway epithelial cells (Fig. 25-1). The cilia are embedded in the periciliary fluid with only the tips of the cilia contacting the mucus. Inhaled material is trapped on the viscoelastic mucus, whereas the watery periciliary fluid allows the cilia to move freely. Effective clearance requires both ciliary activity and the appropriate balance of periciliary fluid and mucus.

PERICILIARY FLUID

The periciliary fluid layer is composed of nonviscous serous fluid, which is produced via active ion transport by the pseudostratified ciliated columnar epithelial cells that line the airways. Several mediators, under basal conditions and in response to inflammation, stimulate Cl⁻ secretion by airway epithelial cells. The balance between Cl⁻ secretion and Na⁺ absorption

determines the volume and ionic composition of the periciliary fluid and maintains the depth of this fluid at about 5 to 6 μm (Fig. 25-1). When net NaCl transport into periciliary fluid is stimulated, diffusive entry of water (i.e., osmosis) into the periciliary fluid is enhanced because of the osmotic gradient that occurs transiently as a result of NaCl transport. Maintaining normal fluid depth and ionic composition in the periciliary fluid is important for rhythmic beating of the cilia and normal mucociliary clearance.

Mucus Layer

The mucus layer lies on top of the periciliary fluid layer and is composed of a complex mixture of macromolecules and electrolytes. Because the mucus layer is in direct contact with air, it entraps inhaled substances. The mucus layer is predominantly water (95% to 97%), 5 to 10 μm thick, and exists as a discontinuous blanket (i.e., islands of mucus). Mucus has low viscosity and high elastic properties and is composed of glycoproteins with groups of oligosaccharides attached to a protein backbone. Healthy individuals produce approximately 100 mL of mucus each day.

Cells That Produce Mucus

Four cell types contribute to the quantity and composition of the mucus layer: **goblet cells, mucous cells,** and **serous cells** within the submucosal tracheobronchial glands, as well as **Clara cells.** Goblet cells, also referred to as surface secretory cells, are present every five to six ciliated cells in the respiratory epithelium. They can be found up to the 5th tracheobronchial division and disappear beyond the 12th division. In many diseases, goblet cells appear further down the tracheobronchial tree, thus making the smaller airways more susceptible to obstruction by mucus plugging.

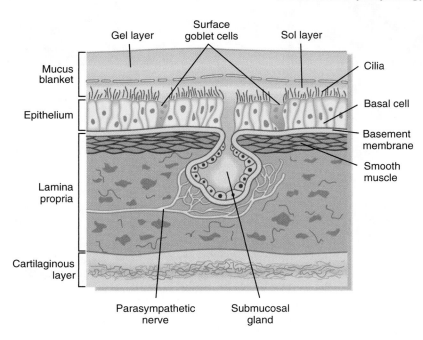

● **Figure 25-1.** Epithelial lining of the tracheobronchial tree. The cilia of the epithelial cell reside in the periciliary fluid layer with the mucus on top. Interspersed between the ciliated epithelial cells are surface secretory (goblet) cells and submucosal glands.

● **Table 25-1.**
Properties of Submucosal Gland Cells

	Serous Cells	Mucous Cells
Granules	Small, electron dense	Large, electron lucent
Glycoproteins	Neutral Lysozyme, lactoferrin	Acidic
Hormones	α- > β-Adrenergic	β- > α-Adrenergic
Receptors	Muscarinic	Muscarinic
Degranulation	α-Adrenergic Cholinergic Substance P	β-Adrenergic Cholinergic

IN THE CLINIC

Sputum is expectorated mucus. However, in addition to mucus, sputum contains serum proteins, lipids, electrolytes, Ca^{++}, DNA from degenerated white cell nuclei (collectively known as bronchial secretions), and extrabronchial secretions, including nasal, oral, lingual, pharyngeal, and salivary secretions. The color of sputum correlates more closely with the amount of time that it has been present in the lower respiratory tract than with the presence of infection.

Goblet cells secrete neutral and acidic glycoproteins rich in sialic acid in response to chemical stimuli. In the presence of infection or cigarette smoke or in patients with chronic bronchitis, goblet cells can increase in size and number, and they secrete copious amounts of mucus. Injury and infection change the properties of the mucus secreted by goblet cells by increasing its viscosity.

Submucosal tracheobronchial glands are present wherever there is cartilage in the upper regions of the conducting airways, and they secrete water, ions, and mucus into the airway lumen through a ciliated duct. The secretory cells of the submucosal gland include mucous cells located near the distal end of the duct and serous cells located at the most distal end of the duct. Although both cell types secrete mucus, their cellular morphology and mucus composition are distinctly different (Table 25-1). Mucous cells secrete acidic glycoproteins, whereas serous cells secrete neutral glycoproteins and bactericidal compounds, including **lysozyme, lactoferrin,** and **antileukoprotease.** Submucosal glands increase in number and size and can extend to the bronchioles in diseases such as

chronic bronchitis (i.e., inflammation of the bronchi). This leads to increased mucus production, alterations in the chemical composition of the mucus (i.e., increased viscosity and decreased elasticity), and the formation of plugs that are manifested clinically as airway obstruction. Mucus secretion from submucosal tracheobronchial glands is under parasympathetic (cholinergic), sympathetic (adrenergic), and peptidergic (vasoactive intestinal polypeptide) neural control. Local inflammatory mediators such as histamine and arachidonic acid metabolites also stimulate mucus production.

Clara cells, located in the epithelium of bronchioles, also contribute to the composition of mucus via secretion of a nonmucinous material containing carbohydrates and proteins. These cells play a role in bronchial regeneration after injury.

Cilia

There are approximately 250 cilia per airway epithelial cell, and each is 2 to 5 μm in length. Cilia are composed of nine microtubular doublets that surround two central microtubules held together by dynein arms, nexin links, and spokes. The central microtubule doublet contains an ATPase that is responsible for the contractile beat of the cilium. Cilia beat with a coordinated oscillation in a characteristic, biphasic, and wavelike rhythm called **metachronism.** They beat at approximately 1000 strokes/min, with a power forward stroke and a slow return or recovery stroke. During their power forward stroke, the tips of the cilia extend upward into the viscous mucus layer and thereby move it and the entrapped particles. On the reverse beat, the cilia release the mucus and withdraw completely into the sol layer. Cilia in the nasopharynx beat in the direction that propels the mucus into the pharynx, whereas cilia in the trachea propel mucus upward toward the pharynx, where it is swallowed.

Particle Deposition and Clearance

Deposition of particles in the lung depends on particle size and density, the distance over which the particle travels, and the relative humidity of the air. In general, particles larger than 10 μm are deposited by **impaction** in the nasal passages and do not penetrate into the lower respiratory tract. Particles 2 to 10 μm in size are deposited in the lower respiratory tract predominantly by inertial impaction at points of turbulent flow (i.e., nasopharynx, trachea, and bronchi) and at airway bifurcations because their inertia (i.e., tendency to move in a straight direction) prevents them from changing directions rapidly. The greater the mass and velocity of a particle, the greater its inertia and likelihood of impacting on a surface directly in front of it. In more distal areas, where airflow is slower, smaller particles (0.2 to 2 μm) are deposited on the surface by **sedimentation** secondary to gravity. Particle size and density, as well as airway diameter, are major factors that influence deposition of particles in the airway via sedimentation. For substances with elongated shapes (i.e., asbestos, silica), another important mechanism of deposition is **interception.** The elongated particle's center of gravity is compatible with the flow of air; however, when the distal tip of the particulate comes in contact with a cell or mucus layer, deposition is facilitated. Particles less than 0.2 μm are deposited by diffusion via brownian motion in the smaller airways and alveoli. The particle's diffusion coefficient is a major influence on the deposition of small particles. Unlike the deposition of larger particles in the upper airways, particle density does not influence diffusion. Diffusion deposition is enhanced with decreased particle size. These small particles come in contact with the alveolar epithelium in the terminal respiratory units where cilia and the mucociliary transport system do not exist. Thus, small particles can be cleared only by lymphatic drainage or phagocytosis by alveolar macrophages. Macrophages migrate through the alveoli and engulf foreign or effete autologous materials in the airway lumen. Clearance of material by alveolar macrophages is usually rapid (<24 hours).

In the conducting airways, the mucociliary clearance system transports deposited particles from the terminal bronchioles to the major airways, where they are coughed up and either expectorated or swallowed. Deposited particles can be removed in a matter of minutes to hours. In the trachea and main bronchi, the rate of particle clearance is 5 to 20 μm/min, but it is slower in the bronchioles (0.5 to 1 μm/min). In general, the longer inhaled material remains in the airways, the greater the probability that the material will cause lung damage because of slow clearance. The region from the terminal bronchioles to the alveoli is devoid of ciliated cells and is considered the "Achilles heel" in what is otherwise a highly effective system. In individuals with the occupational lung disease **pneumoconiosis,** the "black lung" disease of coal miners, the highest concentration of coal dust particles is usually seen just beyond the terminal bronchioles. The relatively slow rate of particle clearance in this area renders the terminal respiratory unit the most common location of airway damage for all types of occupational lung disease.

METABOLIC FUNCTIONS OF THE LUNG

The endothelial cells that line the capillaries of the lungs are exposed to the total cardiac output. Such exposure provides an ideal environment to metabolize substances and modify venous blood before its entry into the systemic circulation. The endothelial cells of the pulmonary capillary bed have developed a variety of metabolic processing mechanisms and cell surface receptors to carry out their unique role in metabolism. Endothelial cells within the pulmonary capillary bed metabolize many substances, including vasoactive amines, cytokines, lipid mediators, and proteins. Metabolism occurs through either intracellular or extracellular processing of substances as they pass through the capillaries or via direct synthesis and secretion by endothelial cells. For example, circulating inactivated **angiotensin I** is activated by extracellular enzymes on the surface of endothelial cells.

Serotonin, a vasoconstrictor, binds to a specific receptor on the surface of the endothelial cell and is internalized and metabolized by intracellular mechanisms. Approximately 80% of the serotonin entering the lung is metabolized in a single pass through the pulmonary capillary bed. Endothelial cells also have surface receptors for **bradykinin, tumor necrosis factor** (TNF), components of complement, immunoglobulin Fc fragments, and adhesion molecules. In addition, endothelial cells synthesize and secrete prostacyclin, endothelin, clotting factors, nitric oxide, prostaglandins, and cytokines. Vascular endothelial cells, however, lack 5-lipoxygenase and are not able to synthesize leukotrienes. Compounds not metabolized by the pulmonary capillary bed include epinephrine, dopamine, histamine, isoproterenol, angiotensin II, and substance P.

IMMUNE DEFENSE SYSTEM

To deal with inhaled viruses, bacteria, and noxious agents, the respiratory system has developed special-

● **Table 25-2.   Innate and Adaptive Immune Cells in the Respiratory System**

Cell Type	Location	Function
TCRγδ lymphocytes	Intraepithelial	Selective antigen recognition Immunoregulation (decreased IgE)
TCRαβ lymphocytes	Lamina propria	Specific adaptive immunity Immunoregulation (T_H1/T_H2 cytokines)
B lymphocytes	Submucosa	IgA antibody synthesis
Dendritic cells	Diffuse in the lung interstitium	Antigen presentation Immunoregulation (tolerance)
Alveolar macrophages	Alveoli and alveolar ducts	Phagocytosis Immunoregulation (cytokines)
NK cells	Diffuse in the lung interstitium	Targeted cytotoxicity Immunoregulation (tolerance)
NK/T cells	Diffuse in the lung interstitium	Immunoregulation (IL-4)

▶ **IN THE CLINIC**

Any process that interferes with normal ciliary beating will interfere with clearance of particles in the lung. Kartagener's syndrome is associated with immotile cilia and comprises the triad of situs inversus with bronchiectasis and sinusitis, which causes a chronic infection.

Patients with asthma have increased mucus production and viscosity. This causes abnormalities in mucociliary clearance in the absence of infection.

▶ **IN THE CLINIC**

An important feature that distinguishes lymph nodes in the systemic immune system from MALT is that true lymph nodes are encapsulated and have an afferent (entering) and efferent (leaving) pattern of lymphatic fluid drainage that is not present in MALT (Fig. 25-2). Once an antigen is processed through a lymph node, it can be assumed that systemic sensitization has or will soon occur. In contrast, although MALT is organized, it is not encapsulated and there is only afferent lymph drainage. It appears that there is direct communication between organs of MALT and that sensitization via one organ is transposed to all MALT tissues via a "lymphatic-like" drainage network. The systemic immune system and MALT may work independently of each other, and sensitization of one may not transpose to the other. This may serve as a defense mechanism in limiting sensitization only to mucosal tissue.

ized defense mechanisms that form the basis of the **mucosal immune system** in the lung. To avoid a continuous inflammatory state, which can cause lung damage, the lung must discriminate between what is harmful and what is not. Although inflammation is a protective response to injury or to an invading pathogen, inflammation usually disrupts the normal physiology. Accordingly, the lung has evolved "first-line" defense mechanisms that are designed to handle the offending agent with minimal or no inflammation. If the first-line defense mechanisms fail, an inflammatory response is initiated. The mucosa of the lung contains specialized adaptive immune cells (e.g., T lymphocytes with limited antigen recognition abilities and plasma cells that synthesize a non–complement-binding antibody, IgA) and innate immune cells (e.g., alveolar macrophages, natural killer [NK] cells, and dendritic cells) (Table 25-2). These cells limit the immunological and inflammatory responses to foreign substances that enter the respiratory system.

Mucosa-Associated Lymphoid Tissue (MALT)

The respiratory, gastrointestinal, and urinary systems are part of the body's **mucosal immune system,** which can function independently of the systemic immune system. In nonmucosal tissues (e.g., spleen, liver, kidney), the adaptive immune response is the body's primary defense. However, the lung and other mucosal tissues are unique in that the adaptive immune response is initiated only after the insulting agent has bypassed the innate immune response.

The lymphatic system and the lymphoid tissue in the lungs filter fluids and particulates through lymph nodes and bronchus-associated lymphoid tissue known as **BALT** (e.g., lymph nodules, lymph aggregates). Solitary lymphocytes and dendritic cells are scattered throughout the respiratory tract in a diffuse submucosal network and play an important role in defense of the lung. Because inhaled particles are broadly dispersed throughout the respiratory tract, each type of lymphoid tissue plays an important and unique role in the overall defense of the lung.

Immunoglobulin A (IgA)

The lung also has several unique defense features that limit airway inflammation. One of the specialized features is a unique antibody system that uses specialized functional features of the IgA antibody. In submucosal areas, **plasma cells** synthesize and secrete IgA, which migrates to the submucosal surface of epithelial cells, where it binds to a surface protein receptor, poly-Ig (Fig. 25-3). The poly-Ig receptor aids in pinocytosis of IgA into the epithelial cell and eventual secretion (exocytosis) of IgA into the airway lumen.

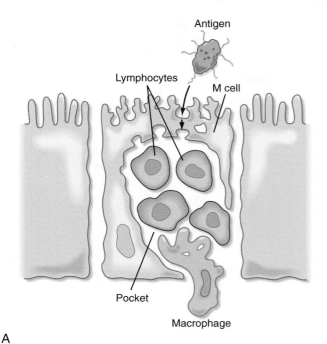

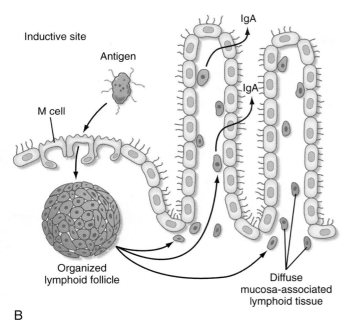

● **Figure 25-2.** Representation of MALT, M cells, and IgA synthesis. **A,** M cells located in mucosal epithelium endocytose antigen in the lumen and transport it for processing to submucosal pockets of immune cells. **B,** Diagram of a mucous membrane showing secretion of IgA antibodies in response to antigen endocytosed by M cells at an inductive site. Activated B cells migrate from the lymphoid follicle to nearby MALT, where they differentiate into IgA-producing plasma cells.

During exocytosis of the IgA complex, the poly-Ig is enzymatically cleaved, and a portion of it, the secretory piece, is still associated with the complex. The secretory piece remains attached to the IgA complex in the airway, and it helps protect the IgA complex

from proteolytic cleavage in the lumen. The IgA-antibody system is very effective in binding particulates and viruses before they invade epithelial cells, and it aids in removal of these substances through the mucociliary clearance system. The IgA-antigen immune complex does not bind complement in the same classic manner as other immune complexes do; this limits its proinflammatory properties.

Adaptive and Innate Immune Cells

The vast majority of T lymphocytes are CD3+ cells with T cell receptors (TCRs) that are composed of α and β chains (TCRαβ cells). Another class of T lymphocytes with a TCR expressing γ and δ chains (TCRγδ cells) has been identified more recently. TCRαβ and TCRγδ cells can secrete similar mediators: interferon-γ (IFN-γ), interleukin-2 (IL-2), IL-4, and IL-5. TCRγδ cells represent a minority of T cells in the peripheral blood and systemic lymphoid tissue; however, they preferentially localize to mucosal sites (i.e., skin, intestine, and lung). TCRγδ cells are the "first line of defense" of epithelial surfaces, and they prevent the development of inflammation mediated by antigen-specific T cells. These cells provide a bridge between adaptive and innate immunity. TCRγδ cells also suppress the IgE response to inhaled antigen.

Natural Killer Cells

Resident populations of functionally active NK cells are present in the lung interstitium. NK cells are a major component of the body's innate immune defense system against invading pathogens such as herpesviruses and various bacterial infections. NK cells are named for their ability to kill target cells without previous sensitization. The mechanism of killing is through the release of granular enzymes, perforins, and serine esterases. These enzymes create holes or pores within

STRUCTURE OF SECRETORY IgA

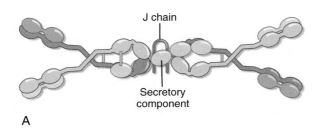

● **Figure 25-3.** Structure and formation of secretory IgA. **A,** Secretory IgA consists of at least two IgA molecules that are covalently linked via a J chain and covalently associated with the secretory component. The secretory component contains five Ig-like domains and is linked to dimeric IgA between its fifth domain and one of the IgA heavy chains. **B,** Secretory IgA is formed during transport through epithelial cells.

FORMATION OF SECRETORY IgA

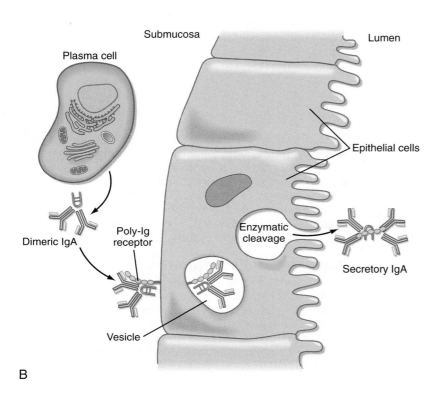

the target cell membranes that lead to cell death. In addition to their cytotoxic activity, they produce cytokines (i.e., IL-4, IL-5, IL-13, IFN-γ, and TNF-α) that are similar to those of lymphocytes. NK cells increase in number and cellular activity in humans with asthma.

Dendritic Cells and Alveolar Macrophages
Dendritic cells and alveolar macrophages are the first nonepithelial cells to respond to a foreign substance. If the foreign material stays within the air space in the lower respiratory system (alveolar ducts and alveoli), it will be phagocytized by alveolar macrophages and removed by the lymphatic system. However, if it penetrates and reaches the interstitial areas, it will come in contact with dendritic cells. Dendritic cells capture, process, and present antigen to T cells, as well as activate or suppress the T cell response.

Alveolar macrophages are found in the alveolus adjacent to the epithelium and, less frequently, in the terminal airways and interstitial space. They migrate freely throughout the alveolar spaces and serve as a first line of defense in the terminal air spaces. They phagocytize foreign particles and substances, as well as surfactant and cellular debris from dead cells. Once a particle is engulfed, the major mechanisms for destruction include the formation of O_2 radicals, enzymatic activity, and halogen derivatives within lysosomes. The phagocytic activity of the alveolar macrophage inhibits the binding of particulates to the

In certain circumstances, such as the inhalation of silica particles, alveolar macrophages phagocytize the particles but are unable to destroy them and the macrophages eventually die. The result is that alveolar macrophages now have localized and concentrated silica particles in the "Achilles heel" region of the lung. The silica particles are not removed from this region by the mucociliary transport system and thus accumulate there and enter the lung interstitium, which leads to a granulomatous-like inflammatory response, fibrosis, and restrictive lung disease. Silica is present in many work environments, including foundries, mining, and photography. There is concern that silicosis may become a leading problem in occupationally related lung disease.

alveolar epithelium and their subsequent penetration into the interstitium. The alveolar macrophage transports engulfed particles to ciliated regions of the mucociliary transport system for elimination. Thus, the alveolar macrophage provides an important link between the alveolar spaces, the "Achilles heel" postterminal bronchiole region, and the mucociliary clearance system. In addition, the alveolar macrophage can suppress T cell activity by direct contact with the T cell or by the secretion of soluble factors such as nitric oxide, prostaglandin E_2, and the immunosuppressive cytokines IL-10 and transforming growth factor β (TGF-β). The ability of the alveolar macrophage to dispose of foreign material rapidly and without mounting an inflammatory response enhances the lung defense system and is a major contributor to the overall defense system.

Toll-like Receptors

Because most inhaled substances are nonpathogenic, the body has developed a recognition system to identify potentially harmful pathogenic substances. The system is based on the recognition of pathogen-associated molecular patterns (PAMPs) on the organism or substance, which are then recognized by a family of receptors on host cells called **Toll-like receptors** (TLRs). Activation of this system initiates inflammatory host defense mechanisms to fight off the pathogen. The TLRs are a family of transmembrane proteins with different specificities for various pathogens. TLR-4 is specific for the gram-negative bacterial product lipopolysaccharide, whereas TLR-2 is specific for lipoproteins associated with gram-positive bacteria. In the lung, bronchial epithelial cells and alveolar type II epithelial cells express TLR-2 and TLR-4. Macrophages and dendritic cells in the lung and other organs also express TLRs. Thus, in addition to classic phagocytic cells, bronchial and alveolar epithelial cells play active roles in host defense via the PAMP-TLR recognition system.

CLINICAL MANIFESTATIONS ASSOCIATED WITH ABNORMALITIES IN INNATE AND ADAPTIVE IMMUNITY

By far the most common pathological conditions associated with mucosal tissue are allergic responses (e.g., allergic asthma, allergic rhinitis, and food and skin allergies). As previously described, the predominant antibody response in MALT is IgA. However, in an allergic response, IgE is the predominant antibody synthesized. Sensitized $CD4^+$ T cells and IL-4 are required for this to occur. IgE binds to the surface of tissue mast cells, and antigen stimulation leads to the degranulation of mast cells (Fig. 25-4). The released granules contain eosinophil chemotactic factors and leukotrienes that induce bronchoconstriction. Symptoms of wheezing, coughing, and shortness of breath occur within minutes as a result of the intense eosinophilia and airway edema. Resolution of the inflammatory response can occur spontaneously or in response to therapy (bronchodilator or antiinflammatory drugs). Low-grade inflammation may persist and result in a process called airway remodeling, manifested by permanent, nonreversible structural changes such as submucosal fibrosis and airway smooth muscle hypertrophy. The mechanisms responsible for airway remodeling in allergic diseases are not clearly understood, but chemokines and cytokines such as TGF-β, a potent profibrotic cytokine, play important roles.

■ KEY CONCEPTS

1. The respiratory system has developed unique structural (mucociliary transport system) and immunological (mucosal immune system) features to cope with the constant environmental exposure to foreign substances in a manner that inhibits or limits an inflammatory response.

2. The three components of the mucociliary transport system are the sol phase (periciliary fluid), the gel phase (mucus), and cilia.

3. The depth of the periciliary fluid layer is maintained by the balance between Cl^- secretion and Na^+ absorption and is essential to normal ciliary beating.

4. Mucus is a complex macromolecule composed of glycoproteins, proteins, electrolytes, and water with low viscous and high elastic mechanical properties.

5. Goblet cells, Clara cells, and the mucous and serous cells residing in the tracheobronchial glands produce mucus.

6. BALT is part of the mucosa-associated lymphoid tissue system and is mainly composed of nonencapsulated aggregates of lymph nodules throughout the conducting airways.

7. Specialized innate immune cells, which play important roles in host defense in the lung, are NK

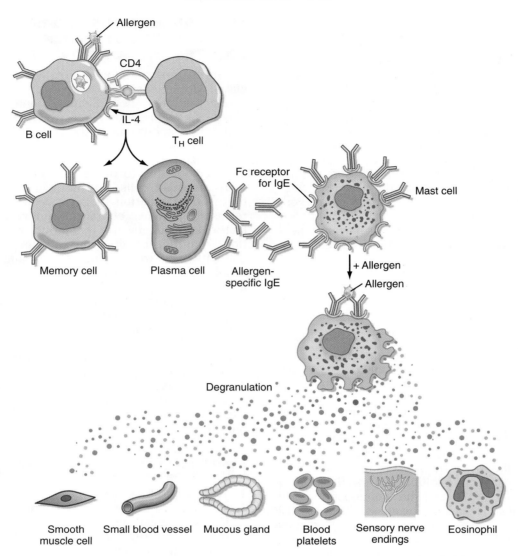

● Figure 25-4 General mechanism underlying an allergic reaction. Exposure to an allergen activates B cells to form IgE-secreting plasma cells. The secreted IgE molecules bind to IgE-specific Fc receptors on mast cells and basophils. After a second exposure to the allergen, the bound IgE is cross-linked, which triggers the release of pharmacologically active mediators from mast cells and basophils. The mediators cause smooth muscle contraction, increased vascular permeability, and vasodilation.

cells, NK/T cells, dendritic cells, and alveolar macrophages.

8. TCRγδ cells and IgA-synthesizing plasma cells are highly specialized adaptive immune cells unique to the lung and other mucosal tissues.

9. The nonciliated lymphoepithelium of BALT establishes a break in the mucociliary blanket that acts as a "drain" to facilitate the collection and immune processing of foreign particles through BALT.

GASTROINTESTINAL PHYSIOLOGY

Kim E. Barrett and Helen E. Raybould

Functional Anatomy and General Principles of Regulation in the Gastrointestinal Tract

The gastrointestinal (GI) tract consists of the alimentary tract from the mouth to the anus and includes the associated glandular organs that empty their contents into the tract. The overall function of the GI tract is to absorb nutrients and water into the circulation and eliminate waste products. The major physiological processes that occur in the GI tract are **motility, secretion, digestion,** and **absorption.** Most of the nutrients in the diet of mammals are taken in as solids and as macromolecules that are not readily transported across cell membranes to enter the circulation. Thus, digestion consists of physical and chemical modification of food such that absorption can occur across intestinal epithelial cells. Digestion and absorption require motility of the muscular wall of the GI tract to move the contents along the tract and to mix the food with secretions. Secretions from the GI tract and associated organs consist of enzymes, biological detergents, and ions that provide an intraluminal environment optimized for digestion and absorption. These physiological processes are highly regulated to maximize digestion and absorption, and the GI tract is endowed with complex regulatory systems to ensure that this occurs. In addition, the GI tract absorbs drugs administered by the oral or rectal routes.

The GI tract also serves as an important organ for the **excretion** of substances. The GI tract stores and excretes waste substances from ingested food materials and excretes products from the liver such as cholesterol, steroids, and drug metabolites (all sharing the common property of being lipid-soluble molecules).

When considering the physiology of the GI tract it is important to remember that it is a long tube that is in contact with the body's external environment. As such, it is vulnerable to infectious microorganisms that can enter along with food and water. To protect itself, the GI tract possesses a complex system of defense consisting of immune cells and other nonspecific defense mechanisms. In fact, the GI tract represents the largest immune organ of the body. This chapter provides an overview of the functional anatomy and general principles of regulation in the GI system.

FUNCTIONAL ANATOMY

The structure of the GI tract varies greatly from region to region, but there are common features in the overall organization of the tissue. Essentially, the GI tract is a **hollow tube** divided into major functional segments; the major structures along the tube are the **mouth** and **pharynx, esophagus, stomach, duodenum, jejunum, ileum, colon, rectum,** and **anus** (Fig. 26-1). Together, the duodenum, jejunum, and ileum make up the small intestine, and the colon is sometimes referred to as the large intestine. Associated with the tube are blind-ending glandular structures that are invaginations of the lining of the tube; these glands empty their secretions into the gut lumen (e.g., Brunner's glands in the duodenum, which secrete copious amounts of HCO_3^-). Additionally, there are glandular organs attached to the tube via ducts through which secretions empty into the gut lumen, for example, the salivary glands and the pancreas.

The major structures along the GI tract have many functions. One important function is storage; the stomach and colon are important storage organs for processed food (sometimes referred to as chyme) and exhibit specialization in terms of both their functional anatomy (e.g., their shape and size) and control mechanisms (characteristics of smooth muscle to produce tonic contractions) that enable them to perform this function efficiently. The predominant function of the small intestine is digestion and absorption; the major specialization of this region of the GI tract is a large surface area over which absorption can occur. The colon reabsorbs water and ions to ensure that they do not get eliminated from the body. Ingested food is moved along the GI tract by the action of muscle in its walls; separating the regions of the GI tract are also specialized muscle structures called **sphincters.** These function to isolate one region from the next and provide selective retention of contents or prevent backflow, or both.

The blood supply to the intestine is important for carrying absorbed nutrients to the rest of the body. Unlike other organ systems of the body, venous drainage from the GI tract does not return directly to the heart but first enters the **portal circulation** leading to the liver. Thus, the liver is unusual in receiving a considerable part of its blood supply from other than the arterial circulation. GI blood flow is also notable for its dynamic regulation; splanchnic blood flow receives about 25% of cardiac output, an amount disproportionate to the mass of the GI tract that it supplies. After a meal, blood can also be diverted from muscle to the GI tract to subserve the metabolic needs of the gut wall and also to remove absorbed nutrients.

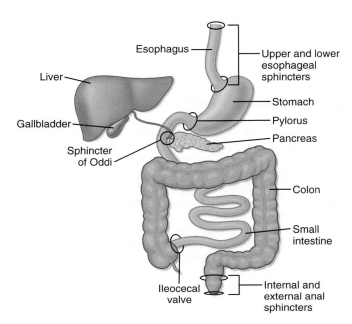

● **Figure 26-1.** General anatomy of the GI system and its division into functional segments.

The **lymphatic drainage** of the GI tract is important for the transport of lipid-soluble substances that are absorbed across the GI tract wall. As we will see later, lipids and other lipid-soluble molecules (including some vitamins and drugs) are packaged into particles that are too large to pass into the capillaries and instead pass into lymph vessels in the intestinal wall. These lymph vessels drain into larger lymph ducts, which finally drain into the thoracic duct and thus into the systemic circulation on the arterial side. This has major physiological implications in lipid metabolism and also in the ability of drugs to be delivered straight into the systemic circulation.

Cellular Specialization

The wall of the tubular gut is made up of layers consisting of specialized cells (Fig. 26-2).

Mucosa

The **mucosa** is the innermost layer of the GI tract. It consists of the **epithelium,** the **lamina propria,** and the **muscularis mucosae.** The epithelium is a single layer of specialized cells that line the lumen of the GI tract. It forms a continuous layer along the tube and with the glands and organs that drain into the lumen of the tube. Within this cell layer are a number of specialized epithelial cells; the most abundant are cells termed absorptive **enterocytes,** which express many proteins important for the digestion and absorption of macronutrients. **Enteroendocrine cells** contain secretory granules that release regulatory peptides and amines to help regulate GI function. In addition, cells in the gastric mucosa are specialized for the production of protons, and mucin-producing cells throughout the GI tract produce a glycoprotein, mucin, that helps protect the GI tract and lubricate the luminal contents.

● **Figure 26-2.** General organization of the layers composing the wall of the GI tract.

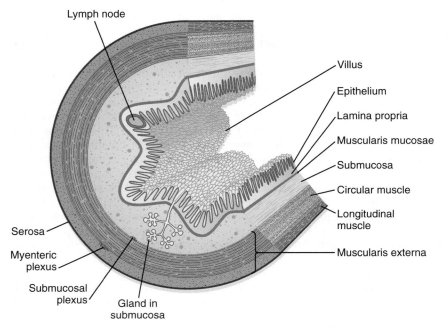

The columnar epithelial cells are linked together by intercellular connections called **tight junctions.** These junctions are complexes of intracellular and transmembrane proteins, and the tightness of these junctions is regulated throughout the postprandial period. The nature of the epithelium varies greatly from one part of the digestive tract to another, depending on the predominant function of that region. For example, the intestinal epithelium is designed for absorption; these cells mediate selective uptake of nutrients, ions, and water. In contrast, the esophagus has a squamous epithelium that has no absorptive role. It is a conduit for the transportation of swallowed food and thus needs some protection from rough food such as fiber, which is provided by the squamous epithelium.

The surface area of the epithelium is arranged into **villi** and **crypts** (Fig. 26-3). Villi are finger-like projections that serve to increase the surface area of the mucosa. Crypts are invaginations or folds in the epithelium. The epithelium lining the GI tract is continuously renewed and replaced by dividing cells; in humans, this process takes about 3 days. These proliferating cells are localized to the crypts, where there is a proliferative zone of intestinal **stem cells.**

The lamina propria immediately below the epithelium consists largely of loose connective tissue that contains collagen and elastin fibrils. The lamina propria is rich in several types of glands and contains lymph vessels and nodules, capillaries, and nerve fibers. The muscularis mucosae is the thin, innermost layer of intestinal smooth muscle. When seen through an endoscope, the mucosa has folds and ridges that are caused by contractions of the muscularis mucosae.

SMALL INTESTINE

Lumen

Villus

Crypt

COLON

Lumen

Surface

Crypt

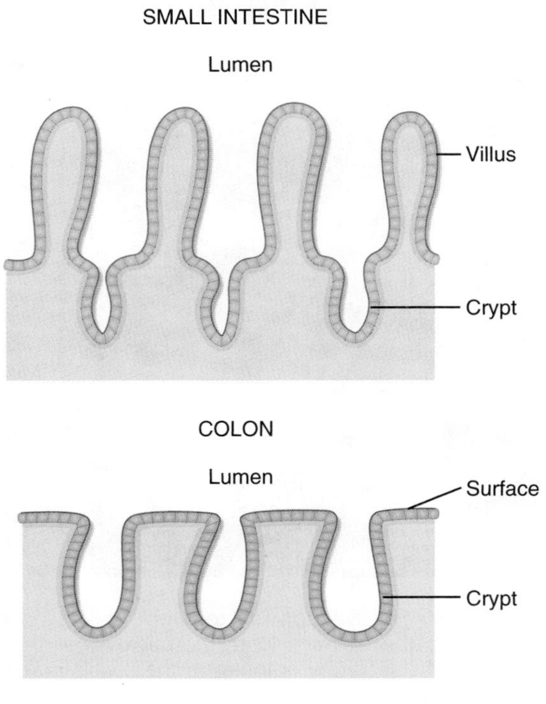

● **Figure 26-3.** Comparison of the morphology of the epithelium of the small intestine and colon.

Submucosa

The next layer is the **submucosa.** The submucosa consists largely of loose connective tissue with collagen and elastin fibrils. In some regions of the GI tract, **glands** (invaginations or folds of the mucosa) are present in the submucosa. The larger nerve trunks, blood vessels, and lymph vessels of the intestinal wall lie in the submucosa, together with one of the plexuses of the enteric nervous system (ENS), the **submucosal plexus.**

Muscle Layers

The **muscularis externa** or **muscularis propria** typically consists of two substantial layers of smooth muscle cells: an inner circular layer and an outer longitudinal layer. Muscle fibers in the **circular muscle layer** are oriented circumferentially, whereas muscle fibers in the **longitudinal muscle layer** are oriented along the longitudinal axis of the tube. In humans and most mammals, the circular muscle layer of the small intestine is subdivided into an inner dense circular layer, which consists of smaller, more closely packed cells, and an outer circular layer. Between the circular and longitudinal layers of muscle lies the other plexus of the ENS, the **myenteric plexus.** Contractions of the muscularis externa mix and circulate the contents of the lumen and propel them along the GI tract.

The wall of the GI tract contains many interconnected neurons. The submucosa contains a dense network of nerve cells called the submucosal plexus (sometimes referred to as **Meissner's plexus**). The prominent myenteric plexus **(Auerbach's plexus)** is located between the circular and longitudinal smooth muscle layers. These intramural plexuses constitute the ENS. The ENS helps integrate the motor and secretory activities of the GI system. If the sympathetic and parasympathetic nerves to the gut are cut, many motor and secretory activities continue because these processes are directly controlled by the ENS.

Serosa

The **serosa,** or **adventitia,** is the outermost layer of the GI tract and consists of a layer of squamous mesothelial cells. It is part of the **mesentery** that lines the surface of the abdominal wall and suspends the organs within the abdominal cavity. The mesenteric membranes secrete a thin, viscous fluid that helps lubricate the abdominal organs so that movement of the organs can occur as the muscle layers contract and relax.

REGULATORY MECHANISMS IN THE GASTROINTESTINAL TRACT

Before we examine the physiology of the GI tract in detail, we will look at the control mechanisms by which function is regulated. Unlike the cardiovascular or respiratory systems, the GI tract undergoes periods of relative quiescence (intermeal period) and periods of intense activity after the intake of food (postprandial period). Consequently, the GI tract has to detect and respond appropriately to the intake of food. In addition, the macronutrient content of a meal can vary considerably, and there have to be mechanisms that can detect this and mount appropriate physiological responses. Thus, the GI tract has to communicate with associated organs such as the pancreas. Finally, because the GI tract is essentially a long tube, there have to be mechanisms by which events occurring in the proximal portion of the GI tract are signaled to the more distal parts, and vice versa.

There are three principal control mechanisms involved in the regulation of GI function: **endocrine, paracrine,** and **neural** (Fig. 26-4).

Endocrine Regulation

Endocrine regulation describes the process whereby the sensing cell in the GI tract, an **enteroendocrine cell (EEC),** responds to a stimulus by secreting a regulatory peptide or hormone that travels via the bloodstream to target cells removed from the point of secretion. Cells responding to a GI hormone express specific receptors for the hormone. Hormones released from the GI tract have effects on cells located in other regions of the GI tract and also on glandular structures associated with the GI tract, such as the pancreas. In addition, GI hormones have effects on other tissues that have no direct role in digestion and absorption, including endocrine cells in liver and brain.

EECs are packed with secretory granules, the products of which are secreted from the cell in response to chemical and mechanical stimuli to the wall of the GI tract (Fig. 26-5). In addition, EECs can be stimulated by neural input or other factors not associated with a meal. The most common EECs in the gut wall are referred to as the "open" type; these cells have an apical membrane that is in contact with the lumen of the GI tract (generally regarded as the location where

THREE MECHANISMS OF COMMUNICATION MEDIATE RESPONSES IN THE GI TRACT

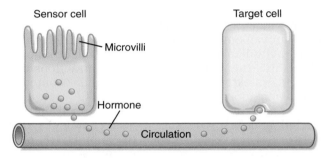

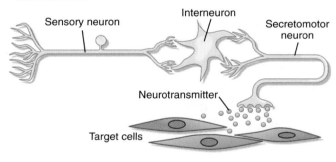

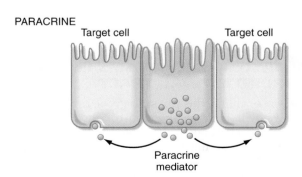

● **Figure 26-4.** The three mechanisms by which function in the GI tract is regulated in the integrated response to a meal.

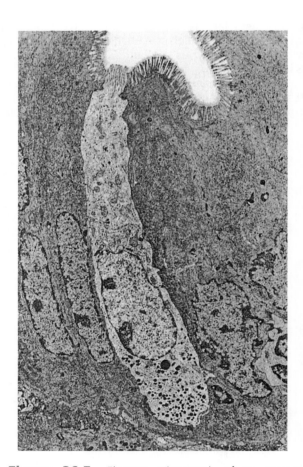

● **Figure 26-5.** Electron micrograph of an open-type endocrine cell in the GI tract. Note the microvilli at the apical projection and the secretory granules in the basolateral portion of the cell. (From Barrett K: Gastrointestinal Physiology [Lange Physiology Series]. New York, McGraw-Hill, 2005.) (Courtesy of Leonard R. Johnson, Ph.D.)

sensing occurs) and a basolateral membrane through which secretion occurs. There are also "closed"-type EECs that do not have part of their membrane in contact with the luminal surface of the gut; an example is the **enterochromaffin-like** (ECL) cell in the gastric epithelium, which secretes histamine.

There are many examples of hormones secreted by the GI tract (Table 26-1); it is worth remembering that the first hormone ever identified was the GI hormone **secretin.** One of the most well characterized GI hormones is **gastrin,** which is released from endocrine cells located in the wall of the distal part of the stomach. Release of gastrin is stimulated by activation of parasympathetic outflow to the GI tract, and gastrin potently stimulates gastric acid secretion in the postprandial period.

Paracrine Regulation

Paracrine regulation describes the process whereby a chemical messenger or regulatory peptide is released from a sensing cell, often an EEC, in the intestinal wall that acts on a nearby target cell by diffusion through the interstitial space. Paracrine agents exert their actions on several different cell types in the wall of the GI tract, including smooth muscle cells, absorptive enterocytes, secretory cells in glands, and even on other EECs. There are several important paracrine agents and they are listed in Table 26-1, along with their site of production, site of action, and function. An important paracrine mediator in the gut wall is histamine. In the stomach, histamine is stored and released by ECL cells located in the gastric glands. Histamine diffuses through the interstitial space in the lamina propria to neighboring parietal cells and stimulates the production of acid. **Serotonin** (5-hydroxytryptamine [5-HT]), released from enteric neurons, mucosal mast cells, and specialized EECs called **enterochromaffin cells,** regulates smooth muscle function and water absorption across the intestinal wall. There are other paracrine mediators in the gut wall, including prostaglandins, adenosine, and nitric oxide (NO); the functions of these mediators are not well described, but they are capable of producing changes in GI function.

Many substances can be both paracrine and endocrine regulators of GI function. For example, **cholecystokinin,** which is released from the duodenum in response to dietary protein and lipid, acts locally on nerve terminals in a paracrine fashion and also affects the pancreas. This will be discussed in more detail in Chapter 29.

Neural Regulation of Gastrointestinal Function

Nerves and neurotransmitters play an important role in regulating the function of the GI tract. In its simplest form, neural regulation occurs when a neurotransmitter is released from a nerve terminal located in the GI tract and the neurotransmitter has an effect on the cell that is innervated. However, in some cases there are no synapses between motor nerves and effector cells in the GI tract. Neural regulation of GI function is very important within an organ, as well as between distant parts of the GI tract.

● AT THE CELLULAR LEVEL

Posttranslational modification of peptide hormones confers receptor selectivity.

There are multiple receptor subtypes for the regulatory peptide hormones released from endocrine cells in the wall of the gut. Their selectivity of action is determined by posttranslational modification of peptide hormones, which then confers receptor selectivity. An example of this is peptide YY (PYY). There are multiple receptor subtypes for PYY, classified as Y1 to Y7. However, not all of them are localized to the gut; Y2 and Y5 are expressed in the GI tract. PYY is released from endocrine cells in the wall of the gut, mainly in response to fatty acids. It is released as a 36–amino acid peptide; however, it can be cleaved to PYY3-36 by the enzyme dipeptidyl peptidase IV, a membrane peptidase. This form of the peptide is selective for the Y2 receptor. Thus, the presence of the enzyme that cleaves the peptide can alter the biological response to PYY secretion.

● Table 26-1. **Hormonal and Paracrine Mediators in the GI Tract**

GI Hormone	Source	Stimulus for Release	Pathway of Action	Targets	Effect
Gastrin	Gastric antrum (G cells)	Oligopeptides	Endocrine	ECL cells and parietal cells of the gastric corpus	Stimulation of parietal cells to secrete H^+ and ECL cells to secrete histamine
Cholecystokinin	Duodenum (I cells)	Fatty acids, hydrolyzed protein	Paracrine, endocrine	Vagal afferent terminals, pancreatic acinar cells	Inhibition of gastric emptying and H^+ secretion; stimulation of pancreatic enzyme secretion, gallbladder contraction, inhibition of food intake
Secretin	Duodenum (S cells)	Protons	Paracrine, endocrine	Vagal afferent terminals, pancreatic duct cell	Stimulation of pancreatic duct secretion (H_2O and HCO_3^-)
Gluco-insulinotropic peptide (GIP)	Intestine (K cells)	Fatty acids, glucose	Endocrine	Beta cells of the pancreas	Stimulation of insulin secretion
Peptide YY (PYY)	Intestine (L cells)	Fatty acids, glucose, hydrolyzed protein	Endocrine, paracrine	Neurons, smooth muscle	Inhibition of gastric emptying, pancreatic secretion, gastric acid secretion, intestinal motility, food intake
Proglucagon-derived peptides 1/2 (GLP-1/2)	Intestine (L cells)	Fatty acids, glucose, hydrolyzed protein	Endocrine, paracrine	Neurons, epithelial cells	Glucose homeostasis, epithelial cell proliferation

GUT STIMULI EVOKE DIGESTIVE RESPONSES VIA THE
ENTERIC AND THE CENTRAL NERVOUS SYSTEMS

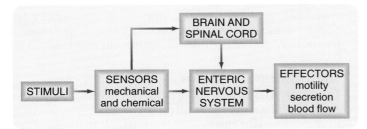

● **Figure 26-6.** Hierarchical neural control of GI function. Stimuli to the GI tract from the meal (e.g., chemical, mechanical, osmotic) will activate both the intrinsic and extrinsic sensory (afferent) pathways, which in turn will activate the extrinsic and intrinsic neural reflex pathways.

IN THE CLINIC

Glucagon-like peptide 1 (GLP-1) is a regulatory peptide released from EECs cells in the gut wall in response to the presence of luminal carbohydrate and lipids. GLP-1 arises from differential processing of the glucagon gene, the same gene that is expressed in the pancreas and that gives rise to glucagon. GLP-1 is involved in regulation of the blood glucose level via stimulation of insulin secretion and also insulin biosynthesis. Agonists of the GLP-1 receptor improve insulin sensitivity in diabetic animal models and human subjects. Administration of GLP-1 also reduces appetite and food intake and delays gastric emptying, responses that may contribute to improving glucose tolerance. Long-acting agonists for the GLP-1 receptor, such as exanatide, have been approved for the treatment of type 2 diabetes.

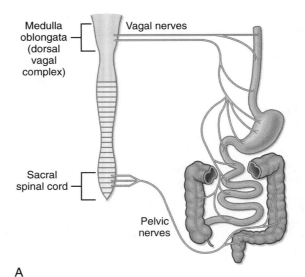

A

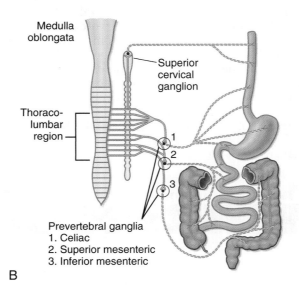

B

● **Figure 26-7.** The extrinsic innervation of the GI tract consisting of the parasympathetic **(A)** and sympathetic **(B)** subdivisions of the autonomic nervous system.

Neural regulation of the GI tract is surprisingly complex. The gut is innervated by two sets of nerves, the extrinsic and intrinsic nervous systems. The **extrinsic nervous system** is defined as nerves that innervate the gut, with cell bodies located outside the gut wall; these extrinsic nerves are part of the autonomic nervous system (ANS). The **intrinsic nervous system,** also referred to as the **enteric nervous system,** has cell bodies that are contained within the wall of the gut (submucosal and myenteric plexuses). Some GI functions are highly dependent on the extrinsic nervous system, yet others can take place independently of the extrinsic nervous system and are mediated entirely by the ENS. However, extrinsic nerves can often modulate intrinsic nervous system function (Fig. 26-6).

Extrinsic Nervous System

Extrinsic neural innervation to the gut is via the two major subdivisions of the ANS, namely, parasympathetic and sympathetic innervation (Fig. 26-7). **Parasympathetic innervation** to the gut is via the vagus and pelvic nerves. The **vagus** nerve, the 10th cranial nerve, innervates the esophagus, stomach, gallbladder, pancreas, first part of the intestine, cecum, and the proximal part of the colon. The **pelvic** nerves innervate the distal part of the colon and the anorectal region, in addition to the other pelvic organs that are not part of the GI tract.

Consistent with the typical organization of the parasympathetic nervous system, the **preganglionic** nerve cell bodies lie in the brainstem (vagus) or the sacral spinal cord (pelvic). Axons from these neurons run in the nerves to the gut (vagus and pelvic nerves, respectively), where they synapse with **postganglionic** neurons in the wall of the organ, which in this case are enteric neurons in the gut wall. There is no direct innervation of these efferent nerves to effector cells within the wall of the gut; the transmission pathway is always via a neuron in the ENS.

Consistent with transmission in the ANS, the synapse between preganglionic and postganglionic neurons is an obligatory nicotinic synapse. That is, the synapse between preganglionic and postganglionic neurons is mediated via acetylcholine released from the nerve terminal and acting at nicotinic receptors localized on the postganglionic neuron, which in this case is an intrinsic neuron.

Sympathetic innervation is supplied by cell bodies in the spinal cord and fibers that terminate in the **prevertebral ganglia** (celiac, superior, and inferior mesenteric ganglia); these are the preganglionic neurons. These nerve fibers synapse with postganglionic neurons in the ganglia, and the fibers leave the ganglia and reach the end organ along the major blood vessels and their branches. Rarely, there is a synapse in the **paravertebral** (chain) ganglia, as seen with sympathetic innervation of other organ systems. Some vasoconstrictor sympathetic fibers directly innervate blood vessels of the GI tract, and other sympathetic fibers innervate glandular structures in the wall of the gut.

The ANS, both parasympathetic and sympathetic, also carries the fibers of **afferent** (toward the central nervous system [CNS]) neurons; these are **sensory** in nature. The cell bodies for the **vagal afferents** are in the nodose ganglion. These neurons have a central projection terminating in the **nucleus of the tractus solitarius** in the brainstem and the other terminal in the gut wall. The cell bodies of the **spinal afferent** neurons that run with the sympathetic pathway are segmentally organized and are found in the dorsal root ganglia. Peripheral terminals of the spinal and vagal afferents are located in all layers of the gut wall, where they detect information about the state of the gut. Afferent neurons send this information to the CNS. Information sent to the CNS relays the nature of the luminal contents, such as acidity, nutrient content, and osmolality of the luminal contents, as well as the degree of stretch or contraction in smooth muscle. Afferent innervation is also responsible for transmitting painful stimuli to the CNS.

The components of a **reflex** pathway—afferents, interneurons, and efferent neurons—exist within the extrinsic innervation to the GI tract. These reflexes can be mediated entirely via the vagus nerve (termed a **vagovagal reflex**), which has both afferent and efferent fibers. The vagal afferents send sensory information to the CNS, where they synapse with an interneuron, which then drives activity in the efferent motor neuron. These extrinsic reflexes are very important in the regulation of GI function after the ingestion of a meal. An example of an important vagovagal reflex is the gastric receptive relaxation reflex, in which distention of the stomach results in relaxation of the smooth muscle in the stomach; this allows filling of the stomach to occur without an increase in intraluminal pressure.

In general, as with other visceral organ systems, the parasympathetic and sympathetic nervous systems tend to work in opposition. However, this is not as simple as in the cardiovascular system, for example. Activation of the parasympathetic nervous system is important in the integrative response to a meal, and we will look at many examples of this in the following chapters. The parasympathetic nervous system generally results in the activation of physiological processes in the gut wall, although there are notable exceptions. In contrast, the sympathetic nervous system tends to be inhibitory to GI function and is more frequently activated in pathophysiological circumstances. Overall, sympathetic activation inhibits smooth muscle function; the exception to this is the sympathetic innervation of GI sphincters, in which sympathetic activation tends to induce contraction of smooth muscle. Moreover, the sympathetic nervous system is notably important in regulation of blood flow in the GI tract.

Intrinsic Neural Innervation

The ENS is made up of two major plexuses, which are collections of nerve cell bodies (ganglia) and their fibers, all originating in the wall of the gut (Fig. 26-8). The **myenteric plexus** lies between the longitudinal and circular muscle layers and the **submucosal plexus** lies in the submucosa. Neurons in the two plexuses are linked by interganglionic strands.

Neurons in the ENS are characterized functionally as afferent neurons, interneurons, or efferent neurons, similar to neurons in the extrinsic part of the ANS. Thus, all components of a reflex pathway can be contained within the ENS. Stimuli in the wall of the gut are detected by afferent neurons, which activate interneurons and then efferent neurons to alter function. In this way the ENS can act autonomously from extrinsic innervation. However, neurons in the ENS, as we have already seen, are innervated by extrinsic neurons, and thus the function of these reflex pathways can be modulated by the extrinsic nervous system. Because the ENS is capable of performing its own integrative functions and complex reflex pathways, it is sometimes referred to as the "little brain in the gut" as a result of its importance and complexity. It is estimated that there are as many neurons in the ENS as in the spinal cord. In addition, many GI hormones also act as neurotransmitters in the ENS and in the brain in regions involved in autonomic outflow. These mediators and regulatory peptides are thus referred to as **"brain-gut peptides,"** and the extrinsic and intrinsic components innervating the gut are sometimes referred to as the **"brain-gut axis."**

RESPONSE OF THE GI TRACT TO A MEAL

This introductory chapter provides a broad overview of the anatomy and regulatory mechanisms in the GI tract. In the following chapters there will be discussion

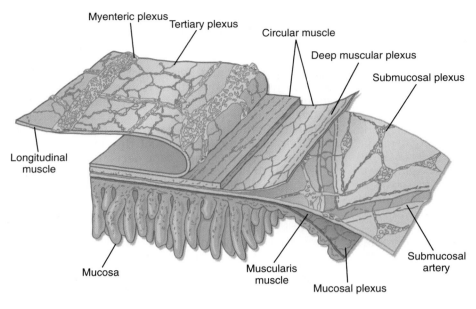

Myenteric plexus
Tertiary plexus
Circular muscle
Deep muscular plexus
Submucosal plexus
Longitudinal muscle
Mucosa
Muscularis muscle
Mucosal plexus
Submucosal artery

● **Figure 26-8.** The enteric nervous system in the wall of the GI tract.

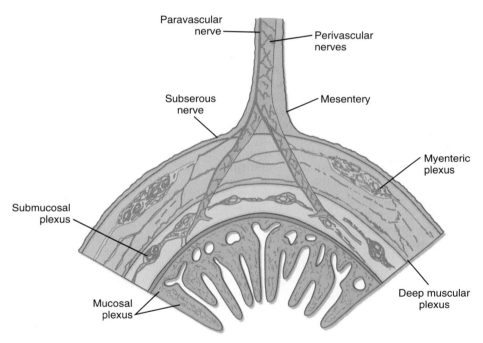

Paravascular nerve
Perivascular nerves
Subserous nerve
Mesentery
Myenteric plexus
Submucosal plexus
Mucosal plexus
Deep muscular plexus

▶ IN THE CLINIC

Hirschsprung's disease is a congenital disorder of the enteric nervous system characterized by failure to pass meconium at birth or severe chronic constipation in infancy. The typical features are absence of myenteric and submucosal neurons in the distal part of the colon and rectum. It is a polygenic disorder with characteristic mutations in at least three different classes of genes involved in neuronal development and differentiation.

of the **integrated response to a meal** in order to provide the details of GI physiology. The response to a meal is classically divided into phases: cephalic, oral, esophageal, gastric, duodenal, and intestinal. In each phase the meal presents certain **stimuli** (e.g., chemical, mechanical, and osmotic) that activate different **pathways** (neural, paracrine, and humoral reflexes) that result in changes in **effector function** (secretion and motility). There is considerable crosstalk between the regulatory mechanisms that have been outlined, and this will be discussed in the next chapters. As with maintenance of homeostasis in other systems of the body, control of GI function requires complex regulatory mechanisms to sense and act in a dynamic fashion.

■ KEY CONCEPTS

1. The GI tract is a tube subdivided into regions that subserve different functions associated with digestion and absorption.

2. The lining of the GI tract is subdivided into layers—the mucosal, submucosal, and muscle layers.

3. There are three major control mechanisms: hormonal, paracrine, and neural.

4. The innervation of the GI tract is particularly interesting because it consists of two interacting components, extrinsic and intrinsic.

5. Extrinsic innervation (cell bodies outside the wall of the GI tract) consists of the two subdivisions of the ANS: parasympathetic and sympathetic. Both have an important sensory (afferent) component.

6. The intrinsic or enteric nervous system (cell bodies in the wall of the GI tract) can act independently of extrinsic neural innervation.

7. When a meal is in different regions of the tract, sensory mechanisms detect the presence of the nutrients and mount appropriate physiological responses in that region of the tract, as well as in more distal regions. These responses are mediated by endocrine, paracrine, and neural pathways.

CHAPTER 27

The Cephalic, Oral, and Esophageal Phases of the Integrated Response to a Meal

In this chapter we will look at the processes that occur in the gastrointestinal (GI) tract in the early stages of the integrated response to a meal. Even before food is ingested there are changes in the physiology of the GI tract, and in this so-called cephalic phase, as well as in the oral phase (when ingested food is in the mouth), the responses of the GI tract to the presence of food are mainly associated with preparing the GI tract for digestion and absorption. We will also look at the transfer of food from the mouth to the esophagus, the esophageal phase of the meal.

CEPHALIC AND ORAL PHASES

The main feature of the **cephalic phase** is activation of the GI tract in readiness for the meal. The stimuli involved are cognitive and include anticipation or thinking about the consumption of food, olfactory input, visual input (seeing or smelling appetizing food when hungry), and auditory input. The latter may be an unexpected link but was clearly demonstrated in the classic conditioning experiments of Pavlov, in which he paired an auditory stimulus to the presentation of food to dogs; eventually, the auditory stimulus alone could stimulate secretion. A real-life analogy is presumably being told that dinner is ready. All these stimuli result in an increase in excitatory parasympathetic neural outflow to the gut. Sensory input, such as smell, stimulates sensory nerves that activate parasympathetic outflow from the brainstem. Higher brain sites are also involved (such as the limbic system, hypothalamus, and cortex) in the cognitive components of this response. The response can be both positive and negative; thus, anticipation of food and a person's psychological status, such as anxiety, can alter the cognitive response to a meal. However, the final common pathway is activation of the dorsal motor nucleus in the brainstem, the region where the cell bodies of the vagal preganglionic neurons arise; activation of the nucleus leads to increased activity in efferent fibers passing to the GI tract in the vagus nerve. In turn, the efferent fibers activate the postganglionic motor neurons (referred to as motor because their activation results in change of function of an effector cell). Increased parasympathetic outflow enhances salivary secretion, gastric acid secretion, pancreatic enzyme secretion, gallbladder contraction, and relaxation of the sphincter of Oddi (the sphincter between the common bile duct and the duodenum). All these responses enhance the ability of the GI tract to receive and digest the incoming food. The salivary response is mediated via the ninth cranial nerve; the remaining responses are mediated via the vagus nerve.

Many of the features of the **oral phase** are indistinguishable from the cephalic phase. The only difference is that food is in contact with the surface of the GI tract. Thus, there are additional stimuli generated from the mouth, both mechanical and chemical **(taste).** However, many of the responses that are initiated by the presence of food in the oral cavity are identical to those initiated in the cephalic phase because the efferent pathway is the same. Here we will discuss the responses specifically initiated in the mouth, which consist mainly of the stimulation of salivary secretion.

The mouth is important for the mechanical disruption of food and for the initiation of digestion. Chewing subdivides and mixes the food with the enzymes salivary amylase and lingual lipase and with the glycoprotein mucin, which lubricates the food for chewing and swallowing. Minimal absorption occurs in the mouth, although alcohol and some drugs are absorbed from the oral cavity and this can be clinically important. However, as with the cephalic phase, it is important to realize that stimulation of the oral cavity initiates responses in the more distal GI tract, including increased gastric acid secretion, increased pancreatic enzyme secretion, gallbladder contraction, and relaxation of the sphincter of Oddi, mediated via the efferent vagal pathway.

Properties of Secretion
General Considerations

Secretions in the GI tract come from glands associated with the tract (the salivary glands, pancreas, and liver), from glands formed by the gut wall itself (e.g., Brunner's glands in the duodenum), and from the intestinal mucosa itself. The exact nature of the secretory products can vary tremendously, depending on the function of that region of the GI tract. However, these secretions have several characteristics in common. Secretions from the GI tract and associated glands include **water, electrolytes, protein,** and **humoral agents.** Water is essential for generating an aqueous environment for the efficient action of enzymes. Secretion of electrolytes is important for the generation of osmotic gradients to drive the movement of water. Digestive enzymes in secreted fluid catalyze the breakdown of macronutrients in ingested food. Moreover, many additional proteins secreted along the GI tract have specialized functions, some of which are fairly well understood, such as those of mucin and immunoglobulins, and others that are only just beginning to be understood, such as those of trefoil peptides.

Secretion is initiated by multiple signals associated with the meal, including chemical, osmotic, and mechanical components. Secretion is elicited by the action of specific effector substances, called **secretagogues,** acting on secretory cells. Secretagogues work in one of the three ways that have already been described in the previous chapter—endocrine, paracrine, and neurocrine.

Constituents of Secretions

Inorganic secretory components are region or gland specific, depending on the particular conditions required in that part of the GI tract. The inorganic components are electrolytes, including H^+ and HCO_3^-. Two examples of different secretions include acid (HCl) in the stomach, which is important to activate pepsin and to start protein digestion, and HCO_3^- in the duodenum, which neutralizes gastric acid and provides optimal conditions for the action of digestive enzymes in the small intestine.

Organic secretory components are also gland or organ specific and depend on the function of that region of the gut. The organic constituents are enzymes (for digestion), mucin (for lubrication and mucosal protection), and other factors such as growth factors, immunoglobulins, and absorptive factors.

Salivary Secretion

During the cephalic and the oral phase of the meal, considerable stimulation of salivary secretion takes place. Saliva has a variety of functions, including those important for the integrative responses to a meal and for other physiological processes (Table 27-1). The main functions of saliva in digestion include lubrication and moistening of food for swallowing, solubilization of material for taste, initiation of carbohydrate digestion, and clearance and neutralization of refluxed gastric secretions in the esophagus. Saliva also has antibacterial actions that are important for overall health of the oral cavity and teeth.

Functional Anatomy of the Salivary Glands

There are three pairs of major salivary glands: parotid, submandibular, and sublingual. In addition, many smaller glands are found on the tongue, lips, and palate. These glands are the typical **tubuloalveolar**

● **Table 27-1. Functions of Saliva and Chewing**

Disruption of food to produce smaller particles
Formation of a bolus for swallowing
Initiation of starch and lipid digestion
Facilitation of taste
Production of intraluminal stimuli in the stomach
Regulation of food intake and ingestive behavior
Cleansing of the mouth and selective antibacterial action
Neutralization of refluxed gastric contents
Mucosal growth and protection in the rest of the GI tract
Aid in speech

structures of glands located in the GI tract (Fig. 27-1). The acinar portion of the gland is classified according to its major secretion: serous ("watery"), mucous, or mixed. The parotid gland produces mainly serous secretion, the sublingual gland secretes mainly mucus, and the submandibular gland produces a mixed secretion.

Cells in the secretory end pieces, or acini, are called acinar cells and are characterized by basally located nuclei, abundant rough endoplasmic reticulum, and apically located secretory granules that contain the enzyme amylase and other secreted proteins. There are also mucous cells in the acinus; the granules in these cells are larger and contain the specialized glycoprotein **mucin.** There are three kinds of ducts in the gland that transport secretions from the acinus to the opening in the mouth and also modify the secretion: intercalated ducts drain acinar fluid into larger ducts, the striated ducts, which then empty into even larger excretory ducts. A single large duct from each gland drains saliva to the mouth. The ductal cells lining the striated ducts, in particular, modify the ionic composition and osmolarity of saliva.

Composition of Saliva

The important properties of saliva are a large flow rate relative to the mass of gland, low osmolarity, high K^+ concentration, and organic constituents, including enzymes (amylase, lipase), mucin, and growth factors. The later are not important in the integrated response to a meal but are essential for long-term maintenance of the lining of the GI tract.

The inorganic composition is entirely dependent on the stimulus and the rate of salivary flow. In humans, salivary secretion is always hypotonic. The major components are Na^+, K^+, HCO_3^-, Ca^{++}, Mg^{++}, and Cl^-. Fluoride can be secreted in saliva, and fluoride secretion forms the basis of oral fluoride treatment for the prevention of dental caries. The concentration of ions varies with the rate of secretion, which is stimulated during the postprandial period.

The **primary secretion** is produced by acinar cells in the secretory end pieces (acini) and is modified by duct cells as saliva passes through the ducts. The primary secretion is isotonic, and the concentration of the major ions is similar to that in plasma. Secretion is driven predominantly by Ca^{++}-dependent signaling,

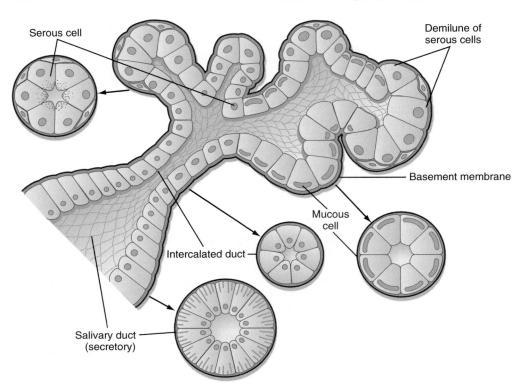

Serous cell

Demilune of serous cells

● **Figure 27-1.** General structure of tubuloalveolar secretory glands associated with the digestive tract, for example, the salivary glands and the pancreas.

Basement membrane

Mucous cell

Intercalated duct

Salivary duct (secretory)

which opens apical Cl⁻ channels in the acinar cells. Cl⁻ therefore flows out into the duct lumen and establishes an osmotic and electrical gradient. Because the epithelium of the acinus is relatively leaky, Na⁺ and water then follow across the epithelium via the tight junctions (i.e., via **paracellular transport**). Transcellular water movement may also occur, mediated by aquaporin 5 water channels. The amylase content and rate of fluid secretion vary with the type and level of stimulus. The excretory duct cells and the striated duct cells modify the primary secretion to produce the secondary secretion. The duct cells reabsorb Na⁺ and Cl⁻ and secrete K⁺ and HCO_3^- into the lumen. At rest, the final salivary secretion is hypotonic and slightly alkaline. Na⁺ is exchanged for protons, but some of the secreted protons are then reabsorbed in exchange for K⁺. HCO_3^-, on the other hand, is secreted only in exchange for Cl⁻, thereby providing excess base equivalents. The alkalinity of saliva is probably important in restricting microbial growth in the mouth, as well as in neutralizing refluxed gastric acid once the saliva is swallowed. When salivary secretion is stimulated, moreover, there is a decrease in K⁺ (but it always remains above plasma concentrations), Na⁺ increases toward plasma levels, Cl⁻ and HCO_3^- increase, and thus the secretion becomes even more alkaline. Note that HCO_3^- secretion can be directly stimulated by the action of secretagogues on duct cells. The duct epithelium is relatively tight and lacks expression of aquaporin, and therefore water cannot follow the ions rapidly enough to maintain isotonicity at moderate or high flow rates during stimulated salivary secretion. Thus, with an increase in the secretion rate, there is less time

for modification by the ducts, and the resulting saliva more closely resembles the primary secretion and therefore plasma. However, $[HCO_3^-]$ remains high because it is secreted by duct and possibly acinar cells by the action of secretagogues (Fig. 27-2).

The organic constituents of saliva, proteins and glycoproteins, are synthesized, stored, and secreted by the acinar cells. The major products are amylase (an enzyme that initiates starch digestion), lipase (important for lipid digestion), glycoprotein (mucin, which forms mucus when hydrated), and lysozyme (attacks bacterial cell walls to limit colonization of bacteria in the mouth). Although salivary amylase begins the process of digestion of carbohydrates, it is not required in healthy adults because of the excess of pancreatic amylase. Similarly, the importance of lingual lipase is unclear.

Metabolism and Blood Flow of Salivary Glands

The salivary glands produce a prodigious flow of saliva. The maximal rate of saliva production in humans is about 1 mL/min/g of gland; thus, at this rate, the glands are producing their own weight in saliva each minute. Salivary glands have a high rate of metabolism and high blood flow; both are proportional to the rate of saliva formation. The blood flow to maximally secreting salivary glands is approximately 10 times that of an equal mass of actively contracting skeletal muscle. Stimulation of the parasympathetic nerves to salivary glands increases blood flow by dilating the vasculature of the glands. Vasoactive intestinal polypeptide (VIP) and acetylcholine are released from

● **Figure 27-2.** **A,** The composition of salivary secretion as a function of the salivary flow rate compared with the concentration of ions in plasma. Saliva is hypotonic to plasma at all flow rates. [HCO_3^-] in saliva exceeds that in plasma except at very low flow rates. **B,** Schematic representation of the two-stage model of salivary secretion. The primary secretion containing amylase and electrolytes is produced in the acinar cell. The concentration of electrolytes in plasma is similar to that in the primary secretion, but it is modified as it passes through ducts that absorb Na^+ and Cl^- and secrete K^+ and HCO_3^-.

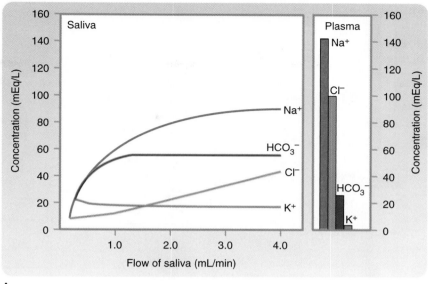

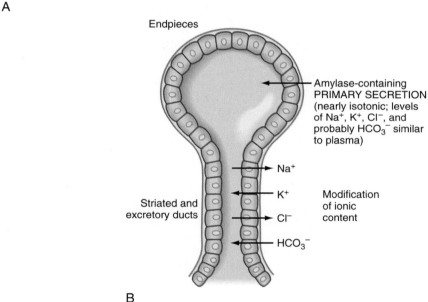

parasympathetic nerve terminals in the salivary glands and are vasodilatory during secretion.

Regulation of Salivary Secretion

Control of salivary secretion is exclusively neural. In contrast, control of most other GI secretions is primarily hormonal. Salivary secretion is stimulated by both the sympathetic and parasympathetic subdivisions of the autonomic nervous system. The primary physiological control of the salivary glands is by the parasympathetic nervous system. Excitation of either sympathetic or parasympathetic nerves to the salivary glands stimulates salivary secretion. If the parasympathetic supply is interrupted, salivation is severely impaired and the salivary glands atrophy.

Sympathetic fibers to the salivary glands stem from the superior cervical ganglion. Preganglionic parasympathetic fibers travel via branches of the facial and

glossopharyngeal nerves (cranial nerves VII and IX, respectively). These fibers form synapses with postganglionic neurons in ganglia in or near the salivary glands. The acinar cells and ducts are supplied with parasympathetic nerve endings.

Parasympathetic stimulation increases the synthesis and secretion of salivary amylase and mucins, enhances the transport activities of the ductular epithelium, greatly increases blood flow to the glands, and stimulates glandular metabolism and growth.

Ionic Mechanisms of Salivary Secretion

Ion Transport in Acinar Cells. Figure 27-3 shows a simplified view of the mechanisms of ion secretion by serous acinar cells. The basolateral membrane of the cell contains **Na^+,K^+-ATPase** and an **Na^+-K^+-$2Cl^-$ symporter.** The concentration gradient for Na^+ across the basolateral membrane, which is dependent on Na^+,K^+-

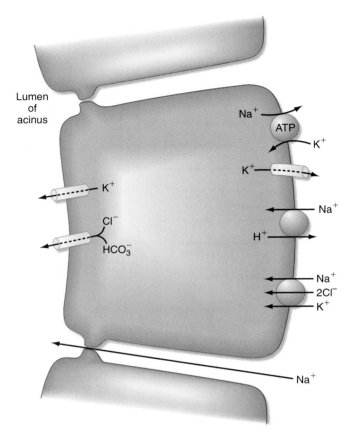

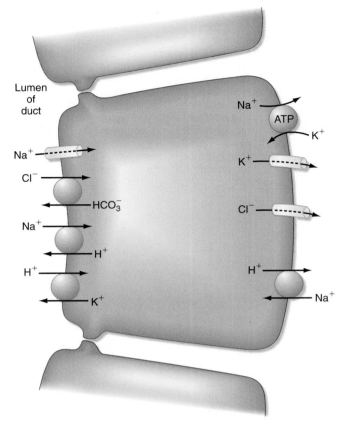

● **Figure 27-3.** Ionic transport mechanism involved in the secretion of amylase and electrolytes in salivary acinar cells.

● **Figure 27-4.** Ionic transport mechanism involved in secretion and absorption in epithelial cells of the striated and excretory duct of the salivary gland.

ATPase, provides the driving force for entry of Na⁺, K⁺, and Cl⁻ into the cell. Cl⁻ and HCO₃⁻ leave the acinar cell and enter the lumen via an anion channel located in the apical membrane of the acinar cell. This secretion of anions drives the entry of Na⁺ and thus water into the acinar lumen via the relatively leaky tight junctions.

Acinar cell fluid secretion is strongly enhanced in response to elevations in intracellular [Ca⁺⁺] as a result of activation of the muscarinic receptor for acetylcholine.

Ion Transport in Ductular Cells. Figure 27-4 shows a simplified model of ion transport processes in epithelial cells of the excretory and striated ducts. Na⁺,K⁺-ATPase, located in the basolateral membrane, maintains the electrochemical gradients for Na⁺ and K⁺ that drive most of the other ionic transport processes of the cell. In the apical membrane, the parallel operation of Na⁺, H⁺, Cl⁻, HCO₃⁻, and H⁺-K⁺ antiporters results in absorption of Na⁺ and Cl⁻ from the lumen and secretion of K⁺ and HCO₃⁻ into the lumen. The relative impermeability of the ductular epithelium to water prevents the ducts from absorbing too much water by osmosis.

Swallowing

Swallowing can be initiated voluntarily, but thereafter it is almost entirely under reflex control. The **swallowing reflex** is a rigidly ordered sequence of events that

● AT THE CELLULAR LEVEL

The acinar cells and duct cells of the salivary glands respond to both cholinergic and adrenergic agonists. Nerves stimulate the release of acetylcholine, norepinephrine, substance P, and VIP by salivary glands, and these hormones increase the secretion of amylase and the flow of saliva. These neurotransmitters act mainly by elevating the intracellular concentration of cAMP and by increasing the concentration of Ca⁺⁺ in the cytosol. Acetylcholine and substance P, acting on muscarinic and tachykinin receptors, respectively, increase the cytosolic concentration of Ca⁺⁺ in serous acinar cells. In contrast, norepinephrine, acting on β receptors, and VIP, acting at its receptor, elevate the cAMP concentration in acinar cells. Agonists that elevate the cAMP concentration in serous acinar cells elicit a secretion that is rich in amylase; agonists that mobilize Ca⁺⁺ elicit a secretion that is more voluminous but has a lower concentration of amylase. Ca⁺⁺-mobilizing agonists may also elevate the concentration of cGMP, which may mediate the trophic effects evoked by these agonists.

Xerostomia, or dry mouth, is caused by impaired salivary secretion. It can be congenital or develop as part of an autoimmune process. The decrease in secretion reduces pH in the oral cavity, which causes tooth decay and is associated with esophageal erosions. Reduced secretion also causes difficulty swallowing.

The ability to measure and monitor a wide range of molecular components that are indicative of overall health is useful in diagnosis and monitoring. Saliva is easy to access, and collection of it is noninvasive. It is used to identify individuals with disease (presence of biomarkers) and to monitor the progress of affected individuals under treatment. In endocrinology, levels of steroids can be measured in the free form rather than as the free and bound form as in plasma (e.g., the stress hormone cortisol and the sex hormones estradiol, progesterone, and testosterone). Viral infections such as human immunodeficiency virus (HIV), herpes, hepatitis C, and Epstein-Barr virus infection can be detected by polymerase chain reaction (PCR) techniques. Bacterial infections, such as *Helicobacter pylori,* can likewise be detected in saliva, and saliva is also used for monitoring of levels of drugs.

BOLUS TRANSFER FROM THE MOUTH TO THE
ESOPHAGUS REQUIRES MULTIPLE EVENTS

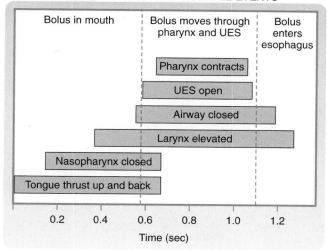

● **Figure 27-5.** Timing of motor events in the pharynx and upper esophageal sphincter (UES) during a swallow.

Gastroesophageal reflux disease (GERD) is commonly referred to as heartburn or indigestion. It occurs when the lower esophageal sphincter allows the acidic contents of the stomach to reflux back into the distal part of the esophagus. This region of the esophagus, unlike the stomach, does not have a robust system to protect the mucosal lining. Thus, the acid will activate pain fibers and thereby result in discomfort and pain. This is not an uncommon phenomenon, even in healthy individuals. In the long term, continual reflux can result in damage to the esophageal mucosa. In this case, this condition is classed as GERD and can be treated by H$_2$ receptor antagonists that reduce gastric acid secretion, such as ranitidine, or by proton pump inhibitors, such as omeprazole.

propel food from the mouth to the pharynx and from there to the stomach. This reflex also inhibits respiration and prevents the entrance of food into the trachea during swallowing. The afferent limb of the swallowing reflex begins when touch receptors, most notably those near the opening of the pharynx, are stimulated. Sensory impulses from these receptors are transmitted to an area in the medulla and lower pons called the swallowing center. Motor impulses travel from the swallowing center to the musculature of the pharynx and upper esophagus via various cranial nerves and to the remainder of the esophagus by vagal motor neurons.

The timing of events in swallowing is shown in Figure 27-5. The voluntary phase of swallowing is initiated when the tip of the tongue separates a bolus of food from the mass of food in the mouth. First the tip of the tongue and later the more posterior portions of the tongue press against the hard palate. The action of the tongue moves the bolus upward and then backward into the mouth. The bolus is forced into the pharynx, where it stimulates the touch receptors that initiate the swallowing reflex. The pharyngeal phase of swallowing involves the following sequence of events, which occur in less than 1 second: (1) the soft palate is pulled upward and the palatopharyngeal folds move inward toward one another; these movements prevent reflux of food into the nasopharynx and open a narrow passage through which food moves into the pharynx; (2) the vocal cords are pulled together and the larynx is moved forward and upward against the epiglottis; these actions prevent food from entering the trachea and help open the upper esophageal sphincter (UES); (3) the UES relaxes to receive the bolus of food; and (4) the superior constrictor muscles of the pharynx then contract strongly to force the bolus deeply into the pharynx. A peristaltic wave is initiated with contraction of the pharyngeal superior constrictor muscles, and the wave moves toward the esophagus. This wave forces the bolus of food through the relaxed UES. During the pharyngeal stage of swallowing, respiration is also reflexively inhibited. After the bolus of food passes the UES, a reflex action causes the sphincter to constrict.

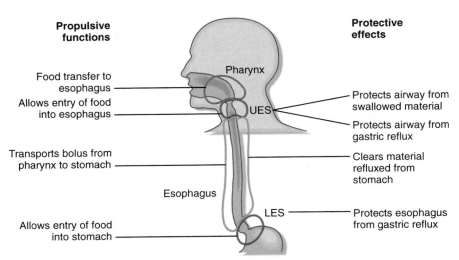

Propulsive functions

Food transfer to esophagus

Allows entry of food into esophagus

Transports bolus from pharynx to stomach

Allows entry of food into stomach

Pharynx

UES

Esophagus

LES

Protective effects

Protects airway from swallowed material

Protects airway from gastric reflux

Clears material refluxed from stomach

Protects esophagus from gastric reflux

● **Figure 27-6.** The esophagus and associated sphincters have multiple functions involved in movement of food from the mouth to the stomach and also in protection of the airway and esophagus.

ESOPHAGEAL PHASE

The **esophagus,** the **UES,** and the **lower esophageal sphincter (LES)** serve two main functions (Fig. 27-6). First, they propel food from the mouth to the stomach. Second, the sphincters protect the airway during swallowing and protect the esophagus from acidic gastric secretions.

The stimuli that initiate the changes in smooth muscle activity that result in these **propulsive** and **protective** functions are mechanical and consist of pharyngeal stimulation during swallowing and distention of the esophageal wall itself. The pathways are exclusively neural and involve both extrinsic and intrinsic reflexes. Mechanosensitive afferents in both the extrinsic (vagus) nerves and intrinsic neural pathways respond to esophageal distention. These pathways include activated reflex pathways via the brainstem (extrinsic, vagus) or solely intrinsic pathways. The striated muscle is regulated from the nucleus ambiguus in the brainstem, and the smooth muscle is regulated by parasympathetic outflow via the vagus nerve. The changes in function resulting from mechanosensitive stimuli and activation of reflex pathways are peristalsis of striated and smooth muscle, relaxation of the LES, and relaxation of the proximal portion of the stomach.

Functional Anatomy of the Esophagus and Associated Structures

The esophagus, like the rest of the GI tract, has two muscle layers—circular and longitudinal—but the esophagus is one of two places in the gut where striated muscle occurs, the other being the external anal sphincter. The type of muscle (striated or smooth) in the esophagus varies along its length. The UES and LES are formed by thickening of striated or circular smooth muscle, respectively.

Motor Activity during the Esophageal Phase

The UES, esophagus, and LES act in a coordinated manner to propel material from the pharynx to the stomach. At the end of a swallow, a bolus passes through the UES, and the presence of the bolus, via stimulation of mechanoreceptors and reflex pathways, initiates a peristaltic wave (alternating contraction and relaxation of the muscle) along the esophagus that is called **primary peristalsis** (Fig. 27-7). This wave moves down the esophagus slowly (3 to 5 cm/sec). Distention of the esophagus by the moving bolus initiates another wave called secondary peristalsis. Frequently, repetitive **secondary peristalsis** is required to clear the esophagus of the bolus. Stimulation of the pharynx by the swallowed bolus also produces reflex relaxation of the LES and the most proximal region of the stomach. Thus, when the bolus reaches the LES, it is already relaxed to allow passage of the bolus into the stomach. Similarly, the portion of the stomach that receives the bolus is relaxed. In addition, esophageal distention produces further receptive relaxation of the stomach. The proximal part of the stomach relaxes at the same time as the LES; this occurs with each swallow and its function is to allow the stomach to accommodate large volumes with a minimal rise in intragastric pressure. This process is called **receptive relaxation** (Fig. 27-8).

The LES also has important protective functions. It is involved in the prevention of acid reflux from the stomach back into the esophagus; an insufficient tonic contraction of the LES is associated with reflux disease, a gradual erosion of the esophageal mucosa, which is not as well protected as the gastric and duodenal mucosa. There is also some evidence that peristalsis in the absence of swallowing (secondary peristalsis) is important for clearing refluxed gastric contents.

■ KEY CONCEPTS

1. The cephalic and oral phases of the meal share many characteristics and ready the remainder of the GI tract for the meal; these responses are neurally mediated, predominantly by the efferent vagus nerve.

● **Figure 27-7.** Changes in pressure in the different regions of the pharynx, esophagus, and associated sphincters initiated during a swallow. The pressure trace is a diagrammatic representation from that obtained during manometry in an awake human. Stimulation of the pharynx by the presence of a bolus initiates a decrease in pressure (= opening) of the UES and a peristaltic wave of contraction along the esophagus. Stimulation of the pharynx also relaxes the smooth muscle of the LES to prepare for entry of food.

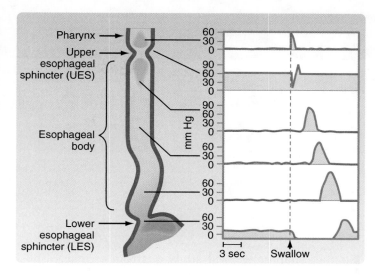

● **Figure 27-8.** Swallowing in the form of pharyngeal stimulation induces neural reflex relaxation of the LES and the proximal part of the stomach to allow entry of food.

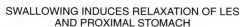
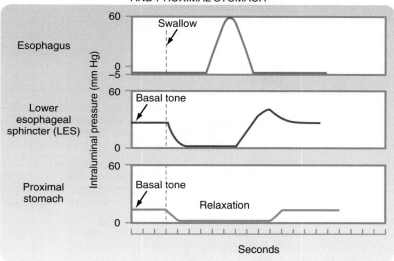

2. Salivary secretion has important functions and, together with chewing of the food, allows the formation of a bolus that can be swallowed and passed along the esophagus to the stomach.

3. The ionic composition of salivary secretion varies with the flow rate, which is stimulated during a meal. The primary secretion comes from cells in the acini and is modified by epithelial cells as it passes through the ducts.

4. Regulation of salivary secretion is exclusively neural; parasympathetic innervation is most important in the response to food.

5. The swallowing reflex is a rigidly ordered sequence of events that propel food from the mouth to the pharynx and from there to the stomach.

6. The major function of the esophagus is to propel food from the mouth to the stomach. The esophagus has sphincters at either end that are involved in protective functions important in swallowing and preserving the integrity of the esophageal mucosa.

7. Esophageal peristalsis (primary) is stimulated by mechanical stimulation of the pharynx, and secondary peristalsis is stimulated by distention of the esophageal wall.

8. Esophageal function and the associated sphincters are regulated by extrinsic and intrinsic neural pathways.

CHAPTER 28

The Gastric Phase of the Integrated Response to a Meal

In this chapter we will study gastrointestinal (GI) tract physiology when food is in the stomach (i.e., the gastric phase of digestion). This chapter discusses gastric function and its regulation, in addition to changes in function that occur in more distal regions of the GI tract. The main functions of the stomach are to act as a temporary reservoir for the meal and to initiate protein digestion through the secretion of acid and the enzyme precursor pepsinogen. Other functions are listed in Table 28-1.

Food entering the stomach from the esophagus causes mechanical stimulation of the gastric wall via distention and stretching of smooth muscle. Food, predominantly oligopeptides and amino acids, also provides chemical stimulation when present in the gastric lumen. Regulation of gastric function during the gastric phase is dependent on endocrine, paracrine, and neural pathways. These pathways are activated by mechanical and chemical stimuli, which result in both intrinsic and extrinsic neural reflex pathways that are important for the regulation of gastric function. Afferent neurons that pass from the GI tract to the central nervous system (and to a lesser extent to the spinal cord) via the vagus nerve respond to these mechanical and chemical stimuli and activate parasympathetic outflow.

The endocrine pathways include the release of **gastrin,** which stimulates gastric acid secretion, and the release of **somatostatin,** which inhibits gastric secretion. Important paracrine pathways include **histamine** release, which stimulates gastric acid secretion. The responses elicited by activation of these pathways include both secretory and motor responses; secretory responses include secretion of acid, pepsinogen, mucus, intrinsic factor, gastrin, lipase, and HCO_3^-. Overall, these secretions initiate protein digestion and protect the gastric mucosa. Motor responses (changes in activity of smooth muscle) include inhibition of motility of the proximal part of the stomach (receptive relaxation) and stimulation of motility of the distal part of the stomach, which causes antral peristalsis. These changes in motility play important roles in storage and mixing of the meal with secretions and are also involved in regulating the flow of contents out of the stomach.

FUNCTIONAL ANATOMY OF THE STOMACH

The stomach is divided into three regions: the **cardia,** the **corpus** (also referred to as the fundus or body), and the **antrum** (Fig. 28-1). However, when discussing the physiology of the stomach, it is helpful to think of it as subdivided into two *functional* regions: the **proximal** and **distal** parts of the stomach. The proximal portion of the stomach (called proximal because it is the most cranial) and the distal portion of the stomach (furthest away from the mouth) have quite different functions in the postprandial response to a meal, which will be discussed later.

The lining of the stomach is covered with a columnar epithelium folded into **gastric pits;** each pit is the opening of a duct into which one or more gastric glands empty (Fig. 28-2). The gastric pits account for a significant fraction of the total surface area of the gastric mucosa. The gastric mucosa is divided into three distinct regions based on the structure of the glands. The small cardiac glandular region, located just below the lower esophageal sphincter (LES), primarily contains mucus-secreting gland cells. The remainder of the gastric mucosa is divided into the **oxyntic** or **parietal** (acid-secreting) **gland region,** located above the gastric notch (equivalent to the proximal part of the stomach), and the pyloric gland region, located below the notch (equivalent to the distal part of the stomach).

The structure of a gastric gland from the oxyntic glandular region is illustrated in Figure 28-2. Surface epithelial cells extend slightly into the duct opening. The opening of the gland is called the **isthmus** and is lined with surface mucous cells and a few parietal cells. Mucous neck cells are located in the narrow **neck** of the gland. Parietal or oxyntic cells, which secrete HCl and intrinsic factor (involved in absorption of vitamin B_{12}), and **chief** or **peptic cells,** which secrete pepsinogens, are located deeper in the gland. Oxyntic glands also contain **enterochromaffin-like** (ECL) cells, which secrete histamine, and D cells, which secrete somatostatin. Parietal cells are particularly numerous in glands in the fundus, whereas mucus-secreting cells are more numerous in glands of the pyloric (antral)

● **Figure 28-1.** The three functional regions of the stomach. The regions have different luminal secretions and patterns of smooth muscle activity indicative of their unique functions in response to food.

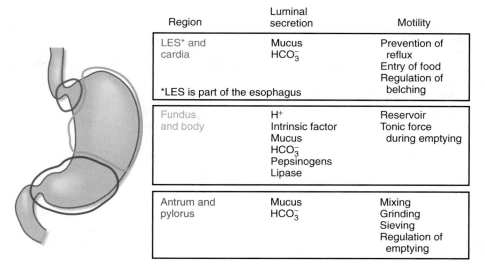

Region	Luminal secretion	Motility
LES* and cardia *LES is part of the esophagus	Mucus HCO_3^-	Prevention of reflux Entry of food Regulation of belching
Fundus and body	H^+ Intrinsic factor Mucus HCO_3^- Pepsinogens Lipase	Reservoir Tonic force during emptying
Antrum and pylorus	Mucus HCO_3^-	Mixing Grinding Sieving Regulation of emptying

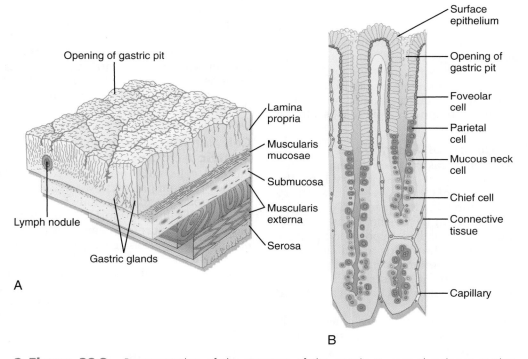

A

B

● **Figure 28-2.** Representation of the structure of the gastric mucosa showing a section through the wall of the stomach **(A)** and detail of the structure of gastric glands and cell types in the mucosa **(B).**

● **Table 28-1. Functions of the Stomach**

Storage—acts as temporary reservoir for the meal

Secretion of H^+ to kill microorganisms and convert pepsinogen to its active form

Secretion of intrinsic factor to absorb vitamin B_{12} (cobalamin)

Secretion of mucus and HCO_3^- to protect the gastric mucosa

Secretion of water for lubrication and to provide aqueous suspension of nutrients

Motor activity for mixing secretions (H^+ and pepsin) with ingested food

Coordinated motor activity to regulate the emptying of contents into the duodenum

glandular region. In addition, the pyloric glands contain G cells, which secrete the hormone gastrin. The parietal glands can also be divided into regions: the neck (mucous neck cells and parietal cells) and the base (peptic/chief and parietal cells). Endocrine cells are scattered throughout the glands.

GASTRIC SECRETION

The fluid secreted into the stomach is called gastric juice. Gastric juice is a mixture of the secretions of the surface epithelial cells and the secretions of gastric glands. One of the most important components of gastric juice is H^+, a secretion that occurs in the face of a very large concentration gradient. Thus, H^+ secretion by the parietal mucosa is an energy-intensive process. The cytoplasm of the parietal cell is densely packed with mitochondria, which have been estimated to fill 30% to 40% of the cell's volume. One major function of H^+ is conversion of inactive pepsinogen (the major enzyme product of the stomach) to pepsins, which initiate protein digestion in the stomach. Additionally, ions are important for preventing invasion and colonization of the gut by bacteria and other pathogens that may be ingested with food. The stomach also secretes significant amounts of HCO_3^- and mucus, important for protection of the gastric mucosa against the acidic and peptic luminal environment. However, in a healthy human the only gastric secretion required is intrinsic factor, which is necessary for the absorption of vitamin B_{12} (**cobalamin**). The functions of other components of gastric juice are redundant with secretions provided more distally in the GI tract.

Composition of Gastric Secretions

Like other GI secretions, gastric juice consists of inorganic and organic constituents together with water. Among the important components of gastric juice are HCl, salts, pepsins, intrinsic factor, mucus, and HCO_3^-. Secretion of all these components increases after a meal.

Inorganic Constituents of Gastric Juice

The ionic composition of gastric juice depends on the rate of secretion. The higher the secretory rate, the higher the concentration of H^+ ions. At lower secretory rates, $[H^+]$ decreases and $[Na^+]$ increases. $[K^+]$ is always higher in gastric juice than in plasma. Consequently, prolonged vomiting may lead to hypokalemia. At all rates of secretion, Cl^- is the major anion of gastric juice. At high rates of secretion, gastric juice resembles an isotonic solution of HCl. Gastric HCl converts pepsinogens to active pepsins and provides the acid pH at which pepsins are active.

The rate of gastric H^+ secretion varies considerably among individuals. In humans, basal (unstimulated) rates of gastric H^+ production typically range from about 1 to 5 mEq/hr. During maximal stimulation, HCl production rises to 6 to 40 mEq/hr. The basal rate is greater at night and lowest in the early morning. The total number of parietal cells in the stomach of normal individuals varies greatly, and this variation is partly responsible for the wide range in basal and stimulated rates of HCl secretion.

Organic Constituents of Gastric Juice

The predominant organic constituent of gastric juice is **pepsinogen,** the inactive proenzyme of pepsin. Pepsins, often collectively called "pepsin," are a group of proteases secreted by the chief cells of the gastric glands. Pepsinogens are contained in membrane-bound zymogen granules in the chief cells. Zymogen granules release their contents by exocytosis when chief cells are stimulated to secrete (Table 28-2). Pep-

● **Table 28-2.**

Stimulation of Chief Cells in the Integrated Response to a Meal

Stimulant	Source
Acetylcholine (ACh)	Enteric neurons
Gastrin	G cells in the gastric antrum
Histamine	ECL cells in the gastric corpus
Cholecystokinin (CCK)	I cells in the duodenum
Secretin	S cells in the duodenum

sinogens are converted to active pepsins by the cleavage of acid-labile linkages. The lower the pH, the more rapid the conversion. Pepsins also act proteolytically on pepsinogens to form more pepsin. Pepsins are most proteolytically active at pH 3 and below. Pepsins may digest as much as 20% of the protein in a typical meal but are not required for digestion because their function can be replaced by that of pancreatic proteases. When the pH of the duodenal lumen is neutralized, pepsins are inactivated by the neutral pH.

Intrinsic factor, a glycoprotein secreted by parietal cells of the stomach, is required for the normal absorption of vitamin B_{12}. Intrinsic factor is released in response to the same stimuli that elicit the secretion of HCl by parietal cells. Secretion of intrinsic factor is the only gastric function that is essential for human life.

Cellular Mechanisms of Gastric Acid Secretion

Parietal cells have a distinctive ultrastructure (Fig. 28-3). Branching secretory canaliculi course through the cytoplasm and are connected by a common outlet to the cell's luminal surface. Microvilli line the surfaces of the **secretory canaliculi.** The cytoplasm of unstimulated parietal cells contains numerous tubules and vesicles, which is called the tubulovesicular system. The membranes of tubulovesicles contain the transport proteins responsible for secretion of H^+ and Cl^- into the lumen of the gland. When parietal cells are stimulated to secrete HCl (Fig. 28-3), **tubulovesicular membranes** fuse with the plasma membrane of the secretory canaliculi. This extensive membrane fusion greatly increases the number of H^+-K^+ antiporters in the plasma membrane of the secretory canaliculi. When parietal cells secrete gastric acid at the maximal rate, H^+ is pumped against a concentration gradient that is about 1 million–fold. Thus, the pH is 7 in the parietal cell cytosol and 1 in the lumen of the gastric gland.

The cellular mechanism of H^+ secretion by the parietal cell is depicted in Figure 28-4. Cl^- enters the cell across the basolateral membrane in exchange for HCO_3^- generated in the cell by the action of carbonic anhydrase, which produces HCO_3^- and H^+. H^+ is secreted across the luminal membrane by H^+,K^+-ATPase in exchange for K^+. Cl^- enters the lumen via an ion channel (a ClC Cl^- channel) located in the luminal membrane. Increased intracellular Ca^{++} and cAMP stimulate luminal membrane conduction of Cl^- and K^+.

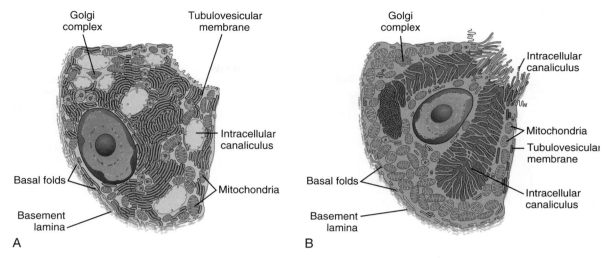

● **Figure 28-3.** Parietal cell ultrastructure. **A,** A resting parietal cell showing the tubulovesicular apparatus in the cytoplasm and the intracellular canaliculus. **B,** An activated parietal cell that is secreting acid. The tubulovesicles have fused with the membranes of the intracellular canaliculus, which is now open to the lumen of the gland and lined with abundant long microvilli.

● **Figure 28-4.** Mechanism of H^+ and Cl^- secretion by an activated parietal cell in the gastric mucosa.

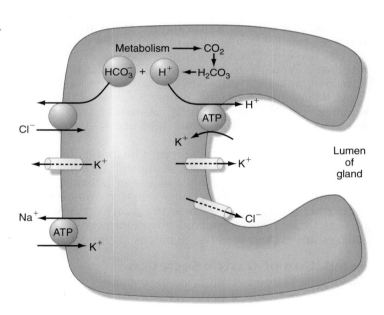

Increased K^+ conductance hyperpolarizes the luminal membrane potential, which increases the driving force for efflux of Cl^- across the luminal membrane. The K^+ channel in the basolateral membrane also mediates the efflux of K^+ that accumulates in the parietal cell via the activity of H^+,K^+-ATPase. In addition, cAMP and Ca^{++} promote the trafficking of Cl^- channels into the luminal membrane and the fusion of cytosolic tubulovesicles containing H^+,K^+-ATPase with the membrane of the secretory canaliculi (Figs. 28-3 and 28-4). Parietal cell secretion of H^+ is also accompanied by transport of HCO_3^- into the bloodstream to maintain intracellular pH.

Secretion of HCO_3^-

The surface epithelial cells also secrete a watery fluid that contains Na^+ and Cl^- in concentrations similar to those in plasma, but with higher K^+ and HCO_3^- concentrations. HCO_3^- is entrapped by the viscous mucus that coats the surface of the stomach; thus, the mucus secreted by the resting mucosa lines the stomach with a sticky, alkaline coat. When food is eaten, moreover, rates of secretion of both mucus and HCO_3^- increase.

Secretion of Mucus

Secretions that contain **mucins** are viscous and sticky and are collectively termed mucus. Mucins are secreted by mucous neck cells located in the necks of gastric glands and by the surface epithelial cells of the stomach. Mucus is stored in large granules in the apical cytoplasm of mucous neck cells and surface epithelial cells and is released by exocytosis.

Gastric mucins are about 80% carbohydrate by weight and consist of four similar monomers of about

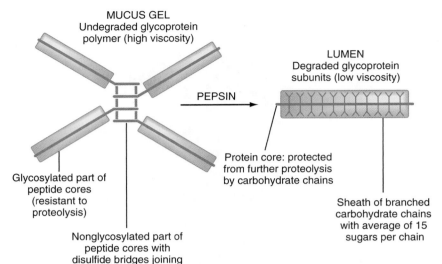

MUCUS GEL
Undegraded glycoprotein
polymer (high viscosity)

PEPSIN

LUMEN
Degraded glycoprotein
subunits (low viscosity)

Glycosylated part of
peptide cores
(resistant to
proteolysis)

Nonglycosylated part of
peptide cores with
disulfide bridges joining
subunits (site of proteolysis)

Protein core: protected
from further proteolysis
by carbohydrate chains

Sheath of branched
carbohydrate chains
with average of 15
sugars per chain

● **Figure 28-5.** Schematic representation of the structure of gastric mucins before and after hydrolysis by pepsin. Intact mucins are tetramers of four similar monomers of about 500,000 Da. Each monomer is largely covered by carbohydrate side chains that protect it from proteolytic degradation. The central portion of the mucin tetramer, near the disulfide cross-links, is more susceptible to proteolytic digestion. Pepsins cleave bonds near the center of the tetramers to release fragments about the size of monomers.

500,000 Da each that are linked together by disulfide bonds (Fig. 28-5). These tetrameric mucins form a sticky gel that adheres to the surface of the stomach. However, this gel is subject to proteolysis by pepsins, which cleave disulfide bonds near the center of the tetramers. Proteolysis releases fragments that do not form gels and thus dissolves the protective mucus layer. Maintenance of the protective mucus layer requires continuous synthesis of new tetrameric mucins to replace the mucins that are cleaved by pepsins.

Mucus is secreted at a significant rate in the resting stomach. Secretion of mucus is stimulated by some of the same stimuli that enhance acid and pepsinogen secretion, especially acetylcholine released from parasympathetic nerve endings near the gastric glands. If the gastric mucosa is mechanically deformed, neural reflexes are evoked to enhance mucus secretion.

Regulation of Gastric Secretion

Parasympathetic innervation via the vagus nerve is the strongest stimulant of gastric H^+ secretion. Extrinsic efferent fibers terminate on intrinsic neurons that innervate parietal cells, ECL cells that secrete the paracrine mediator histamine, and endocrine cells that secrete the hormone gastrin. In addition, vagal stimulation results in the secretion of pepsinogen, mucus, HCO_3^-, and intrinsic factor. Stimulation of the parasympathetic nervous system also occurs during the cephalic and oral phase of the meal. However, the gastric phase produces the largest stimulation of gastric secretion of the postprandial period (Fig. 28-6).

Stimulation of gastric acid secretion is an excellent example of a "feed forward" (or cascade) response that uses endocrine, paracrine, and neural pathways. Activation of intrinsic neurons by vagal efferent activity results in the release of acetylcholine from nerve terminals, which activates cells in the gastric epithelium. Parietal cells express muscarinic receptors and are activated to secrete H^+ in response to vagal effer-

ent nerve activity. In addition, parasympathetic activation, via gastrin-releasing peptide from intrinsic neurons, releases gastrin from G cells located in the gastric glands in the gastric antrum (Fig. 28-6). Gastrin enters the bloodstream and, via an endocrine mechanism, further stimulates the parietal cell to secrete H^+. Parietal cells express cholecystokinin type 2 (CCK2) receptors for gastrin. Histamine is also secreted in response to vagal nerve stimulation, and ECL cells express muscarinic and gastrin receptors. Thus, gastrin and vagal efferent activity induce the release of histamine, which potentiates the effects of both gastrin and acetylcholine on the parietal cell. Hence, activation of parasympathetic (vagal) outflow to the stomach is very efficient at stimulating the parietal cell to secrete acid (Fig. 28-7).

In the gastric phase, the presence of food in the stomach is detected and activates **vagovagal reflexes** to stimulate secretion. Food in the stomach results in distention and stretch, which are detected by afferent (or sensory) nerve endings in the gastric wall. These are the peripheral terminals of vagal afferent nerves that transmit information to the brainstem and thereby drive activity in vagal efferent fibers, a vagovagal reflex (Fig. 28-6). In addition, digestion of proteins increases the concentration of oligopeptides and free amino acids in the lumen, which are detected by **chemosensors** in the gastric mucosa. Oligopeptides and amino acids also stimulate vagal afferent activity. The exact nature of the chemosensors is not clear but may involve endocrine cells that release their contents to activate nerve endings. This topic will be discussed in more detail in Chapter 29.

There is also an important negative-feedback mechanism whereby the presence of acid in the distal part of the stomach (antrum) induces a feedback loop to inhibit the parietal cell such that meal-stimulated H^+ secretion does not go unchecked. When the concentration of H^+ in the lumen reaches a certain threshold (below pH 3), somatostatin is released from endocrine

● **Figure 28-6.** Neural regulation of gastric acid secretion in the gastric phase of the meal is mediated by the vagus nerve. The stimulation that occurs in the cephalic and oral phases, before food reaches the stomach, results in stimulation of parietal cells to secrete acid and chief cells to secrete pepsinogen. Thus, when food reaches the stomach, protein digestion is initiated by generating protein hydrolysate, which further stimulates the secretion of gastrin from the mucosa of the gastric antrum. In addition, gastric distention activates a vagovagal reflex that further stimulates gastric acid and pepsinogen secretion.

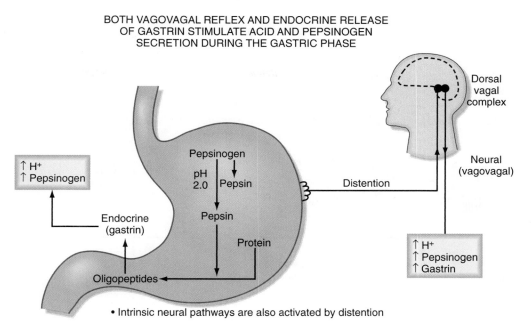

BOTH VAGOVAGAL REFLEX AND ENDOCRINE RELEASE OF GASTRIN STIMULATE ACID AND PEPSINOGEN SECRETION DURING THE GASTRIC PHASE

• Intrinsic neural pathways are also activated by distention

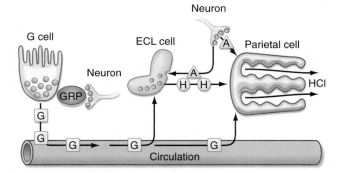

● **Figure 28-7.** The parietal cell is regulated by neural, hormonal, and paracrine pathways. Activation of vagal parasympathetic preganglionic outflow to the stomach acts in three ways to stimulate gastric acid secretion. There is direct neural innervation and activation of the parietal cell via release of acetylcholine (ACh) from enteric neurons, which acts on the parietal cell via muscarinic receptors. In addition, neural activation of the ECL cell stimulates the release of histamine, which acts via a paracrine pathway to stimulate the parietal cell. Finally, G cells located in gastric glands in the gastric antrum are activated by the release of gastrin-releasing peptide from enteric neurons, which acts on the G cell to stimulate the release of gastrin. Gastrin thereafter acts via a humoral pathway to stimulate the parietal cell.

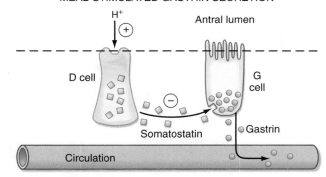

● **Figure 28-8.** Feedback regulation of gastric acid secretion by release of somatostatin and its action on G cells in the gastric antrum. Endocrine cells in the mucosa of the gastric antrum sense the presence of H^+ and secrete somatostatin. This in turn acts on specific receptors on G cells to inhibit the release of gastrin and thus bring about inhibition of gastric acid secretion.

cells in the antral mucosa. Somatostatin has a paracrine action on neighboring G cells to decrease the release of gastrin and thereby decrease gastric acid secretion (Fig. 28-8).

The receptors on the parietal cell membrane for acetylcholine, gastrin, and histamine, as well as the intracellular second messengers by which these secre-

tagogues act, are shown in Figure 28-9. Histamine is the strongest agonist of H^+ secretion, whereas gastrin and acetylcholine are much weaker agonists. However, histamine, acetylcholine, and gastrin potentiate one another's actions on the parietal cell. Antagonists of H_2 histamine receptors, such as cimetidine, block secretagogue-stimulated acid secretion. Thus, much of the response to gastrin results from gastrin-stimulated release of histamine. Gastrin also has important trophic effects: elevation of gastrin levels causes ECL cells to increase in size and number. Binding of histamine to H_2 receptors on parietal cell plasma membranes activates adenylyl cyclase and elevates the

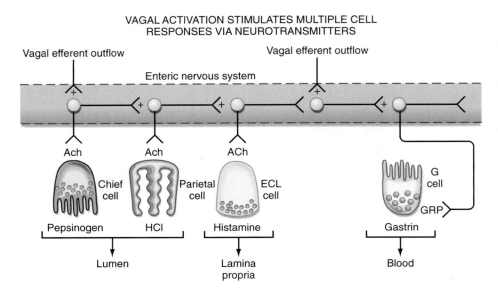

VAGAL ACTIVATION STIMULATES MULTIPLE CELL
RESPONSES VIA NEUROTRANSMITTERS

● **Figure 28-9.** Vagal parasympathetic stimulation of gastric secretions via enteric neurons. Vagal preganglionic neurons innervate the myenteric and submucosal plexus; the terminals of the vagal preganglionic neurons innervate many enteric neurons and thus bring about changes in function as described in Figure 28-7.

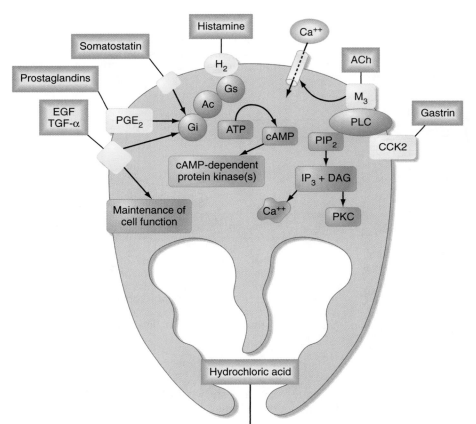

● **Figure 28-10.** Signal transduction mechanisms showing the mechanism of action of agonists (secretagogues) and antagonists that regulate secretion in parietal cells. Acetylcholine (ACh) binds to muscarinic M_3 receptors. Histamine acts via the H_2 receptor. Gastrin binds to the cholecystokinin type 2 (CCK2) receptor. Activation of M_2 and CCK2 receptors results in opening of Ca^{++} channels and release of Ca^{++} from intracellular stores and thus an increase in cytosolic [Ca^{++}]. Activation of H_2 receptors activates adenylyl cyclase to increase intracellular levels of cAMP. Ac, adenylyl cyclase; ACh, acetylcholine; CCK, cholecystokinin; DAG, diacylglycerol; EGF, epidermal growth factor; IP_3, inositol triphosphate; PGE_2, prostaglandin E_2; PIP_2, phosphatidylinositol 4,5-diphosphate; PKC, protein kinase C; PLC, protein lipase C; TGF-α, transforming growth factor α.

cytosolic concentration of cAMP. These events stimulate H^+ secretion by activating basolateral K^+ channels and apical Cl^- channels and by causing more H^+,K^+-ATPase molecules and Cl^- channels to be inserted into the apical plasma membrane (Fig. 28-4). Acetylcholine binds to M_3 muscarinic receptors and opens Ca^{++} channels in the apical plasma membrane. Acetylcholine

also elevates intracellular [Ca^{++}] by promoting the release of Ca^{++} from intracellular stores, which enhances H^+ secretion by activating basolateral K^+ channels and by causing more H^+,K^+-ATPase molecules and Cl^- channels to be inserted into the apical plasma membrane. Gastrin enhances acid secretion by binding to CCK2 receptors (Fig. 28-10).

DIGESTION IN THE STOMACH

Some digestion of nutrients occurs in the stomach. However, this is not required for full digestion of a meal because intestinal digestion is sufficient. Some amylase-mediated digestion of carbohydrates occurs in the stomach. Amylase is sensitive to pH and is inactivated at low pH; however, some amylase is active even in the acidic gastric environment of the stomach because of substrate protection. Thus, when carbohydrate occupies the active site of amylase, it protects the enzyme from degradation.

The digestion of lipids also starts in the stomach. The mixing patterns of gastric motility result in the formation of an emulsion of lipids and **gastric lipase,** which attaches to the surface of lipid droplets in the emulsion and generates free fatty acids and monoglyceride from dietary triglyceride. However, the extent of hydrolysis of triglyceride is approximately 10%, and such hydrolysis is not essential for normal digestion and absorption of dietary lipids. Moreover, as discussed in the next chapter, the products of lipolysis are not available for absorption in the stomach because of its low luminal pH.

Gastric Mucosal Protection and Defense

Mucus and HCO_3^- protect the surface of the stomach from the effects of H^+ and pepsins. The protective mucus gel that forms on the luminal surface of the stomach, as well as alkaline secretions entrapped within it, constitute a **gastric mucosal barrier** that prevents damage to the mucosa by the gastric contents (Fig. 28-11). The mucus gel layer, which is about 0.2 mm thick, effectively separates the HCO_3^--rich

secretions of the surface epithelial cells from the acidic contents of the gastric lumen. The mucus allows the pH of epithelial cells to be maintained at nearly neutral despite a luminal pH of about 2. Mucus also slows the diffusion of acid and pepsins to the epithelial cell surface. Protection of the gastric epithelium depends on both mucus and HCO_3^- secretion.

GASTROINTESTINAL MOTILITY

To understand GI motility, it is necessary to review some properties of smooth muscle function. The motion of the gut wall governs the flow of the luminal contents along its length; the main patterns of motility are mixing **(segmentation)** and propulsion **(peristalsis).** In addition, smooth muscle activity in the stomach and colon subserves a storage function.

Functional Anatomy of Gastrointestinal Smooth Muscle

The smooth muscle in the GI tract is similar in structure to other smooth muscle found in the body. Fusiform cells are packed together in bundles surrounded by a connective tissue sheath. Gap junctions functionally couple the smooth muscle cells so that contraction of bundles occurs synchronously. The **interstitial cells of Cajal** (ICCs) are a specialized group of cells in the intestinal wall that are involved in the transmission of information from enteric neurons to smooth muscle cells (Fig. 28-12). It is also thought that ICCs are **"pacemaker"** cells that have the capacity to generate the basic electrical rhythm, or "slow wave" activ-

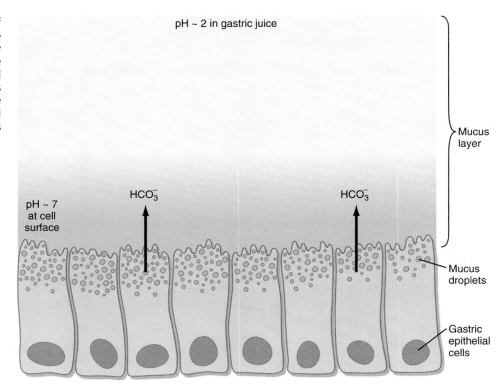

● **Figure 28-11.** The surface of the stomach is protected by the gastric mucosal barrier. Buffering by the HCO_3^--rich secretions and the restraint to convective mixing caused by the high viscosity of the mucus layer allow the pH at the cell surface to remain near 7, whereas the pH in the gastric juice in the lumen is 1 to 2.

pH ~ 2 in gastric juice

pH ~ 7 at cell surface

HCO_3^-

HCO_3^-

Mucus layer

Mucus droplets

Gastric epithelial cells

There are times when the gastric mucosal barrier fails. Superficial breakdowns of the GI lining not involving the submucosa are called erosions. They generally heal without intervention. In contrast, breakdowns of the GI lining involving the muscularis and deeper layers are called ulcers. Gastric and duodenal erosions and ulcers occur as a result of an imbalance between the mechanisms that protect the mucosa and aggressive factors that can break it down. A healthy stomach/duodenum has ample natural protection against the destructive effects of H⁺. Factors that magnify the harmful effect of H⁺ on the stomach/duodenum or act separately from H⁺ include pepsin, bile, the bacterium *Helicobacter pylori*, and the class of drugs known as nonsteroidal antiinflammatory drugs (NSAIDs). Indeed, ulcer disease is becoming more common as the population ages and has more need of NSAIDs for non-GI complaints such as arthritis. Alcohol, tobacco, and caffeine are also risk factors for ulcers. Infectious agents can also cause gastritis (inflammation of the gastric epithelium). *H. pylori* is a spiral bacterium that has now become widely recognized as one factor that can lead to gastritis, ulcer formation, and in humans, gastric carcinoma. *H. pylori* exists in the stomach because it secretes an enzyme, urease, that converts urea to NH_3, which is used to buffer H⁺ by forming NH_4^+. An aggressive regimen of antibiotic treatment, sometimes in combination with an H^+,K^+-ATPase inhibitor, can often eliminate the infection, after which the gastritis and ulcer symptoms improve.

ity, that is a consistent feature of GI smooth muscle (Fig. 28-13).

Electrophysiology of Gastrointestinal Smooth Muscle

The resting membrane potential of GI smooth muscle varies characteristically with time—the basic electrical rhythm, or slow wave. The frequency of slow waves is 3 to 5 per minute in the stomach and about 12 to 20 per minute in the small intestine; it decreases to 6 to 8 per minute in the colon. The frequency of the slow

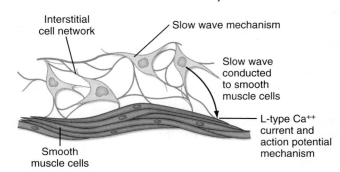

INTERSTITIAL CELLS OF CAJAL (ICC)
ARE THE PACEMAKERS OF THE GUT

Slow waves are generated in interstitial cells of Cajal

● **Figure 28-12.** Diagrammatic representation of the interstitial cells of Cajal network in the smooth muscle wall of the GI tract.

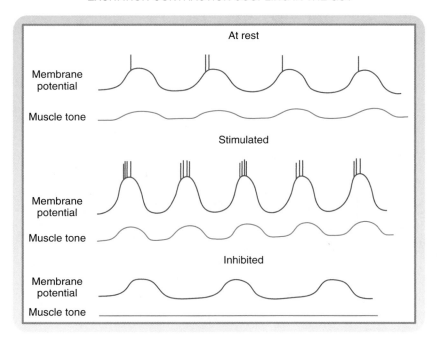

EXCITATION-CONTRACTION COUPLING IN THE GUT

● **Figure 28-13.** Excitation coupling in GI smooth muscle. The slow wave will initiate a contraction in smooth muscle when it reaches a threshold amplitude. The amplitude of the slow wave is altered by release of neurotransmitters from enteric neurons.

wave is set by a pacemaker region in the different regions of the GI tract (Fig. 28-13). The slow wave of that particular region of the GI tract will entrain to the fastest frequency of the slow wave as it is transmitted through the adjacent muscle bundles via gap junctions. Slow waves are thought to be generated by ICCs. These cells are located in a thin layer between the longitudinal and circular layers of the muscularis externa and in other places in the wall of the GI tract. Interstitial cells have properties of both fibroblasts and smooth muscle cells. Their long processes form gap junctions with the longitudinal and circular smooth muscle cells; the gap junctions enable the slow waves to be conducted rapidly to both muscle layers. Because gap junctions electrically and chemically couple the smooth muscle cells of both longitudinal and circular layers, the slow wave spreads throughout the smooth muscle of each segment of the GI tract.

The amplitude and, to a lesser extent, the frequency of the slow wave can be modulated by the activity of intrinsic and extrinsic nerves and by hormones and paracrine substances. If the depolarization of the slow wave exceeds the threshold, a train of action potentials may be triggered during the peak of the slow wave. Action potentials in GI smooth muscle are more prolonged (10 to 20 msec) than those in skeletal muscle and have little or no overshoot. The rising phase of the action potential is caused by flow of ions through channels that conduct both Ca^{++} and Na^+ and are relatively slow to open. The Ca^{++} that enters the cell during the action potential helps initiate contraction. The extent of depolarization of the cells and the frequency of action potentials are enhanced by some hormones and paracrine agonists and by neurotransmitters from excitatory enteric nerve endings (e.g., acetylcholine and substance P). Inhibitory hormones and neuroeffector substances (e.g., vasoactive intestinal polypeptide and nitric oxide) hyperpolarize the smooth muscle cells and may diminish or abolish action potential spikes.

Slow waves that are not accompanied by action potentials elicit little or no contraction of the smooth muscle cells. Much stronger contractions are evoked by the presence of action potentials. The greater the number of action potentials that occur at the peak of a slow wave, the more intense the contraction of the smooth muscle. Because smooth muscle cells contract rather slowly (about a 10th as fast as skeletal muscle cells), the individual contractions caused by each action potential in a train do not cause distinct twitches; rather, they sum temporally to produce a smoothly increasing level of tension.

Between the trains of action potentials, the tension developed by GI smooth muscle falls, but not to zero. This nonzero resting, or baseline, tension of smooth muscle is called **tone.** The tone of GI smooth muscle is altered by neuroeffectors, hormones, paracrine substances, and drugs and is important in the sphincters and also in regions where storage of contents is important, such as the stomach and the colon.

Specialized Patterns of Motility

Peristalsis is a moving ring of contraction that propels material along the GI tract. It involves neurally mediated contraction and relaxation of both muscle layers. Peristalsis occurs in the pharynx, esophagus, gastric antrum, and the small and large intestine.

Segmental contractions produce narrow areas of contracted segments between relaxed segments. These movements allow mixing of the luminal contents with GI tract secretions and increase exposure to the mucosal surfaces where absorption occurs. Segmentation occurs predominantly in the small and large intestine.

There are also characteristic pathological patterns of motility. During **spasm,** maximal contractile activity occurs continuously in a dysregulated manner. In **ileus,** contractile activity is markedly decreased or absent; it often results from irritation of the peritoneum, such as occurs in surgery, peritonitis, and pancreatitis.

GASTRIC MOTILITY

Functional Anatomy of the Stomach

As discussed, the stomach is divided into two functional regions—proximal and distal, with sphincters at either end. The LES and cardia (defined as the region of the stomach immediately surrounding the LES) have important functions. Relaxation of the LES and cardia allows entry of food from the esophagus into the stomach and the release of gas, called belching. By maintaining tone, reflux of contents from the stomach back into the esophagus is prevented.

The proximal part of the stomach (the fundus together with the corpus or body) produces slow changes in tone compatible with its reservoir function. It is important for receiving and storing food and for mixing the contents with gastric juice (Table 28-3). Generation of tone in the proximal portion of the stomach is also an important driving force in the regulation of gastric emptying. Low tone and consequently low intragastric pressure are associated with delayed or slow gastric emptying, and an increase in tone in this region is required for gastric emptying to occur.

The distal part of the stomach is important in the mixing of gastric contents and for propulsion through

● **Table 28-3.**

The Stomach Alters the Physical and Chemical Characteristics of the Meal

Input	Output
Bolus	Emulsion, suspension (particles <2 mm)
Triglyceride	Triglyceride plus small amounts of 2-monoglycerides and free fatty acids
Protein	Protein plus small amounts of peptides and amino acids
Starch	Starch plus oligosaccharides
Water, ions	Addition of large amounts of water and ions of low pH

the pylorus and into the duodenum. The muscle layers in the region of the gastric antrum are much thicker than in the more proximal regions of the stomach, and thus the antrum is capable of producing strong phasic contractions. Contractions, initiated by the slow wave, begin in the midportion of the stomach and move toward the pylorus. The strength of these contractions varies during the postprandial period. In the gastric phase of the meal, the pylorus is usually closed, and these antral contractions serve to mix the gastric contents and reduce the size of solid particles (grinding). However, eventually these antral contractions are also important in emptying the stomach of its contents.

The pyloric sphincter is the **gastroduodenal junction** and is defined as an area of thickened circular muscle. This is a region of high pressure generated by tonic smooth muscle contraction. It is important in regulating gastric emptying.

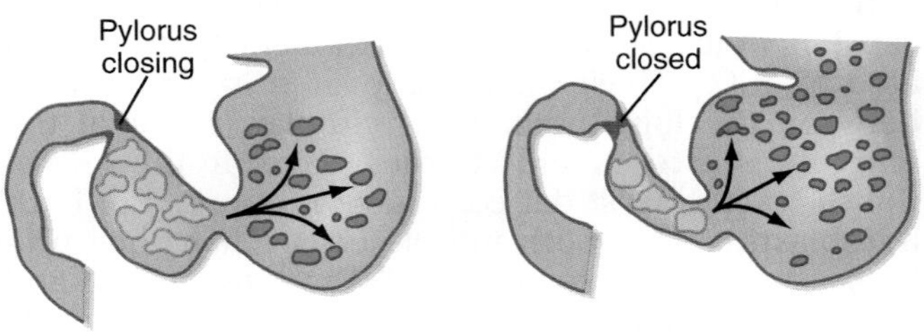

Control of Gastric Motility in the Gastric Phase

Gastric motility is highly regulated and coordinated to perform the functions of storage and mixing. Regulation of emptying of contents into the small intestine, an important part of gastric motor function, will be considered in detail in the discussion of the duodenal phase of the meal because the controls are generated in the duodenum.

The stimuli regulating gastric motor function that result from the presence of the meal in the stomach are both mechanical and chemical and include distention and the presence of products of protein digestion (amino acids and small peptides). The pathways regulating these processes are predominantly neural and consist of vagovagal reflexes initiated by extrinsic vagal afferent fibers that terminate in the muscle and mucosa. Mucosal afferents respond to chemical stimuli, and mechanosensitive afferents respond to distention and contraction of smooth muscle. This afferent stimulation results in reflex activation of vagal efferent (parasympathetic) outflow and activation of enteric neurons that innervate the smooth muscle. Activation of enteric neurons produces both inhibitory and excitatory effects on gastric smooth muscle; these effects vary, depending on the region of the stomach. Thus, distention of the gastric wall results in inhibition of smooth muscle in the proximal portion of the stomach and subsequent reflex accommodation, which allows entry and storage of the meal to occur with minimal increase in intragastric pressure.

In contrast, the predominant motor pattern of the distal part of the stomach in the gastric phase of the meal is activation of smooth muscle to produce and strengthen the antral contractions. The rate of antral contractions is set by the gastric pacemaker; however, the magnitude of the contractions is regulated by the release of neurotransmitters from enteric neurons, including substance P and acetylcholine, which increase the level of depolarization of the smooth

JETLIKE RETROPULSION THROUGH THE ORIFICE OF THE ANTRAL CONTRACTION TRITURATES SOLID PARTICLES

Onset of terminal antral contraction — Pylorus closing

Complete terminal antral contraction — Pylorus closed

• Force for retropulsion is increased pressure in terminal antrum as the antral contraction approaches the closed pylorus.

● **Figure 28-14.** Coordinated activity in the smooth muscle of the proximal and distal portions of the stomach and the pyloric sphincter results in mixing and grinding in the gastric antrum. The peristaltic wave moves down the gastric body and antrum toward the pylorus. If the pylorus is closed, the contents of the gastric antrum are retropulsed back into the more proximal part of the stomach. This pattern of motility results in grinding and mixing of the food with secretions from the gastric wall and eventually leads to a reduction in particle size and the presence of digestive products that will empty into the duodenum.

muscle and therefore produce stronger contractions. In this phase of the meal the pylorus is mostly closed. Thus, antral contractions will tend to move the contents toward the pylorus; however, because the pylorus is closed, the contents will be returned to the more proximal part of the stomach. In this way, the gastric contents will be mixed. In addition, antral contractions can occlude the lumen, and thus larger particles will be dispersed, a process referred to as grinding (Fig. 28-14).

■ KEY CONCEPTS

1. The main functions of the stomach are storage and initiation of protein digestion.

2. Regulation of gastric function is driven by extrinsic and intrinsic neural pathways, together with key humoral (gastrin) and paracrine (histamine) mediators.

3. The key secretions from the stomach are acid and pepsinogen, which together begin protein digestion.

4. H^+ is secreted across the apical plasma membrane of parietal cells via H^+,K^+-ATPase, the proton pump.

5. The only secretion by the stomach that is required is intrinsic factor, which is involved in the absorption of vitamin B_{12}.

6. The gastric epithelium secretes HCO_3^- and mucus to form a gel-like mucosal barrier that protects it against the acidic and peptic luminal contents.

7. The smooth muscle of the gut wall undergoes cyclic changes in membrane potential, termed the basic electrical rhythm or the slow wave.

8. The interstitial cells of Cajal are pacemakers in the gut wall, and they set the frequency of the slow wave.

9. The proximal part of the stomach undergoes a slow change in tone compatible with its storage function.

10. The distal part of the stomach undergoes phasic contractions that can vary considerably in strength.

11. Gastric emptying is regulated by vagovagal reflexes.

CHAPTER 29

The Small Intestinal Phase of the Integrated Response to a Meal

The small intestine is the critical portion of the intestinal tract for assimilation of nutrients. In this site the meal is mixed with a variety of secretions that permit its digestion and absorption, and motility functions serve to ensure adequate mixing and exposure of the intestinal contents **(chyme)** to the absorptive surface. The small intestine has many specializations that enable it to perform its functions efficiently. One of the most obvious specializations is the substantial surface area of the mucosa. This is achieved in a number of different ways: the small intestine is essentially a long tube that is coiled inside the abdominal cavity, there are folds of the full thickness of the mucosa and submucosa, the mucosa has finger-like projections called villi, and finally, each epithelial cell has microvilli on its apical surface. Thus, a large surface area exists over which digestion and absorption occur.

The main characteristic of the small intestinal phase of the response to a meal is controlled delivery of chyme from the stomach to match the digestive and absorptive capacity of the intestine. In addition, there is further stimulation of pancreatic and biliary secretion and emptying of these secretions into the small intestine. Therefore, the function of this region is highly regulated by feedback mechanisms that involve hormonal, paracrine, and neural pathways.

The stimuli that regulate these processes are both mechanical and chemical and include distention of the intestinal wall and the presence of protons, high osmolarity, and nutrients in the intestinal lumen. These stimuli result in a set of changes that represent the intestinal phase of the response to the meal: (1) increased pancreatic secretion, (2) increased gallbladder contraction, (3) relaxation of the sphincter of Oddi, (4) regulation of gastric emptying, (5) inhibition of gastric acid secretion, and (6) interruption of the migrating motor complex (MMC). The goal of this chapter is to discuss how such changes are brought about and how they result ultimately in the assimilation of nutrients. Changes in small intestinal function that occur after the meal has passed through will also be touched on.

GASTRIC EMPTYING IN THE SMALL INTESTINAL PHASE

Immediately after a meal, the stomach may contain up to a liter of material, which will empty slowly into the small intestine. The rate of gastric emptying is dependent on the macronutrient content of the meal and the

amount of solids contained in the meal. Thus, solids and liquids of similar nutritional composition will empty at different rates. Liquids empty rapidly but solids do so only after a lag phase, which means that after a solid meal, there is a period of time during which little or no emptying occurs (Fig. 29-1).

Regulation of gastric emptying is achieved by alterations in motility of the proximal part of the stomach (fundus and corpus) and distal part of the stomach (pylorus and duodenum). Motor function in these regions is highly coordinated. Recall that during the esophageal and gastric phase of the meal, the predominant reflex response is receptive relaxation. At the same time, peristaltic movements in the more distal part of the stomach (antrum) mix the gastric contents with gastric secretions. The pyloric sphincter is largely closed. Even if it opens periodically, little emptying will occur because the proximal portion of the stomach is relaxed and the **antral pump** (antral contractions) is not very strong. Subsequently, gastric emptying is brought about by an increase in tone (intraluminal pressure) in the proximal portion of the stomach, increased strength of antral contractions (increased strength of the antral pump), opening of the pylorus to allow the contents to pass, and simultaneous inhibition of duodenal segmental contractions. Liquids and

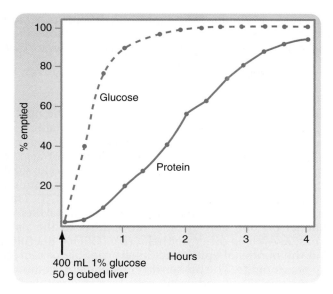

● **Figure 29-1.** Rates of emptying of different meals from a dog's stomach. A solution (1% glucose) is emptied faster than a digestible solid (cubed liver). Note the lag phase for emptying of the solids, which is related to the time needed to reduce particles below 2 mm in size. (Adapted from Hinder RA, Kelly KA: Am J Physiol 233:E335, 1977.)

the semiliquid chyme flow down the pressure gradient from the stomach to the duodenum.

As the meal enters the small intestine, it feeds back via both neural and hormonal pathways to regulate the rate of gastric emptying based on the chemical and physical composition of the chyme. Afferent neurons, predominantly of vagal origin, respond to nutrients, H^+, and the hyperosmotic content of chyme as it enters the duodenum. Reflex activation of vagal efferent outflow decreases the strength of antral contractions, contracts the pylorus, and decreases proximal gastric motility (with a decrease in intragastric pressure), thereby resulting in inhibition (slowing) of gastric emptying. This same pathway is probably responsible for the inhibition of gastric acid secretion that occurs when nutrients are in the duodenal lumen. Cholecystokinin (CCK) is released from endocrine cells in the duodenal mucosa in response to such nutrients. This hormone is physiologically important, in addition to its role in neural pathways, in the regulation of gastric emptying, gallbladder contraction, relaxation of the sphincter of Oddi, and pancreatic secretion. Recent experimental evidence suggests that CCK may act as a hormone not only to inhibit gastric emptying but also to stimulate vagal afferent fiber discharge to produce a vagovagal reflex–mediated decrease in gastric emptying.

How then can gastric emptying proceed in the face of these inhibitory pathways? The amount of chyme in the duodenum decreases as it passes further down the small intestine into the jejunum; thus, the strength of intestinal feedback inhibition fades as there is less activation of the sensory mechanisms in the duodenum by nutrients. At this time, intragastric pressure

in the proximal portion of the stomach increases, thereby moving material into the antrum and toward the antral pump. Antral peristaltic contractions again deepen and culminate in opening of the pylorus and release of gastric contents into the duodenum.

Pancreatic Secretion

Most of the nutrients ingested by humans are in the chemical form of macromolecules. However, such molecules are too large to be assimilated across the epithelial cells that line the intestinal tract and must therefore be broken down into their smaller constituents by processes of chemical and enzymatic digestion. Secretions arising from the pancreas are quantitatively the largest contributors to enzymatic digestion of the meal. The pancreas also provides additional important secretory products that are vital for normal digestive function. Such products include substances that regulate the function or secretion (or both) of other pancreatic products, as well as water and bicarbonate ions. The latter are involved in neutralizing gastric acid so that the small intestinal lumen has a pH approaching 7.0. This is important because pancreatic enzymes are inactivated by high levels of acidity and also because neutralization of gastric acid reduces the likelihood that the small intestinal mucosa will be injured by such acid acting in combination with pepsin. Quantitatively, the pancreas is the largest contributor to the supply of bicarbonate ions needed to neutralize the gastric acid load, although the biliary ductules and duodenal epithelial cells themselves also contribute.

As in the salivary glands, the pancreas has a structure that consists of ducts and **acini.** The pancreatic acinar cells line the blind ends of a branching ductular system that eventually empties into the main pancreatic duct and from there into the small intestine under control of the **sphincter of Oddi.** Also in common with salivary glands, a primary secretion arises in the acini and is then modified as it passes through the pancreatic ducts. In general, the acinar cells supply the organic constituents of the pancreatic juice in a primary secretion whose ionic composition is comparable to that of plasma, whereas the ducts dilute and alkalinize the pancreatic juice while reabsorbing chloride ions (Fig. 29-2). The major constituents of pancreatic juice, which amounts to approximately 1.5 L/day in adult humans, are listed in Table 29-1. This list also outlines the functions of pancreatic secretory products. Many of the digestive enzymes produced by the pancreas, particularly the proteolytic enzymes, are produced as inactive, precursor forms. Storage in these inactive forms appears to be critically important in preventing the pancreas from digesting itself.

Characteristics and Control of Ductular Secretion

In this section we consider how the pancreatic ductular cells contribute to the flow and composition of pancreatic juice in the postprandial period. The ducts of the pancreas can be considered the effector arm of a pH regulatory system designed to respond to luminal acid in the small intestine and secrete just enough bicarbonate to restore pH to neutrality (Fig. 29-3). This regulatory function also requires mechanisms to sense luminal pH and convey this information to the pancreas, as well as other epithelia (e.g., biliary ductules and the duodenal epithelium itself) capable of secreting bicarbonate. The pH-sensing mechanism is embodied in specialized endocrine cells localized within the small intestinal epithelium, known as **S cells.** When luminal pH falls below approximately 4.5, S cells are

---

● AT THE CELLULAR LEVEL

Pancreatitis can result when enzymes secreted by pancreatic acinar cells become proteolytically activated before they have reached their appropriate site of action in the small intestinal lumen. Indeed, pancreatic juice contains a variety of trypsin inhibitors to reduce the risk of such premature activation because trypsin is the activator of other pro-forms of enzymes secreted in pancreatic juice. A second level of protection lies in the fact that trypsin can itself be degraded by other trypsin molecules. However, in some individuals, pancreatitis still arises spontaneously in the absence of known risk factors, as well as in an inherited pattern. This has been mapped to a specific mutation in trypsin that renders it resistant to degradation by other trypsin molecules. In such individuals, if other defenses have been breached and trypsin becomes active prematurely, a vicious cycle of enzyme activation ensues and bouts of pancreatitis follow.

● **Table 29-1.**
Products of Pancreatic Acinar Cells

Precursors of Proteases
Trypsinogen
Chymotrypsinogen
Proelastase
Procarboxypeptidase A
Procarboxypeptidase B
Starch-Digesting Enzymes
Amylase
Lipid-Digesting Enzymes or Precursors
Lipase
Nonspecific esterase
Prophospholipase A$_2$
Nucleases
Deoxyribonuclease
Ribonuclease
Regulatory Factors
Procolipase
Trypsin inhibitors
Monitor peptide

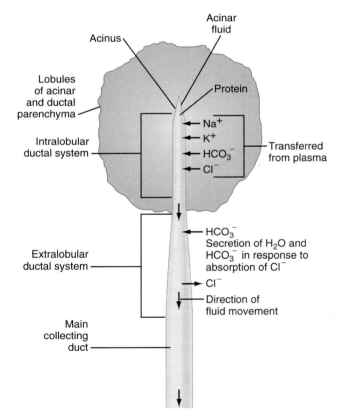

● **Figure 29-2.** Locations of important transport processes involved in the elaboration of pancreatic juice. Acinar fluid is isotonic and resembles plasma in its concentrations of Na$^+$, K$^+$, Cl$^-$, and HCO$_3^-$. Secretion of acinar fluid and the proteins that it contains is stimulated primarily by cholecystokinin. The hormone secretin stimulates secretion of water and electrolytes from the cells that line the extralobular ducts. The secretin-stimulated secretion is richer in HCO$_3^-$ than the acinar secretion because of Cl$^-$/HCO$_3^-$ exchange. (Adapted from Swanson CH, Solomon AK: J Gen Physiol 62:407, 1973.)

triggered to release **secretin,** presumably in response to protons. The components of this regulatory loop constitute a self-limited system. Thus, as secretin evokes secretion of bicarbonate, pH in the small intestinal lumen will rise and the signal for release of secretin from S cells will be terminated.

At the cellular level, secretin directly stimulates epithelial cells to secrete bicarbonate ions into the ductular lumen, with water following via the paracellular route to maintain osmotic equilibrium. Secretin increases cAMP in the ductular cells and thereby opens CFTR Cl^- channels (Fig. 29-4) and causes an outflow of Cl^- into the duct lumen. This secondarily

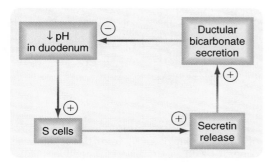

● **Figure 29-3.**   Participation of secretin and HCO_3^- secretion in a classic negative-feedback loop that responds to a fall in luminal pH in the duodenum.

● **Figure 29-4.**   Ion transport pathways in pancreatic duct cells. CA, carbonic anhydrase; CFTR, cystic fibrosis transmembrane conductance regulator; NBC-1, sodium/bicarbonate cotransporter (symporter) type 1; NHE-1, sodium-hydrogen exchanger (antiporter) type 1.

drives the activity of an adjacent antiporter that exchanges the chloride ions for bicarbonate. There is also emerging evidence that CFTR itself may be permeable to some extent to bicarbonate ions when opened. In either case, the bicarbonate secretory process is dependent on CFTR, which provides a rationale for the defects in pancreatic function that are seen in the disease of **cystic fibrosis,** in which CFTR is mutated. The bicarbonate needed for this secretory process is derived from two sources. Some is taken up across the basolateral membrane of the ductular epithelial cells via the symporter NBC-1 (for sodium-bicarbonate cotransporter type 1). Recall that the process of gastric acid secretion results in an increase in circulating bicarbonate ions, which can serve as a source of bicarbonate to be secreted by the pancreas. However, bicarbonate can also be generated intracellularly via the activity of the enzyme carbonic anhydrase. The net effect is to move HCO_3^- into the lumen and thereby increase pH and the volume of pancreatic juice.

Characteristics and Control of Acinar Secretion

In contrast to the pancreatic ductules, where secretin is the most important physiological agonist, CCK plays the predominant role at the level of the acinar cells. Thus, it is important to understand how release of CCK is controlled during the small intestinal phase of the response to a meal.

CCK is the product of **I cells,** which are also localized to the small intestinal epithelium. These classic enteroendocrine cells release CCK into the interstitial

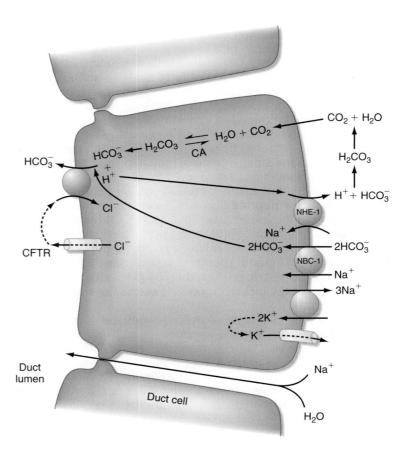

IN THE CLINIC

Cystic fibrosis (CF) is a genetic disease that affects the function of a variety of epithelial organs, including the lung, intestine, biliary system, and pancreas. Previously, the disease was almost uniformly fatal during adolescence as a result of severe respiratory infections, but improved antibiotics can now extend life even into the fifth decade or later in some patients. The disease is caused by a mutation in CFTR, which apparently impairs the ability to hydrate and thus alkalinize the luminal contents. In the gastrointestinal system, specifically, this can result in intestinal obstruction, duodenal mucosal injury, and damage to the liver and biliary system, as well as the pancreas. In some patients the endocrine pancreas will be destroyed even before birth, and these patients are stated to be "pancreatic insufficient" and must be given digestive enzyme supplements to maintain adequate levels of nutrient digestion. In other patients with milder mutations, pancreatitis may develop later in life in the absence of other classic CF symptoms, presumably because of failure to wash digestive enzymes out through the pancreatic ducts. In either case, improved recognition and treatment of the pulmonary complications of CF mean that gastrointestinal symptoms, such as liver failure, reduced bile flow, pancreatitis, obstruction, and maldigestion/malabsorption of nutrients, are acquiring increased importance as facets of the disease that must be managed in adults.

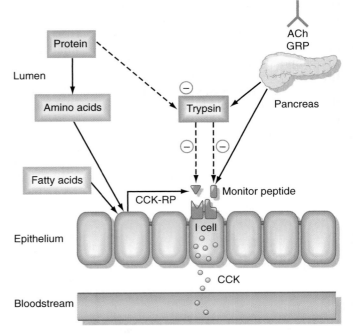

● **Figure 29-5.** Mechanisms responsible for controlling the release of cholecystokinin (CCK) from duodenal I cells. ACh, acetylcholine; CCK-RP, CCK-releasing peptide; GRP, gastrin-releasing peptide. Solid arrows represent stimulatory effects, whereas dashed arrows indicate inhibition. (Redrawn from Barrett KE: Gastrointestinal Physiology. New York, McGraw-Hill, 2006.)

space when specific food components are present in the lumen, particularly free fatty acids and certain amino acids. Release of CCK from I cells may occur as a result of a direct interaction of fatty acids or amino acids, or both, specifically with the I cells themselves. Release of CCK is also regulated by two luminally acting releasing factors that can stimulate the I cell. The first of these, referred to as **CCK-releasing factor** (or **peptide**), is secreted by paracrine cells within the epithelium into the small intestinal lumen, probably in response to products of fat or protein digestion (or both). The second releasing factor, likewise a peptide, is called **monitor peptide** and is released by pancreatic acinar cells into pancreatic juice. Both CCK-releasing factor and monitor peptide can also be released in response to neural input, which is probably particularly important in initiating pancreatic secretion during the cephalic and gastric phases, thereby preparing the system to digest the meal as soon as it enters the small intestine.

What is the significance of these peptide-releasing factors? Their primary role appears to be to match CCK release, as well as the resulting availability of pancreatic enzymes, to the need for these enzymes to digest the meal in the small intestinal lumen (Fig. 29-5). Because the releasing factors are peptides, they will be subject to proteolytic degradation by enzymes such as pancreatic trypsin in exactly the same way as dietary protein. However, when dietary protein is ingested, it is present in much greater amounts in the lumen than the releasing factors and thus "competes" with the releasing factors for proteolytic degradation. The net effect is that the releasing factors will be protected from breakdown while the meal is in the small intestine and are therefore available to continue stimulation of CCK release from I cells. However, once the meal has been digested and absorbed, the releasing factors are degraded and the signal for release of CCK is shut off.

CCK evokes secretion by pancreatic acinar cells in two ways. First, it is a classic hormone that travels through the bloodstream to encounter acinar cell CCK1 receptors. However, CCK also stimulates neural reflex pathways that impinge on the pancreas. Vagal afferent nerve endings in the wall of the small intestine are responsive to CCK by virtue of their expression of CCK1 receptors. As described earlier for the effect of CCK on gastric emptying, binding of CCK activates a vagovagal reflex that can further enhance acinar cell secretion via activation of pancreatic enteric neurons and release of a series of neurotransmitters such as acetylcholine, gastrin-releasing peptide, and vasoactive intestinal polypeptide (VIP).

The secretory products of pancreatic acinar cells are largely presynthesized and stored in granules that cluster toward the apical pole of acinar cells (Fig. 29-6). The most potent stimuli of acinar cell secretion, including CCK itself, acetylcholine, and gastrin-

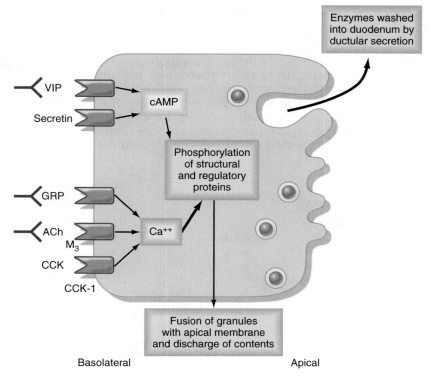

● **Figure 29-6.** Receptors of the pancreatic acinar cell and regulation of secretion. The block arrow indicates that Ca⁺⁺-dependent signaling pathways play the most prominent role. ACh, acetylcholine; CCK, cholecystokinin; GRP, gastrin-releasing peptide; VIP, vasoactive intestinal polypeptide. (Redrawn from Barrett KE: Gastrointestinal Physiology. New York, McGraw-Hill, 2006.)

releasing peptide, act by mobilizing intracellular Ca⁺⁺. Stimulation of acinar cells results in phosphorylation of a series of regulatory and structural proteins within the cell cytosol that serve to move the granules closer to the apical membrane, where fusion of granule and plasma membranes can occur. The contents of the granule are then discharged into the acinar lumen and subsequently washed out of the pancreas by an exudate of plasma crossing the tight junctions linking the acinar cells together and ultimately by ductular secretions. In the period between meals, in contrast, the granule constituents are resynthesized by the acinar cells and then stored until needed to digest the next meal. The signals that mediate granule resynthesis are less well understood, but resynthesis may be stimulated by the same agonists that evoke the initial secretory response.

Biliary Secretion

Another important digestive juice that is mixed with the meal when it is present in the small intestinal lumen is **bile.** Bile is produced by the liver, and the mechanisms that are involved, as well as the specific constituents, will be discussed in greater detail in Chapter 31 when we address the transport and metabolic functions of the liver. However, for purposes of the current discussion, bile is a secretion that serves to aid in the digestion and absorption of lipids. Bile flowing out of the liver is stored and concentrated in the **gallbladder** until it is released in response to ingestion of a meal. Contraction of the gallbladder, as

well as relaxation of the sphincter of Oddi, are evoked predominantly by CCK. Indeed, its ability to contract the gallbladder gave CCK its name.

When considering the small intestinal phase of meal assimilation, the bile constituents that we are most concerned with are the bile acids. These acids form structures known as micelles that serve to shield the hydrophobic products of lipid digestion from the aqueous environment of the lumen. Bile acids are in essence biological detergents, and large quantities are needed on a daily basis for optimal lipid absorption—as much as 1 to 2 g/day. The majority of the bile acid pool is recycled from the intestine back to the liver after each meal via the **enterohepatic circulation** (Fig. 29-7). Thus, bile acids are synthesized in a conjugated form that limits their ability to passively cross the epithelium lining the intestine so that they are retained in the lumen to participate in lipid assimilation (see later). However, when the meal contents reach the terminal ileum, after lipid absorption has been completed, the conjugated bile acids are reabsorbed by a symporter that specifically takes up conjugated bile acids in association with sodium ions, known as the **apical Na⁺-dependent bile acid transporter** (asbt). Only a minor portion of the bile acid pool is left to spill over into the colon in health, and here bile acids become deconjugated and subject to passive reabsorption (Fig. 29-7). The net effect is to cycle the majority of the bile acid pool between the liver and intestine on a daily basis, coincident with signals arising in the postprandial period. For example, CCK is a potent agonist of gallbladder contraction.

CARBOHYDRATE ASSIMILATION

Of course, the most important physiological function of the small intestine is to take up the products of digestion of ingested nutrients. Quantitatively, the most significant nutrients **(macronutrients)** fall into three classes: carbohydrates, proteins, and lipids. The small intestine is critical not only for absorption of such nutrients into the body but also for the final stages of their digestion into molecules that are simple enough to be transported across the intestinal epithe-

lium. We will consider the processes involved in the assimilation of each of these nutrients in turn, beginning with carbohydrates. Carbohydrate digestion occurs in two phases: in the lumen of the intestine and then on the surface of enterocytes in a process known as **brush border digestion.** The latter is thought to be important in generating simple, absorbable sugars only at the point where they can finally be absorbed. This may therefore limit their exposure to the small number of bacteria present in the small intestinal lumen that might otherwise use these sugars as nutrients.

Digestion of Carbohydrates

Dietary **carbohydrates** are composed of several different molecular classes. Starch, the first of these, is a mixture of both straight- and branched-chain polymers of glucose. The straight-chain polymers are called **amylose** and the branched-chain molecules are called **amylopectin** (Fig. 29-8). Starch is a particularly important source of calories, especially in developing countries, and is found predominantly in cereal products. Disaccharides are a second class of carbohydrate nutrients that includes **sucrose** (consisting of glucose and fructose) and **lactose** (consisting of glucose and galactose), which is an important caloric source in infants. It is, however, a key principle that the intestine can absorb only monosaccharides and not larger carbohydrates. Finally, many food items of vegetable origin contain dietary fiber, which consists of carbohydrate polymers that cannot be digested by human enzymes. These polymers are instead digested by bacteria present largely in the colonic lumen (see Chapter 30), thereby allowing salvage of their caloric value.

Dietary disaccharides are hydrolyzed to their component monomers directly on the surface of small intestinal epithelial cells in a process known as brush border digestion, mediated by a family of membrane-bound, heavily glycosylated hydrolytic enzymes synthesized by small intestinal epithelial cells. Brush border hydrolases critical to the digestion of dietary carbohydrates include **sucrase, isomaltase, glucoamylase,** and **lactase** (Table 29-2). Glycosylation of these

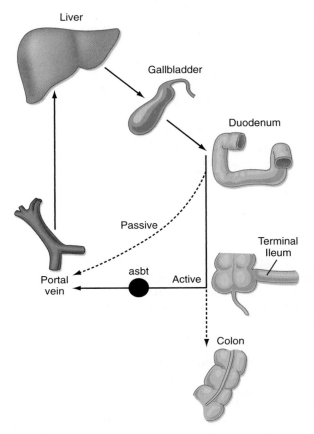

● **Figure 29-7.** Enterohepatic circulation of bile acids.

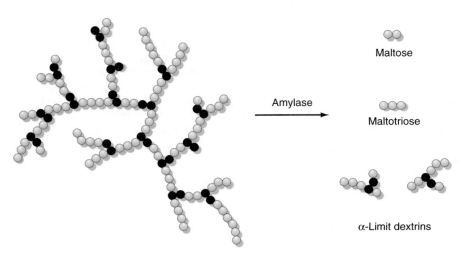

● **Figure 29-8.** Structure of amylopectin and the action of amylase. The colored circles represent glucose monomers linked by α-1,4 bonds. The black circles represent glucose units linked by α-1,6 bonds at the branch points.

Maltose

Maltotriose

α-Limit dextrins

● **Table 29-2.**
Brush Border Carbohydrate Hydrolases

Enzyme	Specificity/Substrates	Products
Sucrase	α-1,4 bonds of maltose, maltotriose, and sucrose	Glucose, fructose
Isomaltase	α-1,4 bonds of maltose, maltotriose; α-1,6 bonds of α-limit dextrins	Glucose
Glucoamylase	α-1,4 bonds of maltose, maltotriose	Glucose
Lactase	Lactose	Glucose, galactose

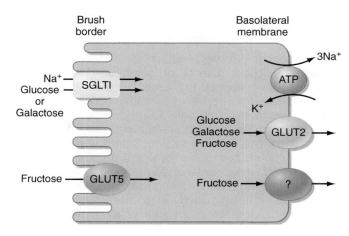

● **Figure 29-9.** Absorption of glucose, galactose, and fructose in the small intestine.

> ### ▶ IN THE CLINIC
>
> Lactose intolerance is relatively common in adults from specific ethnic groups, such as Asians, African Americans, and Hispanics. The disorder reflects a normal developmental decline in the expression of lactase by enterocytes, particularly when lactose is not a consistent component of the diet. In such individuals, consumption of foods containing large quantities of lactose, such as milk and ice cream, can result in abdominal cramping, gas, and diarrhea. These symptoms reflect a relative inability to digest lactose; thus it remains in the lumen and water is retained. Some patients are benefited by administration of a bacterially derived lactase enzyme given in tablet form, before the ingestion of dairy products.

bonds nor the α-1,6 bonds that form the branch points in the amylopectin molecule (Fig. 29-8). Thus, digestion of starch by amylase is of necessity incomplete and results in short oligomers of glucose, including dimers (maltose) and trimers (maltotriose), as well as the simplest branching structures, which are called α-limit dextrins. Thus, to allow absorption of its constituent monosaccharides, starch must also undergo brush border digestion.

At the brush border, straight-chain glucose oligomers can be digested by the hydrolases glucoamylase, sucrase, or isomaltase (Table 29-2). All yield free glucose monomers, which can then be absorbed by the mechanisms discussed later. For α-limit dextrins, on the other hand, isomaltase activity is critical because it is the only enzyme that can cleave not only α-1,4 bonds but also the α-1,6 bonds that make up the branch points.

Uptake of Carbohydrates

Water-soluble monosaccharides resulting from digestion must next be transported across the hydrophobic membrane of the enterocyte. The **sodium/glucose transporter 1** (SGLT1) is a symporter that takes up glucose (and galactose) against its concentration gradient by coupling its transport to that of Na^+ (Fig. 29-9). Once inside the cytosol, glucose and galactose can be retained for the epithelium's metabolic needs or can exit the cell across its basolateral pole via a transporter known as GLUT2. Fructose, in contrast, is taken up across the apical membrane by GLUT5. However, because fructose transport is not coupled to that of Na^+, its uptake is relatively inefficient and can easily be overwhelmed if large quantities of food containing this sugar are ingested. The symptoms that occur from this malabsorption are similar to those experienced by a lactose-intolerant patient who consumes lactose.

PROTEIN ASSIMILATION

Proteins are also water-soluble polymers that must be digested into their smaller constituents before absorption is possible. Their absorption is more complicated

hydrolases is believed to protect them to some extent from degradation by luminal pancreatic proteases. However, between meals, the hydrolases are degraded and must therefore be resynthesized by the enterocyte to participate in digesting the next carbohydrate meal. Sucrase/isomaltase and glucoamylase are synthesized in quantities that are in excess of requirements, and assimilation of their products into the body is limited by the availability of specific membrane transporters for these monosaccharides, as discussed later. Lactase, in contrast, shows a developmental decline in expression after weaning. The relative paucity of lactase means that digestion of lactose, rather than uptake of the resulting products, is rate limiting for assimilation. If lactase levels fall below a certain threshold, the disease of lactose intolerance results.

Digestion of starch occurs in two phases. The first takes place in the lumen and is actually initiated in the oral cavity via the activity of salivary amylase, as discussed in Chapter 27. Salivary amylase, however, is not essential for starch digestion, although it may assume greater importance in neonates or patients in whom the output of pancreatic enzymes is impaired by disease. Quantitatively, the most significant contributor to the luminal digestion of starch is pancreatic amylase. Both enzymes hydrolyze internal α-1,4 bonds in both amylose and amylopectin, but not external

AT THE CELLULAR LEVEL

A rare genetic disorder results in an inability of the intestine to absorb glucose or galactose. This disease state has been mapped to a variety of mutations in the *SGLT1* gene that result in a faulty or unexpressed protein or, more commonly, failure of the protein to traffic appropriately to the apical membrane of enterocytes. In patients carrying such mutations, malabsorbed glucose contributes to diarrheal and other symptoms, as discussed earlier for lactose intolerance. Despite the rarity of the disease, it is important in terms of the insight that it has provided into a critical process of intestinal epithelial transport. Finally, additional, milder mutations in *SGLT1* that reduce transport activity of the protein only partially may nevertheless account for gastrointestinal symptoms and have been implicated in at least some cases of irritable bowel syndrome.

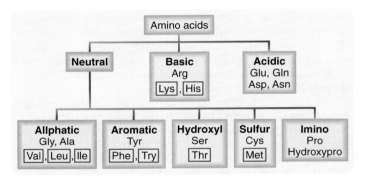

● **Figure 29-10.** Naturally occurring dietary amino acids. Those in boxes are essential amino acids that cannot be synthesized by humans and thus must be obtained from the diet. (Redrawn from Barrett KE: Gastrointestinal Physiology. New York, McGraw-Hill, 2006.)

than that of carbohydrates because they contain 20 different amino acids and short oligomers of these amino acids (dipeptides, tripeptides, and perhaps even tetrapeptides) can also be transported by enterocytes. The body, particularly the liver (see Chapter 31), has substantial ability to interconvert various amino acids subject to the body's needs. However, some amino acids, termed the **essential amino acids,** cannot be synthesized by the body either de novo or from other amino acids and thus must be obtained from the diet. The amino acids that must be obtained in this way in humans are designated in Figure 29-10.

Digestion of Proteins

Proteins can be hydrolyzed to long peptides simply by virtue of the acidic pH that exists in the gastric lumen. However, for assimilation of proteins into the body, three phases of enzymatically mediated digestion are required (Fig. 29-11). Like acid hydrolysis, the first of these phases takes place in the gastric lumen and is

mediated by pepsin, the product of chief cells localized to the gastric glands. When gastric secretion is activated by signals coincident with the ingestion of a meal, pepsin is released from the chief cells as the inactive precursor pepsinogen. At acidic pH, this precursor is autocatalytically cleaved to yield the active enzyme. Pepsin is highly specialized to act in the stomach in that it is activated rather than inhibited by low pH. The enzyme cleaves proteins at sites of neutral amino acids, with a preference for aromatic or large aliphatic side chains. Because such amino acids occur only relatively infrequently in a given protein, pepsin is not capable of digesting protein fully into a form that can be absorbed by the intestine and instead yields a mixture of intact protein, large peptides (the majority), and a limited number of free amino acids.

On moving into the small intestine, the partially digested protein next encounters the proteases provided in pancreatic juice. Recall that these enzymes are secreted in inactive forms. How then are they activated to begin the process of protein digestion? In fact, activation of proteases is delayed until these enzymes are in the lumen by virtue of the localized presence of an activating enzyme, enterokinase, only on the brush border of small intestinal epithelial cells (Fig. 29-12). Enterokinase cleaves trypsinogen to yield active trypsin. Trypsin, in turn, is capable of cleaving all the other protease precursors secreted by the pancreas, thereby resulting in a mixture of enzymes that can almost completely digest the vast majority of dietary proteins. Trypsin is a so-called **endopeptidase** that is capable of cleaving such proteins only at internal bonds within the peptide chain rather than releasing individual amino acids from the end of the chain. Trypsin is specific for cleavage at basic amino acids, and such cleavage results in a set of shorter peptides with a basic amino acid at their C-terminus. The two other pancreatic endopeptidases, chymotrypsin and elastase, on the other hand, have a similar mechanism of action but cleave at sites of neutral amino acids. The peptides that result from endopeptidase activity are then acted on by pancreatic **ectopeptidases.** These enzymes cleave single amino acids from the end of a peptide chain, and those present in pancreatic juice are specific for either neutral **(carboxypeptidase A)** or basic **(carboxypeptidase B)** amino acids situated at the C-terminus. Thus, the products that result overall after digestion of a protein meal by gastric and pancreatic secretions include neutral and basic amino acids, as well as short peptides that have acidic amino acids at their C-termini and thus are resistant to carboxypeptidase A or B (Fig. 29-13).

The final phase of protein digestion then takes place at the brush border. Mature enterocytes express a variety of peptidases on their brush borders, including both aminopeptidases and carboxypeptidases, that generate products suitable for uptake across the apical membrane (Fig. 29-11). However, it should be noted that even with the substantial complement of active proteolytic enzymes, some dietary peptides are either relatively or totally resistant to hydrolysis. In particular, peptides containing either proline or glycine are

● Figure 29-11. Hierarchy of proteases and peptidases that function in the stomach and small intestine to digest dietary protein. Proteins are absorbed as either single amino acids (70%) or short peptides (30%). (Adapted from Van Dyke RW: In Sleisenger MH, Fordtran JS [eds]: Gastrointestinal Disease, 4th ed. Philadelphia, Saunders, 1989.)

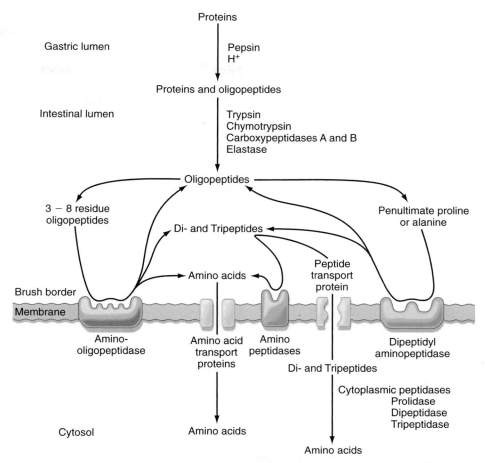

Proteins

Gastric lumen

Pepsin
H+

Proteins and oligopeptides

Intestinal lumen

Trypsin
Chymotrypsin
Carboxypeptidases A and B
Elastase

Oligopeptides

3 − 8 residue oligopeptides

Penultimate proline or alanine

Di- and Tripeptides

Peptide transport protein

Amino acids

Brush border

Membrane

Amino-oligopeptidase

Amino acid transport proteins

Amino peptidases

Di- and Tripeptides

Dipeptidyl aminopeptidase

Cytoplasmic peptidases
Prolidase
Dipeptidase
Tripeptidase

Cytosol

Amino acids

Amino acids

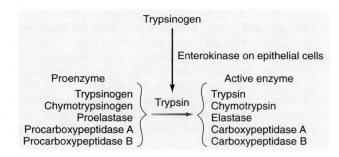

Trypsinogen

Enterokinase on epithelial cells

Proenzyme		Active enzyme
Trypsinogen		Trypsin
Chymotrypsinogen	Trypsin	Chymotrypsin
Proelastase		Elastase
Procarboxypeptidase A		Carboxypeptidase A
Procarboxypeptidase B		Carboxypeptidase B

● Figure 29-12. Conversion of the inactive proenzymes of pancreatic juice to active enzymes by the action of trypsin. Trypsinogen in pancreatic juice is proteolytically converted to active trypsin by enterokinase expressed on the surface of epithelial cells of the duodenum and jejunum. Trypsin then activates the other proenzymes as shown.

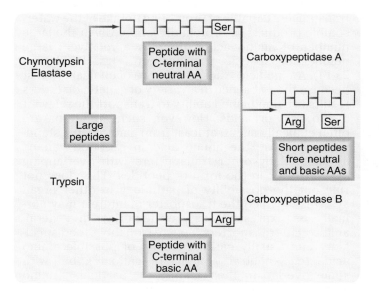

Chymotrypsin
Elastase

Peptide with C-terminal neutral AA

Ser

Carboxypeptidase A

Large peptides

Arg   Ser

Short peptides free neutral and basic AAs

Trypsin

Arg

Carboxypeptidase B

Peptide with C-terminal basic AA

● Figure 29-13. Luminal digestion of peptides resulting from partial proteolysis in the stomach. AA, amino acid. (Redrawn from Barrett KE: Gastrointestinal Physiology. New York, McGraw-Hill, 2006.)

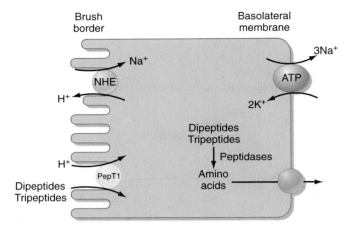

● **Figure 29-14.** A wide variety of dipeptides and tripeptides are taken up across the brush border membrane by the proton-coupled symporter known as PepT1. The proton gradient is created by the action of sodium/hydrogen exchangers (NHEs) in the apical membrane.

digested very slowly. Fortunately, the intestine can take up not only single amino acids but also short peptides. Peptides that are taken up into the enterocyte in their intact form are then subjected to a final stage of digestion in the cytosol of the enterocyte to liberate their constituent amino acids for use in the cell or elsewhere in the body (Fig. 29-14).

UPTAKE OF PEPTIDES AND AMINO ACIDS

The body is also endowed with a series of membrane transporters capable of promoting uptake of the water-soluble products of protein digestion. Given the large number of amino acids, there is a relatively large number of specific transporters (Figs. 29-11 and 29-14). Amino acid transporters are of clinical interest because their absence in a variety of genetic disorders results in a diminished ability to transport the relevant amino acid or acids. However, such mutations are often clinically silent, at least from a nutritional standpoint, because the amino acid in question can be assimilated by other transporters with overlapping specificity or in the form of peptides. This does not rule out the possibility of pathology in other organ systems in which the transporter of interest may normally be expressed (e.g., cysteinuria). In general, amino acid transporters have reasonably broad specificity and usually carry a subset of possible amino acids (e.g., neutral, anionic, or cationic), but with some overlap in their affinity for particular amino acids. Furthermore, some (but not all) of the amino acid transporters are symporters that carry their substrate amino acids in conjunction with obligatory uptake of Na^+.

The small intestine is also notable for its ability to take up short peptides (Fig. 29-14). The primary transporter responsible for such uptake is called PepT1 (for **peptide transporter 1**) and is a symporter that carries

AT THE CELLULAR LEVEL

The redundancy in uptake mechanisms for the products of protein digestion underscores the importance of this process and also means that deficiencies in specific amino acid assimilation across the intestine are relatively rare. However, under certain circumstances, mutations in proteins responsible for specific amino acid transport can lead to pathology in other organs. One example is the disease of cysteinuria, which is a molecularly heterogeneous disease involving mutations in a variety of amino acid transporters capable of transporting cysteine. Because cysteine can also be assimilated across the gut in the form of peptides, nutritional deficiencies do not occur despite a lack of intestinal uptake mechanisms for this particular amino acid. In contrast, cysteine can only be poorly reabsorbed from the urine of patients suffering from cysteinuria, and kidney stones can form because this amino acid is relatively insoluble. Pathophysiology can likewise arise secondary to mutations in SLC6A19, a Na^+-independent transporter of neutral amino acids, and result in a condition known as Hartnup's disease. Again, nutritional deficiencies are relatively rare, but such patients may lose neutral amino acids in urine and display symptoms related to the importance of such amino acids in the brain and skin.

peptides in conjunction with protons. Peptides taken up into enterocytes are then immediately hydrolyzed by a series of cytosolic peptidases into their constituent amino acids. Amino acids not required by the enterocyte are in turn exported across the basolateral membrane and enter blood capillaries to be transported to the liver via the portal vein. PepT1 is also of clinical interest because it can mediate the uptake of so-called **peptidomimetic drugs,** which include a variety of antibiotics, as well as cancer chemotherapeutic agents. The mechanisms by which amino acids and peptidomimetic drugs exit the enterocyte are not fully understood but are presumed to involve additional transport proteins.

LIPID ASSIMILATION

Lipids, defined as substances that are more soluble in organic solvents than in water, are the third major class of macronutrients making up the human diet. Lipids supply more significant calories on a per-gram basis than proteins or carbohydrates do and are thus of major nutritional significance, as well as having a propensity to contribute to obesity if consumed in excessive amounts. Lipids also dissolve volatile compounds that contribute to the food's taste and aroma.

The predominant form of lipid in the human diet is triglyceride, found in oils and other fats. The majority of these triglycerides have long-chain fatty acids (carbon chains longer than 12 carbons) esterified to the glycerol backbone. Additional lipid is supplied in the form of phospholipids and cholesterol, mostly arising from cell membranes. It is also important to consider that the intestine is presented daily not only with dietary lipid but also with lipid originating from the liver in biliary secretions, as described in more detail in Chapter 31. Indeed, the cholesterol supplied in bile exceeds that provided in the diet on a daily basis in all but the most egg-loving individuals. Finally, though present in only trace amounts, the fat-soluble vitamins (A, D, E and K) are essential nutrients that should be supplied in the diet to avoid disease. These substances are almost entirely insoluble in water and thus require special handling to promote their uptake into the body.

Emulsification and Solubilization of Lipids

When a fatty meal is ingested, the lipid becomes liquefied at body temperature and floats on the surface of the gastric contents. This would limit the area of the interface between the aqueous and lipid phases of the gastric contents and thus restrict access of enzymes capable of breaking down the lipid to forms that can be absorbed because the lipolytic enzymes, as proteins, reside in the aqueous phase. Therefore, an early stage in the assimilation of lipid is its emulsification. The mixing action of the stomach churns the dietary lipid into a suspension of fine droplets, which vastly increases the surface area of the lipid phase.

Lipid absorption is also facilitated by the formation of a micellar solution with the aid of bile acids supplied in biliary secretions. Details of this process will be discussed subsequently.

Digestion of Lipids

Lipid digestion begins in the stomach. Gastric lipase is released in large quantities from gastric chief cells; it adsorbs to the surface of fat droplets dispersed in the gastric contents and hydrolyzes component triglycerides to diglycerides and free fatty acids. However, little lipid assimilation can take place in the stomach because of the acidic pH of the lumen, which results in protonation of the free fatty acids released by gastric lipase. Lipolysis is also incomplete in the stomach because gastric lipase, despite its optimum catalytic activity at acidic pH, is not capable of hydrolyzing the second position of the triglyceride ester, which means that the molecule cannot be fully broken down into components that can be absorbed into the body. There is also little if any breakdown of cholesterol esters or the esters of fat-soluble vitamins. Indeed, gastric lipolysis is dispensable in healthy individuals because of the marked excess of pancreatic enzymes.

The majority of lipolysis takes place in the small intestine in health. Pancreatic juice contains three important lipolytic enzymes that are optimized for activity at neutral pH. The first of these is pancreatic lipase. This enzyme differs from the stomach enzyme in that it is capable of hydrolyzing both the 1 and 2 positions of triglyceride to yield a large quantity of free fatty acids and monoglycerides. At neutral pH, the head groups of the free fatty acids are charged, and thus these molecules migrate to the surface of the oil droplets. Lipase also displays an apparent paradox in that it is inhibited by bile acids, which also form part of the small intestinal contents. Bile acids adsorb to the surface of the oil droplets and would thereby cause lipase to dissociate. However, lipase activity is sustained by an important cofactor, colipase, which is also supplied in pancreatic juice. Colipase is a bridging molecule that binds both to bile acids and to lipase; it anchors lipase to the oil droplet even in the presence of bile acids.

Pancreatic juice also contains two additional enzymes that are important in fat digestion. The first of these is phospholipase A_2, which hydrolyzes phospholipids such as those present in cell membranes. Predictably, this enzyme would be quite toxic in the absence of dietary substrates, and thus it is secreted as an inactive pro-form that is activated only when it reaches the small intestine. Furthermore, pancreatic juice contains a relatively nonspecific, so-called cholesterol esterase that can break down not only esters of cholesterol, as its name implies, but also esters of fat-soluble vitamins and even triglycerides. Interestingly, this enzyme *requires* bile acids for activity (contrast with lipase, discussed earlier), and it is related to an enzyme produced in breast milk that plays an important role in lipolysis in neonates.

As lipolysis proceeds, the products are abstracted from the lipid droplet, first into a lamellar, or membrane, phase and subsequently into mixed micelles composed of lipolytic products, as well as bile acids. The amphipathic (meaning that they have both a hydrophobic and hydrophilic face) bile acids serve to shield the hydrophobic regions of lipolytic products from water while presenting their own hydrophilic faces to the aqueous environment (Fig. 29-15). Micelles are truly in solution and thus markedly increase the solubility of lipid in the intestinal contents. This increases the rate at which molecules such as fatty acids can diffuse to the absorptive epithelial surface. Nevertheless, given the very large surface area of the small intestine and the appreciable solubility of the products of triglyceride hydrolysis, micelles are not essential for the absorption of triglyceride. Thus, patients who have insufficient output of bile acids (caused, for example, by a gallstone that obstructs bile output) do not normally show fat malabsorption. On the other hand, cholesterol and the fat-soluble vitamins are almost totally insoluble in water and accordingly require micelles to be absorbed even after they have been digested. Thus, if luminal bile acid concentrations fall below the critical micellar concentration, patients can become deficient in fat-soluble vitamins.

Uptake of Lipids and Subsequent Handling

The products of fat digestion are believed to be capable of crossing cell membranes readily because of their lipophilicity. However, recent evidence suggests that their uptake may alternatively or additionally be regulated via the activity of specific membrane transporters. A microvillus membrane fatty acid–binding protein (MVM-FABP) provides for the uptake of long-chain fatty acids across the brush border. Likewise, Niemann

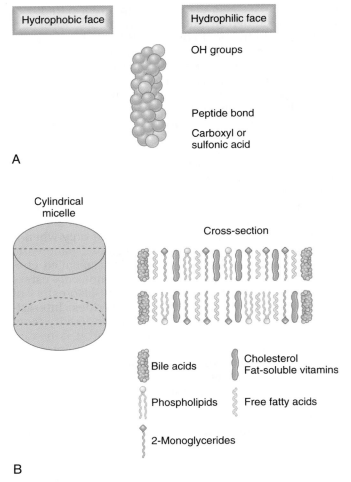

Hydrophobic face

Hydrophilic face

OH groups

Peptide bond

Carboxyl or
sulfonic acid

A

Cylindrical
micelle

Cross-section

Bile acids

Cholesterol
Fat-soluble vitamins

Phospholipids

Free fatty acids

2-Monoglycerides

B

● **Figure 29-15.** Schematic depiction of bile acids **(A)** and mixed micelles **(B).** Bile acids in solution are amphipathic. Mixed micelles are cylindrical assemblages of bile acids with other dietary lipids.

IN THE CLINIC

A relatively new treatment of hypercholesterolemia targets absorption of cholesterol, either derived from the diet or in bile, across the small intestinal epithelium. Ezetimibe is a drug that specifically blocks uptake of cholesterol by inhibiting the activity of the NPC1L1 protein expressed in the apical membrane of enterocytes. In conjunction with other drugs designed to counter atherosclerosis, this may be a useful adjunct in that it can interrupt the enterohepatic circulation, as well as prevent the absorption of dietary cholesterol. Clinical studies suggest that ezetimibe may synergistically improve the efficacy of other strategies designed to reduce circulating levels of low-density lipoprotein cholesterol in those at risk for cardiovascular disease.

Pick C1 like 1 (NPC1L1) has recently been identified as an uptake pathway for cholesterol and may be a therapeutic target in patients who suffer from pathological increases in circulating cholesterol (hypercholesterolemia). However, uptake of cholesterol overall is relatively inefficient because this molecule, along with plant sterols, can also be actively effluxed from enterocytes back into the cytosol by a heterodimeric complex of two so-called "ABC" (ATP-binding cassette) transporters termed ABC G5 and G8.

Lipids also differ from carbohydrates and proteins in terms of their fate after absorption into the enterocyte. Unlike monosaccharides and amino acids, which leave the enterocyte in molecular form and enter the portal circulation, the products of lipolysis are reesterified in the enterocyte to form triglycerides, phospholipids, and cholesterol esters. These metabolic events take place in the smooth endoplasmic reticulum. Concurrently, the enterocyte synthesizes a series of proteins known as apolipoproteins in the rough endoplasmic reticulum. These proteins are then combined with the resynthesized lipids to form a structure known as a **chylomicron,** which consists of a lipid core (predominantly triglyceride with much less cholesterol, phospholipid, and fat-soluble vitamin esters) coated by the apolipoproteins. The chylomicrons are then exported from the enterocyte by a process of exocytosis. However, on entering the lamina propria, they are too large (approximately 750 to 5000 Å in diameter) to permeate through the intercellular spaces of the mucosal capillaries. Instead, they are taken up into lymphatics in the lamina propria and as such bypass the portal circulation and, at least for their first pass, the liver. Eventually, chylomicrons in the lymph enter the bloodstream via the thoracic duct and then serve as the vehicle to transport lipids around the body for use by cells in other organs. The only exception to this chylomicron-mediated transport is for medium-chain fatty acids. These acids are relatively water soluble and can also permeate enterocyte tight junctions appreciably, which means that they bypass the intracellular processing steps described earlier and are not packaged into chylomicrons. They therefore enter the portal circulation and are more readily available to other tissues. A diet rich in medium-chain triglycerides may be of particular benefit in patients with inadequate bile acid pools.

WATER AND ELECTROLYTE SECRETION AND ABSORPTION

The foregoing description of digestion has stressed that these processes take place in the small intestine in an aqueous milieu. The fluidity of intestinal contents, especially in the small intestine, is important in allowing the meal to be propelled along the length of the intestine and to permit digested nutrients to diffuse to their site of absorption. Part of this fluid is derived from oral intake, but in most adults this consists of only about 1 or 2 L/day derived from both food and drink (Fig. 29-16). Additional fluid is supplied by the stomach and the small intestine themselves, as well as

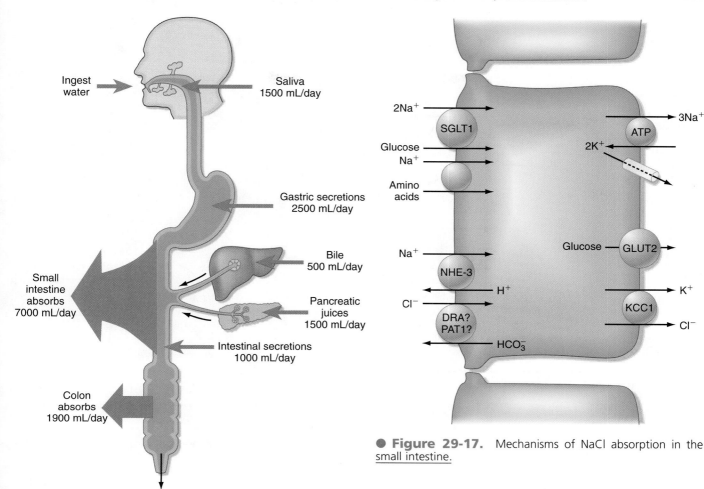

Ingest water

Saliva
1500 mL/day

Gastric secretions
2500 mL/day

Bile
500 mL/day

Pancreatic
juices
1500 mL/day

Intestinal secretions
1000 mL/day

Small
intestine
absorbs
7000 mL/day

Colon
absorbs
1900 mL/day

Water excreted

● **Figure 29-16.** Overall fluid balance in the human gastrointestinal tract. About 2 L of water is ingested and 7 L of various secretions enters the gastrointestinal tract. Of this total, most is absorbed in the small intestine. About 2 L is passed onto the colon, the vast majority of which is absorbed in health. (From Vander AJ et al: Human Physiology, 6th ed. New York, McGraw-Hill, 1994.)

● **Figure 29-17.** Mechanisms of NaCl absorption in the small intestine.

the organs that drain into the gastrointestinal tract. In total, these secretions add another 8 L, which means that the intestine is presented with approximately 9 L of fluid on a daily basis. However, in health only about 2 L of this load is passed to the colon for reabsorption, and eventually only 100 to 200 mL exits in stool. Thus, the transport vector for fluid throughout the intestine emphasizes absorption. During the postprandial period, such absorption is promoted in the small intestine predominantly via the osmotic effects of nutrient absorption. An osmotic gradient is established across the intestinal epithelium that simultaneously drives the movement of water across the tight junctions. The generic mechanism for nutrient-driven Na^+ and water absorption in the small intestine is diagrammed in Figure 29-17. Moreover, in the period between meals, when nutrients are absent, fluid absorption can still occur via the coupled uptake of Na^+ and Cl^- mediated

by the cooperative interaction of the NHE-3 Na^+-H^+ antiporter and a Cl^--HCO_3^- antiporter (see Fig. 29-17).

Even though net water and electrolyte transport in the small intestine predominantly follows an absorptive vector, this does not imply that the tissue fails to participate in electrolyte secretion. Secretion is regulated in response to signals derived from the luminal contents and in response to deformation of the mucosa or intestinal distention, or both. Critical secretagogues include acetylcholine, VIP, prostaglandins, and serotonin. Secretion makes sure that the intestinal contents are appropriately fluid while digestion and absorption are still ongoing and may be important to lubricate the passage of food particles along the length of the intestine. For example, some clinical evidence suggests that constipation and intestinal obstruction, the latter being seen in the disease of cystic fibrosis, can result when secretion is abnormally low. The majority of the intestinal secretory flow of fluid into the lumen is driven by the active secretion of chloride ions via the mechanism diagrammed in Figure 29-18. Some segments of the intestine may engage in additional secretory mechanisms, such as secretion of bicarbonate ions via the mechanisms shown in Figure 29-19. Presumably, this local bicarbonate protects the epithelium, particularly in the most proximal portions of the duodenum immediately downstream from the pylorus, from damage caused by acid and pepsin.

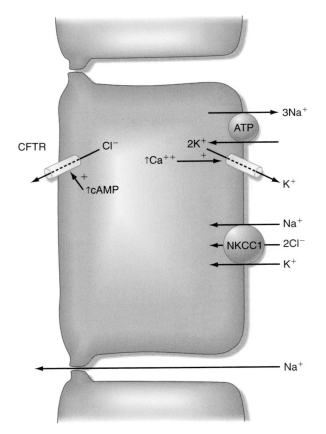

● **Figure 29-18.** Mechanism of Cl⁻ secretion in the small and large intestines.

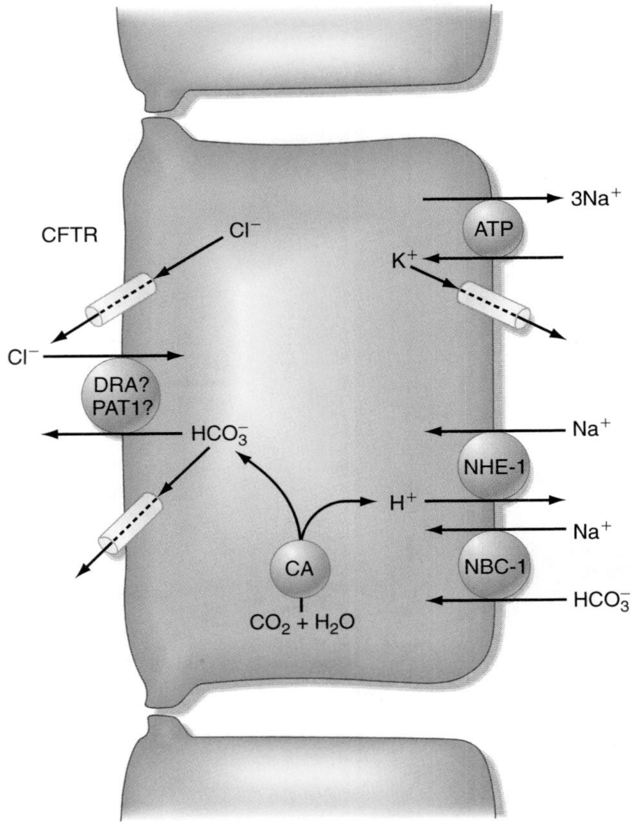

● **Figure 29-19.** Mechanisms of bicarbonate secretion in the duodenum. CA, carbonic anhydrase.

MOTOR PATTERNS OF THE SMALL INTESTINE

Based on the discussions in preceding chapters of this section, it should be possible to predict that the smooth muscle layers of the small intestine act to mix chyme with the various digestive secretions and to move it along the length of the intestine so that its nutrients (along with water and electrolytes) can be absorbed. Motor patterns of the small intestine during the postprandial period are directed predominantly toward mixing and consist largely of segmenting and retropulsive contractions that retard the meal while digestion is still ongoing. **Segmentation** is a stereotypical pattern of rhythmic contractions that is displayed in Figure 29-20 and presumably reflects programmed activity of the enteric nervous system superimposed on the basic electrical rhythm. Hormonal mediators of the fed pattern of motility are poorly defined, although CCK probably contributes. CCK also plays important roles in slowing gastric emptying when the meal is in the small intestine, as described at the beginning of this chapter. This makes sense as a mechanism to match nutrient delivery to the available capacity to digest and absorb the components of the meal.

After the meal has been digested and absorbed, it is desirable to clear any undigested residues from the lumen to prepare the intestine for the next meal. Such clearance is effected by **peristalsis** (Fig. 29-21), a coordinated sequence of contraction occurring above the intestinal contents and relaxation below that permits the contents to be conveyed over considerable distances. Peristalsis reflects the action of acetylcholine and substance P released orad to a site of intestinal distention, which serves to contract the circular muscle, as well as the inhibitory effects of VIP and nitric oxide on the caudad side. Like segmentation, peristalsis originates when action potentials generated by intrinsic innervation are superimposed on sites of cellular depolarization dictated by the basic electrical rhythm. The peristaltic motor patterns that occur during fasting, moreover, are organized into a sequence of phases known as the **migrating motor complex** (Fig. 29-22). Phase I of the MMC is characterized by relative quiescence, whereas small disorganized contractions begin to occur during phase II. During phase III, which lasts about 10 minutes, large contractions that propagate along the length of the intestine are stimulated by the hormone motilin and sweep any remaining gastric and intestinal contents out into the colon. The pylorus and ileocecal valve open fully during this phase, so even large undigested items can eventually pass from the body. Motility of the intestine then reverts to phase I of the MMC, with the entire cycle taking about 90 minutes in adults

---

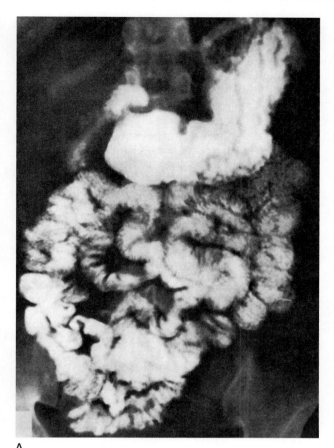

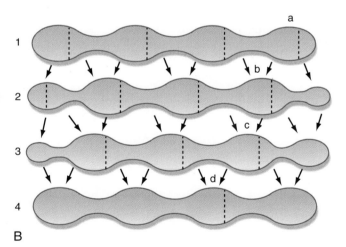

● Figure 29-20. **A,** Radiographic view showing the stomach and small intestine filled with barium contrast medium in a normal individual. Note the segmentation of the intestine. **B,** Sequence of segmental contractions in the small intestine. Lines 1 to 4 represent sequential time points. The dotted lines indicate where contractions will occur next; the arrows depict the direction of movement of the intestinal contents. (**A,** From Gardener EM et al: Anatomy: A Regional Study of Human Structure, 4th ed. Philadelphia, Saunders, 1975; **B,** redrawn from Cannon WB: Am J Physiol 6:251, 1902.)

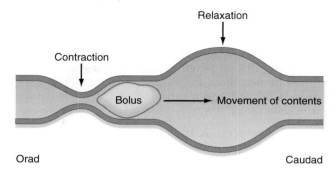

● Figure 29-21. Peristaltic motility in the intestine propels the intestinal contents along the length of the small intestine.

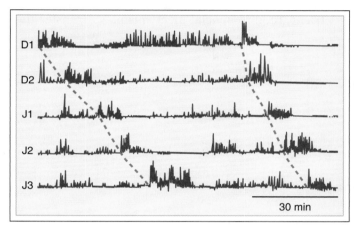

● Figure 29-22. Migrating motor complexes in the duodenum and jejunum as recorded from a fasting human subject by manometry. D1, D2, J1, J2, and J3 indicate sequential recording points along the length of the duodenum and jejunum. The intense contractions (phase III) propagate aborally. (Redrawn from Soffer EE et al: Am J Gastroenterol 93:1318, 1998.)

unless a meal is ingested, in which case the MMC is suspended. After the meal, motilin levels fall (although the mechanisms are unclear), and the MMC cannot be resumed until they rise again.

■ KEY CONCEPTS

1. On leaving the stomach, the meal enters the small intestine, which consists (sequentially) of the duodenum, jejunum, and ileum. The principal function of the small intestine is to digest and absorb the nutrients contained in the meal.

2. The presence of chyme in the duodenum retards additional gastric emptying, thus helping match nutrient delivery to the ability of the small intestine to digest and absorb such substances.

3. Digestion and absorption in the small intestine are aided by two digestive juices derived from the pancreas (pancreatic juice) and liver (bile). These secretions are triggered by hormonal and neural

signals activated by the presence of the meal in the small intestine.

4. Pancreatic secretions arise from the acini and contain various proteins capable of digesting the meal or acting as important cofactors. The secretion is diluted and alkalinized as it passes through the pancreatic ducts.

5. Bile is produced by the liver and stored in the gallbladder until needed in the postprandial period. Bile acids, important components of bile, are biological detergents that solubilize the products of lipid digestion.

6. Carbohydrates and proteins, water-soluble macromolecules, are digested and absorbed by broadly analogous mechanisms. Lipids, the third macronutrient, require special mechanisms to transfer the products of lipolysis to the epithelial surface, where they can be absorbed.

7. The small intestine transfers large volumes of fluid into and out of the lumen on a daily basis to facilitate the digestion and absorption of nutrients, driven by the active transport of ions and other electrolytes.

8. The motor patterns of the small intestine vary depending on whether a meal has been ingested. Immediately after a meal, motility is directed to retaining the meal in the small intestine, mixing it with digestive juices, and providing sufficient time for absorption of nutrients. During fasting, a "housekeeper" complex of intense contractions (the migrating motor complex) sweeps periodically along the length of the stomach and small intestine to clear them of undigested residues.

CHAPTER 30

The Colonic Phase of the Integrated Response to a Meal

OVERVIEW OF THE LARGE INTESTINE

The most distal segment of the gastrointestinal tract is called the **large intestine,** which is composed of the **cecum;** ascending, transverse, and descending portions of the **colon;** the **rectum;** and the **anus** (Fig. 30-1). The primary functions of the large intestine are to digest and absorb components of the meal that cannot be digested or absorbed more proximally, reabsorb the remaining fluid that was used during movement of the meal along the gastrointestinal tract, and store the waste products of the meal until they can conveniently be eliminated from the body. In fulfilling these functions, the large intestine uses characteristic motility patterns and expresses transport mechanisms that drive the absorption of fluid, electrolytes, and other solutes from the stool. The large intestine also contains a unique biological ecosystem consisting of many trillions of so-called **commensal bacteria** that engage in a life-long symbiotic relationship with their human host. These bacteria can metabolize components of the meal that are not digested by host enzymes and make their products available to the body via a process known as **fermentation.** Colonic bacteria also metabolize other endogenous substances such as bile acids and bilirubin, thereby influencing their disposition. There is emerging evidence that the colonic flora is critically involved in promoting development of the normal colonic epithelium and in stimulating its differentiated functions. In addition, these bacteria detoxify xenobiotics (substances originating outside the body, such as drugs) and protect the colonic epithelium from infection by invasive pathogens. Finally, the colon is both the recipient and the source of signals that allow it to communicate with other gastrointestinal segments to optimally integrate function. For example, when the stomach is filled with freshly masticated food, the presence of the meal triggers a long reflex arc that results in increased colonic motility (the **gastrocolic reflex**) and eventually evacuation of the colonic contents to make way for the residues of the next meal. Similarly, the presence of luminal contents in the colon causes the release of both endocrine and neurocrine mediators that slow propulsive motility and decrease electrolyte secretion in the small intestine. This negative-feedback mechanism matches the rate of delivery of colonic contents to the segment's capacity to process and absorb the useful components. Details

of the signals that mediate this crosstalk between the colon and other components of the gastrointestinal system are reviewed in the next section.

Signals That Regulate Colonic Function

The colon is regulated primarily, though not exclusively, by neural pathways. Colonic motility is influenced by local reflexes that are generated by filling of the lumen, thereby initiating distention and the activation of stretch receptors. These regulatory pathways exclusively involve the enteric nervous system. Local reflexes, triggered by distortion of the colonic epithelium and produced, for example, by the passage of a bolus of fecal material, stimulate short bursts of Cl⁻ and fluid secretion mediated by 5-hydroxytryptamine (5-HT) from enteroendocrine cells and acetylcholine from enteric secretomotor nerves. On the other hand, colonic function and motility responses in particular are also regulated by long reflex arcs originating more proximally in the gastrointestinal tract or in other body systems. One example of such a reflex is the gastrocolic reflex. Distention of the stomach activates a generalized increase in colonic motility and mass movement of fecal material, as described in more detail later. This reflex has both chemosensitive and mechanosensitive components at its site of origin and involves the release of 5-HT and acetylcholine. Similarly, the **orthocolic reflex** is activated on rising from bed and promotes a morning urge to defecate in many individuals.

The colon is relatively poorly supplied with cells that release bioactive peptides and other regulatory factors. Exceptions are **enterochromaffin cells,** which release 5-HT, and cells that synthesize **peptide YY,** so named because its sequence contains two adjacent tyrosine residues (Y is the single letter code for amino acids). Peptide YY is synthesized by enteroendocrine cells localized in the terminal ileum and colon and is released in response to lipid in the lumen. It decreases gastric emptying and intestinal propulsive motility. Peptide YY also reduces Cl⁻ and thus fluid secretion by intestinal epithelial cells. Thus, peptide YY has been characterized as an **"ileal brake"** in that it is released if nutrients, especially fat, are not absorbed by the time that the meal reaches the terminal ileum and proximal part of the colon. By reducing propulsion of the intestinal contents, in part by limiting their fluidity and distention-induced motility, peptide YY

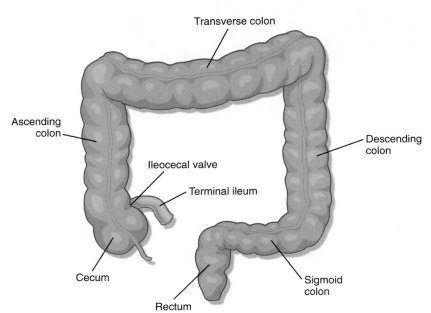

● **Figure 30-1.** Major anatomic subdivisions of the colon.

Transverse colon

Ascending colon

Ileocecal valve

Terminal ileum

Descending colon

Cecum

Rectum

Sigmoid colon

provides more time for the meal to be retained in the small intestine, where its constituent nutrients can be digested and absorbed.

Patterns of Colonic Motility

To appreciate colonic motility, the functional anatomy of the colonic musculature will be reviewed first, followed by a discussion of the regulation of colonic motility.

Functional Anatomy of the Colonic Musculature

As in other segments of the intestine, the colon consists of functional layers with a columnar epithelium most closely opposed to the lumen, which is then underlaid by the lamina propria, serosa, and muscle layers. Similarly, the colonic mucosa is surrounded by continuous layers of circular muscle that can occlude the lumen. Indeed, at intervals, the circular muscle contracts to divide the colon into segments called **haustra.** These haustra are readily appreciated if the colon is viewed at laparotomy or by x-ray imaging as shown in Figure 30-2. The arrangement of the majority of the longitudinal muscle fibers, however, is distinct from that in the small intestine. Three nonoverlapping bands of longitudinal muscle, known as the **taeniae coli,** extend along the length of the colon.

Although the circular and longitudinal muscle layers of the colon are electrically coupled, this process is less efficient than in the small intestine. Thus, propulsive motility in the colon is less effective than in the small intestine. Activity of the enteric nervous system also provides for the segmenting contractions that form the haustra. Contents can be moved back and forward between haustra, which is a means of retarding passage of the colonic contents and maximizing their contact time with the epithelium. In contrast, when rapid propulsion is called for, the contractions

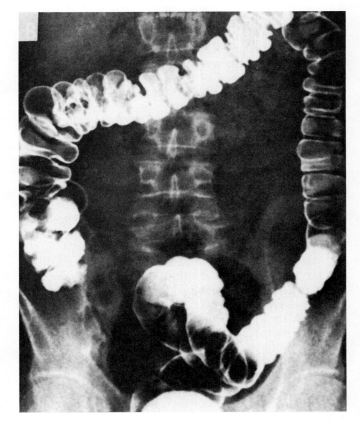

● **Figure 30-2.** Radiograph showing a prominent haustral pattern in the colon of a normal individual. (From Keats TE: An Atlas of Normal Roentgen Variants, 2nd ed. St Louis, Mosby–Year Book, 1979.)

forming the haustra relax, and the contour of the colon is smoothened.

The colon terminates in the **rectum,** which is joined to the colon at an acute angle (the **rectosigmoid junction**) (Fig. 30-3). The rectum lacks circular muscle and

AT THE CELLULAR LEVEL

Hirschsprung's disease is a condition in which a segment of the colon remains permanently contracted and results in obstruction. It is typically diagnosed in infancy and affects up to 1 in 5000 live births in the United States. The basis of the disease is failure of the enteric nervous system to develop normally during fetal life. During organogenesis, cells destined to become enteric neurons migrate out from the neural crest and populate the gut sequentially from mouth to anus. In some individuals, this migration terminates prematurely because of abnormalities in the mechanisms that would otherwise drive this process. Mutations in glial-derived neurotrophic factor and endothelin III, as well as in their receptors, have been described in individuals suffering from this disease, and the affected segment completely lacks the plexuses of the enteric nervous system and associated ganglia. A relative deficiency of interstitial cells of Cajal is also seen in the affected segment, and overall control of motility is markedly impaired. In most individuals, the symptoms can be completely alleviated by surgical excision of the affected segment.

is surrounded only by longitudinal muscle fibers. It is a reservoir wherein feces can be stored before defecation. Muscular contractions also form functional "valves" in the rectum that retard the movement of feces and are important in delaying the loss of feces until it is convenient, at least in adults. The rectum, in turn, joins the anal canal, distinguished by the fact that it is surrounded not only by smooth muscle but also by striated (skeletal) muscle. The combination of these muscle layers functionally accounts for two key sphincters that control the evacuation of solid waste and flatus from the body. The **internal anal sphincter** is composed of a thickened band of circular muscle, whereas the **external anal sphincter** is made up of three different striated muscle structures in the pelvic cavity that wrap around the anal canal. These latter muscles are distinctive because they maintain a significant level of basal tone and can be contracted further either voluntarily or reflexively when abdominal pressure increases abruptly (such as when lifting a heavy object).

Contraction of the smooth muscle layers in the proximal part of the colon is stimulated by vagal input, as well as by the enteric nervous system. On the other hand, the remainder of the colon is innervated by the pelvic nerves, which also control the caliber of the internal anal sphincter. Voluntary input from the spinal cord via branches of the pudendal nerves regulates contraction of the external anal sphincter and muscles of the pelvic floor. The ability to control these structures is learned during toilet training. This voluntary

● **Figure 30-3.** Anatomy of the rectum and anal canal.

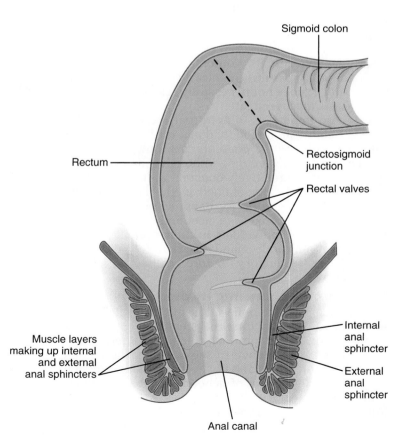

control distinguishes the anal canal from most of the gastrointestinal system, with the exception of the striated muscle in the esophagus that regulates swallowing.

Colonic Motility Responses

Consistent with its primary function, the two predominant motility patterns of the large intestine are directed not to propulsion of the colonic contents but rather to mixing of the contents and retarding their movement, thereby providing them with ample time in contact with the epithelium. Two distinctive forms of colonic motility have been identified. The first is referred to as short-duration contractions, which are designed to provide for mixing. These contractions originate in the circular muscle and are stationary pressure waves that persist for approximately 8 seconds on average. Long-duration contractions, in contrast, are produced by the taeniae coli, last for 20 to 60 seconds, and may propagate over short distances. Notably, however, propagation may move orally as well as aborally, particularly in the more proximal segments of the colon. Both these motility patterns are thought to originate largely in response to local conditions, such as distention. Note that the basal electrical rhythm that governs the rate and origination sites of smooth muscle contraction in the small intestine does not traverse the ileocecal valve to continue into the colon.

On the other hand, probably as a result of both local influences and long reflex arcs, approximately 10 times per day in healthy individuals the colon engages in a motility pattern that is of high intensity and sweeps along the length of the large intestine from the cecum to the rectum. Such contractions, which are labeled **"high-amplitude propagating contractions,"** move exclusively in an aboral direction and are designed to clear the colon of its contents. However, although such a motility pattern can clearly be associated with defecation, it does not necessarily result in defecation for reasons discussed later.

It is also important to note that there is considerable variability among individuals with respect to the rate at which colonic contents are transported from the cecum to the rectum. Although small intestinal transit times are relatively constant in healthy adults, the contents may be retained in the large intestine anywhere from hours to days without signifying dysfunction. This likewise accounts for significant variation among individuals in their normal patterns of defecation and mandates careful elicitation of a patient's history before diagnosing bowel dysfunction.

Transport Mechanisms in the Colon

The surface cells are renewed from stem cells located at the base of the crypts; the stem cells give rise to migrating cells that gradually acquire differentiated properties as they move to the surface. The colonic epithelium turns over rapidly even in health, thus limiting the accumulation of genetic damage that might otherwise be caused by exposure to toxins in the lumen. However, the rapid turnover also increases the risk for malignancy. The major role of the colonic

> ## IN THE CLINIC

Irritable bowel syndrome is the name given to a heterogeneous collection of disorders whose sufferers complain of diarrhea, constipation, or alternating patterns of both, often with accompanying pain and distention. The precise cause or causes of these disorders are still not fully understood but may involve, in part, a condition of **visceral hypersensitivity** in which the individual perceives normal signals originating from the bowel (such as in response to distention) as painful. This hypersensitivity may be at the level of the enteric or central nervous system (or both) and can be triggered by a variety of factors such as previous infections, childhood abuse, or psychiatric disorders. Most treatments focus on symptomatic relief, but there is the promise of more effective therapies as we learn more about the underlying causes of the condition. Treatment of patients with irritable bowel disorders, which are often refractory to therapy, forms a major part of the practice of many gastroenterologists in the community.

> ## IN THE CLINIC

The rapid turnover of the colonic epithelium, as well as frequent/prolonged exposure to bacterially synthesized or environmental toxins, or both, makes the large intestine especially vulnerable to malignancy. Colon cancer is second in prevalence only to lung cancer in men in the United States and third behind lung and breast cancer in women. With the decreased incidence of cigarette smoking, colon cancer may assume even greater significance. Colon cancer arises when normal genetic controls on the rate of epithelial proliferation are subverted; initially, this leads to growth of a polyp and, eventually, if not removed, to an invasive tumor that may metastasize to other parts of the body. Colon cancer can be subdivided according to the basic nature of the underlying molecular defect, which can include overexpression of growth stimulatory factors or a mutation that prevents the cells from responding to factors that would normally be growth suppressive. However, colon cancer mortality can be reduced very substantially by early detection and removal of polyps with malignant potential. This has driven current guidelines for increased screening of even asymptomatic middle-aged individuals for colonic abnormalities via colonoscopy (in which a flexible fiberoptic tube is inserted into the colon to inspect its interior), screening for the presence of so-called occult (or hidden) blood in the stool derived from a bleeding polyp or tumor, or noninvasive imaging techniques such as computed tomography scans.

epithelium is to either absorb or secrete electrolytes and water rather than nutrients. Secretion, which is confined to the crypts, maintains the sterility of the crypts, which might otherwise become stagnant. However, the colonic epithelium absorbs short-chain fatty acids salvaged from nonabsorbed carbohydrates by colonic bacteria. Indeed, one such short-chain fatty acid, butyrate, is a critical energy source for colonocytes. A reduction in butyrate levels in the lumen (as a result of changes in colonic flora caused by the administration of broad-spectrum antibiotics) may induce epithelial dysfunction.

The colon receives 2 L of fluid each day and absorbs 1.8 L, thus leaving 200 mL of fluid to be lost in stool. The colon has a considerable reserve capacity for fluid absorption and can absorb up to three times its normal fluid load without loss of excessive fluid into stool. Therefore, any illness that results in the stimulation of active fluid secretion in the small intestine will cause diarrhea only when the reserve capacity of 4 to 6 L is exceeded.

Absorption and secretion of water by the colon are passive processes driven by the absorption or secretion of electrolytes and other solutes. Quantitatively, fluid absorption by the colon is driven by three transport processes. The first is electroneutral NaCl absorption, which is mediated by the same mechanism that drives NaCl absorption in the intestine (see Fig. 29-17). NaCl absorption is stimulated by various growth factors, such as epidermal growth factor, and is inhibited by hormones and neurotransmitters that increase levels of cAMP in colonic surface epithelial cells.

The second transport process that drives fluid absorption in the colon is the absorption of **short-chain fatty acids,** including acetate, propionate, and butyrate. These molecules are absorbed from the lumen by surface (and perhaps crypt) epithelial cells in an Na^+-dependent fashion by a family of symporters related to the Na^+-glucose symporter in the small intestine known as **sodium-monocarboxylate transporters** (SMCTs). Uptake of short-chain fatty acids by SMCTs located in the apical plasma membrane is driven by the low intracellular $[Na^+]$ established by the basolateral Na^+,K^+-ATPase (Fig. 30-4). These short-chain fatty acids are used for energy by colonocytes. In addition, butyrate regulates the expression of specific genes in colonic epithelial cells and may suppress the development of a malignant phenotype. Expression of **SMCT1** (also identified as SLC5A8) is reduced in some colon cancers, thereby leading to a reduction in butyrate uptake, which may contribute to malignant transformation.

The third absorptive process of major significance in the colon is the absorption of Na^+ (Fig. 30-5). This transport process is predominantly localized to the distal part of the colon and is driven by the epithelial Na^+ channel ENaC, which is also involved in reabsorption of Na^+ in the kidney. When the channel is opened in response to activation by neurotransmitters or hormones, or both, Na^+ flows into the colonocyte cytosol and is then transported across the basolateral membrane by Na^+,K^+-ATPase. Water and Cl^- ions follow passively via the intercellular tight junctions to maintain electrical neutrality. This mode of Na^+ absorption is the last line of defense to prevent excessive loss of water in stool, given its strategic location in the distal part of the colon. Indeed, patients suffering from bowel

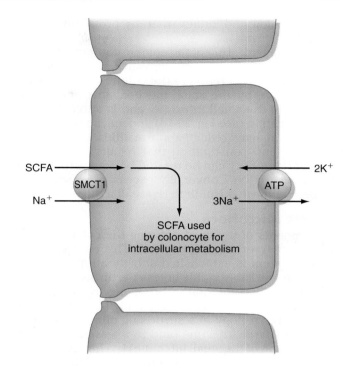

● **Figure 30-4.** Mechanism of short-chain fatty acid (SCFA) uptake by colonocytes.

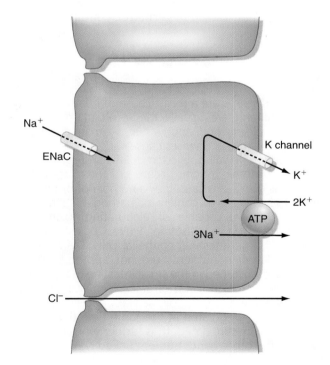

● **Figure 30-5.** Electrogenic Na^+ absorption in the colon.

inflammation often show markedly diminished expression of ENaC, perhaps accounting for their diarrheal symptoms. We also know that expression of ENaC can be acutely regulated in response to whole-body Na^+ balance. Thus, in situations of reduced Na^+ intake, the hormone aldosterone increases ENaC expression in both the colon and kidney, thereby promoting retention of Na^+.

Adequate hydration of the colonic contents is determined by the balance between water absorption and secretion. Fluid secretion in the colon is driven by Cl^- ion secretion, by the same mechanism driving fluid secretion in the small intestine, and is subject to the same regulation (see Fig. 29-18). Indeed, some cases of constipation may reflect abnormalities in epithelial transport, and constipation that results from abnormally slow motility can be treated by agents that stimulate Cl^- secretion. Conversely, excessive Cl^- secretion can be one mechanism underlying diarrhea.

Colonic Microflora

The remnants of the meal entering the colon interact with a vast assortment of bacteria. This **enteric bacterial ecosystem** is established shortly after birth and remains remarkably stable unless perturbed by antibiotics or the introduction of an aggressive pathogen. The enteric bacterial ecosystem contributes to gastrointestinal physiology in a surprising number of ways. Indeed, the large intestine (and to a lesser extent the distal portion of the small intestine) is a highly unusual organ in that it maintains a symbiotic relationship with the bacterial ecosystem, whereas other body compartments are largely sterile.

The colonic microflora is not essential to life because animals raised in germ-free conditions apparently develop normally and are able to reproduce. However, in such animals the mucosal immune system is immature, and intestinal epithelial cells differentiate more slowly. However, the colonic flora provides benefits to the host in that the constituent bacteria are capable of performing metabolic reactions that do not take place in mammalian cells. Bacterial enzymes act on both endogenous and exogenous substrates. They form secondary bile acids and deconjugate any bile acids that have escaped uptake in the terminal ileum so that they can be reabsorbed. They convert bilirubin into urobilinogen (see Chapter 31) and salvage nutrients that are resistant to pancreatic and brush border hydrolases, such as dietary fiber. A summary of the metabolic contributions of the colonic microflora is provided in Table 30-1. Bacterial metabolism can also be exploited for pharmacological purposes. A drug targeted to the colon, for example, can be conjugated in such a way that it will become bioavailable only after it is acted on by bacterial enzymes. Bacterial enzymes may also detoxify some dietary carcinogens, but equally, they may generate toxic or carcinogenic compounds from dietary substrates.

Commensal microorganisms also play a critical role in limiting the growth or invasion (or both) of pathogenic microorganisms. They fulfill this antimicrobial role via a number of different mechanisms—by synthesizing and secreting compounds that inhibit the growth of competitor organisms or that are microbicidal, by

---

▶ IN THE CLINIC

Diarrheal diseases are a major cause of infant mortality worldwide and are usually the result of inadequate access to clean food and water. Even in developed countries, diarrheal diseases cause substantial suffering and occasional, well-publicized deaths and carry a substantial economic burden because of their prevalence. Infectious diarrhea is caused by a number of organisms, with several (such as cholera or pathogenic strains of *Escherichia coli*) capable of elaborating toxins that trigger excessive increases in active Cl^- secretion by small and large intestinal epithelial cells. Diarrhea can also result when nutrients are not appropriately digested and absorbed in the small intestine (e.g., lactose intolerance) or as a result of colonic inflammation. In most diarrheal diseases, colonic NaCl and Na^+ absorption are down-regulated at the same time that Cl^- secretion may be stimulated, thus further worsening fluid loss. On the other hand, nutrient-linked Na^+ absorptive processes typically remain intact. This provides the rationale for the effectiveness of so-called oral rehydration solutions, which are prepackaged mixtures of salt and glucose. Uptake of Na^+ and glucose from these solutions, mediated by SGLT1 (see Chapter 29), drives water back into the body to balance osmotic forces. These solutions save lives in areas where diarrhea is prevalent and the ability to rehydrate patients with sterile intravenous solutions is limited or absent.

● AT THE CELLULAR LEVEL

A toxin known as heat-stable toxin of *E. coli,* or STa, is a major causative agent of traveler's diarrhea, which can be contracted by the consumption of infected food or water. This toxin binds to a receptor on the apical surface of intestinal epithelial cells known as guanylyl cyclase C (GC-C). In turn, this enzyme generates large quantities of intracellular cGMP that trigger increased Cl^- secretion via activation of the cystic fibrosis transmembrane conductance regulator (CFTR) Cl^- channel. However, one could, of course, question, why humans express a receptor for this toxin in a site that would be accessible to luminal bacteria and their products. Indeed, this led to the hypothesis that there is a native ligand for GC-C that could play a physiological role. This hypothesis led to purification and identification of guanylin, a hormone synthesized in the intestine. Together with a related molecule, uroguanylin, secreted by the kidney, guanylin is an important regulator of salt and water homeostasis in the body. STa has structural similarities to guanylin, but it has modifications that permit it to persist in the intestinal lumen for prolonged periods. This is an example of molecular mimicry in which a bacterial product hijacks a receptor and associated signaling for its own purposes (presumably to propagate the toxin-producing bacteria to additional hosts).

● **Table 30-1.** **Metabolic Effects of Enteric Bacteria**

Substrate	Enzymes	Products	Disposition
Endogenous Substrates			
Urea	Urease	Ammonia	Passive absorption or excretion as ammonium
Bilirubin	Reductases	Urobilinogen Stercobilins	Passive reabsorption Excreted
Primary bile acids	Dehydroxylases	Secondary bile acids	Passive reabsorption
Conjugated bile acids (primary or secondary)	Deconjugases	Unconjugated bile acids	Passive reabsorption
Exogenous Substrates			
Fiber	Glycosidases	Short-chain fatty acids Hydrogen, CO_2, and methane	Active absorption Excreted in breath or flatus
Amino acids	Decarboxylases and deaminases	Ammonia and bicarbonate	Reabsorbed or excreted (ammonia) as ammonium
Cysteine, methionine	Sulfatases	Hydrogen sulfide	Excreted in flatus

Adapted from Barrett KE: Gastrointestinal Physiology. New York, McGraw-Hill, 2006.

functioning as a physical barrier to prevent attachment of pathogens and their subsequent entry into colonic epithelial cells, and by triggering patterns of gene expression in the epithelium that counteract the adverse effects of pathogens on epithelial function. These mechanisms provide a basis for understanding why patients who have received broad-spectrum antibiotics, which temporarily disrupt the colonic microflora, are susceptible to overgrowth of pathogenic organisms and associated intestinal and systemic infections. They may also shed light on the efficacy of **probiotics,** commensal bacteria selected for their resistance to gastric acid and proteolysis that are intentionally ingested to prevent or treat a variety of digestive disorders.

The colonic microflora is also notable for its contribution to the formation of **intestinal gas.** Although large volumes of air may be swallowed in conjunction with meals, the majority of this gas returns up the esophagus via belching. However, during fermentation of unabsorbed dietary components, the microflora generates large volumes of nitrogen, hydrogen, and carbon dioxide. Approximately 1 L of these nonodorous gases is excreted on a daily basis via the anus in all individuals, even those who do not complain of flatulence. Some individuals may generate appreciable concentrations of methane. Trace amounts of odorous compounds are also present, such as hydrogen sulfide, indole, and skatole.

Defecation

The final stage in the journey taken by a meal after its ingestion is expulsion of its indigestible residues from the body in the process known as **defecation.** The feces also contain the remnants of dead bacteria; dead and dying epithelial cells that have been desquamated from the lining of the intestine; biliary metabolites specifically targeted for excretion, such as conjugates of xenobiotics (see Chapter 31); and a small amount of water. In health, the stool contains little, if any useful nutrients. The presence of such nutrients in stool, particularly lipid (known as **steatorrhea**), signifies maldigestion, malabsorption, or both. Fat in the stool is a sensitive marker of small intestinal dysfunction because it is poorly used by the colonic microflora, but loss of carbohydrate and protein in stool can also be seen if the underlying condition worsens.

The process of defecation requires coordinated action of the smooth and striated muscle layers in the rectum and anus, as well as surrounding structures such as the pelvic floor muscles. During the mass movement of feces produced by high-amplitude propagating contractions, the rectum fills with fecal material. Expulsion of this material from the body is controlled by the internal and external anal sphincters, which contribute approximately 70% to 80% and 20% to 30% of anal tone at rest, respectively. Filling of the rectum causes relaxation of the internal anal sphincter via the release of vasoactive intestinal polypeptide and the generation of nitric oxide. Relaxation of the inner sphincter permits the **anal sampling mechanism,** which can distinguish whether the rectal contents are solid, liquid, or gaseous in nature. After toilet training, sensory nerve endings in the anal mucosa then generate reflexes that initiate appropriate activity of the external sphincter to either retain the rectal contents or permit voluntary expulsion (e.g., of flatus). If defecation is not convenient, the external sphincter contracts to prevent the loss of stool. Then, with time, the rectum accommodates to its new volume, the internal anal sphincter contracts again, and the external anal sphincter relaxes (Fig. 30-6).

When defecation is desired, on the other hand, adoption of a sitting or squatting position alters the relative orientation of the intestine and surrounding muscular structures by straightening the path for the exit of either solid or liquid feces. Relaxation of the puborectalis muscle likewise increases the rectoanal angle. After voluntary relaxation of the external anal sphincter, rectal contractions move the fecal material out of the body, sometimes followed by additional mass movements of feces from more proximal segments of the colon (Fig. 30-7). Evacuation is assisted by simultaneous contraction of muscles that increase abdominal pressure, such as the diaphragm. The voluntary expulsion of flatus, on the other hand, involves

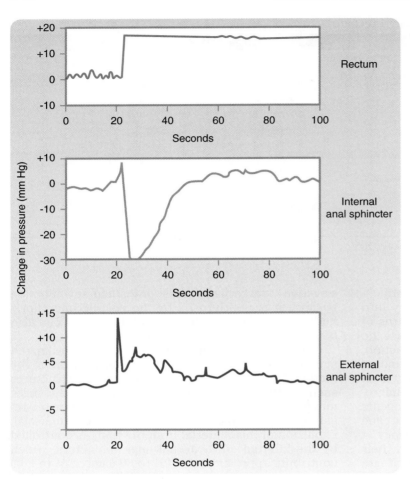

● **Figure 30-6.** Responses of the internal and external anal sphincters to prolonged distention of the rectum. Note that the responses of the sphincters are transient because of accommodation. (Redrawn from Shuster MM et al: Bull Johns Hopkins Hosp 116:79, 1965.)

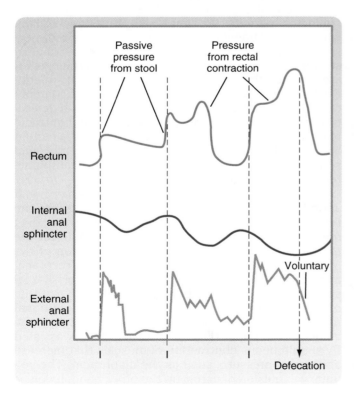

● **Figure 30-7.** Motility of the rectum and anal sphincters in response to rectal filling and during defecation. Note that filling of the rectum causes an initial decrease in internal sphincter tone that is counterbalanced by contraction of the external sphincter. The internal sphincter then accommodates to the new rectal volume, thereby allowing the external sphincter to relax. Finally, defecation occurs when the external anal sphincter is relaxed voluntarily. (Data from Chang EB et al: Gastrointestinal, Hepatobiliary and Nutritional Physiology. Philadelphia, Lippincott-Raven, 1996.)

a similar sequence of events, except that there is no relaxation of the puborectalis muscle. This permits flatus to be squeezed past the acute rectoanal angle while retaining fecal material.

Cooperative activity of the external anal sphincter, puborectalis muscle, and sensory nerve endings in the anal canal is required to delay defecation until it is appropriate, even if the rectum is acutely distended with stool or intraabdominal pressure rises sharply. This explains why incontinence can develop in individuals in whom the integrity of such structures has been compromised, such as after trauma, surgical or obstetrical injuries, prolapse of the rectum, or neuropathic diseases such as long-standing diabetes. Surgical intervention may be necessary to correct muscle abnormalities in patients with the distressing condition of fecal incontinence, although many can be helped to increase the tone of their external anal sphincter with the use of biofeedback exercises.

■ KEY CONCEPTS

1. The final segment of the intestine through which the meal traverses is the large intestine, which is composed of the cecum, colon, rectum, and anus. The primary role of the large intestine is to reclaim water used during the process of digestion and absorption and to store the residues of the meal until defecation is socially convenient.

2. Colonic motility primarily serves to mix and delay passage of the luminal contents, other than during periodic large-amplitude contractions that convey fecal material to the rectum.

3. The colon is highly active in transporting water and electrolytes, as well as products salvaged from undigested components of the meal by colonic bacteria.

4. The colon maintains a life-long, mutually beneficial relationship with a vast bacterial ecosystem that metabolizes endogenous substances, nutrients, and drugs and protects the host from infection with pathogens.

5. Defecation involves both involuntary and voluntary relaxation of muscle structures surrounding the anus and reflex pathways that control these structures.

CHAPTER 31

Transport and Metabolic Functions of the Liver

OVERVIEW OF THE LIVER AND ITS FUNCTIONS

The liver is a large, multilobed organ located in the abdominal cavity whose function is intimately associated with that of the gastrointestinal system. The liver serves as the first site of processing for most absorbed nutrients and also secretes bile acids, which as we learned in Chapter 29, plays a critical role in the absorption of lipids from the diet. In addition, the liver is a metabolic powerhouse, critical for disposing of a variety of metabolic waste products and xenobiotics from the body by converting them to forms that can be excreted. The liver stores or produces numerous substances needed by the body, such as glucose, amino acids, and plasma proteins. In general, key functions of the liver can be divided into three areas: (1) contributions to whole-body metabolism, (2) detoxification, and (3) excretion of protein-bound/lipid-soluble waste products. In this chapter we discuss the structural and molecular features of the liver and the biliary system that subserve these functions, as well as their regulation. However, although the liver contributes in a pivotal way to the maintenance of whole-body biochemical status, a complete discussion of all of the underpinning reactions is beyond the scope of the present text. We will confine our discussion primarily to hepatic functions that relate to gastrointestinal physiology.

Metabolic Functions of the Liver

Hepatocytes contribute to metabolism of the major nutrients: carbohydrates, lipids, and proteins. Thus, the liver plays an important role in glucose metabolism by engaging in **gluconeogenesis,** the conversion of other sugars to glucose. The liver also stores glucose as glycogen at times of glucose excess (such as in the postprandial period) and then releases stored glucose into the bloodstream as it is needed. This process is referred to as the **"glucose buffer function of the liver."** When hepatic function is impaired, glucose concentrations in blood may rise excessively after the ingestion of carbohydrate; conversely, between meals, hypoglycemia may be seen because of an inability of the liver to contribute to carbohydrate metabolism and interconversion of one sugar to another.

Hepatocytes also participate in lipid metabolism. They are a particularly rich source of the metabolic enzymes engaged in **fatty acid oxidation** to supply energy for other body functions. Hepatocytes also convert products of carbohydrate metabolism to lipids that can be stored in adipose tissue and synthesize large quantities of lipoproteins, cholesterol, and phospholipids, the latter two being important in the biogenesis of cell membranes. In addition, hepatocytes convert a considerable portion of synthesized cholesterol to bile acids, of which we will discuss more later in this chapter.

The liver also plays a vital role in protein metabolism. The liver synthesizes all of the so-called **nonessential amino acids** (see Chapter 29) that do not need to be supplied in the diet, in addition to participating in interconverting and deaminating amino acids so that the products can enter biosynthetic pathways for the synthesis of carbohydrates. With the exception of immunoglobulins, the liver synthesizes almost all of the proteins present in plasma, especially **albumin,** which determines plasma oncotic pressure, as well as most of the important **clotting factors.** Patients suffering from liver disease may develop peripheral edema secondary to hypoalbuminemia and are also susceptible to bleeding disorders. Finally, the liver is the critical site for disposal of the ammonia generated from protein catabolism. This is accomplished by converting ammonia to urea, which can then be excreted by the kidneys. The details of this process will be discussed later.

The Liver and Detoxification

The liver serves both as a gatekeeper, by limiting the entry of toxic substances into the bloodstream, and as a garbage disposal, by extracting potentially toxic metabolic products produced elsewhere in the body and converting them to chemical forms that can be excreted. The liver fulfills these functions, in part, because of its unusual blood supply. Unlike all other organs, the majority of blood arriving at the liver is venous in nature and is supplied via the **portal vein** from the intestine (Fig. 31-1). As such, the liver is strategically located to receive not only absorbed nutrients but also potentially harmful absorbed molecules such as drugs and bacterial toxins. Depending on the efficiency with which these molecules are extracted by hepatocytes and subjected to so-called **first-pass metabolism,** little or none of the absorbed substance may make it into the systemic circulation. This is a major reason why not all pharmaceutical agents can

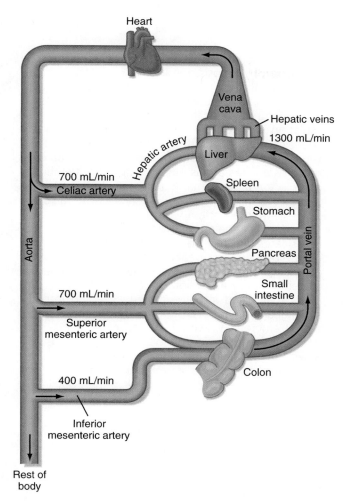

● **Figure 31-1.** Typical blood flow through the splanchnic circulation in a fasting adult human.

● **Table 31-1.**
Key Transporters of Hepatocytes

Name	Basolateral	Canalicular	Substrate/Function
NTCP	Yes	No	Uptake of conjugated bile acids
OATP	Yes	No	Uptake of bile acids and xenobiotics
BSEP	No	Yes	Secretion of conjugated bile acids
MDR3	No	Yes	Secretion of phosphatidylcholine
MDR1	No	Yes	Secretion of cationic xenobiotics
ABC5/ABC8	No	Yes	Secretion of cholesterol
cMOAT/MRP2	No	Yes	Secretion of sulfated lithocholic acid and conjugated bilirubin

achieve therapeutic concentrations in the bloodstream if administered orally.

The liver has two levels at which it removes and metabolizes/detoxifies substances originating from the portal circulation. The first of these is physical. Blood arriving in the liver percolates among cells of macrophage lineage, known as **Kupffer cells.** These cells are phagocytic and are particularly important in removing particulate material from portal blood, including bacteria that may enter blood from the colon even under normal conditions. The second level of defense is biochemical. Hepatocytes are endowed with a broad array of enzymes that metabolize and modify both endogenous and exogenous toxins so that the products are, in general, more water soluble and less susceptible to reuptake by the intestine. The metabolic reactions involved are broadly divided into two classes. **Phase I reactions** (oxidation, hydroxylation, and other reactions catalyzed by cytochrome P-450 enzymes) are followed by **phase II reactions** that conjugate the resulting products with another molecule, such as glucuronic acid, sulfate, amino acids, or glutathione, to promote their excretion. The products of these reactions are then excreted into bile or returned to the bloodstream to ultimately be excreted by the kidneys. We will return to the precise mechanisms involved in the detoxification of some key metabolic waste products later.

Role of the Liver in Excretion

The kidneys play an important role in the excretion of water-soluble catabolites, as discussed in the renal section. Only relatively small water-soluble catabolites can be excreted by the process of glomerular filtration. However, larger water-soluble catabolites and molecules bound to plasma proteins, including lipophilic metabolites and xenobiotics, steroid hormones, and heavy metals, cannot be filtered by the glomerulus. All these substances are potentially harmful if allowed to accumulate, so a mechanism must exist for their excretion. The mechanism for excretion involves the liver, which excretes these substances in bile. Hepatocytes take up these substances with high affinity by virtue of the presence of an array of basolateral membrane transporters, and the substances are subsequently metabolized at the level of microsomes and in the cytosol (Table 31-1). Ultimately, substances destined for excretion in bile are exported across the canalicular membrane of hepatocytes via a different array of transporters. The features of bile allow solubilization of even lipophilic substances, which can then be excreted into the intestine and ultimately leave the body in feces.

STRUCTURAL FEATURES OF THE LIVER AND BILIARY SYSTEM

Hepatocytes, the major cell type in the liver, are arranged in anastomosing cords that form plates around which large volumes of blood circulate (Fig. 31-2). The liver receives a high blood flow that is disproportionate to its mass, which ensures that hepatocytes receive high quantities of both O_2 and nutrients. Hepatocytes receive more than 70% of their blood supply at rest via the portal vein (rising to more than 90% in the postprandial period).

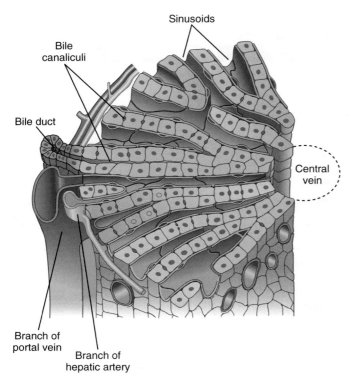

● Figure 31-2. Diagrammatic representation of a hepatic lobule. Plates of hepatocytes are arrayed radially around a central vein. Branches of the portal vein and hepatic artery are located on the periphery of the lobule and form the "portal triad" together with the bile duct. Blood from the portal vein and hepatic artery percolates around the hepatocytes via the sinusoids before draining into the central vein. (Modified from Bloom W, Fawcett DW: A Textbook of Histology, 10th ed. Philadelphia, Saunders, 1975.)

The plates of hepatocytes that constitute the **liver parenchyma** are supplied by a series of **sinusoids,** which are low-resistance cavities supplied by branches of both the portal vein and the **hepatic artery.** The sinusoids are unlike the capillaries that perfuse other organs. During fasting, many sinusoids are collapsed, but more can gradually be recruited as portal blood flow increases during the period after a meal when absorbed nutrients are transported to the liver. The low resistance of the sinusoidal cavities means that blood flow through the liver can increase considerably without a concomitant increase in pressure. Eventually, the blood drains into central branches of the **hepatic vein.**

The sinusoids are also unusual in the endothelial cells that line their walls (Fig. 31-3). Hepatic endothelial cells contain specialized openings, known as **fenestrations,** that are large enough to permit the passage of molecules as big as albumin. Sinusoidal endothelial cells also lack a basement membrane, which might otherwise pose a diffusion barrier. These features allow access of albumin-bound substances to the hepatocytes that will eventually take them up. The sinusoids also contain Kupffer cells. Beneath the sinusoidal endothelium and separating the endothelium

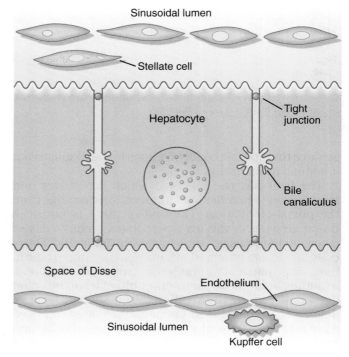

● Figure 31-3. Interrelationships of the major cell types in the liver.

from the hepatocytes is a thin layer of loose connective tissue called the **space of Disse,** which likewise poses little resistance to the movement of molecules even as large as albumin in health. The space of Disse is also the location of another important hepatic cell

Infection of the liver with certain viruses or overexposure to toxic substances such as alcohol kills hepatocytes and activates hepatic stellate cells, which synthesize excessive amounts of collagen that result in the histologic appearance of fibrosis. If the insult is chronic, the fibrosis eventually becomes irreversible, a condition known as **cirrhosis.** The fibrotic, scarred areas crowd out the hepatocyte mass, thereby reducing the synthetic, metabolic, and excretory capacity of the liver. Fibrotic masses press on the sinusoids and prevent them from expanding as portal blood flow to the liver increases during the postprandial period. Edema may develop in patients with chronic liver injury as a result of reduced levels of albumin in blood, and a condition known as **ascites** may then develop, in which fluid accumulates in the peritoneal cavity secondary to increased portal pressure. Eventually, the accumulation of toxic substances in the bloodstream can lead to jaundice, itching, and neurological complications. If hepatic function becomes compromised beyond a certain level, the only effective treatment is liver transplantation.

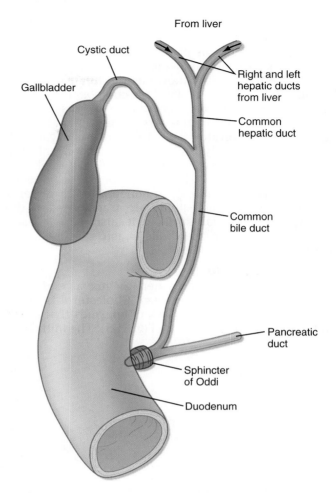

● **Figure 31-4.** Functional anatomy of the biliary system.

type, the **stellate cell.** Stellate cells serve as storage sites for retinoids and in addition are the source of key growth factors for hepatocytes. Under abnormal conditions, stellate cells are activated to synthesize large quantities of collagen, which contributes to the hepatic dysfunction.

Hepatocytes are also the origination point for the **biliary system.** Although hepatocytes are considered to be epithelial cells with basolateral and apical membranes, the spatial arrangement of these two cell domains differs from that seen in simple columnar epithelium, such as that lining the gastrointestinal tract. Rather, in the liver the apical surface of the hepatocyte occupies only a small fraction of the cell membrane, and the apical membranes of adjacent cells oppose each other to form a channel between the cells known as the **canaliculus** (Fig. 31-3). The role of canaliculi is to drain bile from the liver, and these canaliculi drain into biliary ductules, which are lined by classic columnar epithelial cells known as **cholangiocytes.** Ultimately, the biliary ductules drain into large bile ducts that coalesce into the right and left hepatic ducts to permit exit of bile from the liver. These, in turn, form the common hepatic duct, from which bile can flow into either the gallbladder, via the cystic duct, or the intestine, via the common bile duct (Fig. 31-4), on the basis of prevailing pressure relationships.

One other feature of the structural organization of the liver bears emphasis because of its clinical significance. Branches of the hepatic vein, hepatic artery, and bile ducts run in parallel in the so-called **hepatic triad.** Hepatocytes lying closest to this triad are referred to as periportal, or "zone 1," and have the greatest supply of oxygen and nutrients. In contrast,

hepatocytes lying closest to branches of the hepatic vein are referred to as pericentral, or "zone 3." The latter cells are more sensitive to ischemia, whereas the former are more sensitive to oxidative injury. Thus, the location of damaged cells on biopsy may provide clues to the cause of a given case of liver injury. Zone 1 cells are most active in detoxification functions in normal circumstances, but zone 2 (intermediate between zones 1 and 3) and zone 3 cells can progressively be recruited in cases of liver disease, comparable to the concept of the anatomic reserve that we considered for lipid assimilation in the small intestine. Conversely, zone 3 cells are thought to be most active in bile acid synthesis.

BILE FORMATION AND SECRETION

Bile is the excretory fluid of the liver that plays an important role in lipid digestion. Bile formation begins in hepatocytes, which actively transport solutes into bile canaliculi across their apical membranes. Bile is a **micellar solution** in which the major solutes are bile acids, phosphatidylcholine, and cholesterol in an approximate ratio of 10:3:1, respectively. Secretion of these solutes drives the concomitant movement of water and electrolytes across the tight junctions that link adjacent hepatocytes to form canalicular bile. The majority of bile flow is driven by the secretion of bile acids across the apical membrane of hepatocytes via an ATPase transporter known as the **bile salt export pump** (BSEP; Table 31-1). The composition of the resulting fluid can be modified further as it flows through the biliary ductules (resulting in hepatic bile) and still further on storage in the gallbladder (gallbladder bile). Ultimately, bile becomes a concentrated solution of biological detergents that aids in solubilization of the products of lipid digestion in the aqueous environment of the intestinal lumen, thereby enhancing the rate at which lipids are transferred to the absorptive epithelial surface. It also serves as a medium in which metabolic waste products are exported from the body.

Bile Acid Synthesis

Bile acids are produced by hepatocytes as end products of cholesterol metabolism. Cholesterol is selectively metabolized by a series of enzymes that result in the formation of bile acid (Fig. 31-5). The initial and

● AT THE CELLULAR LEVEL

Though rare, a variety of familial syndromes that are manifested as progressive cholestasis have taught us a great deal about the molecular nature of the transporters that deliver bile constituents into the canaliculus. For example, **type II progressive familial intrahepatic cholestasis** (PFIC II) has been mapped to a mutation in BSEP, which results in an almost total absence of bile acids in bile. Cholestasis develops in patients with this disorder, but they have relatively little, if any, evidence of bile duct injury. PFIC III, on the other hand, is a much more aggressive disease in which cholestasis is accompanied by early increases in circulating γ-glutamyl transpeptidase. The molecular culprit is a mutation that abolishes expression of MDR3. In the absence of this transporter, phosphatidylcholine is no longer able to enter bile, thus illustrating the importance of this lipid in protecting cholangiocytes from the injurious effects of bile acids because mixed micelles cannot form in its absence.

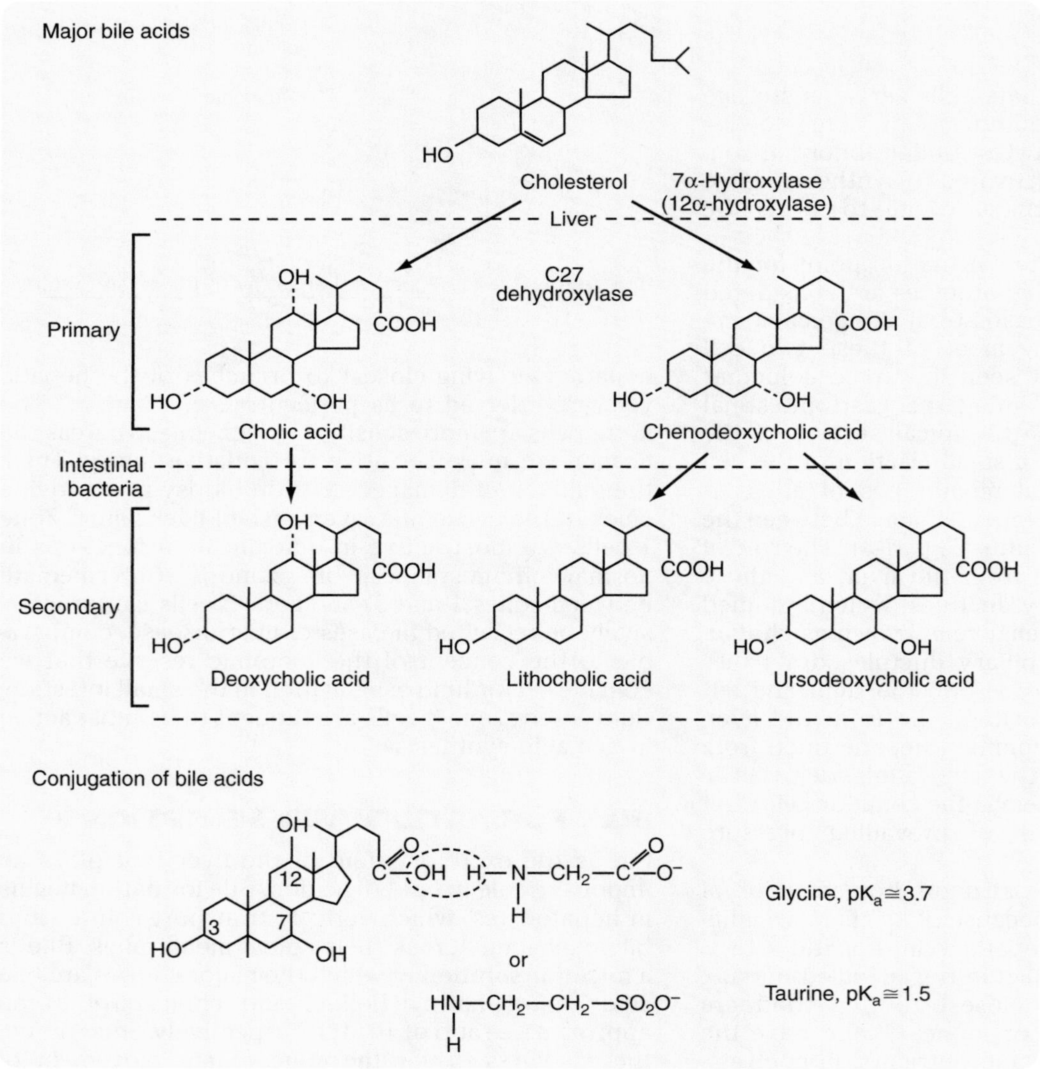

● **Figure 31-5.** Structures and sites of production of the major primary and secondary bile acids of bile. At the bottom of the figure, the conjugation of cholic acid with glycine or taurine is shown.

rate-limiting step is addition of a hydroxyl group to the 7 position of the steroid nucleus by the enzyme **cholesterol 7α-hydroxylase.** The side chain of the product of this reaction is then shortened and a carboxylic acid function added by C27 dehydroxylase to yield chenodeoxycholic acid, a dihydroxy bile acid. Alternatively, the product is further hydroxylated at the 12 position and then acted on by C27 dehydroxylase to yield cholic acid, a trihydroxy bile acid. Bile acid synthesis can be up- or down-regulated, depending on the body's requirements (Fig. 31-6). For example, if bile acid levels are reduced in the blood flowing to the liver, synthesis can be increased up to 10-fold. Conversely, feeding of bile acids profoundly suppresses the new synthesis of bile acids by hepatocytes. The mechanisms underlying these changes in bile acid synthesis relate to changes in expression of the enzymes involved, and bile acids have been shown to be able to directly activate specific transcription factors that mediate such regulation.

Chenodeoxycholic acid and cholic acid are referred to as **primary bile acids** because they are synthesized by the hepatocyte (Fig. 31-5). However, each can be acted on in the colonic lumen by bacterial enzymes to yield ursodeoxycholic and deoxycholic acid, respectively. Chenodeoxycholic acid is also converted by bacterial enzymes to form lithocholic acid, which is relatively cytotoxic. Collectively, these three products of bacterial metabolism are referred to as **secondary bile acids.** One additional important biochemical modification occurs in both primary and secondary bile acids in the hepatocyte (Fig. 31-5). These molecules are conjugated with either glycine or taurine, which significantly depresses their pKa. The result is

that conjugated bile acids are almost totally ionized at the pH prevailing in the small intestinal lumen and thus cannot passively traverse cell membranes. Consequently, the conjugated bile acids are retained in the intestinal lumen until they are actively absorbed in the terminal ileum via the **apical sodium-dependent bile salt transporter (ASBT).** Conjugated bile acids that escape this uptake step are deconjugated by bacterial enzymes in the colon, and the resulting unconjugated forms are passively reabsorbed across the colonic epithelium because they are no longer charged.

Hepatic Aspects of the Enterohepatic Circulation of Bile Acids

Bile acids assist in the digestion and absorption of lipids by acting as detergents rather than enzymes, and thus a significant mass of these molecules is required to solubilize all dietary lipids. Via the **enterohepatic circulation,** actively reabsorbed conjugated bile acids travel through the portal blood back to the hepatocyte, where they are efficiently taken up by basolateral transporters that may be Na^+ dependent or independent (Table 31-1). Similarly, bile acids that are deconjugated in the colon also return to the hepatocyte, where they are reconjugated to be secreted into bile. In this way we acquire a pool of circulating primary and secondary bile acids, and daily synthesis is then equal only to the minor fraction (approximately 10%/day, or 200 to 400 mg) that escapes uptake and is lost in stool (Fig. 31-7). The only exception to this rule is lithocholic acid, which is preferentially sulfated in the hepatocyte rather than being conjugated with

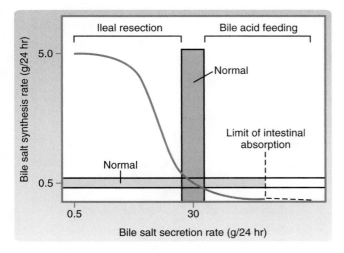

● **Figure 31-6.** Relationship between rates of bile acid synthesis and secretion. Increased secretion normally increases the rate of return of bile acids to the liver via portal blood, which exerts a negative feedback on synthesis. Conversely, interruption of the enterohepatic circulation, such as after ileal resection, can increase synthesis to values more than 10-fold higher than normal. (From Carey MC, Cahalane MJ. In Arias IM et al [eds]: The Liver: Biology and Pathobiology, 2nd ed. New York, Raven Press, 1988.)

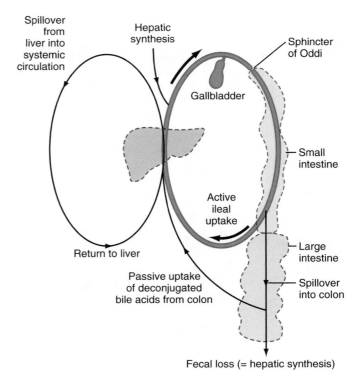

● **Figure 31-7.** Relative amounts of bile acids in different body pools and the enterohepatic circulation.

glycine or taurine. The majority of such conjugates are lost from the body after each meal because they are not substrates for ASBT, thereby avoiding accumulation of a potentially toxic molecule.

Some comment should also be made with respect to the role of bile acids in whole-body cholesterol homeostasis. The pool of cholesterol in the body reflects its daily synthesis, as well as the relatively minor component derived from inefficient dietary uptake, balanced against loss from the body, which can only occur via bile in health (Fig. 31-8). Cholesterol can be excreted in two forms, either as the native molecule or after its conversion to bile acids. The latter account for up to a third of the cholesterol excreted per day despite enterohepatic recycling. Thus, one strategy for the treatment of hypercholesterolemia is to interrupt the enterohepatic circulation of bile acids, which drives increased conversion of cholesterol to bile acids; the bile acids are then lost from the body in feces.

Other Bile Constituents

As noted earlier, bile also contains cholesterol and phosphatidylcholine. Cholesterol transport across the canalicular membrane is mediated, at least in part, by a heterodimer of the active transporters we discussed in Chapter 29 as participating in the efflux of cholesterol from the small intestinal epithelial cells, namely, ABC5 and ABC8 (Table 31-1). Phosphatidylcholine derives from the inner leaflet of the canalicular membrane and is specifically "flipped" across the membrane by another ABC family transporter called **multidrug resistance protein 3** (MDR3). Furthermore, because mixed micelles composed of bile acids, phosphatidylcholine, and cholesterol are osmotically active and the tight junctions that link adjacent hepatocytes are relatively leaky, water is drawn into the canalicular lumen, as well as other plasma solutes, such as Ca^{++}, glucose, glutathione, amino acids, and urea, at concentrations essentially approximating those in plasma

(Fig. 31-9). Finally, conjugated bilirubin, which is water soluble, and a variety of additional organic anions and cations formed from endogenous metabolites and xenobiotics are secreted into bile across the apical membrane of the hepatocyte.

Bile Modification in the Ductules

The cholangiocytes lining the biliary ductules are specifically designed to modify the composition of bile (Fig. 31-10). Useful solutes, such as glucose and amino acids, are reclaimed by the activity of specific transporters. Chloride ions in bile are also exchanged for HCO_3^-, thus rendering the bile slightly alkaline and reducing the risk of precipitation of Ca^{++}. Glutathione is broken down on the surface of cholangiocytes into its constituent amino acids by the enzyme γ-glutamyl transpeptidase (GGT), and the products are reabsorbed. The bile is also diluted at this site, in concert with ingestion of a meal, in response to hormones, such as secretin, that increase HCO_3^- secretion and stimulate the insertion of **aquaporin water channels** into the cholangiocyte's apical membrane. Flow of bile is thereby increased during the postprandial period, when bile acids are needed to aid in assimilation of lipid.

Role of the Gallbladder

Finally, bile enters the ducts and is conveyed toward the intestine. However, in the period between meals, outflow is blocked by constriction of the **sphincter of Oddi,** and thus bile is redirected to the **gallbladder.** The gallbladder is a muscular sac lined with high-resistance epithelial cells. During gallbladder storage, bile becomes concentrated because sodium ions are

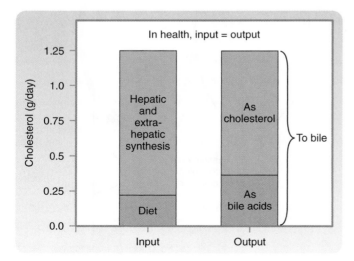

● **Figure 31-8.** Daily cholesterol balance in healthy adult humans.

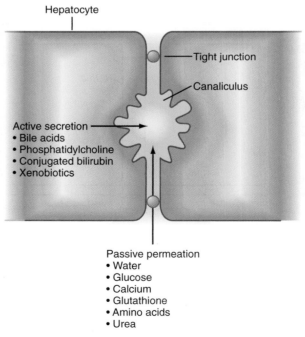

● **Figure 31-9.** Pathways for entry of solutes into bile. (Modified from Barrett KE: Gastrointestinal Physiology. New York, McGraw-Hill, 2006.)

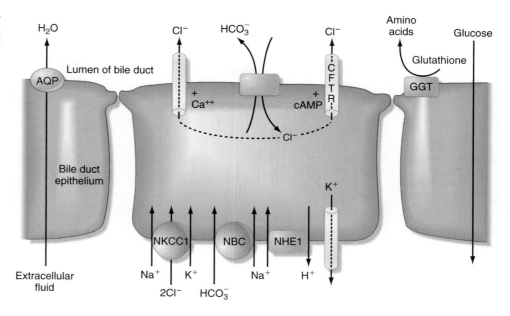

● **Figure 31-10.** The major transport processes of cholangiocytes that secrete an alkaline-rich fluid and reclaim useful substances.

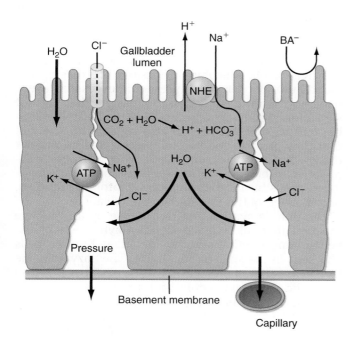

● **Figure 31-11.** Mechanisms accounting for concentration of bile during storage in the gallbladder.

IN THE CLINIC

Humans are unusually susceptible to **gallstones,** which represent precipitated bile constituents that accumulate in the gallbladder or elsewhere in the biliary tree. Gallstones are composed predominantly of cholesterol or Ca^{++} bilirubinate (cholesterol versus pigment stones, respectively). Their significance lies in their propensity to obstruct biliary flow and thereby result in pain, poor tolerance of large fatty meals, retention of biliary constituents, and (if left untreated) liver injury. In susceptible individuals, mechanisms that normally prevent nucleation of saturated bile are either defective or overcome, and small crystals form and can grow into gallstones. Human bile is often supersaturated in terms of its cholesterol content, thus increasing the risk for stone formation, particularly during prolonged fasting. Gallstones are especially common in middle-aged women who are obese, particularly those who have borne children, for unknown reasons. In severe cases, the gallbladder may be removed surgically, which is usually accomplished laparoscopically. Small gallstones that have lodged in the biliary tree can sometimes be retrieved endoscopically by inserting a small snare through the sphincter of Oddi from an endoscope.

actively absorbed in exchange for protons, and bile acids, as the major anions, are too large to exit across the gallbladder epithelial tight junctions (Fig. 31-11). However, although the concentration of bile acids can rise more than 10-fold, bile remains isotonic because a single micelle acts as only one osmotically active particle. Any additional bile acid monomers that become available as a result of concentration are thus immediately incorporated into existing mixed micelles. This also reduces, to some extent, the risk that cho-

lesterol will precipitate from bile. However, cholesterol is supersaturated in the bile of many adults, with precipitation normally being inhibited by the presence of antinucleating proteins. Prolonged storage of bile increases the chance that nucleation can occur, thus making a good case for never skipping breakfast and perhaps explaining why gallstone disease is relatively prevalent in humans.

Bile is secreted from the gallbladder in response to signals that simultaneously relax the sphincter of Oddi

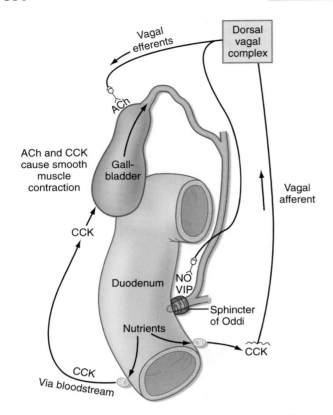

● **Figure 31-12.** Neurohumoral control of gallbladder contraction and biliary secretion. The pathway also involves relaxation of the sphincter of Oddi to permit outflow of bile into the duodenum. ACh, acetylcholine; CCK, cholecystokinin; NO, nitric oxide; VIP, vasoactive intestinal polypeptide.

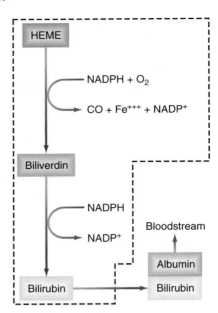

● **Figure 31-13.** Conversion of heme to bilirubin. The reactions inside the dashed box occur in cells of the reticuloendothelial system.

and contract the smooth muscle that encircles the gallbladder epithelium (Fig. 31-12). A critical mediator of this response is cholecystokinin—indeed, this hormone was named for its ability to contract the gallbladder. In addition, intrinsic neural reflexes and vagal pathways, some of which themselves are stimulated by the ability of cholecystokinin to bind to vagal afferents, probably also contribute to gallbladder contractility. The net result is ejection of a concentrated bolus of bile into the duodenal lumen, where the constituent mixed micelles can aid in lipid uptake. Then, when no longer needed, the bile acids are reclaimed and reenter the enterohepatic circulation to begin the cycle again. However, the other components of bile are largely lost in stool, thus providing for their excretion from the body.

Bilirubin Formation and Excretion by the Liver

The liver is also important for excretion of **bilirubin,** which is a metabolite of heme that is potentially toxic to the body. Bilirubin has recently been shown to act as an antioxidant, but it also serves as a way to eliminate the excess heme released from the hemoglobin of senescent red blood cells. Indeed, red blood cells account for 80% of bilirubin production, with the remainder coming from additional heme-containing

proteins in other tissues such as skeletal muscle and the liver itself. Bilirubin is capable of crossing the blood-brain barrier and, if present in excessive levels, results in brain dysfunction for reasons that are not well understood; it can be fatal if left untreated. Bilirubin and its metabolites are also notable for the fact that they provide color to bile, feces, and to a lesser extent, urine. By the same token, when bilirubin accumulates in the circulation as a result of liver disease, it is responsible for the common symptom of **jaundice,** or yellowing of the skin and conjunctiva.

Bilirubin is synthesized from heme by a two-stage reaction that takes place in phagocytic cells of the **reticuloendothelial system,** including Kupffer cells and cells in the spleen (Fig. 31-13). The enzyme heme oxygenase that is present in these cells liberates iron from the heme molecule and produces the green pigment **biliverdin.** This, in turn, can be reduced to form yellow bilirubin. Because this molecule is essentially insoluble in aqueous solutions at neutral pH, it is transported through the bloodstream bound to albumin. When this complex reaches the liver, it enters the space of Disse, where bilirubin is selectively taken up across the basolateral membrane of hepatocytes via an **OATP** transporter (Table 31-1). In the microsomal compartment, bilirubin is then conjugated with one or two molecules of glucuronic acid to enhance its aqueous solubility. The reaction is catalyzed by **UDP glucuronyl transferase** (UGT). This enzyme is synthesized only slowly after birth, which explains why mild jaundice is relatively common in newborn infants. The bilirubin conjugates are then secreted into bile by a multidrug-related protein (MRP2) located in the canalicular membrane. Notably, the conjugated forms of bilirubin cannot be reabsorbed from the intestine, thereby ensuring that they can be excreted.

However, transport of bilirubin across the hepatocyte, and indeed its initial uptake from the bloodstream, is relatively inefficient, so some conjugated and unconjugated bilirubin is present in plasma even under normal conditions. Both circulate bound to albumin, but the conjugated form is bound more loosely and thus can enter the urine.

In the colon, bilirubin conjugates are deconjugated by bacterial enzymes, whereupon the bilirubin liberated is metabolized by bacteria to yield urobilinogen, which is reabsorbed, and urobilins and stercobilins, which are excreted. Absorbed urobilinogen, in turn, can be taken up by hepatocytes and reconjugated, thus giving the molecule yet another chance to be excreted.

Measurement of bilirubin in plasma, as well as assessment of whether it is unconjugated or conjugated, is an important tool in the evaluation of liver disease. The presence of unconjugated bilirubin, which is essentially fully albumin bound and cannot be excreted in urine, reflects either loss of UGT (or a normal, temporary delay in its maturation in infants) or a sudden oversupply of heme that overwhelms the conjugation mechanism (such as occurs in transfusion reactions or in Rhesus-incompatible newborns). Conjugated bilirubinemia, on the other hand, is characterized by the presence of bilirubin in urine, to which it imparts a dark coloration. This is indicative of genetic defects in the transporter that mediates bilirubin glucuronide/diglucuronide secretion into the canaliculus, or it may be due to blockage to flow of bile, perhaps caused by an obstructing gallstone. In both cases, bilirubin conjugates are formed in the liver, but with no means of exit, they regurgitate back into plasma for urinary excretion.

AT THE CELLULAR LEVEL

Crigler-Najjar syndrome is a condition associated with mutations in the hepatocyte enzyme UGT. In type I Crigler-Najjar syndrome, a congenital missense mutation results in complete lack of this enzyme, whereas patients with type II Crigler-Najjar syndrome have a milder mutation that reduces UGT levels to about 10% of those seen in normal individuals. Thus, with varying degrees of severity, Crigler-Najjar syndrome impairs the ability of hepatocytes to conjugate bilirubin. The unconjugated bilirubin regurgitates back into the circulation and binds to albumin, with an associated risk of neurological injury if levels rise precipitously. The only effective treatment of type I Crigler-Najjar syndrome at present is liver transplantation; those with type II disease can sometimes be managed effectively with blue light. This converts circulating unconjugated bilirubin to forms that are more water soluble and thus less firmly bound to albumin, which can be excreted in urine.

AMMONIA HANDLING BY THE LIVER

Ammonia (NH_3) is a small, neutral metabolite that arises from protein catabolism and bacterial activity and is highly membrane permeant. The liver is a critical contributor to the prevention of ammonia accumulation in the circulation, which is important because like bilirubin, ammonia is toxic to the central nervous system. The liver eliminates ammonia from the body by converting it to urea via a series of enzymatic reactions known as the **urea,** or **Krebs-Henseleit, cycle** (Fig. 31-14). The liver is the only tissue in the body that can convert ammonia to urea.

Ammonia is derived from two major sources. Approximately 50% is produced in the colon by bacterial ureases. Because the colonic lumen is normally slightly acidic, some of this ammonia is converted to the ammonium ion (NH_4^+), which renders it impermeant to the colonic epithelium and therefore allows it to be excreted in stool. However, the remainder of the ammonia generated crosses the colonic epithelium passively and is transported to the liver via the portal

● **Figure 31-14.** The urea cycle.

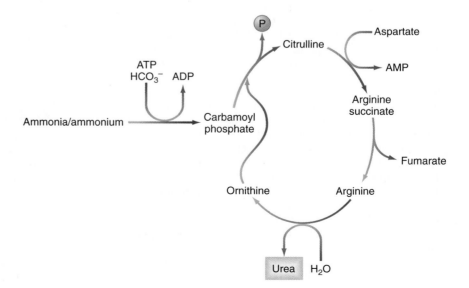

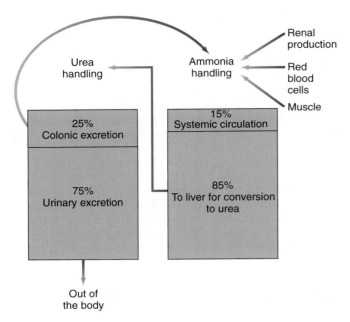

● **Figure 31-15.** Ammonia homeostasis in health.

circulation. The other major source of ammonia (approximately 40%) is the kidney (see Chapter 36). A small amount of ammonia (approximately 10%) is derived from deamination of amino acids in the liver itself, by metabolic processes in muscle cells, and via the release of glutamine from senescent red blood cells.

The "mass balance" for ammonia handling in a healthy adult is presented in Figure 31-15. As just noted, ammonia is a small, neutral molecule that readily crosses cell membranes without the benefit of a specific transporter, although some membrane proteins transport ammonia, including certain aquaporins. Whatever the mechanism for transport, the physicochemical properties of ammonia ensure that it is efficiently extracted from the portal and systemic circulation by hepatocytes, where it then enters the urea cycle to be converted to urea (Fig. 31-14) and is subsequently transported back into the systemic circulation. Urea is a small, neutral molecule that is readily filtered at the glomerulus, and it is reabsorbed by the kidney tubules such that approximately 50% of the filtered urea is excreted in urine (see Chapter 36). Urea that enters the colon is either excreted or metabolized to ammonia via colonic bacteria, with the resulting ammonia being reabsorbed or excreted.

If the metabolic capacity of the liver is compromised acutely, coma and death can rapidly ensue. In chronic liver disease, patients may experience a gradual decline in mental function that reflects the action of both ammonia and other toxins that cannot be cleared by the liver, in a condition known as **hepatic encephalopathy.** The development of confusion, dementia, and eventually coma in a patient with liver disease is evidence of significant progression, and these symptoms can prove fatal if left untreated.

CLINICAL ASSESSMENT OF LIVER FUNCTION

Given the importance of the liver for homeostasis, tests of liver function are a mainstay of clinical diagnosis. Such tests have several goals: (1) to assess whether hepatocytes have been injured or are dysfunctional, (2) to determine whether bile excretion has been interrupted, and (3) to evaluate whether cholangiocytes have been injured or are dysfunctional. **Liver function tests** are also used to monitor responses to therapy or rejection reactions after liver transplantation. However, not all such tests measure function directly. Nevertheless, liver function tests are discussed briefly because of their link to hepatic physiology.

Tests for hepatocyte injury rely on markers that are specific for this cell type. When hepatocytes are killed by necrotic responses to inflammation or infection, for example, they release enzymes, including alanine aminotransferase (ALT) and aspartate aminotransferase (AST). These enzymes, which are essential to interconvert amino acids, are easily measured in serum and indicate hepatocyte injury, although AST may also be released after injury to other tissues, including the heart. Two other tests are markers of injury to the biliary system. Alkaline phosphatase is expressed in the canalicular membrane, and elevations of this enzyme in plasma suggest localized obstruction to bile flow. Similarly, increased levels of GGT are seen when there is damage to cholangiocytes.

Measurement of bilirubin in the circulation or in urine also provides an insight into liver function. In addition, measurement of any of the other characteristic secreted products of the liver can be used to diagnose liver disease. Clinically, the most common tests are measurements of serum albumin and a blood clotting parameter, the prothrombin time. If results of these tests are abnormal, when considered together with other aspects of the clinical picture, a diagnosis of liver disease may be established. Blood glucose and ammonia levels are frequently monitored in patients with chronic liver disease. Finally, imaging tests and histological examination of biopsy specimens of liver parenchyma, usually obtained percutaneously, are also important in the evaluation and monitoring of patients with suspected or proven liver disease.

■ KEY CONCEPTS

1. Vital functions of the liver include carbohydrate, lipid, and protein metabolism and synthesis; detoxification of unwanted substances; and excretion of circulating substances that are lipid soluble and carried in the bloodstream bound to albumin. The liver also synthesizes the majority of plasma proteins, including albumin.

2. Liver function depends on its unique anatomy, its constituent cell types (especially hepatocytes), and the unusual arrangement of its blood supply.

3. Substances are excreted from the liver in bile. Bile flow is driven by the presence of bile acids, which are amphipathic end products of cholesterol metabolism that are produced by hepatocytes. Bile acids circulate between the liver and intestine to conserve their mass, and water-insoluble metabolites, such as cholesterol, are carried in bile in the form of mixed micelles.

4. Bile is stored in the gallbladder between meals, where it is concentrated and released when hormonal and neural signals simultaneously contract the gallbladder and relax the sphincter of Oddi.

5. The liver is critical for disposing of certain substances that would be toxic if allowed to accumulate in the bloodstream, including bilirubin and ammonia.

THE RENAL SYSTEM

Bruce A. Stanton and Bruce M. Koeppen

CHAPTER 32

Elements of Renal Function

OVERVIEW OF RENAL FUNCTION

The kidney presents in the highest degree the phenomenon of sensibility, the power of reacting to various stimuli in a direction which is appropriate for the survival of the organism; a power of adaptation which almost gives one the idea that its component parts must be endowed with intelligence.

E. STARLING—1909

Certainly, mental integrity is a sine qua non of the free and independent life. But let the composition of our internal environment suffer change, let our kidneys fail for even a short time to fulfill their tasks, and our mental integrity, or personality is destroyed.

HOMER W. SMITH—1939

As both Starling and Smith recognized, the kidneys are regulatory rather than excretory organs. However, it is clear that the excretory function of the kidneys is central to their ability to regulate the composition and volume of body fluids. The kidneys regulate (1) body fluid osmolality and volumes, (2) electrolyte balance, and (3) acid-base balance. In addition, the kidneys excrete metabolic products and foreign substances and produce and secrete hormones.

Control of body fluid osmolality is important for maintenance of normal cell volume in all tissues of the body. Control of body fluid volume is necessary for normal function of the cardiovascular system. The kidneys are also essential in regulating the amount of several important inorganic ions in the body, including Na^+, K^+, Cl^-, bicarbonate (HCO_3^-), hydrogen (H^+), Ca^{++}, and inorganic phosphate (P_i). Excretion of these electrolytes must be equal to daily intake of them to maintain appropriate balance. If intake of an electrolyte exceeds its excretion, the amount of this electrolyte in the body increases, and the individual is in positive balance for that electrolyte. Conversely, if excretion of an electrolyte exceeds its intake, its amount in the body decreases, and the individual is in negative balance for that electrolyte. For many electrolytes the kidneys are the sole or primary route for excretion from the body.

Another important function of the kidneys is regulation of acid-base balance. Many of the metabolic functions of the body are exquisitely sensitive to pH. Thus, the pH of body fluids must be maintained within narrow limits. The pH is maintained by buffers within the body fluids and by the coordinated action of the lungs, liver, and kidneys.

The kidneys excrete a number of the end products of metabolism. These waste products include urea (from amino acids), uric acid (from nucleic acids), creatinine (from muscle creatine), end products of hemoglobin metabolism, and metabolites of hormones. The kidneys eliminate these substances from the body at a rate that matches their production. Thus, the kidneys regulate hormone concentrations within the body fluids. The kidneys also represent an important route for the elimination of foreign substances such as drugs, pesticides, and other chemicals from the body.

Finally, the kidneys are important endocrine organs that produce and secrete renin, calcitriol, and erythropoietin. Renin activates the renin-angiotensin-aldosterone system, which helps regulate blood pressure and Na^+ and K^+ balance. Calcitriol, a metabolite of vitamin D_3, is necessary for the normal absorption of Ca^{++} by the gastrointestinal tract and for its deposition in bone (see also Chapter 35). In patients with renal disease, the kidneys' ability to produce calcitriol is impaired, and levels of this hormone are reduced. As a result, Ca^{++} absorption by the intestine is decreased. This reduced intestinal Ca^{++} absorption contributes to the bone formation abnormalities seen in patients with chronic renal disease. Another consequence of many kidney diseases is a reduction in erythropoietin production and secretion. Erythropoietin stimulates red blood cell formation by the bone marrow. Decreased erythrocyte production contributes to the anemia that occurs in chronic renal failure.

A large variety of diseases impair the function of the kidneys and result in renal failure. In some instances the impairment in renal function is transient, but in many cases renal function declines progressively. Patients in whom the glomerular filtration rate (GFR) is less than 10% of normal are said to have end-stage renal disease (ESRD) and must undergo renal replacement therapy to survive.

To understand the mechanisms that contribute to renal disease, it is first necessary to understand the normal physiology of renal function. Thus, in the following chapters in this section of the book various aspects of renal function are considered.

IN THE CLINIC

Kidney disease is a major health problem. In the United States:

- Kidney disease affects over 20 million patients and accounts for more than 80,000 deaths per year.
- Each year kidney disease is diagnosed in more than 3 million new patients.
- Over 500,000 people are treated for **ESRD** every year.
- Approximately 275,000 patients with ESRD are maintained on either hemodialysis or peritoneal dialysis.
- Diabetes, hypertension, glomerulonephritis, and polycystic kidney disease are the leading causes of ESRD.
- ESRD secondary to diabetes is increasing at an annual rate of more than 11% per year.
- The health care cost for ESRD is more than $19 billion dollars per year.
- More than 14,000 kidney transplants are performed each year. Unfortunately, in excess of 54,000 patients are awaiting kidney transplants.
- Urinary tract infections, kidney stones (i.e., urolithiasis), and interstitial cystitis (i.e., inflammation of the urinary bladder) are also major health care problems. Interstitial cystitis (700,000 patients), urinary stones (1.3 million visits annually), urinary tract infections (8.3 million visits annually), and urinary incontinence (13 million adults affected, mostly older than 65) are serious health concerns.

Individuals with ESRD must undergo renal replacement therapy. Such therapy includes peritoneal dialysis, hemodialysis, and renal transplantation. Both peritoneal dialysis and hemodialysis, as their names indicate, are based on the process of dialysis whereby small molecules are removed from the blood by diffusion across a selectively permeable membrane into a solution that lacks these small molecules. In peritoneal dialysis, the peritoneal membrane acts as a dialyzing membrane. Several liters of a solution are introduced into the abdominal cavity, and small molecules in blood diffuse across the peritoneal membrane into the solution, which is then removed from the abdominal cavity. In hemodialysis, a patient's blood is pumped through an artificial kidney machine. In the kidney machine blood is separated from an artificial solution by a dialysis membrane, which allows small molecules to diffuse from blood into the dialysis solution, thereby removing the small molecules from the blood. Patients who are candidates for renal transplantation are treated with dialysis until an appropriate donor kidney can be obtained. Although anemia also used to be a significant problem because of reduced erythropoietin production in ESRD, patients undergoing chronic dialysis now receive recombinant human erythropoietin.

FUNCTIONAL ANATOMY OF THE KIDNEYS

Structure and function are closely linked in the kidneys. Consequently, an appreciation of the gross anatomic and histological features of the kidneys is a prerequisite for understanding their function.

Gross Anatomy

The kidneys are paired organs that lie on the posterior wall of the abdomen behind the peritoneum on either side of the vertebral column. In an adult human, each kidney weighs between 115 and 170 g and is approximately 11 cm long, 6 cm wide, and 3 cm thick.

The gross anatomic features of the human kidney are illustrated in Figure 32-1. The medial side of each kidney contains an indentation through which pass the renal artery and vein, nerves, and pelvis. If a kidney were cut in half, two regions would be evident: an outer region called the **cortex** and an inner region called the **medulla.** The cortex and medulla are composed of **nephrons** (the functional units of the kidney), blood vessels, lymphatics, and nerves. The medulla in the human kidney is divided into conical masses called **renal pyramids.** The base of each pyramid originates at the corticomedullary border, and the apex terminates in a **papilla,** which lies within a **minor calyx.** Minor calyces collect urine from each papilla. The numerous minor calyces expand into two or three open-ended pouches, the **major calyces.** The major calyces in turn feed into the **pelvis.** The pelvis represents the upper, expanded region of the **ureter,** which carries urine from the pelvis to the urinary bladder. The walls of the calyces, pelvis, and ureters contain smooth muscle that contracts to propel the urine toward the **urinary bladder.**

Blood flow to the two kidneys is equivalent to about 25% (1.25 L/min) of the cardiac output in resting individuals. However, the kidneys constitute less than 0.5% of total body weight. As illustrated in Figure 32-2 *(left),* the **renal artery** branches progressively to form the **interlobar artery,** the **arcuate artery,** the **interlobular artery,** and the **afferent arteriole,** which leads into the **glomerular capillaries** (i.e., **glomerulus**). The glomerular capillaries come together to form the **efferent arteriole,** which leads into a second capillary network, the **peritubular capillaries,** which supply blood to the nephron. The vessels of the venous system run parallel to the arterial vessels and progressively form the **interlobular vein, arcuate vein, interlobar vein,** and **renal vein,** which courses beside the ureter.

Ultrastructure of the Nephron

The functional unit of the kidneys is the nephron. Each human kidney contains approximately 1.2 million nephrons, which are hollow tubes composed of a single cell layer. The nephron consists of a **renal corpuscle, proximal tubule, loop of Henle, distal tubule,** and **collecting duct system*** (Fig. 32-3; also

---

*Organization of the nephron is actually more complicated than presented here. However, for simplicity and clarity of presentation in subsequent chapters, the nephron is divided into five segments. The collecting duct system is not actually part of the nephron. However, again for simplicity, we consider the collecting duct system part of the nephron.

● Figure 32-1. Structure of a human kidney, cut open to show the internal structures. (Modified from Marsh DJ: Renal Physiology. New York, Raven, 1983.)

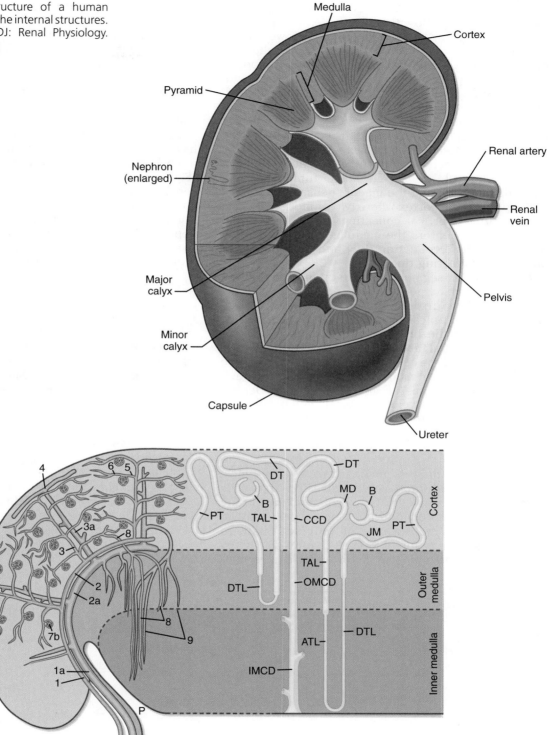

● Figure 32-2. Left, Organization of the vascular system of the human kidney. 1, interlobar arteries; 1a, interlobar vein; 2, arcuate arteries; 2a, arcuate veins; 3, interlobular arteries; 3a, interlobular veins; 4, stellate vein; 5, afferent arterioles; 6, efferent arterioles; 7a, 7b, glomerular capillary networks; 8, descending vasa recta; 9, ascending vasa recta. **Right,** Organization of the human nephron. A superficial nephron is illustrated on the left and a juxtamedullary (JM) nephron is illustrated on the right. The loop of Henle includes the straight portion of the proximal tubule (PT), descending thin limb (DTL), ascending thin limb (ATL), and thick ascending limb (TAL). B, Bowman's capsule; CCD, cortical collecting duct; DT, distal tubule; IMCD, inner medullary collecting duct; MD, macula densa; OMCD, outer medullary collecting duct; P, pelvis. (Modified from Kriz W, Bankir LA: Am J Physiol 254:F1, 1988; and Koushanpour E, Kriz W: Renal Physiology: Principles, Structure, and Function, 2nd ed. New York, Springer-Verlag, 1986.).

see Fig. 32-4). The renal corpuscle consists of glomerular capillaries and **Bowman's capsule.** The proximal tubule initially forms several coils, followed by a straight piece that descends toward the medulla. The next segment is the loop of Henle, which is composed of the straight part of the proximal tubule, the descending thin limb (which ends in a hairpin turn), the ascending thin limb (only in nephrons with long loops of Henle), and the thick ascending limb. Near the end of the thick ascending limb, the nephron passes between the afferent and efferent arterioles of the same nephron. This short segment of the thick ascending limb is called the **macula densa.** The distal tubule begins a short distance beyond the macula densa and extends to the point in the cortex where two or more nephrons join to form a cortical collecting duct. The **cortical collecting duct** enters the medulla and becomes the outer **medullary collecting duct** and then the **inner medullary collecting duct.**

Each nephron segment is made up of cells that are uniquely suited to perform specific transport functions (Fig. 32-3). Proximal tubule cells have an extensively amplified apical membrane (the urine side of the cell) called the **brush border,** which is present only in the proximal tubule. The basolateral membrane (the blood side of the cell) is highly invaginated. These invaginations contain many mitochondria. In contrast, the descending and ascending thin limbs of Henle's loop have poorly developed apical and basolateral surfaces and few mitochondria. The cells of the thick ascending limb and the distal tubule have abundant mitochondria and extensive infoldings of the basolateral membrane.

The collecting duct is composed of two cell types: principal cells and intercalated cells. **Principal cells** have a moderately invaginated basolateral membrane and contain few mitochondria. Principal cells play an important role in reabsorption of NaCl (see Chapters 33 and 34) and secretion of K^+ (see Chapter 35). **Intercalated cells,** which play an important role in regulating acid-base balance, have a high density of mitochondria. One population of intercalated cells secretes H^+ (i.e., reabsorbs HCO_3^-), and a second population secretes HCO_3^- (see Chapter 36). The final segment of the nephron, the inner medullary collecting duct, is composed of inner medullary collecting duct cells. Cells of the inner medullary collecting duct have poorly developed apical and basolateral surfaces and few mitochondria.

All cells in the nephron, except intercalated cells, have in their apical plasma membrane a single nonmotile primary cilium that protrudes into the tubule fluid (Fig. 32-4). Primary cilia are mechanosensors (i.e., they sense changes in the rate of flow of tubule fluid) and chemosensors (i.e., they sense or respond to compounds in the surrounding fluid), and they initiate Ca^{++}-dependent signaling pathways, including those that control kidney cell function, proliferation, differentiation, and apoptosis (i.e., programmed cell death).

AT THE CELLULAR LEVEL

Polycystin 1 (encoded by the *PKD1* gene) and **polycystin 2** (encoded by the *PKD2* gene) are expressed in the membrane of primary cilia and mediate entry of Ca^{++} into cells. PKD1 and PKD2 are thought to play an important role in flow-dependent K^+ secretion by principal cells of the collecting duct. As described in more detail in Chapter 35, increased flow of tubule fluid in the collecting duct is a strong stimulus for secretion of K^+. Increased flow bends the primary cilium in principal cells, which activates the PKD1/PKD2 Ca^{++} conducting channel complex and allows Ca^{++} to enter the cell and increase intracellular $[Ca^{++}]$. The increase in $[Ca^{++}]$ activates K^+ channels in the apical plasma membrane, which enhances secretion of K^+ from the cell into the tubule fluid.

● **Figure 32-3.** Diagram of a nephron, including the cellular ultrastructure.

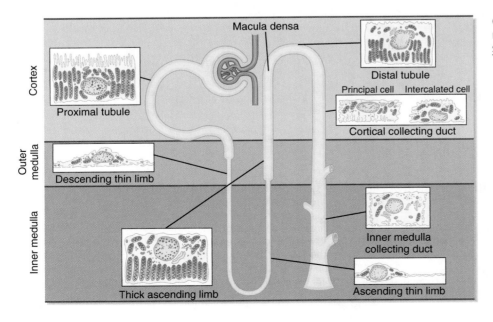

Cortex

Macula densa

Proximal tubule

Distal tubule

Principal cell   Intercalated cell

Cortical collecting duct

Outer medulla

Descending thin limb

Inner medulla

Inner medulla collecting duct

Thick ascending limb

Ascending thin limb

Polycystic kidney disease (PKD) is a genetic disease that occurs in about 1 in 800 people. Approximately 4 to 6 million people worldwide (600,000 in the United States) have PKD, which is caused primarily by mutations in PKD1 (85% to 90% of cases) and PKD2 (10% to 15% of cases). The major phenotype of PKD is enlargement of the kidneys because of the presence of hundreds to thousands of renal cysts that can be as large as 20 cm in diameter. Cysts are also seen in the liver and other organs. PKD causes renal failure, usually in the fifth decade of life, and accounts for 10% of patients with end-stage renal failure. Although it is not clear how mutations in PKD1 and PKD2 cause PKD, renal cyst formation may result from defects in uptake of Ca^{++} that lead to alterations in Ca^{++}-dependent signaling pathways, including those that control kidney cell proliferation, differentiation, and apoptosis.

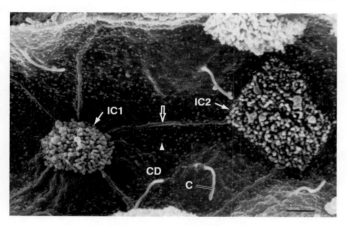

● **Figure 32-4.** Scanning electron micrograph illustrating primary cilia (C) in the apical plasma membrane of principal cells in the cortical collecting duct. Note that intercalated cells do not have cilia. Primary cilia are approximately 2 to 30 μm long and 0.5 μm in diameter. CD, collecting duct principal cells with short microvilli *(arrowhead);* the straight ridges *(open arrow)* represent the cell borders between principal cells; IC1 and IC2, intercalated cells with numerous long microvilli in the apical membrane. (From Kriz W, Kaissling B: Structural organization of the mammalian kidney. In Seldin DW, Giebisch G [eds]: The Kidney: Physiology and Pathophysiology, 3rd ed. Philadelphia, Lippincott Williams & Wilkins, 2000.)

Nephrons may be subdivided into superficial and juxtamedullary types (Fig. 32-2). The renal corpuscle of each superficial nephron is located in the outer region of the cortex. Its loop of Henle is short, and its efferent arteriole branches into peritubular capillaries that surround the nephron segments of its own and adjacent nephrons. This capillary network conveys oxygen and important nutrients to the nephron segments in the cortex, delivers substances to the nephron for secretion (i.e., movement of a substance from blood into tubular fluid), and serves as a pathway for return of reabsorbed water and solutes to the circulatory system. A few species, including humans, also possess very short superficial nephrons whose loops of Henle never enter the medulla.

The renal corpuscle of each **juxtamedullary nephron** is located in the region of the cortex adjacent to the medulla (Fig. 32-2, *right*). When compared with superficial nephrons, juxtamedullary nephrons differ anatomically in two important ways: the loop of Henle is longer and extends deeper into the medulla, and the efferent arteriole forms not only a network of peritubular capillaries but also a series of vascular loops called the **vasa recta.**

As shown in Figure 32-2, the vasa recta descend into the medulla, where they form capillary networks that surround the collecting ducts and ascending limbs of the loop of Henle. The blood returns to the cortex in the ascending vasa recta. Although less than 0.7% of the renal blood flow (RBF) enters the vasa recta, these vessels subserve important functions in the renal medulla, including (1) conveying oxygen and important nutrients to nephron segments, (2) delivering substances to the nephron for secretion, (3) serving as a pathway for the return of reabsorbed water and solutes to the circulatory system, and (4) concentrating and diluting the urine (urine concentration and dilution are discussed in more detail in Chapter 34).

Ultrastructure of the Renal Corpuscle

The first step in urine formation begins with passive movement of a plasma ultrafiltrate from the glomerular capillaries (i.e., glomerulus) into **Bowman's space.** The term ultrafiltration refers to the passive movement of an essentially protein-free fluid from the glomerular capillaries into Bowman's space. To appreciate the process of ultrafiltration one must understand the anatomy of the renal corpuscle. The glomerulus consists of a network of capillaries supplied by the afferent arteriole and drained by the efferent arteriole (Figs. 32-5 and 32-6). During embryological development, the glomerular capillaries press into the closed end of the proximal tubule to form the Bowman capsule of a renal corpuscle. The capillaries are covered by epithelial cells called podocytes that form the visceral layer of Bowman's capsule (Figs. 32-7 through 32-9). The visceral cells face outward at the vascular pole (i.e., where the afferent and efferent arterioles enter and exit Bowman's capsule) to form the parietal layer of Bowman's capsule. The space between the visceral layer and the parietal layer is Bowman's space, which at the urinary pole (i.e., where the proximal tubule joins Bowman's capsule) of the glomerulus becomes the lumen of the proximal tubule.

The endothelial cells of glomerular capillaries are covered by a basement membrane that is surrounded by **podocytes** (Figs. 32-5 and 32-7 to 32-9). The capillary endothelium, basement membrane, and foot processes of podocytes form the so-called **filtration barrier** (Figs. 32-5 and 32-7 to 32-9). The endothelium is fenestrated (i.e., contains 700-Å holes, where 1 Å = 10^{-10} m) and freely permeable to water, small solutes (such as Na$^+$, urea, and glucose), and most proteins but is not permeable to red blood cells, white blood cells, or platelets. Because endothelial cells express

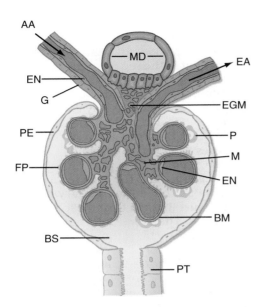

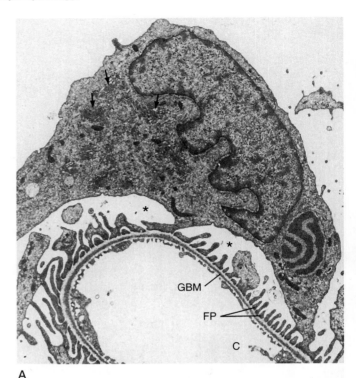

A

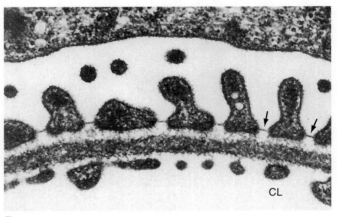

B

● **Figure 32-5.** Anatomy of the renal corpuscle and juxtaglomerular apparatus. The juxtaglomerular apparatus is composed of the macula densa (MD) of the thick ascending limb, extraglomerular mesangial cells (EGM), and renin- and angiotensin II–producing granular cells (G) of the afferent arterioles (AA). BM, basement membrane; BS, Bowman's space; EA, efferent arteriole; EN, endothelial cell; FP, foot processes of the podocyte; M, mesangial cells between capillaries; P, podocyte cell body (visceral cell layer); PE, parietal epithelium; PT, proximal tubule cell. (Modified from Kriz W, Kaissling B. In Seldin DW, Giebisch G [eds]: The Kidney: Physiology and Pathophysiology, 2nd ed. New York, Raven, 1992.)

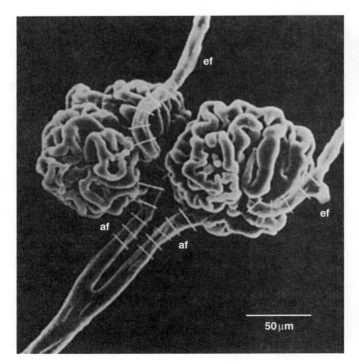

● **Figure 32-6.** Scanning electron micrograph of the interlobular artery, afferent arteriole (af), efferent arteriole (ef), and glomerulus. The white bars on the afferent and efferent arterioles indicate that they are about 15 to 20 μm wide. (From Kimura K et al: Am J Physiol 259:F936, 1990.)

● **Figure 32-7.** **A,** Electron micrograph of a podocyte surrounding a glomerular capillary. The cell body of the podocyte contains a large nucleus with three indentations. Cell processes of the podocyte form the interdigitating foot processes (FP). The arrows in the cytoplasm of the podocyte indicate the well-developed Golgi apparatus, and the asterisks indicate Bowman's space. C, capillary lumen; GBM, glomerular basement membrane. **B,** Electron micrograph of the filtration barrier of a glomerular capillary. The filtration barrier is composed of three layers: the endothelium, basement membrane, and foot processes of the podocytes. Note the filtration slit diaphragm bridging the floor of the filtration slits (*arrows*). CL, capillary lumen. (From Kriz W, Kaissling B. In Seldin DW, Giebisch G [eds]: The Kidney: Physiology and Pathophysiology, 2nd ed. New York, Raven, 1992.)

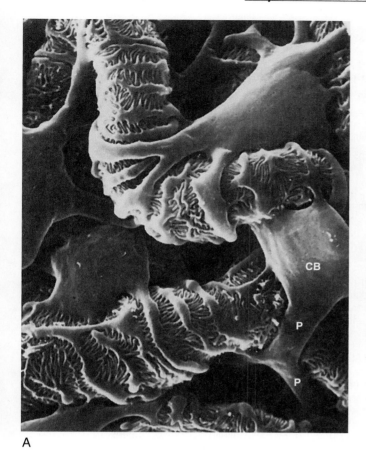

A

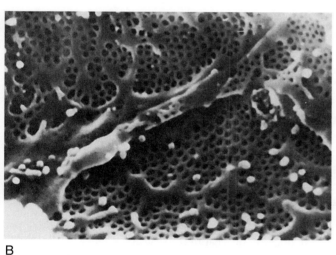

B

● **Figure 32-8.**   **A,** Scanning electron micrograph showing the outer surface of glomerular capillaries. This is the view that would be seen from Bowman's space. Processes (P) of podocytes run from the cell body (CB) toward the capillaries, where they ultimately split into foot processes. Interdigitation of the foot processes creates the filtration slits. **B,** Scanning electron micrograph of the inner surface (blood side) of a glomerular capillary. This view would be seen from the lumen of the capillary. The fenestrations of the endothelial cells are seen as small 700-Å holes. (From Kriz W, Kaissling B. In Seldin DW, Giebisch G [eds]: The Kidney: Physiology and Pathophysiology, 2nd ed. New York, Raven, 1992.).

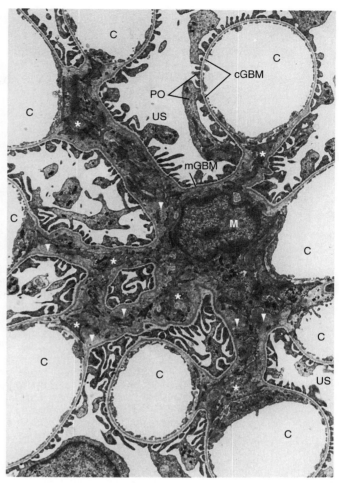

● **Figure 32-9.**   Electron micrograph of the mesangium, the area between the glomerular capillaries containing mesangial cells. C, glomerular capillaries; cGBM, capillary glomerular basement membrane surrounded by foot processes of podocytes (PO) and endothelial cells; M, mesangial cell that gives rise to several processes, some marked by stars; mGBM, mesangial glomerular basement membrane surrounded by foot processes of podocytes and mesangial cells; US, urinary space. Note the extensive extracellular matrix surrounded by mesangial cells *(triangles)* (×4100). (From Kriz W, Kaissling B. In Seldin DW, Giebisch G [eds]: The Kidney: Physiology and Pathophysiology, 2nd ed. New York, Raven, 1992.)

negatively charged glycoproteins on their surface, they may retard the filtration of very large anionic proteins into Bowman's space. In addition to their role as a barrier to filtration, the endothelial cells synthesize a number of vasoactive substances (e.g., nitric oxide [NO], a vasodilator, and endothelin-1 [ET-1], a vasoconstrictor) that are important in controlling renal plasma flow (RPF).

The basement membrane, which is a porous matrix of negatively charged proteins, including type IV collagen, laminin, the proteoglycans agrin and perlecan, and fibronectin, is an important filtration barrier to plasma proteins. The basement membrane is thought to function primarily as a charge-selective filter in

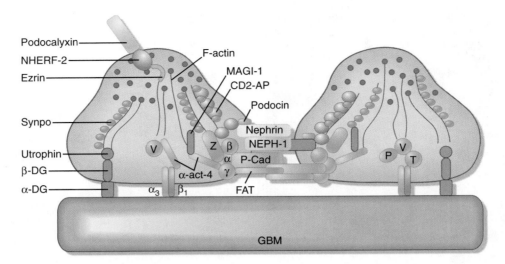

● **Figure 32-10.** Anatomy of podocyte foot processes. This figure illustrates the proteins that make up the slit diaphragm between two adjacent foot processes. Nephrin and NEPH1 are membrane-spanning proteins that have large extracellular domains that interact. Podocin, also a membrane-spanning protein, organizes nephrin and NEPH1 in specific microdomains in the plasma membrane, which is important for signaling events that determine the structural integrity of podocyte foot processes. Many of the proteins that compose the slit diaphragm interact with adapter proteins inside the cell, including CD2-AP. The adapter proteins bind to the filamentous actin (F-actin) cytoskeleton, which in turn binds either directly or indirectly to proteins such as α3β1 and MAGI-1 that interact with proteins expressed by the glomerular basement membrane (GBM). α-act-4, α-actinin 4; α3β1, α3β1 integrin; α-DG, α-dystroglycan; CD2-AP, an adapter protein that links nephrin and podocin to intracellular proteins; FAT, a protocadherin that organizes actin polymerization; MAGI-1, a membrane-associated guanylate kinase protein; NHERF-2, Na$^+$-H$^+$ exchanger regulatory factor 2; P, paxillin; P-Cad, P-cadherin; Synpo, synaptopodin; T, talin; V, vinculin; Z, zona occludens. (Adapted from Mundel P, Shankland SJ: J Am Soc Nephrol 13:3005, 2002.)

which the ability of proteins to cross the filter is based on charge.*

The podocytes, which are endocytic, have long finger-like processes that completely encircle the outer surface of the capillaries (Fig. 32-8). The processes of the podocytes interdigitate to cover the basement membrane and are separated by apparent gaps called **filtration slits.** Each filtration slit is bridged by a thin diaphragm that contains pores with a dimension of 40 × 140 Å. The **filtration slit diaphragm,** which appears as a continuous structure when viewed by electron microscopy (Fig. 32-7, *B*), is composed of several proteins, including **nephrin (NPHS1), NEPH-1, podocin (NPHS2), α-actinin 4 (ACTN4),** and **CD2-AP** (Figs. 32-10 and 32-11). Filtration slits, which function primarily as a size-selective filter, keep the proteins and macromolecules that cross the basement membrane from entering Bowman's space.

Another important component of the renal corpuscle is the **mesangium,** which consists of **mesangial cells** and the **mesangial matrix** (Fig. 32-9). Mesangial cells, which possess many properties of smooth muscle cells, surround the glomerular capillaries, provide structural support for the glomerular capillar-

---

*Because the basement membrane and filtration slits contain negatively charged glycoproteins, some proteins are held back (i.e., not filtered into Bowman's space) on the basis of size and charge. For molecules with an effective molecular radius between 20 and 42 Å, cationic molecules are filtered more readily than anionic molecules.

IN THE CLINIC

Nephrotic syndrome is produced by a variety of disorders and is characterized by an increase in permeability of the glomerular capillaries to proteins and by loss of normal podocyte structure, including effacement (i.e., thinning) of the foot processes. The augmented permeability to proteins results in an increase in urinary protein excretion **(proteinuria).** Thus, the appearance of proteins in urine can indicate kidney disease. Hypoalbuminemia often develops in individuals with this syndrome as a result of the proteinuria. In addition, generalized edema is commonly seen in individuals with nephrotic syndrome. Mutations in several genes that encode slit diaphragm proteins (Figs. 32-10 and 32-11), including **nephrin, NEPH-1, podocin, CD2-AP,** and **α-actinin 4,** or knockout of these genes in mice causes proteinuria and kidney disease. For example, mutations in the nephrin gene (*NPHS1*) lead to abnormal or absent slit diaphragms, which causes massive proteinuria and renal failure (i.e., congenital nephrotic syndrome). In addition, mutations in the podocin gene (*NPHS2*) cause autosomal recessive, steroid-resistant nephrotic syndrome. These naturally occurring mutations and knockout studies in mice demonstrate that nephrin, NEPH-1, podocin, CD2-AP, and α-actinin 4 play a key role in podocyte structure and function.

● **Figure 32-11.** Overview of the major proteins that form the slit diaphragm. Nephrins (red) from opposite foot processes interdigitate in the center of the slit. In the slit, nephrin interacts with NEPH1 and NEPH2 *(blue)*, FAT1 and FAT2 *(green)*, and P-cadherin. The intracellular domains of nephrin, NEPH1, and NEPH2 interact with podocin and CD2-AP, which connect these slit diaphragm proteins with ZO-1, α-actinin 4, and actin. (Modified from Tryggvason K et al: N Engl J Med 354:1387, 2006.)

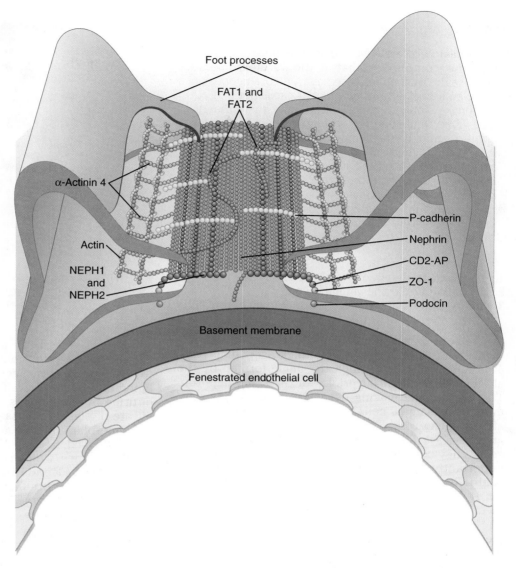

IN THE CLINIC

Alport's syndrome is characterized by hematuria (i.e., blood in urine) and progressive glomerulonephritis (i.e., inflammation of the glomerular capillaries) and accounts for 1% to 2% of all cases of ESRD. Alport's syndrome is caused by defects in type IV collagen (encoded by the *COL4A5* gene), a major component of the glomerular basement membrane. In about 85% of patients with Alport's syndrome, the disease is X-linked with mutations in the *COL4A5* gene. The remaining 15% of patients also have mutations in type IV collagen genes; six have been identified, but the mode of inheritance is autosomal recessive. In Alport's syndrome the glomerular basement membrane becomes irregular in thickness and fails to serve as an effective filtration barrier to blood cells and protein.

ies, secrete the extracellular matrix, exhibit phagocytic activity by removing macromolecules from the mesangium, and secrete prostaglandins and proinflammatory cytokines. Because they also contract and are adjacent to glomerular capillaries, mesangial cells may influence the GFR by regulating blood flow through the glomerular capillaries or by altering the capillary surface area. Mesangial cells located outside the glomerulus (between the afferent and efferent arterioles) are called **extraglomerular mesangial cells.**

Ultrastructure of the Juxtaglomerular Apparatus

The **juxtaglomerular apparatus** is one component of an important feedback mechanism described later in the chapter, the tubuloglomerular feedback mechanism. Structures that make up the juxtaglomerular apparatus include the following (Fig. 32-5):

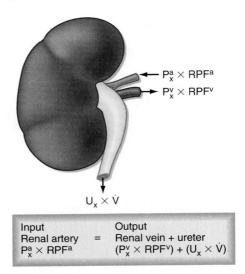

● **Figure 32-12.** Mass balance relationships for the kidney. See text for definition of symbols.

1. The **macula densa** of the thick ascending limb
2. Extraglomerular mesangial cells
3. Renin- and angiotensin II–producing **granular cells** of the afferent arteriole

The cells of the macula densa represent a morphologically distinct region of the thick ascending limb. This region passes through the angle formed by the afferent and efferent arterioles of the same nephron. The cells of the macula densa contact the extraglomerular mesangial cells and the granular cells of the afferent arterioles. The granular cells of the afferent arterioles are derived from metanephric mesenchymal cells. They contain smooth muscle myofilaments, and importantly, they manufacture, store, and release **renin.** Renin is involved in the formation of **angiotensin II** and ultimately in the secretion of **aldosterone** (see Chapter 34). The juxtaglomerular apparatus is one component of the tubuloglomerular feedback mechanism that is involved in the autoregulation of RBF and GFR.

Innervation of the Kidneys

Renal nerves regulate RBF, GFR, and salt and water reabsorption by the nephron. The nerve supply to the kidneys consists of sympathetic nerve fibers that originate in the celiac plexus. There is no parasympathetic innervation. Adrenergic fibers that innervate the kidneys release norepinephrine and dopamine. The adrenergic fibers lie adjacent to the smooth muscle cells of the major branches of the renal artery (interlobar, arcuate, and interlobular arteries) and the afferent and efferent arterioles. Moreover, sympathetic nerves innervate the renin-producing granular cells of the afferent arterioles. Renin secretion is stimulated by increased sympathetic activity. Nerve fibers also innervate the proximal tubule, loop of Henle, distal tubule, and collecting duct; activation of these nerves enhances Na^+ reabsorption by these nephron segments.

ASSESSMENT OF RENAL FUNCTION

The coordinated actions of the nephron's various segments determine the amount of a substance that appears in urine. This represents three general processes: (1) glomerular filtration, (2) reabsorption of the substance from tubular fluid back into blood, and (3) (in some cases) secretion of the substance from blood into tubule fluid. The first step in the formation of urine by the kidneys is the production of an ultrafiltrate of plasma across the glomerulus. The process of glomerular filtration and regulation of GFR and RBF are discussed later in this chapter. The concept of renal clearance, which is the theoretical basis for measurement of GFR and RBF, is presented in the following section. Reabsorption and secretion are discussed in subsequent chapters.

Renal Clearance

The concept of renal **clearance** is based on the Fick principle (i.e., mass balance or conservation of mass). Figure 32-12 illustrates the various factors required to describe the mass balance relationships of a kidney. The renal artery is the single input source to the kidney, whereas the renal vein and ureter constitute the two output routes. The following equation defines the mass balance relationship:

● **Equation 32-1**

$$P_x^a \times RPF^a = (P_x^v \times RPF^v) + (U_x \times \dot{V})$$

where

P_x^a and P_x^v are the concentrations of substance x in the renal artery and renal vein plasma, respectively
RPF^a and RPF^v are **renal plasma flow** rates in the artery and vein, respectively
U_x is the concentration of substance x in urine
$\dot{V}$ is the urine flow rate

This relationship permits quantification of the amount of substance x excreted in urine versus the amount returned to the systemic circulation in renal venous blood. Thus, for any substance that is neither synthesized nor metabolized, the amount that enters the kidneys is equal to the amount that leaves the kidneys in urine plus the amount that leaves the kidneys in renal venous blood.

The principle of renal clearance emphasizes the excretory function of the kidneys; it considers only the rate at which a substance is excreted into urine and not its rate of return to the systemic circulation in the renal vein. Therefore, in terms of mass balance (Equation 32-1), the urinary excretion rate of substance x $(U_x \times \dot{V})$ is proportional to the plasma concentration of substance x (P_x^a):

● **Equation 32-2**

$$P_x^a \propto U_x \times \dot{V}$$

To equate the urinary excretion rate of substance x to its renal arterial plasma concentration, it is necessary to determine the rate at which it is removed from plasma by the kidneys. This removal rate is the clearance (C_x).

● **Equation 32-3**

$$P_x^a \times C_x = U_x \times \dot{V}$$

If Equation 32-3 is rearranged and the concentration of substance x in renal artery plasma (P_x^a) is assumed to be identical to its concentration in a plasma sample from any peripheral blood vessel (P_x), the following relationship is obtained:

● **Equation 32-4**

$$C_x = \frac{U_x \times \dot{V}}{P_x}$$

Clearance has the dimensions of volume/time, and it represents a volume of plasma from which all the substance has been removed and excreted into urine per unit time. This last point is best illustrated by considering the following example. If a substance is present in urine at a concentration of 100 mg/mL and the urine flow rate is 1 mL/min, the excretion rate for this substance is calculated as follows:

● **Equation 32-5**

$$\text{Excretion rate} = U_x \times \dot{V} = 100 \text{ mg/mL}$$
$$\times 1 \text{ mL/min} = 100 \text{ mg/min}$$

If this substance is present in plasma at a concentration of 1 mg/mL, its clearance according to Equation 32-4 is as follows:

● **Equation 32-6**

$$C_x = \frac{U_x \times \dot{V}}{P_x} = \frac{100 \text{ mg/min}}{1 \text{ mg/mL}} = 100 \text{ mL/min}$$

In other words, 100 mL of plasma will be completely cleared of substance x each minute. The definition of clearance as a volume of plasma from which all the substance has been removed and excreted into urine per unit time is somewhat misleading because it is not a real volume of plasma; rather, it is an idealized volume.* The concept of clearance is important because it can be used to measure GFR and RPF and determine whether a substance is reabsorbed or secreted along the nephron.

─────

*For most substances cleared from plasma by the kidneys, only a portion is actually removed and excreted in a single pass through the kidneys.

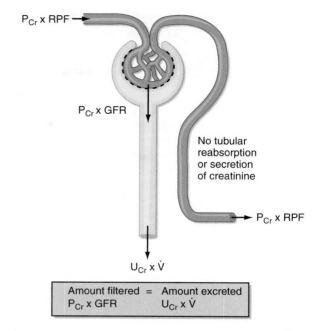

● **Figure 32-13.** Renal handling of creatinine. Creatinine is freely filtered across the glomerulus and is, to a first approximation, not reabsorbed, secreted, or metabolized by the nephron. Note that all the creatinine coming to the kidney in the renal artery does not get filtered at the glomerulus (normally, 15% to 20% of plasma creatinine is filtered). The portion that is not filtered is returned to the systemic circulation in the renal vein. P_{Cr}, plasma creatinine concentration; RPF, renal plasma flow; U_{Cr}, urinary concentration of creatinine; V, urine flow rate.

Glomerular Filtration Rate

The GFR is equal to the sum of the filtration rates of all functioning nephrons. Thus, it is an index of kidney function. A fall in GFR generally means that the kidney disease is progressing, whereas recovery generally suggests recuperation. Thus, knowledge of the patient's GFR is essential in evaluating the severity and course of kidney disease.

Creatinine is a byproduct of skeletal muscle creatine metabolism, and it can be used to measure GFR.* Creatinine is freely filtered across the glomerulus into Bowman's space, and to a first approximation, it is not reabsorbed, secreted, or metabolized by the cells of the nephron. Accordingly, the amount of creatinine excreted in urine per minute equals the amount of creatinine filtered at the glomerulus each minute (Fig. 32-13):

● **Equation 32-7**

$$\text{Amount filtered} = \text{Amount excreted}$$
$$\text{GFR} \times P_{Cr} = U_{Cr} \times \dot{V}$$

where

P_{Cr} = plasma concentration of creatinine
U_{Cr} = urine concentration of creatinine
$\dot{V}$ = urine flow

─────

*Under experimental conditions, GFR is usually measured with inulin, a poly-fructose molecule (MW ≈5000). However, inulin is not produced by the body and must be infused. Therefore, it is not used in most clinical situations.

▶ **IN THE CLINIC**

Creatinine is used to estimate the GFR in clinical practice. It is synthesized at a relatively constant rate, and the amount produced is proportional to the muscle mass. However, creatinine is not a perfect substance for measuring GFR because it is secreted to a small extent by the organic cation secretory system in the proximal tubule (see Chapter 33). The error introduced by this secretory component is approximately 10%. Thus, the amount of creatinine excreted in urine exceeds the amount expected from filtration alone by 10%. However, the method used to measure the plasma creatinine concentration (P_{Cr}) overestimates the true value by 10%. Consequently, the two errors cancel, and in most clinical situations, creatinine clearance provides a reasonably accurate measure of GFR.

▶ **IN THE CLINIC**

A fall in GFR may be the first and only clinical sign of kidney disease. Thus, measuring GFR is important when kidney disease is suspected. A 50% loss of functioning nephrons reduces the GFR only by about 25%. The decline in GFR is not 50% because the remaining nephrons compensate. Because measurements of GFR are cumbersome, kidney function is usually assessed in the clinical setting by measuring P_{Cr}, which is inversely related to GFR (Fig. 32-14). However, as Figure 32-14 shows, GFR must decline substantially before an increase in P_{Cr} can be detected in a clinical setting. For example, a fall in GFR from 120 to 100 mL/min is accompanied by an increase in P_{Cr} from 1.0 to 1.2 mg/dL. This does not appear to be a significant change in P_{Cr}, but the GFR has actually fallen by almost 20%.

If Equation 32-7 is solved for GFR,

● **Equation 32-8**

$$GFR = \frac{U_{Cr} \times \dot{V}}{P_{Cr}}$$

This equation is the same form as that for clearance (Equation 32-4). Thus, clearance of creatinine provides a means for determining the GFR. Clearance has the dimensions of volume/time, and it represents a volume of plasma from which all the substance has been removed and excreted into urine per unit time.

Creatinine is not the only substance that can be used to measure GFR. Any substance that meets the following criteria can serve as an appropriate marker for the measurement of GFR. The substance must

1. Be freely filtered across the glomerulus into Bowman's space
2. Not be reabsorbed or secreted by the nephron
3. Not be metabolized or produced by the kidney
4. Not alter the GFR

Not all of the creatinine (or other substances used to measure GFR) that enters the kidney in renal arterial plasma is filtered at the glomerulus. Likewise, not all of the plasma coming into the kidneys is filtered. Although nearly all of the plasma that enters the kidneys in the renal artery passes through the glomerulus, approximately 10% does not. The portion of filtered plasma is termed the **filtration fraction** and is determined as

● **Equation 32-9**

$$Filtration\ fraction = \frac{GFR}{RPF}$$

Under normal conditions the filtration fraction averages 0.15 to 0.20, which means that only 15% to 20% of the plasma that enters the glomerulus is actually filtered. The remaining 80% to 85% continues on through the glomerular capillaries and into the efferent arterioles and peritubular capillaries. It is finally returned to the systemic circulation in the renal vein.

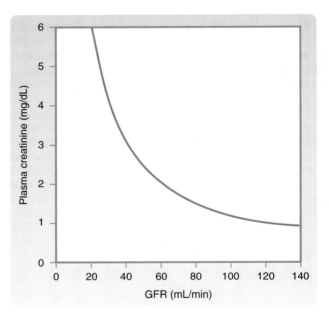

● **Figure 32-14.** Relationship between GFR and plasma [creatinine] (P_{cr}). The amount of creatinine filtered is equal to the amount excreted; thus, GFR × P_{cr} = U_{cr} × V. Because the production of creatinine is constant, excretion must be constant to maintain creatinine balance. Therefore, if the GFR falls from 120 to 60 mL/min, P_{cr} must increase from 1 to 2 mg/dL to keep the filtration of creatinine and its excretion equal to the production rate.

GLOMERULAR FILTRATION

The first step in the formation of urine is ultrafiltration of plasma by the glomerulus. In normal adults, the GFR ranges from 90 to 140 mL/min in males and from 80 to 125 mL/min in females. Thus, in 24 hours as much as 180 L of plasma is filtered by the glomeruli. The plasma ultrafiltrate is devoid of cellular elements (i.e., red and white blood cells and platelets) and is essentially protein free. The concentration of salts and organic molecules, such as glucose and amino acids, is similar

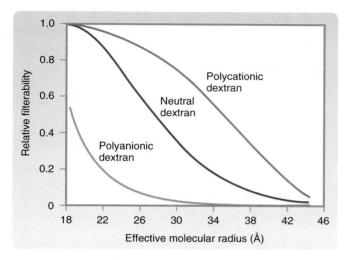

● **Figure 32-15.** Influence of the size and electrical charge of dextran on its filterability. A value of 1 indicates that it is filtered freely, whereas a value of zero indicates that it is not filtered. The filterability of dextrans between approximately 20 and 42 Å depends on charge. Dextrans larger than 42 Å are not filtered regardless of charge, and polycationic dextrans and neutral dextrans smaller than 20 Å are freely filtered. The major proteins in plasma are albumin and immunoglobulins. Because the effective molecular radii of IgG (53 Å) and IgM (>100 Å) are greater than 42 Å, they are not filtered. Although the effective molecular radius of albumin is 35 Å, it is a polyanionic protein, so it does not cross the filtration barrier to a significant degree.

in plasma and the ultrafiltrate. Starling forces drive ultrafiltration across the glomerular capillaries, and changes in these forces alter the GFR. GFR and RPF are normally held within very narrow ranges by a phenomenon called autoregulation. The next sections of this chapter review the composition of the glomerular filtrate, the dynamics of its formation, and the relationship between RPF and GFR. In addition, factors that contribute to autoregulation and regulation of GFR and RBF are discussed.

Determinants of Ultrafiltrate Composition

The glomerular filtration barrier determines the composition of the plasma ultrafiltrate. It restricts the filtration of molecules on the basis of both size and electrical charge (Fig. 32-15). In general, neutral molecules with a radius smaller than 20 Å are filtered freely, molecules larger than 42 Å are not filtered, and molecules between 20 and 42 Å are filtered to various degrees. For example, serum albumin, an anionic protein that has an effective molecular radius of 35.5 Å, is filtered poorly. Because the filtered albumin is normally reabsorbed avidly by the proximal tubule, almost no albumin appears in urine.

Figure 32-15 shows how electrical charge affects the filtration of macromolecules (e.g., dextrans) by the glomerulus. Dextrans are a family of exogenous polysaccharides manufactured in various molecular weights. They can be electrically neutral or have either negative charges (polyanionic) or positive charges (polycationic). As the size (i.e., effective molecular

The importance of the negative charges on the filtration barrier in restricting the filtration of plasma proteins is shown in Figure 32-16. Removal of the negative charges from the filtration barrier causes proteins to be filtered solely on the basis of their effective molecular radius. Hence, at any molecular radius between approximately 20 and 42 Å, filtration of polyanionic proteins will exceed the filtration that prevails in the normal state (in which the filtration barrier has anionic charges). In a number of glomerular diseases the negative charges on the filtration barrier are reduced because of immunological damage and inflammation. As a result, the filtration of proteins is increased, and proteins appear in urine **(proteinuria).**

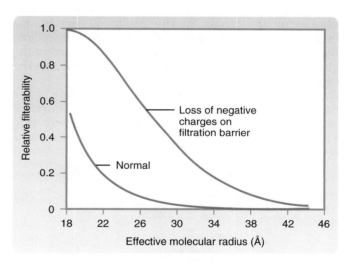

● **Figure 32-16.** Reduction of the negative charges on the glomerular wall results in the filtration of proteins on the basis of size only. In this situation the relative filterability of proteins depends only on the molecular radius. Accordingly, excretion of polyanionic proteins (20 to 42 Å) in urine increases because more proteins of this size are filtered.

radius) of a dextran molecule increases, the rate at which it is filtered decreases. For any given molecular radius, cationic molecules are more readily filtered than anionic molecules. The reduced filtration rate for anionic molecules is explained by the presence of negatively charged glycoproteins on the surface of all components of the glomerular filtration barrier. These charged glycoproteins repel similarly charged molecules. Because most plasma proteins are negatively charged, the negative charge on the filtration barrier restricts the filtration of proteins that have a molecular radius of 20 to 42 Å or greater.

Dynamics of Ultrafiltration

The forces responsible for the glomerular filtration of plasma are the same as those in all capillary beds. Ultrafiltration occurs because the Starling forces (i.e., hydrostatic and oncotic pressure) drive fluid from the lumen of glomerular capillaries, across the filtration barrier, and into Bowman's space (Fig. 32-17). The hydrostatic pressure in the glomerular capillary (P_{GC}) is oriented to promote the movement of fluid from the glomerular capillary into Bowman's space. Because the reflection coefficient (σ) for proteins across the glomerular capillary is essentially 1, the glomerular ultrafiltrate is protein free, and the oncotic pressure in Bowman's space (π_{BS}) is near zero. Therefore, P_{GC} is the only force that favors filtration. The hydrostatic pressure in Bowman's space (P_{BS}) and the oncotic pressure in the glomerular capillary (π_{GC}) oppose filtration.

As shown in Figure 32-17, a net ultrafiltration pressure (P_{UF}) of 17 mm Hg exists at the afferent end of the glomerulus, whereas at the efferent end it is 8 mm Hg (where $P_{UF} = P_{GC} - P_{BS} - \pi_{GC}$). Two additional points concerning Starling forces and this pressure change are important. First, P_{GC} decreases slightly along the length of the capillary because of the resistance to flow along the length of the capillary. Second, π_{GC} increases along the length of the glomerular capillary. Because water is filtered and protein is retained in the glomerular capillary, the protein concentration in the capillary rises, and π_{GC} increases.

GFR is proportional to the sum of the Starling forces that exist across the capillaries [$(P_{GC} - P_{BS}) - \sigma(\pi_{GC} - \pi_{BS})$] multiplied by the ultrafiltration coefficient (K_f). That is,

● Equation 32-10

$$GFR = K_f[(P_{GC} - P_{BS}) - \sigma(\pi_{GC} - \pi_{BS})]$$

K_f is the product of the intrinsic permeability of the glomerular capillary and the glomerular surface area available for filtration. The rate of glomerular filtration is considerably greater in glomerular capillaries than in systemic capillaries, mainly because K_f is approximately 100 times greater in glomerular capillaries. Furthermore, P_{GC} is approximately twice as great as the hydrostatic pressure in systemic capillaries.

GFR can be altered by changing K_f or by changing any of the Starling forces. In normal individuals, the GFR is regulated by alterations in P_{GC} that are mediated mainly by changes in afferent or efferent arteriolar resistance. P_{GC} is affected in three ways:

1. Changes in afferent arteriolar resistance: A decrease in resistance increases P_{GC} and GFR, whereas an increase in resistance decreases them.
2. Changes in efferent arteriolar resistance: A decrease in resistance reduces P_{GC} and GFR, whereas an increase in resistance elevates them.
3. Changes in renal arteriolar pressure: An increase in blood pressure transiently increases P_{GC} (which enhances GFR), whereas a decrease in blood pressure transiently decreases P_{GC} (which reduces GFR).

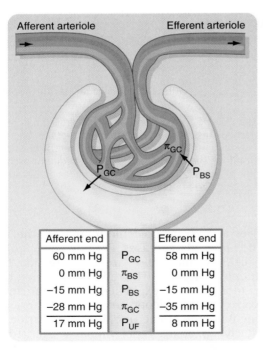

● **Figure 32-17.** Idealized glomerular capillary and the Starling forces across it. The reflection coefficient (σ) for protein across the glomerular capillary is 1. P_{BS}, hydrostatic pressure in Bowman's space; P_{GC}, hydrostatic pressure in the glomerular capillary; P_{UF}, net ultrafiltration pressure; π_{BS}, oncotic pressure in Bowman's space; π_{GC}, oncotic pressure in the glomerular capillary. The negative signs for P_{BS} and π_{GC} indicate that these forces oppose formation of the glomerular filtrate.

Afferent end		Efferent end
60 mm Hg	P_{GC}	58 mm Hg
0 mm Hg	π_{BS}	0 mm Hg
−15 mm Hg	P_{BS}	−15 mm Hg
−28 mm Hg	π_{GC}	−35 mm Hg
17 mm Hg	P_{UF}	8 mm Hg

▶ IN THE CLINIC

A reduction in the GFR in disease states is most often due to decreases in K_f because of the loss of filtration surface area. The GFR also changes in pathophysiological conditions because of changes in P_{GC}, π_{GC}, and P_{BS}.

1. Changes in K_f: Increased K_f enhances the GFR, whereas decreased K_f reduces the GFR. Some kidney diseases reduce K_f by decreasing the number of filtering glomeruli (i.e., diminished surface area). Some drugs and hormones that dilate the glomerular arterioles also increase K_f. Similarly, drugs and hormones that constrict the glomerular arterioles also decrease K_f.
2. Changes in P_{GC}: With decreased renal perfusion, the GFR declines because P_{GC} falls. As previously discussed, a reduction in P_{GC} is caused by a decline in renal arterial pressure, an increase in afferent arteriolar resistance, or a decrease in efferent arteriolar resistance.
3. Changes in π_{GC}: An inverse relationship exists between π_{GC} and GFR. Alterations in π_{GC} result from changes in protein synthesis outside the kidneys. In addition, the protein loss in urine caused by some renal diseases can lead to a decrease in the plasma protein concentration and thus in π_{GC}.
4. Changes in P_{BS}: Increased P_{BS} reduces the GFR, whereas decreased P_{BS} enhances the GFR. Acute obstruction of the urinary tract (e.g., a kidney stone occluding the ureter) increases P_{BS}.

RENAL BLOOD FLOW

Blood flow through the kidneys serves several important functions, including the following:

1. Indirectly determines the GFR
2. Modifies the rate of solute and water reabsorption by the proximal tubule
3. Participates in the concentration and dilution of urine
4. Delivers O_2, nutrients, and hormones to the cells of the nephron and returns CO_2 and reabsorbed fluid and solutes to the general circulation
5. Delivers substrates for excretion in urine

Blood flow through any organ may be represented by the following equation:

● **Equation 32-11**

$$Q = \frac{\Delta P}{R}$$

where

Q = blood flow
ΔP = mean arterial pressure minus venous pressure for that organ
R = resistance to flow through that organ

Accordingly, RBF is equal to the pressure difference between the renal artery and the renal vein divided by renal vascular resistance:

● **Equation 32-12**

$$RBF = \frac{Aortic\ pressure - Renal\ venous\ pressure}{Renal\ vascular\ resistance}$$

The afferent arteriole, efferent arteriole, and interlobular artery are the major resistance vessels in the kidneys and thereby determine renal vascular resistance. Like most other organs, the kidneys regulate their blood flow by adjusting vascular resistance in response to changes in arterial pressure. As shown in Figure 32-18, these adjustments are so precise that blood flow remains relatively constant as arterial blood pressure changes between 90 and 180 mm Hg. GFR is also regulated over the same range of arterial pressures. The phenomenon whereby RBF and GFR are maintained relatively constant, namely, **autoregulation,** is achieved by changes in vascular resistance, mainly through the afferent arterioles of the kidneys. Because both GFR and RBF are regulated over the same range of pressures and because RBF is an important determinant of GFR, it is not surprising that the same mechanisms regulate both flows.

Two mechanisms are responsible for the autoregulation of RBF and GFR: one mechanism that responds to changes in arterial pressure and another that responds to changes in [NaCl] in tubular fluid. Both regulate the tone of the afferent arteriole. The pressure-sensitive mechanism, the so-called **myogenic mechanism,** is related to an intrinsic property of vascular smooth muscle: the tendency to contract when stretched. Accordingly, when arterial pressure rises and the renal afferent arteriole is stretched, the smooth muscle contracts. Because the increase in resistance

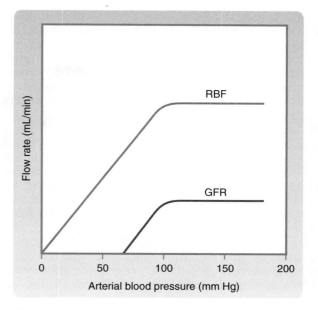

● **Figure 32-18.** Relationship between arterial blood pressure and RBF and between arterial blood pressure and GFR. Autoregulation maintains GFR and RBF relatively constant as blood pressure changes from 90 to 180 mm Hg.

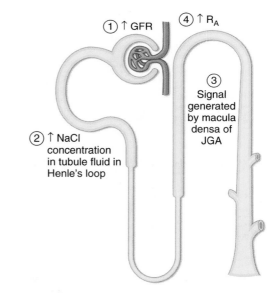

● **Figure 32-19.** Tubuloglomerular feedback. An increase in GFR (1) increases [NaCl] in tubule fluid in the loop of Henle (2). The increase in [NaCl] is sensed by the macula densa and converted to a signal (3) that increases the resistance of the afferent arteriole (R_A) (4), which decreases the GFR. (Modified from Cogan MG: Fluid and Electrolytes: Physiology and Pathophysiology. Norwalk, CT, Appleton & Lange, 1991.)

of the arteriole offsets the increase in pressure, RBF and therefore GFR remain constant. (That is, RBF is constant if $\Delta P/R$ is kept constant [Equation 32-11].)

The second mechanism responsible for the autoregulation of GFR and RBF is the [NaCl]-dependent mechanism known as **tubuloglomerular feedback** (Fig. 32-19). This mechanism involves a feedback loop in which the concentration of NaCl in tubular fluid is sensed by the macula densa of the **juxtaglomerular apparatus** (Fig. 32-20; also see Fig. 32-5) and converted into a signal or signals that affect afferent arteriolar resistance and thus the GFR. When the GFR increases and causes [NaCl] in tubular fluid at the macula densa to rise, more NaCl enters the macula densa cells. This leads to an increase in the formation and release of ATP and adenosine, a metabolite of ATP, by macula densa cells, which causes vasoconstriction of the afferent arteriole. Vasoconstriction of the afferent arteriole returns the GFR to normal levels. In contrast, when the GFR and [NaCl] in tubule fluid decrease, less NaCl enters the macula densa cells, and ATP and adenosine production and release decline. The fall in [ATP] and [adenosine] causes vasodilation of the afferent arteriole, which returns the GFR to normal. NO, a vasodilator produced by the macula densa, attenuates tubuloglomerular feedback, whereas angiotensin II enhances tubuloglomerular feedback. Thus, the macula densa may release both vasoconstrictors (e.g., ATP and adenosine) and a vasodilator (e.g., NO) that oppose each other's action at the level of the afferent arteriole. Production plus release of vasoconstrictors and vasodilators ensures exquisite control over tubuloglomerular feedback.

Figure 32-20 also illustrates the role of the macula densa in controlling the secretion of renin by granular cells of the afferent arteriole. This aspect of function of the juxtaglomerular apparatus is considered in detail in Chapter 34.

Because animals engage in many activities that can change arterial blood pressure, mechanisms that maintain RBF and GFR relatively constant despite changes in arterial pressure are highly desirable. If the GFR and RBF were to rise or fall suddenly in proportion to changes in blood pressure, urinary excretion of fluid and solute would also change suddenly. Such changes in excretion of water and solutes without comparable changes in intake would alter fluid and

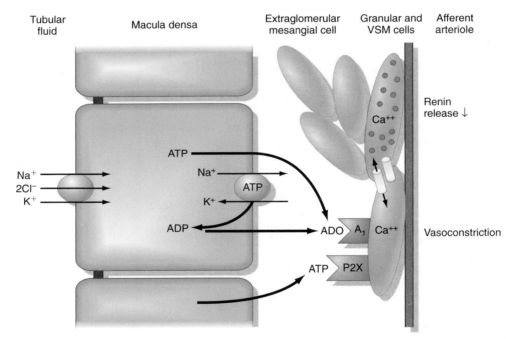

● **Figure 32-20.** Cellular mechanism whereby an increase in the delivery of NaCl to the macula densa causes vasoconstriction of the afferent arteriole of the same nephron (i.e., tubuloglomerular feedback). An increase in GFR elevates [NaCl] in tubule fluid at the macula densa. This in turn enhances uptake of NaCl across the apical cell membrane of macula densa cells via the $1Na^+$-$1K^+$-$2Cl^-$ (NKCC2) symporter, which leads to an increase in [ATP] and [adenosine] (ADO). ATP binds to P2X receptors and adenosine binds to adenosine A_1 receptors in the plasma membrane of smooth muscle cells surrounding the afferent arteriole, both of which increase intracellular $[Ca^{++}]$. The rise in $[Ca^{++}]$ induces vasoconstriction of the afferent arteriole, thereby returning GFR to normal levels. Note that ATP and adenosine also inhibit renin release by granular cells in the afferent arteriole. This too results from an increase in intracellular $[Ca^{++}]$ as a reflection of electrical coupling of the granular and vascular smooth muscle (VSM) cells. When GFR is reduced, [NaCl] in tubule fluid falls, as does uptake of NaCl into macula densa cells. This in turn decreases release of ATP and adenosine, which decreases intracellular $[Ca^{++}]$ and thereby increases GFR and stimulates the release of renin by granular cells. In addition, a decrease in entry of NaCl into macula densa cells enhances the production of PGE_2, which also stimulates renin secretion by granular cells. As discussed in detail in Chapters 4 and 6, renin increases plasma [angiotensin II], a hormone that enhances NaCl and water retention by the kidneys. (Modified from Persson AEG et al: Acta Physiol Scand 181:471, 2004.)

electrolyte balance (the reason for which is discussed in Chapter 34). Accordingly, autoregulation of GFR and RBF provides an effective means for uncoupling renal function from arterial pressure, and it ensures that fluid and solute excretion remain constant.

Three points concerning autoregulation should be noted:

1. Autoregulation is absent when arterial pressure is less than 90 mm Hg.
2. Autoregulation is not perfect; RBF and GFR do change slightly as arterial blood pressure varies.
3. Despite autoregulation, RBF and GFR can be changed by certain hormones and by changes in sympathetic nerve activity (Table 32-1).

REGULATION OF RENAL BLOOD FLOW AND THE GLOMERULAR FILTRATION RATE

Several factors and hormones affect the GFR and RBF (Table 32-1). As discussed, the myogenic mechanism

AT THE CELLULAR LEVEL

Tubuloglomerular feedback (TGF) is absent in mice that do not express the adenosine receptor (A₁). This underscores the importance of adenosine signaling in TGF. Studies have shown that when the GFR increases and causes the concentration of NaCl in tubular fluid at the macula densa to rise, more NaCl enters cells via the $1Na^+$-$1K^+$-$2Cl^-$ symporter (NKCC2) located in the apical plasma membrane (Fig. 32-20). Increased intracellular [NaCl] in turn stimulates the release of ATP via ATP-conducting ion channels located in the basolateral membrane of macula densa cells. In addition, adenosine production is also enhanced. Adenosine binds to A₁ receptors and ATP binds to P2X receptors located on the plasma membrane of smooth muscle cells in the afferent arteriole. Both hormones increase intracellular [Ca⁺⁺], which causes vasoconstriction of the afferent artery and therefore a fall in GFR. Although adenosine is a vasodilator in most other vascular beds, it constricts the afferent arteriole in the kidney.

and tubuloglomerular feedback play key roles in maintaining GFR and RBF constant. In addition, sympathetic nerves, angiotensin II, prostaglandins, NO, endothelin, bradykinin, ATP, and adenosine exert major control over RBF and GFR. Figure 32-21 shows how changes in afferent and afferent arteriolar resistance, mediated by changes in the hormones listed in Table 32-1, modulate GFR and RBF.

Sympathetic Nerves

The afferent and efferent arterioles are innervated by sympathetic neurons; however, sympathetic tone is minimal when the volume of extracellular fluid is normal (see Chapter 34). Sympathetic nerves release norepinephrine and dopamine, and circulating epinephrine (a catecholamine like norepinephrine and dopamine) is secreted by the adrenal medulla. Norepinephrine and epinephrine cause vasoconstriction by binding to α₁-adrenoceptors, which are located mainly on the afferent arterioles. Activation of α₁-adrenoceptors decreases GFR and RBF. Dehydration or strong emotional stimuli, such as fear and pain, activate sympathetic nerves and reduce GFR and RBF.

Renalase, a catecholamine-metabolizing hormone produced by the kidneys, facilitates the degradation of catecholamines.

Angiotensin II

Angiotensin II is produced systemically and locally within the kidneys. It constricts the afferent and effer-

IN THE CLINIC

Individuals with **renal artery stenosis** (narrowing of the lumen of the artery) caused by atherosclerosis, for example, can have elevated systemic arterial blood pressure mediated by stimulation of the renin-angiotensin system (see Chapter 34). Pressure in the renal artery proximal to the stenosis is increased, but pressure distal to the stenosis is normal or reduced. Autoregulation is important in maintaining RBF, P_{GC}, and GFR in the presence of this stenosis. Administration of drugs to lower systemic blood pressure also lowers the pressure distal to the stenosis; accordingly, RBF, P_{GC}, and GFR fall.

● **Table 32-1.**

Major Hormones That Influence the Glomerular Filtration Rate and Renal Blood Flow

	Stimulus	Effect on GFR	Effect on RBF
Vasoconstrictors			
Sympathetic nerves	↓ ECFV	↓	↓
Angiotensin II	↓ ECFV	↓	↓
Endothelin	↑ Stretch, A-II, bradykinin, epinephrine; ↓ ECFV	↓	↓
Vasodilators			
Prostaglandins (PGE₁, PGE₂, PGI₂)	↓ ECFV; ↑ shear stress, A-II	No change/↑	↑
Nitric oxide (NO)	↑ Shear stress, acetylcholine, histamine, bradykinin, ATP	↑	↑
Bradykinin	↑ Prostaglandins, ↓ ACE	↑	↑
Natriuretic peptides (ANP, BNP)	↑ ECFV	↑	No change

A-II, angiotensin II; ECFV, extracellular fluid volume; ACE, angiotensin-converting enzyme.

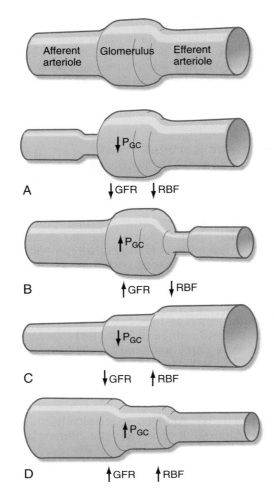

● **Figure 32-21.** Relationship between selective changes in the resistance of either the afferent arteriole or the efferent arteriole on RBF and GFR. Constriction of either the afferent or efferent arteriole increases resistance, and according to Equation 32-11 ($Q = \Delta P/R$), an increase in resistance (R) decreases flow (Q) (i.e., RBF). Dilation of either the afferent or afferent arteriole increases flow (i.e., RBF). Constriction of the afferent arteriole **(A)** decreases P_{GC} because less of the arterial pressure is transmitted to the glomerulus, thereby reducing GFR. In contrast, constriction of the efferent arteriole **(B)** elevates P_{GC} and thus increases GFR. Dilation of the efferent arteriole **(C)** decreases P_{GC} and thus decreases GFR. Dilation of the afferent arteriole **(D)** increases P_{GC} because more of the arterial pressure is transmitted to the glomerulus, thereby increasing GFR. (Modified from Rose BD, Rennke KG: Renal Pathophysiology: The Essentials. Baltimore, Williams & Wilkins, 1994.)

ent arterioles* and decreases RBF and GFR. Figure 32-22 shows how norepinephrine, epinephrine, and angiotensin II act together to decrease RBF and GFR and thereby increase blood pressure and extracellular fluid volume, as would occur, for example, with hemorrhage.

---

*The efferent arteriole is more sensitive to angiotensin II than the afferent arteriole is. Therefore, with low concentrations of angiotensin II, constriction of the efferent arteriole predominates, and GFR increases and RBF decreases. However, with high concentrations of angiotensin II, constriction of both afferent and efferent arterioles occurs, and GFR and RBF both decrease (Fig. 32-21).

Hemorrhage decreases arterial blood pressure and therefore activates the sympathetic nerves to the kidneys via the baroreceptor reflex (Fig. 32-22). Norepinephrine causes intense vasoconstriction of the afferent and efferent arterioles and thereby decreases GFR and RBF. The rise in sympathetic activity also increases the release of epinephrine and angiotensin II, which cause further vasoconstriction and a fall in RBF. The rise in the vascular resistance of the kidneys and other vascular beds increases total peripheral resistance. The resulting tendency for blood pressure to increase (blood pressure = cardiac output × total peripheral resistance) offsets the tendency of blood pressure to decrease in response to hemorrhage. Hence, this system works to preserve arterial pressure at the expense of maintaining normal GFR and RBF.

Prostaglandins

Prostaglandins do not play a major role in regulating RBF in healthy, resting people. However, during pathophysiological conditions such as hemorrhage, prostaglandins (PGI_2, PGE_1, and PGE_2) are produced locally within the kidneys, and they increase RBF without changing GFR. Prostaglandins increase RBF by dampening the vasoconstrictor effects of sympathetic nerves and angiotensin II. This effect is important because it prevents severe and potentially harmful vasoconstriction and renal ischemia. Synthesis of prostaglandins is stimulated by dehydration and stress (e.g., surgery, anesthesia), angiotensin II, and sympathetic nerves. Nonsteroidal antiinflammatory drugs (NSAIDs), such as aspirin and ibuprofen, inhibit the synthesis of prostaglandins. Thus, administration of these drugs during renal ischemia and hemorrhagic shock is contraindicated because by blocking the production of prostaglandins, they decrease RBF and increase renal ischemia. Prostaglandins play an increasingly important role in maintaining RBF and GFR as individuals age. Accordingly, NSAIDs can significantly reduce RBF and GFR in the elderly.

Nitric Oxide

NO, an endothelium-derived relaxing factor, is an important vasodilator under basal conditions, and it counteracts the vasoconstriction produced by angiotensin II and catecholamines. When blood flow increases, greater shear force acts on endothelial cells in the arterioles and increases the production of NO. In addition, a number of vasoactive hormones, including acetylcholine, histamine, bradykinin, and ATP, facilitate the release of NO from endothelial cells. Increased production of NO causes dilation of the afferent and efferent arterioles in the kidneys. Whereas increased levels of NO decrease total peripheral resistance, inhibition of NO production increases total peripheral resistance.

● **Figure 32-22.** Pathway by which hemorrhage activates renal sympathetic nerve activity and stimulates the production of angiotensin II. (Modified from Vander AJ: Renal Physiology, 2nd ed. New York, McGraw-Hill, 1980.)

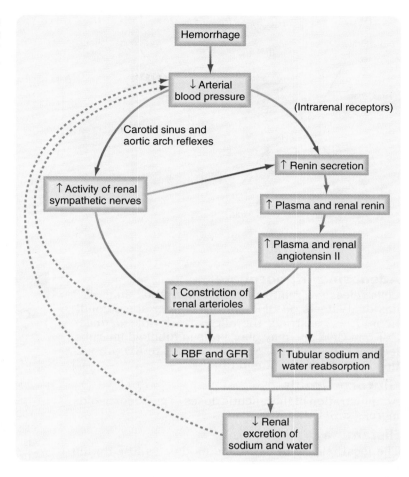

IN THE CLINIC

Abnormal production of NO is observed in individuals with **diabetes mellitus** and **hypertension.** The excess renal NO production in diabetes may be responsible for glomerular hyperfiltration (i.e., increased GFR) and damage to the glomerulus, problems characteristic of this disease. Elevated NO levels increase glomerular capillary pressure secondary to a fall in resistance of the afferent arteriole. The ensuing hyperfiltration is thought to cause glomerular damage. The normal response to an increase in dietary salt intake includes stimulation of renal NO production, which prevents an increase in blood pressure. In some individuals, however, NO production may not increase appropriately in response to an elevation in salt intake, so blood pressure rises.

Endothelin

Endothelin is a potent vasoconstrictor secreted by endothelial cells of the renal vessels, mesangial cells, and distal tubular cells in response to angiotensin II, bradykinin, epinephrine, and endothelial shear stress. Endothelin causes profound vasoconstriction of the afferent and efferent arterioles and decreases GFR and RBF. Although this potent vasoconstrictor may not influence GFR and RBF in resting subjects, production of endothelin is elevated in a number of glomerular disease states (e.g., renal disease associated with diabetes mellitus).

Bradykinin

Kallikrein is a proteolytic enzyme produced in the kidneys. Kallikrein cleaves circulating kininogen to bradykinin, which is a vasodilator that acts by stimulating the release of NO and prostaglandins. Bradykinin increases GFR and RBF.

Adenosine

Adenosine is produced within the kidneys and causes vasoconstriction of the afferent arteriole, thereby reducing GFR and RBF. As previously mentioned, adenosine may play a role in tubuloglomerular feedback.

Natriuretic Peptides

Secretion of atrial natriuretic peptide (ANP) by the cardiac atria and brain natriuretic peptide (BNP) by the cardiac ventricle increases when extracellular fluid volume is expanded. Both ANP and BNP dilate the afferent arteriole and constrict the efferent arteriole. Therefore, ANP and BNP produce a modest increase in GFR with little change in RBF.

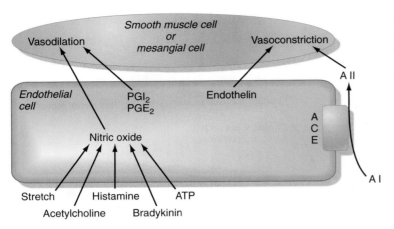

● **Figure 32-23.** Examples of the interactions of endothelial cells with smooth muscle and mesangial cells. ACE, angiotensin-converting enzyme; AI, angiotensin I; AII, angiotensin II. (Modified from Navar LG et al: Physiol Rev 76:425, 1996.)

Adenosine Triphosphate

Cells release ATP into the renal interstitial fluid. ATP has dual effects on GFR and RBF. Under some conditions, ATP constricts the afferent arteriole, reduces RBF and GFR, and may play a role in tubuloglomerular feedback. In contrast, ATP may stimulate NO production and increase GFR and RBF.

Glucocorticoids

Administration of therapeutic doses of glucocorticoids increases GFR and RBF.

Histamine

The local release of histamine modulates RBF during the resting state and during inflammation and injury. Histamine decreases the resistance of the afferent and efferent arterioles and thereby increases RBF without elevating GFR.

Dopamine

The proximal tubule produces the vasodilator substance dopamine. Dopamine has several actions within the kidney, such as increasing RBF and inhibiting renin secretion.

Finally, as illustrated in Figure 32-23, endothelial cells play an important role in regulating the resistance of the renal afferent and efferent arterioles by producing a number of paracrine hormones, including NO, prostacyclin (PGI₂), endothelin, and angiotensin II. These hormones regulate contraction or relaxation of smooth muscle cells in afferent and efferent arterioles and mesangial cells. Shear stress, acetylcholine, histamine, bradykinin, and ATP stimulate the production of NO, which increases GFR and RBF. **Angiotensin-converting enzyme (ACE),** located on the surface of endothelial cells lining the afferent arteriole and glomerular capillaries, converts angiotensin I to angiotensin II, which decreases GFR and RBF. Angiotensin II is also produced locally in granular cells in the afferent arteriole and proximal tubular cells. Secretion of PGI₂ and PGE₂ by endothelial cells, stimulated by sympathetic nerve activity and angiotensin II, increases GFR and RBF. Finally, the release of endothelin from endothelial cells decreases GFR and RBF.

▶ IN THE CLINIC

ACE degrades and thereby inactivates bradykinin, and it converts angiotensin I, an inactive hormone, to angiotensin II, an active hormone. Thus, ACE increases angiotensin II levels and decreases bradykinin levels. Drugs called **ACE inhibitors** (e.g., enalapril, captopril), which reduce systemic blood pressure in patients with hypertension, decrease angiotensin II levels and elevate bradykinin levels. Both effects lower systemic vascular resistance, reduce blood pressure, and decrease renal vascular resistance, thereby increasing GFR and RBF. **Angiotensin II receptor antagonists** (e.g., losartan) are also used to treat high blood pressure. As their name suggests, they block the binding of angiotensin II to the angiotensin II receptor (AT1). These antagonists block the vasoconstrictor effects of angiotensin II on the afferent arteriole; thus, they increase GFR and RBF. In contrast to ACE inhibitors, angiotensin II receptor antagonists do not inhibit kinin metabolism (e.g., bradykinin).

■ KEY CONCEPTS

1. The first step in urine formation is the passive movement of a plasma ultrafiltrate from the glomerular capillaries into Bowman's space. The term ultrafiltration refers to the passive movement of an essentially protein-free fluid from the glomerular capillaries into Bowman's space. The endothelial cells of glomerular capillaries are covered by a basement membrane that is surrounded by podocytes. The capillary endothelium, basement membrane, and foot processes of podocytes form the so-called filtration barrier.

2. The juxtaglomerular apparatus is one component of an important feedback mechanism (i.e., tubuloglomerular feedback) that regulates RBF and GFR. The structures that make up the juxtaglomerular apparatus include the macula densa, extraglomeru-

lar mesangial cells, and renin- and angiotensin II–producing granular cells.

3. Clinically, the GFR is evaluated by measuring plasma [creatinine].

4. Autoregulation allows GFR and RBF to remain constant despite changes in arterial blood pressure between 90 and 180 mm Hg. Sympathetic nerves, catecholamines, angiotensin II, prostaglandins, NO, endothelin, natriuretic peptides, bradykinin, and adenosine exert substantial control over GFR and RBF.

CHAPTER 33

Solute and Water Transport along the Nephron: Tubular Function

The formation of urine involves three basic processes: (1) **ultrafiltration** of plasma by the glomerulus, (2) **reabsorption** of water and solutes from the ultrafiltrate, and (3) **secretion** of selected solutes into tubular fluid. Although an average of 115 to 180 L/day in women and 130 to 200 L/day in men of essentially protein-free fluid is filtered by the human glomeruli each day,* less than 1% of the filtered water and sodium chloride (NaCl) and variable amounts of other solutes are excreted in urine (Table 33-1). By the processes of reabsorption and secretion, the renal tubules modulate the volume and composition of urine (Table 33-2), which in turn allows the tubules to precisely control the volume, osmolality, composition, and pH of the extracellular and intracellular fluid compartments. Transport proteins in cell membranes of the nephron mediate the reabsorption and secretion of solutes and water in the kidneys. Approximately 5% to 10% of all human genes code for transport proteins, and genetic and acquired defects in transport proteins are the cause of many kidney diseases (Table 33-3). In addition, numerous transport proteins are important drug targets. This chapter discusses NaCl and water reabsorption, transport of organic anions and cations, the transport proteins involved in solute and water transport, and some of the factors and hormones that regulate NaCl transport. Details on acid-base transport and on K^+, Ca^{++}, and inorganic phosphate (P_i) transport and their regulation are provided in Chapters 34 through 36.

SOLUTE AND WATER REABSORPTION ALONG THE NEPHRON

The general principles of solute and water transport across epithelial cells were discussed in Chapter 2.

Quantitatively, reabsorption of NaCl and water represents the major function of nephrons. Approximately 25,000 mEq/day of Na^+ and 179 L/day of water are reabsorbed by the renal tubules (Table 33-1). In addition, renal transport of many other important solutes is linked either directly or indirectly to reabsorption of Na^+. In the following sections, the NaCl and water

*The normal glomerular filtration rate (GFR) averages 115 to 180 L/day in women and 130 to 200 L/day in men. Thus, the volume of the ultrafiltrate represents a volume that is approximately 10 times that of the extracellular fluid (ECF) volume. For simplicity, we assume throughout the remainder of this section that the GFR is 180 L/day.

transport processes of each nephron segment and their regulation by hormones and other factors are presented.

Proximal Tubule

The proximal tubule reabsorbs approximately 67% of filtered water, Na^+, Cl^-, K^+, and other solutes. In addition, the proximal tubule reabsorbs virtually all the glucose and amino acids filtered by the glomerulus. The key element in proximal tubule reabsorption is Na^+,K^+-ATPase in the basolateral membrane. Reabsorption of every substance, including water, is linked in some manner to the operation of Na^+,K^+-ATPase.

Na⁺ Reabsorption

Na^+ is reabsorbed by different mechanisms in the first and the second halves of the proximal tubule. In the first half of the proximal tubule, Na^+ is reabsorbed primarily with bicarbonate (HCO_3^-) and a number of other solutes (e.g., glucose, amino acids, P_i, lactate). In contrast, in the second half, Na^+ is reabsorbed mainly with Cl^-. This disparity is mediated by differences in the Na^+ transport systems in the first and second halves of the proximal tubule and by differences in the composition of tubular fluid at these sites.

In the first half of the proximal tubule, Na^+ uptake into the cell is coupled with either H^+ or organic solutes (Fig. 33-1). Specific transport proteins mediate entry of Na^+ into the cell across the apical membrane. For example, the Na^+-H^+ antiporter (Fig. 33-1, *A*) couples entry of Na^+ with extrusion of H^+ from the cell. H^+ secretion results in reabsorption of sodium bicarbonate ($NaHCO_3$) (see Chapter 36). Na^+ also enters proximal cells via several symporter mechanisms, including Na^+-glucose, Na^+–amino acid, Na^+-P_i, and Na^+-lactate (Fig. 33-1, *B*). The glucose and other organic solutes that enter the cell with Na^+ leave the cell across the basolateral membrane via passive transport mechanisms. Any Na^+ that enters the cell across the apical membrane leaves the cell and enters the blood via Na^+,K^+-ATPase. In brief, reabsorption of Na^+ in the first half of the proximal tubule is coupled to that of HCO_3^- and a number of organic molecules. Reabsorption of many organic molecules is so avid that they are almost completely removed from the tubular fluid in the first half of the proximal tubule (Fig. 33-2). Reabsorption of $NaHCO_3$ and Na^+–organic solutes across the proximal tubule establishes a transtubular osmotic gradient (i.e., the osmolality of the interstitial fluid bathing the basolateral side of the cells is higher than the osmolality of

● Table 33-1.

Filtration, Excretion, and Reabsorption of Water, Electrolytes, and Solutes by the Kidneys

Substance	Measure	Filtered*	Excreted	Reabsorbed	% Filtered Load Reabsorbed
Water	L/day	180	1.5	178.5	99.2
Na^+	mEq/day	25,200	150	25,050	99.4
K^+	mEq/day	720	100	620	86.1
Ca^{++}	mEq/day	540	10	530	98.2
HCO_3^-	mEq/day	4320	2	4318	99.9+
Cl^-	mEq/day	18,000	150	17,850	99.2
Glucose	mmol/day	800	0	800	100.0
Urea	g/day	56	28	28	50.0

*The filtered amount of any substance is calculated by multiplying the concentration of that substance in the ultrafiltrate by the glomerular filtration rate (GFR); for example, the filtered load of Na^+ is calculated as $[Na^+]_{ultrafiltrate}$ (140 mEq/L) × GFR (180 L/day) = 25,200 mEq/day.

● Table 33-2. **Composition of Urine**

Substance	Concentration
Na^+	50-130 mEq/L
K^+	20-70 mEq/L
Ammonium (NH_4^+)	30-50 mEq/L
Ca^{++}	5-12 mEq/L
Mg^{++}	2-18 mEq/L
Cl^-	50-130 mEq/L
Inorganic phosphate (P_i)	20-40 mEq/L
Urea	200-400 mM
Creatinine	6-20 mM
pH	5.0-7.0
Osmolality	500-800 mOsm/kg H_2O
Glucose	0
Amino acids	0
Protein	0
Blood	0
Ketones	0
Leukocytes	0
Bilirubin	0

The composition and volume of urine can vary widely in the healthy state. These values represent average ranges. Water excretion ranges between 0.5 and 1.5 L/day.
Data from Valtin HV: Renal Physiology, 2nd ed. Boston, Little, Brown, 1983.

▶ **IN THE CLINIC**

Fanconi's syndrome, a renal disease that is either hereditary or acquired, results from an impaired ability of the proximal tubule to reabsorb HCO_3^-, P_i, amino acids, glucose, and low-molecular-weight proteins. Because other segments of the nephron cannot reabsorb these solutes and protein, Fanconi's syndrome results in increased urinary excretion of HCO_3^-, amino acids, glucose, P_i, and low-molecular-weight proteins.

tubule fluid) that provides the driving force for the passive reabsorption of water by osmosis. Because more water than Cl^- is reabsorbed in the first half of the proximal tubule, the $[Cl^-]$ in tubular fluid rises along the length of the proximal tubule (Fig. 33-2).

In the second half of the proximal tubule, Na^+ is mainly reabsorbed with Cl^- across both the transcellular and paracellular pathways (Fig. 33-3). Na^+ is primarily reabsorbed with Cl^- rather than organic solutes or HCO_3^- as the accompanying anion because the Na^+ transport mechanisms in the second half of the proximal tubule differ from those in the first half. Furthermore, the tubular fluid that enters the second half contains very little glucose and amino acids, but the high $[Cl^-]$ (140 mEq/L) in tubule fluid exceeds that in the first half (105 mEq/L). The high $[Cl^-]$ is due to the preferential reabsorption of Na^+ with HCO_3^- and organic solutes in the first half of the proximal tubule.

The mechanism of transcellular Na^+ reabsorption in the second half of the proximal tubule is shown in Figure 33-3. Na^+ enters the cell across the luminal membrane primarily via the parallel operation of an Na^+-H^+ antiporter and one or more Cl^--anion antiporters. Because the secreted H^+ and anion combine in the tubular fluid and reenter the cell, operation of the Na^+-H^+ and Cl^--anion antiporters is equivalent to uptake of NaCl from tubular fluid into the cell. Na^+ leaves the cell via Na^+,K^+-ATPase, and Cl^- leaves the cell and enters the blood via a K^+-Cl^- symporter in the basolateral membrane.

NaCl is also reabsorbed across the second half of the proximal tubule via a **paracellular route.** Paracellular NaCl reabsorption occurs because the rise in $[Cl^-]$ in tubule fluid in the first half of the proximal tubule creates a $[Cl^-]$ gradient (140 mEq/L in the tubule lumen and 105 mEq/L in the interstitium). This concentration gradient favors diffusion of Cl^- from the tubular lumen across the tight junctions into the lateral intercellular space. Movement of the negatively charged Cl^- results in the tubular fluid becoming positively charged relative to blood. This positive transepithelial voltage causes the diffusion of positively charged Na^+ out of the tubular fluid across the tight junction into blood. Thus, in the second half of the proximal tubule, some Na^+ and Cl^- are reabsorbed across the tight junctions via passive diffusion. Reabsorption of NaCl establishes a transtubular osmotic gradient that provides the driving force for the passive reabsorption of water by osmosis.

In summary, reabsorption of Na^+ and Cl^- in the proximal tubule occurs across paracellular and transcellular pathways. Approximately 67% of the NaCl filtered each day is reabsorbed in the proximal tubule. Of this, two thirds moves across the transcellular pathway, whereas the remaining third moves across the paracellular pathway (Table 33-4).

● **Table 33-3.** **Some Monogenic Renal Diseases Involving Transport Proteins**

Diseases	Mode of Inheritance	Gene	Transport Protein*	Nephron Segment	Phenotype
Cystinuria, type I	AR	SLC3A1, also known as D2/rBAT	Basic amino acid transporter	Proximal tubule	Increased excretion of basic amino acids, nephrolithiasis (kidney stones)
Cystinuria, types I and III	IAR	SLC7A9, also known as b°, +AT	B°, +AT	Proximal tubule	Increased excretion of basic amino acids, nephrolithiasis
Proximal renal tubular acidosis	AR	SLC4A4, also known as NBCe1	Na+-HCO3− symporter	Proximal tubule	Hyperchloremic metabolic acidosis
X-linked nephrolithiasis (Dent's disease)	XLR	CLC5, also known as ClC-5	Cl− channel	Distal tubule	Hypercalciuria, nephrolithiasis
Bartter's syndrome	AR type I	SLC12A1, also known as NKCC2	1Na+-1K+-2Cl− symporter (furosemide sensitive)	TAL	Hypokalemia, metabolic alkalosis, hyperaldosteronism
	AR type II	KCNJ1, also known as ROMK	K+ channel	TAL	Hypokalemia, metabolic alkalosis, hyperaldosteronism
	AR type III	CLCNKB	Cl− channel (basolateral membrane)	TAL	Hypokalemia, metabolic alkalosis, hyperaldosteronism
	AR type IV	BSND, also known as barttin	Cl− channel (barttin recruits CLCNKB to the basolateral membrane)	TAL	Hypokalemia, metabolic alkalosis, hyperaldosteronism
Hypomagnesemia-hypercalciuria syndrome	AR	CLDN16	Claudin-16, also known as paracellin 1	TAL	Hypomagnesemia, hypercalciuria, nephrolithiasis
Gitelman's syndrome	AR	SLC12A3, also known as NCC/TSC	Thiazide-sensitive symporter	Distal tubule	Hypomagnesemia, hypokalemic metabolic alkalosis, hypocalciuria, hypotension
Pseudohypoaldosteronism	AR	SCNN1A, SCNN1B, and SCNN1G, also known as α-ENaC, β-ENaC and γ-ENaC	α, β, and γ subunit of amiloride-sensitive Na+ channel	Collecting duct	Increased excretion of Na+, hyperkalemia, hypotension
	AD	MR	Mineralocorticoid receptor	Collecting duct	Increased excretion of Na+, hyperkalemia, hypotension
Liddle's syndrome	AD	SCNN1B, SCNN1G, also known as β-ENaC and γ-ENaC	β and γ subunits of amiloride-sensitive Na+ channel	Collecting duct	Decreased excretion of Na+, hypertension
Nephrogenic diabetes insipidus	AR	AQP2	Aquaporin-2 water channel	Collecting duct	Polyuria, polydipsia, plasma hyperosmolality
Distal renal tubular acidosis	AD/AR	SLC4A1, also known as AE1	Cl−-HCO3− antiporter	Collecting duct	Metabolic acidosis, hypokalemia, hypercalciuria, nephrolithiasis
	AR	ATP6V1B1	Subunit of H+-ATPase	Collecting duct	Metabolic acidosis, hypokalemia, hypercalciuria, nephrolithiasis
	AR	ATP6V0A4	Accessory subunit of H+-ATPase	Collecting duct	Metabolic acidosis, hypokalemia, hypercalciuria, nephrolithiasis

*There are 40 different solute transporter families that form the so-called SLC (solute carrier) series.
AD, autosomal dominant; AR, autosomal recessive; IAR, incomplete autosomal recessive; TAL, thick ascending limb of Henle's loop; XLR, X-linked recessive.
Data from Guay-Woodford LM: Semin Nephrol 19:312, 1999.

Water Reabsorption

The proximal tubule reabsorbs 67% of the filtered water (Table 33-5). The driving force for water reabsorption is a transtubular osmotic gradient established by reabsorption of solute (e.g., NaCl, Na+-glucose). Reabsorption of Na+ along with organic solutes, HCO3−, and Cl− from tubular fluid into the lateral intercellular spaces reduces the osmolality of the tubular fluid and increases the osmolality of the lateral intercellular space (Fig. 33-4). Because the proximal tubule is highly permeable to water, water is reabsorbed via osmosis. Because the apical and basolateral membranes of proximal tubule cells express aquaporin water channels, water is primarily reabsorbed across the proximal tubular cells.

Some water is also reabsorbed across the tight junctions. The accumulation of fluid and solutes within the lateral intercellular space increases hydrostatic pressure in this compartment. The increased hydrostatic pressure forces fluid and solutes into the capillaries.* Thus, water reabsorption follows solute reabsorption in the proximal tubule. The reabsorbed fluid is slightly hyperosmotic relative to plasma. However, this difference in osmolality is so small that it is commonly said that proximal tubule reabsorption is isosmotic (i.e.,

---

*In addition, protein oncotic pressure in the peritubular capillaries (π_{pc}) is elevated because of the process of glomerular filtration (see Chapter 32). The elevated π_{pc} facilitates uptake of fluid and solute into the capillary.

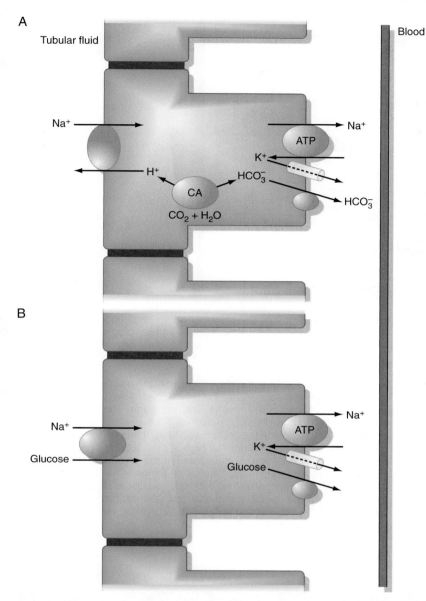

A

Tubular fluid

Na⁺ → → Na⁺

ATP

K⁺

H⁺ ← HCO₃⁻ → K⁺

CA → HCO₃⁻

CO₂ + H₂O

B

Na⁺ →

Glucose →

Na⁺

ATP

K⁺

Glucose →

Blood

● Figure 33-1. Na⁺ transport processes in the first half of the proximal tubule. These transport mechanisms are present in all cells in the first half of the proximal tubule but are separated into different cells to simplify the discussion. **A,** Operation of the Na⁺-H⁺ antiporter (NHE3) in the apical membrane and the Na⁺,K⁺-ATPase and HCO₃⁻ transporters, including the Cl⁻-HCO₃⁻ antiporter (AE2) and the 1Na⁺-3HCO₃⁻ symporter (NBC1; see also Chapter 36) in the basolateral membrane mediates reabsorption of NaHCO₃. Note that a single HCO₃⁻ transporter is illustrated for simplicity. Carbon dioxide and water combine inside the cells to form H⁺ and HCO₃⁻ in a reaction facilitated by the enzyme carbonic anhydrase (CA). **B,** Operation of the Na⁺-glucose symporter (SGLT2) in the apical membrane, in conjunction with Na⁺,K⁺-ATPase and the glucose transporter (GLUT2) in the basolateral membrane, mediates Na⁺-glucose reabsorption. Inactivating mutations in the *GLUT2* gene lead to decreased glucose reabsorption in the proximal tubule and glucosuria (i.e., glucose in the urine). Though not shown, Na⁺ reabsorption is also coupled with other solutes, including amino acids, Pᵢ, and lactate. Reabsorption of these solutes is mediated by the Na⁺–amino acid, Na⁺-Pᵢ, and Na⁺-lactate symporters located in the apical membrane and the Na⁺,K⁺-ATPase, amino acid, Pᵢ, and lactate transporters located in the basolateral membrane. Three classes of amino acid transporters have been identified in the proximal tubule: two that transport Na⁺ in conjunction with either acidic or basic amino acids and one that does not require Na⁺ and transports basic amino acids.

● Figure 33-2. Concentration of solutes in tubule fluid as a function of length along the proximal tubule. [TF] is the concentration of the substance in tubular fluid; [P] is the concentration of the substance in plasma. Values above 100 indicate that relatively less of the solute than water was reabsorbed, and values below 100 indicate that relatively more of the substance than water was reabsorbed.

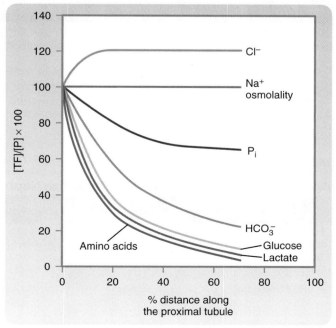

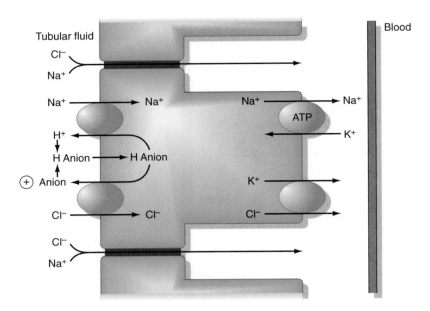

● **Figure 33-3.** Na⁺ transport processes in the second half of the proximal tubule. Na⁺ and Cl⁻ enter the cell across the apical membrane via the operation of parallel Na⁺-H⁺ and Cl⁻-anion antiporters. More than one Cl⁻-anion antiporter may be involved in this process, but only one is depicted. The secreted H⁺ and anion combine in the tubular fluid to form an H⁺-anion complex that can recycle across the plasma membrane. Accumulation of the H⁺-anion complex in tubular fluid establishes an H⁺-anion concentration gradient that favors H⁺-anion recycling across the apical plasma membrane into the cell. Inside the cell, H⁺ and the anion dissociate and recycle back across the apical plasma membrane. The net result is uptake of NaCl across the apical membrane. The anion may be hydroxide ions (OH^-), formate (HCO_2^-), oxalate, HCO_3^-, or sulfate. The positive transepithelial voltage in the lumen, indicated by the plus sign inside the circle in the tubular lumen, is generated by diffusion of Cl⁻ (lumen to blood) across the tight junction. The high [Cl⁻] of tubular fluid provides the driving force for diffusion of Cl⁻. Some glucose is also reabsorbed in the second half of the proximal tubule by a mechanism similar to that described in the first half of the proximal tubule, except that the Na⁺-glucose symporter (*SGLT1* gene) transports 2Na⁺ with one glucose and has higher affinity and lower capacity than the Na⁺-glucose symporter in the first part of the proximal tubule (i.e., SGLT2). In addition, glucose exits the cell across the basolateral membrane via GLUT1 rather than via GLUT2 as in the first part of the proximal tubule.

● **Table 33-4.   NaCl Transport along the Nephron**

Segment	Percentage of Filtrate Reabsorbed	Mechanism of Na⁺ Entry across the Apical Membrane	Major Regulatory Hormones
Proximal tubule	67%	Na⁺-H⁺ antiporter, Na⁺ symporter with amino acids and organic solutes, 1Na⁺-1H⁺-2Cl⁻-anion antiporter, paracellular	Angiotensin II Norepinephrine Epinephrine Dopamine
Loop of Henle	25%	1Na⁺-1K⁺-2Cl⁻ symporter	Aldosterone Angiotensin II
Distal tubule	≈5%	NaCl symporter (early) Na⁺ channels (late)	Aldosterone Angiotensin II
Collecting duct	≈3%	Na⁺ channels	Aldosterone, ANP, BNP, urodilatin, uroguanylin, guanylin, angiotensin II

● **Table 33-5.   Water Transport along the Nephron**

Segment	Percentage of Filtrate Reabsorbed	Mechanism of Water Reabsorption	Hormones That Regulate Water Permeability
Proximal tubule	67%	Passive	None
Loop of Henle	15%	Descending thin limb only; passive	None
Distal tubule	0%	No water reabsorption	None
Late distal tubule and collecting duct	≈8%-17%	Passive	ADH, ANP, BNP*

*Atrial and brain natriuretic peptides inhibit antidiuretic hormone–stimulated water permeability.

● **Figure 33-4.** Routes of reabsorption of water and solute across the proximal tubule. Transport of solutes, including Na+, Cl-, and organic solutes, into the lateral intercellular space increases the osmolality of this compartment, which establishes the driving force for osmotic reabsorption of water across the proximal tubule. This occurs because some Na+,K+-ATPase and some transporters of organic solutes, HCO3-, and Cl- are located on the lateral cell membranes and deposit these solutes between cells. Furthermore, some NaCl also enters the lateral intercellular space via diffusion across the tight junction (i.e., paracellular pathway). An important consequence of osmotic water flow across the transcellular and paracellular pathways in the proximal tubule is that some solutes, especially K+ and Ca++, are entrained in the reabsorbed fluid and thereby reabsorbed by the process of solvent drag.

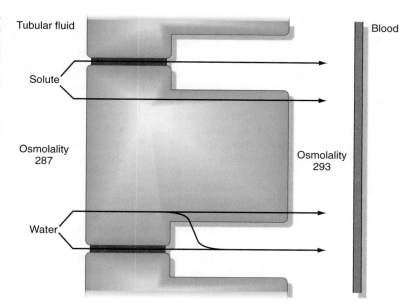

67% of the filtered load of solute and water is reabsorbed). Indeed, there is little difference in the osmolality of tubular fluid at the start and end of the proximal tubule. An important consequence of osmotic water flow across the proximal tubule is that some solutes, especially K+ and Ca++, are entrained in the reabsorbed fluid and thereby reabsorbed by the process of solvent drag (Fig. 33-4). Reabsorption of virtually all organic solutes, Cl- and other ions, and water is coupled to Na+ reabsorption. Therefore, changes in Na+ reabsorption influence the reabsorption of water and other solutes by the proximal tubule.

Protein Reabsorption

Proteins filtered by the glomerulus are reabsorbed in the proximal tubule. As mentioned previously, peptide hormones, small proteins, and small amounts of large proteins such as albumin are filtered by the glomerulus. Overall, only a small percentage of proteins cross the glomerulus and enter Bowman's space (i.e., the concentration of proteins in the glomerular ultrafiltrate is only 40 mg/L). However, the amount of protein filtered per day is significant because the glomerular filtration rate (GFR) is so high:

● **Equation 33-1**

Filtered protein = GFR × [Protein] in the ultrafiltrate

Filtered protein = 180 L/day × 40 mg/L
= 7200 mg/day, or 7.2 g/day

Proteins undergo endocytosis either intact or after being partially degraded by enzymes on the surface of proximal tubule cells. Once the proteins and peptides are inside the cell, enzymes digest them into their constituent amino acids, which then leave the cell across the basolateral membrane by transport proteins and are returned to the blood. Normally, this mechanism reabsorbs virtually all the proteins filtered, and hence the urine is essentially protein free. However, because the mechanism is easily saturated, an increase

● **Table 33-6.**
Some Organic Anions Secreted by the Proximal Tubule

Endogenous Anions	Drugs
cAMP, cGMP	Acetazolamide
Bile salts	Chlorothiazide
Hippurates	Furosemide
Oxalate	Penicillin
Prostaglandins: PGE_2, $PGF_{2\alpha}$	Probenecid
Urate	Salicylate (aspirin)
Vitamins: ascorbate, folate	Hydrochlorothiazide
	Bumetanide
	Nonsteroidal antiinflammatory drugs (NSAIDs): Indomethacin

in filtered proteins causes **proteinuria** (appearance of protein in urine). Disruption of the glomerular filtration barrier to proteins increases the filtration of proteins and results in proteinuria. Proteinuria is frequently seen with kidney disease.

Secretion of Organic Anions and Organic Cations

Cells of the proximal tubule also secrete organic cations and organic anions. Secretion of organic cations and anions by the proximal tubule plays a key role in limiting the body's exposure to toxic compounds derived from endogenous and exogenous sources (i.e., xenobiotics). Many of the organic anions and cations (Tables 33-6 and 33-7) secreted by the proximal tubule are end products of metabolism that circulate in plasma. The proximal tubule also secretes numerous exogenous organic compounds, including numerous drugs and toxic chemicals. Many of these organic compounds can be bound to plasma proteins and are not readily filtered. Therefore, only a small proportion of these potentially toxic substances are eliminated from the body via excretion after filtration alone. Such substances are also secreted from the peritubular capil-

● AT THE CELLULAR LEVEL

Water channels called **aquaporins (AQPs)** mediate the transcellular reabsorption of water across many nephron segments. In 2003, Dr. Peter Agre received the Nobel Prize in Chemistry for his discovery that AQPs regulate and facilitate water transport across cell membranes, a process essential to all living organisms. To date, 12 aquaporins have been identified. The AQP family is divided into two groups based on their permeability characteristics. One group (aquaporins) is permeable to water (AQP0, AQP1, AQP2, AQP4, AQP5, AQP6, and AQP8). The other group (aquaglyceroporins) is permeable to water and small solutes, especially glycerol (AQP3, AQP7, AQP9, AQP5, and AQP10). Aquaporins form tetramers in the plasma membrane of cells, with each subunit forming a water channel. In the kidneys, AQP1 is expressed in the apical and basolateral membranes of the proximal tubule and descending thin limb of Henle's loop. The importance of AQP1 in renal water reabsorption is underscored by studies in which the *AQP1* gene was "knocked out" in mice. These mice had increased urine output (polyuria) and a reduced ability to concentrate urine. In addition, the rate of water reabsorption by the proximal tubule was 50% less in mice lacking APQ1 than in normal mice. AQP7 and AQP8 are also expressed in the proximal tubule. AQP2 is expressed in the apical plasma membrane of principal cells in the collecting duct, and its expression in the membrane is regulated by antidiuretic hormone (ADH) (see Chapter 34). AQP3 and AQP4 are expressed in the basolateral membrane of principal cells in the collecting duct. Mice deficient in AQP3 or AQP4 (i. e., knockout mice) have defects in the ability to concentrate urine (see Chapter 34). AQPs are also expressed in many other organs in the body, including the lung, eye, skin, secretory glands, and brain, where they play key physiological roles. For example, AQP4 is expressed in cells that form the blood-brain barrier. Knockout of AQP4 in mice affects the water permeability of the blood-brain barrier such that brain edema is reduced in AQP4 knockout mice after acute water loading and hyponatremia.

● AT THE CELLULAR LEVEL

Endocytosis of protein by the proximal tubule is mediated by apical membrane proteins that specifically bind luminal proteins and peptides. These peptides, called **multiligand endocytic receptors,** can bind a wide range of peptides and proteins and thereby mediate their endocytosis. **Megalin** and **cubilin** mediate protein and peptide endocytosis in the proximal tubule. Both are glycoproteins, with megalin being a member of the low-density lipoprotein receptor gene family.

lary into tubular fluid. These secretory mechanisms are very powerful and remove virtually all organic anions and cations from plasma that enter the kidneys. Hence, these substances are removed from plasma by both filtration and secretion.

● **Table 33-7.**

Some Organic Cations Secreted by the Proximal Tubule

Endogenous	Drugs
Creatinine	Atropine
Dopamine	Isoproterenol
Epinephrine	Cimetidine
Norepinephrine	Morphine
	Quinine
	Amiloride
	Procainamide

▶ IN THE CLINIC

Urinalysis is an important and routine tool for detection of disease. A thorough analysis of urine includes macroscopic and microscopic assessment. This is performed by visual assessment of the urine, microscopic examination, and chemical evaluation, which is conducted with dipstick reagent strips. The dipstick test is inexpensive and fast (i.e., less than 5 minutes). Dipstick reagent strips test urine for the presence of many substances, including bilirubin, blood, glucose, ketones, protein, and pH. It is normal to find trace amounts of protein in urine. Trace amounts of protein in urine can be derived from two sources: (1) filtration and incomplete reabsorption by the proximal tubule and (2) synthesis by the thick ascending limb of the loop of Henle. Cells in the thick ascending limb produce **Tamm-Horsfall glycoprotein** and secrete it into the tubular fluid. Because the mechanism for protein reabsorption is "upstream" of the thick ascending limb (i.e., proximal tubule), the secreted Tamm-Horsfall glycoprotein appears in urine. However, more than trace amounts of protein in urine are often indicative of renal disease.

Figure 33-5 illustrates the mechanisms of organic anion (OA^-) transport across the proximal tubule. This secretory pathway has a maximum transport rate, low specificity (i.e., it transports many OA^-s), and is responsible for secretion of all the OA^-s listed in Table 33-6. OA^-s are taken up into the cell, across the basolateral membrane, against their chemical gradient in exchange for α-ketoglutarate (α-KG) via several OA^-–α-KG antiporter mechanisms (OAT1, and OAT3). α-KG accumulates inside the cells via metabolism of glutamate and by an Na^+–α-KG symporter (i.e., a Na^+-dicarboxylate transporter [NaDC]) also present in the basolateral membrane. Thus uptake of OA^- into the cell against its electrochemical gradient is coupled to the exit of α-KG out of the cell, down its chemical gradient generated by the Na^+–α-KG symporter mechanism. The resulting high intracellular concentration of OA^- provides a driving force for exit of OA^- across the luminal membrane into tubular fluid via a poorly understood mechanism. However, recent studies suggest that OA^-s are transported across the apical membrane by OAT4, which is electrogenic, and by MRP2 (multidrug resistance–associated protein 2) (Fig. 33-5).

Figure 33-6 illustrates the mechanism of organic cation (OC$^+$) transport across the proximal tubule. OC$^+$s are taken up into the cell, across the basolateral membrane, by several transporters that have different substrate specificities. One mechanism that has not been completely characterized involves passive diffusion. In addition, OC$^+$s are transported into proximal tubule cells across the basolateral membrane by three related transport proteins (OCT1, OCT2, and OCT3).

These transporters mediate the diffusive uptake of OC$^+$s into the cell. Uptake by all four mechanisms is driven by the magnitude of the cell's negative potential difference across the basolateral membrane. OC$^+$ transport across the luminal membrane into tubular fluid, which is the rate-limiting step in secretion, is mediated by several transporters, including two OC$^+$-H$^+$ antiporters (MATEs) and MDR1 (a.k.a. P-glycoprotein). These transport mechanisms mediating secretion of OC$^+$s are nonspecific; several OC$^+$s usually compete for each transport pathway. Secretion of OC$^+$s is stimulated by protein kinase A and C and by testosterone.

Henle's Loop

Henle's loop reabsorbs approximately 25% of the filtered NaCl and 15% of the filtered water. Reabsorption of NaCl in the loop of Henle occurs in both the thin ascending and thick ascending limbs. The descending thin limb does not reabsorb NaCl. Water reabsorption occurs exclusively in the descending thin limb via AQP1 water channels. The ascending limb is impermeable to water. In addition, Ca^{++} and HCO$_3^-$ are also reabsorbed in the loop of Henle (see Chapters 35 and 36 for more details).

The thin ascending limb reabsorbs NaCl by a passive mechanism. Reabsorption of water, but not NaCl, in the descending thin limb increases [NaCl] in the tubule fluid entering the ascending thin limb. As the NaCl-rich fluid moves toward the cortex, NaCl diffuses out of the tubule fluid across the ascending thin limb into the medullary interstitial fluid, down a concentration gradient directed from the tubule fluid to the interstitium.

The key element in the reabsorption of solute by the thick ascending limb is Na$^+$,K$^+$-ATPase in the basolateral membrane (Fig. 33-7). As with reabsorption in the proximal tubule, reabsorption of every solute by

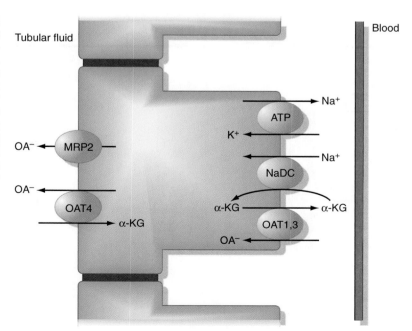

● **Figure 33-5.** Secretion of organic anion (OA$^-$) across the proximal tubule. OA$^-$s enter the cell across the basolateral membrane by one of three OA$^-$–α-ketoglutarate (α-KG) antiporter mechanisms (OAT1, OAT2, OAT3). Uptake of α-KG into the cell, against its chemical concentration gradient, is driven by movement of Na$^+$ into the cell via the Na$^+$-dicarboxylate transporter (NaDC). The [Na$^+$] inside the cell is low because of the Na$^+$,K$^+$-ATPase in the basolateral membrane, which transports Na$^+$ out of the cell in exchange for K$^+$ (not shown). The α-KG recycles across the basolateral membrane on the OATs in exchange for OA$^-$. OA$^-$s leave the cell across the apical membrane, most likely by MRP2 and OAT4.

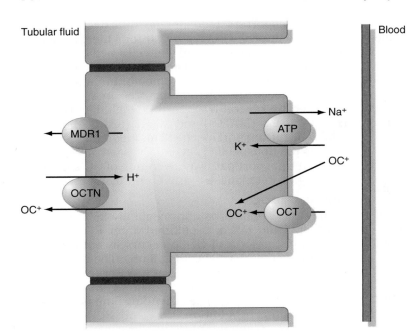

● **Figure 33-6.** Secretion of organic cation (OC⁺) across the proximal tubule. OC⁺s enter the cell across the basolateral membrane by four transport pathways: passive diffusion and three uniporters (OCT1, OCT2, OCT3, illustrated as one transporter for clarity) that mediate electrogenic uptake. Uptake of OC⁺s into the cell, against their chemical concentration gradient, is driven by the cell-negative potential difference. OC⁺s leave the cell across the apical membrane in exchange for H⁺ by two OC⁺-H⁺ antiporters (OCTN1, OCTN2, illustrated as one transporter for clarity) and MDR1.

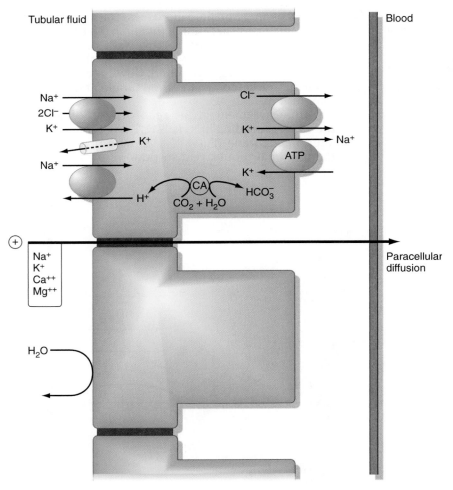

● **Figure 33-7.** Transport mechanisms for reabsorption of NaCl in the thick ascending limb of the loop of Henle. The positive charge in the lumen plays a major role in driving the passive paracellular reabsorption of cations. Mutations in the apical membrane K⁺ channel (ROMK), the apical membrane 1Na⁺-1K⁺-2Cl⁻ symporter (NKCC2), or the basolateral Cl⁻ channel (ClCNKB) cause Bartter's syndrome (see the clinical box on Bartter's syndrome). CA, carbonic anhydrase.

the thick ascending limb is linked to Na$^+$,K$^+$-ATPase. This pump maintains a low intracellular [Na$^+$], which provides a favorable chemical gradient for the movement of Na$^+$ from tubular fluid into the cell. Movement of Na$^+$ across the apical membrane into the cell is mediated by the 1Na$^+$-1K$^+$-2Cl$^-$ symporter (NKCC2), which couples the movement of 1Na$^+$ with 1K$^+$ and 2Cl$^-$. Using the potential energy released by the downhill movement of Na$^+$ and Cl$^-$, this symporter drives the uphill movement of K$^+$ into the cell. The K$^+$ channel in the apical plasma membrane plays an important role in reabsorption of NaCl by the thick ascending limb. This K$^+$ channel allows the K$^+$ transported into the cell via the 1Na$^+$-1K$^+$-2Cl$^-$ symporter to recycle back into tubule fluid. Because the [K$^+$] in tubule fluid is relatively low, this K$^+$ is required for continued operation of the 1Na$^+$-1K$^+$-2Cl$^-$ symporter. An Na$^+$-H$^+$ antiporter in the apical cell membrane also mediates Na$^+$ reabsorption, as well as H$^+$ secretion (HCO$_3^-$ reabsorption), in the thick ascending limb (see also Chapter 36). Na$^+$ leaves the cell across the basolateral membrane via Na$^+$,K$^+$-ATPase, whereas K$^+$, Cl$^-$, and HCO$_3^-$ leave the cell across the basolateral membrane via separate pathways.

The voltage across the thick ascending limb is important for the reabsorption of several cations. The tubular fluid is positively charged relative to blood because of the unique location of transport proteins in the apical and basolateral membranes. Two points are important: (1) increased NaCl transport by the thick ascending limb increases the magnitude of the positive voltage in the lumen, and (2) this voltage is an important driving force for the reabsorption of several cations, including Na$^+$, K$^+$, Mg^{++}, and Ca^{++}, across the paracellular pathway (Fig. 33-7). The importance of the paracellular pathway to solute reabsorption is underscored by the observation that inactivating mutations of the tight junction protein claudin-16 reduce reabsorption of Mg^{++} and Ca^{++} by the ascending thick limb, even in the presence of positive transepithelial voltage in the lumen.

In summary, NaCl reabsorption across the thick ascending limb occurs via the transcellular and paracellular pathways. Fifty percent of NaCl reabsorption is transcellular, and 50% is paracellular. Because the thick ascending limb does not reabsorb water, reabsorption of NaCl and other solutes reduces the osmolality of tubular fluid to less than 150 mOsm/kg H$_2$O. Thus, because the thick ascending limb produces a fluid that is dilute relative to plasma, the ascending limb of Henle's loop is called the **"diluting segment."**

Distal Tubule and Collecting Duct

The distal tubule and collecting duct reabsorb approximately 8% of the filtered NaCl, secrete variable amounts of K$^+$ and H$^+$, and reabsorb a variable amount of water (≈8% to 17%). The initial segment of the distal tubule (early distal tubule) reabsorbs Na$^+$, Cl$^-$, and Ca^{++} and is impermeable to water (Fig. 33-8). Entry of NaCl into the cell across the apical membrane is mediated by an Na$^+$-Cl$^-$ symporter (Fig. 33-8). Na$^+$ leaves the cell via the action of Na$^+$,K$^+$-ATPase, and Cl$^-$

As described in Chapter 1, epithelial cells are joined at their apical surfaces by tight junctions (a.k.a. zonula occludens). A number of proteins have now been identified as components of the tight junction, including proteins that span the membrane of one cell and link to the extracellular portion of the same molecule in the adjacent cell (e.g., occludin and claudins), as well as cytoplasmic linker proteins (e.g., ZO-1, ZO-2, and ZO-3) that link the membrane-spanning proteins to the cytoskeleton of the cell. Of these junctional proteins, claudins appear to be important in determining the permeability characteristics of the tight junction. As noted, claudin-16 is critical for the determining permeability of the tight junctions in the thick ascending limb of Henle's loop to divalent cations. Claudin-4 has been shown in cultured kidney cells to control the permeability of the tight junction to Na$^+$, whereas claudin-15 determines whether a tight junction is permeable to cations or anions. Thus, the permeability characteristics of the tight junctions in different nephron segments are determined, at least in part, by the specific claudins expressed by the cells in that segment.

Bartter's syndrome is a set of autosomal recessive genetic diseases characterized by hypokalemia, metabolic alkalosis, and hyperaldosteronism (Table 33-3). Inactivating mutations in the gene coding for the 1Na$^+$-1K$^+$-2Cl$^-$ symporter (NKCC2 or SLC12A1), the apical K$^+$ channel (KCNJ1 or ROMK), or the basolateral Cl$^-$ channel (ClCNKB) decrease both NaCl reabsorption and K$^+$ reabsorption by the ascending thick limb, which in turn causes hypokalemia (i.e., low plasma [K$^+$]) and a decrease in ECF volume. The fall in ECF volume stimulates aldosterone secretion, which in turn stimulates NaCl reabsorption and H$^+$ secretion by the distal tubule and collecting duct (see later).

leaves the cell via diffusion through Cl$^-$ channels. Thus, dilution of tubular fluid begins in the thick ascending limb and continues in the early segment of the distal tubule.

The last segment of the distal tubule (late distal tubule) and the collecting duct are composed of two cell types: **principal cells** and **intercalated cells.** As illustrated in Figure 33-9, principal cells reabsorb NaCl and water and secrete K$^+$. Intercalated cells secrete either H$^+$ or HCO$_3^-$ and are thus important in regulating acid-base balance (see Chapter 36). Intercalated cells also reabsorb K$^+$ by the operation of an H$^+$,K$^+$-ATPase located in the apical plasma membrane. Both Na$^+$ reabsorption and K$^+$ secretion by principal cells depend on the activity of Na$^+$,K$^+$-ATPase in the basolateral membrane (Fig. 33-9). By maintaining a low intracellular [Na$^+$], this pump provides a favorable chemical gradi-

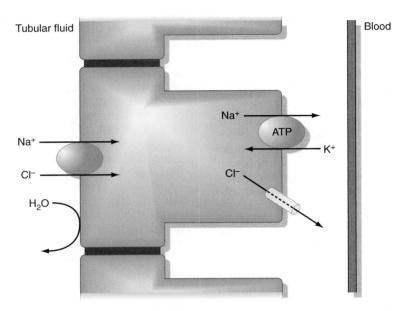

● **Figure 33-8.** Transport mechanism for reabsorption of Na^+ and Cl^- in the early segment of the distal tubule. This segment is impermeable to water.

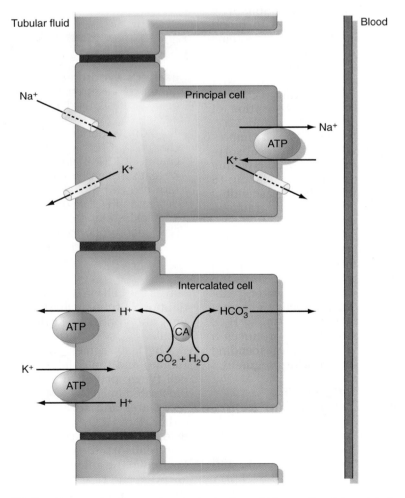

● **Figure 33-9.** Transport pathways in principal cells and H^+-secreting intercalated cells of the distal tubule and collecting duct. CA, carbonic anhydrase.

ent for movement of Na^+ from tubular fluid into the cell. Because Na^+ enters the cell across the apical membrane via diffusion through epithelial Na^+-selective channels (ENaCs) in the apical membrane, the negative charge inside the cell facilitates entry of Na^+. Na^+ leaves the cell across the basolateral membrane and enters the blood via the action of Na^+,K^+-ATPase. Reabsorption of Na^+ generates a negative luminal voltage across the late distal tubule and collecting duct, which provides the driving force for reabsorption of Cl^- across the paracellular pathway. A variable amount of water is reabsorbed across principal cells in the late distal tubule and collecting duct. Water reabsorption is mediated by the AQP2 water channel located in the apical plasma membrane and by AQP3 and AQP4 located in the basolateral membrane of principal cells. In the presence of antidiuretic hormone (ADH), water is reabsorbed. By contrast, in the absence of ADH, the distal tubule and collecting duct reabsorb little water (see Chapter 34).

K^+ is secreted from blood into tubular fluid by principal cells in two steps (Fig. 33-9). First, uptake of K^+ across the basolateral membrane is mediated by the action of Na^+,K^+-ATPase. Second, K^+ leaves the cell via passive diffusion. Because $[K^+]$ inside the cells is high (≈150 mEq/L) and $[K^+]$ in tubular fluid is low (≈10 mEq/L), K^+ diffuses down its concentration gradient through apical cell membrane K^+ channels into tubular fluid. Although the negative potential inside the cells tends to retain K^+ within the cell, the electrochemical gradient across the apical membrane favors secretion of K^+ from the cell into tubular fluid (see Chapter 35). Reabsorption of K^+ by intercalated cells is mediated by an H^+,K^+-ATPase located in the apical cell membrane.

REGULATION OF NaCl AND WATER REABSORPTION

Quantitatively, angiotensin II, aldosterone, catecholamines, natriuretic peptides, and uroguanylin are the most important hormones that regulate NaCl reabsorption and thereby urinary NaCl excretion (Table 33-8). However, other hormones (including dopamine and adrenomedullin), Starling forces, and the phenomenon of glomerulotubular balance influence NaCl reab-

sorption. ADH is the only major hormone that directly regulates the amount of water excreted by the kidneys.

Angiotensin II has a potent stimulatory effect on reabsorption of NaCl and water in the proximal tubule. It has also been shown to stimulate reabsorption of Na^+ in the thick ascending limb of Henle's loop, as well as the distal tubule and collecting duct. A decrease in extracellular fluid (ECF) volume activates the renin-angiotensin-aldosterone system (see Chapter 34 for more details), thereby increasing the plasma concentration of angiotensin II.

Aldosterone is synthesized by the glomerulosa cells of the adrenal cortex, and it stimulates reabsorption of NaCl. It acts on the thick ascending limb of the loop of Henle, distal tubule, and collecting duct. Most of aldosterone's effect on NaCl reabsorption reflects its action on the distal tubule and collecting duct. Aldosterone also stimulates secretion of K^+ by the distal tubule and collecting duct (see Chapter 35). Aldosterone increases the abundance of the Na^+-Cl^- symporter in the early distal tubule. It enhances reabsorption of NaCl across principal cells in the distal tubule and collecting duct by four mechanisms: (1) increasing the amount of Na^+,K^+-ATPase in the basolateral membrane; (2) increasing expression of the sodium channel (ENaC) in the apical cell membrane; (3) elevating Sgk1 (**s**erum **g**lucocorticoid-stimulated **k**inase; see the molecular box) levels, which also increases the expression of ENaC in the apical cell membrane; and (4) stimulating CAP1 (**c**hannel-**a**ctivating **p**rotease, also called "prostatin"), a serine protease that directly activates ENaCs by proteolysis. Taken together, these actions increase uptake of Na^+ across the apical cell membrane and facilitate exit of Na^+ from the cell interior into blood. The increase in reabsorption of Na^+ generates a negative transepithelial luminal voltage across the distal tubule and collecting duct. This negative voltage in the lumen provides the electrochemical driving force for reabsorption of Cl^- across the tight junctions (i.e., paracellular pathway) in the distal tubule and collecting duct. Secretion of aldosterone is increased by hyperkalemia and angiotensin II (after activation of the renin-angiotensin system) and decreased by hypokalemia and natriuretic peptides (see the following text). Through its stimulation of

● **Table 33-8.** **Hormones That Regulate NaCl and Water Reabsorption**

Hormone*	Major Stimulus	Nephron Site of Action	Effect on Transport
Angiotensin II	↑Renin	PT, TAL, DT/CD	↑NaCl and H_2O reabsorption
Aldosterone	↑Angiotensin II, ↑$[K^+]_p$	TAL, DT/CD	↑NaCl and H_2O reabsorption†
ANP, BNP, urodilatin	↑ECFV	CD	↓H_2O and NaCl reabsorption
Uroguanylin, guanylin	Oral ingestion of NaCl	PT, CD	↓H_2O and NaCl reabsorption
Sympathetic nerves	↓ECFV	PT, TAL, DT/CD	↑NaCl and H_2O reabsorption†
Dopamine	↑ECFV	PT	↓H_2O and NaCl reabsorption
ADH	↑P_{osm}, ↓ECFV	DT/CD	↑H_2O reabsorption

*All these hormones act within minutes, except aldosterone, which exerts its action on reabsorption of NaCl with a delay of 1 hour. Aldosterone achieves its maximal effect after a few days.

†The effect on reabsorption of H_2O does not include the thick ascending limb.

ANP, atrial natriuretic peptide; BNP, brain natriuretic peptide, BP, blood pressure; CD, collecting duct; DT, distal tubule; ECFV, extracellular fluid volume; $[K^+]_p$, plasma K^+ concentration; P_{osm}, plasma osmolality; PT, proximal tubule; TAL, thick ascending limb.

NaCl reabsorption in the collecting duct, aldosterone also indirectly increases water reabsorption by this nephron segment.

Atrial natriuretic peptide (ANP) and **brain natriuretic peptide (BNP)** inhibit NaCl and water reabsorption. Secretion of ANP by the cardiac atria and BNP by the cardiac ventricles is stimulated by a rise in blood pressure and an increase in ECF volume. ANP and BNP reduce blood pressure by decreasing total peripheral resistance and enhancing urinary excretion of NaCl and water. These hormones inhibit reabsorption of NaCl by the medullary portion of the collecting duct and inhibit ADH-stimulated water reabsorption across the collecting duct. Moreover, ANP and BNP also reduce the secretion of ADH from the posterior pituitary. These actions of ANP and BNP are mediated by the activation of membrane-bound guanylyl cyclase receptors, which increases intracellular levels of the second messenger cGMP. ANP induces a more profound natriuresis and diuresis than BNP does.

Urodilatin and ANP are encoded by the same gene and have similar amino acid sequences. Urodilatin is a 32–amino acid hormone that differs from ANP by the addition of four amino acids to the amino-terminus.

AT THE CELLULAR LEVEL

Sgk1 (**s**erum **g**lucocorticoid-stimulated **k**inase), a serine/threonine kinase, plays an important role in maintaining NaCl and K^+ homeostasis by regulating excretion of NaCl and K^+ by the kidneys. Studies in Sgk1 knockout mice reveal that this kinase is required for animals to survive severe NaCl restriction and K^+ loading. NaCl restriction and K^+ loading enhance plasma [aldosterone], which rapidly (in minutes) increases Sgk1 protein expression and phosphorylation. Phosphorylated Sgk1 enhances ENaC-mediated Na^+ reabsorption in the collecting duct, primarily by increasing the number of ENaCs in the apical plasma membrane of principal cells and also by increasing the number of Na^+,K^+-ATPase pumps in the basolateral membrane. Phosphorylated Sgk1 inhibits Nedd4-2, a ubiquitin ligase that monoubiquitinylates ENaC subunits, thereby targeting them for endocytic removal from the plasma membrane and subsequent destruction in lysosomes. Inhibition of Nedd4-2 by Sgk1 reduces the monoubiquitinylation of ENaC, thereby reducing endocytosis and increasing the number of channels in the membrane. The mechanism whereby Sgk1 stimulates ROMK-mediated K^+ excretion has not been elucidated. These effects of Sgk1 precede the aldosterone-stimulated increase in ENaC, ROMK, and Na^+,K^+-ATPase expression, which leads to a delayed (>4 hours), secondary increase in NaCl and K^+ transport by the collecting duct. Activating polymorphisms in Sgk1 cause an increase in blood pressure, presumably by enhancing NaCl reabsorption by the collecting duct, which increases ECF volume and thereby blood pressure. As noted, CAP1 is a serine protease that directly activates ENaC by proteolysis of the channel proteins.

Urodilatin is secreted by the distal tubule and collecting duct and is not present in the systemic circulation; thus, urodilatin influences only the function of the kidneys. Secretion of urodilatin is stimulated by a rise in blood pressure and an increase in ECF volume. It inhibits NaCl and water reabsorption across the medullary portion of the collecting duct. Urodilatin is a more potent natriuretic and diuretic hormone than

IN THE CLINIC

Liddle's syndrome is a rare genetic disorder characterized by an increase in blood pressure (i.e., hypertension) secondary to an increase in ECF volume. Liddle's syndrome is caused by activating mutations in either the β or γ subunit of the epithelial Na^+ channel (ENaC, which is composed of three subunits, α, β, and γ). These mutations increase the number of Na^+ channels in the apical cell membrane of principal cells and thereby the amount of Na^+ reabsorbed. In Liddle's syndrome the rate of renal Na^+ reabsorption is inappropriately high, which leads to an increase in ECF volume and hypertension.

There are two different forms of **pseudohypoaldosteronism (PHA)** (i.e., the kidneys reabsorb NaCl as they do when aldosterone levels are low; however, in PHA, aldosterone levels are elevated). The autosomal recessive form is caused by inactivating mutations in the α, β, or γ subunit of ENaC. The cause of the autosomal dominant form is an inactivating mutation in the mineralocorticoid receptor. PHA is characterized by an increase in Na^+ excretion, a reduction in ECF volume, hyperkalemia, and hypotension.

IN THE CLINIC

Some individuals with expanded ECF volume and elevated blood pressure are treated with drugs that inhibit **angiotensin-converting enzyme** (ACE inhibitors [e.g., captopril, enalapril, lisinopril]) and thereby lower fluid volume and blood pressure. The inhibition of ACE blocks the degradation of angiotensin I to angiotensin II and thereby lowers plasma angiotensin II levels (see text for details). The decline in plasma angiotensin II concentration has three effects. First, reabsorption of NaCl and water by the nephron (especially the proximal tubule) falls. Second, aldosterone secretion decreases, thus reducing reabsorption of NaCl in the thick ascending limb, distal tubule, and collecting duct. Third, because angiotensin is a potent vasoconstrictor, a reduction in its concentration permits the systemic arterioles to dilate and thereby lower arterial blood pressure. ACE also degrades the vasodilator hormone bradykinin; ACE inhibitors therefore increase the concentration of bradykinin. Thus, ACE inhibitors decrease ECF volume and arterial blood pressure by promoting the renal excretion of NaCl and water and by reducing total peripheral resistance.

ANP is because some of the ANP that enters the kidneys in blood is degraded by a neutral endopeptidase that has no effect on urodilatin.

Uroguanylin and **guanylin** are produced by neuroendocrine cells in the intestine in response to the oral ingestion of NaCl. These hormones enter the circulation and inhibit NaCl and water reabsorption by the kidneys via the activation of membrane-bound guanylyl cyclase receptors, which increases intracellular [cGMP]. The natriuretic response of the kidneys to an NaCl load is more pronounced when given orally than when delivered intravenously because oral administration of NaCl causes the secretion of uroguanylin and guanylin.

Catecholamines stimulate reabsorption of NaCl. Catecholamines released from the sympathetic nerves (norepinephrine) and the adrenal medulla (epinephrine) stimulate reabsorption of NaCl and water by the proximal tubule, thick ascending limb of the loop of Henle, distal tubule, and collecting duct. Although sympathetic nerves are not active when ECF volume is normal, when ECF volume declines (e.g., after hemorrhage), sympathetic nerve activity rises and stimulates reabsorption of NaCl and water by these four nephron segments.

Dopamine, a catecholamine, is released from dopaminergic nerves in the kidneys and is also synthesized by cells of the proximal tubule. The action of dopamine is opposite that of norepinephrine and epinephrine. Secretion of dopamine is stimulated by an increase in ECF volume, and its secretion directly inhibits reabsorption of NaCl and water in the proximal tubule.

Adrenomedullin is a 52–amino acid peptide hormone that is produced by a variety of organs, including the kidneys. Adrenomedullin induces a marked diuresis and natriuresis, and its secretion is stimulated by congestive heart failure and hypertension. The major effect of adrenomedullin on the kidneys is to increase GFR and renal blood flow and thereby indirectly stimulate the excretion of NaCl and water.

ADH regulates water reabsorption. It is the most important hormone that regulates reabsorption of water in the kidneys (see Chapter 34). This hormone is secreted by the posterior pituitary gland in response to an increase in plasma osmolality (1% or more) or a decrease in ECF volume (>5% to 10% of normal). ADH increases the permeability of the collecting duct to water. It increases reabsorption of water by the collecting duct because of the osmotic gradient that exists across the wall of the collecting duct (see Chapter 34). ADH has little effect on urinary NaCl excretion.

Starling forces regulate reabsorption of NaCl and water across the proximal tubule. As previously described, Na^+, Cl^-, HCO_3^-, amino acids, glucose, and water are transported into the intercellular space of the proximal tubule. Starling forces between this space and the peritubular capillaries facilitate movement of the reabsorbed fluid into the capillaries. Starling forces across the wall of peritubular capillaries consist of hydrostatic pressure in the peritubular capillary (P_{pc}) and lateral intercellular space (P_i) and oncotic pressure in the peritubular capillary (π_{pc}) and lateral intercellular space (π_i). Thus, reabsorption of water as a result of transport of Na^+ from tubular fluid into the lateral intercellular space is modified by the Starling forces. Accordingly,

● **Equation 33-2**

$$J = K_f[(P_i - P_{pc}) + \sigma(\pi_{pc} - \pi_i)]$$

where J is flow (positive numbers indicate flow from the intercellular space into blood). Starling forces that favor movement from the interstitium into the peritubular capillaries are π_{pc} and P_i (Fig. 33-10). The opposing Starling forces are π_i and P_{pc}. Normally, the sum of the Starling forces favors the movement of solute and water from the interstitial space into the capillary.

● **Figure 33-10.** Routes of solute and water transport across the proximal tubule and the Starling forces that modify reabsorption. (1) Solute and water are reabsorbed across the apical membrane. This solute and water then cross the lateral cell membrane. Some solute and water reenter the tubule fluid (3), and the remainder enters the interstitial space and then flows into the capillary (2). The width of the arrows is directly proportional to the amount of solute and water moving by pathways 1 to 3. Starling forces across the capillary wall determine the amount of fluid flowing through pathway 2 versus pathway 3. Transport mechanisms in the apical cell membranes determine the amount of solute and water entering the cell (pathway 1). P_i, interstitial hydrostatic pressure; P_{pc}, peritubular capillary hydrostatic pressure; π_i, interstitial fluid oncotic pressure; π_{pc}, peritubular capillary oncotic pressure. Thin arrows across the capillary wall indicate the direction of water movement in response to each force.

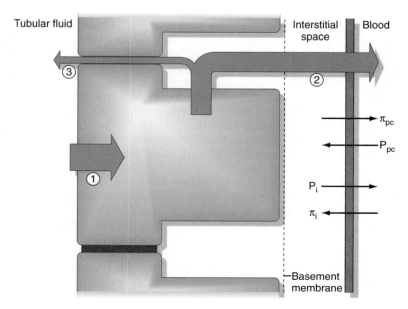

However, some of the solutes and fluid that enter the lateral intercellular space leak back into the proximal tubular fluid. Starling forces do not affect transport by the loop of Henle, distal tubule, and collecting duct because these segments are less permeable to water than the proximal tubule is.

A number of factors can alter the Starling forces across the peritubular capillaries surrounding the proximal tubule. For example, dilation of the efferent arteriole increases P_{pc}, whereas constriction of the efferent arteriole decreases it. An increase in P_{pc} inhibits solute and water reabsorption by increasing back-leak of NaCl and water across the tight junction, whereas a decrease stimulates reabsorption by decreasing back-leak across the tight junction.

Peritubular capillary oncotic pressure (π_{pc}) is partially determined by the rate of formation of the glomerular ultrafiltrate. For example, if one assumes a constant plasma flow in the afferent arteriole, the plasma proteins become less concentrated in the plasma that enters the efferent arteriole and peritubular capillary as less ultrafiltrate is formed (i.e., as GFR decreases). Hence, π_{pc} decreases. Thus π_{pc} is directly related to the **filtration fraction** (FF = GFR/renal plasma flow [RPF]). A fall in the FF resulting from a decrease in GFR, at constant RPF, decreases π_{pc}. This in turn increases the backflow of NaCl and water from the lateral intercellular space into tubular fluid and thereby decreases net reabsorption of solute and water across the proximal tubule. An increase in FF has the opposite effect.

The importance of Starling forces in regulating solute and water reabsorption by the proximal tubule is underscored by the phenomenon of **glomerulotubular (G-T) balance.** Spontaneous changes in GFR markedly alter the filtered load of Na^+ (filtered load = GFR $\times$ [Na^+] in the filtered fluid). Without rapid adjustments in Na^+ reabsorption to counter the changes in filtration of Na^+, urinary excretion of Na^+ would fluctuate widely and disturb the Na^+ balance of the body and thus alter ECF volume and blood pressure (see Chapter 34 for more details). However, spontaneous changes in GFR do not alter Na^+ excretion in urine or Na^+ balance because of the phenomenon of G-T balance. When body Na^+ balance is normal (i.e., ECF volume is normal), G-T balance refers to the fact that reabsorption of Na^+ and water increases in proportion to the increase in GFR and filtered load of Na^+. Thus, a constant fraction of the filtered Na^+ and water is reabsorbed from the proximal tubule despite variations in GFR. The net result of G-T balance is to reduce the impact of changes in GFR on the amount of Na^+ and water excreted in urine.

Two mechanisms are responsible for G-T balance. One is related to the oncotic and hydrostatic pressure differences between the peritubular capillaries and the lateral intercellular space (i.e., Starling forces). For example, an increase in the GFR (at constant RPF) raises the protein concentration in glomerular capillary plasma above normal. This protein-rich plasma leaves the glomerular capillaries, flows through the efferent arterioles, and enters the peritubular capillaries. The increased π_{pc} augments the movement of solute and fluid from the lateral intercellular space into the peritubular capillaries. This action increases net solute and water reabsorption by the proximal tubule.

The second mechanism responsible for G-T balance is initiated by an increase in the filtered load of glucose and amino acids. As discussed earlier, reabsorption of Na^+ in the first half of the proximal tubule is coupled to that of glucose and amino acids. The rate of Na^+ reabsorption therefore partially depends on the filtered load of glucose and amino acids. As the GFR and filtered load of glucose and amino acids increase, reabsorption of Na^+ and water also rises.

In addition to G-T balance, another mechanism minimizes changes in the filtered load of Na^+. As discussed in Chapter 32, an increase in the GFR (and thus in the amount of Na^+ filtered by the glomerulus) activates the tubuloglomerular feedback mechanism. This action returns the GFR and filtration of Na^+ to normal values. Thus, spontaneous changes in GFR (e.g., caused by changes in posture and blood pressure) increase the amount of Na^+ filtered for only a few minutes. The mechanisms that underlie G-T balance maintain urinary Na^+ excretion constant and thereby maintain Na^+ homeostasis (and ECF volume and blood pressure) until the GFR returns to normal.

■ KEY CONCEPTS

1. The four major segments of the nephron (proximal tubule, Henle's loop, distal tubule, and collecting duct) determine the composition and volume of urine by the processes of selective reabsorption of solutes and water and secretion of solutes.

2. Tubular reabsorption allows the kidneys to retain substances that are essential and regulate their levels in plasma by altering the degree to which they are reabsorbed. Reabsorption of Na^+, Cl^-, other anions, and organic anions and cations together with water constitutes the major function of the nephron. Approximately 25,200 mEq of Na^+ and 179 L of water are reabsorbed each day. Proximal tubule cells reabsorb 67% of the glomerular ultrafiltrate, and cells of Henle's loop reabsorb about 25% of the NaCl that was filtered and about 15% of the water that was filtered. The distal segments of the nephron (distal tubule and collecting duct system) have a more limited reabsorptive capacity. However, final adjustments in the composition and volume of urine and most of the regulation by hormones and other factors occur in distal segments.

3. Secretion of substances into tubular fluid is a means for excreting various byproducts of metabolism, and it also serves to eliminate exogenous organic anions and cations (e.g., drugs) and pollutants from the body. Many organic anions and cations are

bound to plasma proteins and are therefore unavailable for ultrafiltration. Thus, secretion is their major route of excretion in urine.

4. Various hormones (including angiotensin II, aldosterone, ADH, natriuretic peptides [ANP, BNP, and urodilatin], uroguanylin, and guanylin), sympathetic nerves, dopamine, and Starling forces regulate reabsorption of NaCl by the kidneys. ADH is the major hormone that regulates water reabsorption.

CHAPTER 34

Control of Body Fluid Osmolality and Volume

The kidneys maintain the osmolality and volume of body fluids within a narrow range by regulating the excretion of water and NaCl, respectively. This chapter discusses the regulation of renal water excretion (urine concentration and dilution) and NaCl excretion. The composition and volumes of the various body fluid compartments are reviewed in Chapter 2.

CONTROL OF BODY FLUID OSMOLALITY: URINE CONCENTRATION AND DILUTION

As described in Chapter 2, water constitutes approximately 60% of the healthy adult human body. Body water is divided into two compartments (i.e., intracellular fluid [ICF] and extracellular fluid [ECF]), which are in osmotic equilibrium. Water intake into the body generally occurs orally. However, in clinical situations, intravenous infusion is an important route of water entry.

The kidneys are responsible for regulating water balance and under most conditions are the major route for elimination of water from the body (Table 34-1). Other routes of water loss from the body include evaporation from cells of the skin and respiratory passages. Collectively, water loss by these routes is termed **insensible water loss** because the individual is unaware of its occurrence. The production of sweat accounts for the loss of additional water. Water loss by this mechanism can increase dramatically in a hot environment, with exercise, or in the presence of fever (Table 34-2). Finally, water can be lost from the gastrointestinal tract. Fecal water loss is normally small (≈100 mL/day) but can increase dramatically with diarrhea (e.g., 20 L/day with cholera). Vomiting can also cause gastrointestinal water loss.

Although water loss from sweating, defecation, and evaporation from the lungs and skin can vary with environmental conditions or during pathological conditions, loss of water by these routes cannot be regulated. In contrast, the renal excretion of water is tightly regulated to maintain whole-body water balance. Maintenance of water balance requires that water intake and loss from the body be precisely matched. If intake exceeds loss, **positive water balance** exists. Conversely, if intake is less than loss, **negative water balance** exists.

When water intake is low or water loss increases, the kidneys conserve water by producing a small volume of urine that is hyperosmotic with respect to plasma. When water intake is high, a large volume of hypoosmotic urine is produced. In a normal individual, urine osmolality (U_{osm}) can vary from approximately 50 to 1200 mOsm/kg H_2O, and the corresponding urine volume can vary from approximately 18 to 0.5 L/day.

It is important to recognize that disorders in water balance are manifested by alterations in body fluid osmolality, which are usually measured by changes in plasma osmolality (P_{osm}). Because the major determinant of plasma osmolality is Na^+ (with its anions Cl^- and HCO_3^-), these disorders also result in alterations in plasma $[Na^+]$. When an abnormal plasma $[Na^+]$ is observed in an individual, it is tempting to suspect a problem in Na^+ balance. However, the problem most often relates to water balance, not Na^+ balance. As described later, changes in Na^+ balance result in alterations in the volume of ECF, not its osmolality.

Under steady-state conditions, the kidneys control water excretion independently of their ability to control the excretion of various other physiologically important substances such as Na^+, K^+, and urea. Indeed, this ability is necessary for survival because it allows water balance to be achieved without upsetting the other homeostatic functions of the kidneys.

The following sections discuss the mechanisms by which the kidneys excrete either hypoosmotic (dilute) or hyperosmotic (concentrated) urine. The control of vasopressin secretion and its important role in regulating excretion of water by the kidneys are also explained (see also Chapter 40).

Antidiuretic Hormone

Antidiuretic hormone (ADH), or **vasopressin,** acts on the kidneys to regulate the volume and osmolality of urine. When plasma ADH levels are low, a large volume of urine is excreted **(diuresis),** and the urine is dilute.* When plasma levels are high, a small volume of urine is excreted **(antidiuresis),** and the urine is concentrated.

---

*Diuresis is simply a large urine output. When the urine contains primarily water, it is referred to as **water diuresis.** This is in contrast to the diuresis seen with diuretic agents. In this latter case urine output is large, but the urine contains solute plus water. This is sometimes termed **solute diuresis.**

● Table 34-1.
Normal Routes of Water Gain and Loss in Adults at Room Temperature (23°C)

Route	mL/Day
Water Intake	
Fluid*	1200
In food	1000
Metabolically produced from food	300
TOTAL	2500
Water Output	
Insensible	700
Sweat	100
Feces	200
Urine	1500
TOTAL	2500

*Fluid intake varies widely for both social and cultural reasons.

● Table 34-2.
Effect of Environmental Temperature and Exercise on Water Loss and Intake (mL/day) in Adults

	Normal Temperature	Hot Weather*	Prolonged Heavy Exercise*
Water Loss			
Insensible Loss			
Skin	350	350	350
Lungs	350	250	650
Sweat	100	1400	5000
Feces	200	200	200
Urine*	1500	1200	500
Total Loss	2500	3400	6700
Water Intake to Maintain Water Balance	2500	3400	6700

*In hot weather and during prolonged heavy exercise, water balance is maintained by increased water ingestion. Decreased excretion of water by the kidneys alone is insufficient to maintain water balance.

IN THE CLINIC

In the clinical setting, **hypoosmolality** (a reduction in plasma osmolality) shifts water into cells, and this process results in cell swelling. Symptoms associated with hypoosmolality are related primarily to swelling of brain cells. For example, a rapid fall in P_{osm} can alter neurological function and thereby cause nausea, malaise, headache, confusion, lethargy, seizures, and coma. When P_{osm} is increased (i.e., **hyperosmolality**), water is lost from cells. The symptoms of an increase in P_{osm} are also primarily neurological and include lethargy, weakness, seizures, coma, and even death.

Symptoms associated with changes in body fluid osmolality vary depending on how quickly the osmolality is changed. Rapid changes in osmolality (i.e., over a period of hours) are less well tolerated than changes that occur more gradually (i.e., over a period of days to weeks). Indeed, individuals in whom alterations in body fluid osmolality have developed over an extended period may be entirely asymptomatic. This reflects the ability of cells over time to either eliminate intracellular osmoles, as occurs with hypoosmolality, or generate new intracellular osmoles in response to hyperosmolality and thus minimize changes in cell volume of the neurons. This has important clinical implications when treating a patient with abnormal plasma osmolality. For example, rapid correction of osmolality of an individual who has had long-standing hypoosmolality of body fluids can lead to demyelination, especially of the pons, the results of which are irreversible. Depending on the extent of pontine demyelination, this condition can be fatal.

AT THE CELLULAR LEVEL

The gene for ADH is found on chromosome 20. It contains approximately 2000 base pairs with three exons and two introns. The gene codes for a preprohormone that consists of a signal peptide, the ADH molecule, neurophysin, and a glycopeptide (copeptin). As the cell processes the preprohormone, the signal peptide is cleaved off in the rough endoplasmic reticulum. Once packaged in neurosecretory granules, the preprohormone is further cleaved into ADH, neurophysin, and copeptin molecules. The neurosecretory granules are then transported down the axon to the posterior pituitary and stored in the nerve endings until released. When the neurons are stimulated to secrete ADH, the action potential opens Ca^{++} channels in the nerve terminal, which raises intracellular $[Ca^{++}]$ and causes exocytosis of the neurosecretory granules. All three peptides are secreted in this process. Neurophysin and copeptin do not have an identified physiological function.

ADH is a small peptide that is nine amino acids in length. It is synthesized in neuroendocrine cells located within the supraoptic and paraventricular nuclei of the hypothalamus.* The synthesized hormone is packaged in granules that are transported down the axon of the cell and stored in nerve terminals located in the neurohypophysis (posterior pituitary). The anatomy of the hypothalamus and pituitary gland is shown in Figure 34-1.

Secretion of ADH by the posterior pituitary can be influenced by several factors. The two primary physiological regulators of ADH secretion are the osmolality of the body fluids (osmotic) and the volume and pressure of the vascular system (hemodynamic). Other factors that can alter ADH secretion include nausea (stimulates), atrial natriuretic peptide (inhibits), and angiotensin II (stimulates). A number of drugs, prescription and nonprescription, also affect secretion of ADH. For example, nicotine stimulates secretion, whereas ethanol inhibits secretion.

*Neurons within the supraoptic and paraventricular nuclei synthesize either ADH or the related peptide oxytocin. ADH-secreting cells predominate in the supraoptic nucleus, whereas oxytocin-secreting neurons are primarily found in the paraventricular nucleus.

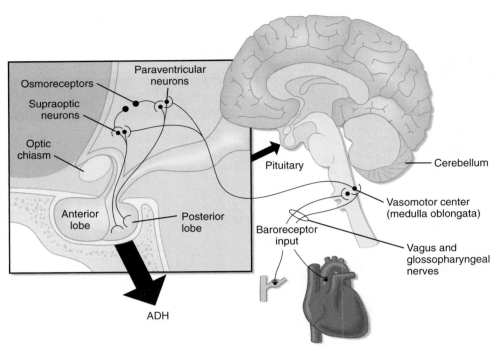

● **Figure 34-1.** Anatomy of the hypothalamus and pituitary gland (midsagittal section). Also shown are pathways involved in regulating secretion of ADH. Afferent fibers from the baroreceptors are carried in the vagus and glossopharyngeal nerves. The closed box is an expanded view of the hypothalamus and pituitary gland.

Osmotic Control of ADH Secretion

Changes in the osmolality of body fluids play the most important role in regulating secretion of ADH; changes as minor as 1% are sufficient to alter it significantly. Although neurons in the supraoptic and paraventricular nuclei respond to changes in body fluid osmolality by altering their secretion of ADH, it is clear that there are separate cells in the anterior hypothalamus that are exquisitely sensitive to changes in body fluid osmolality and therefore play an important role in regulating the secretion of ADH.* These cells, termed osmoreceptors, appear to behave as osmometers and sense changes in body fluid osmolality by either shrinking or swelling. The osmoreceptors respond only to solutes in plasma that are effective osmoles (see Chapter 1). For example, urea is an ineffective osmole when the function of osmoreceptors is considered. Thus, elevation of the plasma urea concentration alone has little effect on ADH secretion.

When the effective osmolality of plasma increases, the osmoreceptors send signals to ADH-synthesizing/secreting cells located in the supraoptic and paraventricular nuclei of the hypothalamus, and synthesis and secretion of ADH are stimulated. Conversely, when the effective osmolality of plasma is reduced, secretion is inhibited. Because ADH is rapidly degraded in plasma, circulating levels can be reduced to zero within minutes after secretion is inhibited. As a result, the ADH system can respond rapidly to fluctuations in body fluid osmolality.

Figure 34-2, _A_, illustrates the effect of changes in plasma osmolality on circulating ADH levels. The slope of the relationship is quite steep and accounts for the sensitivity of this system. The set point of the system is the plasma osmolality value at which ADH secretion begins to increase. Below this set point, virtually no ADH is released. The set point varies among individuals and is genetically determined. In healthy adults, it varies from 275 to 290 mOsm/kg H_2O (average, ≈280 to 285 mOsm/kg H_2O). Several physiological factors can also change the set point in a given individual. As discussed later, alterations in blood volume and pressure can shift it. In addition, pregnancy is associated with a decrease in the set point.

Hemodynamic Control of ADH Secretion

A decrease in blood volume or pressure also stimulates secretion of ADH. The receptors responsible for this response are located in both the low-pressure (left atrium and large pulmonary vessels) and the high-pressure (aortic arch and carotid sinus) sides of the circulatory system. Because the low-pressure receptors are located in the high-compliance side of the circulatory system (i.e., venous) and because the majority of blood is in the venous side of the circulatory system, these low-pressure receptors can be viewed as responding to overall vascular volume. The high-pressure receptors respond to arterial pressure. Both groups of receptors are sensitive to stretch of the wall of the structure in which they are located (e.g., cardiac atrial wall, wall of the aortic arch) and are termed baroreceptors. Signals from these receptors are carried in afferent fibers of the vagus and glossopharyngeal nerves to the brainstem (solitary tract nucleus of the medulla oblongata), which is part of the center that regulates heart rate and blood pressure (see also Chapter 18). Signals are then relayed from the brainstem to the ADH-secreting cells of the supraoptic and paraventricular hypothalamic nuclei. The

---

*Several sites for the location of the osmoreceptors have been identified; one of these sites is the organum vasculosum of the lamina terminalis. In addition, the subfornical organ, which is outside the blood-brain barrier, responds to circulating levels of angiotensin II.

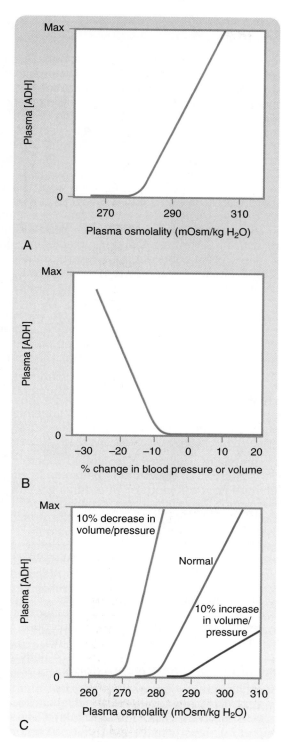

● **Figure 34-2.** Osmotic and hemodynamic control of secretion of ADH. **A,** Effect of changes in plasma osmolality (constant blood volume and pressure) on plasma ADH levels. **B,** Effect of changes in blood volume or pressure (constant plasma osmolality) on plasma ADH levels. **C,** Interactions between osmolality and blood volume and pressure stimuli on plasma ADH levels.

sensitivity of the baroreceptor system is less than that of the osmoreceptors, and a 5% to 10% decrease in blood volume or pressure is required before ADH secretion is stimulated. This is illustrated in Figure 34-2, *B.* A number of substances have been shown to alter the secretion of ADH through their effects on blood pressure, including bradykinin and histamine, which lower pressure and thus stimulate ADH secretion, and norepinephrine, which increases blood pressure and inhibits ADH secretion.

Alterations in blood volume and pressure also affect the response to changes in body fluid osmolality (see Fig. 34-2, *C*). With a decrease in blood volume or pressure, the set point is shifted to lower osmolality values and the slope of the relationship is steeper. In terms of survival of the individual, this means that when faced with circulatory collapse, the kidneys will continue to conserve water, even though by doing so they reduce the osmolality of body fluids. With an increase in blood volume or pressure, the opposite occurs. The set point is shifted to higher osmolality values, and the slope is decreased.

Actions of ADH on the Kidneys

The primary action of ADH on the kidneys is to increase the permeability of the collecting duct to water. In addition and importantly, ADH increases the permeability of the medullary portion of the collecting duct to urea. Finally, ADH stimulates reabsorption of NaCl by the thick ascending limb of Henle's loop, the distal tubule, and the collecting duct.

The actions of ADH on permeability of the collecting duct to water have been studied extensively. ADH binds to a receptor on the basolateral membrane of the cell. This receptor is termed the V_2 receptor (i.e., vasopressin 2 receptor).* Binding to this receptor, which is coupled to adenylyl cyclase via a stimulatory G protein (G_s), increases intracellular levels of cAMP. The rise in intracellular cAMP activates protein kinase A (PKA), which ultimately results in the insertion of vesicles containing aquaporin-2 (AQP2) water channels into the apical membrane of the cell, as well as the synthesis of more AQP2 (Fig. 34-3). With the removal of ADH, these water channels are reinternalized into the cell, and the apical membrane is once again impermeable to water. This shuttling of water channels into and out of the apical membrane provides a rapid mechanism for controlling permeability of the membrane to water. Because the basolateral membrane is freely permeable to water as a result of the presence of AQP3 and AQP4 water channels, any water that enters the cell through apical membrane water channels exits across the basolateral membrane, thereby resulting in net absorption of water from the tubule lumen.

In addition to the acute effects of ADH just described, ADH regulates the expression of AQP2 (and AQP3). When large volumes of water are ingested over an

---

*A different ADH receptor (V_1 receptor) is present on vascular smooth muscle. This receptor mediates the vasoconstrictor response to ADH. It is this action that accounts for its alternative name, vasopressin.

▶ IN THE CLINIC

Inadequate release of ADH from the posterior pituitary results in the excretion of large volumes of dilute urine **(polyuria).** To compensate for this loss of water, the individual must ingest large volumes of water **(polydipsia)** to maintain constant body fluid osmolality. If the individual is deprived of water, the body fluids will become hyperosmotic. This condition is called **central diabetes insipidus** or pituitary diabetes insipidus. Central diabetes insipidus can be inherited, although this is rare. It occurs more commonly after head trauma and with brain neoplasms or infections. Individuals with central diabetes insipidus have a urine-concentrating defect that can be corrected by the administration of exogenous ADH.

The inherited (autosomal dominant) form of central diabetes insipidus has been shown to represent multiple mutations in the ADH gene. In patients with this form of central diabetes insipidus, mutations have been identified in all regions of the ADH gene (i.e., ADH, copeptin, and neurophysin). The most common mutation is found in the neurophysin portion of the gene. In each of these situations there is defective trafficking of the peptide, with abnormal accumulation in the endoplasmic reticulum. It is believed that this abnormal accumulation in the endoplasmic reticulum results in death of the ADH secretory cells of the supraoptic and paraventricular nuclei.

The **syndrome of inappropriate ADH secretion (SIADH)** is a common clinical problem characterized by plasma ADH levels that are elevated above what would be expected on the basis of body fluid osmolality and blood volume and pressure—hence the term inappropriate ADH secretion. Individuals with SIADH retain water, and their body fluids become progressively hypoosmotic. In addition, their urine is more hyperosmotic than expected based on the low body fluid osmolality. SIADH can be caused by infections and neoplasms of the brain, drugs (e.g., antitumor drugs), pulmonary diseases, and carcinoma of the lung. Many of these conditions stimulate secretion of ADH by altering neural input to the ADH secretory cells. However, small cell carcinoma of the lung produces and secretes a number of peptides, including ADH.

● AT THE CELLULAR LEVEL

The gene for the V_2 receptor is located on the X chromosome. It codes for a 371–amino acid protein that is in the family of receptors that have seven membrane-spanning domains and are coupled to heterotrimeric G proteins. As shown in Figure 34-3, binding of ADH to its receptor on the basolateral membrane activates adenylyl cyclase. The increase in intracellular cAMP then activates protein kinase A (PKA), which results in phosphorylation of AQP2 water channels, as well as increased transcription of the AQP2 gene via activation of a cAMP-response element (CRE). Vesicles containing phosphorylated AQP2 move toward the apical membrane along microtubules driven by the molecular motor dynein. Once near the apical membrane, proteins called SNAREs interact with vesicles containing AQP2 and facilitate fusion of these vesicles with the membrane. The addition of AQP2 to the membrane allows water to enter the cell driven by the osmotic gradient (lumen osmolality < cell osmolality). The water then exits the cell across the basolateral membrane through AQP3 and AQP4 water channels, which are constitutively present in the basolateral membrane. When the V_2 receptor is not occupied by ADH, the AQP2 water channels are removed from the apical membrane by clathrin-mediated endocytosis, thus rendering the apical membrane once again impermeable to water. The endocytosed AQP2 molecules may be either stored in cytoplasmic vesicles, ready for reinsertion into the apical membrane when ADH levels in plasma increase, or degraded.

Recently, individuals have been found who have activating (gain-of-function) mutations in the V_2 receptor gene. Thus, the receptor is constitutively activated, even in the absence of ADH. These individuals have laboratory findings similar to those seen in SIADH, including reduced plasma osmolality, **hyponatremia** (reduced plasma $[Na^+]$), and urine more concentrated than would be expected from the reduced body fluid osmolality. However, unlike SIADH, where circulating levels of ADH are elevated and thus responsible for water retention by the kidneys, these individuals have undetectable levels of ADH in their plasma. This new clinical entity has been termed **"nephrogenic syndrome of inappropriate antidiuresis."**

extended period (e.g., psychogenic polydipsia), expression of AQP2 and AQP3 in the collecting duct is reduced. As a consequence, when water ingestion is restricted, these individuals cannot maximally concentrate their urine. Conversely, in states of restricted water ingestion, expression of AQP2 and AQP3 in the collecting duct increases and thus facilitates the excretion of maximally concentrated urine.

It is also clear that expression of AQP2 (and in some instances also AQP3) varies in pathological conditions associated with disturbances in urine concentration

and dilution. As discussed elsewhere, AQP2 expression is reduced in a number of conditions associated with impaired urine-concentrating ability. By contrast, in conditions associated with water retention, such as congestive heart failure, hepatic cirrhosis, and pregnancy, AQP2 expression is increased.

ADH also increases the permeability of the terminal portion of the inner medullary collecting duct to urea. This results in an increase in reabsorption of urea and an increase in the osmolality of the medullary interstitial fluid. The apical membrane of medullary collecting

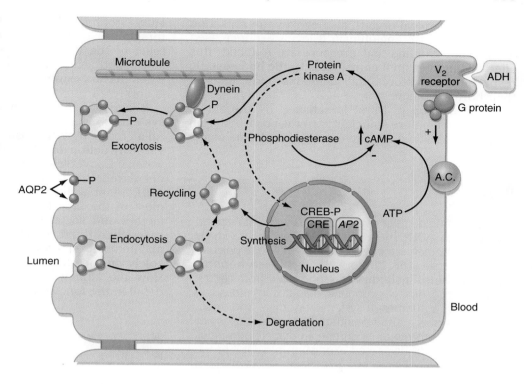

● **Figure 34-3.** Action of ADH via the V_2 receptor on the principal cell of the late distal tubule and collecting duct. See text for details. A.C., adenylyl cyclase; *AP2*, aquaporin-2 gene; AQP2, aquaporin-2; CRE, cAMP response element; CREB-P, phosphorylated cAMP response element–binding protein; -P, phosphorylated proteins. (Adapted and modified from Brown D, Nielsen S. In Brenner BM [ed]: The Kidney, 7th ed. Philadelphia, Saunders, 2004.)

duct cells contains two different urea transporters (UT-A1 and UT-A3).* ADH, acting through the cAMP/ PKA cascade, increases permeability of the apical membrane to urea. This increase in permeability is associated with phosphorylation of UT-A1 and perhaps also UT-A3. Increasing the osmolality of the interstitial fluid of the renal medulla also increases the permeability of the collecting duct to urea. This effect is mediated by the phospholipase C pathway and involves phosphorylation by protein kinase C. Thus, this effect is separate and additive to that of ADH.

In addition to its acute effect on permeability of the collecting duct to urea, ADH also increases the abundance of UT-A1 in states of chronic water restriction. In contrast, with water loading (i.e., suppressed ADH levels), UT-A1 abundance in the collecting duct is reduced.

ADH also stimulates reabsorption of NaCl by the thick ascending limb of Henle's loop and by the distal tubule and cortical segment of the collecting duct. This increase in Na^+ reabsorption is associated with increased abundance of key Na^+ transporters: 1Na^+-1K^+-2Cl^- symporter (thick ascending limb of Henle's loop), Na^+-Cl^- symporter (distal tubule), and the epithelial Na^+ channel (ENaC, in the distal tubule and collecting duct). It is thought that stimulation of NaCl transport by the thick ascending limb may help maintain the hyperosmotic medullary interstitium that is necessary for the absorption of water from the medullary portion of the collecting duct (see later).

---

*Localization of UT-A3 is species specific. In some species it is localized to the apical membrane, whereas in others it is found in the basolateral membrane.

Thirst

In addition to affecting the secretion of ADH, changes in plasma osmolality and blood volume or pressure lead to alterations in the perception of thirst. When body fluid osmolality is increased or blood volume or pressure is reduced, the individual perceives thirst. Of these stimuli, hypertonicity is the more potent. An increase in plasma osmolality of only 2% to 3% produces a strong desire to drink, whereas decreases in blood volume and pressure in the range of 10% to 15% are required to produce the same response.

As already discussed, there is a genetically determined threshold for ADH secretion (i.e., a body fluid osmolality above which ADH secretion increases). Similarly, there is a genetically determined threshold for triggering the sensation of thirst. However, the thirst threshold is higher than the threshold for ADH secretion. On average, the threshold for ADH secretion is approximately 285 mOsm/kg H_2O, whereas the thirst threshold is approximately 295 mOsm/kg H_2O. Because of this difference, thirst is stimulated at a body fluid osmolality at which secretion of ADH is already maximal.

The neural centers involved in regulating water intake (the thirst center) are located in the same region of the hypothalamus involved in regulating ADH secretion. However, it is not certain whether the same cells serve both functions. Indeed, the thirst response, like the regulation of ADH secretion, occurs only in response to effective osmoles (e.g., NaCl). Even less is known about the pathways involved in the thirst response to decreased blood volume or pressure, but it is believed that they are the same as those involved in the volume- and pressure-related regulation of ADH secretion. Angiotensin II, acting on cells of the thirst center (subfornical organ), also evokes the sensation of thirst. Because angiotensin II levels are increased when blood volume and pressure are reduced, this effect of angiotensin II contributes to the homeostatic response that restores and maintains body fluids at their normal volume.

The sensation of thirst is satisfied by the act of drinking even before sufficient water is absorbed from the gastrointestinal tract to correct the plasma osmo-

lality. Oropharyngeal and upper gastrointestinal receptors appear to be involved in this response. However, relief of the thirst sensation via these receptors is short-lived, and thirst is completely satisfied only when plasma osmolality or blood volume or pressure is corrected.

It should be apparent that the ADH and thirst systems work in concert to maintain water balance. An increase in plasma osmolality evokes drinking and, via ADH action on the kidneys, the conservation of water. Conversely, when plasma osmolality is decreased, thirst is suppressed, and in the absence of ADH, renal water excretion is enhanced. However, most of the time fluid intake is dictated by cultural factors and social situations. This is especially the case when thirst is not stimulated. In this situation, maintenance of normal body fluid osmolality relies solely on the ability of the kidneys to excrete water. How the kidney accomplishes this is discussed in detail in the following sections of this chapter.

> ### ▶ IN THE CLINIC
>
> The collecting ducts of some individuals do not respond normally to ADH. These individuals cannot maximally concentrate their urine and consequently have polyuria and polydipsia. This clinical entity is termed **nephrogenic diabetes insipidus** to distinguish it from central diabetes insipidus. Nephrogenic diabetes insipidus can result from a number of systemic disorders and, more rarely, occurs as a result of inherited disorders. Many of the acquired forms of nephrogenic diabetes insipidus are the result of decreased expression of AQP2 in the collecting duct. Decreased expression of AQP2 has been documented in the urine-concentrating defects associated with hypokalemia, lithium ingestion (some degree of nephrogenic diabetes insipidus develops in 35% of individuals who take lithium for bipolar disorder), ureteral obstruction, a low-protein diet, and hypercalcemia. The inherited forms of nephrogenic diabetes insipidus reflect mutations in the ADH receptor (V_2 receptor) or the AQP2 molecule. Of these, approximately 90% of hereditary forms of nephrogenic diabetes insipidus are the result of mutations in the V_2 receptor gene, with the other 10% being the result of mutations in the AQP2 gene. Because the gene for the V_2 receptor is located on the X chromosome, these inherited forms are X-linked. To date, more than 150 different mutations in the V_2 receptor gene have been described. Most of the mutations result in trapping of the receptor in the endoplasmic reticulum of the cell; only a few cases result in the surface expression of a V_2 receptor that will not bind ADH. The gene coding for AQP2 is located on chromosome 12 and is inherited as both an autosomal recessive and an autosomal dominant defect. As noted in Chapter 1, aquaporins exist as homotetramers. This homotetramer formation explains the difference between the two forms of nephrogenic diabetes insipidus. In the recessive form, heterozygotes produce both normal AQP2 and defective AQP2 molecules. The defective AQP2 monomer is retained in the endoplasmic reticulum of the cell, and thus the homotetramers that do form contain only normal molecules. Accordingly, mutations in both alleles are required to produce nephrogenic diabetes insipidus. In the autosomal dominant form, the defective monomers can form tetramers with normal monomers, as well as with defective monomers. However, these tetramers are unable to traffic to the apical membrane.

> ### ▶ IN THE CLINIC
>
> With adequate access to water, the thirst mechanism can prevent the development of hyperosmolality. Indeed, it is this mechanism that is responsible for the polydipsia seen in response to the polyuria of both central and nephrogenic diabetes insipidus.
>
> Water intake is also influenced by social and cultural factors. Thus, individuals will ingest water even in the absence of the thirst sensation. Normally, the kidneys are able to excrete this excess water because they can excrete up to 18 L/day of urine. However, in some instances, the volume of water ingested exceeds the kidneys' capacity to excrete water, especially over short periods. When this occurs, the body fluids become hypoosmotic. An example of how water intake can exceed the capacity of the kidneys to excrete water is long-distance running. A recent study of participants in the Boston Marathon found that hyponatremia developed in 13% of the runners during the course of the race.* This reflected the practice of some runners of ingesting water, or other hypotonic drinks, during the race to remain "well hydrated." In addition, water is produced from the metabolism of glycogen and triglycerides used as fuels by the exercising muscle. Because over the course of the race they ingested, as well as generated through metabolism, more water than their kidneys were able to excrete or was lost by sweating, hyponatremia developed. In some racers the hyponatremia was severe enough to elicit the neurological symptoms described previously.
>
> One can find throughout the popular press the admonition to drink eight 8-oz glasses of water a day (the 8×8 recommendation). Drinking this volume of water is said to provide innumerable health benefits. As a result, it seems that everyone now has a water bottle as a constant companion. Although ingesting this volume of water over the course of a day (approxi-

mately 2 L) will not harm most individuals, there is no scientific evidence to support the beneficial health claims ascribed to the 8 × 8 recommendation.[†] Indeed most individuals get adequate amounts of water through the food that they ingest and the fluids taken with those meals.

The maximum amount of water that can be excreted by the kidneys depends on the amount of solute excreted, which in turn depends on food intake. For example, with maximally dilute urine (U_{osm} = 50 mOsm/kg H_2O), the maximum urine output of 18 L/day will be achieved only if the solute excretion rate is 900 mmol/day.

● **Equation 34-1**

$$U_{osm} = \text{Solute excreted/Volume excreted}$$

$$50 \text{ mOsm/kg } H_2O = 900 \text{ mmol/18 L}$$

If excretion of solute is reduced, as commonly occurs in the elderly with reduced food intake, the maximum urine output will decrease. For example, if solute excretion is only 400 mmol/day, a maximum urine output (at U_{osm} = 50 mOsm/kg H_2O) of only 8 L/day can be achieved. Thus, individuals with reduced food intake have a reduced capacity to excrete water.

*See Almond CS et al: Hyponatremia among runners in the Boston Marathon. N Engl J Med 2005; 352:1150, 2005.)
[†]See Valtin H: "Drink at least eight glasses of water a day." Really? Is there scientific evidence for "8x8"? Am J Physiol Reg Integr Comp Physiol 283: R993, 2002.)

Renal Mechanisms for Dilution and Concentration of Urine

Under normal circumstances, excretion of water is regulated separately from excretion of solutes. For this to occur, the kidneys must be able to excrete urine that is either hypoosmotic or hyperosmotic with respect to body fluids. This ability to excrete urine of varying osmolality in turn requires that solute be separated from water at some point along the nephron. As discussed in Chapter 33, reabsorption of solute in the proximal tubule results in reabsorption of a proportional amount of water. Hence, solute and water are not separated in this portion of the nephron. Moreover, this proportionality between proximal tubule water and solute reabsorption occurs regardless of whether the kidneys excrete dilute or concentrated urine. Thus, the proximal tubule reabsorbs a large portion of the filtered load of solute and water, but it does not produce dilute or concentrated tubular fluid. The loop of Henle, in particular, the thick ascending limb, is the major site where solute and water are separated. Consequently, excretion of both dilute and concentrated urine requires normal function of the loop of Henle.

Excretion of hypoosmotic urine is relatively easy to understand. The nephron must simply reabsorb solute from the tubular fluid and not allow reabsorption of water to also occur. As just noted and as described in

greater detail later, reabsorption of solute without concomitant water reabsorption occurs in the ascending limb of Henle's loop. Under appropriate conditions (i.e., in the absence of ADH), the distal tubule and collecting duct also dilute the tubular fluid.

Excretion of hyperosmotic urine is more complex and thus more difficult to understand. This process in essence involves removing water from the tubular fluid without solute. Because water movement is passive and driven by an osmotic gradient, the kidney must generate a hyperosmotic compartment that then reabsorbs water osmotically from the tubular fluid. The compartment in the kidney that serves this function is the interstitium of the renal medulla. Henle's loop, in particular, the thick ascending limb, is critical for generating the hyperosmotic medullary interstitium. Once established, this hyperosmotic compartment drives reabsorption of water from the collecting duct and thereby concentrates the urine.

Figure 34-4 summarizes the essential features of the mechanisms whereby the kidneys excrete either dilute or concentrated urine. Table 34-3 summarizes the transport and passive permeability properties of the nephron segments involved in these processes.

First, how the kidneys excrete dilute urine **(water diuresis)** when ADH levels are low or zero is considered. The following numbers refer to those encircled in Figure 34-4, *A:*

1. Fluid entering the descending thin limb of the loop of Henle from the proximal tubule is isosmotic with respect to plasma. This reflects the essentially isosmotic nature of solute and water reabsorption in the proximal tubule (see Chapter 33).
2. The descending thin limb is highly permeable to water and much less so to solutes such as NaCl and urea. (*Note:* Urea is an ineffective osmole in many tissues, but it is an effective osmole in many portions of the nephron [Table 34-3]). Consequently, as the fluid in the descending thin limb descends deeper into the hyperosmotic medulla, water is reabsorbed (via AQP1) as a result of the osmotic gradient set up across the descending thin limb by both NaCl and urea, which are present at high concentrations in the medullary interstitium (see later). By this process, tubular fluid at the bend of the loop has an osmolality equal to that of the surrounding interstitial fluid. Although the osmolality of tubular and interstitial fluid is similar at the bend of the loop, their compositions differ. The concentration of NaCl in tubular fluid is greater than that in the surrounding interstitial fluid. However, the concentration of urea in tubular fluid is less than that of interstitial fluid (see later).
3. The ascending thin limb is impermeable to water but permeable to NaCl. Consequently, as tubular fluid moves up the ascending limb, NaCl is passively reabsorbed because the concentration of NaCl in tubular fluid is higher than that in interstitial fluid. As a result, the volume of tubular fluid remains unchanged along the length of the thin ascending limb, but the concentration of NaCl

Water diuresis

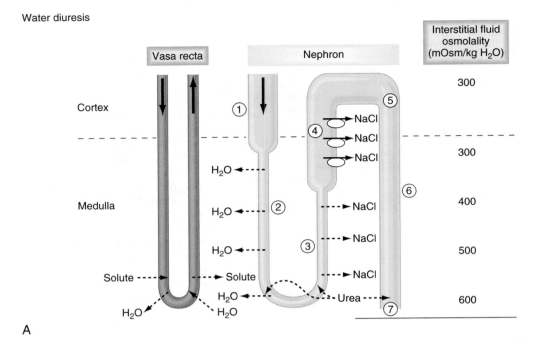

A

Antidiuresis

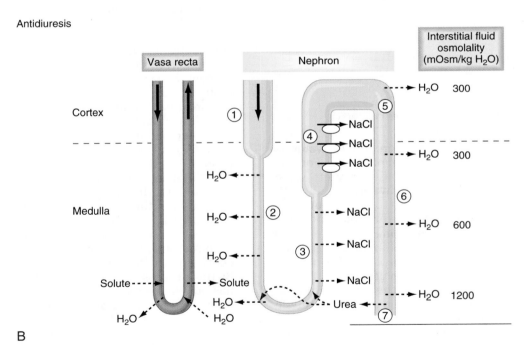

B

● **Figure 34-4.**   Schematic of the nephron segments involved in dilution and concentration of urine. Henle's loops of juxtamedullary nephrons are shown. **A,** Mechanism for the excretion of dilute urine (water diuresis). ADH is absent, and the collecting duct is essentially impermeable to water. Note also that during water diuresis the osmolality of the medullary interstitium is reduced as a result of increased vasa recta blood flow and entry of some urea into the medullary collecting duct. **B,** Mechanism for the excretion of concentrated urine (antidiuresis). Plasma ADH levels are maximal, and the collecting duct is highly permeable to water. Under this condition, the medullary interstitial gradient is maximal.

● **Figure 34-5.** The process of countercurrent multiplication by the loop of Henle. Initially (1), fluid in the loop of Henle and interstitium has an osmolality essentially equal to that of plasma (300 mOsm/kg H_2O). Transport of solute out of the ascending limb into the interstitium represents the single effect of separating solute from water (2 and 5). The osmotic pressure gradient between the interstitium and the descending limb results in passive movement of water out of the descending limb (3 and 6). In the steady state with continuous tubular fluid flow, the single effect is multiplied along the length of the loop to establish an osmotic gradient, with the fluid at the bend of the loop having the highest osmolality.

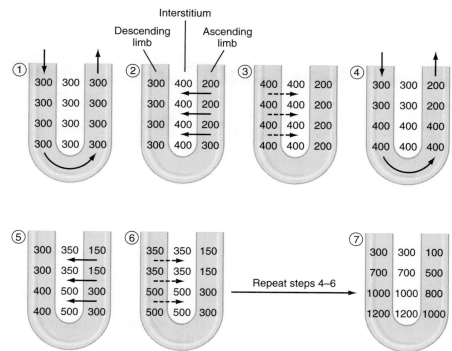

decreases. Thus, as fluid ascends through the thin ascending limb, it becomes less concentrated than the surrounding interstitial fluid (i.e., tubular fluid dilution begins).

4. The thick ascending limb of the loop of Henle is impermeable to water and urea. This portion of the nephron actively reabsorbs NaCl from tubular fluid and thereby dilutes it. Dilution occurs to such a degree that this segment is often referred to as the **diluting segment** of the kidney. Fluid leaving the thick ascending limb is hypoosmotic with respect to plasma (approximately 150 mOsm/kg H_2O).

5. The distal tubule and the cortical portion of the collecting duct actively reabsorb NaCl and are impermeable to urea. In the absence of ADH, these segments are not permeable to water. Thus, when ADH is absent or present at low levels (i.e., decreased plasma osmolality), the osmolality of tubule fluid in these segments is reduced further because NaCl is reabsorbed without water. Under this condition, fluid leaving the cortical portion of the collecting duct is hypoosmotic with respect to plasma (approximately 50 to 100 mOsm/kg H_2O).

6. The medullary collecting duct actively reabsorbs NaCl. Even in the absence of ADH, this segment is slightly permeable to water and urea. Consequently, some urea enters the collecting duct from the medullary interstitium, and a small volume of water is reabsorbed.

7. Urine has an osmolality as low as approximately 50 mOsm/kg H_2O and contains low concentrations of NaCl and urea. The volume of urine excreted can be as much as 18 L/day, or approximately 10% of the glomerular filtration rate (GFR).

Next, how the kidneys excrete concentrated urine **(antidiuresis)** when plasma osmolality and plasma

ADH levels are high is considered. The following numbers refer to those encircled in Figure 34-4, *B:*

1-4. These steps are similar to those for the production of dilute urine. An important point in understanding how concentrated urine is produced is to recognize that although reabsorption of NaCl by the ascending thin and thick limbs of the loop of Henle dilutes the tubular fluid, the reabsorbed NaCl accumulates in the medullary interstitium and raises the osmolality of this compartment. Accumulation of NaCl in the medullary interstitium is crucial for the production of urine hyperosmotic to plasma because it provides the osmotic driving force for reabsorption of water by the medullary collecting duct. The overall process by which the loop of Henle, in particular, the thick ascending limb, generates the hyperosmotic medullary interstitial gradient is termed **countercurrent multiplication*** (Fig. 34-5). As already noted, ADH stimulates reabsorption of NaCl by the thick

---

*The term countercurrent multiplication derives from both the form and function of the loop of Henle. The loop of Henle consists of two parallel limbs with tubular fluid flowing in opposite directions (countercurrent flow). Fluid flows into the medulla in the descending limb and out of the medulla in the ascending limb. The ascending limb is impermeable to water and reabsorbs solute from the tubular fluid. Thus, fluid within the ascending limb becomes diluted. This separation of solute and water by the ascending limb is termed the **single effect** of the countercurrent multiplication process. The solute removed from the tubular fluid in the ascending limb accumulates in the surrounding interstitial fluid and raises its osmolality. Because the descending limb is highly permeable to water, the increased osmolality of the medullary interstitium causes water to be reabsorbed and thereby concentrates the tubular fluid in this segment. The countercurrent flow within the descending and ascending limbs of the loop of Henle magnifies, or "multiplies," the osmotic gradient between the tubule fluid in the descending and ascending limbs of the loop of Henle such that an increasing osmotic gradient is generated throughout the medullary interstitium, as illustrated (Fig. 34-5).

● **Table 34-3.**

Transport and Permeability Properties of Nephron Segments Involved in Urine Concentration and Dilution

Tubule Segment	Active Transport	Passive Permeability*			Effect of ADH
		NaCl	*Urea*	*H₂O*	
Loop of Henle					
Descending thin limb	0	+	+	+++	
Ascending thin limb	0	+++	+	0	
Thick ascending limb	+++	+	0	0	↑ NaCl reabsorption
Distal tubule	++	+	0	0	↑ H₂O permeability (late portion only)
Collecting duct					
Cortex	+	+	0	0	↑ H₂O permeability
Medulla	+	+	++	+	↑ H₂O and urea permeability

*Permeability is proportional to the number of plus signs indicated: +, low permeability; +++, high permeability; 0, impermeable.

ascending limb of Henle's loop. This is thought to maintain the medullary interstitial gradient at a time when water is being added to this compartment from the medullary collecting duct, which would tend to dissipate the gradient.

5. Because of reabsorption of NaCl by the ascending limb of the loop of Henle, the fluid reaching the collecting duct is hypoosmotic with respect to the surrounding interstitial fluid. Thus, an osmotic gradient is established across the collecting duct. In the presence of ADH, which increases the permeability of the last half of the distal tubule and the collecting duct to water, water diffuses out of the tubule lumen, and tubule fluid osmolality increases. This diffusion of water out of the lumen of the collecting duct begins the process of urine concentration. The maximum osmolality that the fluid in the distal tubule and cortical portion of the collecting duct can attain is approximately 290 mOsm/kg H₂O (i.e., the same as plasma), which is the osmolality of the interstitial fluid and plasma within the cortex of the kidney. Although the fluid at this point has the same osmolality as the fluid that entered the descending thin limb, its composition has been altered dramatically. Because of reabsorption of NaCl by the preceding nephron segments, NaCl accounts for a much smaller proportion of total tubular fluid osmolality. Instead, tubule fluid osmolality reflects the presence of urea (filtered urea plus urea added to the descending thin limb of the loop of Henle) and other solutes (e.g., K⁺, NH₄⁺, and creatinine).

6. The osmolality of the interstitial fluid in the medulla progressively increases from the junction between the renal cortex and medulla, where it is approximately 300 mOsm/kg H₂O, to the papilla, where it is approximately 1200 mOsm/kg H₂O. Thus, an osmotic gradient exists between tubule fluid and interstitial fluid along the entire medullary collecting duct. In the presence of ADH, which increases the permeability of the medullary collecting duct to water, the osmolality of tubule

fluid increases as water is reabsorbed. Because the initial portions of the collecting duct (cortical and outer medullary) are impermeable to urea, it remains in the tubular fluid, and its concentration increases. As already noted, in the presence of ADH, the permeability of the last portion of the medullary collecting duct (inner medullary) to urea is increased. Because the concentration of urea in the tubular fluid has been increased by reabsorption of water in the cortex and outer medulla, its concentration in tubular fluid is greater than its concentration in interstitial fluid, and some urea diffuses out of the tubule lumen into the medullary interstitium. The maximal osmolality that the fluid in the medullary collecting duct can attain is equal to that of the surrounding interstitial fluid. The major components of the tubular fluid within the medullary collecting ducts are substances that have either escaped reabsorption or have been secreted into the tubular fluid. Of these, urea is the most abundant.

7. The urine produced when ADH levels are elevated has an osmolality of 1200 mOsm/kg H₂O and contains high concentrations of urea and other nonreabsorbed solutes. Because urea in tubular fluid equilibrates with urea in the medullary interstitial fluid, its concentration in urine is similar to that in the interstitium. Urine volume under this condition can be as low as 0.5 L/day.

As just described, reabsorption of water by the proximal tubule (67% of the filtered amount) and the thin descending limb of the loop of Henle (15% of the filtered amount) is essentially the same regardless of whether the urine is dilute or concentrated. As a result, a relatively constant volume of water is delivered to the distal tubule and collecting duct each day. Depending on the plasma ADH concentration, a variable portion of this water is then reabsorbed (8% to 17% of the filtered amount), with water excretion ranging from less than 1% to 10% of the filtered water.

Movement of water across the various segments of the nephron occurs via water channels (aquaporins). The proximal tubule and the thin descending limb of Henle's loop are highly permeable to water, and these segments express high levels of AQP1 in both the apical and basolateral membrane. The vasa recta are likewise highly permeable to water and express AQP1. AQP7 and AQP8 are also expressed in the proximal tubule. As already discussed, AQP2 is responsible for ADH-regulated water movement across the apical membrane of principal cells of the late distal tubule and collecting duct, and AQP3 and AQP4 are responsible for water movement across the basolateral membrane.

Mice lacking the AQP1 gene have been created. These mice have a urine-concentrating defect with increased urine output. Several individuals have been found who also lack the normal AQP1 gene. Interestingly, these individuals do not have polyuria. However, when challenged by water deprivation, they are able to concentrate their urine to only approximately half of what is seen in a normal individual.

During antidiuresis, most of the water is reabsorbed in the distal tubule and cortical and outer medullary portions of the collecting duct. Thus, a relatively small volume of fluid reaches the inner medullary collecting duct, where it is then reabsorbed. This distribution of water reabsorption along the length of the collecting duct (i.e., cortex > outer medulla > inner medulla) allows maintenance of a hyperosmotic interstitial environment in the inner medulla by minimizing the amount of water entering this compartment.

Medullary Interstitium

As noted, the interstitial fluid of the renal medulla is critically important in concentrating urine. The osmotic pressure of interstitial fluid provides the driving force for reabsorbing water from both the descending thin limb of the loop of Henle and the collecting duct. The principal solutes of medullary interstitial fluid are NaCl and urea, but the concentration of these solutes is not uniform throughout the medulla (i.e., a gradient exists from the cortex to the papilla). Other solutes also accumulate in the medullary interstitium (e.g., NH_4^+ and K^+), but the most abundant solutes are NaCl and urea. For simplicity, this discussion assumes that NaCl and urea are the only solutes.

At the junction of the medulla with the cortex, interstitial fluid has an osmolality of approximately 300 mOsm/kg H_2O, with virtually all osmoles attributable to NaCl. The concentrations of both NaCl and urea increase progressively with increasing depth into the medulla. When maximally concentrated urine is excreted, the osmolality of the medullary interstitial fluid is approximately 1200 mOsm/kg H_2O at the papilla (Fig. 34-4, *B*). Of this value, approximately 600 mOsm/kg H_2O is attributed to NaCl and 600 mOsm/kg H_2O to

urea. As described later, NaCl is an effective osmole in the inner medulla and thus is responsible for driving reabsorption of water from the medullary collecting duct.

The medullary gradient for NaCl results from the accumulation of NaCl reabsorbed by the nephron segments in the medulla during countercurrent multiplication. The most important segment in this regard is the ascending limb (the thick limb more than the thin limb) of the loop of Henle. Accumulation of urea within the medullary interstitium is more complex and occurs most effectively when hyperosmotic urine is excreted (i.e., antidiuresis). When dilute urine is produced, especially over extended periods, the osmolality of the medullary interstitium declines (Fig. 34-4). This reduced osmolality is almost entirely caused by a decrease in the concentration of urea. This decrease reflects washout by the vasa recta (see later) and diffusion of urea from the interstitium into the tubular fluid within the medullary portion of the collecting duct. Recall that the medullary collecting duct is significantly permeable to urea even in the absence of ADH (Table 34-3).

Urea is not synthesized in the kidney but is generated by the liver as a product of protein metabolism. It enters tubular fluid via glomerular filtration. As indicated in Table 34-3, the permeability of most nephron segments involved in urinary concentration and dilution to urea is relatively low. The important exception is the medullary collecting duct, which has relatively high permeability to urea that is further increased by ADH. As fluid moves along the nephron and water is reabsorbed in the collecting duct, the urea concentration in tubular fluid increases. When this urea-rich tubular fluid reaches the medullary collecting duct, where permeability to urea is not only high but also increased by ADH, urea diffuses down its concentration gradient into medullary interstitial fluid, where it accumulates. When ADH levels are elevated, the urea within the lumen of the collecting duct and the interstitium equilibrates. The resultant concentration of urea in urine is equal to that in the medullary interstitium at the papilla, or approximately 600 mOsm/kg H_2O.

Some of the urea within the interstitium enters the descending thin limb of the loop of Henle via the UT-A2 urea transporter. This urea is then trapped in the nephron until it again reaches the medullary collecting duct, where it can reenter the medullary interstitium. Thus, urea recycles from the interstitium to the nephron and back into the interstitium. This process of recycling facilitates the accumulation of urea in the medullary interstitium. Consequently, during antidiuresis, the concentration of urea can reach 600 mOsm/kg H_2O, which is approximately half of the total medullary interstitial concentration (Fig. 34-4, *B*).

As described, the hyperosmotic medullary interstitium is essential for concentrating the tubular fluid within the collecting duct. Because reabsorption of water from the collecting duct is driven by the osmotic gradient established in the medullary interstitium, urine can never be more concentrated than that of the interstitial fluid in the papilla. Thus, any condition that reduces medullary interstitial osmolality impairs the ability of the kidneys to maximally concentrate urine. Urea within the medullary interstitium contributes to the total osmolality of the urine. However, because the inner medullary collecting duct is highly permeable to urea, especially in the presence of ADH, urea cannot drive water reabsorption across this nephron segment (i.e., urea is an ineffective osmole). Instead, the urea in tubular fluid and the medullary interstitium equilibrates, and a small volume of urine with a high concentration of urea is excreted. This, in effect, allows the kidneys to excrete the daily urea load in a relatively small volume of urine. If urine with a high concentration of urea could not be excreted, the need to excrete the daily urea load would obligate the excretion of a much larger volume of urine. It is the medullary interstitial NaCl concentration that is responsible for reabsorbing water from the medullary collecting duct and thereby concentrating the nonurea solutes (e.g., NH_4^+ salts, K^+ salts, creatinine) in urine.

Vasa Recta Function

The **vasa recta,** the capillary networks that supply blood to the medulla, are highly permeable to solute and water (water via AQP1). As with the loop of Henle, the vasa recta form a parallel set of hairpin loops within the medulla (see Chapter 32). Not only do the vasa recta bring nutrients and oxygen to the medullary nephron segments, but more importantly, they also remove the excess water and solute that is continuously being added to the medullary interstitium by these nephron segments. The ability of the vasa recta to maintain the medullary interstitial gradient is flow dependent. A substantial increase in vasa recta blood flow dissipates the medullary gradient (i.e., washout of osmoles from the medullary interstitium). Alternatively, reduced blood flow decreases oxygen delivery to the nephron segments within the medulla. Because transport of salt and other solutes requires oxygen and ATP, reduced medullary blood flow decreases salt and solute transport by nephron segments in the medulla. As a result, the medullary interstitial osmotic gradient cannot be maintained.

Assessment of Renal Diluting and Concentrating Ability

Assessment of renal water handling includes measurement of urine osmolality and the volume of urine excreted. The range of urine osmolality is 50 to 1200 mOsm/kg H_2O. The corresponding range in urine volume is 18 L to as little as 0.5 L/day. These ranges are not fixed, but they vary from individual to individual and, as noted previously, depend on the amount of solute excreted.

As emphasized in this chapter, the ability of the kidneys to dilute or concentrate urine requires the separation of solute and water (i.e., the single effect of the countercurrent multiplication process). This separation of solute and water in essence generates a volume of water that is "free of solute." When the urine is dilute, **solute-free water** is excreted from the body. When the urine is concentrated, solute-free water is returned to the body (i.e., conserved). The concept of **free water clearance** provides a way to calculate the amount of solute-free water generated by the kidneys, either when dilute urine is excreted or when concentrated urine is formed. As its name denotes, free water clearance is directly derived from the concept of renal clearance discussed in Chapter 32.

To determine free water clearance, the clearance of total solute by the kidneys must be calculated. This clearance of total solute (i.e., osmoles, whether effective or ineffective) from plasma by the kidneys is termed **osmolar clearance (C_{osm})** and can be calculated as follows:

● **Equation 34-2**

$$C_{osm} = \frac{U_{osm} \times \dot{V}}{P_{osm}}$$

where U_{osm} is urine osmolality, $\dot{V}$ is the urine flow rate, and P_{osm} is the osmolality of plasma. C_{osm} has units of volume/unit time. Free water clearance (C_{H_2O}) is then calculated as follows:

● **Equation 34-3**

$$C_{H_2O} = \dot{V} - C_{osm}$$

By rearranging Equation 34-3, it should be apparent that

● **Equation 34-4**

$$\dot{V} = C_{H_2O} + C_{osm}$$

In other words, it is possible to partition total urine output ($\dot{V}$) into two hypothetical components. One component contains all the urine solutes and has an osmolality equal to that of plasma (i.e., $U_{osm} = P_{osm}$). This volume is defined by C_{osm} and represents a volume from which there has been no separation of solute and water. The second component is a volume of solute-free water (i.e., C_{H_2O}).

When dilute urine is produced, the value of C_{H_2O} is positive, which indicates that solute-free water is being excreted from the body. When concentrated urine is produced, the value of C_{H_2O} is negative, which indicates that solute-free water is being retained in the body. By convention, negative C_{H_2O} values are expressed as $T^c_{H_2O}$ **(tubular conservation of water).**

Calculation of C_{H_2O} and $T^c_{H_2O}$ can provide important information about the function of portions of the nephron involved in producing dilute and concentrated urine. Whether the kidneys excrete or reabsorb solute-free water depends on the presence of ADH. When ADH is absent or ADH levels are low, solute-free water is excreted. When ADH levels are high, solute-free water is reabsorbed.

The following factors are necessary for the kidneys to excrete a maximal amount of solute-free water (C_{H_2O}):

1. ADH must be absent. Without ADH, the collecting duct does not reabsorb a significant amount of water.
2. The tubular structures that separate solute from water (i.e., dilute the luminal fluid) must function normally. In the absence of ADH, the following nephron segments can dilute the luminal fluid:
   Ascending thin limb of Henle's loop
   Thick ascending limb of Henle's loop
   Distal tubule
   Collecting duct

Because of its high transport rate, the thick ascending limb is quantitatively the most important nephron segment involved in the separation of solute and water.

3. An adequate amount of tubular fluid must be delivered to the aforementioned nephron sites for maximal separation of solute and water. Factors that reduce delivery (e.g., decreased GFR or enhanced proximal tubule reabsorption) impair the kidneys' ability to maximally excrete solute-free water.

Similar requirements also apply to conservation of water by the kidneys ($T^c_{H_2O}$). For the kidneys to conserve water maximally, the following conditions must exist:

1. An adequate amount of tubular fluid must be delivered to the nephron segments that separate solute from water. The important segment in the separation of solute and water is the thick ascending limb of Henle's loop. Delivery of tubular fluid to Henle's loop depends on the GFR and proximal tubule reabsorption.
2. Reabsorption of NaCl by the nephron segments must be normal; again, the most important segment is the thick ascending limb of Henle's loop.
3. A hyperosmotic medullary interstitium must be present. The osmolality of interstitial fluid is maintained via reabsorption of NaCl by Henle's loop

(conditions 1 and 2) and by effective accumulation of urea. Accumulation of urea in turn depends on adequate intake of dietary protein.

4. Maximum levels of ADH must be present and the collecting duct must respond normally to ADH.

CONTROL OF EXTRACELLULAR FLUID VOLUME AND REGULATION OF RENAL NaCl EXCRETION

The major solutes in ECF are the salts of Na^+. Of these, NaCl is the most abundant. Because NaCl is also the major determinant of ECF osmolality, alterations in Na^+ balance are commonly assumed to disturb ECF osmolality. However, under normal circumstances such is not the case because the ADH and thirst systems maintain body fluid osmolality within a very narrow range (see earlier). For example, the addition of NaCl to ECF (without water) increases the $[Na^+]$ and osmolality of this compartment. (ICF osmolality also increases because of osmotic equilibration with ECF.) This increase in osmolality in turn stimulates thirst and release of ADH from the posterior pituitary. The increased ingestion of water in response to thirst, together with the ADH-induced decrease in excretion of water by the kidneys, quickly restores ECF osmolality to normal. However, ECF volume increases in proportion to the amount of water ingested, which in turn depends on the amount of NaCl added to ECF. Thus, in the new steady state, the addition of NaCl to ECF is equivalent to adding an isosmotic solution, and the volume of this compartment increases. Conversely, a decrease in the NaCl content of ECF lowers the volume of this compartment and is equivalent to removing an isosmotic solution.

The kidneys are the major route for the excretion of NaCl from the body. Only about 10% of the Na^+ lost from the body each day does so by nonrenal routes (e.g., in perspiration and feces). As such, the kidneys are critically important in regulating ECF volume. Under normal conditions, the kidneys keep ECF volume constant by adjusting the excretion of NaCl to match the amount ingested in the diet. If ingestion exceeds excretion, ECF volume increases above normal, whereas the opposite occurs if excretion exceeds ingestion.

The typical diet contains approximately 140 mEq/day of Na^+ (8 g of NaCl), and thus daily excretion of Na^+ in urine is also about 140 mEq/day. However, the kidneys can vary the excretion of Na^+ over a wide range. Excretion rates as low as 10 mEq/day can be attained when individuals are placed on a low-salt diet. Conversely, the kidneys can increase their excretion rate to more than 1000 mEq/day when challenged by the ingestion of a high-salt diet. These changes in excretion of Na^+ can occur with only modest changes in ECF volume and the Na^+ content of the body.

The response of the kidneys to abrupt changes in NaCl intake typically takes several hours to several days, depending on the magnitude of the change. During this transition period, intake and excretion of Na^+ are not matched as they are in the steady state.

Thus, the individual experiences either **positive Na⁺ balance** (intake > excretion) or **negative Na⁺ balance** (intake < excretion). However, by the end of the transition period, a new steady state is established, and intake once again equals excretion. Provided that the ADH and thirst systems are intact and normal, alterations in Na⁺ balance change the volume but not the [Na⁺] of the ECF. Changes in ECF volume can be monitored by measuring body weight because 1 L of ECF equals 1 kg of body weight.

This section reviews the physiology of the receptors that monitor ECF volume and explains the various signals that act on the kidneys to regulate excretion of NaCl and thereby ECF volume. In addition, the responses of the various portions of the nephron to these signals are considered.

Concept of Effective Circulating Volume

As described in Chapter 2, the ECF is subdivided into two compartments: blood plasma and interstitial fluid. Plasma volume is a determinant of vascular volume and thus blood pressure and cardiac output. Maintenance of Na⁺ balance, and thus ECF volume, involves a complex system of sensors and effector signals that act primarily on the kidneys to regulate the excretion of NaCl. As can be appreciated from the dependency of vascular volume, blood pressure, and cardiac output on ECF volume, this complex system is designed to ensure adequate tissue perfusion. Because the primary sensors of this system are located in the large vessels

of the vascular system, changes in vascular volume, blood pressure, and cardiac output are the principal factors regulating renal NaCl excretion (see later). In a normal individual, changes in ECF volume result in parallel changes in vascular volume, blood pressure, and cardiac output. Thus, a decrease in ECF volume, a situation termed **volume contraction,** results in reduced vascular volume, blood pressure, and cardiac output. Conversely, an increase in ECF volume, a situation termed **volume expansion,** results in increased vascular volume, blood pressure, and cardiac output. The extent to which these cardiovascular parameters change is dependent on the degree of volume contraction or expansion and the effectiveness of cardiovascular reflex mechanisms (see Chapters 18 and 19). When a person is in negative Na⁺ balance, ECF volume is decreased and renal NaCl excretion is reduced. Conversely, with positive Na⁺ balance there is an increase in ECF volume, which results in enhanced renal NaCl excretion (i.e., **natriuresis**).

However, in some pathological conditions (e.g., congestive heart failure, hepatic cirrhosis), the renal excretion of NaCl does not reflect the ECF volume. In both these situations ECF volume is increased. However, instead of increased renal NaCl excretion, as would be expected, there is a reduction in the renal excretion of NaCl. To explain renal Na⁺ handling in these situations, it is necessary to understand the concept of **effective circulating volume** (ECV). Unlike ECF, ECV is not a measurable and distinct body fluid compartment. ECV refers to the portion of the ECF that is contained within the vascular system and is "effectively" perfusing the tissues (effective blood volume and effective arterial blood volume are other commonly used terms). More specifically, ECV reflects the activity of volume sensors located in the vascular system (see later).

In normal individuals, ECV varies directly with the volume of the ECF and in particular the volume of the vascular system (arterial and venous), arterial blood pressure, and cardiac output. However, as noted, this is not the case in certain pathological conditions. The remaining sections of this chapter examine the relationship between ECF volume and renal NaCl excretion in normal adults, where changes in ECV and ECF volume occur in parallel.

Volume-Sensing Systems

ECF volume (or ECV) is monitored by multiple sensors (Table 34-4). A number of the sensors are located in

---

● AT THE CELLULAR LEVEL

Neuroendocrine cells in the intestine (primarily the jejunum) produce a peptide hormone called **uroguanylin** in response to ingestion of NaCl. A related peptide, **guanylin,** is also produced by the intestine (primarily the colon). These hormones have been shown to cause increased excretion of NaCl and water by the kidneys. Interestingly, both guanylin and uroguanylin are produced by the nephron (guanylin primarily in the proximal tubule and uroguanylin primarily in the collecting duct), thus suggesting a paracrine role for these peptides in the intrarenal regulation of NaCl and water transport. The actions of both uroguanylin and guanylin are mediated via activation of guanylyl cyclase (and also phospholipase A₂). In the proximal tubule, guanylin and uroguanylin decrease the expression of Na⁺,K⁺-ATPase and inhibit the activity of the apical membrane Na⁺-H⁺ antiporter. In the collecting duct these peptides inhibit the K⁺ channel (ROMK) in the apical membrane of the principal cells, which in turn indirectly inhibits reabsorption of Na⁺ by changing the driving force for entry of Na⁺ across the apical membrane. Interestingly, mice lacking the uroguanylin gene have been found to have a blunted natriuretic response to an oral NaCl load. These mice also have increased blood pressure. Thus, uroguanylin (and guanylin) may be important hormones in regulating the renal excretion of NaCl in response to changes in NaCl intake.

● Table 34-4. Volume and Na⁺ Sensors

I. Vascular
A. Low pressure
1. Cardiac atria
2. Pulmonary vasculature
B. High pressure
1. Carotid sinus
2. Aortic arch
3. Juxtaglomerular apparatus of the kidney
II. Central nervous system
III. Hepatic

Patients with congestive heart failure frequently have an increase in ECF volume that is manifested as increased plasma volume and accumulation of interstitial fluid in the lungs **(pulmonary edema)** and peripheral tissues **(generalized edema).** This excess fluid is the result of NaCl and water retention by the kidneys. The kidneys' response (i.e., retention of NaCl and water) is paradoxical because ECF volume is increased. However, this fluid is not in the vascular system but in the interstitial fluid compartment. In addition, blood pressure and cardiac output may be reduced because of poor cardiac performance. Therefore, the sensors located in the vascular system respond as they do in ECF volume contraction and cause retention of NaCl and water by the kidneys. In this situation, ECV, as monitored by volume sensors, is decreased.

Large volumes of fluid accumulate in the peritoneal cavity of patients with advanced hepatic cirrhosis. This fluid, called **ascites,** is a component of ECF and results from retention of NaCl and water by the kidneys. Again, the response of the kidneys in this situation seems paradoxical if only ECF volume is considered. With advanced hepatic cirrhosis, blood pools in the splanchnic circulation (i.e., the damaged liver impedes the drainage of blood from the splanchnic circulation via the portal vein). Thus, volume and pressure are reduced in the portions of the vascular system in which the sensors are found, but venous pressure in the portal system increases, which enhances fluid transudation into the peritoneal cavity. Hence, the kidneys respond as they would during ECF volume contraction: retention of NaCl and water and accumulation of ascites fluid. As with congestive heart failure, ECV in cirrhosis with ascites is decreased.

the vascular system, and they monitor its fullness and pressure. These receptors are typically called volume receptors, or because they respond to pressure-induced stretch of the walls of the receptor (e.g., blood vessels or cardiac atria), they are also referred to as baroreceptors (see earlier). The sensors within the liver and central nervous system (CNS) are less well understood and do not seem to be as important as the vascular sensors in monitoring ECF volume.

Vascular Low-Pressure Volume Sensors

Volume sensors (i.e., baroreceptors) are located within the walls of the cardiac atria, right ventricle, and large pulmonary vessels, and they respond to distention of these structures (see also Chapters 18 and 19). Because the low-pressure side of the circulatory system has high compliance, these sensors respond mainly to "fullness" of the vascular system. These baroreceptors send signals to the brainstem via afferent fibers in the glossopharyngeal and vagus nerves. The activity of these sensors modulates both sympathetic nerve outflow and ADH secretion. For example, a decrease

in filling of the pulmonary vessels and cardiac atria increases sympathetic nerve activity and stimulates secretion of ADH. Conversely, distention of these structures decreases sympathetic nerve activity. In general, 5% to 10% changes in blood volume and pressure are necessary to evoke a response.

The cardiac atria possess an additional mechanism related to control of renal NaCl excretion. The myocytes of the atria synthesize and store a peptide hormone. This hormone, termed **atrial natriuretic peptide** (ANP), is released when the atria are distended, which via mechanisms outlined later in this chapter, reduces blood pressure and increases the excretion of NaCl and water by the kidneys. The ventricles of the heart also produce a natriuretic peptide termed **brain natriuretic peptide** (BNP), so named because it was first isolated from the brain. Like ANP, BNP is released from ventricular myocytes by distention of the ventricles. Its actions are similar to those of ANP.

Vascular High-Pressure Volume Sensors

Baroreceptors are also present in the arterial side of the circulatory system, located in the walls of the aortic arch, carotid sinus, and afferent arterioles of the kidneys. The aortic arch and carotid baroreceptors send input to the brainstem via afferent fibers in the glossopharyngeal and vagus nerves. The response to this input alters sympathetic outflow and ADH secretion. Thus, a decrease in blood pressure increases sympathetic nerve activity and ADH secretion. An increase in pressure tends to reduce sympathetic nerve activity (and activate parasympathetic nerve activity). The sensitivity of the high-pressure baroreceptors is similar to that in the low-pressure side of the vascular system; 5% to 10% changes in pressure are needed to evoke a response.

The **juxtaglomerular apparatus** of the kidneys (see Chapter 32), particularly the afferent arteriole, responds directly to changes in pressure. If perfusion pressure in the afferent arteriole is reduced, renin is released from myocytes. Secretion of renin is suppressed when perfusion pressure is increased. As described later in this chapter, renin determines blood levels of angiotensin II and aldosterone, both of which play an important role in regulating renal NaCl excretion.

Of the two classes of baroreceptors, those on the high-pressure side of the vascular system appear to be more important in influencing sympathetic tone and ADH secretion. For example, patients with congestive heart failure often have increased vascular volume with dilation of the atria and ventricles. This would be expected to decrease sympathetic tone and inhibit ADH secretion via the low-pressure baroreceptors. However, sympathetic tone is often increased and ADH secretion stimulated in these patients (the renin-angiotensin-aldosterone system is also activated). This reflects the activity of the high-pressure baroreceptors in response to reduced blood pressure and cardiac output secondary to the failing heart (i.e., the high-pressure baroreceptors detect a reduced ECV).

▶ **IN THE CLINIC**

Constriction of a renal artery by an atherosclerotic plaque, for example, reduces perfusion pressure to that kidney. This reduced perfusion pressure is sensed by the afferent arteriole of the juxtaglomerular apparatus and results in the secretion of renin. The elevated renin levels increase the production of angiotensin II, which in turn increases systemic blood pressure via its vasoconstrictor effect on arterioles throughout the vascular system. The increased systemic blood pressure is sensed by the juxtaglomerular apparatus of the contralateral kidney (i.e., the kidney without stenosis of its renal artery), and renin secretion from that kidney is suppressed. In addition, the high levels of angiotensin II act to inhibit renin secretion by the contralateral kidney (negative feedback). Treatment of patients with constricted renal arteries includes surgical repair of the stenotic artery, administration of angiotensin II receptor blockers, or administration of an inhibitor of angiotensin-converting enzyme (ACE). The ACE inhibitor blocks the conversion of angiotensin I to angiotensin II.

● **Table 34-5.**

Signals Involved in Control of Renal NaCl and Water Excretion

Renal Sympathetic Nerves (↑ Activity: ↓ NaCl Excretion)
↓ GFR
↑ Renin secretion
↑ Na$^+$ reabsorption along the nephron
Renin-Angiotensin-Aldosterone (↑ Secretion: ↓ NaCl Excretion)
↑ Angiotensin II stimulates reabsorption of Na$^+$ along the nephron
↑ Aldosterone stimulates Na$^+$ reabsorption in the thick ascending limb of Henle's loop, distal tubule, and collecting duct
↑ Angiotensin II stimulates secretion of ADH
Natriuretic Peptides: ANP, BNP, and Urodilatin (↑ Secretion: ↑ NaCl Excretion)
↑ GFR
↓ Renin secretion
↓ Aldosterone secretion (indirect via ↓ in angiotensin II and direct on the adrenal gland)
↓ NaCl and water reabsorption by the collecting duct
↓ ADH secretion and inhibition of ADH action on the distal tubule and collecting duct
ADH (↑ Secretion: ↓ H$_2$O Excretion)
↑ H$_2$O reabsorption by the distal tubule and collecting duct

Hepatic Sensors

Though not as important as the vascular sensors, the liver also contains volume sensors that can modulate renal NaCl excretion. One type of hepatic sensor responds to pressure within the hepatic vasculature and therefore functions in a manner similar to the low- and high-pressure baroreceptors. A second type of sensor also appears to exist in the liver. This sensor responds to the [Na$^+$] of the portal blood entering the liver. Afferent signals from both types of sensors are sent to the same area of the brainstem where afferent fibers from both the low- and high-pressure baroreceptors converge. Increased pressure within the hepatic vasculature or an increase in portal blood [Na$^+$] results in a decrease in efferent sympathetic nerve activity.* As described later, this decreased sympathetic nerve activity leads to an increase in renal NaCl excretion.

Central Nervous System Na$^+$ Sensors

Like the hepatic sensors, the CNS sensors do not appear to be as important as the vascular sensors in monitoring ECF volume and controlling renal NaCl excretion. Nevertheless, alterations in the [Na$^+$] of blood carried to the brain in the carotid arteries or the [Na$^+$] of cerebrospinal fluid (CSF) modulate renal NaCl excretion. For example, if the [Na$^+$] in either carotid artery blood or CSF is increased, there is a decrease in renal sympathetic nerve activity, which in turn leads to an increase in renal NaCl excretion. The hypothalamus appears to be the site where these sensors are located. Angiotensin II and natriuretic peptides are generated in the hypothalamus. These locally generated signals, together with systemically generated

angiotensin II and natriuretic peptides, appear to play a role in modulating the CNS Na$^+$-sensing system.

Of the volume and Na$^+$ sensors just described, those located in the vascular system are better understood. Moreover, their function in health and disease explains quite effectively the regulation of renal NaCl excretion. Therefore, the remainder of this chapter will focus on the vascular volume sensors (i.e., baroreceptors) and their role in regulating renal NaCl excretion.

Volume Sensor Signals

When the vascular volume sensors have detected a change in ECF volume, they send signals to the kidneys, which results in an appropriate adjustment in excretion of NaCl and water. Accordingly, when ECF volume is expanded, renal NaCl and water excretion is increased. Conversely, when ECF volume is contracted, renal NaCl and water excretion is reduced. The signals involved in coupling the volume sensors to the kidneys are both neural and hormonal. These signals are summarized in Table 34-5, as are their effects on renal NaCl and water excretion.

Renal Sympathetic Nerves

As described in Chapter 33, sympathetic nerve fibers innervate the afferent and efferent arterioles of the glomerulus, as well as the cells of the nephron. With ECF volume contraction, activation of the low- and high-pressure vascular baroreceptors results in stimulation of sympathetic nerve activity, including fibers innervating the kidneys. This has the following effects:

1. The afferent and efferent arterioles are constricted (mediated by α-adrenergic receptors). This vasoconstriction (the effect is greater on the afferent arteriole) decreases hydrostatic pressure within the glomerular capillary lumen, which results in a decrease in GFR. With this decrease in GFR, the filtered load of Na$^+$ to the nephrons is reduced.

---

*The hepatic sensors also appear to be involved in the regulation of gastrointestinal NaCl absorption. For example, when the [Na$^+$] of portal vein blood is increased, a reflex reduction in jejunal NaCl absorption is seen.

2. Renin secretion is stimulated by cells of the afferent arterioles (mediated by β-adrenergic receptors). As described later, renin ultimately increases the circulating levels of angiotensin II and aldosterone, both of which stimulate Na^+ reabsorption by the nephron.
3. NaCl reabsorption along the nephron is directly stimulated (mediated by α-adrenergic receptors on cells of the nephron). Because of the large amount of Na^+ reabsorbed by the proximal tubule, the effect of increased sympathetic nerve activity is quantitatively most important for this segment.

As a result of these actions, increased renal sympathetic nerve activity decreases excretion of NaCl, an adaptive response that works to restore ECF volume to normal, a state termed **euvolemia.** With ECF volume expansion, renal sympathetic nerve activity is reduced. This generally reverses the effects just described.

Renin-Angiotensin-Aldosterone System

Cells in the afferent arterioles (juxtaglomerular cells) are the site of synthesis, storage, and release of the proteolytic enzyme renin. Three factors are important in stimulating renin secretion:

1. *Perfusion pressure.* The afferent arteriole behaves as a high-pressure baroreceptor. When perfusion pressure to the kidneys is reduced, renin secretion is stimulated. Conversely, an increase in perfusion pressure inhibits release of renin.
2. *Sympathetic nerve activity.* Activation of the sympathetic nerve fibers that innervate the afferent arterioles increases renin secretion (mediated by β-adrenergic receptors). Renin secretion is decreased as renal sympathetic nerve activity is decreased.
3. *Delivery of NaCl to the macula densa.* Delivery of NaCl to the macula densa regulates the GFR by a process termed **tubuloglomerular feedback** (see Chapter 32). In addition, the macula densa plays a role in

renin secretion. When delivery of NaCl to the macula densa is decreased, renin secretion is enhanced. Conversely, an increase in NaCl delivery inhibits renin secretion. It is likely that macula densa–mediated renin secretion helps maintain systemic arterial pressure under conditions of reduced vascular volume. For example, when vascular volume is reduced, perfusion of body tissues (including the kidneys) decreases. This in turn decreases the GFR and the filtered load of NaCl. The reduced delivery

● AT THE CELLULAR LEVEL

Although many tissues express renin (e.g., brain, heart, adrenal gland), the primary source of circulating renin is the kidneys. Renin is secreted by juxtaglomerular cells located in the afferent arteriole. At the cellular level, secretion of renin is mediated by the fusion of renin-containing granules with the luminal membrane of the cell. This process is stimulated by a decrease in intracellular $[Ca^{++}]$, a response opposite that of most secretory cells, where secretion is stimulated by an increase in intracellular $[Ca^{++}]$. It is also stimulated by an increase in intracellular [cAMP]. Thus, anything that increases intracellular $[Ca^{++}]$ will inhibit renin secretion. This would include stretch of the afferent arteriole (myogenic control of renin secretion), angiotensin II (i.e., feedback inhibition), and endothelin. Conversely, anything that increases intracellular [cAMP] will stimulate renin secretion. This would include norepinephrine acting via β-adrenergic receptors and prostaglandin E_2. Increases in intracellular [cGMP] have been shown to stimulate renin secretion in some situations and to inhibit secretion in others. Importantly, two substances that increase intracellular [cGMP] are ANP and nitric oxide. Both inhibit renin secretion.

Control of renin secretion by the macula densa is complex and appears to involve several paracrine factors. For example, when delivery of NaCl to the macula densa is increased, ATP (and perhaps also adenosine) is released across the basolateral membrane. Binding of ATP to receptors on extraglomerular mesangial cells results in an increase in intracellular $[Ca^{++}]$. Because mesangial cells are coupled to juxtaglomerular cells by gap junctions, the intracellular $[Ca^{++}]$ in juxtaglomerular cells also increases, and renin secretion is suppressed. This increase in the intracellular $[Ca^{++}]$ of mesangial cells also increases the intracellular $[Ca^{++}]$ of vascular smooth muscle cells of the afferent arteriole (again via gap junctions), thereby resulting in constriction and thus a decrease in GFR (see also Chapter 32). When delivery of NaCl to the macula densa is decreased, release of ATP and adenosine is suppressed, and the intracellular $[Ca^{++}]$ of mesangial, juxtaglomerular, and vascular smooth muscle cells decreases. This stimulates secretion of renin by the juxtaglomerular cells, and the afferent arteriole dilates. In addition, with decreased delivery of NaCl, macula densa cells release prostaglandin E_2, which also stimulates renin secretion and causes afferent arteriole dilation.

● AT THE CELLULAR LEVEL

Recently, a new "renal hormone" was discovered: a flavin adenine dinucleotide–dependent amine oxidase named **renalase.** Renalase is similar in structure to monoamine oxidase and metabolizes catecholamines (e.g., dopamine, epinephrine, and norepinephrine). Other tissues also express renalase (e.g., skeletal muscle, heart, small intestine), but the kidneys secrete the enzyme into the circulation. Because individuals with chronic renal failure have very low levels of renalase in their plasma, the kidney is probably the primary source of the circulating enzyme. In experimental animals, infusion of renalase decreases blood pressure and heart contractility. Although the precise role of renalase in regulation of cardiovascular function and blood pressure is not known, it may be important in modulating the effect of the sympathetic nervous system, especially the effects of sympathetic nerves on the kidney.

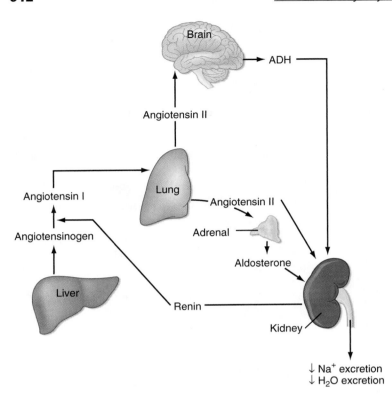

of NaCl to the macula densa then stimulates secretion of renin, which acts through angiotensin II (a potent vasoconstrictor) to increase blood pressure and thereby maintain tissue perfusion.

Figure 34-6 summarizes the essential components of the renin-angiotensin-aldosterone system. Renin alone does not have a physiological function; it functions solely as a proteolytic enzyme. Its substrate is a circulating protein, **angiotensinogen,** which is produced by the liver. Angiotensinogen is cleaved by renin to yield a 10–amino acid peptide, **angiotensin I.** Angiotensin I also has no known physiological function, and it is further cleaved to an eight–amino acid peptide, **angiotensin II,** by a converting enzyme **(ACE)** found on the surface of vascular endothelial cells. (Pulmonary and renal endothelial cells are important sites for the conversion of angiotensin I to angiotensin II.) ACE also degrades bradykinin, a potent vasodilator.* Angiotensin II has several important physiological functions, including

1. Stimulation of aldosterone secretion by the adrenal cortex.
2. Arteriolar vasoconstriction, which increases blood pressure.
3. Stimulation of ADH secretion and thirst.
4. Enhancement of NaCl reabsorption by the proximal tubule, thick ascending limb of Henle's loop, the distal tubule, and the collecting duct. Of these seg-

ments the effect on the proximal tubule is quantitatively the largest.

Angiotensin II is an important secretagogue for **aldosterone.** An increase in plasma [K$^+$] is the other important stimulus for aldosterone secretion (see Chapter 35). Aldosterone is a steroid hormone produced by the glomerulosa cells of the adrenal cortex. It acts in a number of ways on the kidneys (see also Chapters 35 and 36). With regard to the regulation of ECF volume, aldosterone reduces excretion of NaCl by stimulating its reabsorption by the thick ascending limb of the loop of Henle, distal tubule, and collecting duct. The effect of aldosterone on renal NaCl excretion depends mainly on its ability to stimulate reabsorption of Na$^+$ in the distal tubule, as well as the collecting duct. (*Note:* These segments are often referred to collectively as the aldosterone-sensitive distal nephron).

Aldosterone has many cellular actions in responsive cells (see also Chapter 33). Importantly, it increases the abundance of the apical membrane Na$^+$-Cl$^-$ symporter in cells of the early portion of the distal tubule and the abundance of the Na$^+$ channel (ENaC) in the apical membrane of principal cells in the late portion of the distal tubule and collecting duct (the activity of Na$^+$ channels is also increased). These actions of aldosterone increase entry of Na$^+$ into cells across the apical membrane. Extrusion of Na$^+$ from cells across the basolateral membrane occurs by Na$^+$,K$^+$-ATPase, the abundance of which is also increased by aldosterone. Thus, aldosterone increases reabsorption of Na$^+$ from tubular fluid by distal nephron segments, whereas reduced levels of aldosterone decrease the amount of Na$^+$ reabsorbed by these segments.

---

*Endothelial cells express another angiotensin-converting enzyme (ACE2). ACE2 cleaves a single amino acid off angiotensin I. More importantly, ACE2 degrades angiotensin II but not bradykinin. Thus, ACE2 may serve to counterbalance the effect of ACE, which generates the potent vasoconstrictor angiotensin II and degrades the vasodilator bradykinin.

AT THE CELLULAR LEVEL

The response to aldosterone has two phases. In the initial phase, which occurs within minutes, reabsorption of Na^+ in the aldosterone-sensitive distal nephron increases without changes in transporter abundance. This phase reflects the activation of existing transporters, as well as inhibition of the cell's normal process of removal and recycling of membrane transport proteins (see Chapter 1). By slowing the retrieval process, more transporters are retained in the membrane, thereby increasing entry of Na^+ into the cell across the apical membrane (see Chapter 33 for details). In the second phase, which occurs with a lag period of several hours, there is increased synthesis of key Na^+ transport proteins, including the Na^+-Cl^- symporter (NCC/TSC) in the early distal tubule, the α subunit of the Na^+ channel (ENaC)* in the late distal tubule and collecting duct, and the α subunit of Na^+,K^+-ATPase in these same segments.

*ENaC is composed of three subunits (α, β, and γ). The α subunit is rate limiting for assembly. Thus, it is the abundance of this subunit that determines the amount of functional ENaC in the plasma membrane.

IN THE CLINIC

Diseases of the adrenal cortex can alter aldosterone levels and thereby impair the ability of the kidneys to maintain Na^+ balance and euvolemia. With decreased secretion of aldosterone **(hypoaldosteronism)**, reabsorption of Na^+, mainly by the aldosterone-sensitive distal nephron, is reduced, and NaCl is lost in urine. Because urinary NaCl loss can exceed the amount of NaCl ingested in the diet, negative Na^+ balance ensues, and ECF volume decreases. In response to the ECF volume contraction, sympathetic tone is increased, and levels of renin, angiotensin II, and ADH are elevated. With increased aldosterone secretion **(hyperaldosteronism)**, the effects are the opposite: Na^+ reabsorption by the aldosterone-sensitive distal nephron is enhanced, and excretion of NaCl is reduced. Consequently, ECF volume is increased, sympathetic tone is decreased, and levels of renin, angiotensin II, and ADH are decreased. As described later, ANP and BNP levels are also elevated in this setting.

As noted, aldosterone also enhances reabsorption of Na^+ by cells of the thick ascending limb of the loop of Henle, though to a lesser degree than in the aldosterone-sensitive distal nephron. This action probably reflects increased entry of Na^+ into the cell across the apical membrane (most likely by the apical membrane $1Na^+$-$1K^+$-$2Cl^-$ symporter) and increased extrusion from the cell by the basolateral membrane Na^+,K^+-ATPase.

As summarized in Table 34-5, activation of the renin-angiotensin-aldosterone system, as occurs with ECF volume depletion, decreases the excretion of NaCl by the kidneys. This system is suppressed with ECF volume expansion, and renal NaCl excretion is therefore enhanced.

Natriuretic Peptides

The body produces a number of substances that act on the kidneys to increase Na^+ excretion.* Of these, natriuretic peptides produced by the heart and kidneys are best understood and will be the focus of the following discussion.

The heart produces two natriuretic peptides. Atrial myocytes primarily produce and store the peptide hormone ANP, and ventricular myocytes primarily produce and store BNP. Both peptides are secreted when the heart dilates (i.e., during volume expansion and with heart failure), and they act to relax vascular smooth muscle and promote excretion of NaCl and water by the kidneys. The kidneys also produce a related natriuretic peptide termed urodilatin. Its actions are limited to promoting NaCl excretion by the kidneys. In general, the actions of these natriuretic peptides, as they relate to renal NaCl and water excretion, antagonize those of the renin-angiotensin-aldosterone system. These actions include

1. Vasodilation of the afferent and vasoconstriction of the efferent arterioles of the glomerulus. This increases GFR and the filtered load of Na^+.
2. Inhibition of renin secretion by the afferent arterioles.
3. Inhibition of aldosterone secretion by the glomerulosa cells of the adrenal cortex. This occurs via two mechanisms: (a) inhibition of renin secretion by the juxtaglomerular cells and consequently a reduction in angiotensin II–induced aldosterone secretion and (b) direct inhibition of aldosterone secretion by the glomerulosa cells of the adrenal cortex.
4. Inhibition of NaCl reabsorption by the collecting duct, which is also caused in part by reduced levels of aldosterone. However, the natriuretic peptides also act directly on the collecting duct cells. Through the second messenger cGMP, natriuretic peptides inhibit cation channels in the apical membrane and thereby decrease reabsorption of Na^+. This effect occurs predominantly in the medullary portion of the collecting duct.
5. Inhibition of ADH secretion by the posterior pituitary and ADH action on the collecting duct. These effects decrease water reabsorption by the collecting duct and thus increase excretion of water in urine.

The foregoing effects of natriuretic peptides increase the excretion of NaCl and water by the kidneys. Hypothetically, a reduction in circulating levels of these peptides would be expected to decrease NaCl and

*Uroguanylin and adrenomedullin are two examples of these substances. As noted earlier, uroguanylin increases renal NaCl excretion and may serve to regulate the renal excretion of ingested NaCl. Adrenomedullin is produced by many tissues, including the heart, kidneys, and the adrenal medulla (from whence its name is derived). It is secreted in response to a number of factors (e.g., cytokines, angiotensin II, endothelin, and increased shear stress on endothelial cells). Though structurally distinct from ANP and BNP, its actions are similar in that it reduces blood pressure, increases GFR, suppresses angiotensin II–induced secretion of aldosterone, and causes increased NaCl excretion.

water excretion, but convincing evidence for this effect has not been reported.

Antidiuretic Hormone

As discussed previously, a decreased ECF volume stimulates secretion of ADH by the posterior pituitary. The elevated levels of ADH decrease water excretion by the kidneys, which serves to reestablish euvolemia.

Control of NaCl Excretion during Euvolemia

Maintenance of Na^+ balance and therefore euvolemia requires precise matching of the amount of NaCl ingested with the amount excreted from the body. As already noted, the kidneys are the major route for excretion of NaCl. Accordingly, in a euvolemic individual we can equate daily urine NaCl excretion with daily NaCl intake.

The amount of NaCl excreted by the kidneys can vary widely. Under conditions of salt restriction (i.e., low-NaCl diet), virtually no Na^+ appears in the urine. Conversely, in individuals who ingest large quantities of NaCl, renal Na^+ excretion can exceed 1000 mEq/day. The kidneys may require several days to respond maximally to variations in dietary NaCl intake. During the transition period, excretion does not match intake, and the individual is in either positive (intake > excretion) or negative (intake < excretion) Na^+ balance. When Na^+ balance is altered during these transition periods, ECF volume changes in parallel. Water excretion, regulated via the ADH system, is also adjusted to keep plasma osmolality constant, and an isosmotic change in ECF volume results. Thus, with positive Na^+ balance, ECF volume expands (detected as an acute increase in body weight), whereas with negative Na^+ balance, ECF volume contracts (detected as an acute decrease in body weight). Ultimately, renal excretion reaches a new steady state and NaCl excretion once again is matched to intake. The time course for adjustment of renal NaCl excretion varies (hours to days) and depends on the magnitude of the change in NaCl intake. Adaptation to large changes in NaCl intake requires a longer time than adaptation to small changes in intake.

The general features of Na^+ handling along the nephron must be understood to comprehend how renal Na^+ excretion is regulated. (See Chapter 33 for the cellular mechanisms of Na^+ transport along the nephron.) Most (67%) of the filtered load of Na^+ is reabsorbed by the proximal tubule. An additional 25% is reabsorbed by the thick ascending limb of the loop of Henle and the remainder by the distal tubule and collecting duct (Fig. 34-7).

In a normal adult, the filtered load of Na^+ is approximately 25,000 mEq/day.

● **Equation 34-5**

Filtered load of Na^+ = (GFR) × (Plasma [Na^+])
= (180 L/day) × (140 mEq/L)
= 25,200 mEq/day

With a typical diet, less than 1% of this filtered load is excreted in urine (approximately 140 mEq/day).* Because of the large filtered load of Na^+, small changes in Na^+ reabsorption by the nephron can profoundly affect Na^+ balance and, thus, ECF volume. For example, an increase in Na^+ excretion from 1% to 3% of the filtered load represents an additional loss of approximately 500 mEq/day of Na^+. Because [Na^+] in ECF is 140 mEq/L, such an Na^+ loss would decrease ECF volume by more than 3 L (i.e., water excretion would parallel the loss of Na^+ to maintain body fluid osmolality constant: 500 mEq/day/140 mEq/L = 3.6 L/day of fluid loss). Such fluid loss in a 70-kg individual would represent a 26% decrease in ECF volume.

In euvolemic subjects, the nephron segments distal to the loop of Henle (distal tubule and collecting duct) are the main nephron segment where Na^+ reabsorption is adjusted to maintain excretion at a level appropriate for dietary intake. However, this does not mean that the other portions of the nephron are not involved in this process. Because the reabsorptive capacity of the distal tubule and collecting duct is limited, these other portions of the nephron (i.e., proximal tubule and loop of Henle) must reabsorb the bulk of the filtered load of Na^+. Thus, during euvolemia, Na^+ handling by the nephron can be explained by two general processes:

1. Na^+ reabsorption by the proximal tubule and loop of Henle is regulated so that a relatively constant portion of the filtered load of Na^+ is delivered to the distal tubule. The combined action of the proximal tubule and loop of Henle reabsorbs approximately 92% of the filtered load of Na^+, and thus 8% of the filtered load is delivered to the distal tubule.
2. Reabsorption of this remaining portion of the filtered load of Na^+ by the distal tubule and collecting duct is regulated so that the amount of Na^+ excreted in urine matches the amount ingested in the diet. Thus, these later nephron segments make final adjustments in Na^+ excretion to maintain the euvolemic state.

Mechanisms for Maintaining Constant Delivery of NaCl to the Distal Tubule

A number of mechanisms maintain a constant delivery of Na^+ to the beginning of the distal tubule. These processes are autoregulation of the GFR (and thus the filtered load of Na^+), glomerulotubular balance, and dependency of Na^+ reabsorption by the loop of Henle on load.

Autoregulation of the GFR (see Chapter 32) allows maintenance of a relatively constant filtration rate over a wide range of perfusion pressures. Because the filtration rate is constant, the filtered load of Na^+ is also constant.

Despite the autoregulatory control of GFR, small variations occur. If these changes are not compensated for by an appropriate adjustment in Na^+ reabsorption by the nephron, excretion of Na^+ would

---

*The percentage of the filtered load excreted in urine is termed **fractional excretion.** In this example, the fractional excretion of Na^+ is 140 mEq/day ÷ 25,200 mEq/day = 0.005, or 0.5%.

change markedly. Fortunately, Na⁺ reabsorption in the euvolemic state, especially by the proximal tubule, changes in parallel with changes in GFR. This phenomenon is termed **glomerulotubular balance.** Thus, if the GFR increases, the amount of Na⁺ reabsorbed by the proximal tubule also increases. The opposite occurs if the GFR decreases (see Chapter 33 for a more detailed description of glomerulotubular balance).

The final mechanism that helps maintain constant delivery of Na⁺ to the distal tubule involves the ability of the loop of Henle to increase its reabsorptive rate in response to increased delivery of Na⁺.

Regulation of NaCl Reabsorption by the Distal Tubule and Collecting Duct

When delivery of Na⁺ is constant, small adjustments in Na⁺ reabsorption by the distal tubule and, to a lesser degree, by the collecting duct are sufficient to balance excretion with intake. As already noted, as little as a 2% change in fractional Na⁺ excretion produces more than a 3-L change in ECF volume. Aldosterone is the primary regulator of Na⁺ reabsorption by the distal tubule and collecting duct and, thus, the primary regulator of Na⁺ excretion under this condition. When aldosterone levels are elevated, reabsorption of Na⁺ by these segments is increased (excretion decreased). When aldosterone levels are decreased, reabsorption of Na⁺ is decreased (excretion increased).

In addition to aldosterone, a number of other factors, including natriuretic peptides, prostaglandins, uroguanylin, adrenomedullin, and sympathetic nerves, alter reabsorption of Na⁺ by the distal tubule and collecting duct. However, the relative effects of these other factors on regulation of Na⁺ reabsorption by these segments during euvolemia are unclear.

As long as variations in the dietary intake of NaCl are minor, the mechanisms previously described can regulate renal Na⁺ excretion appropriately and thereby maintain euvolemia. However, these mechanisms cannot effectively handle significant changes in NaCl intake. When NaCl intake changes significantly, ECF volume expansion or ECF volume contraction occurs. In such cases, additional factors act on the kidneys to adjust Na⁺ excretion and thereby reestablish the euvolemic state.

Control of NaCl Excretion with Volume Expansion

During ECF volume expansion, the high-pressure and low-pressure vascular volume sensors send signals to the kidneys that result in increased excretion of NaCl and water. The signals acting on the kidneys include

1. Decreased activity of the renal sympathetic nerves
2. Release of ANP and BNP from the heart and urodilatin from the kidneys
3. Inhibition of ADH secretion from the posterior pituitary and decreased ADH action on the collecting duct
4. Decreased renin secretion and thus decreased production of angiotensin II

5. Decreased aldosterone secretion, which is caused by reduced angiotensin II levels, and elevated natriuretic peptide levels

The integrated response of the nephron to these signals is illustrated in Figure 34-8. Three general responses to ECF volume expansion occur (the numbers correlate with those encircled in Fig. 34-8):

1. *The GFR increases.* The GFR increases mainly as a result of the decrease in sympathetic nerve activity. Sympathetic fibers innervate the afferent and efferent arterioles of the glomerulus and control their diameter. Decreased sympathetic nerve activity leads to arteriolar dilation. Because the effect appears to be greater on the afferent arterioles, hydrostatic pressure within the glomerular capillary is increased, thereby increasing the GFR. Because renal plasma flow increases to a greater degree than the GFR does, the filtration fraction decreases. Natriuretic peptides also increase GFR by dilating the afferent and constricting the efferent arterioles. Thus, the increased natriuretic peptide levels that occur during ECF volume expansion contribute to this response. With the increase in GFR, the filtered load of Na⁺ increases.

2. *Reabsorption of Na⁺ decreases in the proximal tubule and loop of Henle.* Several mechanisms may act to reduce Na⁺ reabsorption by the proximal tubule, but the precise role of each of these mechanisms remains controversial. Because activation of the sympathetic nerve fibers that innervate this nephron segment stimulates reabsorption of Na⁺, the decreased sympathetic nerve activity that results from ECF volume expansion decreases Na⁺

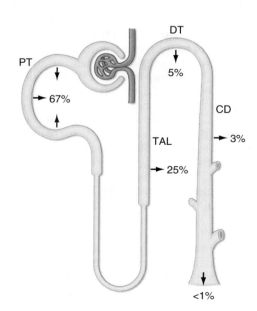

● **Figure 34-7.** Segmental Na⁺ reabsorption. The percentage of the filtered load of Na⁺ reabsorbed by each nephron segment is indicated. CD, cortical collecting duct; DT, distal tubule; PT, proximal tubule; TAL, thick ascending limb.

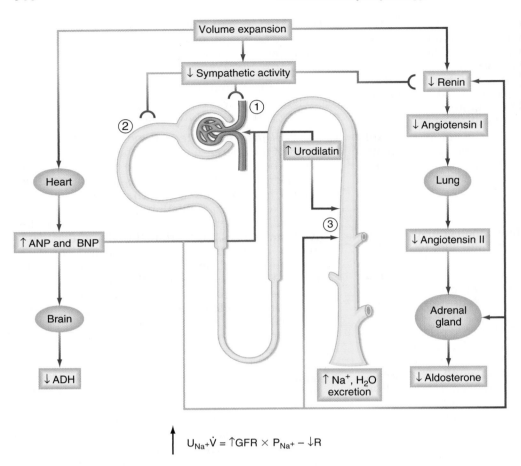

● **Figure 34-8.** Integrated response to ECF volume expansion. Numbers refer to the description of the response in the text. P_{Na^+}, plasma [Na^+]; R, tubular reabsorption of Na^+; $U_{Na^+}V$, Na^+ excretion rate.

$$U_{Na^+}\dot{V} = \uparrow GFR \times P_{Na^+} - \downarrow R$$

reabsorption. In addition, angiotensin II directly stimulates reabsorption of Na^+ by the proximal tubule. Because angiotensin II levels are also reduced under this condition, proximal tubule Na^+ reabsorption decreases as a result. The increased hydrostatic pressure within the glomerular capillaries also tends to increase the hydrostatic pressure within the peritubular capillaries. In addition, the decrease in filtration fraction reduces peritubular oncotic pressure. These alterations in capillary Starling forces reduce the absorption of solute (e.g., NaCl) and water from the lateral intercellular space and thus reduce tubular reabsorption (see Chapter 33 for a complete description of this mechanism). Both the increase in the filtered load and the decrease in NaCl reabsorption by the proximal tubule result in the delivery of more NaCl to the loop of Henle. Because activation of sympathetic nerves and aldosterone stimulates reabsorption of NaCl by the loop of Henle, the reduced nerve activity and low aldosterone levels that occur with ECF volume expansion serve to reduce NaCl reabsorption by this nephron segment. Thus, the fraction of the filtered load delivered to the distal tubule is increased.

3. _Na$^+$ reabsorption decreases in the distal tubule and collecting duct._ As noted, the amount of Na^+ delivered to the distal tubule exceeds that observed in the euvolemic state (i.e., the amount of Na^+ deliv-

ered to the distal tubule varies in proportion to the degree of ECF volume expansion). This increased load of Na^+ overwhelms the reabsorptive capacity of the distal tubule and the collecting duct, and this capacity is even further impaired by the actions of natriuretic peptides and by the decrease in circulating levels of aldosterone.

The final component in the response to ECF volume expansion is the excretion of water. As Na^+ excretion increases, plasma osmolality begins to fall. This decreases the secretion of ADH. ADH secretion is also decreased in response to the elevated levels of natriuretic peptides. In addition, these natriuretic peptides inhibit the action of ADH on the collecting duct. Together, these effects decrease reabsorption of water by the collecting duct and thereby increase excretion of water by the kidneys. Thus, excretion of Na^+ and water occurs in concert; euvolemia is restored, and body fluid osmolality remains constant. The time course of this response (hours to days) depends on the magnitude of the ECF volume expansion. Hence, if the degree of ECF volume expansion is small, the mechanisms just described generally restore euvolemia within 24 hours. However, with large degrees of ECF volume expansion, the response may take several days.

In brief, the renal response to ECF volume expansion involves the integrated action of all parts of the nephron: (1) the filtered load of Na^+ is increased, (2) reabsorption in the proximal tubule and loop of Henle is reduced (GFR is increased, whereas proximal reabsorption is decreased; thus, glomerulotubular balance does not occur under this condition), and (3) delivery of Na^+ to the distal tubule is increased. This increased delivery, along with the inhibition of reabsorption in the distal tubule and collecting duct, results in the excretion of a larger fraction of the filtered load of Na^+ and thus restores euvolemia.

Control of NaCl Excretion with Volume Contraction

During ECF volume contraction, the high-pressure and low-pressure vascular volume sensors send signals to the kidneys that reduce the excretion of NaCl and water. The signals that act on the kidneys include

1. Increased renal sympathetic nerve activity
2. Increased secretion of renin, which results in elevated angiotensin II levels and thus increased secretion of aldosterone by the adrenal cortex
3. Inhibition of ANP and BNP secretion by the heart and urodilatin production by the kidneys
4. Stimulation of ADH secretion by the posterior pituitary

The integrated response of the nephron to these signals is illustrated in Figure 34-9. The general response is as follows (the numbers correlate with those encircled in Fig. 34-9):

1. _The GFR decreases._ Afferent and efferent arteriolar constriction occurs as a result of increased renal sympathetic nerve activity. The effect appears to be greater on the afferent than on the efferent arteriole. This causes hydrostatic pressure in the glomerular capillary to fall and thereby decreases the GFR. Because renal plasma flow decreases more than the GFR, the filtration fraction increases. The decrease in GFR reduces the filtered load of Na^+.

2. Na^+ _reabsorption by the proximal tubule and loop of Henle is increased._ Several mechanisms augment reabsorption of Na^+ in the proximal tubule. For example, increased sympathetic nerve activity and angiotensin II levels directly stimulate Na^+ reabsorption. The decreased hydrostatic pressure within the glomerular capillaries also leads to a decrease in the hydrostatic pressure within the peritubular capillaries. In addition, the increased filtration fraction results in an increase in peritubular oncotic pressure. These alterations in capillary Starling forces facilitate the movement of fluid from the lateral intercellular space into the capillary and thereby stimulate the reabsorption of solute (e.g., NaCl) and water by the proximal tubule (see Chapter 33 for a complete description of this mechanism). The reduced filtered load and enhanced proximal tubule reabsorption decrease the delivery of Na^+ to the loop of Henle. Increased sympathetic nerve activity, as well as elevated levels of angiotensin II

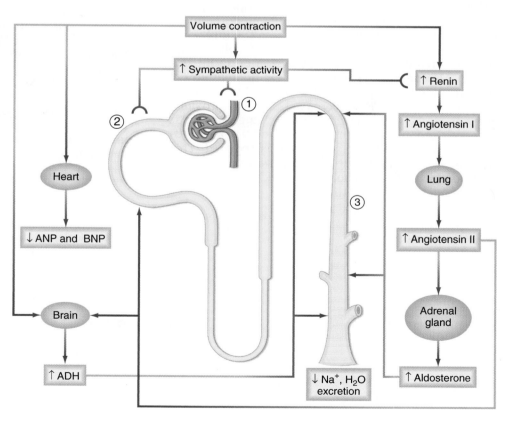

● **Figure 34-9.** Integrated response to ECF volume contraction. Numbers refer to the description of the response in the text. P_{Na^+}, plasma $[Na^+]$; R, tubular reabsorption of Na^+; $U_{Na^+}\dot{V}$; Na^+ excretion rate.

$$U_{Na^+}\dot{V} = \downarrow GFR \times P_{Na^+} - \uparrow R$$

and aldosterone, stimulate reabsorption of Na^+ by the thick ascending limb. Because sympathetic nerve activity is increased and angiotensin II and aldosterone levels are elevated during ECF volume contraction, increased Na^+ reabsorption by this segment is expected. Thus, less Na^+ is delivered to the distal tubule.

3. *Na^+ reabsorption by the distal tubule and collecting duct is enhanced.* The small amount of Na^+ that is delivered to the distal tubule is almost completely reabsorbed because transport in this segment and the collecting duct is enhanced. This stimulation of Na^+ reabsorption by the distal tubule and collecting duct is mainly induced by increased aldosterone levels. In addition, plasma levels of natriuretic peptides, which inhibit reabsorption in the collecting duct, are reduced.

Finally, water reabsorption by the late portion of the distal tubule and the collecting duct is enhanced by ADH, levels of which are elevated through activation of the low- and high-pressure vascular volume sensors, as well as by the elevated levels of angiotensin II. As a result, water excretion is reduced. Because both water and Na^+ are retained by the kidneys in equal proportions, euvolemia is reestablished, and body fluid osmolality remains constant. The time course of this expansion in ECF (hours to days) and the degree to which euvolemia is attained depend on the magnitude of the ECF volume contraction, as well as the dietary intake of Na^+. Thus, the kidneys reduce excretion of Na^+, and euvolemia can be restored more quickly if additional NaCl is ingested in the diet.

In brief, the nephron's response to ECF volume contraction involves the integrated action of all its segments: (1) the filtered load of Na^+ is decreased, (2) reabsorption by the proximal tubule and loop of Henle is enhanced (the GFR is decreased, whereas proximal reabsorption is increased; thus, glomerulotubular balance does not occur under this condition), and (3) delivery of Na^+ to the distal tubule is reduced. This decreased delivery, together with enhanced Na^+ reabsorption by the distal tubule and collecting duct, virtually eliminates Na^+ from the urine.

■ KEY CONCEPTS

1. Regulation of body fluid osmolality (i.e., steady-state balance) requires that the amount of water added to the body exactly match the amount lost from the body. Water is lost from the body by several routes (e.g., during respiration, with sweating, and in feces). The kidneys are the only regulated route of water excretion. Excretion of water by the kidneys is regulated by ADH secreted from the posterior pituitary. When ADH levels are high, the kidneys excrete a small volume of hyperosmotic urine. When ADH levels are low, a large volume of hypoosmotic urine is excreted.

2. Disorders of water balance alter body fluid osmolality. Because Na^+ and its anions are the major determinant of ECF osmolality, disorders in water balance are manifested as changes in ECF $[Na^+]$. Positive water balance (intake > excretion) results in a decrease in body fluid osmolality and hyponatremia. Negative water balance (intake < excretion) results in an increase in body fluid osmolality and hypernatremia.

3. ECF volume is determined by the amount of Na^+ in this compartment. To maintain constant ECF volume (i.e., euvolemia), Na^+ excretion must match Na^+ intake. The kidneys are the major route for regulating excretion of Na^+ from the body. Volume sensors located primarily in the vascular system monitor volume and pressure. When ECF volume expansion occurs, neural and hormonal signals are sent to the kidneys to increase the excretion of NaCl and water and thereby restore euvolemia. When ECF volume contraction occurs, neural and hormonal signals are sent to the kidneys to decrease NaCl and water excretion and thereby restore euvolemia. The sympathetic nervous system, the renin-angiotensin-aldosterone system, and natriuretic peptides are important components of the system needed to maintain steady-state Na^+ balance.

CHAPTER 35

Potassium, Calcium, and Phosphate Homeostasis

K⁺ HOMEOSTASIS

Potassium (K⁺) is one of the most abundant cations in the body, and it is critical for many cell functions, including regulation of cell volume, regulation of intracellular pH, synthesis of DNA and protein, growth, enzyme function, resting membrane potential, and cardiac and neuromuscular activity. Despite wide fluctuations in dietary K⁺ intake, [K⁺] in cells and extracellular fluid (ECF) remains remarkably constant. Two sets of regulatory mechanisms safeguard K⁺ homeostasis. First, several mechanisms regulate [K⁺] in the ECF. Second, other mechanisms maintain the amount of K⁺ in the body constant by adjusting renal K⁺ excretion to match dietary K⁺ intake. It is the kidneys that regulate excretion of K⁺.

Total body [K⁺] is 50 mEq/kg of body weight, or 3500 mEq for a 70-kg individual. Ninety-eight percent of the K⁺ in the body is located within cells, where the average [K⁺] is 150 mEq/L. High intracellular [K⁺] is required for many cell functions, including cell growth and division and volume regulation. Only 2% of total body [K⁺] is located in the ECF, where its normal concentration is approximately 4 mEq/L. A [K⁺] in ECF that exceeds 5.0 mEq/L constitutes **hyperkalemia.** Conversely, a [K⁺] in ECF of less than 3.5 mEq/L constitutes **hypokalemia.**

The large concentration difference of K⁺ across cell membranes (approximately 146 mEq/L) is maintained by the operation of Na⁺,K⁺-ATPase. This [K⁺] gradient is important in maintaining the potential difference across cell membranes. Thus, K⁺ is critical for the excitability of nerve and muscle cells, as well as for the contractility of cardiac, skeletal, and smooth muscle cells (Fig. 35-1).

After a meal, the K⁺ absorbed by the gastrointestinal tract enters the ECF within minutes (see Fig. 35-3). If the K⁺ ingested during a normal meal (≈33 mEq) were to remain in the ECF compartment (14 L), plasma [K⁺] would increase by a potentially lethal 2.4 mEq/L (33 mEq added to 14 L of ECF):

● **Equation 35-1**

$$\frac{33\,mEq/L}{14\,L} = 2.4\,mEq/L$$

This rise in plasma [K⁺] is prevented by the rapid (minutes) uptake of K⁺ into cells. Because excretion of K⁺ by the kidneys after a meal is relatively slow (hours), uptake of K⁺ by cells is essential to prevent life-threatening hyperkalemia. Maintaining total body [K⁺] constant requires that all the K⁺ absorbed by the gastrointestinal tract eventually be excreted by the kidneys. This process requires about 6 hours.

► IN THE CLINIC

Hypokalemia is one of the most common electrolyte disorders in clinical practice and can be observed in as many as 20% of hospitalized patients. The most frequent causes of hypokalemia include administration of diuretic drugs, surreptitious vomiting (e.g., bulimia), and severe diarrhea. Gitelman's syndrome (a genetic defect in the Na⁺-Cl⁻ symporter in the apical membrane of distal tubule cells) also causes hypokalemia (see Chapter 33, Table 33-3). Hyperkalemia is also a common electrolyte disorder and is seen in 1% to 10% of hospitalized patients. Hyperkalemia often occurs in patients with renal failure, in patients taking drugs, including angiotensin-converting enzyme (ACE) inhibitors and K⁺-sparing diuretics, in patients with hyperglycemia (i.e., high blood sugar), and in the elderly. **Pseudohyperkalemia,** a falsely high plasma [K⁺], is caused by traumatic lysis of red blood cells during blood drawing. Red blood cells, like all cells, contain K⁺, and lysis of red blood cells releases K⁺ into plasma, thereby artificially elevating plasma [K⁺].

► IN THE CLINIC

Cardiac arrhythmias are produced by both hypokalemia and hyperkalemia. The electrocardiogram (ECG; see Fig. 35-2 and Chapter 16) monitors the electrical activity of the heart and is a fast and easy way to determine whether changes in plasma [K⁺] influence the heart and other excitable cells. In contrast, measurement of plasma [K⁺] by the clinical laboratory requires a blood sample, and values are often not immediately available. The first sign of hyperkalemia is the appearance of tall, thin T waves on the ECG. Further increases in plasma [K⁺] prolong the PR interval, depress the ST segment, and lengthen the QRS interval of the ECG. Finally, as plasma [K⁺] approaches 10 mEq/L, the P wave disappears, the QRS interval broadens, the ECG appears as a sine wave, and the ventricles fibrillate (i.e., manifest rapid, uncoordinated contractions of muscle fibers). Hypokalemia prolongs the QT interval, inverts the T wave, and lowers the ST segment of the ECG.

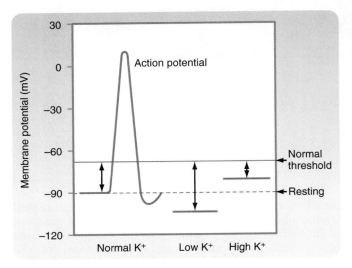

● Figure 35-1. The effects of variations in plasma [K⁺] on the resting membrane potential of skeletal muscle. Hyperkalemia causes the membrane potential to become less negative, which decreases excitability by inactivating the fast Na⁺ channels responsible for the depolarizing phase of the action potential. Hypokalemia hyperpolarizes the membrane potential and thereby reduces excitability.

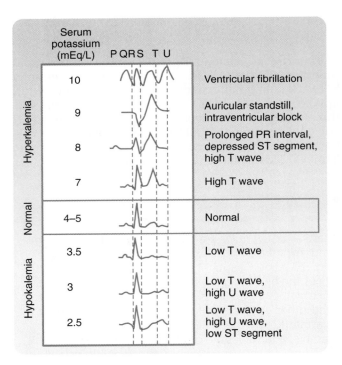

● Figure 35-2. Electrocardiographs from individuals with varying plasma [K⁺]. Hyperkalemia increases the height of the T wave, and hypokalemia inverts the T wave. See text for details. (Modified from Barker L et al: Principles of Ambulatory Medicine, 5th ed. Baltimore, Williams & Wilkins, 1999.)

REGULATION OF PLASMA [K⁺]

As illustrated in Figure 35-3 and Table 35-1, several hormones, including epinephrine, insulin, and aldosterone, increase uptake of K⁺ into skeletal muscle, liver, bone, and red blood cells by stimulating Na⁺,K⁺-ATPase, the 1Na⁺-1K⁺-2Cl⁻ symporter, and the Na⁺-Cl⁻ symporter in these cells. Acute stimulation of K⁺ uptake (i.e., within minutes) is mediated by an increased turnover rate of existing Na⁺,K⁺-ATPase, 1Na⁺-1K⁺-2Cl⁻, and Na⁺-Cl⁻ transporters, whereas a chronic increase in K⁺ uptake (i.e., within hours to days) is mediated by an increase in the quantity of Na⁺,K⁺-ATPase. The rise in plasma [K⁺] that follows K⁺ absorption by the gastrointestinal tract stimulates secretion of insulin from the pancreas, release of aldosterone from the adrenal cortex, and secretion of epinephrine from the adrenal medulla. In contrast, a decrease in plasma [K⁺] inhibits the release of these hormones. Whereas insulin and epinephrine act within a few minutes, aldosterone requires about an hour to stimulate uptake of K⁺ into cells.

Epinephrine

Catecholamines affect the distribution of K⁺ across cell membranes by activating α- and β₂-adrenergic receptors. Stimulation of α-adrenoceptors releases K⁺ from cells, especially in the liver, whereas stimulation of β₂-adrenoceptors promotes K⁺ uptake by cells.

For example, activation of β₂-adrenoceptors after exercise is important in preventing hyperkalemia. The rise in plasma [K⁺] after a K⁺-rich meal is greater if the patient has been pretreated with propranolol, a β₂-adrenoceptor antagonist. Furthermore, the release of epinephrine during stress (e.g., myocardial ischemia) can rapidly lower plasma [K⁺].

Insulin

Insulin also stimulates uptake of K⁺ into cells. The importance of insulin is illustrated by two observations. First, the rise in plasma [K⁺] after a K⁺-rich meal is greater in patients with diabetes mellitus (i.e., insulin deficiency) than in normal people. Second, insulin (and glucose to prevent insulin-induced hypoglycemia) can be infused to correct hyperkalemia. Insulin is the most important hormone that shifts K⁺ into cells after the ingestion of K⁺ in a meal.

Aldosterone

Aldosterone, like catecholamines and insulin, also promotes uptake of K⁺ into cells. A rise in aldosterone levels (e.g., primary aldosteronism) causes hypokalemia, whereas a fall in aldosterone levels (e.g., Addison's disease) causes hyperkalemia. As discussed later, aldosterone also stimulates urinary K⁺ excretion. Thus, aldosterone alters plasma [K⁺] by acting on uptake of K⁺ into cells and altering urinary K⁺ excretion.

ALTERATIONS IN PLASMA [K⁺]

Several factors can alter plasma [K⁺] (Table 35-1). These factors are not involved in the regulation of plasma [K⁺] but rather alter the movement of K⁺ between the intra-

● **Figure 35-3.** Overview of K^+ homeostasis. An increase in plasma insulin, epinephrine, or aldosterone stimulates movement of K^+ into cells and decreases plasma $[K^+]$, whereas a fall in the plasma concentration of these hormones increases plasma $[K^+]$. The amount of K^+ in the body is determined by the kidneys. An individual is in K^+ balance when dietary intake and urinary output (plus output by the gastrointestinal tract) are equal. Excretion of K^+ by the kidneys is regulated by plasma $[K^+]$, aldosterone, and ADH.

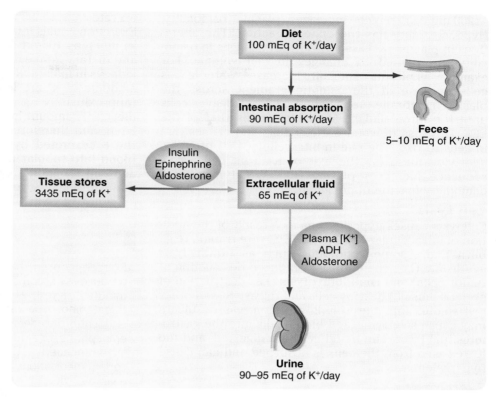

Diet
100 mEq of K^+/day

Intestinal absorption
90 mEq of K^+/day

Feces
5–10 mEq of K^+/day

Insulin
Epinephrine
Aldosterone

Tissue stores
3435 mEq of K^+

Extracellular fluid
65 mEq of K^+

Plasma $[K^+]$
ADH
Aldosterone

Urine
90–95 mEq of K^+/day

● **Table 35-1.**

Major Factors, Hormones, and Drugs Influencing the Distribution of K^+ between the Intracellular and Extracellular Fluid Compartments

Physiological: Keep Plasma $[K^+]$ Constant
Epinephrine
Insulin
Aldosterone
Pathophysiological: Displace Plasma $[K^+]$ from Normal
Acid-base balance
Plasma osmolality
Cell lysis
Exercise
Drugs That Induce Hyperkalemia
Dietary K^+ supplements
ACE inhibitors
K^+-sparing diuretics
Heparin

cellular fluid (ICF) and ECF and thus cause the development of hypokalemia or hyperkalemia.

Acid-Base Balance

Metabolic acidosis increases the plasma $[K^+]$, whereas metabolic alkalosis and respiratory alkalosis decreases it. In contrast, respiratory acidosis has little or no effect on the plasma $[K^+]$. Metabolic acidosis produced by the addition of inorganic acids (e.g., HCl, H_2SO_4) increases plasma $[K^+]$ much more than an equivalent acidosis produced by the accumulation of organic acids (e.g., lactic acid, acetic acid, keto acids). The reduced pH (i.e., increased $[H^+]$) promotes the move-

ment of H^+ into cells and the reciprocal movement of K^+ out of cells to maintain electroneutrality. This effect of acidosis occurs in part because acidosis inhibits the transporters that accumulate K^+ inside cells, including Na^+,K^+-ATPase and the $1Na^+$-$1K^+$-$2Cl^-$ symporter. In addition, movement of H^+ into cells occurs as the cells buffer changes in $[H^+]$ of the ECF (see Chapter 36). As H^+ moves across the cell membranes, K^+ moves in the opposite direction, and thus cations are neither gained nor lost across cell membranes. Metabolic alkalosis has the opposite effect; plasma $[K^+]$ decreases as K^+ moves into cells and H^+ exits.

Although organic acids produce a metabolic acidosis, they do not cause significant hyperkalemia. Two explanations have been suggested for the reduced ability of organic acids to cause hyperkalemia. First, the organic anion may enter the cell with H^+ and thereby eliminate the need for K^+-H^+ exchange across the membrane. Second, organic anions may stimulate insulin secretion, which moves K^+ into cells. This movement may counteract the direct effect of the acidosis, which moves K^+ out of cells.

Plasma Osmolality

The osmolality of plasma also influences the distribution of K^+ across cell membranes. An increase in the osmolality of ECF enhances the release of K^+ by cells and thus increases extracellular $[K^+]$. Plasma $[K^+]$ may increase by 0.4 to 0.8 mEq/L with a 10 mOsm/kg H_2O elevation in plasma osmolality. In patients with diabetes mellitus who do not take insulin, plasma $[K^+]$ is often elevated, in part because of the lack of insulin and in part because of the increase in plasma [glucose] (i.e., from a normal value of ≈100 mg/dL to as high as

≈1200 mg/dL), which increases plasma osmolality. Hypoosmolality has the opposite action. The alterations in plasma [K⁺] associated with changes in osmolality are related to changes in cell volume. For example, as plasma osmolality increases, water leaves cells because of the osmotic gradient across the plasma membrane (see Chapter 1). Water leaves cells until the intracellular osmolality equals that of the ECF. This loss of water shrinks cells and causes [K⁺] in cells to rise. The rise in intracellular [K⁺] provides a driving force for the exit of K⁺ from cells. This sequence increases plasma [K⁺]. A fall in plasma osmolality has the opposite effect.

Cell Lysis

Cell lysis causes hyperkalemia as a result of the addition of intracellular K⁺ to the ECF. Severe trauma (e.g., burns) and some conditions such as **tumor lysis syndrome** (i.e., chemotherapy-induced destruction of tumor cells) and **rhabdomyolysis** (i.e., destruction of skeletal muscle) destroy cells and release K⁺ and other cell solutes into the ECF. In addition, gastric ulcers may cause seepage of red blood cells into the gastrointestinal tract. The blood cells are digested, and the K⁺ released from the cells is absorbed and can cause hyperkalemia.

Exercise

More K⁺ is released from skeletal muscle cells during exercise than during rest. The ensuing hyperkalemia depends on the degree of exercise. In people walking slowly, plasma [K⁺] increases by 0.3 mEq/L. With vigorous exercise, plasma [K⁺] may increase by 2.0 mEq/L.

K⁺ EXCRETION BY THE KIDNEYS

The kidneys play a major role in maintaining K⁺ balance. As illustrated in Figure 35-3, the kidneys excrete 90% to 95% of the K⁺ ingested in the diet. Excretion equals intake even when intake increases by as much as 10-fold. This balance in urinary excretion and dietary intake underscores the importance of the kidneys in maintaining K⁺ homeostasis. Although small amounts of K⁺ are lost each day in feces and sweat (approximately 5% to 10% of the K⁺ ingested in the diet), this amount is essentially constant, is not regulated, and therefore is relatively less important than the K⁺ excreted by the kidneys. K⁺ secretion from blood into tubular fluid by cells of the distal tubule and collecting duct system is the key factor in determining urinary K⁺ excretion (Fig. 35-4).

> ### ▶ IN THE CLINIC
>
> Exercise-induced changes in plasma [K⁺] do not usually produce symptoms and are reversed after several minutes of rest. However, exercise can lead to life-threatening hyperkalemia in individuals (1) who have endocrine disorders that affect the release of insulin, epinephrine, or aldosterone; (2) whose ability to excrete K⁺ is impaired (e.g., renal failure); or (3) who take certain medications, such as β₂-adrenergic blockers. For example, during exercise, plasma [K⁺] may increase by at least 2 to 4 mEq/L in individuals who take β₂-adrenergic receptor antagonists for hypertension.
>
> Because acid-base balance, plasma osmolality, cell lysis, and exercise do not maintain plasma [K⁺] at a normal value, they do not contribute to K⁺ homeostasis (Table 35-1). The extent to which these pathophysiological states alter plasma [K⁺] depends on the integrity of the homeostatic mechanisms that regulate plasma [K⁺] (e.g., secretion of epinephrine, insulin, and aldosterone).

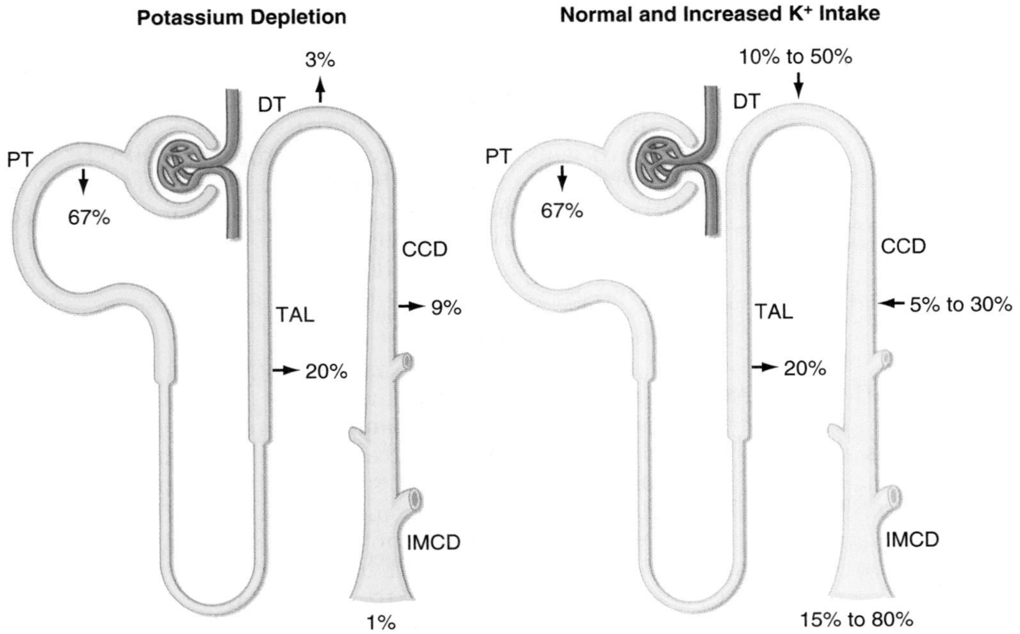

● **Figure 35-4.** K⁺ transport along the nephron. Excretion of K⁺ depends on the rate and direction of K⁺ transport by the distal tubule and collecting duct. Percentages refer to the amount of filtered K⁺ reabsorbed or secreted by each nephron segment. **Left,** Dietary K⁺ depletion. An amount of K⁺ equal to 1% of the filtered load of K⁺ is excreted. **Right,** Normal and increased dietary K⁺ intake. An amount of K⁺ equal to 15% to 80% of the filtered load is excreted. CCD, cortical collecting duct; DT, distal tubule; IMCD, inner medullary collecting duct; PT, proximal tubule; TAL, thick ascending limb.

Because K$^+$ is not bound to plasma proteins, it is freely filtered by the glomerulus. When individuals ingest 100 mEq of K$^+$ per day, urinary K$^+$ excretion is about 15% of the amount filtered. Accordingly, K$^+$ must be reabsorbed along the nephron. When dietary K$^+$ intake increases, however, K$^+$ excretion can exceed the amount filtered. Thus, K$^+$ can also be secreted.

The proximal tubule reabsorbs about 67% of the filtered K$^+$ under most conditions. Approximately 20% of the filtered K$^+$ is reabsorbed by the loop of Henle, and as with the proximal tubule, the amount reabsorbed is a constant fraction of the amount filtered. In contrast to these segments, which can only reabsorb K$^+$, the distal tubule and collecting duct are able to reabsorb or secrete K$^+$. The rate of K$^+$ reabsorption or secretion by the distal tubule and collecting duct depends on a variety of hormones and factors. When 100 mEq/day of K$^+$ is ingested, it is secreted by these nephron segments. A rise in dietary K$^+$ intake increases K$^+$ secretion. K$^+$ secretion can increase the amount of K$^+$ that appears in urine so that it approaches 80% of the amount filtered (Fig. 35-4). In contrast, a low-K$^+$ diet activates K$^+$ reabsorption along the distal tubule and collecting duct so that urinary excretion falls to about 1% of the K$^+$ filtered by the glomerulus (Fig. 35-4). The kidneys cannot reduce K$^+$ excretion to the same low levels as they can for Na$^+$ (i.e., 0.2%). Therefore, hypokalemia can develop in individuals placed on a K$^+$-deficient diet. Because the magnitude and direction of K$^+$ transport by the distal tubule and collecting duct are variable, the overall rate of urinary K$^+$ excretion is determined by these tubular segments.

CELLULAR MECHANISM OF K$^+$ SECRETION BY PRINCIPAL CELLS IN THE DISTAL TUBULE AND COLLECTING DUCT

Figure 35-5 illustrates the cellular mechanisms of K$^+$ secretion by principal cells in the distal tubule and collecting duct. Secretion from blood into the tubule lumen is a two-step process: (1) uptake of K$^+$ from blood across the basolateral membrane by Na$^+$,K$^+$-ATPase and (2) diffusion of K$^+$ from the cell into tubular fluid via K$^+$ channels. Na$^+$,K$^+$-ATPase creates a high intracellular [K$^+$] that provides the chemical driving force for exit of K$^+$ across the apical membrane through K$^+$ channels. Although K$^+$ channels are also present in the basolateral membrane, K$^+$ preferentially leaves the cell across the apical membrane and enters the tubular fluid. K$^+$ transport follows this route for two reasons. First, the electrochemical gradient of K$^+$ across the apical membrane favors its downhill movement into tubular fluid. Second, the permeability of the apical membrane to K$^+$ is greater than that of the basolateral membrane. Therefore K$^+$ preferentially diffuses across the apical membrane into tubular fluid. The three major factors that control the rate of K$^+$ secretion by the distal tubule and the collecting duct are

1. The activity of Na$^+$,K$^+$-ATPase
2. The driving force (electrochemical gradient) for movement of K$^+$ across the apical membrane
3. The permeability of the apical membrane to K$^+$

Every change in K$^+$ secretion results from an alteration in one or more of these factors.

Intercalated cells reabsorb K$^+$ via an H$^+$,K$^+$-ATPase transport mechanism located in the apical membrane (see Chapter 36). This transporter mediates uptake of K$^+$ in exchange for H$^+$. The pathway for exit of K$^+$ from intercalated cells into blood is unknown. Reabsorption of K$^+$ is activated by a low K$^+$-diet.

REGULATION OF K$^+$ SECRETION BY THE DISTAL TUBULE AND COLLECTING DUCT

Regulation of K$^+$ excretion is achieved mainly by alterations in K$^+$ secretion by principal cells of the distal tubule and collecting duct. Plasma [K$^+$] and aldosterone are the major physiological regulators of K$^+$ secretion. Antidiuretic hormone (ADH) also stimulates K$^+$ secretion; however, it is less important than plasma [K$^+$] and aldosterone. Other factors, including the flow rate of tubular fluid and acid-base balance, influence secretion of K$^+$ by the distal tubule and collecting duct. However, they are not homeostatic mechanisms because they disturb K$^+$ balance (Table 35-2).

Plasma [K$^+$]

Plasma [K$^+$] is an important determinant of K$^+$ secretion by the distal tubule and collecting duct. Hyperkalemia (e.g., resulting from a high-K$^+$ diet or from rhabdomyolysis) stimulates secretion of K$^+$ within minutes. Several mechanisms are involved. First,

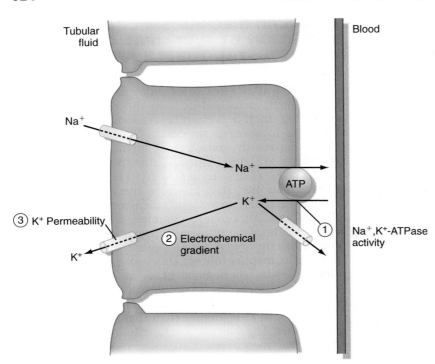

Tubular fluid

Blood

Na⁺

Na⁺

ATP

K⁺

③ K⁺ Permeability

② Electrochemical gradient

① Na⁺,K⁺-ATPase activity

K⁺

● **Figure 35-5.** Cellular mechanism of K⁺ secretion by a principal cell in the distal tubule and collecting duct. The numbers indicate the sites where K⁺ secretion is regulated. 1, Na⁺,K⁺-ATPase; 2, electrochemical gradient of K⁺ across the apical membrane; 3, permeability of the apical membrane to K⁺.

● Table 35-2.
Major Factors and Hormones Influencing K⁺ Excretion

Physiological: Keep K⁺ Balance Constant
Plasma [K⁺]
Aldosterone
ADH
Pathophysiological: Displace K⁺ Balance
Flow rate of tubule fluid
Acid-base balance
Glucocorticoids

hyperkalemia stimulates Na⁺,K⁺-ATPase and thereby increases K⁺ uptake across the basolateral membrane. This uptake raises intracellular [K⁺] and increases the electrochemical driving force for exit of K⁺ across the apical membrane. Second, hyperkalemia also increases the permeability of the apical membrane to K⁺. Third, hyperkalemia stimulates secretion of aldosterone by the adrenal cortex, which as discussed later, acts synergistically with plasma [K⁺] to stimulate secretion of K⁺. Fourth, hyperkalemia also increases the flow rate of tubular fluid, which as discussed later, stimulates secretion of K⁺ by the distal tubule and collecting duct.

Hypokalemia (e.g., caused by a low-K⁺ diet or loss of K⁺ in diarrhea fluid) decreases K⁺ secretion via actions opposite those described for hyperkalemia. Hence, hypokalemia inhibits Na⁺,K⁺-ATPase, decreases the electrochemical driving force for efflux of K⁺ across the apical membrane, reduces permeability of the apical membrane to K⁺, and decreases plasma aldosterone levels.

Chronic hypokalemia (plasma [K⁺] <3.5 mEq/L) occurs most often in patients who receive diuretics for hypertension. Hypokalemia also occurs in patients who vomit, undergo nasogastric suction, have diarrhea, abuse laxatives, or have hyperaldosteronism. Hypokalemia occurs because excretion of K⁺ by the kidneys exceeds the dietary intake of K⁺. Vomiting, nasogastric suction, diuretics, and diarrhea can all decrease ECF volume, which in turn stimulates secretion of aldosterone (see Chapter 34). Because aldosterone stimulates excretion of K⁺ by the kidneys, its action contributes to the development of hypokalemia.

Chronic hyperkalemia (plasma [K⁺] >5.0 mEq/L) occurs most frequently in individuals with reduced urine flow, low plasma aldosterone levels, and renal disease in which the glomerular filtration rate falls below 20% of normal. In these individuals, hyperkalemia occurs because the excretion of K⁺ by the kidneys is less than the dietary intake of K⁺. Less common causes of hyperkalemia occur in people with deficiencies in insulin, epinephrine, and aldosterone secretion or in people with metabolic acidosis caused by inorganic acids.

Aldosterone

Chronically (i.e., ≥24 hours) elevated plasma aldosterone levels enhance secretion of K⁺ across principal cells in the distal tubule and collecting duct via five mechanisms (Fig. 35-6): (1) by increasing the amount of Na⁺, K⁺-ATPase in the basolateral membrane; (2) by increasing expression of the epithelial sodium channel (ENaC) in the apical cell membrane; (3) by elevating

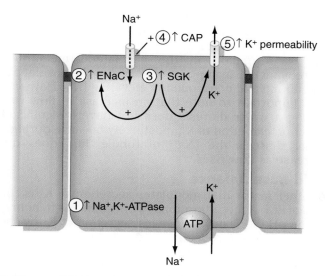

● **Figure 35-6.** Effects of aldosterone on secretion of K⁺ by principal cells in the collecting duct. Numbers refer to the five effects of aldosterone discussed in text.

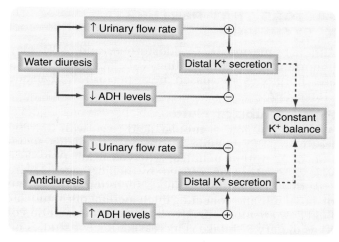

● **Figure 35-7.** Opposing effects of ADH on secretion of K⁺ by the distal tubule and cortical collecting duct. Secretion is stimulated by an increase in the electrochemical gradient for K⁺ across the apical membrane and by an increase in the permeability of the apical membrane to K⁺. In contrast, secretion is reduced by a fall in the flow rate of tubular fluid. Because these effects oppose each other, net K⁺ secretion is not affected by ADH.

SGK1 (**s**erum **g**lucocorticoid-stimulated **k**inase) levels, which also increases expression of ENaC in the apical membrane and activates K⁺ channels; (4) by stimulating CAP1 (**c**hannel-**a**ctivating **p**rotease, also called **prostatin**), which directly activates ENaC; and (5) by stimulating the permeability of the apical membrane to K⁺. The cellular mechanisms by which aldosterone affects the expression and activity of Na⁺,K⁺-ATPase and ENaC (actions 1 to 5 just listed) have been described (see Chapter 33). Aldosterone increases the permeability of the apical membrane to K⁺ by increasing the number of K⁺ channels in the membrane. However, the cellular mechanisms involved in this response are not completely known. Increased expression of Na⁺,K⁺-ATPase facilitates uptake of K⁺ across the basolateral membrane into cells and thereby elevates intracellular [K⁺]. The increase in the number and activity of Na⁺ channels enhances entry of Na⁺ into the cell from tubular fluid, an effect that depolarizes the apical membrane voltage. Depolarization of the apical membrane and increased intracellular [K⁺] enhance the electrochemical driving force for secretion of K⁺ from the cell into the tubule fluid. Taken together, these actions increase uptake of K⁺ into the cell across the basolateral membrane and enhance exit of K⁺ from the cell across the apical membrane. Secretion of aldosterone is increased by hyperkalemia and by angiotensin II (after activation of the renin-angiotensin system). Secretion of aldosterone is decreased by hypokalemia and natriuretic peptides released from the heart.

Although an acute (e.g., within hours) increase in aldosterone levels enhances the activity of Na⁺,K⁺-ATPase, K⁺ excretion does not increase. The reason for this relates to the effect of aldosterone on Na⁺ reabsorption and tubular flow. Aldosterone stimulates reabsorption of Na⁺ and water and thus decreases tubular flow. The reduction in flow in turn decreases

K⁺ secretion (as discussed in more detail later). However, chronic stimulation of Na⁺ reabsorption expands the ECF and thereby returns tubular flow to normal. These actions allow a direct stimulatory effect of aldosterone on the distal tubule and collecting duct to enhance K⁺ excretion.

Antidiuretic Hormone

Although ADH does not affect urinary K⁺ excretion, this hormone does stimulate secretion of K⁺ by the distal tubule and collecting duct (Fig. 35-7). ADH increases the electrochemical driving force for exit of K⁺ across the apical membrane of principal cells by stimulating uptake of Na⁺ across the apical membrane of these cells. The increased Na⁺ uptake reduces the electrical potential difference across the apical membrane (i.e., the interior of the cell becomes less negatively charged). Despite this effect, ADH does not change K⁺ secretion by these nephron segments. The reason for this relates to the effect of ADH on tubular fluid flow. ADH decreases flow of tubular fluid by stimulating water reabsorption. The decrease in tubular flow in turn reduces secretion of K⁺ (explained later). The inhibitory effect of decreased flow of tubular fluid offsets the stimulatory effect of ADH on the electrochemical driving force for exit of K⁺ across the apical membrane (Fig. 35-7). If ADH did not increase the electrochemical gradient favoring K⁺ secretion, urinary K⁺ excretion would fall as ADH levels increased and urinary flow rates decreased. Hence, K⁺ balance would change in response to alterations in water balance. Thus, the effects of ADH on the electrochemical driving force for exit of K⁺ across the apical membrane and on tubule flow enable urinary K⁺ excretion to be maintained constant despite wide fluctuations in water excretion.

FACTORS THAT PERTURB K⁺ EXCRETION

Although plasma [K⁺], aldosterone, and ADH play important roles in regulating K⁺ balance, the factors and hormones discussed next perturb K⁺ balance (Table 35-2).

Flow of Tubular Fluid

A rise in the flow of tubular fluid (e.g., with diuretic treatment, ECF volume expansion) stimulates secretion of K⁺ within minutes, whereas a fall (e.g., ECF volume contraction caused by hemorrhage, severe vomiting, or diarrhea) reduces secretion of K⁺ by the distal tubule and collecting duct. Increments in tubular fluid flow are more effective in stimulating secretion of K⁺ as dietary K⁺ intake is increased. Recent studies on the primary cilium in principal cells have elucidated some of the mechanisms whereby increased flow stimulates secretion of K⁺ (Fig. 35-8). Increased flow bends the primary cilium in principal cells, which activates the PKD1/PKD2 Ca⁺⁺ conducting channel complex. This allows more Ca⁺⁺ to enter principal cells and increases intracellular [Ca⁺⁺]. The increase in [Ca⁺⁺] activates K⁺ channels in the apical plasma membrane, which enhances secretion of K⁺ from the cell into tubule fluid. Increased flow may also stimulate secretion of K⁺ by other mechanisms. As flow increases, such as after the administration of diuretics or as the result of an increase in ECF volume, so does the [Na⁺] of tubule fluid. This increase in [Na⁺] facilitates entry of Na⁺ across the apical membrane of distal tubule and collecting duct cells, thereby decreasing the cells' interior negative membrane potential. This depolarization of the cell membrane potential increases the electrochemical driving force that promotes secretion of K⁺ across the apical cell membrane into tubule fluid. In addition, increased uptake of Na⁺ into cells activates the Na⁺,K⁺-ATPase in the basolateral membrane, thereby increasing uptake of K⁺ across the basolateral membrane and consequently elevating [K⁺]. However, it is important to note that an increase in flow rate during a water diuresis does not have a significant effect on excretion of K⁺, most likely because during a water diuresis the [Na⁺] of tubule fluid does not increase as flow rises.

Acid-Base Balance

Another factor that modulates secretion of K⁺ is the [H⁺] of ECF. Acute alterations (within minutes to hours) in the pH of plasma influences secretion of K⁺ by the distal tubule and collecting duct. Alkalosis (i.e., plasma pH above normal) increases secretion of K⁺, whereas acidosis (i.e., plasma pH below normal) decreases it. An acute acidosis reduces K⁺ secretion via two mechanisms: (1) it inhibits Na⁺,K⁺-ATPase and thereby reduces cell [K⁺] and the electrochemical driving force for exit of K⁺ across the apical membrane, and (2) it reduces the permeability of the apical membrane to K⁺. Alkalosis has the opposite effects.

● AT THE CELLULAR LEVEL

ROMK (KCNJ1) is the primary channel in the apical membrane responsible for secretion of K⁺. Four ROMK subunits make up a single channel. In addition, a maxi-K⁺ channel (rbsol1), which is activated by elevations in intracellular [Ca⁺⁺], is also expressed in the apical membrane. The maxi-K⁺ channel mediates the flow-dependent increase in K⁺ secretion, as discussed earlier. Interestingly, knockout of the *KCNJ1* gene (ROMK) causes increased excretion of NaCl and K⁺ by the kidneys, thereby leading to reduced ECF volume and hypokalemia. Although this effect is somewhat perplexing, it should be noted that ROMK is also expressed in the apical membrane of the thick ascending limb of Henle's loop, where it plays a very important role in recycling of K⁺ across the apical membrane, an effect that is critical for operation of the Na⁺-K⁺-2Cl⁻ symporter (see Chapter 33). In the absence of ROMK, reabsorption of NaCl by the thick ascending limb is reduced, which leads to loss of NaCl in urine. Reduction of NaCl reabsorption by the thick ascending limb also reduces the positive transepithelial luminal voltage, which is the driving force for reabsorption of K⁺ by this nephron segment. Thus, the reduction in paracellular K⁺ reabsorption by the thick ascending limb increases urinary K⁺ excretion, even when the cortical collecting duct is unable to secrete the normal amount of K⁺ because of a lack of ROMK channels. The cortical collecting duct, however, does secrete K⁺ even in ROMK knockout mice via the flow- and Ca⁺⁺-dependent maxi-K⁺ channels and possibly by the operation of a K⁺-Cl⁻ symporter expressed in the apical membrane of principal cells.

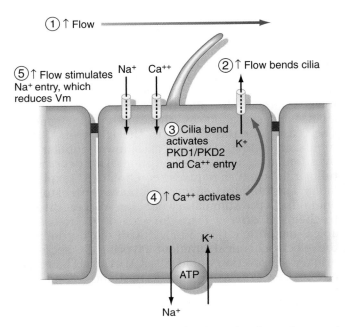

● **Figure 35-8.** Cellular mechanism whereby an increased flow rate of tubule fluid stimulates secretion of K⁺ by principal cells in the collecting duct. See text for details.

The effect of metabolic acidosis on excretion of K$^+$ is time dependent. When metabolic acidosis lasts for several days, urinary K$^+$ excretion is stimulated (Fig. 35-9). This occurs because chronic metabolic acidosis decreases the reabsorption of water and solutes (e.g., NaCl) by the proximal tubule by inhibiting Na$^+$,K$^+$-ATPase. Hence, the flow of tubular fluid is augmented along the distal tubule and collecting duct. The inhibition of water and NaCl reabsorption by the proximal tubule also decreases ECF volume and thereby stimulates secretion of aldosterone. In addition, chronic acidosis, caused by inorganic acids, increases plasma [K$^+$], which stimulates secretion of aldosterone. The rise in tubular fluid flow, plasma [K$^+$], and aldosterone levels offsets the effects of acidosis on cell [K$^+$] and apical membrane permeability, and K$^+$ secretion rises. Thus, metabolic acidosis may either inhibit or stimulate excretion of K$^+$, depending on the duration of the disturbance. Renal K$^+$ excretion remains elevated during chronic metabolic acidosis and may even increase further, depending on the cause of the acidosis.

As noted, acute metabolic alkalosis stimulates excretion of K$^+$. Chronic metabolic alkalosis, especially in association with ECF volume contraction, significantly increases renal K$^+$ excretion because of the associated increased levels of aldosterone.

Glucocorticoids

Glucocorticoids increase urinary K$^+$ excretion. This effect is mediated in part by an increase in the glomerular filtration rate, which enhances the urinary flow rate, a potent stimulus of K$^+$ excretion, and by stimulation of SGK1 activity (see earlier).

As discussed earlier, the rate of urinary K$^+$ excretion is frequently determined by simultaneous changes in hormone levels, acid-base balance, or the flow rate of tubule fluid (Table 35-3). The powerful effect of flow often enhances or opposes the response of the distal tubule and collecting duct to hormones and changes in acid-base balance. This interaction can be beneficial in the case of hyperkalemia, in which the change in flow enhances excretion of K$^+$ and thereby restores K$^+$ homeostasis. However, this interaction can also be detrimental, as in the case of alkalosis, in which changes in flow and acid-base status alter K$^+$ homeostasis.

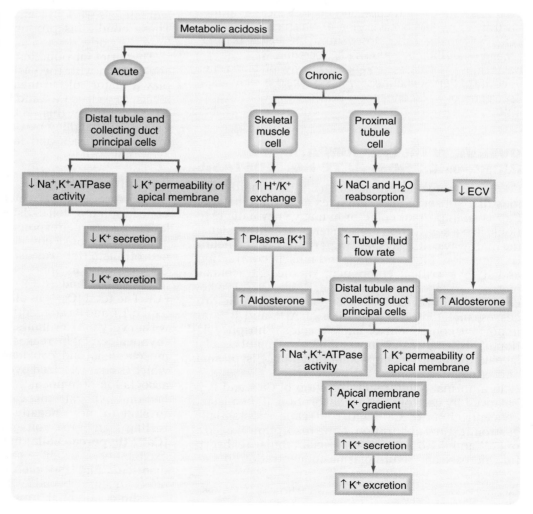

● **Figure 35-9.** Acute versus chronic effect of metabolic acidosis on excretion of K$^+$. See text for details. ECV, effective circulating volume.

● AT THE CELLULAR LEVEL

The cellular mechanisms whereby changes in the K^+ content of the diet and acid-base balance regulate secretion of K^+ by the distal tubule and collecting duct have recently been elucidated. Elevated K^+ intake increases secretion of K^+ by several mechanisms, all related to increased serum $[K^+]$. Hyperkalemia increases the activity of the ROMK channel in the apical plasma membrane of principal cells. Moreover, hyperkalemia inhibits reabsorption of NaCl and water by the proximal tubule, thereby increasing the distal tubule and collecting duct flow rate, a potent stimulus to secretion of K^+. Hyperkalemia also enhances [aldosterone], which increases K^+ secretion by three mechanisms. First, aldosterone increases the number of K^+ channels in the apical plasma membrane. Second, aldosterone stimulates uptake of K^+ across the basolateral membrane by increasing the number of Na^+,K^+-ATPase pumps, thereby enhancing the electrochemical gradient driving secretion of K^+ across the apical membrane. Third, aldosterone increases movement of Na^+ across the apical membrane, which depolarizes the apical plasma membrane voltage and thus increases the electrochemical gradient promoting secretion of K^+.

A low-K^+ diet dramatically reduces secretion of K^+ by the distal tubule and collecting duct by increasing the activity of protein tyrosine kinase, which causes ROMK channels to be endocytosed from the apical plasma membrane, thereby reducing K^+ secretion.

Acidosis decreases secretion of K^+ by inhibiting the activity of ROMK channels, whereas alkalosis stimulates secretion of K^+ by enhancing ROMK channel activity.

OVERVIEW OF CALCIUM AND INORGANIC PHOSPHATE HOMEOSTASIS

Ca^{++} and inorganic phosphate (P_i)* are multivalent ions that subserve many complex and vital functions. Ca^{++} is an important cofactor in many enzymatic reactions; it is a key second messenger in numerous signaling pathways; it plays an important role in neural transduction, blood clotting, and muscle contraction; and it is a critical component of the extracellular matrix, cartilage, teeth, and bone. P_i, like Ca^{++}, is a key component of bone. P_i is essential for metabolic processes, including the formation of ATP, and it is an important component of nucleic acids. Phosphorylation of proteins is an important mechanism of cellular signaling, and P_i is an important buffer in cells, plasma, and urine.

In a normal adult, renal excretion of Ca^{++} and P_i is balanced by gastrointestinal absorption. If the plasma concentrations of Ca^{++} and P_i decline substantially, gastrointestinal absorption, bone resorption (i.e., loss of Ca^{++} and P_i from bone), and renal tubular reabsorption increase and return plasma concentrations of Ca^{++}

● Table 35-3.

Net Effects of Hormones and Other Factors on K^+ Secretion by the Distal Tubule and Collecting Duct

Condition	Direct or Indirect	Flow	Urinary Excretion
Hyperkalemia	Increase	Increase	Increase
Aldosterone			
Acute	Increase	Decrease	No change
Chronic	Increase	No change	Increase
Glucocorticoids	Increase	Increase	Increase
ADH	Increase	Decrease	No change
Acidosis			
Acute	Decrease	No change	Decrease
Chronic	Decrease	Large increase	Increase
Alkalosis	Increase	Increase	Large increase

Modified from Field MJ et al. In Narins R (ed): Textbook of Nephrology: Clinical Disorders of Fluid and Electrolyte Metabolism, 5th ed. New York, McGraw-Hill, 1994.

---

and P_i to normal levels. During growth and pregnancy, intestinal absorption exceeds urinary excretion, and these ions accumulate in newly formed fetal tissue and bone. In contrast, bone disease (e.g., osteoporosis) or a decline in lean body mass increases urinary multivalent ion loss without a change in intestinal absorption. These conditions produce a net loss of Ca^{++} and P_i from the body.

This brief introduction reveals that the kidneys, in conjunction with the gastrointestinal tract and bone, play a major role in maintaining plasma Ca^{++} and P_i levels, as well as Ca^{++} and P_i balance (see also Chapter 39). Accordingly, this section of the chapter discusses Ca^{++} and P_i handling by the kidneys with an emphasis on the hormones and factors that regulate urinary excretion.

Calcium

Cellular processes in which Ca^{++} plays a part include bone formation, cell division and growth, blood coagulation, hormone-response coupling, and electrical stimulus–response coupling (e.g., muscle contraction, neurotransmitter release). Ninety-nine percent of Ca^{++} is stored in bone, approximately 1% is found in intracellular fluid (ICF), and 0.1% is located in the ECF. The total $[Ca^{++}]$ in plasma is 10 mg/dL (2.5 mM or 5 mEq/L), and its concentration is normally maintained within very narrow limits. A low ionized plasma $[Ca^{++}]$ **(hypocalcemia)** increases the excitability of nerve and muscle cells and can lead to hypocalcemic **tetany,** which is characterized by skeletal muscle spasms. The association of hypocalcemia with tetany is due to the fact that hypocalcemia causes the threshold potential to shift to more negative values (i.e., closer to the resting membrane voltage). Elevated ionized plasma $[Ca^{++}]$ **(hypercalcemia)** may decrease neuromuscular excitability or produce cardiac arrhythmias, lethargy, disorientation, and even death. This hypercalcemic effect occurs because hypercalcemia causes the threshold potential to shift to less negative values

---

*At physiological pH, inorganic phosphate exists as HPO_4^- and $H_2PO_4^-$ (pK = 6.8). For simplicity, we collectively refer to these ion species as P_i.

(i.e., further from the resting membrane voltage). Within cells, Ca^{++} is sequestered in the endoplasmic reticulum and mitochondria, or it is bound to proteins. Thus, the free intracellular $[Ca^{++}]$ is very low (≈ 100 nM). The large concentration gradient for $[Ca^{++}]$ across cell membranes is maintained by a Ca^{++}-ATPase pump (PMCa1b) in all cells and by a $3Na^+$-$1Ca^{++}$ antiporter (NCX1) in some cells.

Overview of Calcium Homeostasis

Ca^{++} homeostasis depends on two factors: (1) the total amount of Ca^{++} in the body and (2) the distribution of Ca^{++} between bone and ECF. Total body $[Ca^{++}]$ is determined by the relative amounts of Ca^{++} absorbed by the gastrointestinal tract and excreted by the kidneys (Fig. 35-10). The gastrointestinal tract absorbs Ca^{++} through an active, carrier-mediated transport mechanism that is stimulated by **calcitriol,** a metabolite of vitamin D_3. Net Ca^{++} absorption is normally 200 mg/day, but it can increase to 600 mg/day when calcitriol levels rise. In adults, Ca^{++} excretion by the kidneys equals the amount absorbed by the gastrointestinal tract (200 mg/day), and it changes in parallel with reabsorption of Ca^{++} by the gastrointestinal tract. Thus, in adults, Ca^{++} balance is maintained because the amount of Ca^{++} ingested in an average diet (1500 mg/day) equals the amount lost in feces (1300 mg/day, the amount that escapes absorption by the gastrointestinal tract) plus the amount excreted in urine (200 mg/day).

The second factor that controls Ca^{++} homeostasis is the distribution of Ca^{++} between bone and ECF. Three hormones (**parathyroid hormone [PTH], calcitriol, and calcitonin**) regulate the distribution of Ca^{++} between bone and ECF and thereby regulate plasma $[Ca^{++}]$.

PTH is secreted by the parathyroid glands, and its secretion is regulated by the $[Ca^{++}]$ in ECF. The plasma membrane of the chief cells of the parathyroid glands contains the **calcium-sensing receptor (CaSR),** which monitors the $[Ca^{++}]$ in ECF. A decrease in $[Ca^{++}]$ (i.e., hypocalcemia) increases PTH gene expression and release by the chief cells. In contrast, an increase in $[Ca^{++}]$ (i.e., hypercalcemia) decreases PTH release by the chief cells.

PTH increases plasma $[Ca^{++}]$ by (1) stimulating bone resorption, (2) increasing Ca^{++} reabsorption by the kidneys, and (3) stimulating the production of calcitriol, which in turn increases Ca^{++} absorption by the gastrointestinal tract and facilitates PTH-mediated bone resorption.

The production of calcitriol, a metabolite of vitamin D_3 produced in the proximal tubule of the kidney, is stimulated by hypocalcemia and hypophosphatemia. In addition, hypocalcemia stimulates secretion of PTH, which also stimulates production of vitamin D_3 by the proximal tubule cells. Calcitriol increases plasma $[Ca^{++}]$ primarily by stimulating absorption of Ca^{++} from the gastrointestinal tract. It also facilitates the action of PTH on bone and increases the expression of key Ca^{++} transport and binding proteins in the kidneys.

Calcitonin is secreted by thyroid C cells (a.k.a., parafollicular cells), and its secretion is stimulated by hypercalcemia. Calcitonin decreases plasma $[Ca^{++}]$ mainly by stimulating bone formation (i.e., deposition of Ca^{++} in bone). Figure 35-11 illustrates the relationship between plasma $[Ca^{++}]$ and plasma levels of PTH and calcitonin. Although calcitonin plays an important role in Ca^{++} homeostasis in lower vertebrates, it plays only a minor role in normal Ca^{++} homeostasis in humans.

Approximately 50% of the Ca^{++} in plasma is ionized, 45% is bound to plasma proteins (mainly albumin), and 5% is complexed to several anions, including HCO_3^-, citrate, P_i, and SO_4^{2-}. The pH of plasma influences this distribution. The increase in $[H^+]$ in patients with

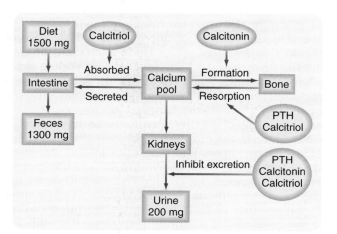

● Figure 35-10. Overview of Ca^{++} homeostasis. See text for details. PTH, parathyroid hormone.

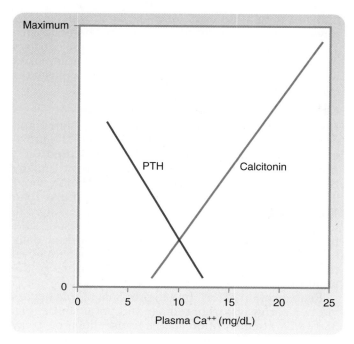

● Figure 35-11. Effect of plasma $[Ca^{++}]$ on plasma levels of PTH and calcitonin. (Modified from Azria M: The Calcitonins: Physiology and Pharmacology. Basel, Karger, 1989.)

▶ IN THE CLINIC

Conditions that lower PTH levels (i.e., hypoparathyroidism after parathyroidectomy for an adenoma) reduce plasma [Ca++], which can cause hypocalcemic tetany (intermittent muscular contractions). In severe cases, **hypocalcemic tetany** can cause death by asphyxiation. Hypercalcemia can also cause lethal cardiac arrhythmias and decreased neuromuscular excitability. Clinically, the most common causes of hypercalcemia are primary hyperparathyroidism and malignancy-associated hypercalcemia. Primary hyperparathyroidism results from the overproduction of PTH by the parathyroid glands. In contrast, malignancy-associated hypercalcemia, which occurs in 10% to 20% of all patients with cancer, is caused by the secretion of **parathyroid hormone–related peptide (PTHrP),** a PTH-like hormone secreted by carcinomas in various organs. Increased levels of PTH and PTHrP cause hypercalcemia and hypercalciuria.

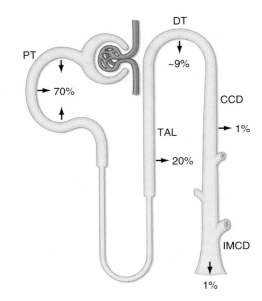

● **Figure 35-12.** Ca++ transport along the nephron. Percentages refer to the amount of filtered Ca++ reabsorbed by each segment. Approximately 1% of the filtered Ca++ is excreted. CCD, cortical collecting duct; DT, distal tubule; IMCD, inner medullary collecting duct; PT, proximal tubule; TAL, thick ascending limb.

metabolic acidosis causes more H^+ to bind to plasma proteins, HCO_3^-, citrate, P_i, and SO_4^{2-}, thereby displacing Ca++. This displacement increases the plasma concentration of ionized Ca++. In alkalosis, the [H^+] of plasma decreases. Some H^+ ions dissociate from plasma proteins, HCO_3^-, citrate, P_i, and SO_4^{2-} in exchange for Ca++, thereby decreasing the plasma concentration of ionized Ca++. In addition, the plasma albumin concentration also affects ionized plasma [Ca++]. Hypoalbuminemia increases ionized [Ca++], whereas hyperalbuminemia decreases ionized plasma [Ca++]. Under both conditions the total plasma [Ca++] may not reflect the total ionized [Ca++], which is the physiologically relevant measure of Ca++ homeostasis. The Ca++ available for glomerular filtration consists of the ionized fraction and the amount complexed with anions. Thus, about 55% of the Ca++ in plasma is available for glomerular filtration.

Calcium Transport along the Nephron

Normally, 99% of the filtered Ca++ (i.e., ionized and complexed) is reabsorbed by the nephron. The proximal tubule reabsorbs about 70% of the filtered Ca++. Another 20% is reabsorbed in the loop of Henle (mainly the cortical portion of the thick ascending limb), about 9% is reabsorbed by the distal tubule, and less than 1% is reabsorbed by the collecting duct. Approximately 1% (200 mg/day) is excreted in urine. This fraction is equal to the net amount absorbed daily in the gastrointestinal tract. Figure 35-12 summarizes the handling of Ca++ by the different portions of the nephron.

Reabsorption of Ca++ by the proximal tubule occurs via two pathways: transcellular and paracellular (Fig. 35-13). Ca++ reabsorption via the transcellular pathway accounts for 20% of proximal reabsorption. Reabsorption of Ca++ through the cell is an active process that occurs in two steps. First, Ca++ diffuses down its electrochemical gradient across the apical membrane

through Ca++ channels and into the cell. Second, at the basolateral membrane, Ca++ is extruded from the cell against its electrochemical gradient by a Ca++-ATPase. In contrast, 80% of Ca++ is reabsorbed between cells across the tight junctions (i.e., the paracellular pathway). This passive, paracellular reabsorption of Ca++ occurs via solvent drag along the entire length of the proximal tubule and is also driven by the positive luminal voltage in the second half of the proximal tubule (i.e., diffusion). Thus, approximately 80% of Ca++ reabsorption is paracellular, and approximately 20% is transcellular in the proximal tubule.

Reabsorption of Ca++ by the loop of Henle is restricted to the cortical portion of the thick ascending limb. Ca++ is reabsorbed by the cellular and paracellular routes via mechanisms similar to those described for the proximal tubule but with one difference (Fig. 35-13): Ca++ is not reabsorbed by solvent drag in this segment. (The thick ascending limb is impermeable to water.) In the thick ascending limb, reabsorption of Ca++ and Na+ occurs in parallel. These processes are parallel because of the significant component of Ca++ reabsorption that occurs via passive paracellular mechanisms secondary to reabsorption of Na+ and via generation of positive transepithelial voltage in the lumen. Loop diuretics inhibit reabsorption of Na+ by the thick ascending limb of the loop of Henle and in so doing reduce the magnitude of the positive transepithelial luminal voltage (see Chapter 33). This action in turn inhibits reabsorption of Ca++ via the paracellular pathway. Thus, loop diuretics are used to increase renal Ca++ excretion in patients with hypercalcemia. Therefore, reabsorption of Na+ also changes in parallel with reabsorption of Ca++ by both

● **Figure 35-13.** Cellular mechanisms for reabsorption of Ca^{++} by the transcellular and cellular pathways. Note that all transport mechanisms are not expressed in every nephron segment. In distal tubule cells, Ca^{++} enters the cells across the apical membrane via Ca^{++}-permeable ion channels (TRPV5 and TRPV6). Inside distal tubule cells, Ca^{++} binds to calbindin (calbindin-D$_{28K}$ and calbindin-D$_{9K}$, CB), and the Ca^{++}-calbindin complex diffuses across the cell to deliver Ca^{++} to the basolateral membrane. Ca^{++} is transported across the basolateral membrane by a 3Na$^+$-1Ca^{++} antiporter (NCX1) and Ca^{++}-ATPase (PMCa1b). In the proximal tubule, reabsorption of Ca^{++} involves uptake across the brush border membrane via a Ca^{++}-permeable ion channel and exit across the basolateral membrane via Ca^{++}-ATPase. A large portion of proximal tubule Ca^{++} reabsorption occurs via the paracellular pathway. This component of proximal tubule Ca^{++} reabsorption is driven by solvent drag. Reabsorption of Ca^{++} via the paracellular pathway in the thick ascending limb of Henle's loop is driven by the transepithelial electrochemical gradient for Ca^{++}. The tight junction protein claudin-16 (CLDCN16) regulates the paracellular diffusion of Ca^{++} (see the molecular box on claudin-16). Ca^{++} reabsorption in the distal tubule occurs exclusively by the transcellular pathway.

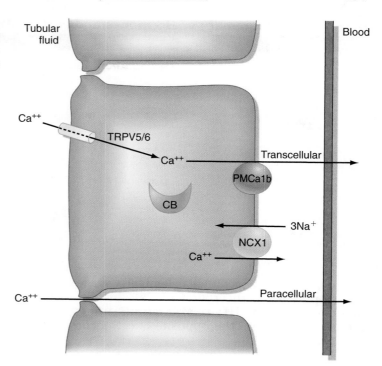

● AT THE CELLULAR LEVEL

Mutations in the tight junction protein, **claudin-16**, alters the diffusive movement of Ca^{++} across tight junctions in the thick ascending limb of Henle's loop (TAL). Familial hypomagnesemic hypercalciuria is caused by mutations in claudin-16, a protein that is a component of the tight junctions in TAL cells. This disorder is characterized by enhanced excretion of Ca^{++} and magnesium (Mg^{++}) because of a fall in the passive reabsorption of these ions across the paracellular pathway in the TAL. The mutation in the claudin-16 gene reduces the permeability of the paracellular pathway to Ca^{++} and Mg^{++}, thereby reducing passive, paracellular reabsorption of both ions.

the proximal tubule and the thick ascending limb of the loop of Henle.

In the distal tubule, where the voltage in the tubule lumen is electrically negative with respect to blood, reabsorption of Ca^{++} is entirely active because Ca^{++} is reabsorbed against its electrochemical gradient (Fig. 35-13). Reabsorption of Ca^{++} by the distal tubule is exclusively transcellular. Calcium enters the cell across the apical membrane through Ca^{++}-permeable epithelial ion channels (TRPV5/TRPV6). Inside the cell, Ca^{++} binds to calbindin. The calbindin-Ca^{++} complex carries Ca^{++} across the cell and delivers Ca^{++} to the basolateral membrane, where it is extruded from the cell by either Ca^{++}-ATPase (PMCA1b) or the 3Na$^+$-1Ca^{++} antiporter

(NCX1). Urinary Na$^+$ and Ca^{++} excretion usually changes in parallel. However, excretion of these ions does not always change in parallel because reabsorption of Ca^{++} and Na$^+$ by the distal tubule is independent and differentially regulated. For example, **thiazide diuretics** inhibit reabsorption of Na$^+$ by the distal tubule and stimulate reabsorption of Ca^{++} by this segment. Accordingly, the net effects of thiazide diuretics are to increase urinary Na$^+$ excretion and reduce urinary Ca^{++} excretion.

Regulation of Urinary Calcium Excretion

Several hormones and factors influence urinary Ca^{++} excretion (Table 35-4). Of these, PTH exerts the most powerful control on renal Ca^{++} excretion, and it is responsible for maintaining Ca^{++} homeostasis. Overall, this hormone stimulates reabsorption of Ca^{++} by the kidneys (i.e., reduces Ca^{++} excretion). Although PTH inhibits reabsorption of NaCl and fluid and therefore reabsorption of Ca^{++} by the proximal tubule, PTH stimulates reabsorption of Ca^{++} by the thick ascending limb of the loop of Henle and the distal tubule. In humans, this effect is greater in the distal tubule. Changes in [Ca^{++}] in ECF also regulate urinary Ca^{++} excretion, with hypercalcemia increasing excretion and hypocalcemia decreasing it. Hypercalcemia increases urinary Ca^{++} excretion by (1) reducing proximal tubule Ca^{++} reabsorption (reduced paracellular reabsorption because of increased interstitial fluid [Ca^{++}]); (2) inhibiting Ca^{++} reabsorption by the thick ascending limb of the loop of Henle, an effect mediated by the CaSR located in the basolateral membrane of these cells (the activity of the 1Na$^+$-1K$^+$-2Cl$^-$ symporter is decreased, thereby reducing the magnitude

● **Table 35-4. Summary of Hormones and Factors Affecting Reabsorption of Ca^{++}**

Factor/Hormone	Nephron Location		
	Proximal Tubule	*Thick Ascending Limb*	*Distal Tubule*
Volume expansion	Decrease	No change	Decrease
Hypercalcemia	Decrease	Decrease (CaSR, ↓PTH)	Decrease (CaSR, ↓PTH)
Hypocalcemia	Increase	Increase (CaSR, ↑PTH)	Increase (CaSR, ↑PTH)
Phosphate loading			Increase (↑PTH)
Phosphate depletion			Decrease (↓PTH)
Acidosis			Decrease
Alkalosis			Increase
PTH	Decrease	Increase	Increase
Vitamin D			Increase
Calcitonin		Increase	Increase

CaSR, calcium-sensing receptor; PTH, parathyroid hormone.
Modified from Yu A. In Brenner BM (ed): Brenner and Rector's The Kidney, 7th ed. Philadelphia, Saunders, 2004.

of the positive transepithelial luminal voltage); and (3) suppressing reabsorption of Ca^{++} by the distal tubule by reducing PTH levels. As a result, urinary Ca^{++} excretion increases. The opposite effect occurs with hypocalcemia.

Calcitonin stimulates reabsorption of Ca^{++} by the thick ascending limb and distal tubule, but it is less effective than PTH, and it is not known how important this effect is in humans. Calcitriol either directly or indirectly enhances Ca^{++} reabsorption by the distal tubule, but it is also less effective than PTH.

Several factors disturb Ca^{++} excretion. An increase in plasma [P_i] (e.g., caused by increased dietary intake of P_i) elevates PTH levels and thereby decreases Ca^{++} excretion. A decline in plasma [P_i] (e.g., caused by dietary P_i depletion) has the opposite effect. Changes in ECF volume alter excretion of Ca^{++} mainly by affecting reabsorption of NaCl and fluid in the proximal tubule. Volume contraction increases NaCl and water reabsorption by the proximal tubule and thereby enhances reabsorption of Ca^{++}. Accordingly, urinary Ca^{++} excretion declines. Volume expansion has the opposite effect. Acidosis increases Ca^{++} excretion, whereas alkalosis decreases it. Regulation of Ca^{++} reabsorption by pH occurs in the distal tubule. Alkalosis stimulates the apical membrane Ca^{++} channel (TRPV5), thereby increasing reabsorption of Ca^{++}. By contrast, acidosis inhibits the same channel, thereby reducing reabsorption of Ca^{++}.

Calcium-Sensing Receptor

The CaSR is a receptor expressed in the plasma membrane of cells involved in regulating Ca^{++} homeostasis. The CaSR senses small changes in extracellular [Ca^{++}]. Ca^{++} binds to CaSRs in PTH-secreting cells of the parathyroid gland, calcitonin-secreting parafollicular cells in the thyroid gland, and calcitriol-producing cells of the proximal tubule. Activation of the receptor by an increase in plasma [Ca^{++}] results in inhibition of PTH secretion and calcitriol production and stimulation of calcitonin secretion. Moreover, the reduction in PTH secretion also contributes to decreased production of calcitriol because PTH is a potent stimulus of calcitriol synthesis. By contrast, a fall in plasma [Ca^{++}] has the

> ### IN THE CLINIC
>
> Mutations in the gene coding for **CaSR** cause disorders in Ca^{++} homeostasis. **Familial hypocalciuric hypercalcemia (FHH)** is an autosomal dominant disease caused by an inactivating mutation of CaSR. The hypercalcemia is caused by deranged Ca^{++}-regulated PTH secretion (i.e., PTH levels are elevated at any level of plasma [Ca^{++}]). Hypocalciuria is caused by enhanced Ca^{++} reabsorption in the thick ascending limb and distal tubule as a result of elevated PTH levels and defective CaSR regulation of Ca^{++} transport in the kidneys. **Autosomal dominant hypocalcemia** is caused by an activating mutation in CaSR. Activation of CaSRs causes deranged Ca^{++}-regulated PTH secretion (i.e., PTH levels are decreased at any level of plasma [Ca^{++}]). Hypercalciuria results and is caused by decreased PTH levels and defective CaSR-regulated Ca^{++} transport in the kidneys.

opposite effect on PTH, calcitriol, and calcitonin secretion. These three hormones act on the kidneys, intestine, and bone to regulate plasma [Ca^{++}] by mechanisms described elsewhere in this chapter.

The CaSR also maintains Ca^{++} homeostasis by directly regulating excretion of Ca^{++} by the kidneys. CaSRs in the thick ascending limb and distal tubule respond directly to changes in plasma [Ca^{++}] and regulate Ca^{++} absorption by these nephron segments. An increase in plasma [Ca^{++}] activates CaSRs in the thick ascending limb and distal tubule and inhibits Ca^{++} absorption in these nephron segments, thereby stimulating urinary Ca^{++} excretion. By contrast, a fall in plasma [Ca^{++}] leads to an increase in Ca^{++} absorption by the thick ascending limb and distal tubule and a corresponding decrease in urinary Ca^{++} excretion. Thus, the direct effect of plasma [Ca^{++}] on CaSRs in the thick ascending limb and distal tubule acts in concert with changes in PTH to regulate urinary Ca^{++} excretion and thereby maintain Ca^{++} homeostasis.

Phosphate

P_i is an important component of many organic molecules, including DNA, RNA, ATP, and intermediates of metabolic pathways. It is also a major constituent of bone. Its concentration in plasma is an important determinant of bone formation and resorption. In addition, urinary P_i is an important buffer (titratable acid) for the maintenance of acid-base balance (see Chapter 36). Eighty-six percent of P_i is located in bone, approximately 14% in ICF, and 0.03% in ECF. The normal plasma $[P_i]$ is 4 mg/dL. Approximately 10% of the P_i in plasma is protein bound and therefore unavailable for ultrafiltration by the glomerulus. Accordingly, the $[P_i]$ in the ultrafiltrate is 10% less than that in plasma.

Overview of Phosphate Homeostasis

A general scheme of P_i homeostasis is shown in Figure 35-14. Maintenance of P_i homeostasis depends on two factors: (1) the amount of P_i in the body and (2) the distribution of P_i between the ICF and ECF compartments. Total body $[P_i]$ is determined by the relative amount of P_i absorbed by the gastrointestinal tract versus the amount excreted by the kidneys. Absorption of P_i by the gastrointestinal tract occurs via active and passive mechanisms; P_i absorption increases as dietary P_i rises, and it is stimulated by calcitriol. Despite variations in P_i intake between 800 and 1500 mg/day, the kidneys keep total body P_i balance constant by excreting an amount of P_i in urine equal to the amount absorbed by the gastrointestinal tract. Thus, renal P_i excretion is the primary mechanism by which the body regulates P_i balance and thereby P_i homeostasis.

The second factor that maintains P_i homeostasis is the distribution of P_i among bone and the ICF and ECF compartments. PTH, calcitriol, and calcitonin regulate the distribution of P_i between bone and the ECF. As with Ca^{++} homeostasis, calcitonin is the least important of the hormones involved in P_i homeostasis in humans. Release of P_i from bone is stimulated by the same hormones (i.e., PTH, calcitriol) that release Ca^{++} from this pool. Thus, release of P_i is always accompanied by a release of Ca^{++}. In contrast, calcitonin increases bone formation and thereby decreases plasma $[P_i]$.

The kidneys also make an important contribution to the regulation of plasma $[P_i]$. A small rise in plasma $[P_i]$ increases the amount of P_i filtered by the glomerulus. Because the kidneys normally reabsorb P_i at a maximum rate, any increase in the amount filtered leads to a rise in urinary P_i excretion. In fact, an increase in the amount of P_i filtered enhances urinary P_i excretion to a value greater than the rate of P_i absorption by the gastrointestinal tract. This process results in net loss of P_i from the body and decreases plasma $[P_i]$. In this way the kidneys regulate plasma $[P_i]$. The maximum reabsorptive rate for P_i varies and is regulated by dietary P_i intake. A diet high in P_i decreases the maximum reabsorptive rate of P_i by the kidneys, and a diet low in P_i increases it. This effect is independent of changes in PTH levels.

Phosphate Transport along the Nephron

Figure 35-15 summarizes P_i transport by the various portions of the nephron. The proximal tubule reabsorbs 80% of the P_i filtered by the glomerulus, and the distal tubule reabsorbs 10%. In contrast, the loop of Henle and the collecting duct reabsorb negligible amounts of P_i. Therefore approximately 10% of the filtered load of P_i is excreted.

Reabsorption of P_i by the proximal tubule occurs mainly, if not exclusively, by means of a transcellular route. Uptake of P_i across the apical membrane occurs via Na^+-P_i symport mechanisms (NPT). Three symport-

---

▶ IN THE CLINIC

In patients with **chronic renal failure,** the kidneys cannot excrete P_i. Because of continued P_i absorption by the gastrointestinal tract, P_i accumulates in the body, and plasma $[P_i]$ rises. The excess P_i complexes with Ca^{++} and reduces plasma $[Ca^{++}]$. Accumulation of P_i also decreases the production of calcitriol. This response reduces absorption of Ca^{++} by the intestine, an effect that further reduces plasma $[Ca^{++}]$. This reduction in plasma $[Ca^{++}]$ increases PTH secretion and Ca^{++} release from bone. These actions result in **osteitis fibrosa cystica** (i.e., increased bone resorption with replacement by fibrous tissue, which renders bone more susceptible to fracture). Chronic hyperparathyroidism (i.e., elevated PTH levels because of the fall in plasma $[Ca^{++}]$) during chronic renal failure can lead to metastatic calcifications in which Ca^{++} and P_i precipitate in arteries, soft tissues, and viscera. Deposition of Ca^{++} and P_i in heart and lung tissue may cause myocardial failure and pulmonary insufficiency, respectively. Prevention and treatment of hyperparathyroidism and P_i retention include a low-P_i diet or the administration of a "phosphate binder" (i.e., an agent that forms insoluble P_i salts and thereby renders P_i unavailable for absorption by the gastrointestinal tract). Supplemental Ca^{++} and calcitriol are also prescribed.

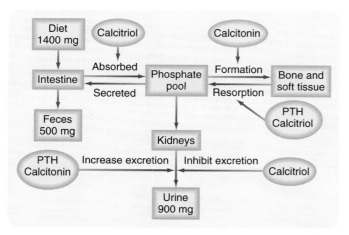

● **Figure 35-14.** Overview of P_i homeostasis. See text for details.

ers have been identified: one transports $2Na^+$ with each P_i (NPT1), whereas the other two transport $3Na^+$ with each P_i (NPT2 and NPT3). NPT2 is the most important symporter involved in reabsorption of P_i by the proximal tubule (Fig. 35-16). P_i exits across the basolateral membrane by a P_i–inorganic anion antiporter. The cellular mechanism of P_i reabsorption by the distal tubule has not been characterized.

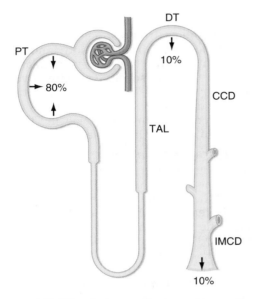

● **Figure 35-15.** P_i transport along the nephron. P_i is reabsorbed primarily by the proximal tubule. Percentages refer to the amount of the filtered P_i reabsorbed by each nephron segment. Approximately 10% of the filtered P_i is excreted. CCD, cortical collecting duct; DT, distal tubule; IMCD, inner medullary collecting duct; PT, proximal tubule; TAL, thick ascending limb.

Regulation of Urinary Phosphate Excretion

Several hormones and factors regulate urinary P_i excretion (Table 35-5). PTH, the most important hormone that controls P_i excretion, inhibits reabsorption of P_i by the proximal tubule and thereby increases P_i excretion. PTH reduces P_i reabsorption by stimulating the endocytic removal of NPT2 from the brush border membrane of the proximal tubule. Dietary P_i intake also regulates P_i excretion by mechanisms unrelated to changes in PTH levels. P_i loading increases excretion, whereas P_i depletion decreases it. Changes in dietary P_i intake modulate P_i transport by altering the transport rate of each NPT2 symporter and the number of transporters.

● **Table 35-5.**

Summary of Hormones and Factors Affecting P_i Reabsorption by the Proximal Tubule

Factor/Hormone	Rate of Occurrence	Proximal Tubule Reabsorption
Volume expansion		Decrease
Hypercalcemia	Acute	Increase
Hypercalcemia	Chronic	Decrease
Phosphate loading		Decrease
Phosphate depletion		Increase
Metabolic acidosis	Chronic	Decrease
Metabolic alkalosis	Chronic	Increase
PTH		Decrease
Vitamin D	Acute	Increase
Vitamin D	Chronic	Decrease
Growth hormone		Increase
FGF-23/FGF-24		Decrease
Glucocorticoids		Decrease

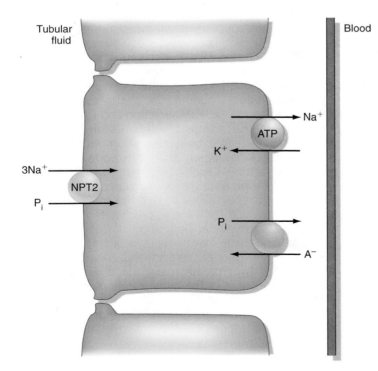

● **Figure 35-16.** Cellular mechanisms of P_i reabsorption by the proximal tubule. The apical transport pathway operates primarily as a $3Na^+$-$1P_i$ symporter (NPT2). P_i leaves the cell across the basolateral membrane by a P_i-anion antiporter. A^- indicates an anion.

ECF volume also affects P_i excretion. Volume expansion increases excretion, and volume contraction decreases it. The effect of ECF volume on P_i excretion is indirect and may involve changes in levels of hormones other than PTH. Acid-base balance also influences P_i excretion; acidosis increases P_i excretion, whereas alkalosis decreases it. Glucocorticoids increase the excretion of P_i. Glucocorticoids increase delivery of P_i to the distal tubule and collecting duct by inhibiting reabsorption of P_i by the proximal tubule. This inhibition enables the distal tubule and collecting duct to secrete more H^+ and generate more HCO_3^- because P_i is an important urinary buffer (see Chapter 36). Finally, growth hormone decreases excretion of P_i. Several phosphaturic factors, also called phosphatonins, including **fibroblast growth factor 23 (FGF-23)** and **frizzled-related protein 4 (FRP-4),** are hormones produced by tumors in patients with osteomalacia that inhibit renal P_i reabsorption. An increase in dietary P_i enhances plasma FGF-23 levels, which by reducing NPT2 expression in the apical membrane of the proximal tubule, enhances urinary P_i excretion and also decreases calcitriol levels. Prolonged increases in plasma $[P_i]$ are associated with increased tissue calcification and a reduced life span.

> ## IN THE CLINIC
>
> In the absence of glucocorticoids (e.g., in **Addison's disease**), excretion of P_i is depressed, as is the ability of the kidneys to excrete titratable acid and to generate new HCO_3^- (see Chapter 36). Growth hormone also has an important effect on P_i homeostasis. Growth hormone increases reabsorption of P_i by the proximal tubule. As a result, growing children have higher plasma $[P_i]$ than adults do, and this elevated $[P_i]$ is important for the formation of bone.

■ KEY CONCEPTS

1. K^+ homeostasis is maintained by the kidneys, which adjust K^+ excretion to match dietary K^+ intake, and by the hormones insulin, epinephrine, and aldosterone, which regulate the distribution of K^+ between the ICF and ECF compartments. Other events, such as cell lysis, exercise, and changes in acid-base balance and plasma osmolality, disturb K^+ homeostasis and plasma $[K^+]$.

2. Excretion of K^+ by the kidneys is determined by the rate and direction of K^+ transport by the distal tubule and collecting duct. Secretion of K^+ by these tubular segments is regulated by plasma $[K^+]$, aldosterone, and ADH. In contrast, changes in tubular fluid flow and acid-base disturbances perturb K^+ excretion by the kidneys. In K^+-depleted states, K^+ secretion is inhibited and the distal tubule and collecting duct reabsorb K^+.

3. The kidneys, in conjunction with the gastrointestinal tract and bone, play a vital role in regulating plasma $[Ca^{++}]$ and $[P_i]$. Plasma $[Ca^{++}]$ is regulated by PTH and calcitriol. Excretion of Ca^{++} by the kidneys is determined by (1) the net rate of intestinal Ca^{++} absorption, (2) the balance between bone formation and resorption, and (3) the net rate of Ca^{++} reabsorption by the distal tubule and thick ascending limb of the loop of Henle. Reabsorption of Ca^{++} by the thick ascending limb and distal tubule is regulated by PTH and calcitriol, both of which stimulate Ca^{++} reabsorption.

4. Plasma $[P_i]$ is regulated by the maximal reabsorptive capacity of P_i by the kidneys. A fall in $[P_i]$ stimulates the production of calcitriol, which releases P_i from bone into ECF and increases P_i absorption by the intestine.

CHAPTER 36

Role of the Kidneys in the Regulation of Acid-Base Balance

The concentration of H^+ in body fluids is low in comparison to the concentration of other ions. For example, Na^+ is present at a concentration some 3 million times greater than that of H^+ ([Na^+] = 140 mEq/L; [H^+] = 40 nEq/L). Because of the low [H^+] of body fluids, it is commonly expressed as the negative logarithm, or pH.

Virtually all cellular, tissue, and organ processes are sensitive to pH. Indeed, life cannot exist outside a range of body fluid pH from 6.8 to 7.8 (160 to 16 nEq/L of H^+). Normally, the pH of extracellular fluid (ECF) is maintained between 7.35 and 7.45. As described in Chapter 2, the pH of intracellular fluid (ICF) is slightly lower (7.1 to 7.2), but also tightly regulated.

Each day, acid and alkali are ingested in the diet. In addition, cellular metabolism produces a number of substances that have an impact on the pH of body fluids. Without appropriate mechanisms to deal with this daily acid and alkali load and thereby maintain acid-base balance, many processes necessary for life could not occur. This chapter reviews the maintenance of whole-body acid-base balance. Although emphasis is on the role of the kidneys in this process, the role of the lungs and liver is also considered. Moreover, the impact of diet and cellular metabolism on acid-base balance is presented. Finally, disorders of acid-base balance are considered, primarily to illustrate the physiological processes involved. Throughout this chapter, **acid** is defined as any substance that adds H^+ to body fluids, whereas **alkali** is defined as a substance that removes H^+ from body fluids.

THE HCO_3^- BUFFER SYSTEM

Bicarbonate (HCO_3^-) is an important buffer of ECF. With a normal plasma [HCO_3^-] of 23 to 25 mEq/L and a volume of 14 L (for a 70-kg individual), ECF can potentially buffer 350 mEq of H^+. The HCO_3^- buffer system differs from other buffer systems of the body (e.g., phosphate) in that it is regulated by both the lungs and the kidneys. This is best appreciated by considering the following reaction:

● **Equation 36-1**

Slow   Fast

$$CO_2 + H_2O \leftrightarrow H_2CO_3 \leftrightarrow H^+ + HCO_3^-$$

As indicated, the first reaction (hydration/dehydration of CO_2) is the rate-limiting step. This normally slow reaction is greatly accelerated in the presence of carbonic anhydrase.* The second reaction, the ionization of H_2CO_3 to H^+ and HCO_3^- is virtually instantaneous.

The Henderson-Hasselbalch equation (36-2) is used to quantitate how changes in CO_2 and HCO_3^- affect pH.

● **Equation 36-2**

$$pH = pK' + \log \frac{[HCO_3^-]}{\alpha P_{CO_2}}$$

or

● **Equation 36-3**

$$pH = 6.1 + \log \frac{[HCO_3^-]}{0.03 P_{CO_2}}$$

In these equations, the amount of CO_2 is determined from the partial pressure of CO_2 (P_{CO_2}) and its solubility (α) in solution. For plasma at $37°C$, α has a value of 0.03. Also, pK' is the negative logarithm of the overall dissociation constant for the reaction in Equation 36-1 and has a value of 6.1 for plasma at $37°C$. Alternatively, the relationship between HCO_3^-, CO_2, and [H^+] can be expressed as follows:

● **Equation 36-4**

$$[H^+] = 24 \times \frac{P_{CO_2}}{HCO_3^-}$$

Inspection of Equations 36-3 and 36-4 show that pH and [H^+] vary when either [HCO_3^-] or P_{CO_2} is altered. Disturbances in acid-base balance that result from a change in [HCO_3^-] are termed metabolic acid-base disorders, whereas those resulting from a change in P_{CO_2} are termed respiratory acid-base disorders. These disorders are considered in more detail in a subsequent section. The kidneys are primarily responsible for regulating [HCO_3^-] in ECF, whereas the lungs control P_{CO_2}.

OVERVIEW OF ACID-BASE BALANCE

The diet of humans contains many constituents that are either acid or alkali. In addition, cellular metabolism produces acid and alkali. Finally, alkali is normally lost each day in feces. As described later, the net effect

---

*Carbonic anhydrase (CA) actually catalyzes the reaction: $H_2O \rightarrow H^+ + OH^- + CO_2 \xrightarrow{CA} HCO_3^- + H^+ \rightarrow H_2CO_3$.

of these processes is the addition of acid to body fluids. For acid-base balance to be maintained, acid must be excreted from the body at a rate equivalent to its addition. If addition of acid exceeds excretion, **acidosis** results. Conversely, if excretion of acid exceeds addition, **alkalosis** results.

The major constituents of the diet are carbohydrates and fats. When tissue perfusion is adequate, O_2 is available to tissues, and insulin is present at normal levels, carbohydrates and fats are metabolized to CO_2 and H_2O. On a daily basis, 15 to 20 mol of CO_2 is generated through this process. Normally, this large quantity of CO_2 is effectively eliminated from the body by the lungs. Therefore, this metabolically derived CO_2 has no impact on acid-base balance. CO_2 is usually termed **volatile acid** because it has the potential to generate H^+ after hydration with H_2O (Equation 36-1). Acid not derived directly from the hydration of CO_2 is termed **nonvolatile acid** (e.g., lactic acid).

The cellular metabolism of other dietary constituents also has an impact on acid-base balance. For example, cysteine and methionine, sulfur-containing amino acids, yield sulfuric acid when metabolized, whereas hydrochloric acid results from the metabolism of lysine, arginine, and histidine. A portion of this nonvolatile acid load is offset by the production of HCO_3^- through metabolism of the amino acids aspartate and glutamate. On average, the metabolism of dietary amino acids yields net nonvolatile acid production. The metabolism of certain organic anions (e.g., citrate) results in the production of HCO_3^-, which offsets the production of nonvolatile acid to some degree. Overall, in individuals ingesting a meat-containing diet, acid production exceeds HCO_3^- production. In addition to the metabolically derived acids and alkalis, the foods ingested contain acid and alkali. For example, the presence of phosphate ($H_2PO_4^-$) in ingested food increases the dietary acid load. Finally, during digestion, some HCO_3^- is normally lost in feces. This loss is equivalent to the addition of nonvolatile acid to the body. Together, dietary intake, cellular metabolism, and fecal HCO_3^- loss result in the addition of approximately 0.7 to 1.0 mEq/kg body weight of nonvolatile acid to the body each day (50 to 100 mEq/day for most adults).

Nonvolatile acids do not circulate throughout the body but are immediately neutralized by the HCO_3^- in ECF.

● **Equation 36-5**

$$H_2SO_4 + 2NaHCO_3 \leftrightarrow Na_2SO_4 + 2CO_2 + 2H_2O$$

● **Equation 36-6**

$$HCl + NaHCO_3 \leftrightarrow NaCl + CO_2 + H_2O$$

This neutralization process yields the Na^+ salts of the strong acids and removes HCO_3^- from ECF. Thus, HCO_3^- minimizes the effect of these strong acids on the pH of ECF. As noted previously, ECF contains approximately 350 mEq of HCO_3^-. If this HCO_3^- were not replenished, the daily production of nonvolatile acids ($\approx$70 mEq/day) would deplete the ECF of HCO_3^- within 5 days. To maintain acid-base balance the kidneys

> ### ▶ IN THE CLINIC
>
> When insulin levels are normal, carbohydrates and fats are completely metabolized to $CO_2 + H_2O$. However, if insulin levels are abnormally low (e.g., **diabetes mellitus**), metabolism of carbohydrates leads to the production of several organic keto acids (e.g., β-hydroxybutyric acid).
>
> In the absence of adequate levels of O_2 **(hypoxia)**, anaerobic metabolism by cells can also lead to the production of organic acids (e.g., lactic acid) rather than $CO_2 + H_2O$. This frequently occurs in normal individuals during vigorous exercise. Poor tissue perfusion, such as that occurring with reduced cardiac output, can also lead to anaerobic metabolism by cells and thus to acidosis. In these conditions organic acids accumulate, and the pH of body fluids decreases (acidosis). Treatment (e.g., administration of insulin in the case of diabetes) or improved delivery of adequate levels of O_2 to tissues (e.g., in the case of poor tissue perfusion) results in the metabolism of these organic acids to $CO_2 + H_2O$, which consumes H^+ and thereby helps correct the acid-base disorder.

must replenish the HCO_3^- that is lost by neutralization of the nonvolatile acids.

NET ACID EXCRETION BY THE KIDNEYS

Under normal conditions the kidneys excrete an amount of acid equal to the production of nonvolatile acids and in so doing replenish the HCO_3^- that is lost by neutralization of the nonvolatile acids. In addition, the kidneys must prevent the loss of HCO_3^- in urine. This latter task is quantitatively more important because the filtered load of HCO_3^- is approximately 4320 mEq/day (24 mEq/L × 180 L/day = 4320 mEq/day), as compared with only 50 to 100 mEq/day needed to balance nonvolatile acid production.

Both reabsorption of the filtered HCO_3^- and excretion of acid are accomplished via H^+ secretion by nephrons. Thus, in a single day the nephrons must secrete approximately 4390 mEq of H^+ into tubular fluid. Most of the secreted H^+ serves to reabsorb the filtered load of HCO_3^-. Only 50 to 100 mEq of H^+, an amount equivalent to the production of nonvolatile acids, is excreted in urine. As a result of this acid excretion, the urine is normally acidic.

The kidneys cannot excrete urine more acidic than pH 4.0 to 4.5. Even at a pH of 4.0 only 0.1 mEq/L of H^+ can be excreted. Therefore, to excrete sufficient acid, the kidneys excrete H^+ with urinary buffers such as phosphate (P_i).* Other constituents of urine can also serve as buffers (e.g., creatinine), although their role is less important than that of P_i. Collectively, the various urinary buffers are termed **titratable acids.**

---

*The titration reaction is $HPO_4^{-2} + H^+ \leftrightarrow H_2PO_4^-$. This reaction has a pK of approximately 6.8.

This term is derived from the method by which these buffers are quantitated in the laboratory. Typically, alkali (OH⁻) is added to a urine sample to titrate its pH to that of plasma (i.e., 7.4). The amount of alkali added is equal to the amount of H^+ titrated by these urine buffers and is termed titratable acid.

Excretion of H^+ as a titratable acid is insufficient to balance the daily nonvolatile acid load. An additional and important mechanism by which the kidneys contribute to the maintenance of acid-base balance is through the synthesis and excretion of **ammonium (NH_4^+).** The mechanisms involved in this process are discussed in more detail later in this chapter. With regard to the renal regulation of acid-base balance, each NH_4^+ excreted in urine results in the return of one HCO_3^- to the systemic circulation, which replenishes the HCO_3^- lost during neutralization of the nonvolatile acids. Thus, production plus excretion of NH_4^+, like the excretion of titratable acid, is equivalent to the excretion of acid by the kidneys.

In brief, the kidneys contribute to acid-base homeostasis by reabsorbing the filtered load of HCO_3^- and excreting an amount of acid equivalent to the amount of nonvolatile acid produced each day. This overall process is termed **net acid excretion (NAE),** and it can be quantitated as follows:

● **Equation 36-7**

$$NAE = [(U_{NH_4^+} \times \dot{V}) + (U_{TA} \times \dot{V})] - (U_{HCO_3^-} \times \dot{V})$$

where $(U_{NH_4^+} \times \dot{V})$ and $(U_{TA} \times \dot{V})$ are the rates of excretion (mEq/day) of NH_4^+ and titratable acid (TA) and $(U_{HCO_3^-} \times \dot{V})$ is the amount of HCO_3^- lost in urine (equivalent to adding H^+ to the body).* Again, maintenance of acid-base balance means that net acid excretion must equal nonvolatile acid production. Under most conditions, very little HCO_3^- is excreted in urine. Thus, net acid excretion essentially reflects titratable acid and NH_4^+ excretion. Quantitatively, titratable acid accounts for approximately a third and NH_4^+ for two thirds of net acid excretion.

HCO_3^- Reabsorption along the Nephron

As indicated by Equation 36-7, net acid excretion is maximized when little or no HCO_3^- is excreted in urine. Indeed, under most circumstances, very little HCO_3^- appears in urine. Because HCO_3^- is freely filtered at the glomerulus, approximately 4320 mEq/day is delivered to the nephrons and then reabsorbed. Figure 36-1 summarizes the contribution of each nephron segment to reabsorption of the filtered HCO_3^-.

The proximal tubule reabsorbs the largest portion of the filtered load of HCO_3^-. Figure 36-2 summarizes the primary transport processes involved. H^+ secretion across the apical membrane of the cell occurs by both an Na^+-H^+ antiporter and H^+-ATPase. The Na^+-H^+ antiporter (NHE3) is the predominant pathway for H^+ secretion and uses the lumen-to-cell [Na^+] gradient to drive this process (i.e., secondary active secretion of H^+). Within the cell, H^+ and HCO_3^- are produced in a reaction

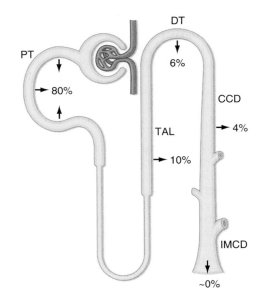

● **Figure 36-1.** Segmental reabsorption of HCO_3^-. The fraction of the filtered load of HCO_3^- reabsorbed by the various segments of the nephron is shown. Normally, the entire filtered load of HCO_3^- is reabsorbed and little or no HCO_3^- appears in urine. CCD, cortical collecting duct; DT, distal tubule; IMCD, inner medullary collecting duct; PT, proximal tubule; TAL, thick ascending limb.

⬤ AT THE CELLULAR LEVEL

Carbonic anhydrases are zinc-containing enzymes that catalyze the hydration of CO_2 (see Equation 36-1). The isoform CA-I is found in red blood cells and is critical for these cells' ability to carry CO_2. Two isoforms, CA-II and CA-IV, play important roles in urine acidification. The CA-II isoform is localized to the cytoplasm of many cells along the nephron, including the proximal tubule, thick ascending limb of Henle's loop, and intercalated cells of the distal tubule and collecting duct. The CA-IV isoform is membrane bound and exposed to the contents of the tubular fluid. It is found in the apical membrane of both the proximal tubule and thick ascending limb of Henle's loop, where it facilitates reabsorption of the large amount of HCO_3^- reabsorbed by these segments. CA-IV has also been demonstrated in the basolateral membrane of the proximal tubule and thick ascending limb of Henle's loop. Its function at this site is thought to facilitate the exit of HCO_3^- from the cell in some way.

catalyzed by carbonic anhydrase. The H^+ is secreted into tubular fluid, whereas HCO_3^- exits the cell across the basolateral membrane and returns to the peritubular blood. Movement of HCO_3^- out of the cell across the basolateral membrane is coupled to other ions. The majority of HCO_3^- exits via a symporter that couples the efflux of $1Na^+$ with $3HCO_3^-$ (sodium bicarbonate cotransporter: NBC1). In addition, some of the HCO_3^- may exit in exchange for Cl^- (via Na^+-independent and/or Na^+-dependent Cl^--HCO_3^- antiporters). As noted in Figure 36-2, carbonic anhydrase is also present in the

---

*This equation ignores the small amount of free H^+ excreted in urine. As already noted, urine with a pH of 4.0 contains only 0.1 mEq/L of H^+.

● **Figure 36-2.** Cellular mechanism for the reabsorption of filtered HCO_3^- by cells of the proximal tubule. Only the primary H^+ and HCO_3^- transporters are shown. CA, carbonic anhydrase.

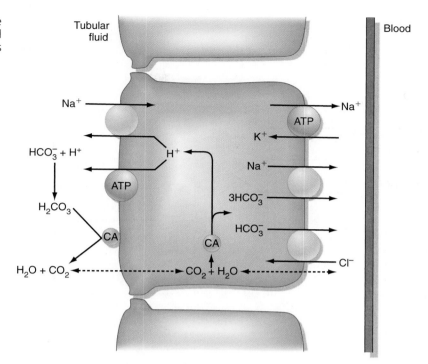

brush border of the proximal tubule cells. This enzyme catalyzes the dehydration of H_2CO_3 in luminal fluid and thereby facilitates reabsorption of HCO_3^-.

The cellular mechanism for reabsorption of HCO_3^- by the thick ascending limb of the loop of Henle is very similar to that in the proximal tubule. H^+ is secreted by an Na^+-H^+ antiporter and H^+-ATPase. As in the proximal tubule, the Na^+-H^+ antiporter is the predominant pathway for secretion of H^+. Exit of HCO_3^- from the cell involves both a $1Na^+$-$3HCO_3^-$ symporter (although the isoform is different from that in the proximal tubule), and a Cl^--HCO_3^- antiporter (anion exchanger: AE-2). A K^+-HCO_3^- symporter in the basolateral membrane may also contribute to exit of HCO_3^- from the cell.

The distal tubule* and collecting duct reabsorb the small amount of HCO_3^- that escapes reabsorption by the proximal tubule and loop of Henle. Figure 36-3 shows the cellular mechanism of H^+/HCO_3^- transport by intercalated cells located within these segments (see Chapter 32).

One type of intercalated cell secretes H^+ (reabsorbs HCO_3^-) and is called the A- or α-intercalated cell. Within this cell, H^+ and HCO_3^- are produced by the hydration of CO_2; this reaction is catalyzed by carbonic anhydrase. H^+ is secreted into tubular fluid via two mechanisms. The first involves an apical membrane H^+-ATPase. The second couples the secretion of H^+ with the reabsorption of K^+ via an H^+,K^+-ATPase similar to that found in the stomach. The HCO_3^- exits the cell across the basolateral membrane in exchange for Cl^- (via a Cl^--

HCO_3^- antiporter: AE-1) and enters the peritubular capillary blood. Other HCO_3^- transporters have been localized to this cell. However, their role in H^+ secretion (HCO_3^- reabsorption) has not been completely defined.

A second population of intercalated cells secrete HCO_3^- rather than H^+ into the tubular fluid (also called B- or β-intercalated cells).[†] In these cells, the H^+-ATPase is located in the basolateral membrane, and the Cl^--HCO_3^- antiporter is located in the apical membrane (Fig. 36-3). However, the apical membrane Cl^--HCO_3^- antiporter is different from the one found in the basolateral membrane of the H^+-secreting intercalated cells and has been identified as pendrin. Other HCO_3^- transporters have been localized to the HCO_3^--secreting intercalated cell, but their precise role in the function of the cell has not been defined. The activity of the HCO_3^--secreting intercalated cell is increased during metabolic alkalosis, when the kidneys must excrete excess HCO_3^-. However, under most conditions (i.e., ingestion of a meat-containing diet), H^+ secretion predominates in these segments.

The apical membrane of collecting duct cells is not very permeable to H^+, and thus the pH of tubular fluid can become quite acidic. Indeed, the most acidic tubular fluid along the nephron (pH of 4.0 to 4.5) is produced there. In comparison, the permeability of the proximal tubule to H^+ and HCO_3^- is much higher, and tubular fluid pH falls to only 6.5 in this segment. As explained later, the ability of the collecting duct to

---

*Here and in the remainder of the chapter we focus on the function of intercalated cells. The early portion of the distal tubule, which does not contain intercalated cells, also reabsorbs HCO_3^-. The cellular mechanism is similar to that already described for the thick ascending limb of Henle's loop, although transporter isoforms may be different.

[†]A third group of intercalated cells shares features of both H^+-secreting and HCO_3^--secreting intercalated cells. The precise function of this cell type is not fully understood.

H⁺-secreting cell

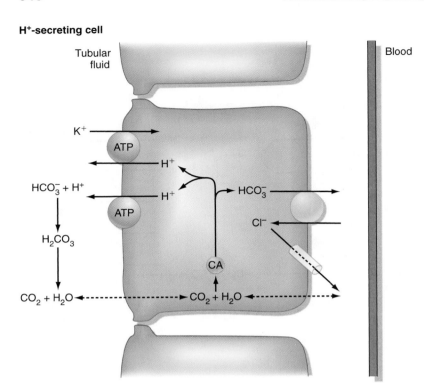

● **Figure 36-3.** Cellular mechanisms for the reabsorption and secretion of HCO_3^- by intercalated cells of the collecting duct. Only the primary H^+ and HCO_3^- transporters are shown. CA, carbonic anhydrase.

HCO₃⁻-secreting cell

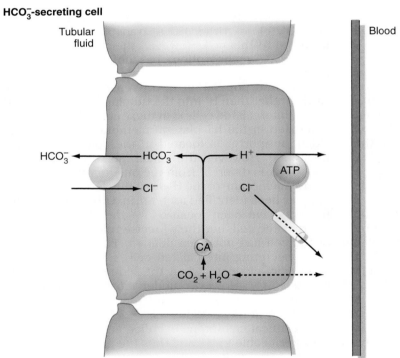

lower the pH of tubular fluid is critically important for the excretion of urinary titratable acids and NH_4^+.

Regulation of H⁺ Secretion

A number of factors regulate secretion of H^+ and thus reabsorption of HCO_3^- by cells of the nephron (Table 36-1). From a physiological perspective, the primary factor that regulates H^+ secretion by the nephron is a change in systemic acid-base balance. Thus, acidosis stimulates H^+ secretion, whereas H^+ secretion is reduced during alkalosis. The response of the kidneys to changes in acid-base balance includes both immediate changes in the activity or number of transporters in the membrane (or both) and longer-term changes in the synthesis of transporters. For example, with metabolic acidosis, whether produced by a decrease

● **Table 36-1.**

Factors Regulating H⁺ Secretion (HCO₃⁻ Reabsorption) by the Nephron

Factor	Primary Site of Action
Increased H⁺ Secretion	
Primary	
Decrease in ECF [HCO_3^-] ($\downarrow$pH)	Entire nephron
Increase in arterial P_{CO_2}	Entire nephron
Cortisol	Proximal tubule*
Endothelin	Proximal tubule*
Secondary	
Increase in the filtered load of HCO_3^-	Proximal tubule
ECF volume contraction	Proximal tubule
Angiotensin II	Proximal and distal tubules
Aldosterone	Distal tubule and collecting duct
Hypokalemia	Proximal tubule
PTH (chronic)	Thick ascending limb; distal tubule
Decreased H⁺ Secretion	
Primary	
Increase in ECF [HCO_3^-] ($\uparrow$pH)	Entire nephron
Decrease in arterial P_{CO_2}	Entire nephron
Secondary	
Decrease in the filtered load of HCO_3^-	Proximal tubule
ECF volume expansion	Proximal tubule
Hypoaldosteronism	Distal tubule and collecting duct
Hyperkalemia	Proximal tubule
PTH (acute)	Proximal tubule

*Effect on the proximal tubule is established. It may also regulate H⁺ secretion in other nephron segments.

in ECF [HCO_3^-] or by an increase in the partial pressure of carbon dioxide (P_{CO_2}), the pH of cells of the nephron decreases. This will stimulate H⁺ secretion by multiple mechanisms, depending on the particular nephron segment. First, the decrease in intracellular pH will create a more favorable cell-to–tubular fluid [H⁺] gradient and thereby make the secretion of H⁺ across the apical membrane more energetically favorable. Second, the decrease in pH may lead to allosteric changes in transport proteins, thereby altering their kinetics. This has been reported for the Na⁺-H⁺ antiporter (NHE3) in the proximal tubule. Finally, transporters may be shuttled to the membrane from intracellular vesicles. This mechanism occurs in both the intercalated cells of the collecting duct, where acidosis stimulates the exocytotic insertion of H⁺-ATPase into the apical membrane, and in the proximal tubule, where insertion of the Na⁺-H⁺ antiporter and H⁺-ATPase into the apical membrane occurs. With long-term acidosis, the abundance of transporters increases, either by increased transcription of appropriate transporter genes or by increased translation of transporter mRNA. Examples include the Na⁺-H⁺ antiporter and the 1Na⁺-3HCO₃⁻ symporter in the proximal tubule and H⁺-ATPase in the intercalated cell.

Although some of the effects just described may be directly attributable to the decrease in intracellular pH, most of these changes in cellular H⁺ transport are mediated by hormones or other factors. Two important mediators of the renal response to acidosis are endothelin and cortisol. **Endothelin-1 (ET-1)** is produced by endothelial and proximal tubule cells, and

thus it exerts its effects via autocrine and paracrine mechanisms. With acidosis, secretion of ET-1 is enhanced. In the proximal tubule, ET-1 stimulates the phosphorylation and subsequent insertion of the Na⁺-H⁺ antiporter into the apical membrane and insertion of the 1Na⁺-3HCO₃⁻ symporter into the basolateral membrane. ET-1 may mediate the response to acidosis in other nephron segments as well. Acidosis also stimulates secretion of the glucocorticoid hormone **cortisol** by the adrenal cortex. Cortisol in turn acts on the kidneys to increase transcription of the Na⁺-H⁺ antiporter and 1Na⁺-3HCO₃⁻ symporter genes in the proximal tubule, as well as increase translation of the mRNA of these transporters.

Alkalosis, caused by an increase in ECF [HCO_3^-] or a decrease in P_{CO_2}, inhibits secretion of H⁺ secondary to an increase in the intracellular pH of nephron cells. Thus, the responses just described for the renal adaptation to acidosis are reversed.

Table 36-1 also lists other factors that influence secretion of H⁺ by cells of the nephron. However, these factors are not directly related to the maintenance of acid-base balance. Because H⁺ secretion in the proximal tubule and thick ascending limb of the loop of Henle is linked to the reabsorption of Na⁺ (via the Na⁺-H⁺ antiporter), factors that alter Na⁺ reabsorption secondarily affect H⁺ secretion. For example, the process of glomerulotubular balance ensures that the reabsorption rate of the proximal tubule is matched to the glomerular filtration rate (GFR) (see Chapter 33). Thus, when the GFR is increased, the filtered load to the proximal tubule is increased, and more fluid (including HCO_3^-) is reabsorbed. Conversely, a decrease in the filtered load results in decreased reabsorption of fluid and thus HCO_3^-.

Alterations in Na⁺ balance, through changes in ECF volume, also have an impact on H⁺ secretion. With volume contraction (negative Na⁺ balance), secretion of H⁺ is enhanced. This occurs via several mechanisms. One mechanism involves the renin-angiotensin-aldosterone system, which is activated by volume contraction and leads to enhanced reabsorption of Na⁺ by the nephron (see Chapter 34). Angiotensin II acts on the proximal tubule to stimulate the apical membrane Na⁺-H⁺ antiporter, as well as the basolateral 1Na⁺-3HCO₃⁻ symporter. This stimulatory effect includes increased activity of the transporters and exocytotic insertion of transporters into the membrane. To a lesser degree, angiotensin II stimulates H⁺ secretion in the early portion of the distal tubule, a process also mediated by the Na⁺-H⁺ antiporter. Aldosterone's primary action on the distal tubule and collecting duct is to stimulate Na⁺ reabsorption by principal cells (see Chapter 33). However, it also stimulates intercalated cells in these segments to secrete H⁺. This effect is both indirect and direct. By stimulating Na⁺ reabsorption by principal cells, aldosterone hyperpolarizes the transepithelial voltage (i.e., the lumen becomes more electrically negative). This change in transepithelial voltage then facilitates the secretion of H⁺ by the intercalated cells. In addition to this indirect effect, aldosterone acts directly on intercalated cells to stimulate

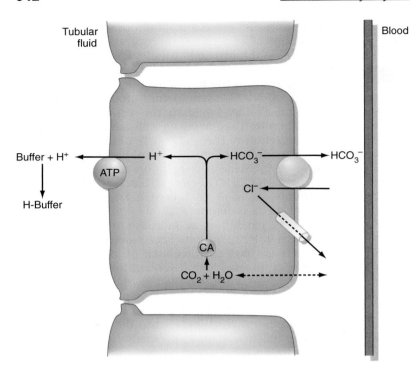

● **Figure 36-4.** General scheme for the excretion of H^+ with non-HCO_3^- urinary buffers (titratable acid). The primary urinary buffer is phosphate (HPO_4^{-2}). An H^+-secreting intercalated cell is shown. For simplicity, only the H^+-ATPase is depicted. H^+ secretion by H^+-K^+-ATPase also titrates luminal buffers. CA, carbonic anhydrase.

H^+ secretion. The precise mechanism or mechanisms for this stimulatory effect are not fully understood.

Another mechanism by which ECF volume contraction enhances H^+ secretion (HCO_3^- reabsorption) is via changes in peritubular capillary Starling forces. As described in Chapters 33 and 34, ECF volume contraction alters the peritubular capillary Starling forces such that overall proximal tubule reabsorption is enhanced. With this enhanced reabsorption, more of the filtered load of HCO_3^- is reabsorbed.

With volume expansion (positive Na^+ balance), secretion of H^+ is reduced because of low levels of angiotensin II and aldosterone, as well as alterations in peritubular Starling forces that reduce overall proximal tubule reabsorption.

Parathyroid hormone (PTH) has both inhibitory and stimulatory effect on renal H^+ secretion. Acutely, PTH inhibits H^+ secretion by the proximal tubule by inhibiting the activity of the Na^+-H^+ antiporter and by also causing the antiporter to be endocytosed from the apical membrane. Long-term, PTH stimulates renal acid excretion by acting on the thick ascending limb of Henle's loop and the distal tubule. Because secretion of PTH is increased during acidosis, this long-term stimulatory effect on renal acid excretion is a component of the renal response to acidosis. The stimulatory effect of PTH on acid excretion is due in part to the delivery of increased amounts of P_i to more distal nephron sites, where it is then titrated and excreted as titratable acid.*

Finally, K^+ balance influences secretion of H^+ by the proximal tubule. Hypokalemia stimulates and hyperkalemia inhibits H^+ secretion. It is thought that K^+-induced changes in intracellular pH are responsible, at least in part, for this effect, with hypokalemia acidifying and hyperkalemia alkalinizing the cells. Hypokalemia also stimulates H^+ secretion by the collecting duct. This occurs as a result of increased expression of H^+-K^+-ATPase in the intercalated cells.

Formation of New HCO_3^-

As discussed previously, reabsorption of the filtered load of HCO_3^- is important for maximizing net acid excretion. However, HCO_3^- reabsorption alone does not replenish the HCO_3^- lost during neutralization of the nonvolatile acids produced during metabolism. To maintain acid-base balance, the kidneys must replace this lost HCO_3^- with new HCO_3^-. Generation of new HCO_3^- is achieved by the excretion of titratable acid and by the synthesis and excretion of NH_4^+.

The production of new HCO_3^- as a result of excretion of titratable acid is depicted in Figure 36-4. Because of HCO_3^- reabsorption by the proximal tubule and loop of Henle, fluid reaching the distal tubule and collecting duct normally contains little HCO_3^-. Thus, when H^+ is secreted, it will combine with non-HCO_3^- buffers (primarily P_i) and be excreted as titratable acid. Because the H^+ was produced inside the cell from the hydration of CO_2, HCO_3^- is also produced. This HCO_3^- is returned to the ECF as new HCO_3^-. As noted, P_i excretion increases with acidosis. However, even with increased P_i available for the formation of titratable acid, this response is insufficient to generate the required amount of new HCO_3^-. The remainder of new HCO_3^- generation occurs as a result of NH_4^+ production and excretion.

---

*As described in Chapter 35, one of the important actions of PTH is to inhibit reabsorption of P_i by the proximal tubule. In so doing, more P_i is delivered to downstream nephron segments, where it is available for titration and excretion as titratable acid.

NH_4^+ is produced by the kidneys, and its synthesis and subsequent excretion add HCO_3^- to the ECF. Importantly, this process is regulated in response to the acid-base requirements of the body.

NH_4^+ is produced in the kidneys via the metabolism of **glutamine.** Essentially, the kidneys metabolize glutamine, excrete NH_4^+, and add HCO_3^- to the body. However, the formation of new HCO_3^- via this process depends on the kidneys' ability to excrete NH_4^+ in urine. If NH_4^+ is not excreted in urine but enters the systemic circulation instead, it is converted to urea by the liver. This conversion process generates H^+, which is then buffered by HCO_3^-. Thus, production of urea from renally generated NH_4^+ consumes HCO_3^- and negates the formation of HCO_3^- through the synthesis and excretion of NH_4^+ by the kidneys.

The process by which the kidneys excrete NH_4^+ is complex. Figure 36-5 illustrates the essential features

of this process. NH_4^+ is produced from glutamine in the cells of the proximal tubule, a process termed **ammoniagenesis.** Each glutamine molecule produces two molecules of NH_4^+ and the divalent anion 2-oxoglutarate^{-2}. Metabolism of this anion ultimately provides two molecules of HCO_3^-. The HCO_3^- exits the cell across the basolateral membrane and enters the peritubular blood as new HCO_3^-. NH_4^+ exits the cell across the apical membrane and enters the tubular fluid. The primary mechanism for secretion of NH_4^+ into tubular fluid involves the Na^+-H^+ antiporter, with NH_4^+ substituting for H^+. In addition, NH_3 can diffuse out of the cell across the plasma membrane into tubular fluid, where it is protonated to NH_4^+.

A significant proportion of the NH_4^+ secreted by the proximal tubule is reabsorbed by the loop of Henle. The thick ascending limb is the primary site of this NH_4^+ reabsorption, with NH_4^+ substituting for K^+ on the

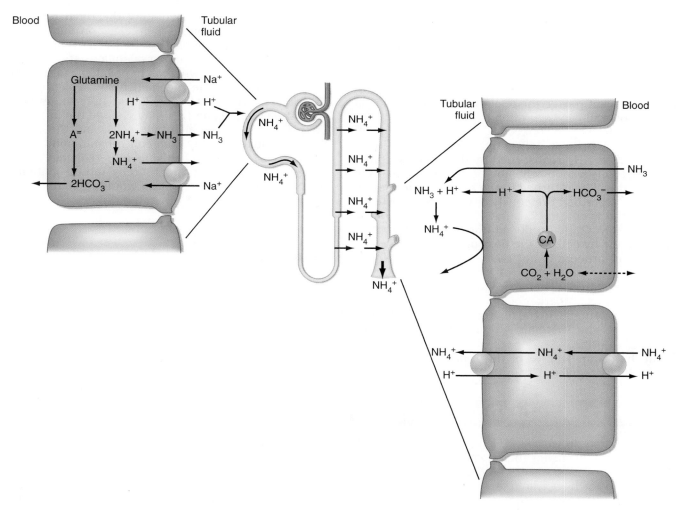

● **Figure 36-5.**   Production, transport, and excretion of NH_4^+ by the nephron. Glutamine is metabolized to NH_4^+ and HCO_3^- in the proximal tubule. The NH_4^+ is secreted into the lumen, and the HCO_3^- enters the blood. The secreted NH_4^+ is reabsorbed in Henle's loop primarily by the thick ascending limb and accumulates in the medullary interstitium. NH_4^+ is secreted by the collecting duct via nonionic diffusion and diffusion trapping, as well as by NH_4^+ antiporters. Both secretory processes require secretion of H^+ by the collecting duct. For each molecule of NH_4^+ excreted in urine, a molecule of "new" HCO_3^- is added back to the ECF. CA, carbonic anhydrase.

$1Na^+$-$1K^+$-$2Cl^-$ symporter. In addition, the positive transepithelial luminal voltage in this segment drives the paracellular reabsorption of NH_4^+.

The NH_4^+ reabsorbed by the thick ascending limb of the loop of Henle accumulates in the medullary interstitium. From there it is then secreted into tubular fluid by the collecting duct. Two mechanisms for secretion of NH_4^+ by the collecting duct have been identified. The first is **nonionic diffusion** and **diffusion trapping.** By this mechanism, NH_3 diffuses from the medullary interstitium into the lumen of the collecting duct. As previously described, H^+ secretion by the intercalated cells of the collecting duct acidifies the luminal fluid (a luminal fluid pH as low as 4.0 to 4.5 can be achieved). Consequently, NH_3 diffusing from the medullary interstitium into the collecting duct lumen (nonionic diffusion) is protonated to NH_4^+ by the acidic tubular fluid. Because the collecting duct is less permeable to NH_4^+ than to NH_3, NH_4^+ is trapped in the tubule lumen (diffusion trapping) and eliminated from the body in urine. The second mechanism involves NH_4^+-H^+ antiporters located in the basolateral and apical membranes of the collecting duct cells (see Fig. 36-5). Because acidification of the tubular fluid drives both nonionic diffusion and diffusion trapping, as well as secretion of NH_4^+ across the apical membrane by the NH_4^+-H^+ antiporter, the relative role of each mechanism to overall NH_4^+ secretion is not known.

H^+ secretion by the collecting duct is critical for the excretion of NH_4^+. If collecting duct H^+ secretion is inhibited, the NH_4^+ reabsorbed by the thick ascending limb of Henle's loop will not be excreted in urine. Instead, it will be returned to the systemic circulation, where as described previously, it will be converted to urea by the liver and consume HCO_3^- in the process. Thus, new HCO_3^- is produced during the metabolism of glutamine by cells of the proximal tubule. However, the overall process is not complete until the NH_4^+ is excreted (i.e., production of urea from NH_4^+ by the liver is prevented). Therefore, NH_4^+ excretion in urine can be used as a "marker" of glutamine metabolism in the proximal tubule. In the net result, one new HCO_3^- is returned to the systemic circulation for each NH_4^+ excreted in urine.

An important feature of the renal NH_4^+ system is that it can be regulated by systemic acid-base balance.

AT THE CELLULAR LEVEL

The NH_4^+ transporters (RhBG and RhCG) are termed rhesus glycoproteins for their homology to the rhesus proteins found on the surface of erythrocytes that are responsible for hemolytic diseases and blood transfusion reactions. These transporters have been localized to the late portion of the distal tubule and the collecting duct. RhBG is localized to the basolateral membrane, whereas RhCG is localized to the apical membrane (in some species, RhCG is also found in the basolateral membrane). Both transporters appear to function as NH_4^+-H^+ antiporters.

An alteration in the pH of the ECF, by affecting the pH of the ICF, changes glutamine metabolism in the cells of the proximal tubule. In addition, as already noted, cortisol levels increase during acidosis and cortisol stimulates ammoniagenesis (i.e., NH_4^+ production from glutamine). During systemic acidosis, the enzymes in the proximal tubule cell that are responsible for the metabolism of glutamine are stimulated. This involves the synthesis of new enzyme and requires several days for complete adaptation. With increased levels of these enzymes, NH_4^+ production is increased, thereby allowing enhanced production of new HCO_3^-. Conversely, glutamine metabolism is reduced with alkalosis.

Acidosis also increases the abundance of RhCG in the medullary portion of the collecting duct. Thus, the ability to secrete NH_4^+ is enhanced.

Other factors also influence ammoniagenesis. Both angiotensin II and PTH stimulate ammoniagenesis, whereas ammoniagenesis is inhibited by prostaglandins. Because PTH levels are increased with acidosis, it may play a role in mediating the renal response, which as noted, includes increased production and excretion of NH_4^+. Finally, the $[K^+]$ of ECF also alters NH_4^+ production. When hyperkalemia exists, NH_4^+ production is inhibited, whereas hypokalemia stimulates NH_4^+ production. The mechanism by which plasma $[K^+]$ alters NH_4^+ production is not fully understood. Alterations in plasma $[K^+]$ may change the intracellular pH of the proximal tubule cells, and the change in intracellular pH may then control glutamine metabolism. Via this mechanism, hyperkalemia would raise intracellular pH and thereby inhibit glutamine metabolism. The opposite would occur during hypokalemia.

IN THE CLINIC

Assessing NH_4^+ excretion by the kidneys is done indirectly because assays of urine NH_4^+ are not routinely available. Consider, for example, the situation of metabolic acidosis. In metabolic acidosis, the appropriate renal response is to increase net acid excretion. Accordingly, little or no HCO_3^- will appear in urine, the urine will be acidic, and NH_4^+ excretion will be increased. To assess this and especially the amount of NH_4^+ excreted, the "urinary net charge" or "urine anion gap" can be calculated by measuring the urinary concentrations of Na^+, K^+, and Cl^-.

$$\text{Urine anion gap} = [Na^+] + [K^+] - [Cl^-]$$

The concept of urine anion gap during metabolic acidosis assumes that the major cations in urine are Na^+, K^+, and NH_4^+ and that the major anion is Cl^- (with urine pH <6.5, virtually no HCO_3^- is present). As a result, the urine anion gap will yield a negative value when adequate amounts of NH_4^+ are being excreted. Indeed, the absence of a urine anion gap or the existence of a positive value indicates a renal defect in NH_4^+ production and excretion.

IN THE CLINIC

Renal tubule acidosis (RTA) refers to conditions in which net acid excretion by the kidneys is impaired. Under these conditions the kidneys are unable to excrete a sufficient amount of net acid to balance non-volatile acid production, and acidosis results. RTA can be caused by a defect in H^+ secretion in the proximal tubule **(proximal RTA)** or distal tubule **(distal RTA)** or by inadequate production and excretion of NH_4^+.

Proximal RTA can be caused by a variety of hereditary and acquired conditions (e.g., **cystinosis, Fanconi's syndrome,** administration of carbonic anhydrase inhibitors). The majority of cases of proximal RTA are acquired and reflect generalized tubule dysfunction rather than a selective defect in one of the proximal tubule acid-base transporters. However, autosomal recessive and autosomal dominant forms of proximal RTA have been identified. An autosomal recessive form of proximal RTA results from a defect in the $1Na^+$-$3HCO_3^-$ symporter (NBC1). Because this transporter is also expressed in the eye, these patients have ocular abnormalities as well. Another autosomal recessive form of proximal RTA occurs in individuals who lack carbonic anhydrase (CA-II). Because CA-II is required for normal distal acidification, this defect also includes a distal RTA component. Finally, an autosomal dominant form of proximal RTA has been identified. However, the transporter involved has not been identified. Regardless of the cause, if H^+ secretion by cells of the proximal tubule is impaired, reabsorption of the filtered load of HCO_3^- is decreased. Consequently, HCO_3^- is lost in urine, plasma $[HCO_3^-]$ decreases, and acidosis ensues.

Distal RTA also occurs in a number of hereditary and acquired conditions (e.g., **medullary sponge kidney,** certain drugs such as **amphotericin B,** and conditions secondary to urinary obstruction). Like the inherited forms of proximal RTA, the inherited forms of distal RTA are rare. Both autosomal dominant and autosomal recessive forms of distal RTA have been identified. An autosomal dominant form results from mutations in the gene coding for the Cl^--HCO_3^- antiporter (AE-1) in the basolateral membrane of the acid-secreting intercalated cell. Autosomal recessive forms are caused by mutations in various subunits of H^+-ATPase. In some patients with Sjögren's syndrome, an autoimmune disease, distal RTA develops as a result of antibodies directed against H^+-ATPase. Finally, H^+ secretion by the distal tubule and collecting duct may be normal, but the permeability of the cells to H^+ is increased. This occurs with the antifungal drug amphotericin B, administration of which also leads to the development of distal RTA. Regardless of the cause of distal RTA, the ability to acidify tubular fluid in the distal tubule and collecting duct is impaired. Consequently, excretion of titratable acid and NH_4^+ is reduced. This in turn decreases net acid excretion, with the subsequent development of acidosis.

Failure to produce and excrete sufficient quantities of NH_4^+ can also reduce net acid excretion by the kidneys. This situation occurs as a result of generalized dysfunction of the distal tubule and collecting duct with impaired secretion of H^+, NH_4^+, and K^+. Generalized distal nephron dysfunction is seen in individuals with mutations in the epithelial Na^+ channel (ENaC), which is inherited in an autosomal recessive pattern. An autosomal dominant form is also seen with mutations in the mineralocorticoid receptor. More commonly, NH_4^+ production and excretion are impaired in patients with hyporeninemic hypoaldosteronism. These patients typically have moderate degrees of renal failure with reduced levels of renin and thus aldosterone. As a result, distal tubule and collecting duct function are impaired. Finally, a number of drugs can also result in distal tubule and collecting duct dysfunction, including drugs that block the Na^+ channel (e.g., amiloride), block the production or action of angiotensin II (angiotensin-converting enzyme inhibitors), or block the action of aldosterone (e.g., spironolactone). Regardless of the cause, the impaired function of the distal tubule and collecting duct results in the development of hyperkalemia, which in turn impairs ammoniagenesis by the proximal tubule. H^+ secretion by the distal tubule and collecting duct and thus NH_4^+ secretion are also impaired by these drugs. Thus, net acid excretion is less than net acid production, and metabolic acidosis develops.

If the acidosis that results from any of these forms of RTA is severe, individuals must ingest alkali (e.g., baking soda or a citrate-containing solution*) to maintain acid-base balance. In this way the HCO_3^- lost each day in the buffering of nonvolatile acid is replenished by the extra HCO_3^- ingested in the diet.

---

*One of the byproducts of citrate metabolism is HCO_3^-. Ingestion of citrate-containing drinks is often more palatable to patients than ingesting baking soda.

RESPONSE TO ACID-BASE DISORDERS

The pH of ECF is maintained within a very narrow range (7.35 to 7.45).* Inspection of Equation 36-3 shows that the pH of ECF varies when either $[HCO_3^-]$ or P_{CO_2} is altered. As already noted, disturbances in acid-base balance that result from a change in ECF $[HCO_3^-]$ are termed **metabolic acid-base disorders,** whereas those resulting from a change in P_{CO_2} are termed **respiratory acid-base disorders.** The kidneys are primarily responsible for regulating $[HCO_3^-]$, whereas the lungs regulate P_{CO_2}.

When an acid-base disturbance develops, the body uses a series of mechanisms to defend against the change in pH of the ECF. These defense mechanisms do not correct the acid-base disturbance but merely

---

*For simplicity of presentation in this chapter, the value of 7.40 for body fluid pH is used as normal, even though the normal range is 7.35 to 7.45. Similarly, the normal range for P_{CO_2} is 35 to 45 mm Hg. However, a P_{CO_2} of 40 mm Hg is used as the normal value. Finally, a value of 24 mEq/L is considered a normal ECF $[HCO_3^-]$, even though the normal range is 22 to 28 mEq/L.

minimize the change in pH imposed by the disturbance. Restoration of blood pH to its normal value requires correction of the underlying process or processes that produced the acid-base disorder. The body has three general mechanisms to compensate for or defend against changes in body fluid pH produced by acid-base disturbances: (1) extracellular and intracellular buffering, (2) adjustments in blood P_{CO_2} via alterations in the ventilatory rate of the lungs, and (3) adjustments in renal net acid excretion.

Extracellular and Intracellular Buffers

The first line of defense against acid-base disorders is extracellular and intracellular buffering. The response of the extracellular buffers is virtually instantaneous, whereas the response to intracellular buffering is slower and can take several minutes.

Metabolic disorders that result from the addition of nonvolatile acid or alkali to body fluids are buffered in both the ECF and ICF compartments. The HCO_3^- buffer system is the principal ECF buffer. When nonvolatile acid is added to body fluids (or alkali is lost from the body), HCO_3^- is consumed during the process of neutralizing the acid load, and the $[HCO_3^-]$ of ECF is reduced. Conversely, when nonvolatile alkali is added to body fluids (or acid is lost from the body), H^+ is consumed, which causes more HCO_3^- to be produced from the dissociation of H_2CO_3. Consequently, $[HCO_3^-]$ increases.

Although the HCO_3^- buffer system is the principal ECF buffer, P_i and plasma proteins provide additional extracellular buffering. The combined action of the buffering processes for HCO_3^-, P_i, and plasma protein accounts for approximately 50% of the buffering of a nonvolatile acid load and 70% of a nonvolatile alkali load. The remainder of the buffering under these two conditions occurs intracellularly. Intracellular buffering involves the movement of H^+ into cells (during buffering of nonvolatile acid) or the movement of H^+ out of cells (during buffering of nonvolatile alkali). H^+ is titrated inside the cell by HCO_3^-, P_i, and the histidine groups on proteins.

Bone represents an additional source of extracellular buffering. With acidosis, buffering by bone results in its demineralization because Ca^{++} is released from bone as Ca^{++}-containing salts bind H^+ in exchange for Ca^{++}.

When respiratory acid-base disorders occur, the pH of body fluid changes as a result of alterations in P_{CO_2}. Virtually all buffering in respiratory acid-base disorders occurs intracellularly. When P_{CO_2} rises (respiratory acidosis), CO_2 moves into the cell, where it combines with H_2O to form H_2CO_3, which then dissociates to H^+ and HCO_3^-. Some of the H^+ is buffered by cellular protein, and HCO_3^- exits the cell and raises ECF $[HCO_3^-]$ (ECF $[H^+]$ is also increased). This process is reversed when P_{CO_2} is reduced (respiratory alkalosis). Under this condition, the hydration reaction ($H_2O + CO_2 \leftrightarrow H_2CO_3$) is shifted to the left by the decrease in P_{CO_2}. As a result, the dissociation reaction ($H_2CO_3 \leftrightarrow H^+ + HCO_3^-$) also shifts to the left, thereby reducing ECF $[HCO_3^-]$ (ECF $[H^+]$ is also decreased). Thus, the CO_2-associated changes in ECF $[HCO_3^-]$ minimize the change in pH.

Respiratory Compensation

The lungs are the second line of defense against acid-base disorders. As indicated by the Henderson-Hasselbalch equation (Equation 36-3), changes in P_{CO_2} alter blood pH: a rise decreases pH, and a reduction increases pH.

The ventilatory rate determines P_{CO_2}. Increased ventilation decreases P_{CO_2}, whereas decreased ventilation increases it. Blood P_{CO_2} and pH are important regulators of the ventilatory rate. Chemoreceptors located in the brainstem (ventral surface of the medulla) and periphery (carotid and aortic bodies) sense changes in P_{CO_2} and $[H^+]$ and alter the ventilatory rate appropriately. Thus, when metabolic acidosis occurs, a rise in $[H^+]$ (decrease in pH) increases the ventilatory rate. Conversely, during metabolic alkalosis, a decrease in $[H^+]$ (increase in pH) leads to a reduced ventilatory rate. With maximal hyperventilation, P_{CO_2} can be reduced to approximately 10 mm Hg. Because hypoxia, a potent stimulator of ventilation, also develops with hypoventilation, the degree to which P_{CO_2} can be increased is limited. In an otherwise normal individual, hypoventilation cannot raise P_{CO_2} above 60 mm Hg. The respiratory response to metabolic acid-base disturbances may be initiated within minutes but could require several hours to complete.

Renal Compensation

The third and final line of defense against acid-base disorders is the kidneys. In response to an alteration in plasma pH and P_{CO_2}, the kidneys make appropriate adjustments in the excretion of HCO_3^- and net acid. The renal response may require several days to reach completion because it takes hours to days to increase the synthesis and activity of the proximal tubule enzymes involved in NH_4^+ production. In the case of acidosis (increased $[H^+]$ or P_{CO_2}), secretion of H^+ by the nephron is stimulated, and the entire filtered load of HCO_3^- is reabsorbed. Excretion of titratable acid is increased, production and excretion of NH_4^+ are also stimulated, and net acid excretion by the kidneys is thus increased (Equation 36-7). The new HCO_3^- generated during the process of net acid excretion is added to the body, and plasma $[HCO_3^-]$ increases.

> ### ▶ IN THE CLINIC
>
> Metabolic acidosis can develop in insulin-dependent diabetic patients secondary to the production of keto acids if insulin dosages are not adequate. As a compensatory response to this acidosis, deep and rapid breathing develops. This breathing pattern is termed Kussmaul respiration. With prolonged Kussmaul respiration, the muscles involved can become fatigued. When fatigue occurs, respiratory compensation is impaired and the acidosis can become more severe.

Loss of gastric contents from the body (i.e., vomiting, nasogastric suction) produces metabolic alkalosis secondary to the loss of HCl. If the loss of gastric fluid is significant, ECF volume contraction occurs. Under this condition, the kidneys cannot excrete sufficient quantities of HCO_3^- to compensate for the metabolic alkalosis. Excretion of HCO_3^- is impaired because ECF volume contraction reduces the filtered load of HCO_3^- (GFR is decreased) and stimulates HCO_3^- reabsorption by the nephron. ECF volume contraction stimulates HCO_3^- reabsorption because of the need for the kidneys to reduce Na^+ excretion (see Chapter 34). Thus, in response to ECF volume contraction, Na^+ reabsorption by the proximal tubule is enhanced and aldosterone levels are increased. These responses in turn limit HCO_3^- excretion because a significant amount of Na^+ reabsorption in the proximal tubule is coupled to H^+ secretion via the Na^+-H^+ antiporter. As a result, HCO_3^- is reabsorbed because of the need to reduce Na^+ excretion. In addition, the elevated aldosterone levels stimulate not only Na^+ reabsorption but also H^+ secretion by the distal tubule and collecting duct. Thus, in individuals who lose gastric contents, the metabolic alkalosis is seen in the setting of a paradoxically acidic urine. Correction of the alkalosis occurs only when euvolemia is reestablished. With restoration of euvolemia, the filtered load of HCO_3^- increases (GFR increases), and HCO_3^- reabsorption by the proximal tubule decreases, as does H^+ secretion by the distal tubule and collecting duct. As a result, HCO_3^- excretion increases, and ECF $[HCO_3^-]$ returns to normal.

● Table 36-2.
Characteristics of Simple Acid-Base Disorders

Disorder	Plasma pH	Primary Alteration	Defense Mechanisms
Metabolic acidosis	↓	↓ECF $[HCO_3^-]$	ICF and ECF buffers Hyperventilation (↓PCO_2) ↑Renal NAE
Metabolic alkalosis	↑	↑ECF $[HCO_3^-]$	ICF and ECF buffers Hypoventilation (↑PCO_2) ↓Renal NAE
Respiratory acidosis	↓	↑PCO_2	ICF buffers ↑Renal NAE
Respiratory alkalosis	↑	↓PCO_2	ICF buffers ↓Renal NAE

ECF, extracellular fluid; ICF, intracellular fluid; NAE, net acid excretion.

nonvolatile acid to the body (e.g., diabetic ketoacidosis), loss of nonvolatile base (e.g., HCO_3^- loss caused by diarrhea), or failure of the kidneys to excrete sufficient net acid to replenish the HCO_3^- used to neutralize nonvolatile acids (e.g., renal tubular acidosis, renal failure). As previously described, buffering of H^+ occurs in both the ECF and ICF compartments. When pH falls, the respiratory centers are stimulated, and the ventilatory rate is increased (respiratory compensation). This reduces PCO_2, which further minimizes the fall in plasma pH. In general, there is a 1.2–mm Hg decrease in PCO_2 for every 1-mEq/L fall in ECF $[HCO_3^-]$. Thus, if $[HCO_3^-]$ were reduced to 14 mEq/L from a normal value of 24 mEq/L, the expected decrease in PCO_2 would be 12 mm Hg and the measured PCO_2 would fall to 28 mm Hg (normal $PCO_2 = 40$ mm Hg).

Finally, in metabolic acidosis, renal net acid excretion is increased. This occurs via the elimination of all HCO_3^- from urine (enhanced reabsorption of filtered HCO_3^-) and via increased excretion of titratable acid and NH_4^+ (enhanced production of new HCO_3^-). If the process that initiated the acid-base disturbance is corrected, the enhanced net acid excretion by the kidneys will ultimately return the pH and $[HCO_3^-]$ to normal. After correction of the pH, the ventilatory rate also returns to normal.

When alkalosis exists (decreased $[H^+]$ or PCO_2), the filtered load of HCO_3^- is increased (plasma $[HCO_3^-]$ is elevated), and secretion of H^+ by the nephron is inhibited. As a result, HCO_3^- excretion is increased, and the excretion of both titratable acid and NH_4^+ is decreased. Thus, net acid excretion is decreased and HCO_3^- appears in urine. In addition, some HCO_3^- is secreted into urine by the HCO_3^--secreting intercalated cells of the distal tubule and collecting duct. With enhanced excretion of HCO_3^-, plasma $[HCO_3^-]$ decreases.

SIMPLE ACID-BASE DISORDERS

Table 36-2 summarizes the primary alterations and the subsequent compensatory or defense mechanisms of the various simple acid-base disorders. In all acid-base disorders the compensatory response does not correct the underlying disorder but simply reduces the magnitude of the change in pH. Correction of the acid-base disorder requires treatment of its cause.

Types of Acid-Base Disorders

Metabolic Acidosis
Metabolic acidosis is characterized by decreased ECF $[HCO_3^-]$ and pH. It can develop via the addition of

Metabolic Alkalosis
Metabolic alkalosis is characterized by increased ECF $[HCO_3^-]$ and pH. It can occur via the addition of nonvolatile base to the body (e.g., ingestion of antacids), as a result of volume contraction (e.g., hemorrhage), or more commonly, from the loss of nonvolatile acid (e.g., loss of gastric HCl because of prolonged vomiting). Buffering occurs predominantly in the ECF compartment and to a lesser degree in the ICF compartment. The increase in pH inhibits the respiratory centers, the ventilatory rate is reduced, and thus PCO_2 is elevated (respiratory compensation). With appropriate respiratory compensation, a 0.7–mm Hg increase in PCO_2 is expected for every 1-mEq/L rise in ECF $[HCO_3^-]$.

The primary renal compensatory response to metabolic alkalosis is to increase the excretion of HCO_3^- by reducing its reabsorption along the nephron.

▶ IN THE CLINIC

When nonvolatile acid is added to body fluids, as in **diabetic ketoacidosis,** [H$^+$] increases (pH decreases), and [HCO$_3^-$] decreases. In addition, the concentration of the anion associated with the nonvolatile acid increases. This change in anion concentration provides a convenient way of analyzing the cause of a metabolic acidosis by calculating what is termed the **anion gap.** The anion gap represents the difference between the concentration of the major ECF cation (Na$^+$) and the major ECF anions (Cl$^-$ and HCO$_3^-$):

$$\text{Anion gap} = [\text{Na}^+] - ([\text{Cl}^-] + [\text{HCO}_3^-])$$

Under normal conditions the anion gap ranges from 8 to 16 mEq/L. It is important to recognize that an anion gap does not actually exist. All cations are balanced by anions. The gap simply reflects the parameters that are measured. In reality,

$$[\text{Na}^+] + [\text{Unmeasured cations}] =$$
$$[\text{Cl}^-] + [\text{HCO}_3^-] + [\text{Unmeasured anions}]$$

If the anion of the nonvolatile acid is Cl$^-$, the anion gap will be normal. (That is, the decrease in [HCO$_3^-$] is matched by an increase in [Cl$^-$].) The metabolic acidosis associated with diarrhea or renal tubular acidosis has a normal anion gap. In contrast, if the anion of the nonvolatile acid is not Cl$^-$ (e.g., lactate, β-hydroxybutyrate), the anion gap will increase (i.e., the decrease in [HCO$_3^-$] is not matched by an increase in [Cl$^-$] but rather by an increase in concentration of the unmeasured anion). The anion gap is increased in metabolic acidosis associated with renal failure, diabetes mellitus (ketoacidosis), lactic acidosis, and the ingestion of large quantities of aspirin. Thus, calculation of the anion gap is a useful way of identifying the cause of metabolic acidosis in the clinical setting.

Excretion of titratable acid and NH$_4^+$ is also reduced. Normally, this occurs quite rapidly (minutes to hours) and effectively. However, as already noted, when alkalosis occurs with ECF volume contraction (e.g., vomiting in which fluid loss occurs with H$^+$ loss), HCO$_3^-$ excretion is impaired. In individuals with ECF volume contraction, renal excretion of HCO$_3^-$ is enhanced, and the alkalosis is corrected only with restoration of euvolemia. Enhanced renal excretion of HCO$_3^-$ eventually returns the pH and [HCO$_3^-$] to normal, provided that the underlying cause of the initial acid-base disturbance is corrected. When the pH is corrected, the ventilatory rate also returns to normal.

Respiratory Acidosis

Respiratory acidosis is characterized by an elevated PCO$_2$ and reduced ECF pH. It results from decreased gas exchange across the alveoli as a result of either inadequate ventilation (e.g., drug-induced depression of the respiratory centers) or impaired gas diffusion (e.g., pulmonary edema, such as occurs in cardiovascular or lung disease). In contrast to the metabolic disorders, buffering during respiratory acidosis occurs almost entirely in the ICF compartment. The increase in PCO$_2$ and the decrease in pH stimulate both reabsorption of HCO$_3^-$ by the nephron and excretion of titratable acid and NH$_4^+$ (renal compensation). Together, these responses increase net acid excretion and generate new HCO$_3^-$. The renal compensatory response takes several days to occur. Consequently, respiratory acid-base disorders are commonly divided into acute and chronic phases. In the acute phase, the time needed for the renal compensatory response to take effect is not sufficient, and the body relies on ICF buffering to minimize the change in pH. During this phase and because of this buffering there is a 1-mEq/L increase in ECF [HCO$_3^-$] for every 10–mm Hg rise in PCO$_2$. In the chronic phase, renal compensation takes place, and a 3.5-mEq/L increase in ECF [HCO$_3^-$] occurs for each 10–mm Hg rise in PCO$_2$. Correction of the underlying disorder returns the PCO$_2$ to normal, and renal net acid excretion decreases to its initial level.

Respiratory Alkalosis

Respiratory alkalosis is characterized by reduced PCO$_2$ and increased ECF pH. It results from increased gas exchange in the lungs, usually caused by increased ventilation from stimulation of the respiratory centers (e.g., via drugs or disorders of the central nervous system). Hyperventilation also occurs at high altitude and as a result of anxiety, pain, or fear. As noted, buffering primarily takes place in the ICF compartment. As with respiratory acidosis, respiratory alkalosis has both acute and chronic phases reflecting the time required for renal compensation to occur. In the acute phase of respiratory alkalosis, which reflects intracellular buffering, ECF [HCO$_3^-$] decreases 2 mEq/L for every 10–mm Hg fall in PCO$_2$. With renal compensation, the elevated pH and reduced PCO$_2$ inhibit reabsorption of HCO$_3^-$ by the nephron and reduce excretion of titratable acid and NH$_4^+$. As a result of these two effects, net acid excretion is reduced. With complete renal compensation there is an expected 5-mEq/L decrease in ECF [HCO$_3^-$] for every 10–mm Hg reduction in PCO$_2$. Correction of the underlying disorder returns the PCO$_2$ to normal, and renal excretion of acid then increases to its initial level.

Analysis of Acid-Base Disorders

Analysis of an acid-base disorder is directed at identifying the underlying cause so that appropriate therapy can be initiated. The patient's medical history and associated physical findings often provide valuable clues about the nature and origin of an acid-base disorder. In addition, analysis of an arterial blood sample is frequently required. Such analysis is straightforward if approached systematically. For example, consider the following data:

$$\text{pH} = 7.35$$
$$[\text{HCO}_3^-] = 16 \text{ mEq/L}$$
$$\text{PCO}_2 = 30 \text{ mm Hg}$$

The acid-base disorder represented by these values, or any other set of values, can be determined by using the following three-step approach (Fig. 36-6):

●**Figure 36-6.**   Approach for the analysis of simple acid-base disorders.

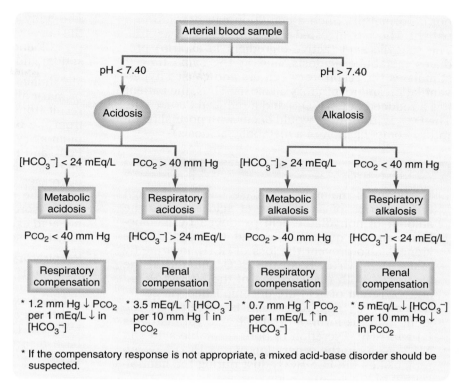

* If the compensatory response is not appropriate, a mixed acid-base disorder should be suspected.

1. *Evaluation of pH:* When the pH is considered first, the underlying disorder can be classified as either an acidosis or an alkalosis. The defense mechanisms of the body cannot correct an acid-base disorder by themselves. Thus, even if the defense mechanisms are completely operative, the change in pH indicates the acid-base disorder. In the example provided, a pH of 7.35 indicates acidosis.

2. *Determination of a metabolic versus a respiratory disorder:* Simple acid-base disorders are either metabolic or respiratory. To determine which disorder is present, the clinician must next examine ECF [HCO_3^-] and P_{CO_2}. As discussed previously, acidosis could be the result of a decrease in [HCO_3^-] (metabolic) or an increase in P_{CO_2} (respiratory). Alternatively, alkalosis could be the result of an increase in ECF [HCO_3^-] (metabolic) or a decrease in P_{CO_2} (respiratory). For the example provided, ECF [HCO_3^-] is reduced from normal (normal = 24 mEq/L), as is the P_{CO_2} (normal = 40 mm Hg). The disorder must therefore be metabolic acidosis; it cannot be a respiratory acidosis because the P_{CO_2} is reduced.

3. *Analysis of a compensatory response:* Metabolic disorders result in compensatory changes in ventilation and thus in P_{CO_2}, whereas respiratory disorders result in compensatory changes in renal net acid excretion and thus in ECF [HCO_3^-]. In an appropriately compensated metabolic acidosis, P_{CO_2} is decreased, whereas it is elevated in compensated metabolic alkalosis. With respiratory acidosis, complete compensation results in an elevation in [HCO_3^-]. Conversely, ECF [HCO_3^-] is reduced in response to respiratory alkalosis. In this example, P_{CO_2} is

reduced from normal, and the magnitude of this reduction (10–mm Hg decrease in P_{CO_2} for an 8-mEq/L increase in ECF [HCO_3^-]) is as expected (Fig. 36-6). Therefore, the acid-base disorder is a simple metabolic acidosis with appropriate respiratory compensation.

If the appropriate compensatory response is not present, a **mixed acid-base disorder** should be suspected. Such a disorder reflects the presence of two or more underlying causes of the acid-base disturbance. A mixed disorder should be suspected when arterial blood gas analysis indicates that appropriate compensation has not occurred. For example, consider the following data:

$$pH = 6.96$$

$$[HCO_3^-] = 12 \text{ mEq/L}$$

$$P_{CO_2} = 55 \text{ mm Hg}$$

When the three-step approach is followed, it is evident that the disturbance is an acidosis that has both a metabolic component (ECF [HCO_3^-] <24 mEq/L) and a respiratory component (P_{CO_2} >40 mm Hg). Thus, this disorder is mixed. Mixed acid-base disorders can occur, for example, in an individual who has a history of a chronic pulmonary disease such as emphysema (i.e., chronic respiratory acidosis) and in whom an acute gastrointestinal illness with diarrhea develops. Because diarrhea fluid contains HCO_3^-, its loss from the body results in the development of a metabolic acidosis.

A mixed acid-base disorder is also indicated when a patient has abnormal P_{CO_2} and ECF [HCO_3^-] values but a normal pH. Such a condition can develop in a patient who has ingested a large quantity of aspirin. The salicylic acid (active ingredient in aspirin) produces metabolic acidosis, and at the same time it stimulates the respiratory centers and causes hyperventilation and respiratory alkalosis. Thus, the patient has a reduced ECF [HCO_3^-] and a reduced P_{CO_2}. (*Note:* The P_{CO_2} is lower than would occur with normal respiratory compensation of a metabolic acidosis).

■ KEY CONCEPTS

1. The kidneys maintain acid-base balance through the excretion of an amount of acid equal to the amount of nonvolatile acid produced by metabolism and the quantity ingested in the diet. The kidneys also prevent the loss of HCO_3^- in urine by reabsorbing virtually all the HCO_3^- filtered at the glomeruli. Both reabsorption of the filtered HCO_3^- and excretion of acid are accomplished via secretion of H^+ by nephrons. Acid is excreted by the kidneys in the form of titratable acid (primarily as P_i) and NH_4^+. Excretion of both titratable acid and NH_4^+ results in the generation of new HCO_3^-, which replenishes the ECF HCO_3^- lost during the neutralization of nonvolatile acids.

2. The body uses three lines of defense to minimize the impact of acid-base disorders on body fluid pH: (1) ECF and ICF buffering, (2) respiratory compensation, and (3) renal compensation.

3. Metabolic acid-base disorders are caused by primary alterations in ECF [HCO_3^-], which in turn result from the addition of acid to or loss of alkali from the body. In response to metabolic acidosis, pulmonary ventilation is increased, which decreases P_{CO_2}, and renal net acid excretion is increased. An increase in ECF [HCO_3^-] causes alkalosis. This decreases pulmonary ventilation, which elevates P_{CO_2}. The pulmonary response to metabolic acid-base disorders occurs in a matter of minutes. Renal net acid excretion is also decreased. This response may take several days.

4. Respiratory acid-base disorders result from primary alterations in P_{CO_2}. Elevation of P_{CO_2} produces acidosis, and the kidneys respond with an increase in net acid excretion. Conversely, a reduction in P_{CO_2} produces alkalosis, and renal net acid excretion is reduced. The kidneys respond to respiratory acid-base disorders over a period of several hours to days.

THE ENDOCRINE AND REPRODUCTIVE SYSTEMS

Bruce A. White

CHAPTER 37

Introduction to the Endocrine System

The ability of cells to communicate with each other represents an underpinning of human biology. As discussed in Chapter 3, cell-to-cell communication exists at various levels of complexity and distance. **Endocrine signaling** involves (1) the **regulated secretion** of an extracellular signaling molecule, called a **hormone,** into the extracellular fluid; (2) diffusion of the hormone into the **vasculature** and its circulation throughout the body; and (3) diffusion of the hormone out of the vascular compartment into the extracellular space and binding to a **specific receptor** within cells of a **target organ.** Because of the spread of hormones throughout the body, one hormone often regulates the activity of several target organs. Conversely, cells frequently express receptors for multiple hormones.

The **endocrine system** is a collection of glands whose function is to regulate multiple organs within the body to (1) meet the growth and reproductive needs of the organism and (2) respond to fluctuations within the internal environment, including various types of stress. The endocrine system comprises the following major glands (Fig. 37-1):

Endocrine pancreas
Parathyroid glands
Pituitary gland (in association with hypothalamic nuclei)
Thyroid gland
Adrenal glands
Gonads (testes or ovaries)

These endocrine glands synthesize and secrete bioactive hormones and, with the exception of gonads, which perform both endocrine and gametogenic functions, are dedicated to hormone production (Table 37-1). A transitory organ, the **placenta,** also performs a major endocrine function.

In addition to dedicated endocrine glands, there are endocrine cells within organs whose primary function is not endocrine (Table 37-1). These include cells within the heart that produce **atrial natriuretic peptide,** liver cells that produce **insulin-like growth factor type I (IGF-I),** cells within the kidney that produce **erythropoietin,** and numerous cell types within the gastrointestinal tract that produce gastrointestinal hormones. There also exist collections of cell bodies (called nuclei) within the hypothalamus that secrete peptides, called neurohormones, into capillaries associated with the pituitary gland.

A third arm of the endocrine system is represented by numerous cell types that express intracellular enzymes, ectoenzymes, or secreted enzymes that modify inactive precursors or less active hormones into highly active hormones (Table 37-1). An example is the generation of **angiotensin II** from the inactive polypeptide angiotensinogen by two subsequent proteolytic cleavages (see Chapter 42). Another example is activation of **vitamin D** by two subsequent hydroxylation reactions in the liver and kidney to produce the highly bioactive hormone 1,25-dihydroxyvitamin D (vitamin D).

CONFIGURATION OF FEEDBACK LOOPS WITHIN THE ENDOCRINE SYSTEM

The predominant mode of a closed feedback loop among endocrine glands is **negative feedback.** In a negative-feedback loop, "hormone A" acts on one or more target organs to induce a change (either a decrease or increase) in circulating levels of "component B," and the change in component B then inhibits secretion of hormone A. Negative-feedback loops confer stability by keeping a physiological parameter (e.g., blood glucose) within a normal range. There are also a few examples of **positive feedback** in endocrine regulation. A positive closed feedback loop, in which hormone X increases levels of component Y and component Y stimulates secretion of hormone X, confers instability. Under the control of positive-feedback loops, something has "got to give." For example, positive-feedback loops control processes that lead to rupture of a follicle through the ovarian wall or expulsion of a fetus from the uterus.

There are two basic configurations of negative-feedback loops within the endocrine system: a **physiological response–driven** feedback loop (referred to simply as "response-driven feedback") and an **endocrine axis–driven** feedback loop (Fig. 37-2). The response-driven feedback loop is observed in endocrine glands that control blood glucose levels (pancreatic islets), blood Ca^{++} and P_i levels (parathyroid glands, kidney), blood osmolarity and volume (hypothalamus/posterior pituitary), and blood Na^+, K^+, and H^+ (zona glomerulosa of the adrenal cortex and atrial cells). In the response-driven configuration, secretion of a hormone is stimulated or inhibited by a change in the level of a specific extracellular parameter (e.g., an increase in blood glucose stimulates insulin secretion). Altered

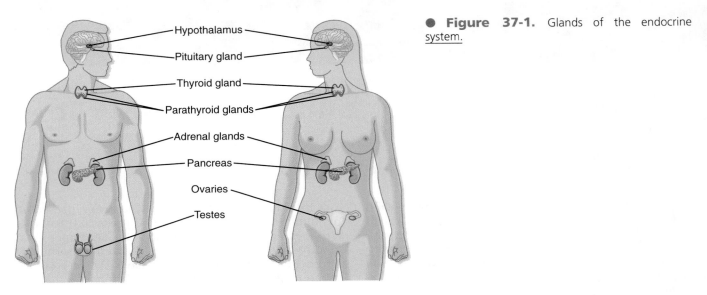

● **Figure 37-1.** Glands of the endocrine system.

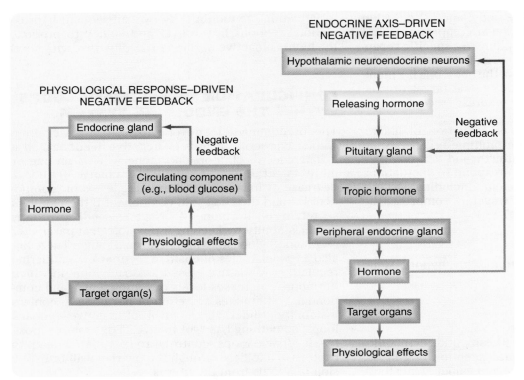

● **Figure 37-2.** Physiological response–driven and endocrine axis–driven negative-feedback loops.

hormone levels lead to changes in the physiology of target organs (e.g., decreased hepatic gluconeogenesis, increased uptake of glucose by muscle) that directly regulate the parameter (i.e., blood glucose) in question. The change in the parameter (i.e., decreased blood glucose) then inhibits further secretion of the hormone (i.e., insulin secretion drops as blood glucose falls).

Much of the endocrine system is organized into **endocrine axes,** with each axis consisting of the hypothalamus and the pituitary and peripheral endocrine glands (Fig. 37-2). Thus, the endocrine axis–driven feedback loop involves a three-tiered configuration.

The first tier is represented by **hypothalamic neuroendocrine neurons** that secrete **releasing hormones.** Releasing hormones stimulate (or, in a few cases, inhibit) the production and secretion of **tropic hormones** from the **pituitary gland** (second tier). Tropic hormones stimulate the production and secretion of hormones from **peripheral endocrine glands** (third tier). The peripherally produced hormones, namely, thyroid hormone, cortisol, sex steroids, and IGF-I, typically have **pleiotropic** actions (e.g., multiple phenotypic effects) on numerous cell types. However, in endocrine axis–driven feedback, the primary feedback loop involves feedback inhibition of pituitary tropic

● **Table 37-1.**

Hormones and Their Sites of Production in Nonpregnant Adults

Gland	Hormone
Hormones Synthesized and Secreted by Dedicated Endocrine Glands	
Pituitary gland	Growth hormone (GH) Prolactin Adrenocorticotropic hormone (ACTH) Thyroid-stimulating hormone (TSH) Follicle-stimulating hormone (FSH) Luteinizing hormone (LH)
Thyroid gland	Tetraiodothyronine (T_4; thyroxine) Triiodothyronine (T_3) Calcitonin
Parathyroid glands	Parathyroid hormone (PTH)
Islets of Langerhans (endocrine pancreas)	Insulin Glucagon Somatostatin
Adrenal gland	Epinephrine Norepinephrine Cortisol Aldosterone Dehydroepiandrosterone sulfate (DHEAS)
Ovaries	Estradiol-17β Progesterone Inhibin
Testes	Testosterone Antimüllerian hormone (AMH) Inhibin
Hormones Synthesized in Organs with a Primary Function Other Than Endocrine	
Brain (hypothalamus)	Antidiuretic hormone (ADH; vasopressin) Oxytocin Corticotropin-releasing hormone (CRH) Thyrotropin-releasing hormone (TRH) Gonadotropin-releasing hormone (GnRH) Growth hormone–releasing hormone (GHRH) Somatostatin Dopamine
Brain (pineal gland)	Melatonin
Heart	Atrial natriuretic peptide (ANP)
Kidney	Erythropoietin
Adipose tissue	Leptin Adiponectin
Stomach	Gastrin Somatostatin Ghrelin
Intestines	Secretin Cholecystokinin Glucagon-like peptide-1 (GLP-1) Glucagon-like peptide-2 (GLP-2) Glucose-dependent insulinotropic peptide (GIP; gastrin inhibitory peptide) Motilin
Liver	Insulin-like growth factor type I (IGF-I)
Hormones Produced to a Significant Degree by Peripheral Conversion	
Lungs	Angiotensin II
Kidney	1,25-Dihydroxyvitamin D (vitamin D)
Adipose, mammary glands, other organs	Estradiol-17β
Liver, sebaceous gland, other organs	Testosterone
Genital skin, prostate, other organs	5-Dihydrotestosterone (DHT)
Many organs	T_3

hormones and hypothalamic releasing hormones by the peripherally produced hormone. In contrast to response-driven feedback, the physiological responses to the peripherally produced hormone play only a minor role in regulation of feedback within endocrine axis–driven feedback loops.

An important aspect of the endocrine axes is the ability of descending and ascending neuronal signals to modulate release of the hypothalamic releasing hormones and thereby control the activity of the axis. A major neuronal input to releasing hormone–secreting neurons comes from another region of the hypothalamus called the **suprachiasmatic nucleus (SCN)**. SCN neurons impose a daily rhythm, called a **circadian rhythm,** on the secretion of hypothalamic releasing hormones and the endocrine axes that they control (Fig. 37-3). SCN neurons represent an intrinsic circadian clock, as evidenced by the fact that they demonstrate a spontaneous peak of electrical activity at the same time every 24 to 25 hours. The 24- to 25-hour cycle can be **"entrained"** by the normal environmental light-dark cycle created by the earth's rotation such that the periodicity of the clock appears to be environmentally controlled (Fig. 37-4). Neural input is generated from specialized light-sensitive retinal cells that are distinct from rods and cones and from signals to the SCN via the retinohypothalamic tract. Under constant conditions of light or dark, however, the SCN clock becomes "free running" and slightly drifts away from a 24-hour cycle each day.

The **pineal gland** forms a neuroendocrine link between the SCN and various physiological processes that require circadian control. This tiny gland, close to the hypothalamus, synthesizes the hormone **melatonin** from the neurotransmitter **serotonin,** of which tryptophan is the precursor. The rate-limiting enzyme for melatonin synthesis is *N*-acetyltransferase. The amount and activity of this enzyme in the pineal gland vary markedly in a cyclic fashion, which accounts for the cycling of melatonin secretion and its plasma levels. Synthesis of melatonin is inhibited by light and markedly stimulated by darkness (Fig. 37-4). Thus, melatonin may transmit the information that nighttime has arrived, and body functions are regulated accordingly. Melatonin feedback to the SCN at dawn or dusk may also help evoke day-night entrainment of the SCN 24- to 25-hour clock. Melatonin has numerous other actions, including induction of sleep.

Another important input to hypothalamic neurons and the pituitary gland is stress, either as **systemic stress** (e.g., hemorrhage, inflammation) or as **processive stress** (e.g., fear, anxiety). Major medical or surgical stress overrides the circadian clock and causes a pattern of persistent and exaggerated hormone release and metabolism that mobilizes endogenous fuels, such as glucose and free fatty acids, and augments their delivery to critical organs. By contrast, growth and reproductive processes are suppressed. Additionally, cytokines released during inflammatory or immune responses, or both, directly regulate the release of hypothalamic releasing hormones and pituitary hormones.

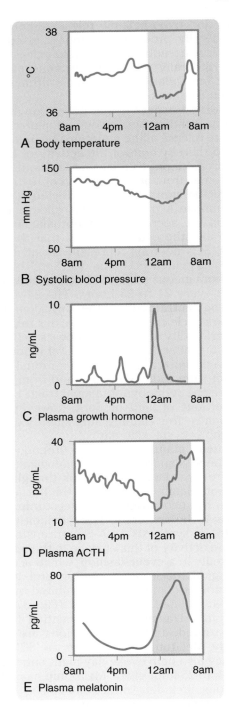

● Figure 37-3. A circadian pacemaker directs numerous endocrine and body functions, each with its own daily profile. The nighttime rise in plasma melatonin may mediate certain other circadian patterns. (Data from Schwartz WJ: Adv Intern Med 38:81, 1994.)

CHEMICAL NATURE OF HORMONES

Hormones are classified biochemically as **proteins/ peptides, catecholamines, iodothyronines,** or **steroid hormones.** The chemical nature of a hormone determines (1) how it is synthesized, stored, and released; (2) how it is transported in blood; (3) its biological

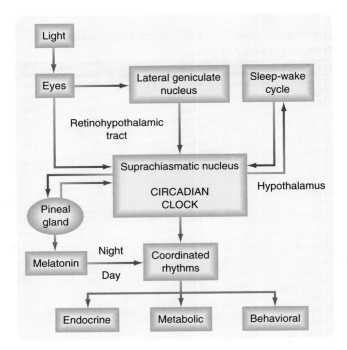

● Figure 37-4. Origin of circadian rhythms in endocrine gland secretion, metabolic processes, and behavioral activity. (Modified from Turek FW: Recent Prog Horm Res 49:43, 1994.)

half-life and mode of clearance; and (4) its cellular mechanism of action.

Proteins/Peptides

Protein and peptide hormones can be grouped into structurally related molecules that are encoded by gene families. Protein/peptide hormones gain their specificity from their primary amino acid sequence and from posttranslational modifications, especially glycosylation.

Because protein/peptide hormones are destined for secretion outside the cell, they are synthesized and processed differently from proteins destined to remain within the cell or to be continuously added to the membrane (Fig. 37-5). These hormones are synthesized on the polyribosome as larger preprohormones or prehormones. The nascent peptides have at their N-terminal a group of 15 to 30 amino acids called the **signal peptide.** The signal peptide interacts with a ribonucleoprotein particle, which ultimately directs the growing peptide chain through a pore in the membrane of the endoplasmic reticulum located on the cisternal (i.e., inner) surface of the endoplasmic reticular membrane. Removal of the signal peptide by a **signal peptidase** generates a hormone or prohormone, which is then transported from the cisternae of the endoplasmic reticulum to the Golgi apparatus, where it is packaged into a membrane-bound secretory vesicle that is subsequently released into the cytoplasm. The carbohydrate moiety of glycoproteins is added in the Golgi apparatus.

Most hormones are produced as **prohormones.** Prohormones harbor the peptide sequence of the

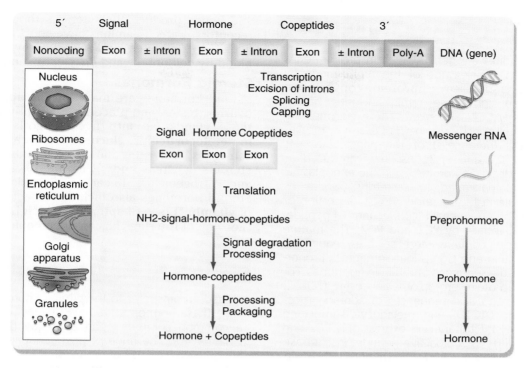

● **Figure 37-5.** Schematic representation of peptide hormone synthesis. In the nucleus the primary gene transcript, a premessenger RNA molecule, undergoes excision of introns, splicing of exons, capping of the 5′ end, and addition of poly(A) at the 3′ end. The resultant mature messenger RNA enters the cytoplasm, where it directs the synthesis of a preprohormone peptide sequence on ribosomes. In this process the N-terminal signal is removed, and the resultant prohormone is transferred vectorially into the endoplasmic reticulum. The prohormone undergoes further processing and packaging in the Golgi apparatus. After final cleavage of the prohormone within the granules, they contain the hormone and copeptides ready for secretion by exocytosis.

active hormone within their primary sequence. However, prohormones are inactive or less active and require the action of endopeptidases to trim away the neighboring inactive sequences.

Protein/peptide hormones are stored in the gland as membrane-bound secretory vesicles and are released by **exocytosis** through the **regulated secretory pathway.** Thus, hormones are not continually secreted. Rather, they are secreted in response to a stimulus through a mechanism of **stimulus-secretion coupling.** Regulated exocytosis requires energy, Ca^{++}, an intact cytoskeleton (microtubules, microfilaments), and the presence of coat proteins that specifically deliver secretory vesicles to the cell membrane. The ultrastructure of protein hormone–producing cells is characterized by abundant rough endoplasmic reticulum and Golgi membranes and the presence of secretory vesicles (Fig. 37-6).

Protein/peptide hormones are soluble in body fluids and, with the notable exceptions of IGFs and growth hormone (GH), circulate in blood predominantly in an unbound form and therefore have short biological half-lives. Protein hormones are removed from blood primarily by endocytosis and lysosomal degradation of hormone-receptor complexes (see later). Many protein hormones are small enough to appear in urine in a physiologically active form. For example, follicle-stimulating hormone (FSH) and luteinizing hormone (LH) are present in urine.

Proteins/peptides are readily digested in the gastrointestinal tract if administered orally. Hence, they must be administered by injection or, in the case of small peptides, through a mucous membrane (sublingually or intranasally). Because proteins/peptides do not cross cell membranes readily, they signal through membrane receptors (see Chapter 3).

Catecholamines

Catecholamines are synthesized by the adrenal medulla and neurons and include **norepinephrine, epinephrine,** and **dopamine** (Fig. 37-7). The primary hormonal product of the adrenal medulla is epinephrine and, to a lesser extent, norepinephrine. Catecholamines gain their specificity through enzymatic modifications of the amino acid tyrosine. Catecholamines are stored in secretory vesicles that are part of the regulated secretory pathway. They are copackaged with ATP, Ca^{++}, and proteins called **chromogranins.** Chromogranins play a role in the biogenesis of secretory vesicles and in the organization of components within the vesicles. Catecholamines are soluble in blood and circulate either unbound or loosely bound to albumin. They are similar to protein/peptide hormones in that they do not cross cell membranes readily

● AT THE CELLULAR LEVEL

Bioactive hormones are generated from prohormones through proteolytic cleavage of the prohormone by **prohormone** (also called **proprotein**) **convertases.** The proprotein convertase family includes hfurin, hPC1, hPC2, hPACE4, and hPLC. These enzymes are expressed in a cell-specific manner. For example, insulin-producing cells (beta cells) of the pancreatic islets express both PC1 and PC2. Insulin is produced as preproinsulin, cleaved to proinsulin in the endoplasmic reticulum, and packaged in secretory vesicles as proinsulin. While in the secretory vesicle, a portion of the center of the single chain (connecting [C] peptide) is cleaved sequentially by PC1 and PC2. The mature secretory vesicle contains and secretes equimolar amounts of insulin and C peptide. Sometimes prohormones contain the sequence of multiple hormones. For example, the protein pro-opiomelanocortin (POMC) contains the amino acid sequences of adrenocortico-tropic hormone (ACTH) and melanocyte-stimulating hormones (MSHs). Pituitary cells express only PC1 and release only ACTH as a bioactive peptide. In contrast, certain neuronal cell types and keratinocytes express both PC1 and PC2 and can produce MSHs. There are also prohormones, called **polyproteins,** that contain multiple copies of the same bioactive peptide. For example, the sequence for thyrotropin-releasing hormone (TRH) is reiterated six times within the prepro-TRH sequence. Rare mutations in PC1 have been identified in humans and are associated with extreme childhood obesity, defects in glucose homeostasis, low glucocorticoid levels, loss of menstrual cycles and hypogonadism, and problems in gastrointestinal function.

and hence produce their actions though membrane receptors. Catecholamines have short biological half-lives (1 to 2 minutes) and are primarily removed from blood by cell uptake and enzymatic modification.

Steroid Hormones

Steroid hormones are made by the **adrenal cortex, ovaries, testes,** and **placenta.** Steroid hormones from these glands fall into five categories: **progestins, mineralocorticoids, glucocorticoids, androgens,** and **estrogens.** Progestins and the corticoids are 21-carbon steroids, whereas androgens are 19-carbon steroids and estrogens are 18-carbon steroids (Table 37-2). Steroid hormones also include the active metabolite of **vitamin D** (see Chapter 39), which is a secosteroid (i.e., one of the rings has an open conformation).

▶ IN THE CLINIC

Gonadotropins refer to the pituitary hormones LH and FSH. These hormones are heterodimers that consist of a common α subunit and a unique β subunit (see Chapter 40). The urine of postmenopausal women is an excellent source of gonadotropins because post-menopausal serum gonadotropin levels are high as a result of the loss of negative feedback by ovarian steroids (see Chapter 43), and the hormones are filtered and excreted as intact molecules in urine. A third gonadotropin is the placental hormone human chorionic gonadotropin (hCG; see Chapter 43). hCG has the same common α subunit and an hCG-specific β subunit. hCG is an extremely stable hormone, and blood hCG levels double every 2 days during the first trimester. Accordingly, urinary levels of hCG also increase rapidly. **Pregnancy tests** are based on immunological detection in urine of the hCG-specific β subunit as part of the intact hCG heterodimer.

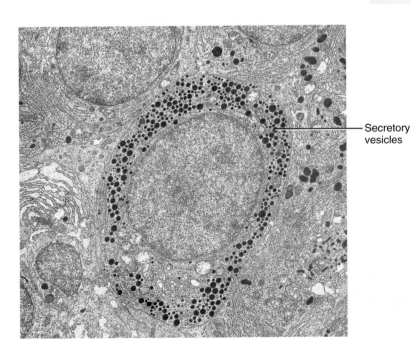

● **Figure 37-6.** Ultrastructure of a protein hormone–producing cell. Note the presence of secretory vesicles and rough endoplasmic reticulum in the protein hormone–secreting cell. (From Kierszenbaum AL: Histology and Cell Biology: An Introduction to Pathology, 2nd ed. Philadelphia, Mosby, 2007.)

Secretory vesicles

● Table 37-2. Steroid Hormones

Family	Number of Carbons	Specific Hormone	Primary Site of Synthesis	Primary Receptor
Progestin	21	Progesterone	Ovary Placenta	Progesterone receptor (PR)
Glucocorticoid	21	Cortisol Corticosterone	Adrenal cortex	Glucocorticoid receptor (GR)
Mineralocorticoid	21	Aldosterone 11-Deoxycorticosterone	Adrenal cortex	Mineralocorticoid receptor (MR)
Androgen	19	Testosterone Dihydrotestosterone	Testis	Androgen receptor (AR)
Estrogen	18	Estradiol-17β Estriol	Ovary Placenta	Estrogen receptor (ER)

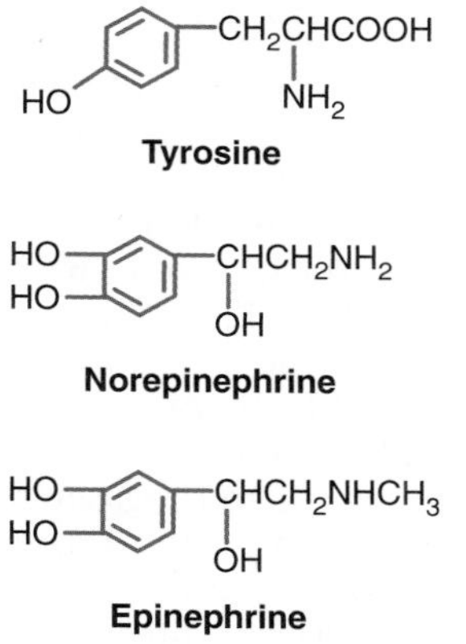

Tyrosine

Norepinephrine

Epinephrine

● **Figure 37-7.** Structure of catecholamines.

Steroid hormones are synthesized by a series of enzymatic modifications of cholesterol and have a cyclopentanoperhydrophenanthrene ring (or a derivative thereof) as their core (Fig. 37-8). The enzymatic modifications of cholesterol are of three general types: hydroxylation, dehydrogenation/reduction, and lyase reactions. The purpose of these modifications is to produce a cholesterol derivative that is sufficiently unique to be recognized by a specific receptor. Thus, progestins bind to the **progesterone receptor (PR),** mineralocorticoids bind to the **mineralocorticoid receptor (MR),** glucocorticoids bind to the **glucocorticoid receptor (GR),** androgens bind to the **androgen receptor (AR),** estrogens bind to the **estrogen receptor (ER),** and the active vitamin D metabolite binds to the **vitamin D receptor (VDR).** The complexity of steroid hormone action is increased by the expression of multiple forms of each receptor. Additionally, there is some degree of nonspecificity between steroid hormones and the receptors that they bind to. For example, glucocorticoids bind to the MR with high affinity, and progestins, glucocorticoids, and androgens can all interact with the PR, GR, and AR to some degree. As discussed later, steroid hormones are hydrophobic and pass through cell membranes easily. Accordingly, classic steroid hormone receptors are localized intracellularly and act by regulating gene expression. Evidence is mounting for the presence of plasma membrane and juxtamembrane steroid hormone receptors that mediate rapid, nongenomic actions of steroid hormones.

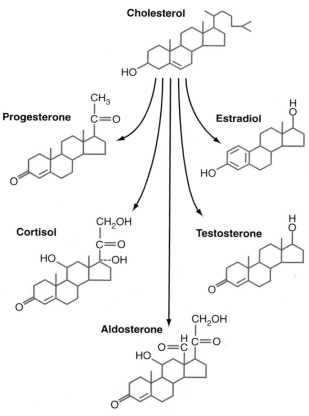

● **Figure 37-8.** **A,** Structure of cholesterol, the precursor of steroid hormones. **B,** Structure of steroid hormones.

Steroidogenic cell types are defined as cells that can convert cholesterol to pregnenolone, which is the first reaction common to all steroidogenic pathways. Steroidogenic cells have some capacity for cholesterol synthesis but often obtain cholesterol from cholesterol-rich lipoproteins (low-density lipoproteins and high-density lipoproteins). Pregnenolone is then further modified by several enzymatic reactions. Because of their hydrophobic nature, steroid hormones and precursors can leave the steroidogenic cell easily and thus are not stored. Therefore, steroidogenesis is regulated at the level of uptake, storage, and mobilization of cholesterol and at the level of steroidogenic enzyme gene expression and activity. Steroids are not regulated at the level of secretion of the preformed hormone. A clinical implication of this mode of secretion is that high levels of steroid hormone precursors are easily released into blood when a steroidogenic enzyme within a given pathway is inactive or absent. The ultrastructure of steroidogenic cells is distinct from protein- and catecholamine-secreting cells. Steroidogenic enzymes reside within the inner mitochondrial membrane or the membrane of the smooth endoplasmic reticulum. Thus, steroidogenic cells typically contain extensive mitochondria and smooth endoplasmic reticulum (Fig. 37-9). These cells also contain lipid droplets, which represent a store of cholesterol esters.

An important feature of steroidogenesis is that steroid hormones often undergo further modifications (apart from those involved in deactivation and excretion) after their release from the original steroidogenic cell. For example, estrogen synthesis by the ovary and placenta requires at least two cell types to complete the conversion of cholesterol to estrogen. This means that one cell secretes a precursor and a second cell converts the precursor to estrogen. There is also considerable **peripheral conversion** of active steroid hormones. For example, the testis secretes little estrogen. However, adipose, muscle, and other tissues express the enzyme for converting testosterone (a potent androgen) to estradiol-17β (a potent estrogen). Thus, the overall production of "steroid hormone X" is equivalent to the sum of the secretion of "steroid hormone X" from a steroidogenic cell type and peripheral conversion of other steroids to "steroid hormone X" (Fig. 37-10). Peripheral conversion can produce (1) a more active, but similar class of hormone (e.g., conversion of 25-hydroxyvitamin D to 1,25-dihydroxyvitamin D); (2) a less active hormone that can be reversibly activated by another tissue (e.g., conversion of cortisol to cortisone in the kidney, followed by conversion of cortisone to cortisol in abdominal adipose tissue); or (3) a different class of hormone (e.g., conversion of testosterone to estrogen). Peripheral conversion of steroids plays an important role in several endocrine disorders (see Chapters 42 and 43).

Because of their nonpolar nature, steroid hormones are not readily soluble in blood. Therefore, steroid hormones circulate bound to **transport proteins,** including albumin, but also the specific transport proteins **sex hormone–binding globulin (SHBG)** and **corticosteroid-binding globulin (CBG)** (see later). Excretion of hormones from the body typically involves inactivating modifications followed by **glucuronide or sulfate conjugation** in the liver. These modifications increase the water solubility of the steroid and decrease its affinity for transport proteins, thereby allowing the inactivated steroid hormone to be excreted by the kidney. Steroid compounds are absorbed fairly readily in the gastrointestinal tract and may therefore be administered orally.

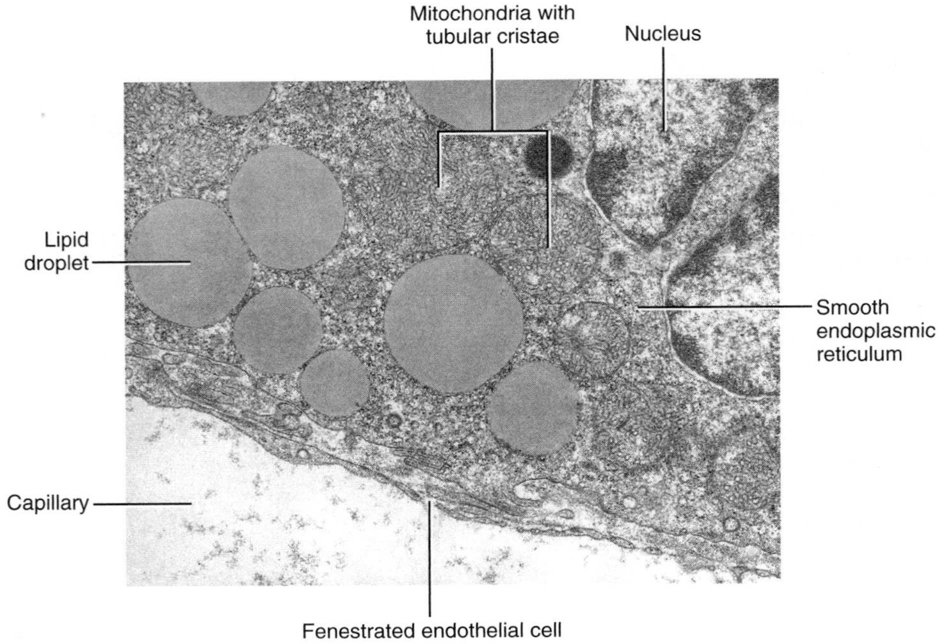

● **Figure 37-9.** Ultrastructure of a steroidogenic cell. Note the abundance of lipid droplets, smooth endoplasmic reticulum, and mitochondria with tubular cristae. (From Kierszenbaum AL: Histology and Cell Biology: An Introduction to Pathology, 2nd ed. Philadelphia, Mosby, 2007.)

Mitochondria with tubular cristae

Nucleus

Lipid droplet

Smooth endoplasmic reticulum

Capillary

Fenestrated endothelial cell

● **Figure 37-10.** Peripheral conversion of steroid hormones.

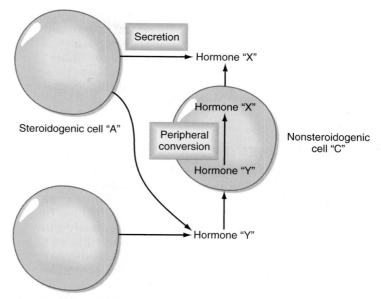

Total production of hormone "X" =
secretion of hormone "X" + peripheral conversion of hormone "Y"
into hormone "X"

Iodothyronines

Thyroid hormones are iodothyronines (Fig. 37-11) that are made by the coupling of iodinated tyrosine residues through an ether linkage. Their specificity is determined by the thyronine structure, as well as by where the thyronine is iodinated. Thyroid hormones cross cell membranes by both diffusion and transport systems. They are stored extracellularly in the thyroid as an integral part of the glycoprotein molecule thyroglobulin. Thyroid hormones are sparingly soluble in blood and aqueous fluids and are transported in blood bound (>99%) to serum-binding proteins. A major transport protein is **thyroid hormone–binding globulin** (TBG). Thyroid hormones have long half-lives ($t_{1/2}$; thyroxine [T_4] = 7 days; triiodothyronine [T_3] = 18 hours). Thyroid hormones are similar to steroid hormones in that the **thyroid hormone receptor (TR)** is intracellular and acts as a transcription factor. In fact, the TR belongs to the same gene family that includes steroid hormone receptors and VDR. Thyroid hormones can be administered orally, and sufficient hormone is absorbed intact to make this an effective mode of therapy.

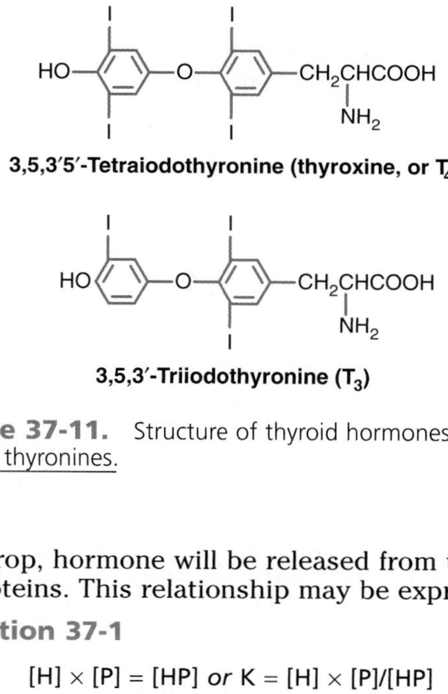

TRANSPORT OF HORMONES IN THE CIRCULATION

A significant fraction of steroid and thyroid hormones is transported in blood bound to plasma proteins that are produced in a regulated manner by the liver. Protein and polypeptide hormones are generally transported free in blood. The concentrations of bound hormone (HP), free hormone (H), and plasma transport protein (P) are in equilibrium. If free hormone

3,5,3′5′-Tetraiodothyronine (thyroxine, or T_4)

3,5,3′-Triiodothyronine (T_3)

● **Figure 37-11.** Structure of thyroid hormones, which are iodinated thyronines.

levels drop, hormone will be released from the transport proteins. This relationship may be expressed as

● **Equation 37-1**

$$[H] \times [P] = [HP] \ or \ K = [H] \times [P]/[HP]$$

where K is the dissociation constant.

Free hormone is the biologically active form for action on the target organ, feedback control, and clearance by cellular uptake and metabolism. Consequently, when evaluating hormonal status, one must sometimes determine free hormone levels rather than just total hormone levels. This is particularly important because hormone transport proteins themselves are regulated by altered endocrine and disease states.

Protein binding serves several purposes. It prolongs the circulating $t_{1/2}$ of the hormone. Many hormones cross cell membranes readily and would either enter cells or be excreted by the kidney were they not protein bound. The bound hormone represents a "reservoir" of hormone and as such can serve to "buffer" acute changes in hormone secretion. Some hormones, such as steroids, are sparingly soluble in blood, and protein binding facilitates their transport.

CELLULAR RESPONSES TO HORMONES

Hormones are also referred to as **ligands,** in the context of ligand-receptor binding, and as **agonists,** in that their binding to the receptor is transduced into a cellular response. Receptor **antagonists** typically bind to a receptor and lock it in an inactive state, unable to induce a cellular response. Loss or inactivation of a receptor results in **hormonal resistance.** Constitutive activation of a receptor leads to unregulated, hormone-independent activation of cellular processes.

Hormones regulate essentially every major aspect of cellular function in every organ system. Hormones control the growth of cells, ultimately determining their size and competency for cell division. Hormones regulate the differentiation of cells and their ability to survive or undergo programmed cell death. They influence cellular metabolism, the ionic composition of body fluids, and cell membrane potential. Hormones orchestrate several complex cytoskeletal-associated events, including cell shape, migration, division, exocytosis, recycling/endocytosis, and cell-cell and cell-matrix adhesion. Hormones regulate the expression and function of cytosolic and membrane proteins, and a specific hormone may determine the level of its own receptor or the receptors for other hormones.

Although hormones can exert coordinated, pleiotropic control on multiple aspects of cell function, any given hormone does not regulate every function in every cell type. Rather, a single hormone controls a subset of cellular functions in only the cell types that express receptors for that hormone. Thus, selective receptor expression determines which cells will respond to a given hormone. Moreover, the differentiated state of a cell will determine how it will respond to a hormone. Thus, the specificity of hormonal responses resides in the structure of the hormone itself, the receptor for the hormone, and the cell type in which the receptor is expressed. Serum hormone concentrations are typically extremely low (10^{-11} to 10^{-9} M). Therefore, a receptor must have high affinity, as well as specificity, for its cognate hormone.

How does hormone-receptor binding get transduced into a cellular response? Hormone binding to a receptor induces conformational changes in the receptor. This is referred to as a **signal.** The signal is transduced into the activation of one or more **intracellular messengers.** Messenger molecules then bind to **effector proteins,** which in turn modify specific cellular functions. The combination of hormone-receptor binding (signal), activation of messengers (transduction), and regulation of one or more effector proteins is referred to as a **signal transduction pathway** (also called simply a **signaling pathway**), and the final outcome is referred to as the **cellular response.** Signaling pathways are usually characterized by the following:

1. Multiple, hierarchical steps in which "downstream" effector proteins are dependent on and driven by "upstream" receptors, transducers, and effector proteins. This means that loss or inactivation of one or more components within the pathway leads to general resistance to the hormone, whereas constitutive activation or overexpression of components can drive a pathway in an unregulated manner.
2. Amplification of the initial hormone-receptor binding. Amplification can be so great that maximal response to a hormone is achieved on binding of hormone to a small percentage of receptors.
3. Activation of multiple pathways, or at least regulation of multiple cell functions, from one hormone-receptor binding event. For example, binding of insulin to its receptor activates three separate signaling pathways. Even in fairly simple pathways (e.g., glucagon activation of adenylyl cyclase), divergent downstream events allow the regulation of multiple functions (e.g., posttranslational activation of glycogen phosphorylase and increased phosphoenolpyruvate carboxykinase [PEPCK] gene transcription).
4. Antagonism by constitutive and regulated negative-feedback reactions. This means that a signal is dampened or terminated (or both) by opposing reactions and that loss or gain of function of opposing components can cause hormone-independent activation of a specific pathway, or hormone resistance.

As discussed in Chapter 3, hormones signal to cells through membrane or intracellular receptors. Membrane receptors have rapid effects on cellular processes (e.g., enzyme activity, cytoskeletal arrangement) that are independent of the synthesis of new protein. Membrane receptors can also rapidly regulate gene expression through either mobile kinases (e.g., PKA, MAPKs) or mobile transcription factors (e.g., STATs, Smads). Steroid hormones have slower, longer-term effects that involve chromatin remodeling and changes in gene expression. Increasing evidence points to rapid, nongenomic effects of steroid hormones as well, but these pathways are still being elucidated.

The presence of a functional receptor is an absolute requirement for hormone action, and loss of a receptor produces essentially the same symptoms as loss of hormone. In addition to the receptor, there are fairly complex pathways involving numerous intracellular messengers and effector proteins. Accordingly, endocrine diseases can arise from abnormal expression or activity, or both, of any of these signal transduction pathway components. Finally, hormonal signals can be terminated in several ways, including hormone/receptor internalization, phosphorylation/dephosphorylation, proteosomal destruction of receptor, and generation of feedback inhibitors.

Endocrine diseases can be broadly categorized as hyperfunction or hypofunction of a specific hormonal pathway. Hypofunction can be caused by lack of active hormone or by **hormone resistance** as a result of inactivation of hormone receptors or postreceptor defects. **Testicular feminization syndrome** is a dramatic form of hormone resistance in which the androgen receptor is mutated and cannot be activated by androgens. In patients in whom the diagnosis is not made before puberty, the testis becomes hyperstimulated because of abrogation of the negative feedback between the testis and the pituitary gland. The increased androgen levels have no direct biological effect as a result of the receptor defect. However, the androgens are peripherally converted to estrogens. Thus, individuals who are genetically male (i.e., 46,XY) have a strongly feminized external phenotype, a female sexual identity, and usually a sexual preference for males (i.e., heterosexual relative to sexual identity). Treatment involves removal of the hyperstimulated testes (which reside in the abdomen and pose a risk for cancer), estrogen replacement therapy, and counseling for the patient and, if one exists, the partner/spouse to address infertility and social/psychological distress.

■ **KEY CONCEPTS**

1. Endocrine signaling involves (1) regulated secretion of an extracellular signaling molecule, called a hormone, into the extracellular fluid; (2) diffusion of the hormone into the vasculature and circulation throughout the body; and (3) diffusion of the hormone out of the vascular compartment into the extracellular space and binding to a specific receptor within cells of a target organ.

2. The endocrine system is composed of the endocrine pancreas, the parathyroid glands, the pituitary gland, the thyroid gland, the adrenal glands, and the gonads (testes or ovaries).

3. Negative feedback represents an important control mechanism that confers stability on endocrine systems. Hormonal rhythms are imposed on negative-feedback loops.

4. Protein/peptide hormones are produced on ribosomes and stored in endocrine cells in membrane-bound secretory granules. They typically do not cross cell membranes readily and act through membrane-associated receptors.

5. Catecholamines are synthesized in the cytosol and secretory granules and do not readily cross cell membranes. They act through cell membrane–associated receptors.

6. Steroid hormones are not stored in tissues and generally cross cell membranes relatively readily. They act through intracellular receptors.

7. Thyroid hormones are synthesized in follicular cells and stored in follicular colloid as thyroglobulin. They cross cell membranes and associate with nuclear receptors.

8. Some hormones act through membrane receptors, with their responses being mediated by G protein–associated systems (adenylyl cyclase and phosphatidylinositol), calcium-calmodulin, tyrosine kinase–containing receptor, tyrosine kinase–associated systems, or serine/threonine kinase receptor.

9. Other hormones bind to nuclear receptors and act by directly regulating gene transcription.

CHAPTER 38

Hormonal Regulation of Energy Metabolism

This chapter considers the role of hormones in maintaining a constant supply of energy to cells in the body during the digestive and interdigestive periods and during fasting and exercise.

OVERVIEW OF ENERGY METABOLISM

Adenosine Triphosphate

Cells continually perform work to maintain their integrity and internal environment, respond to stimuli, and perform their differentiated functions (Fig. 38-1). The absolute minimal amount of energy expenditure is called the basal metabolic rate (BMR) or resting metabolic rate (RMR).

In an adult, other forms of energy expenditure involve

1. Ingestion of food. This causes a small obligate increase in energy expenditure, referred to as diet-induced thermogenesis.
2. Nonshivering thermogenesis. This refers to energy expended to produce heat, either in an obligatory manner to maintain a constant thermoneutral state or in a facultative manner when an individual is acutely exposed to cold. All tissues contribute to the obligatory thermogenic process.
3. Spontaneous unconscious physical activity such as "fidgeting."
4. Occupational labor and purposeful exercise (Table 38-1), which vary greatly among individuals, as well as from day to day and from season to season. Labor and exercise generate the greatest need for variations in daily caloric intake, thus underscoring the importance of energy stores to buffer temporary discrepancies between energy output and intake.

Of a total average daily expenditure of 2300 kcal (9700 kJ) in a sedentary adult, basal metabolism accounts for 60% to 70%, dietary and obligatory thermogenesis for 5% to 15%, and spontaneous physical activity for 20% to 30%. An additional 4000 kcal may be expended in daily physical work. During short periods of occupational or recreational exercise, energy expenditure can increase more than 10-fold over basal levels. Transient and longer-term changes in an individual's physiology, including pregnancy, growth and aging, or infection and cancer, significantly alter energy demands.

Cells derive their energy to perform this work primarily from **ATP,** which is not stored. Thus, cells need a continual supply of ATP to the extent that humans synthesize well over half their own weight in ATP daily. This is done by oxidizing glucose, free fatty acids (FFAs), amino acids (AAs), and ketone bodies. On average, the process of oxidizing fuels to form ATP is 40% efficient, with 60% lost as heat (Fig. 38-1). All fuels originally come from the diet—humans must eat to stay alive. Normally, people eat intermittently. Consequently, the use and distribution of fuels change over time.

Metabolic Phases

In general, there are four metabolic phases (Fig. 38-1): (1) the **digestive** or **absorptive** phase, which occurs during the 2 to 3 hours that it takes to digest a discrete meal; (2) the **interdigestive** or **postabsorptive** phase, which normally occurs between meals; (3) **fasting**, which most commonly occurs between the last snack before bedtime and breakfast (in fact, physicians refer to a blood value as "fasting," e.g., "fasting blood glucose," if the patient abstains from eating after midnight and has blood drawn about 8 AM; prolonged fasting and starvation are extreme forms of fasting); and (4) **strenuous exercise** or physical labor, which usually imposes an intense energy demand for a relatively short period (e.g., 1 hour).

A central feature of the utilization of different nutrients is the nature of cell-specific needs and capabilities. Cells with no or very few mitochondria cannot utilize AAs and FFAs for energy but must rely entirely on anaerobic glycolysis (see later). The brain, which continually accounts for about 20% of O_2 consumption, cannot efficiently access circulating FFAs for energy. The brain converts most of its AA pool into neurotransmitters instead of oxidizing them for energy. This means that the brain and some other tissues are obligate glucose users. In other words, the function of the brain is critically dependent on circulating levels of blood glucose, much as it is on a continuous supply of O_2. An acute fall in blood glucose levels below 50 mg/100 mL (i.e., **hypoglycemia**) leads to impaired central nervous system functions, including vision, cognition, and muscle coordination, as well as lethargy and weakness (Fig. 38-2). Severe hypoglycemia can ultimately lead to coma and death. Thus, a major role of the hormones involved in metabolic homeostasis is to maintain blood glucose levels above

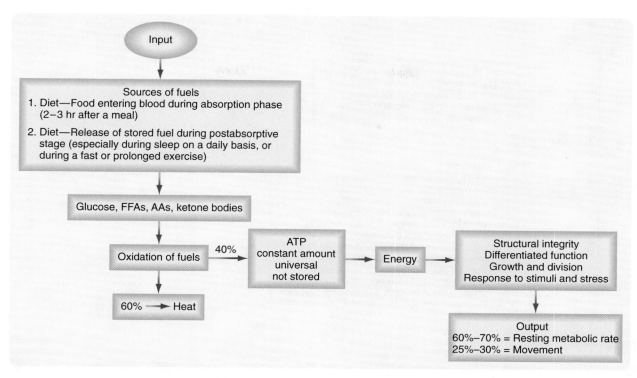

● **Figure 38-1.** Overview of energy metabolism.

● **Table 38-1.**
Estimates of Energy Expenditure in Adults

Activity	Caloric Expenditure (kcal/min)
Basal	1.1
Sitting	1.8
Walking, 2.5 miles/hr	4.3
Walking, 4.0 miles/hr	8.2
Climbing stairs	9.0
Swimming	10.9
Bicycling, 13 miles/hr	11.1
Household domestic work	2-4.5
Factory work	2-6
Farming	4-6
Building trades	4-9

Data from Kottke FJ. In Altman PL (ed): Metabolism. Bethesda, MD, Federation of American Society for Experimental Biology, 1968.

60 mg/100 mL. Conversely, it is important that fasting blood glucose levels remain below 110 mg/100 mL. Indeed, the complications associated with poorly controlled diabetes mellitus have shown not only that too little blood glucose is incompatible with life but also that too much blood glucose imposes various stresses on cell function, increases morbidity, and shortens life (Fig. 38-2).

Thus, a balance must be struck in which a discontinuous caloric intake is matched to the utilization or storage of energy substrates as required by an ever-present but fluctuating energy demand. This balance is achieved through the differential activation and inactivation of selective metabolic pathways during the fed state (i.e., during caloric surplus) versus during the interdigestive period, prolonged fasting, or exer-

cise (i.e., during caloric deficit). Importantly, all organs and tissues cannot simply transport glucose from blood and oxidize it to the same extent at all times. In the following sections we briefly review the primary metabolic pathways involved in the utilization and storage of glucose, FFAs, and AAs. We also discuss a nondietary fuel, ketone bodies, which are made by the liver for use by other organs during fasting.

ATP SYNTHESIS
Making ATP from Carbohydrates
ATP is generated from the oxidation of carbohydrates, FFAs, and AAs. The primary carbohydrate used by cells is the six-carbon (hexose) monosaccharide **glucose.** Three main phases are involved in the process of oxidizing glucose to the full extent: (1) transport and trapping of glucose inside the cell; (2) **glycolysis** (i.e., splitting [lysis] of the six-carbon molecule glucose [glyco]) to the three-carbon molecules pyruvate (aerobic) or lactate (anaerobic); and (3) the **tricarboxylic acid (TCA) cycle,** which occurs in the inner mitochondrial matrix in close proximity to components of the electron transport chain, and **oxidative phosphorylation.**

In the first phase (Fig. 38-3), glucose is transported across the cell membrane by bidirectional facilitative glucose transporters called **GLUTs.** Once inside the cell, glucose is prevented from exiting by phosphorylation to **glucose-6-phosphate (G6P).** This phosphorylation is catalyzed by **hexokinases.** The hexokinase that is expressed in the liver and pancreatic beta cells

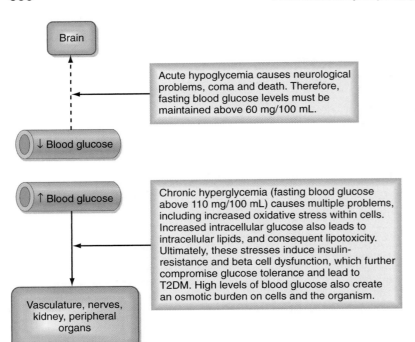

● **Figure 38-2.** Importance of maintaining blood glucose within the normal range. (Modified from Porterfield SP, White BA: Endocrine Physiology, 3rd ed. Philadelphia, Mosby, 2007.)

● AT THE CELLULAR LEVEL

Glucose is a hydrophilic molecule and, as such, cannot diffuse across cell membranes. The two families of glucose transporters are the sodium-glucose cotransporters (SGLTs) and the facilitated-diffusion GLUT transporters. SGLTs are localized in the apical membranes of simple epithelia (intestine and proximal tubules of the kidney) and are involved in the transepithelial transport of glucose. GLUTs provide for sodium-independent transmembrane transport of glucose by facilitated diffusion. **GLUT1** and **GLUT3** are widely expressed and are high-affinity, low-capacity transporters. These GLUT isoforms are linked to high-affinity **hexokinases.** Hexokinases phosphorylate glucose to form glucose-6-phosphate (G6P). Because G6P does not bind to GLUTs, G6P cannot leave the cell. Consequently, the hexokinase reaction commits glucose to metabolic pathways. **GLUT2** is a low-affinity, high-capacity isoform expressed in the liver, pancreatic islet beta cell, and basolateral side of intestinal

and renal tubule cells. In the liver and beta cells, GLUT2 is coupled to a low-affinity isoform of hexokinase called **glucokinase.** GLUT2 and glucokinase play critical roles during the digestive phase, when blood glucose levels are high. Expression and membrane localization of GLUT1, GLUT2, and GLUT3 are independent of insulin. In contrast, **GLUT4** is an **insulin-dependent GLUT** that is expressed primarily in skeletal muscle and adipose tissue. It resides in the membranes of cytoplasmic vesicles. In response to insulin signaling, GLUT4 is inserted into the plasma membrane. GLUT4 plays a central role in **"glucose tolerance,"** which is the ability of insulin to prevent excessive increases in blood glucose during and after a meal. In muscle, GLUT4 is coupled to the activity of hexokinase I and II. Hexokinase II gene expression is rapidly increased by insulin. Thus, insulin promotes the uptake of glucose by muscle and its rapid phosphorylation to G6P.

has low affinity for glucose (i.e., it transports glucose only when glucose is available at elevated concentrations) and is designated **glucokinase.**

The second phase involves **glycolysis** (Fig. 38-3), which occurs in the cytoplasm. Glycolysis yields a net production of 2 mol of ATP/mol of glucose while consuming the required cofactor NAD^+ by reducing it to NADH. In the presence of robust oxidative phosphorylation (relative to the rate of glycolysis), NADH is converted back to NAD^+ in an O_2-dependent manner, and pyruvate is the primary product of glycolysis (oxidative glycolysis). If the cell has no or very few mitochondria (e.g., erythrocytes, lens of the eye), oxidative phosphorylation cannot be carried out and used to oxidize NADH back to NAD^+. In this case, the cell regen-

erates NAD^+ by reducing pyruvate to lactate by the process of anaerobic glycolysis.

During the third process (Fig. 38-3), pyruvate enters the mitochondria and is converted to acetyl coenzyme A (acetyl CoA). Acetyl CoA is then further metabolized in the **TCA cycle** and the closely coupled process of **oxidative phosphorylation** via the **electron transport chain.** This second stage of oxidation yields almost 20 times more ATP than glycolysis does. Thus, the TCA cycle and oxidative phosphorylation are very efficient means of generating ATP from glucose. However, molecular O_2 is required. This is why humans need to breathe air, and oxidative phosphorylation can proceed only as fast as the respiratory and cardiovascular systems can deliver O_2 to tissues. Therefore, even

● **Figure 38-3.** ATP is made from glucose, AAs, FFAs, and ketone bodies. (Modified from Porterfield SP, White BA: Endocrine Physiology, 3rd ed. Philadelphia, Mosby, 2007.)

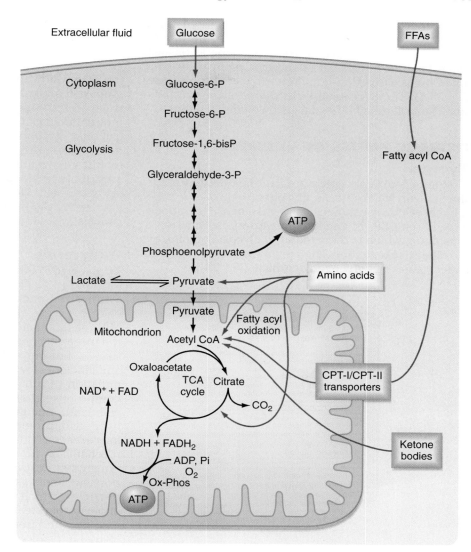

tissues with mitochondria rely on anaerobic glycolysis for some needs. The process of oxidative phosphorylation is also a major contributor to the generation of **reactive oxygen species (ROS),** which impose oxidative stress that is harmful to cells.

Making ATP from Free Fatty Acids

The other two energy substrates, FFAs and AAs, bypass glycolysis and ultimately enter the TCA cycle/oxidative phosphorylation as pyruvate, acetyl CoA, or different components of the TCA cycle. FFAs are released from adipose tissue by lipolysis and circulate in blood bound to serum albumin. Transport proteins then translocate FFAs into cells. FFAs are metabolized in mitochondria by the repetitive, cyclic process of β **oxidation** (Fig. 38-3). This requires the transport of FFAs into the inner mitochondrial matrix by the **carnitine palmitoyltransferase** (**CPT-I** and **CPT-II**) system of transporters. Each cycle of β oxidation removes two carbon moieties at a time from FFA chains and generates a molecule of acetyl CoA, which is oxidized through the TCA cycle and oxidative phosphorylation. In addition to the generation of acetyl CoA, each cycle

of β oxidation generates 1 molecule each of $FADH_2$ and NADH, thereby producing up to 17 ATP molecules via oxidative phosphorylation. Thus, FFAs are a more efficient source of energy storage than carbohydrates in that the cell can obtain more ATPs per carbon from FFAs than from glucose.

Making ATP from Amino Acids

AAs can also be oxidized after transamination (transfer of their amino group to another molecule). The carbon skeletons of AAs converge on the TCA cycle by conversion to intermediates, including pyruvate, acetyl CoA, α-ketoglutarate, succinyl CoA, fumarate, and oxaloacetate (Fig. 38-3). The amino group of AAs can give rise to ammonia, a highly toxic substance. Thus, the use of AAs for energy must be coupled to the urea cycle in the liver, which converts ammonia to urea.

Making ATP from Ketone Bodies

Ketone bodies are four-carbon molecules that include **acetoacetate** and **β-hydroxybutyrate.** Ketone bodies do not exist in the diet at significant levels, as do carbohydrates, fats, and AAs. Rather, ketone bodies represent a fourth class of fuel that is synthesized from acetyl CoA in the liver and exported into the bloodstream for other organs to use. Extrahepatic tissues convert ketone bodies back to acetyl CoA by using succinyl CoA as a CoA donor and the enzyme **thiophorase** (Fig. 38-4). The liver itself lacks thiophorase and thus cannot use ketone bodies for its own energy needs.

STORAGE FORMS OF ENERGY

Glycogen

In general, nutrients are stored during the fed state. Glucose can be stored as **glycogen,** which is a large polymer of glucose molecules. Once glucose is trapped in cells as G6P, it can be converted to glucose-1-phosphate, which is then added to glycogen chains by two repetitive reactions. The primary, regulated enzyme in glycogenesis is **glycogen synthase** (Fig. 38-5).

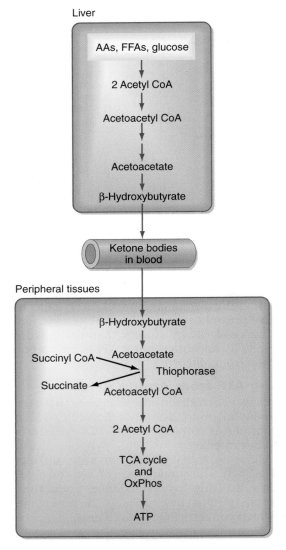

Liver

AAs, FFAs, glucose

↓

2 Acetyl CoA

↓

Acetoacetyl CoA

↓

Acetoacetate

↓

β-Hydroxybutyrate

↓

Ketone bodies in blood

↓

Peripheral tissues

β-Hydroxybutyrate

↓

Succinyl CoA → Acetoacetate

Thiophorase

Succinate → Acetoacetyl CoA

↓

2 Acetyl CoA

↓

TCA cycle and OxPhos

↓

ATP

● **Figure 38-4.** Production of ketone bodies in the liver and their utilization by peripheral tissues. (Modified from Porterfield SP, White BA: Endocrine Physiology, 3rd ed. Philadelphia, Mosby, 2007.)

During the interdigestive period, individual glucose moieties can be cleaved from glycogen and metabolized back to G6P (Fig. 38-5). The primary enzyme in glycogenolysis is called **glycogen phosphorylase.** In the liver, G6P can be further converted to glucose by **glucose-6-phosphatase (G6Pase),** and the glucose that is generated can be transported out of the cell by the bidirectional GLUT2 transporter. Thus, liver glycogen can directly contribute to blood glucose levels. Muscle does not express G6Pase, so glycogenolysis is linked to intramyocellular glycolysis. Muscle glycogen can contribute to blood glucose indirectly. Muscle glycolysis generates lactate, which is converted back to glucose by the liver through the process of gluconeogenesis (see later).

Triglyceride

Triglyceride (TG) represents the storage form of nutrient lipid (e.g., FFAs). TG is obtained from the diet or synthesized endogenously by the liver in the face of caloric excess. Each molecule of TG is composed of three fatty acid chains in an ester linkage to each of the three carbons of glycerol. TG can be stored in most tissues, but only **adipose tissue** has evolved as a safe and efficient storage depot for TG. Significant TG accumulation in other organs (cardiac muscle, liver) can compromise their physiological functions and cause cell death. Accumulation of TG in skeletal muscle and liver also promotes insulin resistance and glucose intolerance. Thus, the body has developed transport mechanisms for the delivery of dietary and endogenously synthesized TGs to adipose tissue. These transport mechanisms involve the assembly of **lipoprotein particles,** which entails coating hydrophobic TG and cholesterol esters with relatively more hydrophilic (or amphipathic) free cholesterol and phospholipids (Fig. 38-6). Lipid-soluble vitamins (e.g., vitamins E, A, D, and K) also associate with lipoproteins. Specific apoproteins, as well as enzymes and transfer proteins, become associated with the surface of lipoprotein particles both before secretion and during transit in blood. The protein complement of lipoprotein particles is absolutely required for their specific function or functions and metabolic clearance. Lipoproteins are summarized in Table 38-2.

Dietary Triglyceride

Most of the TG stored in adipose tissue originates from the diet. Dietary TGs are digested by lipases in the intestinal lumen and are absorbed by intestinal cells as FFAs and 2-monoglycerides. These components are reassembled into TGs within enterocytes. The intestinal cells package TGs into a lipoprotein particle called a **chylomicron,** which enters the villar lymphatics (Fig. 38-7). The intestinal lymphatics bypass the hepatic portal circulation and the liver and empty into the general circulation. Once in blood, chylomicrons travel to adipose tissue, skeletal muscle, and cardiac muscle, where TGs are unloaded as FFAs and glycerol.

A primary apoprotein on chylomicrons is **apo B-48.** Secreted chylomicrons acquire additional apoproteins

● **Figure 38-5.** Glycogen synthesis and breakdown serve different needs in liver versus muscle. (Modified from Porterfield SP, White BA: Endocrine Physiology, 3rd ed. Philadelphia, Mosby, 2007.)

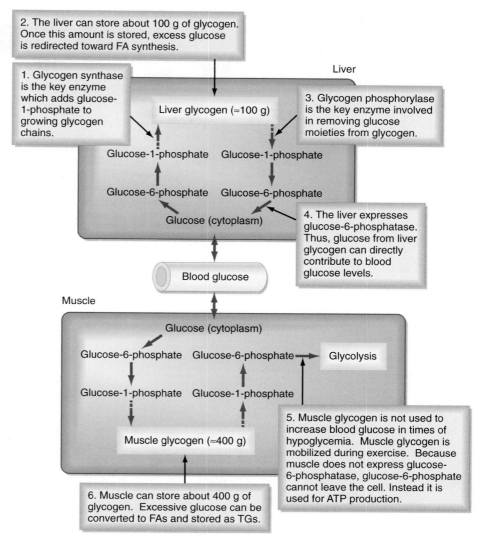

2. The liver can store about 100 g of glycogen. Once this amount is stored, excess glucose is redirected toward FA synthesis.

1. Glycogen synthase is the key enzyme which adds glucose-1-phosphate to growing glycogen chains.

3. Glycogen phosphorylase is the key enzyme involved in removing glucose moieties from glycogen.

4. The liver expresses glucose-6-phosphatase. Thus, glucose from liver glycogen can directly contribute to blood glucose levels.

5. Muscle glycogen is not used to increase blood glucose in times of hypoglycemia. Muscle glycogen is mobilized during exercise. Because muscle does not express glucose-6-phosphatase, glucose-6-phosphate cannot leave the cell. Instead it is used for ATP production.

6. Muscle can store about 400 g of glycogen. Excessive glucose can be converted to FAs and stored as TGs.

LIPOPROTEIN STRUCTURE

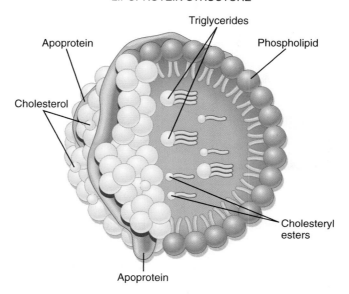

● **Figure 38-6.** The lipoprotein particle. The external monolayer of the particle contains free cholesterol, phospholipids, and apoproteins. The very hydrophobic cholesterol esters and TGs concentrate within the particle core. Lipoproteins also carry fat-soluble vitamins. (From Baynes JW, Dominiczak MH: Medical Biochemistry, 2nd ed. Philadelphia, Mosby, 2005.)

● Table 38-2.   **Characteristics of Different Lipoprotein Particles**

Particle	Main Lipid Component	Apoproteins	Function	Promotes Atherosclerosis
Chylomicron	TG	B-48 (A, C, E)	Transports dietary TG to adipose (and other) tissue	No
Chylomicron remnant	TG	B-48 (A, C, E)	Delivers leftover dietary TG to the liver Exchanges TG for CE from HDL and delivers CE to the liver	Yes
VLDL	TG	B-100 (A, C, E)	Transports endogenously synthesized TG to adipose tissue and skeletal and cardiac muscle Exchanges TG for CE from HDL	No
IDL (VLDL remnant)	TG and cholesterol	B-100, E	Delivers leftover TG and cholesterol to the liver Exchanges TG for CE from HDL and delivers CE to the liver	Yes
LDL	Cholesterol	B-100	Delivers cholesterol to the liver, steroidogenic cells, and dividing cells	Yes
HDL	Cholesterol	As (C, E)	Accepts cholesterol from peripheral cells, esterifies it, and transports cholesterol esters to the liver	No
			Exchanges cholesterol esters for TG in VLDL, IDL, and chylomicron remnants Atheroprotective through several mechanisms, including carrying enzymes (paraoxonase) that inhibit LDL oxidation Acts as a reservoir of circulating apolipoproteins (A, C, and E) for transfer to other lipoprotein particles	Atheroprotective

CE, cholesterol ester.

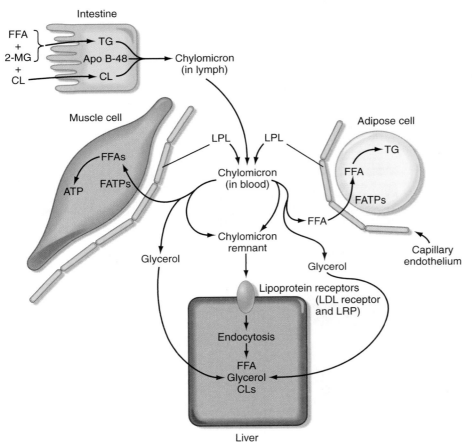

● **Figure 38-7.** Dietary fats are conveyed from the small intestine to adipose tissue as chylomicron particles. Dietary FFAs and 2-monoglycerides (2-MGs) are transported into the enterocyte and reesterified into TG. Other complex lipids (cholesterol [CL], cholesterol esters, phospholipids) are complexed with TG and apolipoprotein B-48 (Apo B-48) into chylomicrons. In the capillary beds of adipose tissue, chylomicrons are digested by lipoprotein lipase (LPL), and the released FFAs are transported into adipocytes by fatty acid transporters (FATPs) and reesterified into TGs. In skeletal and cardiac muscle, FFAs are used for energy. The partially digested chylomicron remnants bind to the LDL receptor (LDLR) and its related protein (LRP; via apo E) and are endocytosed by hepatocytes.

by transfer of proteins from **high-density lipoproteins (HDLs)** in blood. For example, **Apo C-II** is an apoprotein that is exchanged between HDL and chylomicrons. Apo C-II acts as an activator/cofactor of the enzyme **lipoprotein lipase (LPL),** which digests circulating chylomicrons. LPL is synthesized by adipocytes and muscle cells. It is secreted and ultimately translocated to the apical surface of the endothelium lining neigh-

boring capillaries, to which LPL remains noncovalently attached by heparin sulfate proteoglycans. Dozens of LPL molecules attach to and digest lipoprotein particles, thereby releasing FFAs and glycerol (Fig. 38-7). Several fatty acid transport proteins are involved in the transport of FFAs from the apical surface of endothelial cells to the cytoplasm of neighboring cells. Once FFAs enter a cell, they are immediately converted to fatty acyl CoAs. In skeletal and cardiac muscle, fatty acyl CoAs are oxidized for production of ATP. In adipocytes, FFAs are stored in the form of TG. Esterification of the first fatty acyl chain requires glycerol-3-phosphate (G3P). Adipocytes do not express glycerol kinase and consequently cannot synthesize G3P directly from the glycerol released from chylomicrons. Instead, adipocytes generate G3P from intermediates of glycolysis. Partially digested, TG-depleted chylomicrons are called **chylomicron remnants.** These are cleared by the liver through the process of receptor-mediated endocytosis, which requires another apoprotein, **apo E.** Multiple apo E proteins are transferred to a chylomicron from HDL and bind to the **low-density lipoprotein (LDL)** receptor and LDL receptor–related protein (LRP) on hepatocyte membranes.

Endogenously Synthesized Triglyceride

TGs can also be synthesized from glucose and other precursors of acetyl CoA (Fig. 38-8). This occurs during high caloric intake when liver and muscle glycogen stores are saturated and the supply of glucose exceeds the need for synthesis of ATP (e.g., during the development of diet-induced obesity). The primary site of endogenous FFA and TG synthesis in humans is the liver, usually in response to high levels of glucose. Glucose is metabolized to acetyl CoA and then to citrate in the first reaction of the TCA cycle. However, the presence of high ATP and NADH levels in the well-fed state inhibits progression of the TCA cycle and

> ## IN THE CLINIC
>
> Familial hyperchylomicronemia syndrome is due to inactivating mutations in **LPL** or its cofactor **apo C-II.** In these individuals, TGs cannot be efficiently digested and unloaded from chylomicrons after a lipid-containing meal. Chylomicrons are normally cleared from blood by 12 hours after a meal. In individuals with LPL or apo C-II deficiency, TG-laden chylomicrons persist for days after a single meal. Fasting plasma TG levels are normally below 160 mg/dL, but in affected individuals, plasma TG is typically greater than 1000 mg/dL. **Pancreatitis, hepatosplenomegaly** (i.e., enlarged liver and spleen because of phagocytosis of chylomicrons by the reticuloendothelial cells of these organs), **lipemia retinalis** (i.e., opalescent blood vessels in the retina), and **eruptive xanthomas** (i.e., clusters of yellowish white bumps on the skin) develop in many, but not all patients with familial hyperchylomicronemia syndrome. VLDL (see later) is also increased, but to a lesser extent than chylomicrons. Primary clinical management of this syndrome is **dietary fat restriction.** Because chylomicrons also deliver lipid-soluble vitamins to the body, **vitamin supplementation** is also called for.

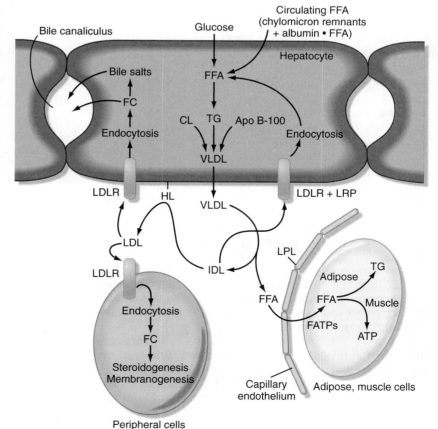

● **Figure 38-8.** Endogenously synthesized fats are conveyed from the hepatocyte to adipose tissue as very-low-density lipoprotein (VLDL) particles. VLDL is digested by LPL in the capillary beds of adipose tissue, skeletal muscle, and other tissues. Partially digested VLDL (intermediate-density lipoproteins [IDLs]) are further digested by hepatic lipase (HL), thereby generating LDL particles, which are endocytosed via the LDL receptor (LDLR) on peripheral cells and hepatocytes. IDLs are also endocytosed by hepatocytes after binding to the LDLR and LRP. CL, complex lipids; FC, free cholesterol; FFA, free fatty acids; TG, triglycerides.

causes intramitochondrial levels of citrate to accumulate. Citrate is then translocated to the cytoplasm, where it is converted back to cytosolic acetyl CoA and oxaloacetate. Once in the cytoplasm, acetyl CoA can enter fatty acyl CoA and TG synthesis (see later). Fatty acyl CoAs are esterified to G3P to form monoglycerides, diglycerides, and finally TGs. TGs are not normally stored in the liver to a large extent but are transferred to adipose tissue. Thus, TGs must be packaged by the liver into lipoprotein particles called **very-low-density lipoproteins (VLDLs)** before being secreted into blood. Like chylomicrons, VLDLs contain a core of very hydrophobic TG and cholesterol esters and a covering of amphipathic phospholipids and free cholesterol. The VLDL particle also contains **apo B-100.** After secretion, VLDLs acquire other proteins from circulating HDL particles, including apo C-II and apo E, and are digested by LPL within the capillary beds of adipose tissue, as well as skeletal and cardiac muscle (Fig. 38-8).

Partially LPL-digested VLDL particles are called **VLDL remnants,** or **intermediate-density lipoprotein (IDL) particles** (Fig. 38-8). IDL has two fates. First, IDL is removed from the circulation by receptor-mediated endocytosis by the LDL receptor (via binding to apo B-100 and apo E) and LRP (via binding to apo E) at the liver. Efficient endocytosis of IDL is dependent on multiple copies of apo E being associated with the remnant particle. Second, IDL is further digested by the ecto-enzyme **hepatic lipase.** This delivers FFAs and glycerol to the liver and transforms the IDL into a TG-poor, cholesterol-rich **LDL particle.**

Low-Density Lipoprotein and Cholesterol Economy

With the formation of LDL, the nutritional role of lipoproteins (i.e., delivery of TG to adipose tissue or muscle) has largely been completed. This is due to the fact that cholesterol cannot be metabolized by humans for energy. However, cholesterol is used as the backbone for certain molecules and is an important component in cell membranes. Although most cells can synthesize some cholesterol from acetate, LDL is an important source of cholesterol, particularly for cells with a high demand for cholesterol. Quantitatively, hepatocytes that synthesize **bile salts** have the greatest need for cholesterol and endocytose the largest amount of LDL. Other cell types that have a high demand for cholesterol include steroidogenic cells and growing and proliferating cells that need to synthesize new cell membrane. In fact, some aggressively growing cancers import LDL cholesterol to the extent that circulating levels of cholesterol fall well below normal **(hypocholesterolemia).**

LDL particles deliver cholesterol to cells through binding of apo B-100 to the **LDL receptor,** followed by receptor-mediated endocytosis. In the transition of IDL to LDL, the LDL loses apo E. This means that LDL cannot be cleared from blood through apo E–dependent binding to LRP, only through apo B-100–dependent binding to the LDL receptor. Quantitatively, the primary site of LDL endocytosis is the liver, which is

Familial hypertriglyceridemia is due to increased VLDL production, decreased VLDL clearance, or both. This condition is associated with elevated plasma TG (250 to 1000 mg/dL), reduced HDL, but *not* usually an increased risk of peripheral or coronary atherosclerosis or cardiovascular disease (see later). In some cases, familial hypertriglyceridemia progresses to decreased clearance of chylomicrons (i.e., hyperchylomicronemia). In the latter case, patients experience eruptive xanthomas and pancreatitis, but not usually cardiovascular disease. **Diet-induced obesity, alcoholism, insulin resistance, and type 2 diabetes** (see later) are factors that increase VLDL production by the liver and can exacerbate this condition.

Abetalipoproteinemia is due to a mutation in the gene encoding **microsomal transfer protein (MTP).** MTP is required for proper packaging of lipids with apoproteins during the formation of chylomicrons and VLDL. Affected individuals have extremely low plasma TG and cholesterol and no circulating chylomicrons, VLDL, or apo B. The inability to synthesize chylomicrons leads to **fat malabsorption** and **diarrhea** in early childhood. In affected individuals, neurological disorders such as **spinocerebellar degeneration** and **pigmented retinopathy** can develop and cause several neurological symptoms, including **ataxia** (i.e., loss of coordination) and a **spastic gait.** The neurological disorders are due to malabsorption of fat-soluble vitamins, especially **vitamin E** (but also vitamins A and K). Thus, early diagnosis and early vitamin supplementation, along with a high-calorie, low-fat diet, can prevent the development of neurological sequelae.

Diet-induced obesity, especially when associated with central (visceral) obesity, can overwhelm the liver with an influx of FFAs via the hepatic portal vein. This is further exacerbated by the insulin resistance of obesity, which allows increased lipolysis and release of FFAs from adipose tissue. Diet-induced obesity and the associated insulin resistance also lead to an inability of skeletal muscle to effectively lower the typically high carbohydrate load after a meal (i.e., **glucose intolerance**). Thus, the liver, which always accepts glucose via the insulin-independent, high-capacity GLUT2 transporter (coupled to a high-capacity glucokinase), is exposed to an increased burden of intrahepatic glucose that is converted to FFAs and TG. The influx of FFAs and glucose can exceed the ability of the liver to package lipids into VLDL for secretion and transport to adipose tissue. Under these conditions, the liver begins to store increasing amounts of TG, which leads to **hepatic steatosis (fatty liver)** and can progress to **nonalcoholic steatotic hepatitis (NASH).**

also the site of cholesterol excretion. About 1 g of cholesterol is excreted daily by the liver—50% as cholesterol and 50% as bile salts. The liver is also the primary site of cholesterol synthesis. Importantly, the synthesis of cholesterol and uptake of LDL cholesterol are highly regulated in a negative-feedback loop. Therefore, the daily amount of cholesterol synthesis (about 1 g) is modulated by the amount absorbed from the diet (about 250 mg/day), so changes in dietary cholesterol normally have a relatively small effect on total circulating and LDL cholesterol.

High-Density Lipoprotein and Reverse Cholesterol Transport

Because cells cannot break cholesterol down, they intermittently need to discharge cholesterol (Fig. 38-9). There is also a need for macrophages that ingest oxidized LDL to rid themselves of excess cholesterol before they become foam cells and die. The efflux of cholesterol from cells is facilitated by **ATP-binding cassette (ABC) proteins,** most notably **ABCA1.** The cholesterol that is transferred out of cells is accepted by **nascent HDL.** Nascent HDL is produced by the liver and small intestine and is composed of **apo A-I,** phospholipids (primarily lecithin), and the enzyme **lecithin-cholesterol acyltransferase (LCAT).** LCAT esterifies cholesterol, and the cholesterol esters accumulate within the center of the maturing spherical HDL (**HDL₃**). Mature HDL can return cholesterol to the liver for excretion (i.e., reverse cholesterol transport) via two pathways. First, HDL can transfer cholesterol esters to TG-rich VLDL, IDL, and chylomicron remnants through the action of an HDL-associated protein, **cholesterol ester transfer protein (CETP).** This is done in exchange for TG, which produces a larger HDL particle (**HDL₂**). The cholesterol-enriched IDL and chylomicron remnants are then endocytosed by the liver through apo E–dependent binding to the LDL receptor and LRP (A in Fig. 38-9). The second pathway involves apo A-I–dependent binding to the scavenger receptor BI (SR-BI) on the hepatocyte membrane (B in Fig. 38-9). This allows the transfer of cholesterol esters from HDL into the hepatocyte membrane. Cholesterol esters are then cleaved by **hepatic hormone-sensitive lipase,** and the free cholesterol enters the bile salt pathway or is excreted as cholesterol. Larger, TG-enriched HDL is first processed by **hepatic lipase,** which decreases its size and enhances its binding to SR-BI.

In addition to the role of HDL in reverse cholesterol transport, HDL has several other atheroprotective actions. For example, other enzymes associated with HDL (e.g., paraoxonase) inhibit oxidation of LDL in the intima of blood vessels. HDL also increases nitric oxide synthesis by endothelial cells. Thus, HDL plays a major atheroprotective role, which explains why the ratio of LDL to HDL is an important consideration when assessing a patient's blood chemistry in terms of risk for cardiovascular disease.

Catabolism of Triglycerides in Adipose Cells

During a fast, TGs are catabolized back to FFAs and glycerol. This is initiated by the action of a **hormone-sensitive lipase,** followed by additional lipases that remove the second and third fatty acyl groups. The net amount of TG versus FFAs in adipose tissue is thus determined by the balance of TG synthesis and lipolysis, which is extremely sensitive to hormonal signals.

IN THE CLINIC

LDL is relatively small (about 30 nm in diameter). As such, LDL can gain entry into the subendothelial intima of blood vessels at sites of minimal endothelial damage. In this environment, the outer components of LDL (i.e., phospholipids, cholesterol, apo B-100) become oxidized. Oxidized LDL has several direct effects on endothelial cells, including a reduction in endothelial viability and their production of the potent vasodilator and atheroprotective substance nitric oxide. Additionally, oxidized apo B-100 binds to scavenger receptors on macrophages, which then endocytose oxidized LDL. Scavenger receptors are not down-regulated by their cargo (oxidized LDL) or by the intracellular byproducts of oxidized LDL. As a consequence, macrophages can become engorged with oxidized LDL. These cholesterol-filled macrophages, called **foam cells,** eventually die and release large amounts of cholesterol into the intima. The released pools of cholesterol from many foam cells promote the development of **atherosclerotic plaque.** Oxidized LDL may also contribute to a mounting inflammatory reaction within the intima involving movement of immune cells into the intima, release of cytokines and chemoattractants, and proliferation and migration of vascular smooth muscle cells into the intima.

Familial hypercholesterolemia is due to mutations in the **LDL receptor.** These mutations (many hundreds have been characterized) impair the ability of the liver to clear LDL cholesterol from blood. Thus, total cholesterol and LDL cholesterol are elevated, whereas TG is normal. Affected individuals are prone to the development of cutaneous xanthomas and are at extreme risk for atherosclerosis and cardiovascular disease. In fact, untreated, homozygous patients rarely survive to 30 years of age. Treatment is LDL apheresis, which involves physical removal of LDL from blood. **Autosomal recessive hypercholesterolemia** is due to mutations in the **ARH protein,** a scaffolding protein that links the LDL receptor to clathrin-dependent endocytosis.

Insulin resistance and type 2 diabetes mellitus (see later) are often characterized by dyslipidemia, especially in association with central (visceral) obesity, hypertension, and cardiovascular disease. This constellation of metabolic derangements is collectively referred to as **metabolic syndrome.** The liver produces larger than normal VLDL particles, which are very efficiently processed by LPL and hepatic lipase and ultimately give rise to **small, dense LDL particles** that are highly atherogenic. Atherosclerosis is key to development of the hypertension (decreased nitric oxide synthesis, decreased arterial compliance) and coronary heart disease (blockage of coronary arteries by plaque) of metabolic syndrome. A major pharmacological treatment to lower LDL cholesterol is the use of **statins.** These drugs inhibit the rate-limiting enzyme in cholesterol biosynthesis (i.e., HMG-CoA reductase). Less intracellular cholesterol is sensed by the transcription factor **sterol responsive element–binding protein (SREBP-2),** which up-regulates the expression of HMG-CoA reductase, as well as the LDL receptor. On balance, less LDL cholesterol is made, and more LDL cholesterol is cleared by the liver.

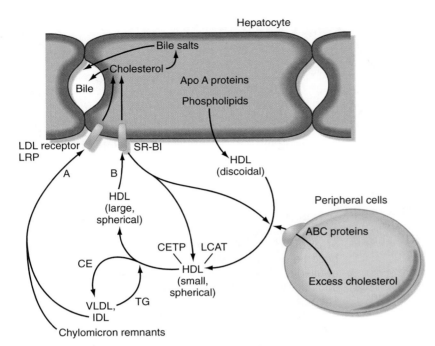

● **Figure 38-9.** Reverse cholesterol transport is mediated by HDL particles. Excess cholesterol in extrahepatic cells is transported out of the cell by ATP-binding cassette (ABC) proteins and onto discoidal HDL particles, thereby generating small, spherical HDL particles. Cholesterol is esterified by the enzyme lecithin-cholesterol acyltransferase (LCAT). Cholesterol esters (CEs) and TGs are exchanged between VLDL, IDL, and chylomicron remnants and HDL through the activity of cholesterol ester transfer protein (CETP). As HDLs take on TG, they become large, spherical HDL particles. HDL transfers its CEs to the liver through interaction with the HDL receptor, called scavenger receptor B1 (SR-B1). Cholesterol is then secreted in bile, either as cholesterol or as bile salts. The HDL particles are recycled.

> ### IN THE CLINIC
>
> **Mutations in apo A-I** result in complete absence of HDL, which gives rise to increased coronary heart disease. Because apo A-I is a cofactor for LCAT, total blood and cellular free cholesterol is increased and leads to **corneal opacities** and **planar xanthomas.** Other mutations in apo A-I increase the rate of clearance of HDL. Interestingly, these patients have low plasma HDL and HDL cholesterol but are not at increased risk for cardiovascular disease. **Fibrates** are ligands for the transcription factor **peroxisome proliferation activator receptor α (PPARα)** (see later), which stimulates hepatic synthesis of apo A-I. Thus, fibrates can be used to increase circulating HDL. A more recently discovered member of the PPAR family, PPARδ/β, also strongly increases apo A production. However, exogenous ligands for PPARδ/β are not yet approved for use in humans.

Hydrophobic FFAs are transported in blood mostly in FFA-albumin complexes. FFAs are actively transported into cells, which divert FFAs into β oxidative pathways for energy or, in the case of the liver, into ketone bodies (Fig. 38-4). This latter fate of FFAs is important during a prolonged fast because unlike FFAs, ketone bodies in sufficient levels can cross the blood-brain barrier.

Protein

Unlike TG stored in depot fat, proteins perform many dynamic functions other than storage of energy. Nevertheless, proteins are metabolically active and can be hydrolyzed when needed to produce AAs, which can then be oxidized for energy or used to make glucose (see the following section on gluconeogenesis), FFAs, or ketone bodies. Under fasting conditions, protein synthesis is reduced, whereas protein breakdown is enhanced. For AAs to be used for energy, their amino groups must be converted to urea to prevent buildup of toxic ammonia.

GLUCONEOGENESIS: SYNTHESIZING GLUCOSE FROM GLYCEROL, LACTATE, AND AMINO ACIDS

Breakdown of glycogen is a transient way by which the liver can contribute directly to blood glucose levels. The liver and, to a lesser extent, the kidney can also produce glucose for a much longer period by converting glycerol, lactate, and AAs into glucose. Pyruvate or TCA intermediates that can generate oxaloacetate are glucogenic. A major glucogenic molecule is pyruvate, which is directly converted to oxaloacetate by **pyruvate carboxylase** (Fig. 38-10). Oxaloacetate escapes the mitochondria as malate, which is then reoxidized to oxaloacetate. Oxaloacetate is converted to phosphoenolpyruvate (PEP) by the enzyme **PEP carboxykinase (PEPCK).** PEP is subsequently converted to fructose-1,6-bisphosphate via the reversible reactions of glycolysis. In the presence of a high ATP/AMP ratio, the enzyme **fructose-1,6-bisphosphatase** is active; it generates fructose-6-phosphate (F6P) and then reversibly converts it to G6P, which is dephosphorylated by **G6Pase** and released into blood through the bidirectional GLUT2 transporter.

Importantly, acetyl CoA cannot be used to make glucose. This means that FFAs, ketone bodies, and certain AAs cannot directly contribute to blood glucose levels. However, the utilization of FFAs has a **glucose-sparing** effect because during prolonged fasting, ketone bodies eventually reach levels sufficient to be used by the brain, thereby reducing the glucose required for the brain.

● **Figure 38-10.** Gluconeogenesis. The liver expresses key enzymes that can use AAs, glycerol, and lactate to synthesize glucose in order to maintain blood glucose levels. (Modified from Porterfield SP, White BA: Endocrine Physiology, 3rd ed. Philadelphia, Mosby, 2007.)

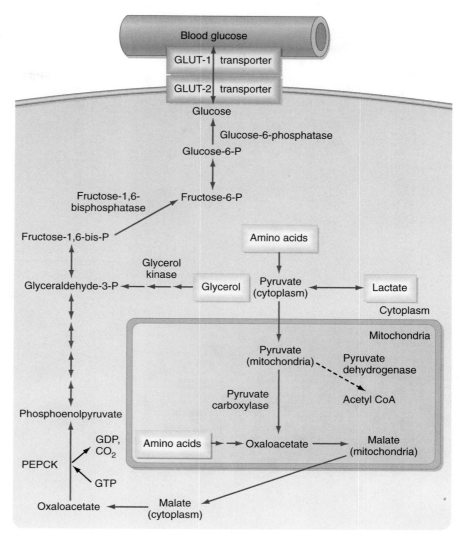

SUMMARY OF KEY METABOLIC PATHWAYS

ATP is the primary source of energy in all cells. The body can make ATP from carbohydrates, FFAs, AAs, and ketone bodies. However, the brain is exclusively dependent on glucose, except after days of fasting, when it can metabolize ketone bodies. As hunter-gatherers, humans evolved to efficiently store excess calories as glycogen, TGs, and protein during a meal and release stored energy substrates as needed during fasting or for physical activity (or both). Additionally, in times of a fast, the liver can convert substrates to ketone bodies for use by other organs (especially the brain). The enzymatic pathways that coordinate the partitioning of energy stores during a meal and their utilization between meals and during exercise are regulated by nutrient status, autonomic innervation, and key hormones. Before discussing how hormones regulate these pathways, we first need to learn about the hormones themselves.

KEY HORMONES INVOLVED IN METABOLIC HOMEOSTASIS

Endocrine Pancreatic Hormones

The islets of Langerhans constitute the endocrine portion of the pancreas (Fig. 38-11). Approximately 1 million islets, making up about 1% to 2% of the pancreatic mass, are spread throughout the pancreas. The islets are composed of several cell types, each producing a different hormone. In islets situated in the body, tail, and anterior portion of the head of the pancreas, the most abundant cell type is the beta cell (also called B cell). Beta cells make up about three fourths of the cells of the islets and produce the hormone **insulin.** Alpha (A) cells account for about 10% of these islets and secrete **glucagon.** The third major cell type of the islets within these regions is the delta (D) cell, which makes up about 5% of the cells and produces the peptide **somatostatin.** A fourth cell type, the F cell, constitutes about 80% of the cells in the islets situated within the posterior portion of the head of the pan-

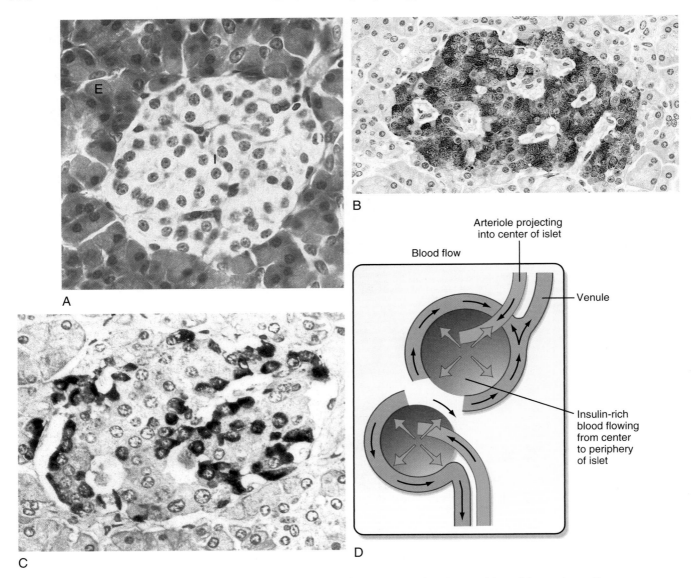

● **Figure 38-11.** **A,** Histological section of a pancreas showing an islet of Langerhans (I) surrounded by the exocrine pancreas (E). (From Young B et al: Wheater's Functional Histology, 5th ed. London, Churchill Livingstone, 2006). A human islet stained by immunohistochemical methods shows the predominance and central core location of **(B)** beta cells (insulin) and **(C)** the peripheral distribution of alpha cells (glucagon). (From Stevens A, Lowe J: Human Histology, 3rd ed. Philadelphia, Mosby, 2004.) **D,** Drawing showing arterial blood flowing into the center of an islet and then percolating centrifugally toward the periphery of the islet.

creas (including the uncinate process); it secretes the peptide **pancreatic polypeptide.** Because the physiological function of pancreatic polypeptide in humans remains obscure, it will not be discussed further.

Blood flow to the islets is somewhat autonomous from blood flow to the surrounding exocrine pancreatic tissue. Blood flow through the islets passes from beta cells, which predominate in the center of the islet, to alpha and delta cells, which predominate in the periphery (Fig. 38-11). Consequently, the first cells affected by circulating insulin are the alpha cells, in which insulin inhibits glucagon secretion.

Insulin

Insulin is the primary anabolic hormone that is responsible for maintaining the upper limit of blood glucose and FFA levels. Insulin achieves this objective by promoting glucose uptake and utilization by muscle and adipose tissue, increasing glycogen storage in liver and muscle, and reducing glucose output by the liver. Insulin promotes protein synthesis from AAs and inhibits protein degradation in peripheral tissues. Insulin also promotes TG synthesis in the liver and adipose tissue and represses lipolysis of adipose TG stores. Finally, insulin regulates metabolic homeostasis through effects on satiety. Partial or complete loss of insulin's action results in severe hyperglycemia, dyslipidemia, and diabetes mellitus.

Structure, Synthesis, and Secretion

Insulin is a protein hormone that belongs to the gene family that includes **insulin-like growth factors I and II (IGF-I, IGF-II), relaxin,** and several insulin-like peptides. The insulin gene encodes preproinsulin. Insulin is synthesized on the polyribosome as preproinsulin, and microsomal enzymes cleave the N-terminal signal peptide to produce proinsulin as the peptide enters the endoplasmic reticulum. **Proinsulin** is packaged in the Golgi apparatus into membrane-bound secretory granules. Proinsulin contains the AA sequence of insulin plus the 31–amino acid **C (connecting) peptide**

and four linking AAs. The proteases that cleave proinsulin (proprotein convertases 1/3 and 2) are packaged with proinsulin within the secretory granule. The mature hormone consists of two chains, an α chain and a β chain, connected by two disulfide bridges (Fig. 38-12). A third disulfide bridge is contained within the α chain. Insulin is stored in secretory granules in zinc-bound crystals. On stimulation, the granule's contents are released to the outside of the cell by exocytosis.

Insulin has a half-life of 5 to 8 minutes and is cleared rapidly from the circulation. It is degraded by insulinase in the liver, kidney, and other tissues. Because insulin is secreted into the portal vein, it is exposed to liver insulinase before it enters the peripheral circulation. Consequently, almost half the insulin is degraded

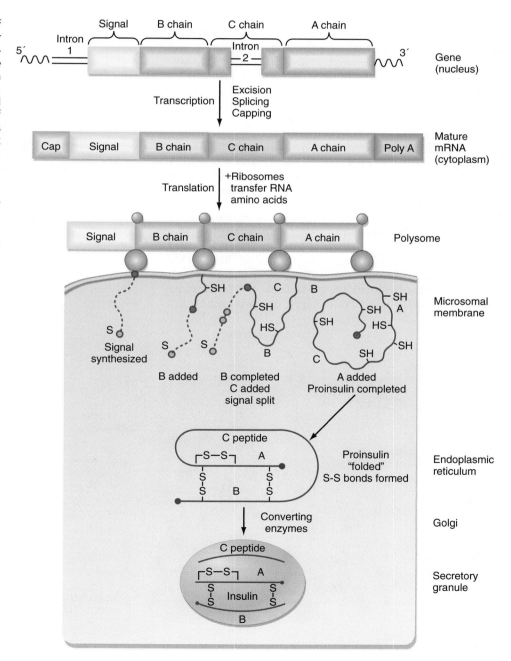

● **Figure 38-12.** Synthesis of insulin. The insulin gene codes for preproinsulin. The mature messenger RNA initiates synthesis of the N-terminal signal peptide (S) in ribosomes, followed by the B, C, and A chains. The signal is degraded during the course of completion of the proinsulin molecule. The latter is folded into a conformation that permits disulfide linkages to form between the A and B chains. Within the Golgi and secretory granule, converting enzymes cleave off the C chain, known as C peptide, thereby completing the synthesis of insulin. The insulin molecules are concentrated in the electron-dense core of the granule, whereas the C peptide molecules are in the peripheral halo areas of the granule. (Data from Permutt M et al: Diabetes Care 7:386, 1984; and Steiner DF et al. In Degroot LJ et al [eds]: Endocrinology, vol 2. New York, Grune & Stratton, 1979.)

before leaving the liver. Thus, peripheral tissues are exposed to only half the serum insulin concentration as the liver. Recombinant human insulin and insulin analogues with different characteristics of onset and duration of action and peak activity are now available.

Serum insulin levels normally begin to rise within 10 minutes after ingestion of food and reach a peak in 30 to 45 minutes. The higher serum insulin level rapidly lowers blood glucose to baseline values.

When insulin secretion is stimulated, insulin is released within minutes. If the stimulus is maintained, insulin secretion falls within 10 minutes and then slowly rises over a period of about 1 hour (Fig. 38-13). The latter phase is referred to as the **late phase of insulin release.** The **early phase of insulin release** probably involves the release of preformed insulin, whereas the late phase represents the release of newly formed insulin.

Glucose is the primary stimulus of insulin secretion. Entry of glucose into beta cells is facilitated by the GLUT2 transporter. Once glucose enters the beta cell, it is phosphorylated to G6P by the low-affinity hexokinase **glucokinase.** Glucokinase is referred to as the **"glucose sensor"** of the beta cell because the rate of glucose entry is correlated to the rate of glucose phosphorylation, which in turn is directly related to insulin secretion. Metabolism of G6P by beta cells increases the intracellular ATP/ADP ratio and closes an **ATP-sensitive K$^+$ channel** (Fig. 38-14). This results in depolarization of the beta cell membrane, which opens **voltage-gated Ca^{++} channels.** Increased intracellular [Ca^{++}] activates microtubule-mediated exocytosis of insulin/proinsulin-containing secretory granules. The ATP-sensitive K$^+$ channel is a protein complex that contains an ATP-binding subunit called **SUR.** This subunit is also activated by **sulfonylurea drugs,** which are widely used as oral agents to treat hyperglycemia in patients with partially impaired beta cell function.

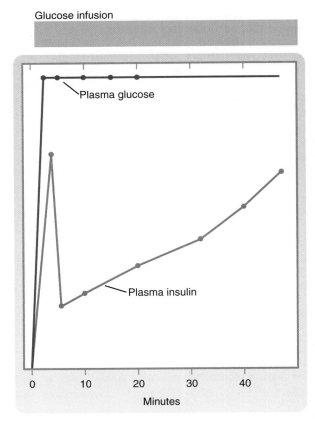

● **Figure 38-13.** The insulin response to glucose infusion shows a rapid first phase of insulin release followed by a fall and a later, slower second phase.

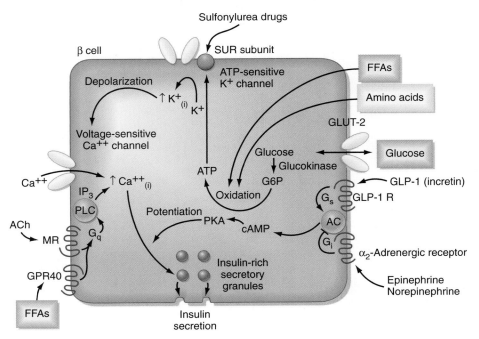

● **Figure 38-14.** Regulation of insulin secretion by the energy substrates glucose (primary secretagogue), AAs, and FFAs and by the neurotransmitters and hormones acetylcholine (ACh), norepinephrine, epinephrine, and glucagon-like peptide-1 (GLP-1). AC, adenylyl cyclase; GPR40, G protein–coupled receptor 40; MR, muscarinic receptor; PLC, phospholipase C. (Modified from Porterfield SP, White BA: Endocrine Physiology, 3rd ed. Philadelphia, Mosby, 2007.)

Several AAs and vagal (parasympathetic) cholinergic innervation (i.e., in response to a meal) also stimulate insulin through increasing intracellular [Ca^{++}] (Fig. 38-14). In addition, long-chain FFAs increase insulin secretion, though to a lesser extent than glucose and AAs. FFAs may act through a G protein–coupled receptor (GPR40) on the beta cell membrane or as a nutrient that increases ATP through oxidation (Fig. 38-14).

Nutrient-dependent stimulation of insulin release is enhanced by the incretin hormones glucagon-like peptide-1 (GLP-1) and gastric inhibitory polypeptide (GIP) and possibly by other gastrointestinal hormones. These hormones act primarily by raising intracellular cAMP, which amplifies the intracellular effects of Ca^{++} on glucose (Fig. 38-14). However, these agents do not increase insulin secretion in the absence of glucose.

Insulin secretion is inhibited by α_2-adrenergic receptors, which are activated by epinephrine (from the adrenal medulla) and norepinephrine (from postganglionic sympathetic fibers). α_2-Adrenergic receptors act by decreasing cAMP and possibly by closing Ca^{++} channels (Fig. 38-14). Adrenergic inhibition of insulin serves to protect against hypoglycemia, especially during exercise. Although somatostatin from D cells inhibits both insulin and glucagon, its physiological role in pancreatic islet function in humans is unclear.

The Insulin Receptor

The **insulin receptor (IR)** is a member of the **receptor tyrosine kinase (RTK)** family (see Chapter 3). The IR is expressed on the cell membrane as a homodimer composed of α/β monomers (Fig. 38-15). The α/β monomer is synthesized as one protein, which is then proteolytically cleaved, with the two fragments connected by a disulfide bond. The two α/β monomers are also held together by a disulfide bond between the α subunits. The α subunits are external to the cell membrane and contain the hormone binding sites. The β subunits span the membrane and contain a tyrosine kinase domain on the cytosolic surface. Binding of insulin to the receptor induces the β subunits to cross-phosphorylate each other on three tyrosine residues. These phosphotyrosine residues recruit three classes of adapter proteins: **insulin receptor substrates (IRSs),**

> ### ◢ IN THE CLINIC
>
> Insulin gene expression and islet cell biogenesis are dependent on several transcription factors that are specific to the pancreas, liver, and kidney. These transcription factors include **hepatocyte nuclear factor-4α (HNF-4α), HNF-1α, insulin promoter factor-1 (IPF-1), HNF-1β,** and **neurogenic differentiation 1/beta cell E-box trans-activator 2 (NeuroD1/β$_2$).** Heterozygous mutation of one of these factors results in progressively inadequate production of insulin and maturity-onset diabetes of the young (MODY) before the age of 25. MODY is characterized by nonketotic hyperglycemia, often asymptomatic, that begins in childhood or adolescence. In addition to the five transcription factors, mutations in **glucokinase** give rise to MODY.

● **Figure 38-15.** Intracellular signaling pathways coupled to the insulin receptor. Grb2, adapter protein that links the SH2 domain on tyrosine kinase receptors to the SH3 domain of SOS, which is a Ras guanosine nucleotide exchange factor; GLUT4, glucose transporter 4; I, insulin; IRS, insulin receptor substrate; MAPK, mitogen-activated protein kinase; MEK, MAPK kinase; PI3K, phosphoinositide-3-kinase; PKB, protein kinase B (also called Akt); PIP$_2$, phosphatidylinositol 4,5-bisphosphate; PIP$_3$, phosphatidylinositol 3,4,5-trisphosphate; pY, phosphorylated tyrosine residue; Raf, MAPK kinase kinase. (Modified from Porterfield SP, White BA: Endocrine Physiology, 3rd ed. Philadelphia, Mosby, 2007.)

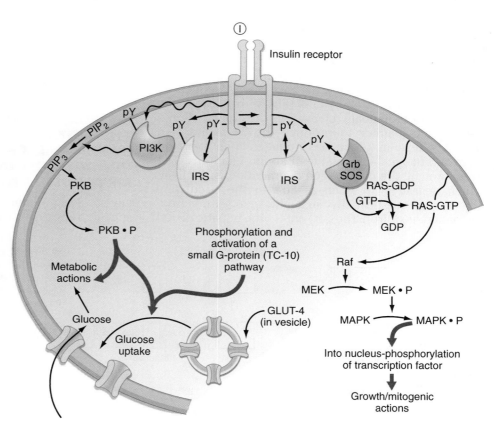

Shc protein, and **APS protein.** The IRS proteins are phosphorylated, and phosphoinositide-3-kinase (PI3K) is then recruited to the membrane, where it phosphorylates its substrates and activates a pleiotropic **protein kinase B (PKB)-dependent pathway** that is largely involved in the metabolic effects of insulin. One important effect of insulin is to induce insertion of the glucose transporter GLUT4 into the cell membranes of muscle and adipose tissue (see later). This action requires both IRS/PI3K-dependent signaling and an additional APS adapter protein–dependent pathway that activates a small GTPase pathway. The Shc protein is linked to the mitogen-activated protein kinase (MAPK) pathway, which mediates the growth and mitogenic actions of insulin.

The termination of insulin/IR signaling is a topic of interest because these mechanisms potentially play a role in **insulin resistance** and **type 2 diabetes mellitus (T2DM).** Insulin induces the down-regulation of its own receptor by receptor-mediated endocytosis and degradative pathways. Additionally, there are several serine/threonine protein kinases that are activated by insulin and that subsequently inactivate IR and IRS proteins. A third mechanism appears to involve activation of the **"suppressor of cytokine signaling" (SOCS)** family of proteins, which reduces the activity or levels (or both) of the IR and IRS proteins.

Glucagon

Glucagon is the primary "counterregulatory" hormone that increases blood glucose levels through its effects on liver glucose output. Glucagon promotes the production of glucose through elevated glycogenolysis and gluconeogenesis and through decreased glycolysis and glycogenolysis. Glucagon also inhibits the synthesis of hepatic lipid from glucose.

Structure, Synthesis, and Secretion

Glucagon is a member of the secretin gene family. The precursor preproglucagon harbors the AA sequences for glucagon, **GLP-1** and **GLP-2** (Fig. 38-16). Preproglucagon is proteolytically cleaved in the alpha cell in a cell-specific manner to produce the 29–amino acid peptide glucagon. Glucagon circulates in an unbound form and has a short half-life of about 6 minutes. The predominant site of glucagon degradation is the liver, which degrades as much as 80% of the circulating glucagon in one pass. Because glucagon (either from the pancreas or from the gut) enters the hepatic portal vein and is carried to the liver before reaching the systemic circulation, a large portion of the hormone never reaches the systemic circulation. The liver is the primary target organ of glucagon, with only small effects on peripheral tissues.

Several factors that stimulate insulin inhibit glucagon. Indeed, it is the **insulin-glucagon ratio** that determines the net flow of hepatic metabolic pathways. A major stimulus for secretion of glucagon is a drop in blood glucose, which is primarily an indirect effect of the removal of inhibition by insulin (Fig. 38-17). Circulating catecholamines, which inhibit the secretion of insulin via α_2-adrenergic receptors, stimulate the secretion of glucagon via β_2-adrenergic receptors (Fig. 38-17). Serum AAs promote the secretion of glucagon. This means that a protein meal will increase postprandial levels of both insulin and glucagon, which protects against hypoglycemia, whereas a carbohydrate meal stimulates only insulin.

Epinephrine and Norepinephrine

The other major counterregulatory factors are the catecholamines **epinephrine** and **norepinephrine.** Epinephrine and norepinephrine are secreted by the adrenal medulla (see Chapter 42), whereas only norepinephrine is released from postganglionic sympathetic nerve endings. The direct metabolic actions of catecholamines are mediated primarily by β-adrenergic receptors located on muscle, adipose, and liver tissue (Fig. 38-17). Like the glucagon receptor, β-adrenergic receptors (β_2 and β_3) increase intracellular cAMP. Catecholamines are released from sympathetic nerve endings and the adrenal medulla in response to decreased glucose concentrations, stress, and exercise. Decreased glucose levels (i.e., hypoglycemia) are primarily sensed by hypothalamic neurons, which initiate a sympathetic response to release catecholamines.

METABOLIC HOMEOSTASIS: THE INTEGRATED OUTCOME OF HORMONAL AND SUBSTRATE/ PRODUCT REGULATION OF METABOLIC PATHWAYS

Levels of blood glucose must be maintained within a specific range and are determined by the absorption

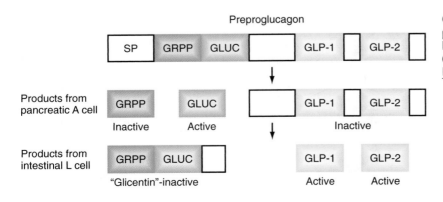

Preproglucagon

Products from pancreatic A cell

Products from intestinal L cell

● **Figure 38-16.** Cell-specific processing of preproglucagon. GLUC, glucagon; GLP, glucagon-like peptide; GRPP, glicentin-related polypeptide. (Modified from Porterfield SP, White BA: Endocrine Physiology, 3rd ed. Philadelphia, Mosby, 2007.)

● **Figure 38-17.** Feedback loops between blood glucose and insulin, glucagon, and sympathoadrenal catecholamines.

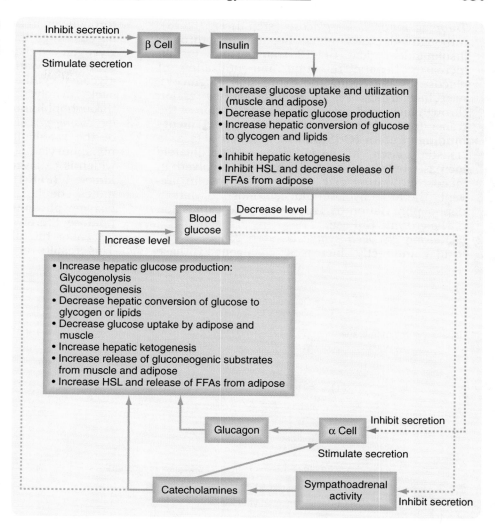

of food and the flow of recently absorbed or stored energy substrates through different metabolic pathways, which must also meet the energy demands of all cells. The relative flow of carbon through different pathways is determined by key enzymatic reactions. The enzymes involved are regulated by substrate and product concentrations and by endocrine and autonomic regulation of enzyme gene expression or activity, or both. The hormonal regulation of these key enzymatic steps will be emphasized in this section.

Fasting-to-Fed State Transition Involving Anabolic Pathways That Store Energy

Insulin and the Storage of Glucose as Glycogen and Triglycerides in the Liver

Ingestion of a mixed meal stimulates beta cells to release insulin, and insulin rapidly inhibits release of glucagon from the adjacent alpha cells (Fig. 38-17). This results in an increased insulin-glucagon ratio in the hepatic portal vein as it enters the liver. The liver responds to this signal by increasing hepatic glucose utilization—first through enhanced glycogen synthesis. Once hepatic glycogen stores (80 to 100 g) are

replenished, excess glucose is used for the synthesis of TG (the liver meets its own energy needs primarily from the oxidation of unbranched AAs in the fed state). Glucose is directed into glycolysis, which in the liver can be thought of as an accessory pathway for the synthesis of TG. Glycolysis promotes the accumulation of citrate, which serves to transport the acetyl group of acetyl CoA into the cytoplasm, where fatty acyl CoA synthesis is performed. Glucose is also directed into the nonoxidative pathway, the hexose monophosphate shunt, which is a major supplier of the NADPH required for fatty acyl CoA synthesis. In addition to these glucose-utilizing, anabolic pathways of glycogen synthesis and lipogenesis, the high insulin-glucagon ratio inhibits the hepatic glucose–producing pathways of glycogenolysis and gluconeogenesis and inhibits hepatic fatty acyl CoA oxidation. This is achieved by the stimulation of key enzymes and the concomitant inhibition of opposing enzymes. This coordinated process of activation and repression minimizes the generation of futile cycles.

Some of the key metabolic steps that are regulated by insulin in the liver are as follows:

1. *Trapping intracellular glucose* (step 1; Fig. 38-18). Although glucose enters hepatocytes through insulin-independent GLUT2 transporters, insulin increases hepatic retention and utilization of glucose by increasing the expression of **glucokinase.** Insulin increases glucokinase gene expression through increased expression and activation of the transcription factor **sterol regulatory element– binding protein-1C (SREBP-1C),** which acts as a "master switch" in the fed state to coordinately increase levels of several enzymes involved in glucose utilization and TG synthesis. Insulin prevents the futile cycle of glucose phosphorylation- dephosphorylation by repressing gene expression of the enzyme **G6Pase.**

2. *Increasing glycogen synthesis* (step 2; Fig. 38-18). Insulin indirectly increases glycogen synthase

through increased expression of glucokinase because high levels of G6P allosterically increase glycogen synthase activity. Insulin promotes the dephosphorylation and thereby the activation of **glycogen synthase.** Insulin also prevents the futile cycle of glycogen synthesis ↔ glycogenolysis through inhibition of **glycogen phosphorylase.**

3. *Increasing glycolysis.* Insulin increases the activity of the rate-limiting and irreversible reaction of phosphorylating F6P to fructose-1,6-bisphosphate, which is catalyzed by the enzyme **phosphofructo- kinase-1 (PFK-1)** (step 3; Fig. 38-18). Insulin promotes dephosphorylation of the bifunctional enzyme **phosphofructokinase-2/fructose bisphos- phatase,** thereby activating the kinase function and lessening the phosphatase function (Fig. 38-19). This results in increased levels of **fructose-2,6-**

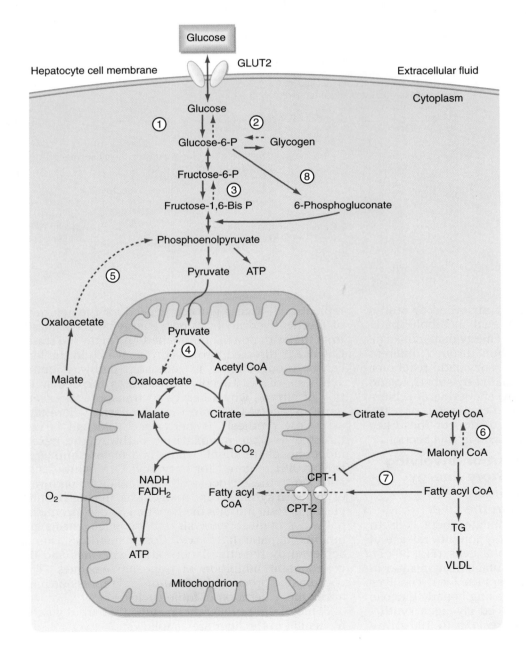

● **Figure 38-18.** Key hormonally regulated steps in glucose metabolism by the liver. See text for details on individual reactions. (Modified from Porterfield SP, White BA: Endocrine Physiology, 3rd ed. Philadelphia, Mosby, 2007.)

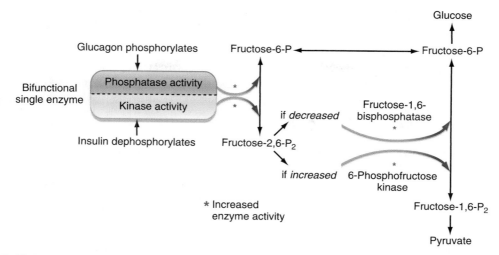

● **Figure 38-19.** Regulation of the relative rates of gluconeogenesis and glycolysis by the actions of islet hormones on a single bifunctional enzyme. Insulin causes dephosphorylation of the enzyme, thus making it a kinase, which raises the level of fructose-2,6-bisphosphate. This intermediate stimulates the activity of 6-phosphofructose kinase and shifts metabolism toward pyruvate (glycolysis). Phosphorylation of the bifunctional enzyme by glucagon makes it a phosphatase, which lowers the level of fructose-2,6-bisphosphate and thereby increases the activity of fructose-1,6-bisphosphatase and shifts metabolism toward glucose (gluconeogenesis).

bisphosphate, which is an allosteric activator of PFK-1. Fructose-2,6-bisphosphatase also competitively inhibits the gluconeogenic enzyme **fructose-1,6-bisphosphatase,** thereby blocking the futile cycle of F6P ↔ fructose-1,6-bisphosphate. In addition, fructose-1,6-bisphosphate activates the downstream irreversible reaction of converting phosphoenolpyruvate to pyruvate, which is catalyzed by **pyruvate kinase.** Thus, insulin activates pyruvate kinase indirectly through a feed-forward mechanism that is initiated by dephosphorylation of phosphofructokinase-2/fructose bisphosphatase. Insulin also promotes the dephosphorylation of pyruvate kinase, thereby increasing the activity of the enzyme. Insulin increases pyruvate dehydrogenase activity (step 4, Fig. 38-18), which converts pyruvate to acetyl CoA, an important building block for fatty acid synthesis. Insulin represses gene expression of the gluconeogenic enzyme **PEPCK** (step 5, Fig. 38-18), which converts pyruvate, by way of oxaloacetate-malate-oxaloacetate transfer out of the mitochondria, to phosphoenolpyruvate. By repressing PEPCK, insulin blocks the futile cycle of pyruvate ↔ phosphoenolpyruvate.

4. *Increasing synthesis of TG* (steps 6–8; Fig. 38-18). In the presence of excess amounts of glucose and AAs, the excess acetyl CoA is not used for ATP synthesis by the liver. Instead, acetyl CoA is transferred from the mitochondria to the cytosol in the form of citrate, which is then converted back to acetyl CoA and oxaloacetate by the cytosolic enzyme **ATP-citrate lyase.** Insulin increases ATP-citrate lyase gene expression through the transcription factor SREBP-1C. Once in the cytoplasm, acetyl CoA can enter fatty acid synthesis. The first step involves the conversion of acetyl CoA to malonyl CoA by the enzyme **acetyl-CoA carboxylase.** Insulin stimulates acetyl-CoA carboxylase gene expression through the transcription factor SREBP-1C. Insulin also promotes the dephosphorylation of acetyl-CoA carboxylase, which activates the enzyme. Finally, by promoting pathways (especially glycolysis) that generate high levels of citrate, insulin increases acetyl-CoA carboxylase activity indirectly through allosteric activation by citrate.

Malonyl CoA is converted to the 16-carbon fatty acid palmitate by repetitive additions of acetyl groups (contributed by malonyl CoA) by the **fatty acid synthase (FAS) complex.** FAS gene expression is enhanced by insulin through the transcription factor SREBP-1C. Palmitate synthesis also requires NADPH. A major source of NADPH is the **pentose phosphate shunt.** The first reaction of this pathway converts G6P to 6-phosphogluconolactone by the enzyme **G6P dehydrogenase (G6PD)** and generates NADPH. Insulin increases G6PD gene expression through the transcription factor SREBP-1C. Insulin also stimulates **palmitoyl-CoA desaturase,** which produces unsaturated fatty acids.

By activating steps that lead to the generation of malonyl CoA, insulin indirectly inhibits the oxidation of FFAs. Malonyl CoA inhibits CPT-I activity. As a result, FFAs that are synthesized cannot be transported into mitochondria, where they undergo β oxidation. Thus, increased malonyl CoA prevents the futile cycle of FFA synthesis to FFA oxidation.

FFAs are converted to TGs by the liver and are either stored in the liver or transported to adipose tissue and muscle in the form of VLDL. Synthesis of TG requires the presence of G3P. In the liver, G3P is

● AT THE CELLULAR LEVEL

SREBP-2 was discovered as a transcription factor that resides in the membrane of the endoplasmic reticulum (ER). In the presence of high intracellular cholesterol, SREBP-2 is held in the ER by a lipid-sensing protein called SCAP (SREBP cleavage–activating protein). In response to depleted sterols, SCAP escorts SREBP-2 to the Golgi, where SREBP is cleaved sequentially by proteases and released into the cytoplasm. SREBP-2 then translocates to the nucleus and increases the transcription of genes involved in synthesis and uptake of cholesterol. A more recently discovered member of this transcription factor family is **SREBP-1C,** which is highly expressed in adipose and liver. In contrast to SREBP-2, SREBP-1C stimulates genes involved in the synthesis of fatty acid and TG. Regulation of SREBP-1C occurs at the transcriptional level of the SREBP-1C gene, with cleavage induced by polyunsaturated fatty acids and activation by the MAPK pathway.

Peroxisome proliferation activator receptors (PPARs) belong to the nuclear hormone receptor superfamily that also includes steroid hormone receptors and thyroid hormone receptors. PPARs heterodimerize with the **retinoid X receptors** (RXRs). Unlike steroid and thyroid hormone receptors, PPARs bind to ligands in the micromolar range (i.e., with lower affinity). PPARs bind saturated and unsaturated fatty acids, as well as natural and synthetic prostanoids. **PPARγ** is highly expressed in adipose tissue and at a lower level in skeletal muscle and liver. Its natural ligands include several polyunsaturated fatty acids. PPARγ regulates genes that promote the storage of fat. It also synergizes with SREBP-1C to promote differentiation of adipocytes from preadipocytes. Tissue-specific knockout of PPARγ in mice and PPARγ dominant negative mutations in humans give rise to **lipodystrophy** (i.e., lack of white adipose tissue), which leads to deposits of TG in muscle and liver (called steatosis), insulin resistance, diabetes, and hypertension. The **thiazolidinediones** are exogenous ligands for PPARγ. Although they promote weight gain, moderate levels of thiazolidinediones significantly improve insulin sensitivity. PPARγ also stimulates secretion of **adiponectin,** which promotes the oxidation of lipids in muscle and fat and thereby improves insulin sensitivity. **PPARα** is abundantly expressed in liver and to a lesser extent in skeletal and cardiac muscle and kidney. PPARα promotes the uptake and oxidation of FFAs. Thus, PPARα is an antisteatotic molecule. The **fibrates** are exogenous ligands of PPARα and are used to reduce TG deposits in muscle and liver, thereby improving insulin sensitivity. A third member, **PPARδ,** similarly promotes fatty acid oxidation in adipose and muscle tissue. PPARδ promotes the development of slow-twitch, oxidative muscle fibers and increases muscle stamina. PPARδ has a positive effect on lipoprotein metabolism by increasing the production of apo A apoproteins and the number of HDL particles.

Another family of lipid-sensing transcription factors is the **liver X receptor (LXR)** family, which is composed of LXRα and LXRβ. LXRα is expressed primarily in adipose tissue, liver, intestine, and kidney, whereas LXRβ is ubiquitously expressed. LXRs are related to PPARs in that they are members of the nuclear hormone receptor family and heterodimerize with RXR. LXRs are cholesterol sensors. In high-cholesterol conditions, LXRs up-regulate the expression of ATP-binding cassette (ABC) proteins. In the face of excess cholesterol, LXRs also increase ABC protein expression in the gastrointestinal tract, which promotes the efflux of cholesterol from enterocytes to the lumen for excretion. Mutations in these transporters (ABCG5 and ABCG8) cause **sitosterolemia,** characterized by excessive absorption of cholesterol and plant sterols. In the liver, LXRs promote the conversion of cholesterol to bile acids for excretion or to cholesterol esters for storage. In the latter action, LXRs increase SREBP-1C expression, thereby increasing the fatty acyl CoAs needed for esterification.

---

derived from insulin-enhanced glycolysis or from the phosphorylation of glycerol by the enzyme **glycerol kinase.** Insulin acutely promotes degradation of the VLDL apoprotein apo B-100. This keeps the liver from secreting VLDL during a meal, when the blood is rich with chylomicrons. Thus, the lipid made in response to insulin during a meal is released as VLDL during the interdigestive period and provides an important source of energy to skeletal and cardiac muscle.

Insulin and Utilization of Glucose by Skeletal Muscle and Adipose Tissue

The glucose that is not captured by the liver contributes to the postprandial rise in glucose levels in the peripheral circulation (Fig. 38-20). **Glucose tolerance** refers to the ability of an individual to minimize the increase in blood glucose concentration after a meal. A primary way by which insulin promotes glucose tolerance is activation of glucose transporters in skeletal muscle. Insulin stimulates the translocation of preexisting GLUT4 transporters to the cell membrane and promotes the storage of glucose in muscle by stimulating synthesis of glycogen. However, the relative amount of glucose used for replenishing glycogen stores versus the amount used for energy is dependent on the amount of physical activity that an individual is engaged in during or soon after a meal.

Insulin also stimulates GLUT4-dependent uptake of glucose and subsequent glycolysis in adipose tissue (Fig. 38-20). Adipose tissue utilizes glycolysis for energy needs, but also for the generation of G3P, which is required for the reesterification of FFAs into TGs. As in the liver and skeletal muscle, excessive intake of carbohydrate can also lead to insulin-stimulated lipogenesis in adipose tissue.

● **Figure 38-20.** Partitioning of glucose and TG during the digestive period (high insulin-glucagon ratio). Highlighted (*red*) pathways are stimulated by insulin.

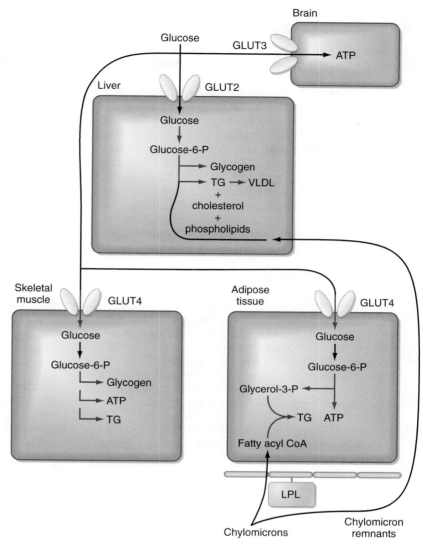

Insulin and Storage of Ingested Lipids in Adipose Tissue

Insulin stimulates the expression of **LPL** within adipose cells and its migration to the apical side of endothelia in adipose capillaries (Fig. 38-20). This action of insulin promotes the release of FFAs from chylomicrons within adipose tissue. Insulin also stimulates the translocation of fatty acid transport proteins into the cell membrane that facilitate the movement of FFAs into adipocytes and the activation of FFAs by their conversion to fatty acyl CoAs. Insulin stimulates glycolysis in adipocytes, which generates the G3P required for reesterification of FFAs into TGs. Insulin also inhibits **hormone-sensitive lipase**.

Insulin and Protein Synthesis

Insulin promotes protein synthesis in muscle and adipose tissue by stimulating AA uptake and mRNA translation. Insulin also inhibits proteolysis. Although the liver utilizes AAs for the synthesis of ATP, insulin also promotes the synthesis of proteins during the digestive period and attenuates the activity of urea cycle enzymes in the liver.

> ## IN THE CLINIC

Diabetes mellitus is a disease in which insulin levels or responsiveness of tissues to insulin (or both) is insufficient to maintain normal levels of plasma glucose. Although the diagnosis of diabetes is based primarily on plasma glucose, diabetes also promotes imbalances in the circulating levels of lipids and lipoproteins (i.e., **dyslipidemia**). With normal fasting (i.e., no caloric intake for at least 8 hours), plasma glucose levels should be below 110 mg/dL. A patient is considered to have impaired glucose control if fasting plasma glucose levels are between 110 and 126 mg/dL, and the diagnosis of diabetes is made if fasting plasma glucose exceeds 126 mg/dL on 2 successive days. Another approach to the diagnosis of diabetes is the oral glucose tolerance test. After overnight fasting, the patient is given a bolus of glucose (usually 75 g) orally, and blood glucose levels are measured at 2 hours. A 2-hour plasma glucose concentration greater than 200 mg/dL on 2 consecutive days is sufficient to make the diagnosis of diabetes.

The diagnosis of diabetes is also indicated if the patient has symptoms associated with diabetes and has a non-fasting plasma glucose level greater than 200 mg/dL.

Diabetes mellitus is currently classified as **type 1 (T1DM)** or **type 2 (T2DM)**. **T2DM** is by far the more common form and accounts for 90% of diagnosed cases. However, T2DM is usually a progressive disease that remains undiagnosed in a significant percentage of patients for several years. T2DM is often associated with visceral obesity and lack of exercise—indeed, obesity-related T2DM is reaching epidemic proportions worldwide. Usually, there are multiple causes for the development of T2DM in a given individual that are associated with defects in the ability of target organs to respond to insulin (i.e., **insulin resistance**), along with some degree of **beta cell deficiency.** Insulin sensitivity can be compromised at the level of the insulin receptor (IR) or at the level of postreceptor signaling. T2DM appears to be the consequence of insulin resistance, followed by reactive hyperinsulinemia, but ultimately by **relative hypoinsulinemia** (i.e., inadequate release of insulin to compensate for the end-organ resistance; Fig. 38-21) and **beta cell failure.**

The underlying causes of insulin resistance differ among patients. Three major underlying causes of obesity-induced insulin resistance are as follows:

1. Decreased ability of insulin to increase GLUT4-mediated uptake of glucose, especially by skeletal muscle. This function, which is specifically a part of the **glucometabolic** regulation by insulin, may be due to excessive accumulation of TG in muscle in obese individuals. Excessive caloric intake induces hyperinsulinemia. Initially, this leads to excessive glucose uptake into skeletal muscle. Just as in the liver, excessive calories in the form of glucose promote lipogenesis and, through the generation of malonyl CoA, repression of fatty acyl CoA oxidation. Byproducts of fatty acid and TG synthesis, such as diacylglycerol and ceramide, may accumulate and stimulate signaling pathways (e.g., protein kinase C–dependent pathways) that antagonize signaling from the IR or IRS proteins, or both. Thus, insulin resistance in the skeletal muscle of obese individuals may be due to **lipotoxicity.**

2. Decreased ability of insulin to repress hepatic glucose production. The liver makes glucose by glycogenolysis in the short term and by gluconeogenesis in the long term. The ability of insulin to repress key hepatic enzymes in both these pathways (Fig. 38-18) is attenuated in insulin-resistant individuals. Insulin resistance in the liver may also be due to lipotoxicity in obese individuals (e.g., **fatty liver** or **hepatic steatosis**). Visceral adipose tissue is likely to affect insulin signaling at the liver in several ways, in addition to the effects of lipotoxicity. For example, visceral adipose tissue releases the cytokine **tumor necrosis factor-α (TNF-α)**, which has been shown to antagonize insulin signaling pathways. Also, TG in visceral adipose tissue has a high rate of turnover (possibly because of rich sympathetic innervation), so the liver is exposed to high levels of FFAs, which further exacerbates hepatic lipotoxicity.

3. Inability of insulin to repress hormone-sensitive lipase or increase LPL in adipose tissue (or both). High HSL and low LPL are major factors in the dyslipidemia associated with insulin resistance and diabetes. Although the factors that resist the actions of insulin on HSL and LPL are not completely understood, there is evidence for the increased production of paracrine diabetogenic factors in adipose tissue, such as TNF-α. The dyslipidemia is characterized as hypertriglyceridemia with large TG-rich VLDL particles produced by the liver. Because of their high TG content, large VLDLs and IDLs are digested very efficiently, thereby giving rise to small dense LDL particles, which are very atherogenic. In addition, HDL takes on excess TG in exchange for cholesterol esters, which appears to shorten the circulating half-life of HDL and apo A proteins. Thus, there are lower levels of HDL particles, which normally play a protective role against vascular disease.

Type 1 diabetes mellitus is characterized by the destruction, almost always by an autoimmune mechanism, of beta cells. T1DM is also termed "insulin-dependent diabetes mellitus."

Characteristics of T1DM include the following:

1. People with T1DM need exogenous insulin to maintain life and prevent ketosis; virtually no pancreatic insulin is produced.

2. There is pathological damage to the pancreatic beta cells. Insulinitis with pancreatic mononuclear cell infiltration is a characteristic feature at the onset of the disorder. Cytokines may be involved in the early destruction of the pancreas.

3. People with T1DM are prone to ketosis.

4. Ninety percent of cases begin in childhood, mostly between 10 and 14 years of age. This common observation led to application of the term "juvenile diabetes" to the disorder. This term is no longer used because T1DM can arise at any time of life, although juvenile onset is the typical pattern.

5. Islet cell autoantibodies are frequently present around the time of onset. If T1DM is induced by a virus, the autoantibodies are transient. Occasionally, antibodies will persist long-term, particularly if they are associated with other autoimmune disorders.

About 50% of T1DM is related to problems with the major histocompatibility complex on chromosome 6. It is correlated with an increased frequency of certain human leukocyte antigen (HLA) alleles. The HLA types DR3 and DR4 are most commonly associated with diabetes.

● **Figure 38-21.** Twenty-four-hour profiles of plasma glucose, C peptide, and insulin in normal-weight *(blue lines)* and obese *(red lines)* humans. Note the parallel increases with each meal, the rapid return toward baseline, and the exaggerated beta cell responses in obesity. (Data from Polonsky K et al: J Clin Invest 81:442, 1988.)

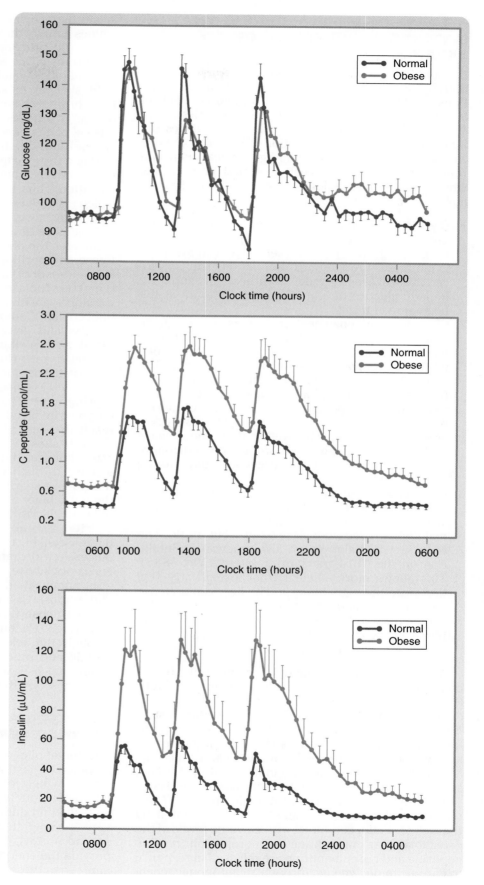

RELEASE OF ENERGY DURING THE INTERDIGESTIVE PERIOD OR AN EXTENDED FAST

Nutrient levels in blood fall several hours after a meal, thereby leading to lower levels of insulin secretion. Consequently, the stimulatory and inhibitory effects of insulin on hepatic, muscle, and adipose tissue are attenuated. The decrease in insulin also relieves the inhibition of glucagon secretion. Thus, the liver is exposed to an increasingly larger glucagon-insulin ratio during the interdigestive period and fasting, which has the following effects on hepatic metabolism:

1. Glycogen phosphorylase is activated through protein kinase A (PKA) and phosphorylase kinase (step 2, Fig. 38-18). Conversely, glycogen synthase is inhibited through phosphorylation. Thus, glycogenolysis exceeds glycogen synthesis and supports hepatic glucose output for about 12 hours at the beginning of a fast.
2. Gluconeogenic enzymes are increased over glycolytic enzymes (steps 1, 3, 4, 5, Fig. 38-18). Glucagon increases PEPCK at a transcriptional level while inhibiting pyruvate kinase by phosphorylation. The increased glucagon-insulin ratio also increases fructose-1,6-bisphosphatase and G6Pase while inhibiting the opposing enzymes phosphofructokinase-1 and glucokinase, respectively. Gluconeogenesis takes over after glycogenolysis as the primary pathway of hepatic glucose production and continues to support blood glucose levels for days during an extended fast.
3. Lipogenesis is inhibited, in part, by the phosphorylation-dependent inhibition of acetyl-CoA carboxylase and activation of the opposing enzyme malonyl-CoA decarboxylase (step 6, Fig. 38-18). The reduction in malonyl CoA also relieves the inhibition on the CPT-I transporter (step 7, Fig. 38-18). This allows more efficient transport of fatty acyl CoAs into the mitochondria. The liver can then use circulating FFAs for energy, but also to synthesize ketone bodies (Fig. 38-4). Ketogenesis supplements blood glucose in that the brain can use ketone bodies after several days of a fast.

As liver glycogen is depleted, the liver shifts to gluconeogenesis to maintain blood glucose levels. However, the ability of the liver to generate glucose is dependent on the ability of the liver to obtain a sufficient level of substrates (lactate, AAs, and glycerol) for gluconeogenesis. These substrates originate primarily from skeletal muscle and adipose tissue (Fig. 38-22). Most of the glucagon is inactivated by the liver, so the hormone has a small effect on adipose tissue. There are no glucagon receptors in muscle. Thus, release of gluconeogenic substrates is promoted by the lack of insulin combined with elevated levels of the catecholamines epinephrine and norepinephrine. Epinephrine and norepinephrine are released in response to chronic hypoglycemia through an autonomic mechanism that originates in the hypothalamus. Catecholamines amplify the effects of glucagon on the liver and act as the primary counterregulatory hormones (or neurotransmitter in the case of norepinephrine) at skeletal muscle and adipose tissue.

In skeletal muscle, a high catecholamine-insulin ratio promotes increased proteolysis and decreased protein synthesis (Fig. 38-22). This results in the release of gluconeogenic and ketogenic AAs. Because skeletal muscle shifts to the use of FFAs for energy during a fast, pyruvate dehydrogenase is inhibited by the relatively abundant acetyl CoA generated by β oxidation. Thus, more pyruvate is converted to lactate, which is released to be used by the liver for gluconeogenesis.

In adipose tissue, a high catecholamine-insulin ratio stimulates the phosphorylation of **hormone-sensitive lipase** and **perilipin proteins** that surround fat droplets. Phosphorylated perilipins dissociate from the TG-cytoplasm interface and allow access to hormone-sensitive lipase, which is activated by phosphorylation. Complete deesterification of TGs results in FFAs and glycerol (Fig. 28-22). FFAs circulate in blood as FFA-albumin complexes and are used by several tissues (including skeletal muscle, liver, and adipose tissue) for energy. This use of FFAs, especially by skeletal muscle, plays an essential **"glucose-sparing"** role. This means that FFAs compete for the enzymes involved in the oxidation of glucose, with the result that less glucose is consumed by muscle and other tissues. The high catecholamine-insulin ratio also minimizes the ability of skeletal muscle to take up glucose through GLUT4 transporters. Consequently, the glucose-sparing action of FFAs indirectly increases the availability of blood glucose to cell types that are obligate glucose users.

After several days of fasting, circulating ketone bodies can be used by the brain (Fig. 38-22). This places less demand on the liver to maintain normal levels of glucose.

In summary, during fasting, both skeletal muscle and adipose tissue contribute directly to circulating blood glucose through the release of gluconeogenic substrates (lactate, AAs, glycerol) and indirectly through the release of FFAs, which allow skeletal muscle and other tissues to consume less glucose. Finally, release of FFAs and ketogenic AAs supports ketogenesis by the liver.

RELEASE OF ENERGY DURING EXERCISE

The metabolic response to exercise resembles the response to fasting in that the mobilization and generation of fuels for oxidation are dominant factors. The type and amounts of expended substrate vary with the intensity and duration of the exercise (Fig. 38-23). For very intense, short-term exercise (e.g., a 10- to 15-second sprint), stored creatine phosphate and ATP provide the energy at a rate of approximately 50 kcal/min. When these stores are depleted, additional inten-

● **Figure 38-22.** Utilization of glucose, TG, and protein during the interdigestive period or fasting (low insulin-glucagon ratio). Highlighted steps (in red) are promoted by glucagon or epinephrine/norepinephrine, or both.

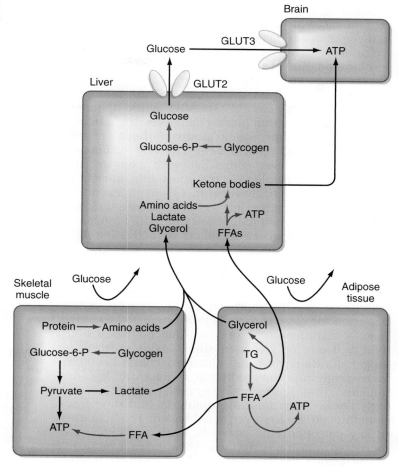

● **Figure 38-23.** Energy sources during exercise. Note the sequential use of stored high-energy phosphate bonds, glycogen, circulating glucose, and circulating FFAs. The latter dominate in sustained exercise.

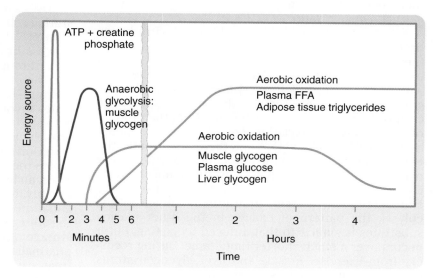

sive exercise for up to 2 minutes can be sustained by breakdown of muscle glycogen to G6P, with glycolysis yielding the necessary energy (at a rate of 30 kcal/min). This anaerobic phase is not limited by depletion of muscle glycogen, but rather by the rapid accumulation of lactic acid in the exercising muscles and circulation.

After several minutes of exhaustive anaerobic exercise, an O_2 debt of 10 to 12 L can be built up. This must be repaid before the exercise can be repeated. From 6 to 8 L of O_2 is required either to resynthesize the accumulated lactic acid back into glucose in the liver or to oxidize it to CO_2. About 2 L of O_2 is required to replenish normal muscle ATP and creatine phosphate stores.

An additional 2 L of O_2 will replenish the O_2 normally present in the lungs and body fluids and the O_2 bound to myoglobin and hemoglobin.

For less intense but longer periods of exercise, aerobic oxidation of substrates is required to produce the necessary energy (at a maximum of about 12 kcal/min). Substrates from the circulation are added to muscle glycogen (Fig. 38-23). After a few minutes, uptake of glucose from plasma increases dramatically, up to 30-fold in some muscle groups. Although resting glucose uptake by muscle is regulated by insulin and this effect increases somewhat with exercise, the major increase in glucose transport into muscle is mediated by an entirely separate insulin-independent factor. During exercise, intracellular glucose and ATP levels initially fall and AMP levels rise. AMP then markedly stimulates glucose transport by activating AMP kinase. To offset this drain on extracellular glucose and to maintain a normal plasma glucose level, hepatic glucose production must increase up to fivefold. Initially, this occurs largely from glycogenolysis. Indeed, endurance can be improved by high carbohydrate ingestion for several days before prolonged exercise (e.g., a marathon run) because this increases both liver and muscle glycogen stores. With exercise of longer duration, however, gluconeogenesis becomes increasingly important as liver glycogen stores become depleted. To support gluconeogenesis, AAs are increasingly released by muscle proteolysis, and their fractional uptake by the liver is enhanced. The activities of key gluconeogenic enzymes, such as PEPCK, are increased, and transcription of their genes is induced. These events are coordinated by increased sympathetic neural activity and by the relative effects of the glucagon-insulin ratio.

Eventually, fatty acids liberated from TGs in adipose tissue form the predominant energy substrate, and they supply two thirds of the needs during sustained exercise. The increased AMP levels noted earlier activate AMP kinase, which phosphorylates and thereby greatly reduces the activity of the enzyme acetyl-CoA carboxylase. Thus, levels of malonyl CoA, the product of acetyl CoA carboxylation, fall. This releases inhibition of CPT by malonyl CoA and thereby promotes the entry of fatty acids into the mitochondria, where their oxidation provides energy for sustained muscle work. Except for increases in circulating levels of pyruvate and lactate, which result from greatly enhanced glycolysis, the pattern of change in the other plasma substrates is similar to that induced by fasting, but it occurs over a much shorter time frame. During recovery from exercise, muscle and liver glycogen stores must be rebuilt, which requires input of energy. Some energy is also needed during this period to recycle the unexpended FFA back into TGs.

LEPTIN AND ADIPOSE TISSUE

Adipose tissue is not contiguous, but spread throughout the body. There are two forms of adipose tissue, **brown adipose tissue (BAT)** and **white adipose tissue**

> ### IN THE CLINIC
>
> Several diseases that affect muscle function and exercise capacity result from genetic defects in energy-generating steps. (1) In **McArdle's disease,** or **muscle phosphorylase deficiency,** glycogen cannot be rapidly broken down to G6P, and hence pain and weakness occur even during brief exercise. The impairment in glycolysis from lack of substrate is demonstrated by failure of lactate levels to rise in a draining vein after anaerobic forearm muscle exercise with arterial inflow occluded. (2) In **von Gierke's disease,** or **G6Pase deficiency,** hepatic glucose release is impaired, and this limits the supply of glucose during the early phase of exercise. (3) Deficiencies of the β oxidation enzymes carnitine or CPT (required to transfer FFA into mitochondria) prevent efficient use of FFA. This restricts exercise capacity and produces muscle weakness and pain. Conditions (2) and (3) also lead to hypoglycemia during fasting because hepatic glucose production is decreased.

(WAT). BAT plays an important role in thermogenesis in the newborn, but BAT is reduced in adult humans. WAT plays three general roles. First, WAT is used for cushioning (e.g., in the orbits surrounding the eyeballs). Second, the vast majority of WAT is used as a metabolic storage depot that can be called on to release FFAs and glycerol in times of fasting. Third, the WAT involved in nutrient storage also functions as a classic endocrine organ.

WAT is composed of several cell types. The TG-storing cell is called the **adipocyte.** These cells develop from preadipocytes during gestation in humans. This process of adipocyte differentiation, which may continue throughout life, is promoted by several transcription factors. One of these factors is **sterol regulatory element–binding protein 1C.** SREBP-1C regulates genes involved in FFA and TG synthesis. SREBP-1C is activated by lipids, as well as by insulin and several growth factors and cytokines. Another important transcription factor in WAT is **PPARγ.** Activated PPARγ promotes the expression of genes involved in TG storage. Thus, an increase in food consumption leads to activation of SREBP-1C and PPARγ, which increase the differentiation of preadipocytes into small adipocytes and the up-regulation of enzymes within these cells to allow storage of the excess fat. The **thiazolidinediones** are pharmacological activators of PPARγ that are used to treat insulin resistance and T2DM.

Adipose tissue produces paracrine and endocrine factors, including adiponectin, TNF-α, resistin, interleukin-6, angiotensinogen, and acylation-stimulating protein. The roles of these factors in humans are uncertain, and thus they will not be considered in detail.

Leptin

Leptin is an adipocyte-derived protein that signals information to the hypothalamus about the degree of adiposity and nutrition, which in turn controls eating behavior and energy expenditure. Leptin-deficient mice and humans become morbidly obese. These findings originally raised hope that leptin therapy could be used to combat morbid obesity. However, administration of leptin to individuals who suffer from diet-induced obesity does not have a significant anorectic or energy-consuming effect. In fact, obese individuals already have elevated endogenous circulating levels of leptin and appear to have developed **leptin resistance.**

Leptin has an important role in liporegulation in peripheral tissues. Leptin protects peripheral tissues (e.g., the liver, skeletal muscle, cardiac muscle, beta cells) from the accumulation of too much lipid by directing storage of excess caloric intake into adipose tissue. This action of leptin, though opposing the lipogenic actions of insulin, contributes significantly to the maintenance of insulin sensitivity (as defined by insulin-dependent glucose uptake) in peripheral tissues. Leptin also acts as a signal that the body has sufficient energy stores to allow reproduction and to enhance erythropoiesis, lymphopoiesis, and myelopoiesis. For example, in women suffering from anorexia nervosa, leptin levels are extremely low and result in low ovarian steroids, amenorrhea (lack of menstrual bleeding), anemia from low red blood cell production, and immune dysfunction.

Structure, Synthesis, and Secretion

Leptin, a 16-kDa protein secreted by mature adipocytes, is structurally related to cytokines. Thus, it is sometimes referred to as an **adipocytokine.** Circulating levels of leptin have a direct relationship with adiposity and nutritional status. Leptin output is increased by insulin, which prepares the body for the correct partitioning of incoming nutrients. Leptin is inhibited by fasting and weight loss and by lipolytic signals (e.g., increased cAMP and β_3-agonists).

Diet-induced obesity, advanced age, and T2DM are associated with leptin resistance. Thus, mechanisms that turn off leptin signaling are potential therapeutic targets.

Energy Storage

The amount of energy stored by an individual is determined by caloric intake and calories expended as energy per day. In many individuals, input and output are in balance, so weight remains relatively constant. However, the abundance of inexpensive high-fat, high-carbohydrate food, along with more sedentary lifestyles, is currently contributing to a pandemic of obesity and the pathological sequelae of obesity, including T2DM and cardiovascular disease.

The preponderance of stored energy consists of fat, and individuals vary greatly in the amount and percentage of body weight that is accounted for by adipose tissue. About 25% of the variance in total body fat appears to be due to genetic factors. A genetic influence on fat mass is supported by (1) the tendency for the body mass of adopted children to correlate better with that of their biological parents than with that of their adoptive parents; (2) the greater similarity of adipose stores in identical (monozygotic) twins, whether reared together or apart, than in fraternal (dizygotic) twins; (3) the greater correlation between gains in body weight and abdominal fat in identical twins than in fraternal twins when they are fed a caloric excess; and (4) the discovery of several genes that cause obesity.

In addition, the gestational environment has a profound effect on body mass of the adult. The effect of maternal diet on the weight and body composition of offspring is called **fetal programming.** Low birth weights correlate with increased risk for obesity, cardiovascular disease, and diabetes. These findings suggest that the efficiency of fetal metabolism has plasticity and can be altered by the in utero environment. The development of a "thrifty" metabolism would be advantageous to an individual born to a mother who received poor nutrition and into a life that meant chronic undernourishment.

Body Mass Index

A measure of adiposity is the body mass index (BMI). The BMI of an individual is calculated as

● **Equation 38-1**

$$BMI = Weight\ (kg)/Height\ (m)^2$$

The BMI of healthy lean individuals ranges from 20 to 25. A BMI greater than 25 indicates that the individual is overweight, whereas a BMI higher than 30 indicates obesity. The condition of being overweight or obese is a risk factor for multiple pathologies, including insulin resistance, dyslipidemia, diabetes, cardiovascular disease, and hypertension.

WAT tissue is divided into subcutaneous and intraabdominal (visceral) depots. Intraabdominal WAT refers primarily to omental and mesenteric fat and is the smaller of the two depots. These depots receive different blood supplies that are drained in a fundamentally different way in that venous return from intraabdominal fat leads into the hepatic portal system. Thus, intraabdominally derived FFAs are mostly cleared by the liver, whereas subcutaneous fat is the primary site for providing FFAs to muscle during exercise or fasting. The regulation of intraabdominal and subcutaneous adipose tissue also differs. Abdominal fat is highly innervated by autonomic neurons and has a greater turnover rate. Furthermore, these two depots display differences in hormone production and enzyme activity.

Men tend to gain fat in the intraabdominal depot **(android [apple-shaped] adiposity),** whereas women tend to gain fat in the subcutaneous depot, particularly in the thighs and buttocks **(gynecoid [pear-shaped] adiposity).** Clearly, an excess of abdominal fat poses a greater risk factor for the pathologies mentioned earlier. Thus, another indicator of body composition is circumference of the waist (measured in inches around the narrowest point between the ribs and hips when viewed from the front after exhaling) divided by the circumference of the hips (measured at the point where the buttocks are largest when viewed from the side). This **waist-hip ratio** may be a better indicator of body fat than BMI, especially as it relates to the risk for the development of diseases. A waist-hip ratio of greater than 0.95 in men or 0.85 in women is linked to a significantly higher risk for the development of diabetes and cardiovascular disease.

In recent years, numerous hormones and neuropeptides have been implicated in the chronic and acute regulation of appetite, satiety, and energy expenditure in humans (Table 38-3). One simplified model involves two peptide hormones, leptin and insulin (Fig. 38-24). Leptin acts on at least two neuron types in the arcuate nucleus of the hypothalamus. In the first, leptin represses the production of **neuropeptide Y (NPY),** a very potent stimulator of food-seeking behavior (energy intake) and an inhibitor of energy expenditure. Norepinephrine, another appetite stimulator, colocalizes with NPY in some of these neurons. At the same time, leptin represses the production of agouti-related peptide (AGRP), an endogenous antagonist that acts on MC4R, a hypothalamic receptor for the anorexigenic peptide α-melanocyte–stimulating hormone (α-MSH), which inhibits food intake. In another type of arcuate neuron, leptin stimulates the production of proopiomelanocortin (POMC) products, one of which is α-MSH, and the production of cocaine-amphetamine–regulated transcript (CART), both of which inhibit food intake. Thus, leptin decreases food consumption and increases energy expenditure by simultaneously inhibiting NPY and the α-MSH antagonist AGRP and by stimulating α-MSH and CART (Fig. 38-24). These second-order neuropeptides are transmitted to and interact with receptors in neurons of the paraventricular hypothalamic nucleus ("satiety" neurons) and lateral hypothalamic nucleus ("hunger" neurons). In turn, these hypothalamic neurons generate signals that coordinate feeding behavior and autonomic

● **Table 38-3.** **Modulators of Feeding Behavior**

Stimulate Orexigenic Behavior	Inhibit Anorexigenic Behavior
Neuropeptide Y (NPY)	Leptin
Agouti-related peptide (AGRP)	Insulin
Melanin-concentrating hormone (MCH)	α-Melanocyte–stimulating hormone (α-MSH)
Orexin A and B (hypocretin 1 and 2)	Corticotropin-releasing hormone (CRH)
Galanin	Urocortin
Norepinephrine	Cocaine-amphetamine–regulated transcript (CART)
Ghrelin	GLP-1
Cortisol	Cholecystokinin (CCK)
	Interleukin-1β
	Serotonin
	Enterostatin
	Calcitonin
	Bombesin

● **Figure 38-24.** Current concept of the effects of leptin in the brain. One target neuron transmits the proorexigenic peptide NPY and the peptide AGRP, which antagonizes the anorexigenic peptide α-MSH. Neuronal expression of these two genes is inhibited by leptin. Another target neuron transmits α-MSH, synthesized by expression of the POMC gene, and CART. This neuron's activity is stimulated by leptin. The cumulative effect of all four actions is to decrease food intake. (Modified from Schwartz MW et al: Nature 404:661, 2000.).

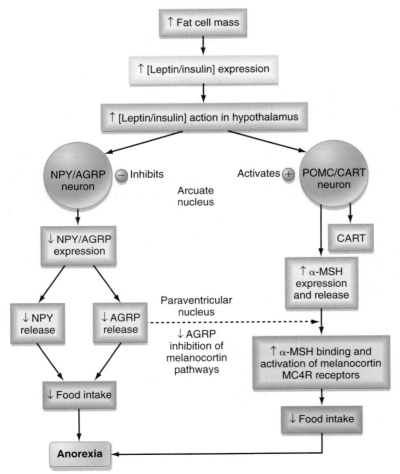

nervous system activity (especially sympathetic outflow) with diverse endocrine actions on thyroid gland function, reproduction, and growth.

Another regulator of food intake and body energy stores is **melanin-concentrating hormone (MCH).** This neuropeptide increases food seeking and adipose tissue by antagonizing the satiety effect of α-MSH downstream from the interaction of α-MSH with its MC4R receptor. The probable importance of this molecule is demonstrated by the fact that it is the only regulator whose ablation by gene knockout actually results in leanness.

To maintain overall energy homeostasis, the system must also balance specific nutrient intake and expenditure, for example, carbohydrate (CHO) intake with CHO oxidation. This may account for some specificity in neuropeptide and neurotransmitter responses to meals. Serotonin produces satiety after the ingestion of glucose. Gastrointestinal hormones such as cholecystokinin and GLP-1 (Table 38-3) produce satiety by humoral effects, but their local production in the brain may participate in nutrient and caloric regulation. The recently discovered hormone **ghrelin** is an acylated peptide with potent orexigenic activity that arises in cells of the oxyntic glands in the stomach. Plasma levels of ghrelin rise in humans in the 1 to 2 hours that precede their normal meals. Plasma levels of ghrelin fall drastically to minimum values about 1 hour after eating. Ghrelin appears to stimulate food intake by reacting with its receptor in hypothalamic neurons that express NPY.

▷ IN THE CLINIC

Hyperglycemia leads to elevated intracellular glucose and cellular toxicity, notably in endothelial cells in the retina, kidney, and capillaries associated with peripheral nerves. This **glucotoxicity** alters cell function in several ways that may contribute to pathological changes, including increased synthesis of **polyols, hexosamines,** and **diacylglycerol** (which activates protein kinase C). Although the exact mechanisms by which intracellular accumulation of these molecules causes abnormal cell function remain unclear, current thinking indicates that these changes lead to increased **oxidative stress** within the cell. Additionally, intracellular **nonenzymatic glycation** of proteins gives rise to **advanced glycation end products (AGEs).** Intracellular AGEs have altered function, whereas AGEs secreted in the extracellular matrix interact abnormally with other matrix components and matrix receptors on cells. Finally, some secreted AGEs interact with receptors on macrophages and endothelial cells. Endothelial **receptors for AGEs (RAGEs)** lead to proinflammatory gene expression.

An important circulating product of glycation is **hemoglobin A$_{1c}$ (HbA$_{1c}$),** which is a useful marker for long-term glucose regulation. A red blood cell has a 120-day life span; once glycation occurs, the hemoglobin remains glycated for the remainder of the red blood cell's life span. The proportion of HbA$_{1c}$ present in a nondiabetic person is low. However, a diabetic patient who has had prolonged periods of hyperglycemia (8 to 12 weeks) has elevated levels of HbA$_{1c}$; thus measurements of HbA$_{1c}$ are clinically useful for determining compliance with treatment.

1. **Retinopathies** (e.g., retinal abnormalities) frequently develop in diabetic patients. Retinopathies are the major cause of new-onset blindness in preretirement adults in the United States. Hyperglycemia results in high intracellular glucose concentrations in retinal endothelial cells and pericytes (capillary supportive cells). This is due to an inability of these cells to adapt to hyperglycemia by decreasing GLUT2 expression. Elevated intracellular glucose initiates multiple mechanisms that ultimately result in **endothelial cell dysfunction** and, as a result, decreased nitric oxide production, increased vascular resistance, hypertensive-induced changes, and cell death. These microvascular changes lead to microaneurysms, increased capillary permeability, small retinal hemorrhages, and excessive microvascular proliferation. Proliferative retinopathy is caused by impaired blood flow to the retina and the resultant tissue hypoxia. Subsequent vascular degeneration can produce vitreal hemorrhage, retinal detachment, and neovascular glaucoma, all of which can lead to severe visual loss.

2. Peripheral nerve damage **(neuropathy)** can occur as a result of metabolic, oxidative, or immune-related damage to neurons or Schwann cells. Additionally, the microvasculature of peripheral nerves undergoes changes similar to those seen in retinopathy and may represent an event that is concurrent with or causal to the peripheral neuropathy. Schwann cells (supportive cells involved in myelination) are among those shown to accumulate sorbitol in response to hyperglycemia. Diabetic patients can exhibit sensory loss, paresthesias, and even pain as a result of the neurologic damage. Neuropathy of the autonomic nerves also develops in diabetics and can lead to numerous symptoms in multiple organ systems, including erectile dysfunction, postural hypotension, and heat intolerance. The sensory loss is more apparent in the extremities, particularly the lower portions of the legs and feet. This poses particular problems because as diabetic patients lose cutaneous sensation in their feet, they become unaware of poorly fitting shoes and are more prone to injuries. Poor peripheral circulation aggravates this problem. Because diabetic patients have impaired wound healing, foot ulcerations can become a serious threat.

3. Diabetes is a common cause of reduced renal function **(nephropathy)** and is the greatest cause of end-stage renal disease in North America. Clinical or overt diabetic nephropathy is characterized by the loss of greater than 300 mg of albumin in urine over a 24-hour period **(albuminuria)** and a progressive decline in renal function. Nephropathies develop

from microvascular changes that occur in the glomerular capillaries. The glomerular capillary basement membrane thickens, and as a result the walls are thicker, the lumens are narrower **(glomerulosclerosis),** and the supportive mesangial cells are expanded. Poor renal filtration also leads to activation of the renin-angiotensin system, which induces hypertension.

4. Atherosclerosis develops in diabetic patients at an accelerated rate **(macroangiopathy).** Diabetic patients are more likely to have coronary artery disease and myocardial infarction than nondiabetic individuals are. Many diabetics with coronary artery disease have the additional risk factors of hypertension, abdominal obesity, insulin resistance, and dyslipidemia. This cluster of factors has been identified as **metabolic syndrome** (also called **syndrome X, insulin resistance syndrome, and cardiovascular dysmetabolic syndrome**). Some of the consequences of visceral obesity, insulin resistance, and dyslipidemia have been discussed earlier.

5. **Nonretinal visual problems** result as blood glucose and therefore blood osmolarity rise; the volume of the lens changes, thereby distorting vision. Diabetic patients commonly have cataracts, and accumulations of sorbitol and glycosylated protein have been proposed as mechanisms for inducing cataract formation.

■ KEY CONCEPTS

1. Cells make ATP to meet their energy needs. ATP is made by glycolysis and by the TCA cycle coupled to oxidative phosphorylation.

2. Cells can oxidize carbohydrate (primarily in the form of glucose), AAs, and FFAs to make ATP. Additionally, the liver makes ketone bodies for other tissues to oxidize for energy in times of fasting.

3. Some cell types are limited in the energy substrates that they can oxidize for energy. The brain is normally exclusively dependent on glucose for energy. Thus, blood glucose must be maintained above 60 mg/dL for normal autonomic and central nervous system function. Conversely, inappropriately high levels of glucose (i.e., fasting glucose above 110 mg/dL) promote glucotoxicity and thereby lead to the long-term complications of diabetes.

4. The endocrine pancreas produces the hormones insulin, glucagon, somatostatin, gastrin, and pancreatic polypeptide.

5. Insulin is an anabolic hormone that is secreted in times of excess nutrient availability. It allows the body to use carbohydrates as energy sources and store nutrients.

6. Major stimuli for insulin secretion include increased serum glucose and some AAs. Activation of cholinergic (muscarinic) receptors also increases insulin secretion, whereas activation of α_2-adrenergic receptors inhibits insulin secretion. The gastrointestinal tract releases incretin hormones that stimulate pancreatic insulin secretion. GLP-1 and GIP are particularly potent in augmenting glucose-dependent stimulation of insulin secretion.

7. Insulin binds to the insulin receptor, which is linked to multiple pathways that mediate the metabolic and growth effects of insulin.

8. During the digestive period, insulin acts on the liver to promote trapping of glucose as G6P. Insulin also increases glycogenesis, glycolysis, and fatty acid synthesis in the liver. Insulin regulates hepatic metabolism both by regulating gene expression and by posttranslational dephosphorylation events.

9. Insulin increases GLUT4-mediated glucose uptake in muscle and adipose tissue. It increases glycogenesis, glycolysis, and in the presence of caloric excess, lipogenesis in muscle and adipose tissue. Insulin increases muscle AA uptake and protein synthesis. It also increases fatty acid esterification and lipoprotein lipase activity and decreases hormone-sensitive lipase activity in adipocytes.

10. Glucagon is a catabolic hormone. Its secretion increases during periods of food deprivation, and it acts to mobilize nutrient reserves. It also mobilizes glycogen, fat, and even protein.

11. Glucagon is released in response to decreased serum glucose (and therefore insulin) and increased serum AA levels and β-adrenergic signaling.

12. Glucagon binds to the glucagon receptor, which is linked to PKA-dependent pathways. The primary target organ for glucagon is the liver. Glucagon increases liver glucose output by increasing glycogenolysis and gluconeogenesis. It increases β oxidation of fatty acids and ketogenesis.

13. Glucagon regulates hepatic metabolism both by regulation of gene expression and through posttranslational PKA-dependent pathways.

14. The major counterregulatory factors in muscle and adipose tissue are the adrenal hormone epinephrine and the sympathetic neurotransmitter norepinephrine. These two factors act through β_2- and β_3-adrenergic receptors to increase cAMP levels. Epinephrine and norepinephrine enhance glycogenolysis and fatty acyl oxidation in muscle and increase hormone-sensitive lipase in adipose tissue.

15. Diabetes mellitus is classified as type 1 (T1DM) and type 2 (T2DM). T1DM is characterized by the destruction of pancreatic beta cells, and exogenous insulin is required for treatment. T2DM can be due to numerous factors but is usually characterized as insulin resistance coupled to some degree of beta cell deficiency. Patients with T2DM

may require exogenous insulin at some point to maintain blood glucose levels.

16. Obesity-associated T2DM is currently at epidemic proportions worldwide and is characterized by insulin resistance because of lipotoxicity, hyperinsulinemia, and inflammatory cytokines produced by adipose tissue. T2DM is often associated with obesity, insulin resistance, hypertension, and coronary artery disease. This constellation of risk factors is referred to as the metabolic syndrome.

17. Major symptoms of diabetes mellitus include hyperglycemia, polyuria, polydipsia, polyphagia, muscle wasting, electrolyte depletion, and ketoacidosis (in T1DM).

18. The long-term complications of poorly controlled diabetes are due to excess intracellular glucose (glucotoxicity), especially in the retina, kidney, and peripheral nerves. This leads to retinopathy, nephropathy, and neuropathy.

19. Adipose tissue has an endocrine function, especially in terms of energy homeostasis. Hormones produced by adipose tissue include leptin and adiponectin. Leptin acts on the hypothalamus to promote satiety.

CHAPTER 39

Hormonal Regulation of Calcium and Phosphate Metabolism

Calcium (**Ca^{++}**) and phosphate are essential to human life because they play important structural roles in hard tissues (i.e., bones and teeth) and important regulatory roles in metabolic and signaling pathways. In blood, most phosphate exists in the ionized form of phosphoric acid, which is called **inorganic phosphate (P$_i$).** The two primary sources of circulating Ca^{++} and P$_i$ are the diet and the skeleton (Fig. 39-1). Two hormones, **1,25-dihydroxyvitamin D** (also called **calcitriol**) and **parathyroid hormone (PTH),** regulate intestinal absorption of Ca^{++} and P$_i$ and release of Ca^{++} and P$_i$ into the circulation after bone resorption. The primary processes for removal of Ca^{++} and P$_i$ from blood are renal excretion and bone formation (Fig. 39-1). 1,25-Dihydroxyvitamin D and PTH regulate both processes. Other hormones and paracrine growth factors also regulate Ca^{++} and P$_i$ homeostasis.

CRUCIAL ROLES OF CALCIUM AND PHOSPHATE IN CELLULAR PHYSIOLOGY

Calcium is an essential dietary element. In addition to obtaining Ca^{++} from the diet, humans contain a vast store (i.e., >1 kg) of Ca^{++} in their bones, which can be called on to maintain normal circulating levels of Ca^{++} in times of dietary restriction and during the increased demands of pregnancy and nursing. Circulating Ca^{++} exists in three forms (Table 39-1): free ionized Ca^{++}, protein-bound Ca^{++}, and Ca^{++} complexed with anions (e.g., phosphates, HCO$_3^-$, citrate). The ionized form represents about 50% of circulating Ca^{++}, and because this form is so critical to many cellular functions, [Ca^{++}] in both the extracellular and intracellular compartments is tightly controlled. Circulating Ca^{++} is under direct hormonal control and normally maintained in a relatively narrow range. Either too little Ca^{++} (**hypocalcemia;** total serum [Ca^{++}] below 8.5 mg/dL [4.2 mEq/L]) or too much Ca^{++} (**hypercalcemia;** total serum [Ca^{++}] above 10.5 mg/dL [5.2 mEq/L]) in blood can lead to a broad range of pathophysiological changes, including neuromuscular dysfunction, central nervous system dysfunction, renal insufficiency, calcification of soft tissue, and skeletal pathology.

P$_i$ is also an essential dietary element, and it is stored in large quantities in bone complexed with Ca^{++}. Most circulating P$_i$ is in the free ionized form, but some

P$_i$ (<20%) circulates as a protein-bound form or is complexed with cations (Table 39-1). Because soft tissues contain 10-fold more P$_i$ than Ca^{++}, tissue damage (e.g., crush injury with massive muscle cell death) can result in **hyperphosphatemia,** whereupon the increased P$_i$ complexes with Ca^{++} to cause acute hypocalcemia.

P$_i$ is a key intracellular component. Indeed, it is the high-energy phosphate bonds of ATP that maintain life. Phosphorylation and dephosphorylation of proteins, lipids, second messengers, and cofactors represent key regulatory steps in numerous metabolic and signaling pathways, and phosphate also serves as the backbone for nucleic acids.

PHYSIOLOGICAL REGULATION OF CALCIUM AND PHOSPHATE: PARATHYROID HORMONE AND 1,25-DIHYDROXYVITAMIN D

PTH and **1,25-dihydroxyvitamin D** are the two physiologically most important hormones that are dedicated to maintenance of normal blood [Ca^{++}] and [P$_i$] in humans. As such, they are referred to as **calciotropic hormones.** The structure, synthesis, and secretion of these two hormones and their receptors will be discussed first. In the following section, the detailed actions of PTH and 1,25-dihydroxyvitamin D on the three key sites of Ca^{++}/P$_i$ homeostasis (i.e., gut, bone, and kidney) are discussed.

Parathyroid Glands

The predominant parenchymal cell type in the parathyroid gland is the **principal** (also called **chief**) **cell** (Fig. 39-2).

Parathyroid Hormone

PTH is the primary hormone that protects against hypocalcemia. The primary targets of PTH are bone and the kidneys. PTH also functions in a positive feedforward loop by stimulating production of 1,25-dihydroxyvitamin D.

Structure, Synthesis, and Secretion

PTH is secreted as an 84–amino acid polypeptide and is synthesized as a **prepro-PTH,** which is proteolytically processed to **pro-PTH** in the endoplasmic reticulum and then to PTH in the Golgi and secretory vesicles. Unlike proinsulin, all intracellular pro-PTH is normally

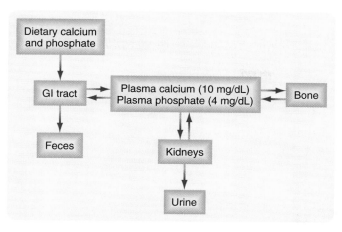

● **Figure 39-1.** Daily Ca^{++} and P$_i$ flux.

● **Table 39-1.** **Forms of Ca^{++} and P$_i$ in Plasma**

Ion	mg/dL	Ionized	Protein Bound	Complexed
Ca^{++}	10	50%	45%	5%
P$_i$	4	84%	10%	6%

Ca^{++} is bound (i.e., complexed) to various anions in plasma, including HCO$_3^-$, citrate, and SO$_4^{-2}$. P$_i$ is complexed to various cations, including Na$^+$ and K$^+$. (From Koeppen BM, Stanton BA: Renal Physiology, 4th ed. Philadelphia, Mosby, 2007.)

● AT THE CELLULAR LEVEL

PTH is proteolytically cleaved into biologically inactive N-terminus and C-terminus fragments that are excreted by the kidney. Older PTH assays detected both intact 1-84 PTH and inactive C-terminus fragments and therefore detected active and inactive PTH, especially in patients with renal disease. Current assays use two antibodies that recognize epitopes from both ends of the molecule, thereby more accurately measuring the intact 1-84 form of PTH.

converted to PTH before secretion. PTH has a short half-life (<5 minutes).

The primary signal that stimulates PTH secretion is low circulating [Ca^{++}] (Fig. 39-3). The extracellular [Ca^{++}] is sensed by the parathyroid chief cell through a **Ca^{++}-sensing receptor (CaSR).** In the parathyroid gland, increasing amounts of extracellular Ca^{++} bind to the CaSR and activate signaling pathways that repress PTH secretion.

Although the CaSR binds to extracellular Ca^{++} with relatively low affinity, the CaSR is extremely sensitive to changes in extracellular [Ca^{++}]. A 0.2-mEq/L drop in blood [Ca^{++}] produces an increase in circulating PTH levels from basal (5% of maximum) to maximum levels (Fig. 39-4). Thus, the CaSR regulates PTH output in response to subtle fluctuations in [Ca^{++}] on a minute-to-minute basis.

PTH production is also regulated at the level of gene transcription (Fig. 39-3). The PTH gene is repressed by

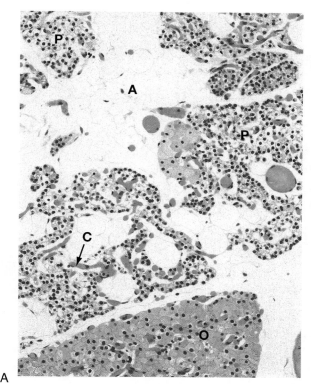

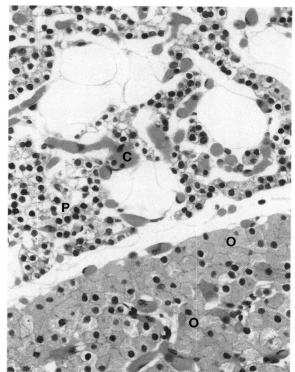

● **Figure 39-2.** **A** and **B,** Histology of parathyroid glands. A, adipose tissue within parathyroid glands; C, capillaries; O, oxyphil cells; P, principal or chief cells. (From Young B et al: Wheater's Functional Histology, 5th ed. Philadelphia, Churchill Livingstone, 2006.)

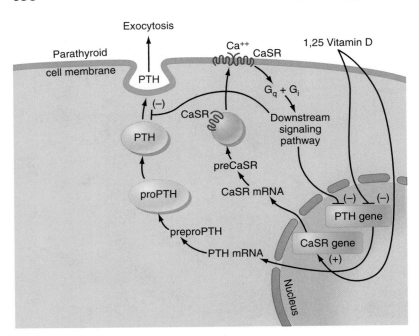

● **Figure 39-3.** Regulation of PTH gene expression and secretion. (Modified from Porterfield SP, White BA: Endocrine Physiology, 3rd ed. Philadelphia, Mosby, 2007.)

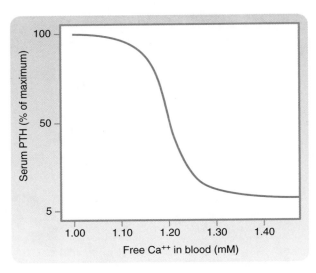

● **Figure 39-4.** Ca^{++}/PTH secretion dose-response curve. (Modified from Porterfield SP, White BA: Endocrine Physiology, 3rd ed. Philadelphia, Mosby, 2007.)

⬤ AT THE CELLULAR LEVEL

PTHrP is a peptide paracrine hormone produced by several tissues. PTHrP is also expressed in several developing tissues, including the growth plate of bones and in the mammary glands, and may play several roles in adults (e.g., regulation of uterine contractions). The 30 amino acids at the N-terminus of PTHrP have significant structural homology with PTH. Thus, PTHrP binds to and signals through the PTH/PTHrP receptor. PTHrP is not regulated by circulating Ca^{++} and normally does not play a role in Ca^{++}/P$_i$ homeostasis in adults. However, certain tumors secrete high levels of PTHrP, which causes **hypercalcemia of malignancy** and symptoms that resemble hyperparathyroidism.

▷ IN THE CLINIC

Patients with **familial benign hypocalciuric hypercalcemia (FBHH)** or **neonatal severe hyperparathyroidism** are heterozygous or homozygous, respectively, for inactivating mutations of the CaSR. In these patients the CaSR fails to appropriately inhibit PTH secretion in response to high blood levels of Ca^{++}. The CaSR also plays a direct role in Ca^{++} reabsorption in the kidney. The hypocalciuria (i.e., inappropriately low Ca^{++} excretion in the face of high circulating [Ca^{++}]) in patients with FBHH is due to the lowered ability of the CaSR to monitor blood calcium and respond by increasing urinary Ca^{++} excretion.

a **calcium response element** within the promoter of this gene. Thus, the signaling pathway that is activated by binding of Ca^{++} to the CaSR ultimately leads to repression of PTH gene expression and synthesis. The PTH gene is also repressed by 1,25-dihydroxyvitamin D (acting through vitamin D response elements—see later). The ability of 1,25-dihydroxyvitamin D to hold PTH gene expression in check is reinforced by the coordinated up-regulation of CaSR gene expression by positive vitamin D response elements in the promoter region of the CaSR gene (Fig. 39-3).

Parathyroid Hormone Receptor. Because the PTH receptor also binds PTH-related peptide (PTHrP), it is usually referred to as the **PTH/PTHrP receptor.** The PTH/PTHrP receptor is expressed on osteoblasts in bone and in the proximal and distal tubules of the kidney, and it is the receptor that mediates the systemic actions of PTH. However, the PTH/PTHrP receptor is also expressed in many developing organs, in which PTHrP has an important paracrine function.

Vitamin D

Vitamin D is actually a prohormone that must undergo two successive hydroxylation reactions to become the active form **1,25-dihydroxyvitamin D** (Fig. 39-5). Vitamin D plays a critical role in Ca^{++} absorption and, to a lesser extent, P_i absorption by the small intestine. Vitamin D also regulates bone remodeling and renal reabsorption of Ca^{++} and P_i.

Structure, Synthesis, and Transport of Active Vitamin D Metabolites

Vitamin D_3 (also called **cholecalciferol**) is synthesized via the conversion of 7-dehydrocholesterol by ultraviolet B light (UVB) in the more basal layers of the skin (Fig. 39-6). Vitamin D_3 is therefore referred to as a **secosteroid,** which is a class of steroids in which one of the cholesterol rings is opened (Fig. 39-5). **Vitamin D_2** is produced in plants. Vitamin D_3 and, to a lesser extent, vitamin D_2 are absorbed from the diet and are equally effective after conversion to active hydroxylated forms. The balance between UVB-dependent, endogenously synthesized vitamin D_3 and absorption of the dietary forms of vitamin D becomes important in certain situations. Individuals with higher epidermal melanin content who live in higher latitudes convert less 7-dehydrocholesterol to vitamin D_3 and thus are more dependent on dietary sources of vitamin D_3. Dairy products are enriched with vitamin D_3, but not all individuals tolerate or enjoy dairy products. Institutionalized, sedentary elderly patients who stay indoors and avoid dairy products are particularly at risk for the development of **vitamin D_3 deficiency.**

Vitamin D_3 is transported in blood from the skin to the liver. Dietary vitamin D_3 and vitamin D_2 reach the liver directly via transport in the portal circulation and indirectly via chylomicrons (Fig. 39-6). In the liver, vitamin D_2 and vitamin D_3 are hydroxylated at the 25-carbon position to yield **25-hydroxyvitamin D** (at this juncture, no distinction will be made between D_3 and D_2 metabolites because they are equipotent). Hepatic 25-hydroxyvitamin D is expressed at a relatively constant and high level, so circulating levels largely reflect the amount of precursor available for 25-hydroxylation. Because the hydroxyl group at the 25 carbon represents the second hydroxyl group on the molecule, 25-hydroxyvitamin D is also referred to as **calcifediol.**

25-Hydroxyvitamin D is further hydroxylated in the proximal tubules of the kidney (Figs. 39-5 and 39-6). Hydroxylation of 25-hydroxyvitamin D in the 1 position generates **1,25-dihydroxyvitamin D,** which is the most active form of vitamin D. Hydroxylation of 25-hydroxyvitamin D at the 24 position generates **24,25-dihydroxyvitamin D.**

Vitamin D and its metabolites circulate in blood primarily bound to **vitamin D–binding protein (DBP).** DBP is a serum glycoprotein that is synthesized by the liver. DBP binds more than 85% of 1,25-hydroxyvitamin D and 24,25-dihydroxyvitamin D. Because of binding to other proteins, only 0.4% of 1,25-dihydroxyvitamin D circulates as free hormone. DBP transports the highly lipophilic vitamin D in blood and provides a reservoir

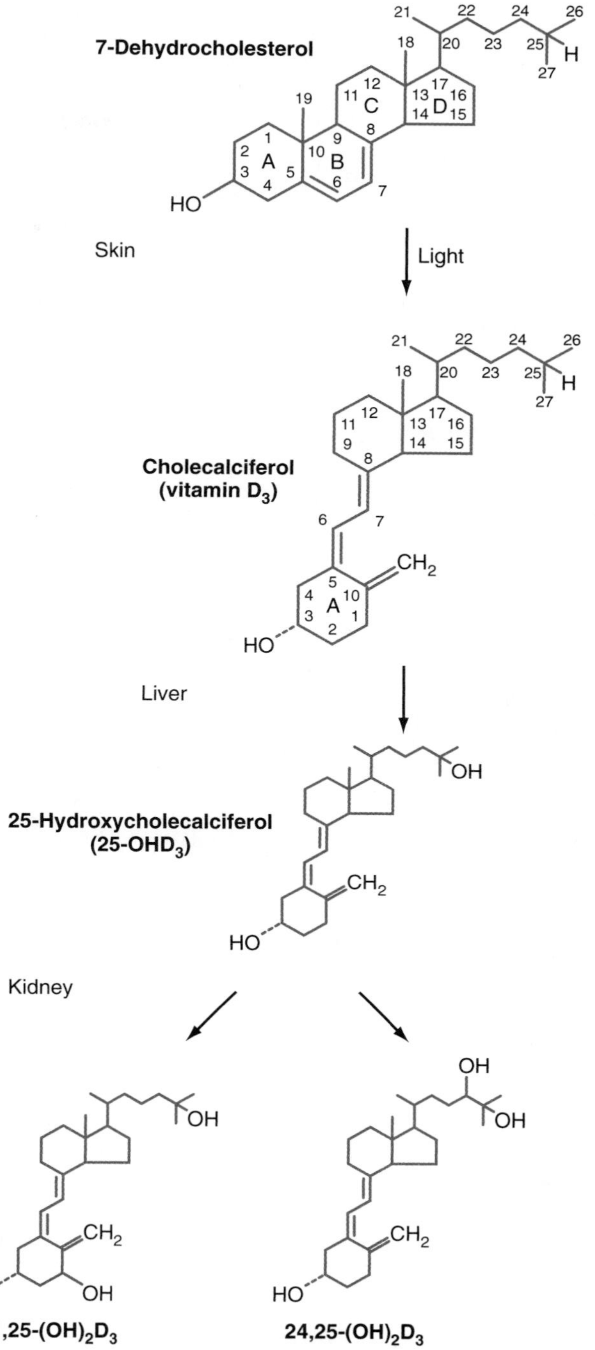

● **Figure 39-5.** Biosynthesis of 1,25-dihydroxyvitamin D. (Modified from Porterfield SP, White BA: Endocrine Physiology, 3rd ed. Philadelphia, Mosby, 2007.)

of vitamin D that protects against vitamin D deficiency. DBP-bound vitamin D metabolites have a circulating half-life of several hours.

The kidney 1α-hydroxylase enzyme (encoded by the Cyp1α gene) is tightly regulated at the transcriptional level (Fig. 39-7). 1,25-Dihydroxyvitamin D inhibits 1α-hydroxylase expression and stimulates 24-hydroxylase expression. Ca^{++} is also an important reg-

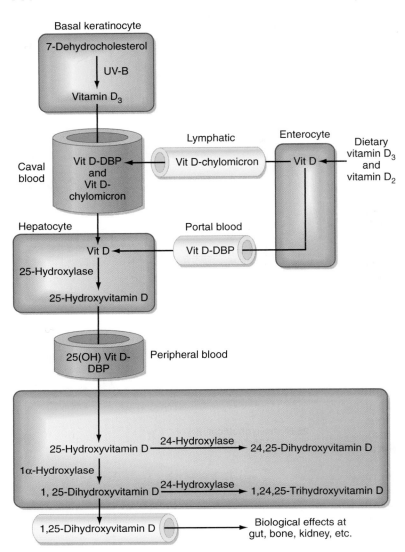

● **Figure 39-6.** Vitamin D metabolism. (Modified from Porterfield SP, White BA: Endocrine Physiology, 3rd ed. Philadelphia, Mosby, 2007.)

ulator of renal 1α-hydroxylase. Low circulating [Ca^{++}] indirectly stimulates renal 1α-hydroxylase expression through increased PTH levels, whereas elevated [Ca^{++}] inhibits 1α-hydroxylase activity directly through the CaSR in the proximal tubule. A low-P$_i$ diet also stimulates renal 1α-hydroxylase activity in a PTH-independent manner.

1,25-Dihydroxyvitamin D Receptor

1,25-Dihydroxyvitamin D exerts its actions primarily through binding to the **nuclear vitamin D receptor (VDR),** which is a member of the nuclear hormone receptor family. The VDR is a transcription factor that binds to DNA sequences **(vitamin D response elements)** as a heterodimer with the **retinoid X receptor** (RXR). Thus, the primary action of 1,25-dihydroxyvitamin D is to regulate gene expression in its target tissues, including the small intestine, bone, kidneys, and parathyroid gland.

The genomic actions of 1,25-dihydroxyvitamin D, as mediated by the VDR, occur over a period of hours or days. 1,25-Dihydroxyvitamin D also has rapid effects (seconds to 10 minutes). For example, 1,25-dihy-droxyvitamin D rapidly induces absorption of Ca^{++} by the duodenum **(transcaltachia).** The VDR is also expressed in the plasma membrane of cells and is linked to rapid signaling pathways (e.g., G proteins, phosphatidylinositol-3′-kinase). Current molecular modeling has led to the development of ligands that specifically bind to the nuclear- versus the membrane-localized VDR, thus paving the way for the selective treatment of disorders related to the rapid versus slow actions of 1,25-dihydroxyvitamin D with synthetic vitamin D analogues.

REGULATION OF [CA^{++}] AND [P$_i$] BY THE SMALL INTESTINE AND BONE

An overview of the regulation of [Ca^{++}] and [P$_i$] by the action of PTH and 1,25-dihydroxyvitamin D on the small intestine, bone, and parathyroid glands is summarized in Table 39-2 and in the following paragraphs. For details on the renal handling of Ca^{++}, consult Chapter 35.

● **Figure 39-7.** Regulation of the renal Cyp1α gene expression by Ca⁺⁺ and hormones. (Modified from Porterfield SP, White BA: Endocrine Physiology, 3rd ed. Philadelphia, Mosby, 2007.)

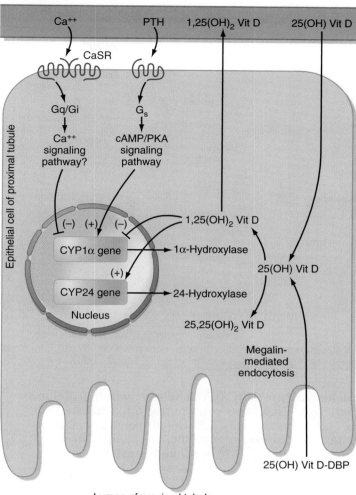

AT THE CELLULAR LEVEL

The primary actions of **calcitonin** are on bone and kidney. Calcitonin lowers serum [Ca⁺⁺] and [P$_i$], primarily by inhibiting bone resorption; however, this effect occurs only at high circulating levels. There are no complications caused by calcitonin deficiency or excess in humans. For this reason, it is unlikely that calcitonin has an important physiological role in humans. Medical interest in calcitonin stems from the fact that potent forms of calcitonin can be used therapeutically in the treatment of bone disorders. Calcitonin is also a useful histochemical marker of medullary thyroid cancer.

The **calcitonin receptor** is closely related to the PTH/PTHrP receptor. In contrast to the PTH/PTHrP receptor, the calcitonin receptor is expressed in osteoclasts. Calcitonin acts rapidly and directly on osteoclasts to suppress bone resorption. **Paget's disease** is characterized by excessive bone turnover that is driven by large, bizarre osteoclasts. Because these osteoclasts retain the calcitonin receptor, active forms of calcitonin can be used to suppress aberrant osteoclastic activity in patients with this disease.

Ca⁺⁺ and P$_i$ Transport by the Small Intestine

Dietary intake of Ca⁺⁺ can vary, but in general, North Americans consume about 1.5 g of Ca⁺⁺ per day. Of this, about 200 mg is absorbed by the proximal part of the small intestine. Importantly, absorption of Ca⁺⁺ is stimulated by 1,25-dihydroxyvitamin D, so absorption is more efficient in the face of declining dietary Ca⁺⁺.

Ca⁺⁺ is absorbed from the duodenum and jejunum by both a Ca⁺⁺-regulated and a hormonally regulated transcellular route and by a passive, paracellular route. The transcellular route of Ca⁺⁺ absorption is summarized in Figure 39-8. Movement of Ca⁺⁺ from the lumen of the gastrointestinal tract into the enterocyte, which is favored by both chemical and electrical gradients, is facilitated by apical **epithelial calcium channels** called **TRPV5** and **TRPV6**. Inside the cell Ca⁺⁺ ions bind to **calbindin-D$_{9K}$**, which maintains a low cytoplasmic [Ca⁺⁺], thus preserving the favorable lumen-to-enterocyte [Ca⁺⁺] gradient. Calbindin-D$_{9K}$ also plays a role in apical-to-basolateral shuttling of Ca⁺⁺, which is transported across the basolateral membrane against an electrochemical gradient by **plasma membrane**

● **Table 39-2.** **Actions of PTH and 1,25-Dihydroxyvitamin D on Ca⁺⁺/Pᵢ Homeostasis**

	Small Intestine	Bone	Kidney	Parathyroid Gland
PTH	No direct action	Promotes osteoblastic growth and survival Regulates M-CSF, RANKL, and OPG production by osteoblasts Chronic high levels promote net Ca⁺⁺ and Pᵢ release from bone	Stimulates 1α-hydroxylase activity Stimulates Ca⁺⁺ reabsorption by the thick ascending limb of Henle's loop and the distal tubule Inhibits Pᵢ reabsorption by proximal nephrons (represses NPT2a expression)	No direct action
1,25-Dihydroxyvitamin D	Increases Ca⁺⁺ absorption by increasing TRPV channels, calbindin-D and PMCA expression Marginally increases Pᵢ absorption	Sensitizes osteoblasts to PTH Regulates osteoid production and calcification	Minimal actions on Ca⁺⁺ reabsorption Promotes Pᵢ reabsorption by proximal nephrons (stimulates NPT2a expression)	Directly inhibits PTH gene expression Directly stimulates CaSR gene expression

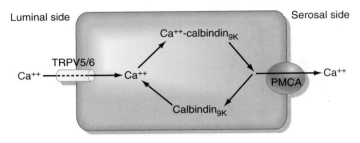

● **Figure 39-8.** Intestinal absorption of Ca⁺⁺ via the transcellular route. (Modified from Porterfield SP, White BA: *Endocrine Physiology*, 3rd ed. Philadelphia, Mosby, 2007.)

calcium ATPase (PMCA). The **Na⁺-Ca⁺⁺ sodium/calcium exchanger (NCX)** also contributes to the transport of Ca⁺⁺ out of enterocytes. 1,25-Dihydroxyvitamin D stimulates the expression of all the components involved in absorption of Ca⁺⁺ by the small intestine.

The fraction of dietary Pᵢ absorbed by the jejunum remains relatively constant at about 70% and is under minor hormonal control by 1,25-dihydroxyvitamin D. The limiting process in transcellular Pᵢ absorption is transport across the apical brush border, which is mediated by the **Na⁺-Pᵢ cotransporter (NPT2).**

Handling of Ca⁺⁺ and Pᵢ by Bone

Bone stores a large amount of Ca⁺⁺ and Pᵢ. Once maximal bone mass has been achieved in an adult, the skeleton is constantly remodeled through the concerted activities of bone cells. The processes of **bone formation (accretion)** and **bone resorption** are in balance in a healthy, physically active, and well-nourished individual. Of the 1 kg of Ca⁺⁺ immobilized in bone, about 500 mg (i.e., 0.5% of skeletal Ca⁺⁺) is mobilized from and deposited in bone each day. However, the process of bone remodeling can be modulated to provide a net gain or loss of Ca⁺⁺ and Pᵢ into blood and is responsive to physical activity (or lack thereof), diet, age, and hormonal regulation. Because the integrity of bone is absolutely dependent on Ca⁺⁺ and Pᵢ, chronic dysregulation of [Ca⁺⁺] and [Pᵢ] or the hormones that regulate [Ca⁺⁺] and [Pᵢ] lead to pathological changes in bone.

PHYSIOLOGY OF BONE

The process of biogenesis, growth, and remodeling of bone is complex and beyond the scope of this chapter.

The key features required to understand the role of adult bone in the hormonal regulation of Ca⁺⁺/Pᵢ metabolism are discussed in this section.

In adults, bone remodeling involves (1) destruction of preformed bone with the release of Ca⁺⁺, Pᵢ, and hydrolyzed fragments of the proteinaceous matrix (called **osteoid**) into blood and (2) new synthesis of osteoid at the site of resorption and subsequent calcification of the osteoid, primarily with Ca⁺⁺ and Pᵢ from blood. Bone remodeling occurs continually in about 2 million discrete sites involving subpopulations of bone cells called **basic multicellular units.**

The cells involved in bone remodeling fall into two major classes: cells that promote the formation of bone **(osteoblasts)** and cells that promote the resorption of bone **(osteoclasts).** The process of bone remodeling is a highly integrated process (Fig. 39-9). Osteoblasts express factors that induce differentiation of osteoclasts from cells of the monocyte/macrophage lineage and then fully activate osteoclast function. Osteoblasts release **monocyte colony-stimulating factor (M-CSF),** which induces the earliest differentiating processes that lead to osteoclast precursors. M-CSF also acts in concert with another factor, **RANKL** (named for **r**eceptor **a**ctivator of NF-κB **l**igand), to promote osteoclastogenesis. RANKL binds to its receptor **RANK** on osteoclast precursor membranes and induces osteoclastogenesis. This process involves the clustering and fusion of several osteoclast precursors and gives rise to a fused, polykaryonic osteoclast. The perimeter of the osteoclast membrane facing the bone adheres tightly to the bone and essentially seals off the area of osteoclast-bone contact (Fig. 39-9). The osteoclast cell membrane facing the bone secretes hydrolytic enzymes and HCl. The acidic enzyme-rich microenvironment dissolves the calcified crystals, thereby releasing Ca⁺⁺ and Pᵢ into blood. After about 2 weeks, osteoclasts receive a different signal from neighboring osteoblasts. This signal is **osteoprotegerin (OPG),** which acts as a soluble decoy receptor for RANKL (Fig. 39-9). Consequently, the proosteoclastic signal from osteoblasts is terminated.

During a reversal phase, adjacent osteoblasts migrate into the resorbed area (now vacated by osteoclasts) and begin to lay down osteoid. Some of the components in osteoid promote its calcification, a process that removes Ca⁺⁺ and Pᵢ from blood. As the

● **Figure 39-9.** Osteoblast regulation of osteoclast differentiation and function. (Modified from Porterfield SP, White BA: Endocrine Physiology, 3rd ed. Philadelphia, Mosby, 2007.)

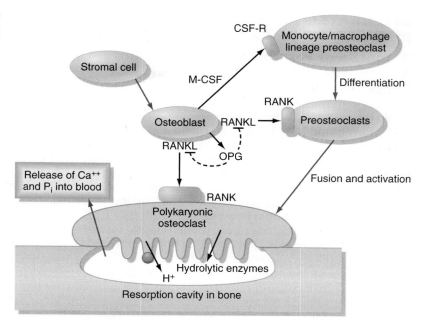

● AT THE CELLULAR LEVEL

The importance of the RANK/RANKL/OPG system is underscored by mutations in the human genes for RANK and OPG, which are associated with bone deformities. Loss of RANKL in mice causes **osteopetrosis** (i.e., excessive bone density) because of the loss of osteoclasts. Conversely, loss of OPG causes **osteoporosis** (reduced bone density) because of a high number of overly active osteoclasts.

▶ IN THE CLINIC

In vitamin D–deficient individuals, osteoid is not properly calcified and the bone is weak. Vitamin D deficiency produces hypocalcemia and hypomagnesemia and decreases gastrointestinal absorption of Ca^{++} and P_i. The drop in serum $[Ca^{++}]$ stimulates secretion of PTH, which stimulates excretion of P_i by the kidney, thereby aggravating the loss of P_i in serum. Because the Ca^{++}/P_i product in serum is low, bone mineralization is impaired and demineralization is increased. In children, this leads to **rickets,** in which the growth of long bones is abnormal and the weakened bones lead to bowing of the extremities and collapse of the rib cage. In adults, vitamin D deficiency leads to **osteomalacia,** which is characterized by poorly calcified osteoid associated with pain, increased risk for fracture, and vertebral collapse. The secondary elevation in PTH can produce osteoporosis.

osteoblasts become surrounded by and entrapped within bone, they become **osteocytes** that sit within small spaces, called haversian lacunae. Osteocytes remain interconnected through cell processes that run within canaliculi and form communicating junctions with adjacent cell processes. The new concentric layers of bone, along with the interconnected osteocytes and the central canal, are referred to collectively as an **osteon.** The exact function or functions of osteocytes are presently unclear, although evidence exists for a role of osteocytes in sensing mechanical stress in bones.

As a calciotropic hormone, PTH is the primary endocrine regulator of bone remodeling in adults. The PTH/PTHrP receptor is expressed on osteoblasts, but not on osteoclasts. Therefore, PTH directly stimulates osteoblastic activity and stimulates osteoclastic activity indirectly through osteoblast-derived paracrine factors (i.e., M-CSF, RANKL). Intermittent administration of low doses of PTH promotes osteoblast survival and bone anabolic functions, increases bone density, and reduces the risk of fracture in humans. In contrast, sustained elevated levels of PTH shift the balance to a relative increase in osteoclast activity, thereby increasing bone turnover and reducing bone density.

Regulation of bone remodeling by PTH requires normal levels of 1,25-dihydroxyvitamin D. In vitamin D–deficient individuals, the Ca^{++}-PTH secretion curve is shifted to the right. Thus, normal Ca^{++} levels are less effective in suppressing PTH secretion, and elevated PTH levels and increased bone turnover result. The VDR is expressed in osteoblasts, and normal 1,25-dihydroxyvitamin D levels are also required for coordination of osteoid production with its calcification.

INTEGRATED PHYSIOLOGICAL REGULATION OF CA⁺⁺/Pᵢ METABOLISM

Response of Parathyroid Hormone and 1,25-Dihydroxyvitamin D to a Hypocalcemic Challenge

The integrated response of PTH and 1,25-dihydroxyvitamin D to a hypocalcemic challenge is shown in Figure 39-10. Low blood [Ca⁺⁺], detected by the CaSR on parathyroid chief cells, stimulates secretion of PTH. In the kidney, PTH increases Ca⁺⁺ reabsorption in the thick ascending limb of Henle's loop and the distal tubule. Hypocalcemia also stimulates Ca⁺⁺ reabsorption by activating the CaSR and, to a lesser extent, by increasing 1,25-dihydroxyvitamin D levels. PTH inhibits NPT2, thereby increasing excretion of Pᵢ. The relative loss of Pᵢ increases ionized [Ca⁺⁺] in blood. In bone, PTH stimulates osteoblasts to secrete RANKL, which in turn rapidly increases osteoclast activity and leads to increased bone resorption and release of Ca⁺⁺ and Pᵢ into blood.

In a slower phase of the response to hypocalcemia, PTH and low [Ca⁺⁺] directly stimulate 1α-hydroxylase (CYP1α) expression in the proximal renal tubule, thereby increasing 1,25-dihydroxyvitamin D levels. In the small intestine, 1,25-dihydroxyvitamin D stimulates absorption of Ca⁺⁺. These effects occur over a period of hours and days and involve increased expression of TRPV5 and TRPV6 Ca⁺⁺ channels, calbindin-D₉ₖ, and PMCA. 1,25-Dihydroxyvitamin D also stimulates osteoblast release of RANKL, thereby amplifying the effect of PTH.

1,25-Dihydroxyvitamin D, along with the CaSR, plays a key role in a negative-feedback mechanism. Elevated PTH stimulates the production of 1,25-dihydroxyvitamin D, which inhibits PTH gene expression directly and indirectly by up-regulating the CaSR. 1,25-Dihydroxyvitamin D also represses renal 1α-hydroxylase activity while increasing 24-hydroxylase activity. Thus, as blood [Ca⁺⁺] returns to normal, PTH secretion and 1α-hydroxylase activity fall.

Regulation by Gonadal and Adrenal Steroid Hormones

Gonadal and **adrenal steroid hormones** have profound effects on Ca⁺⁺ and Pᵢ metabolism and on bone. **Estradiol-17β (E₂;** see Chapter 43) has bone anabolic and calciotropic effects and stimulates intestinal Ca⁺⁺ absorption. E₂ is also one of the most potent regulators of osteoblast and osteoclast function. Estrogen promotes the survival of osteoblasts and apoptosis of osteoclasts, thereby favoring bone formation over resorption. In postmenopausal women, estrogen deficiency results in an initial phase of rapid bone loss that lasts about 5 years, followed by a second phase of slower bone loss that results in hypocalcemia because of inefficient Ca⁺⁺ absorption and renal Ca⁺⁺ wasting. This can result in secondary hyperparathyroidism, which further exacerbates the bone loss. **Androgens** also have bone anabolic and calciotropic effects, although some of these effects are due to the peripheral conversion of testosterone to E₂ (see Chapter 43).

In contrast to gonadal steroids, the **glucocorticoids** (e.g., **cortisol**) promote bone resorption and renal Ca⁺⁺ wasting and inhibit intestinal Ca⁺⁺ absorption. Patients treated with high levels of a glucocorticoid (e.g., as an antiinflammatory and immunosuppressive drug) can have glucocorticoid-induced osteoporosis.

● **Figure 39-10.** Integrated response to a hypocalcemic challenge. (Modified from Porterfield SP, White BA: Endocrine Physiology, 3rd ed. Philadelphia, Mosby, 2007.)

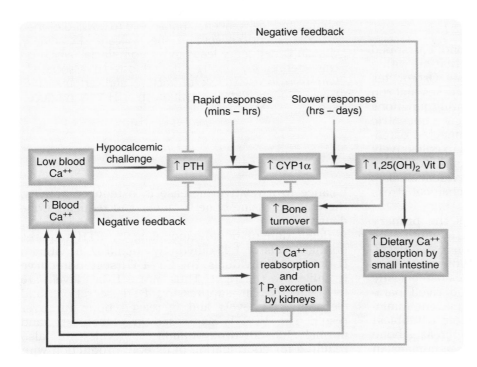

▶ IN THE CLINIC

Primary hyperparathyroidism is caused by excessive production of PTH by the parathyroid glands. It is frequently caused by a single **adenoma** confined to one of the parathyroid glands.

Patients with primary hyperparathyroidism have high serum [Ca^{++}] and, in most cases, low serum [P$_i$]. **Hypercalcemia** is a result of bone demineralization, increased gastrointestinal Ca^{++} absorption (mediated by 1,25-dihydroxyvitamin D), and increased renal Ca^{++} reabsorption. The major symptoms of the disorder are directly related to increased bone resorption, hypercalcemia, and **hypercalciuria**. High serum [Ca^{++}] decreases neuromuscular excitability. People with hyperparathyroidism often show psychological disorders, particularly depression. Other neurological symptoms include fatigue, mental confusion, and at very high levels (>15 mg/dL), coma. Hypercalcemia can cause cardiac arrest and peptic ulcer formation because Ca^{++} increases gastrin secretion. Kidney stones **(nephrolithiasis)** are common because hypercalcemia eventually leads to hypercalciuria and increased P$_i$ clearance leads to **phosphaturia**. The high urinary [Ca^{++}] and [P$_i$] increase the tendency for precipitation of Ca^{++}/P$_i$ salts in soft tissues of the kidney. When serum [Ca^{++}] exceeds about 13 mg/dL with a normal phosphate level, the Ca^{++}/P$_i$ **solubility product** is exceeded. At this level, insoluble Ca^{++}/P$_i$ salts form, which results in calcification of soft tissues such as blood vessels, skin, lungs, and joints.

People with hyperparathyroidism have evidence of increased bone turnover, such as increased urinary hydroxyproline levels, which is indicative of high bone resorptive activity. Hydroxyproline is an amino acid characteristically found in type I collagen. When the collagen is degraded, urinary excretion of hydroxyproline increases. Although hyperparathyroidism will eventually cause **osteoporosis** (bone loss involving both osteoid and mineral), it is not necessarily the initial symptom. However, bone demineralization is apparent.

■ KEY CONCEPTS

1. Serum [Ca^{++}] is determined by the rate of Ca^{++} absorption by the gastrointestinal tract, bone formation and resorption, and renal excretion. Serum [Ca^{++}] is normally maintained within a narrow range.

2. Serum [P$_i$] is determined by the rate of P$_i$ absorption by the gastrointestinal tract, soft tissue influx and efflux, bone formation and resorption, and renal excretion. Serum [P$_i$] normally fluctuates over a relatively wide range.

3. The major physiological hormones regulating serum [Ca^{++}] and [P$_i$] are PTH and 1,25-dihydroxyvitamin D (calcitriol).

4. Vitamin D is synthesized from 7-dehydrocholesterol in skin in the presence of UVB light. It is hydroxylated to 25-hydroxycholecalciferol in the liver and activated by renal 1α-hydroxylase to 1,25-dihydroxyvitamin D.

5. 1,25-Dihydroxyvitamin D promotes intestinal Ca^{++} absorption and weakly increases P$_i$ absorption.

6. The flux of Ca^{++} and P$_i$ into and out of bone is determined by the relative activities of osteoblasts versus osteoclasts.

7. The PTH/PTHrP receptor is expressed on osteoblasts, not on osteoclasts. PTH promotes osteoblast differentiation, proliferation, and survival, and intermittent administration of PTH promotes bone formation.

8. 1,25-Dihydroxyvitamin D binds to the VDR in osteoblasts to increase osteoblast differentiation, promote the secretion of osteoid components, and sensitize osteoblasts to PTH.

CHAPTER 40

The Hypothalamus and Pituitary Gland

The **pituitary gland** (also called the **hypophysis**) is a small (about 0.5 g in weight), yet complex endocrine structure at the base of the forebrain (Fig. 40-1). It is composed of an epithelial component called the **adenohypophysis** and a neural structure called the **neurohypophysis.** The adenohypophysis is composed of five cell types that secrete six hormones. The neurohypophysis releases several neurohormones. All endocrine functions of the pituitary gland are regulated by the hypothalamus and by negative- and positive-feedback loops.

ANATOMY

Microscopic examination of the pituitary reveals two distinct types of tissue: epithelial and neural (Fig. 40-2). The epithelial portion of the human pituitary gland is called the **adenohypophysis.** The adenohypophysis makes up the anterior portion of the pituitary and is often referred to as the **anterior lobe of the pituitary,** and its hormones are referred to as **anterior pituitary hormones.** The adenohypophysis is composed of three parts: (1) the **pars distalis,** which makes up about 90% of the adenohypophysis; (2) the pars tuberalis, which wraps around the stalk; and (3) the pars intermedia, which regresses and is absent in adult humans.

The neural portion of the pituitary is called the **neurohypophysis** and it represents a down-growth of the hypothalamus. The lowest portion of the neurohypophysis is called the **pars nervosa,** which is also called the **posterior lobe of the pituitary** (or simply, the **"posterior pituitary"**). At the superior end of the neurohypophysis, a funnel-shaped swelling called the **median eminence** develops. The rest of the neurohypophysis, which extends from the median eminence down to the pars nervosa, is called the **infundibulum.** The infundibulum and the pars tuberalis make up the pituitary stalk—a physical connection between the hypothalamus and the pituitary gland (Fig. 40-2).

The pituitary gland (anterior and posterior lobes) is situated within a depression of the sphenoid bone called the **sella turcica.** Generally, cancers of the pituitary have only one way to expand, which is up into the brain and against the optic nerves. Thus, any increase in size of the pituitary is often associated with dizziness or vision problems, or both. The sella turcica is sealed off from the brain by a membrane called the **diaphragma sellae.**

THE NEUROHYPOPHYSIS

The pars nervosa is a **neurovascular** structure that is the site of release of neurohormones adjacent to a rich bed of fenestrated capillaries. The peptide hormones that are released are **antidiuretic hormone** (**ADH,** or arginine vasopressin) and **oxytocin.** The cell bodies of the neurons that project to the pars nervosa are located in the **supraoptic nuclei (SON)** and **paraventricular nuclei (PVN)** of the **hypothalamus** (in this context, a "nucleus" refers to a collection of neuronal cell bodies residing within the central nervous system [CNS]—a "ganglion" is a collection of neuronal cell bodies residing outside the CNS). The cell bodies of these neurons are described as **magnocellular** (i.e., large cell bodies), and they project axons down the infundibular stalk as the **hypothalamohypophyseal tracts.** These axons terminate in the pars nervosa (Fig. 40-3). In addition to axonal processes and termini from the SON and PVN, there are glial-like supportive cells called **pituicytes.** The posterior pituitary is extensively vascularized and the capillaries are fenestrated, thereby facilitating diffusion of hormones into the vasculature.

Synthesis of ADH and Oxytocin

ADH and oxytocin are nonapeptides (nine amino acids) that are similar in structure, differing in only two amino acids. They have limited overlapping activity. ADH and oxytocin are synthesized as preprohormones (Fig. 40-4). Each prohormone harbors the structure of oxytocin or ADH and a cosecreted peptide: either **neurophysin I** (associated with ADH) or **neurophysin II** (associated with oxytocin). These preprohormones are called **preprovasophysin** and **preprooxyphysin.** The N-signal peptide is cleaved as the peptide is transported into the endoplasmic reticulum. The prohormone is packaged in the endoplasmic reticulum and Golgi apparatus in a membrane-bound secretory granule in cell bodies within the SON and PVN (Fig. 40-5). The secretory granules are conveyed intraaxonally through a "fast" (i.e., millimeters per hour) ATP-dependent transport mechanism down the infundibular stalk to axonal termini in the pars nervosa. During

● **Figure 40-1.** Cross-sectional image of the head demonstrating the proximity of the hypothalamus and pituitary gland and their connection by a neurohypophyseal (pituitary) stalk.

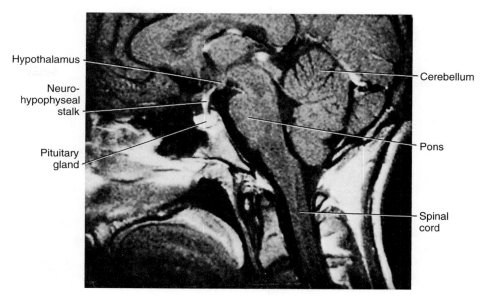

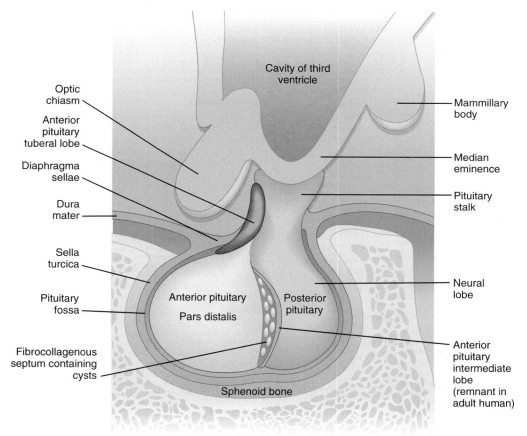

A

● **Figure 40-2.** **A,** Gross structure of the pituitary gland. The pituitary gland is below the hypothalamus and is connected to it by the pituitary stalk. The gland sits within the sella turcica, a fossa within the sphenoid bone, and is covered by a dural reflection, the diaphragma sellae. The pars distalis makes up most of the anterior pituitary. (Modified from Stevens A. In Lowe JS [ed]: Human Histology, 3rd ed. Philadelphia, Elsevier, 2005.)

(Continued)

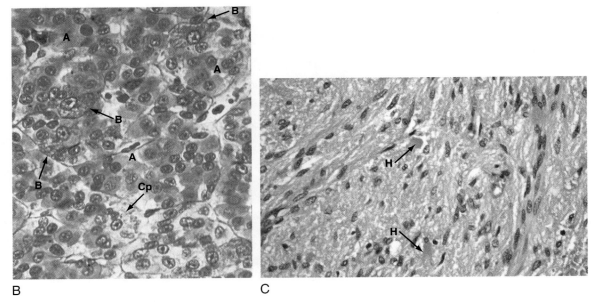

B C

● **Figure 40-2—cont'd** **B,** The pars distalis is derived from epithelial tissue that is composed of acidophils (A) (somatotropes and lactotropes) and basophils (B) (thyrotropes, gonadotropes, and corticotropes). The posterior pituitary is derived from neural tissue and has a histological appearance of nonmyelinated nerves **(C).** Cp, chromophobes; H, Herring bodies. (From Young B et al [eds]: Wheater's Functional Histology, 5th ed. Philadelphia, Churchill Livingstone, 2006.)

● **Figure 40-3.** Magnocellular neurons of the hypothalamus (paraventricular and supraoptic nuclei) project their axons down the infundibular process and terminate in the pars nervosa (posterior lobe), where they release their hormones (either ADH or oxytocin) into a capillary bed. (Modified from Larsen PR et al [eds]: Williams Textbook of Endocrinology, 10th ed. Philadelphia, Saunders, 2003.)

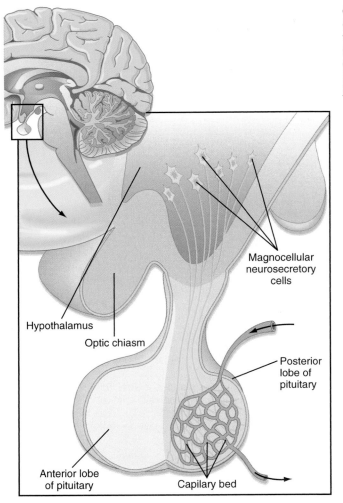

Magnocellular neurosecretory cells

Hypothalamus

Optic chiasm

Posterior lobe of pituitary

Anterior lobe of pituitary

Capilary bed

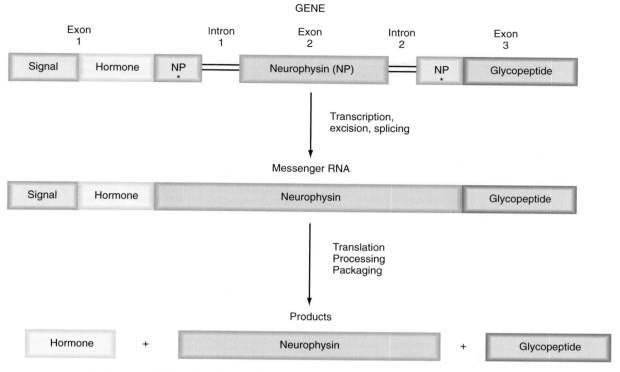

GENE

● **Figure 40-4.** Synthesis and processing of preprovasopressin or preprooxytocin.

transit of the secretory granule, the prohormones are proteolytically cleaved to produce equimolar amounts of hormone and neurophysin. Secretory granules containing fully processed peptides are stored in the axonal termini. Axonal swelling because of the storage of secretory granule can be observed by light microscopy and is termed **Herring bodies.**

ADH and oxytocin are released from the pars nervosa in response to stimuli that are primarily detected at the cell body and its dendrites in the SON and PVN of the hypothalamus. The stimuli are mainly in the form of neurotransmitters released from hypothalamic interneurons. With sufficient stimulus, the neurons will depolarize and propagate an action potential down the axon. At the axonal termini, the action potential increases intracellular $[Ca^{++}]$ and results in a stimulus-secretion response, with the exocytosis of ADH or oxytocin, along with neurophysins, into the extracellular fluid of the pars nervosa (Fig. 40-5). Hormones and neurophysins enter the peripheral circulation, and both can be measured in blood.

Actions and Regulation of ADH and Oxytocin

ADH primarily acts at the kidney to retain water (antidiuresis). The actions of ADH and regulation of ADH secretion were described in Chapter 34. Oxytocin primarily acts on the pregnant uterus (labor inducing) and myoepithelial cells of the breast (milk let-down during nursing). The actions and regulation of oxytocin are discussed in Chapter 43.

▶ IN THE CLINIC

Because posterior pituitary hormones are synthesized in the hypothalamus rather than the pituitary, **hypophysectomy** (pituitary removal) does not necessarily permanently disrupt synthesis and secretion of these hormones. Immediately after hypophysectomy, secretion of the hormones decreases. However, over a period of weeks, the severed proximal end of the tract will show histological modification and pituicytes will form around the neuron terminals. Secretory vacuoles are seen, and secretion of hormone resumes from this proximal end. Secretion of hormone can even potentially return to normal levels. In contrast, a lesion higher up on the pituitary stalk can lead to loss of neuronal cell bodies in the PVN and SON.

THE ADENOHYPOPHYSIS

The pars distalis is composed of five endocrine cell types that produce six hormones (Table 40-1). Because of the histological characteristics of the cell types, the corticotropes, thyrotropes, and gonadotropes are referred to as pituitary **basophils,** whereas the somatotropes and lactotropes are referred to as pituitary **acidophils** (Fig. 40-2, *B*).

Endocrine Axes

Before discussing the individual hormones of the adenohypophysis, it is important to understand the

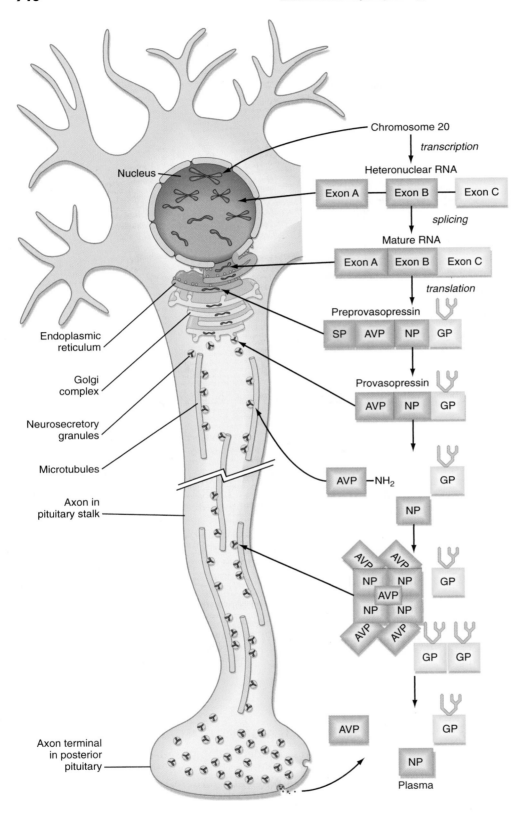

● **Figure 40-5.** Synthesis, processing, and transport of preprovasopressin. Human ADH (also called arginine vasopressin or AVP) is synthesized in the hypothalamic magnocellular cell bodies and packaged into neurosecretory granules. During intraaxonal transport of the granules down the infundibular process to the pars nervosa, provasopressin is proteolytically cleaved into the active hormone (AVP = ADH), neurophysin (NP), and a C-terminal glycoprotein (GP). NP arranges into tetramers that bind five AVP molecules. All three fragments are secreted from axonal termini in the pars nervosa (posterior pituitary) and enter the systemic blood. Only AVP (ADH) is biologically active. (Modified from Larsen PR et al [eds]: Williams Textbook of Endocrinology, 10th ed. Philadelphia, Saunders, 2003.)

● AT THE CELLULAR LEVEL

Significant progress has been made in understanding the differentiation of the five endocrine cells of the pars distalis from one precursor cell. The homeodomain transcription factor **Prop-1** is expressed soon after Rathke's pouch forms and promotes the cell lineages of somatotropes, lactotropes, thyrotropes, and gonadotropes. In humans, rare mutations in the Prop-1 gene result in a type of **combined pituitary hormone deficiency.** These individuals display dwarfism because of lack of GH, mental retardation secondary to hypothyroidism, and infertility as a result of a lack of gonadotropins. A subsequently expressed, pituitary-specific gene product called **Pit-1** was identified in mice. Pit-1 and its human homologue **POUF1** are also homeodomain transcription factors. POUF1 is absolutely required for the differentiation of thyrotropes, somatotropes, and lactotropes, and it directly stimulates the transcription and expression of TSH, GH, and prolactin. Affected individuals with POUF1 mutations have dwarfism and mental retardation. The orphan nuclear hormone receptor–related transcription factor **steroidogenic factor-1 (SF-1)** was originally identified in the adrenal cortex and gonads as a regulator of steroidogenic enzyme gene expression. However, SF-1 is also expressed in GnRH neurons in the hypothalamus and pituitary gonadotropes. SF-1 regulates the transcription of LH and FSH. Mutations in the SF-1 gene disrupt adrenal and gonadal function, including the loss of gonadotropes in the pituitary gland. **Tpit** is a transcription factor involved in the differentiation of corticotropes. Tpit interacts with other transcription factors to promote the differentiation of corticotropes and expression of the POMC gene (see later). Mutations in the human Tpit gene result in **isolated ACTH deficiency** (i.e., other cell types in the body that also express the POMC gene are not affected). This results in a form of **secondary adrenal insufficiency** that requires lifelong replacement with glucocorticoids (see Chapter 42).

structural and functional organization of the adenohypophysis within the **endocrine axes** (discussed briefly in Chapter 37; also refer to Table 40-1 and Fig. 40-6). Each endocrine axis is composed of three levels of endocrine cells: (1) hypothalamic neurons, (2) anterior pituitary cells, and (3) peripheral endocrine glands. Hypothalamic neurons release specific **hypothalamic releasing hormones** (XRHs) that stimulate the secretion of specific **pituitary tropic hormones** (XTHs). In some cases, production of a pituitary tropic hormone is secondarily regulated by a **release-inhibiting hormone** (XIH). Pituitary tropic hormones then act on specific peripheral target endocrine glands and stimulate them to release peripheral hormones (X). The peripheral hormone X has two general functions: it regulates several aspects of human physiology, and it negatively feeds back on the pituitary gland and

hypothalamus to inhibit the production and secretion of tropic hormones and releasing hormones, respectively (Fig. 40-6).

The hypothalamic level of regulation is neurohormonal. Collections of neuronal cell bodies (called **nuclei**) reside in several regions of the hypothalamus and are collectively referred to as the **hypophysiotropic** (i.e., "stimulatory to the hypophysis" [= pituitary]) region of the hypothalamus. These nuclei are distinguished from the magnocellular neurons of the PVN and SON that project to the pars nervosa in that they have small, or **parvicellular,** neuronal cell bodies that project axons to the median eminence. Parvicellular neurons secrete **releasing hormones** from their axonal termini at the median eminence (Fig. 40-7). The releasing hormones enter a primary plexus of fenestrated capillaries and are then conveyed to a second capillary plexus located in the pars distalis by the **hypothalamohypophyseal portal vessels** (a "portal" vessel is defined as a vessel that begins and ends in capillaries without going through the heart). At the secondary capillary plexus, the releasing hormones diffuse out of the vasculature and bind to their specific receptors on specific cell types within the pars distalis. The neurovascular link (i.e., the pituitary stalk) between the hypothalamus and pituitary is somewhat fragile and can be disrupted by physical trauma, surgery, or hypothalamic disease. Damage to the stalk and subsequent functional isolation of the anterior pituitary result in a decline in all anterior pituitary tropic hormones except prolactin (see later).

The cells of the adenohypophysis make up the intermediate level of an endocrine axis. The adenohypophysis secretes protein hormones that are referred to as **tropic hormones—ACTH, TSH, FSH, LH, GH,** and **PRL** (Table 40-1). With a few exceptions, tropic hormones bind to their cognate receptors on peripheral endocrine glands. Because of this arrangement, pituitary tropic hormones generally do not directly regulate physiological responses (see Chapter 37).

The endocrine axes have the following important features:

1. The activity of a specific axis is normally maintained at a **set point,** which varies from individual to individual, usually within a normal range. The set point is determined primarily by the integration of hypothalamic stimulation and peripheral hormone negative feedback. Importantly, the negative feedback is not exerted primarily by the physiological responses regulated by a specific endocrine axis, but from the peripheral hormone acting on the pituitary and hypothalamus (Fig. 40-6). Thus, if the level of a peripheral hormone drops, secretion of hypothalamic releasing hormones and pituitary tropic hormones will increase. As the level of peripheral hormone rises, the hypothalamus and pituitary will decrease secretion because of negative feedback. Although certain nonendocrine physiological parameters (e.g., acute hypoglycemia) can regulate some endocrine axes, the axes function semiautonomously with respect to the physiological changes

● Table 40-1.

Cell Types of the Adenohypophysis: Hormonal Production and Action, Hypothalamic Regulation, and Feedback Regulation

	Basophils			Acidophils	
	Corticotrope	*Thyrotrope*	*Gonadotrope*	*Somatotrope*	*Lactotrope*
Primary hypothalamic regulation	Corticotropin-releasing hormone (CRH): 41–amino acid peptide, stimulatory	Thyrotropin-releasing hormone (TRH): tripeptide, stimulatory	Gonadotropin-releasing hormone (GnRH): decapeptide, stimulatory	Growth hormone–releasing hormone (GHRH): 44–amino acid peptide, stimulatory Somatostatin: tetradecapeptide, inhibitory	Dopamine (catecholamine): inhibitory PRL-releasing factor?: stimulatory
Tropic hormone secreted	Adrenocorticotropic hormone (ACTH): 4.5-kDa protein	Thyroid-stimulating hormone (TSH): 28-kDa glycoprotein hormone	Follicle-stimulating hormone and luteinizing hormone (FSH, LH): 28- and 33-kDa glycoprotein hormones	Growth hormone (GH): ≈22-kDa protein	Prolactin (PRL): ≈23-kDa protein)
Receptor	MC2R (G_s-linked GPCR)	TSH receptor (G_s-linked GPCR)	FSH and LH receptors (G_s-linked GPCRs)	GH receptor (JAK/STAT-linked cytokine receptor)	PRL receptor (JAK/STAT-linked cytokine receptor)
Target endocrine gland	Zona fasciculata and zona reticularis of the adrenal cortex	Thyroid epithelium	Ovary (theca and granulosa*) Testis (Leydig and Sertoli cells)	Liver (but also direct actions—especially in terms of metabolic effects)	No endocrine target organ—not part of an endocrine axis
Peripheral hormone involved in negative feedback	Cortisol	Triiodothyronine	Estrogen,[†] progesterone, testosterone, and inhibin[‡]	IGF-I GH (short loop)	None

*Both follicular and luteinized thecal and granulosa cells.
[†]Estrogen can also have a positive feedback in women.
[‡]Inhibin selectively inhibits release of FSH from the gonadotrope.

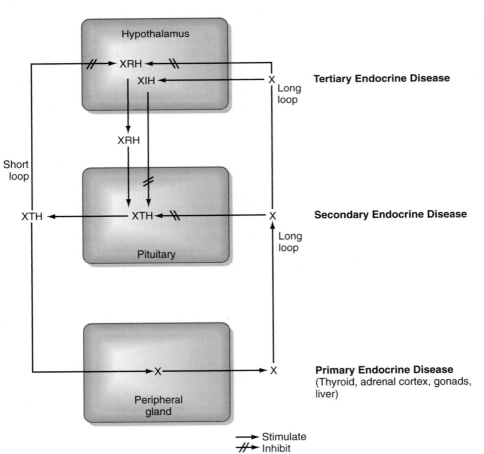

● **Figure 40-6.** Negative-feedback loops regulating hormone secretion in a typical hypothalamus-pituitary-peripheral gland axis. X, peripheral gland hormone; XIH, hypothalamic-inhibiting hormone; XRH, hypothalamic-releasing hormone; XTH, pituitary tropic hormone.

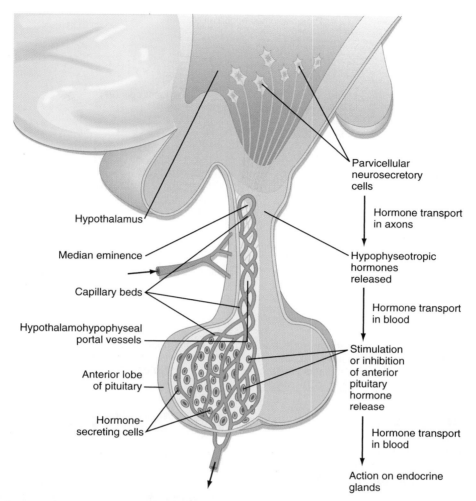

Hypothalamus

Median eminence

Capillary beds

Hypothalamohypophyseal portal vessels

Anterior lobe of pituitary

Hormone-secreting cells

Parvicellular neurosecretory cells

Hormone transport in axons

Hypophyseotropic hormones released

Hormone transport in blood

Stimulation or inhibition of anterior pituitary hormone release

Hormone transport in blood

Action on endocrine glands

● **Figure 40-7.** Neurovascular link between the hypothalamus and the anterior lobe (pars distalis) of the pituitary. Parvicellular "hypophysiotropic" neurosecretory neurons within various hypothalamic nuclei project axons to the median eminence, where they secrete releasing hormones (RHs). RHs flow down the pituitary stalk in the hypothalamohypophyseal portal vessels to the anterior pituitary. RHs (and release-inhibiting hormones—see text) regulate the secretion of tropic hormones from the five cell types of the anterior pituitary. (From Larsen PR et al [eds]: Williams Textbook of Endocrinology, 10th ed. Philadelphia, Saunders, 2003.)

that they produce. This configuration means that a peripheral hormone (e.g., thyroid hormone) can regulate multiple organ systems without these organ systems exerting competing negative-feedback regulation on the hormone. Clinically, this partial autonomy means that multiple aspects of a patient's physiology are at the mercy of whatever derangements exist within a specific axis.

2. Hypothalamic hypophysiotropic neurons are often secreted in a **pulsatile** manner and are entrained to daily and seasonal rhythms through CNS input. Additionally, hypothalamic nuclei receive a variety of neuronal input from higher and lower levels of the brain. These can be short-term (e.g., various stress/infections) or long-term (e.g., onset of reproductive function at puberty). Thus, inclusion of the hypothalamus in an endocrine axis allows the integration of a considerable amount of information for determining or changing the set point of that axis

(or both). Clinically, this means that a broad range of complex neurogenic states can alter pituitary function. **Psychosocial dwarfism** is a striking example in which children who are abused or under intense emotional stress have lower growth rates as a result of decreased growth hormone secretion by the pituitary gland.

3. Abnormally low or high levels of a peripheral hormone (e.g., thyroid hormone) may be due to a defect at the level of the peripheral endocrine gland (e.g., thyroid), the pituitary gland, or the hypothalamus. Such lesions are referred to as **primary, secondary,** and **tertiary endocrine disorders,** respectively (Fig. 40-6). A thorough understanding of the feedback relationships within an axis allows the physician to determine where the defect lies. Primary endocrine deficiencies tend to be the most severe because they often involve complete absence of the peripheral hormone.

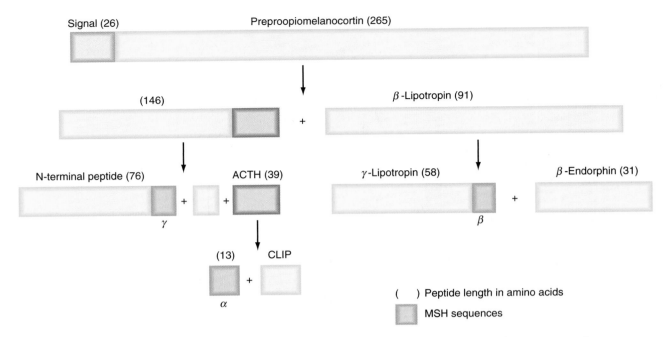

● **Figure 40-8.** The original gene transcript of proopiomelanocortin contains structures of multiple bioactive compounds. ACTH, adrenocorticotropic hormone; CLIP, corticotropin-like intermediate peptide; MSH, melanocyte-stimulating hormone. Note that ACTH is the only bioactive peptide released by the human corticotrope.

Endocrine Function of the Adenohypophysis

The adenohypophysis consists of the following endocrine cell types: **corticotropes, thyrotropes, gonadotropes, somatotropes,** and **lactotropes** (Table 40-1).

Corticotropes

Corticotropes stimulate (i.e., are "tropic to") the adrenal cortex as part of the **hypothalamic-pituitary-adrenal (HPA) axis.** Corticotropes produce the hormone **adrenocorticotropic hormone (ACTH;** also called **corticotropin**), which stimulates two zones of the adrenal cortex (see Chapter 42). ACTH is a 39–amino acid peptide that is synthesized as part of a larger prohormone, **proopiomelanocortin (POMC).** Thus, corticotropes are also referred to as **POMC cells.** POMC harbors the peptide sequence for ACTH, forms of melanocyte-stimulating hormone (MSH), endorphins (endogenous opioids), and enkephalins (Fig. 40-8). The human corticotrope expresses only the prohormone convertase, which produces ACTH as the sole active hormone secreted from these cells. The other fragments that are cleaved from POMC are the N-terminal fragment and β-lipotropic hormone (β-LPH). Neither of these fragments play a physiological role in humans.

ACTH circulates as an unbound hormone and has a short half-life of about 10 minutes. It binds to the **melanocortin 2 receptor (MC2R)** on cells in the adrenal cortex (Fig. 40-9). ACTH acutely increases cortisol and adrenal androgen production, increases the expression of steroidogenic enzyme genes, and in the long term, promotes the growth and survival of two zones in the adrenal cortex (see Chapter 42).

● AT THE CELLULAR LEVEL

At supraphysiological levels, **ACTH** causes darkening of light-colored skin (e.g., Cushing's disease). Normally, keratinocytes express the POMC gene but process it to α-MSH instead of ACTH. Keratinocytes secrete α-MSH in response to ultraviolet light, and α-MSH acts as a paracrine factor on neighboring melanocytes to darken the skin. α-MSH binds to the **MC1R** on melanocytes. However, at high levels, ACTH can also cross-react with the MC1R receptor on skin melanocytes (Fig. 40-9). Thus, **darkening of skin** is one indicator of excessive ACTH levels.

ACTH is under stimulatory control by the hypothalamus. A subset of parvicellular hypothalamic neurons expresses the peptide **procorticotropin-releasing hormone (pro-CRH)** (Table 40-1). Pro-CRH is processed to an amidated 41–amino acid peptide, **CRH.** CRH acutely stimulates ACTH secretion and increases transcription of the POMC gene. The parvicellular neurons that express CRH also coexpress ADH, and ADH potentiates the action of CRH on corticotropes.

ACTH secretion has a pronounced diurnal pattern, with a peak in early morning and a valley in late afternoon (Fig. 40-10). In addition, secretion of CRH—and hence secretion of ACTH—is pulsatile.

There are multiple regulators of the HPA axis, and many of them are mediated through the CNS (Fig. 40-11). Many types of stress, both neurogenic (e.g., fear) and systemic (e.g., infection), stimulate secretion

● **Figure 40-9.** Normal levels of ACTH act on the MC2R to increase cortisol. Supraphysiological levels of ACTH due to decreased cortisol production act on both the MC2R and the MC1R on melanocytes and cause skin darkening. (Modified from Porterfield SP, White BA: Endocrine Physiology, 3rd ed. Philadelphia, Mosby, 2007.)

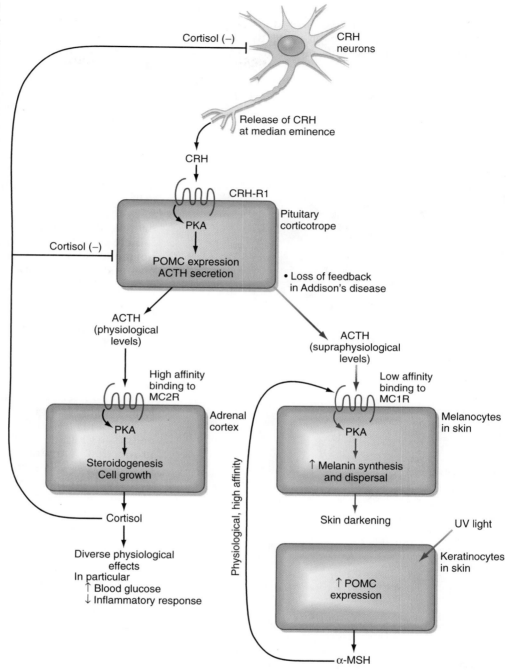

● **Figure 40-10.** Diurnal pattern of serum ACTH. (Modified from Porterfield SP, White BA: Endocrine Physiology, 3rd ed. Philadelphia, Mosby, 2007.)

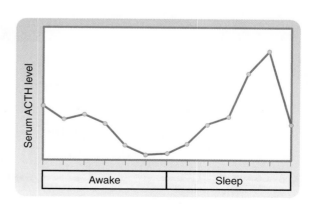

of ACTH. The stress effects are mediated through CRH and ADH and the CNS. The response to many forms of severe stress can persist despite negative feedback from high cortisol levels. This means that the hypothalamus has the ability to reset the "set point" of the HPA axis in response to stress. Severe, chronic depression can reset the HPA axis as a result of hypersecre-

tion of CRH and is a factor in the development of **tertiary hypercortisolism.** Cortisol exerts negative feedback on the pituitary, where it suppresses POMC gene expression and ACTH secretion, and on the hypothalamus, where it decreases pro-CRH gene expression and release of CRH. Because cortisol has profound effects on the immune system (see Chapter 42), the HPA axis and the immune system are closely coupled. Moreover, cytokines, particularly interleukin-1 (IL-1), IL-2, and IL-6, stimulate the HPA axis.

Thyrotropes

Thyrotropes regulate thyroid function by secreting the hormone **thyroid-stimulating hormone (TSH;** also called **thyrotropin**) as part of the **hypothalamic-pituitary-thyroid axis.** TSH is one of three **pituitary glycoprotein hormones** (Table 40-1), which also include **follicle-stimulating hormone (FSH)** and **luteinizing hormone (LH)** (see later). TSH is a heterodimer composed of an α subunit, called the **α-glycoprotein subunit (α-GSU),** and a β subunit **(β-TSH)** (Fig. 40-12). The α-GSU is common to TSH, FSH, and LH, whereas the β subunit is specific to the hormone (i.e., β-TSH, β-FSH, and β-LH are all unique). Glycosylation of the subunits increases their stability in circulation and enhances the affinity and specificity of the hormones for their receptors. The half-lives of TSH, FSH, and LH (and an LH-like placental glycoprotein hormone, **human chorionic gonadotropin [hCG]**) are relatively long, ranging from tens of minutes to several hours.

TSH binds to the TSH receptor on thyroid epithelial cells (see Chapter 41). As discussed in Chapter 41, the production of thyroid hormones is a complex, multistep process. TSH stimulates essentially every aspect of thyroid function. TSH also has a strong tropic effect and stimulates hypertrophy, hyperplasia, and survival of thyroid epithelial cells. In geographical regions where the availability of iodide is limited (iodide is required for the synthesis of thyroid hormone), TSH levels are elevated because of reduced negative feedback. Elevated TSH levels can produce noticeable growth of the thyroid and a bulge in the neck called a **goiter.**

The pituitary thyrotrope is stimulated by the releasing hormone **thyrotropin-releasing hormone (TRH)** (Table 40-1). TRH, produced by a subset of parvicellular hypothalamic neurons, is a tripeptide with cyclization of a glutamine at its N-terminus (pyro-Glu) and an amidated C-terminus. TRH is synthesized as a larger

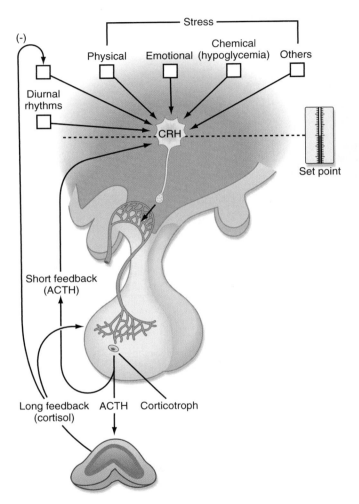

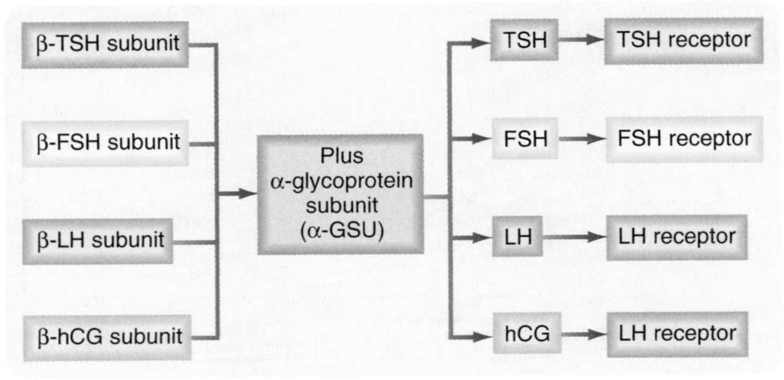

● **Figure 40-11.** Hypothalamic-pituitary-adrenal axis illustrating factors regulating the secretion of corticotropin-releasing hormone (CRH). ACTH, adrenocorticotropic hormone. (Modified from Porterfield SP, White BA: Endocrine Physiology, 3rd ed. Philadelphia, Mosby, 2007.)

● **Figure 40-12.** Pituitary glycoprotein hormones. hCG is made by the placenta (see Chapter 43) and binds to the LH receptor. FSH, follicle-stimulating hormone; hCG, human chorionic gonadotropin; LH, luteinizing hormone; TSH, thyroid-stimulating hormone.

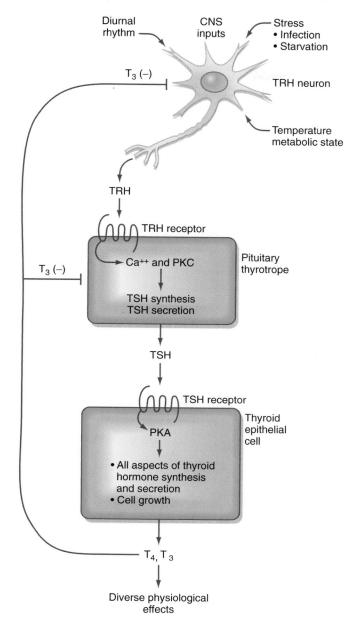

● **Figure 40-13.** Hypothalamic-pituitary-thyroid axis. PKA, protein kinase A; PKC, protein kinase C; T_3, triiodothyronine (active form of thyroid hormone); T_4, tetraiodothyronine; TRH, thyrotropin-releasing hormone; TSH, thyroid-stimulating hormone. (Modified from Porterfield SP, White BA: Endocrine Physiology, 3rd ed. Philadelphia, Mosby, 2007.)

prohormone that contains six copies of TRH within its sequence. It binds to the TRH receptor on thyrotropes (Fig. 40-13). TRH neurons are regulated by numerous CNS-mediated stimuli, and TRH is released according to a diurnal rhythm (highest during overnight hours, lowest around dinnertime). TRH is regulated by various types of stress, but unlike CRH, stress inhibits secretion of TRH. Such stress includes physical stress, starvation, and infection. The active form of thyroid hormone, triiodothyronine (T_3), negatively feeds back on both pituitary thyrotropes and TRH-producing

neurons. T_3 represses both β-TSH expression and the sensitivity of thyrotropes to TRH. T_3 also inhibits TRH production and secretion.

The Gonadotrope

The gonadotrope secretes FSH and LH (also called gonadotropins) and regulates the function of gonads in both sexes. As such, the gonadotrope plays an integral role in the **hypothalamic-pituitary-testis axis** and the **hypothalamic-pituitary-ovarian axis** (Fig. 40-14).

FSH and LH are segregated into different secretory granules and are not cosecreted in equimolar amounts (in contrast to ADH and neurophysin, for example). This allows independent secretion of FSH/LH by gonadotropes. The actions of FSH and LH on gonadal function are complex, especially in women, and will be discussed in detail in Chapter 43. In general, gonadotropins promote testosterone secretion in men and estrogen and progesterone secretion in women. FSH also increases the secretion of a transforming growth factor-β (TGF-β)-related protein hormone called **inhibin** in both sexes.

FSH and LH secretion are regulated by one hypothalamic releasing hormone, **gonadotropin-releasing hormone (GnRH; also called LHRH).** GnRH is a 10–amino acid peptide produced by a subset of parvicellular hypothalamic GnRH neurons (Fig. 40-14). GnRH is produced as a larger prohormone and, as part of its processing to a decapeptide, is modified with a cyclized glutamine (pyro-Glu) at its N-terminus and an amidated C-terminus.

GnRH is released in a pulsatile manner (Fig. 40-15), and both the pulsatile secretion and the frequency of the pulses have important effects on the gonadotrope. Continuous infusion of GnRH down-regulates the GnRH receptor, thereby resulting in a decrease in FSH and LH secretion. In contrast, pulsatile secretion does not desensitize the gonadotrope to GnRH, and FSH and LH secretion is normal. At a frequency of one pulse per hour, GnRH preferentially increases LH secretion (Fig. 40-16). At a slower frequency of one pulse per 3 hours, GnRH preferentially increases FSH secretion. Gonadotropins increase sex steroid synthesis (Fig. 40-14). In men, testosterone and estrogen negatively feed back at the level of the pituitary and the hypothalamus. Exogenous progesterone also inhibits gonadotropin function in men and is being considered as a possible ingredient in a male contraceptive pill. Additionally,

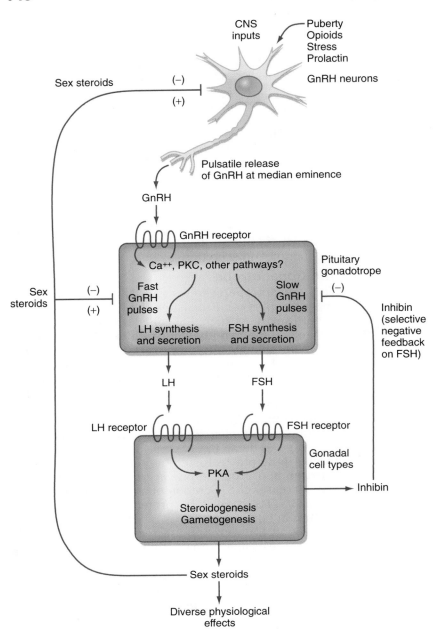

● **Figure 40-14.** Hypothalamic-pituitary-gonadal axis. FSH, follicle-stimulating hormone; GnRH, gonadotropin-releasing hormone; LH, luteinizing hormone. (Modified from Porterfield SP, White BA: Endocrine Physiology, 3rd ed. Philadelphia, Mosby, 2007.)

inhibin negatively feeds back selectively on FSH secretion in men and women. In women, progesterone and testosterone negatively feed back on gonadotropic function at the level of the hypothalamus and pituitary. At low doses, estrogen also exerts negative feedback on FSH and LH secretion. However, high estrogen levels maintained for 3 days cause a surge in LH and, to a lesser extent, FSH secretion. This positive feedback is observed at the hypothalamus and pituitary. At the hypothalamus, GnRH pulse amplitude and frequency increase. At the pituitary, high estrogen levels greatly increase the sensitivity of the gonadotrope to GnRH, both by increasing GnRH receptor levels and by enhancing postreceptor signaling pathway components (see Chapter 43).

The Somatotrope

The somatotrope produces **growth hormone** (**GH**, also called **somatotropin**) and is part of the hypothalamic-pituitary-liver axis (Fig. 40-17). A major target of GH is the liver, where it stimulates the production of **insulin-like growth factor type I (IGF-I).** GH is a 191–amino acid protein that is similar to **prolactin (PRL)** and **human placental lactogen (hPL);** accordingly, there is some overlap in activity among these hormones. Multiple forms of GH are present in serum and constitute a "family of hormones," with the 191–amino acid (22-kDa) form representing approximately 75% of the circulating GH. The GH receptor is a member of the cytokine/GH/PRL/erythropoietin receptor family and, as such, is linked to the JAK/STAT signaling

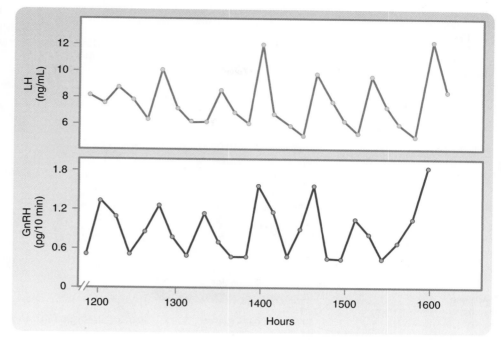

● **Figure 40-15.** Fluctuation of peripheral vein plasma LH levels and portal vein plasma GnRH levels in unanesthetized, ovariectomized female sheep. Each pulse of LH is coordinated with a pulse of GnRH. This supports the view that pulsatility of LH release is dependent on pulsatile stimulation of the pituitary by GnRH. (From Levine J et al: Endocrinology 111:1449, 1982.)

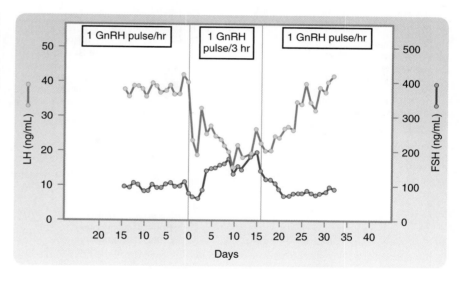

● **Figure 40-16.** Frequency-encoded regulation of FSH and LH secretion from gonadotropes. A high frequency of GnRH (1 pulse/hr) preferentially stimulates LH secretion, whereas a slower frequency of GnRH promotes FSH secretion. (From Larsen PR et al [eds]: Williams Textbook of Endocrinology, 10th ed. Philadelphia, Saunders, 2003.)

pathway (see Chapter 3). Human GH can also act as an agonist for the PRL receptor. About 50% of the 22-kDa form of GH in serum is bound to the N-terminal portion (the extracellular domain) of the GH receptor and is called **GH-binding protein (GHBP). Laron dwarfs,** who lack normal GH receptors but have normal GH secretion, do not have detectable GHBP in their serum. GHBP reduces renal clearance and thus increases the biological half-life of GH, which is about 20 minutes. The liver and kidney are major sites of GH degradation.

GH secretion is under dual control by the hypothalamus (Fig. 40-17). The hypothalamus predominantly stimulates GH secretion via the peptide **growth hormone-releasing hormone (GHRH).** This hormone is a member of the vasoactive intestinal polypeptide (VIP)/secretin/glucagon family and is processed into a 44–amino acid peptide with an amidated C-terminus

from a larger prohormone. GHRH enhances GH secretion and GH gene expression. The hypothalamus inhibits pituitary GH synthesis and release via the peptide **somatostatin.** Somatostatin, in the anterior pituitary, inhibits the release of GH and TSH. GH secretion is also regulated by **ghrelin,** which is primarily produced by the stomach but is also expressed in the hypothalamus. Ghrelin increases appetite and may serve as a signal to coordinate nutrient acquisition with growth.

The primary negative feedback on the somatotrope is exerted by IGF-I (Fig. 40-17). GH stimulates IGF-I production by the liver, and IGF-I then inhibits GH synthesis and secretion by the pituitary and hypothalamus in a classic "long" feedback loop. In addition, GH itself exerts negative feedback on release of GHRH through a "short" feedback loop. GH also increases somatostatin release.

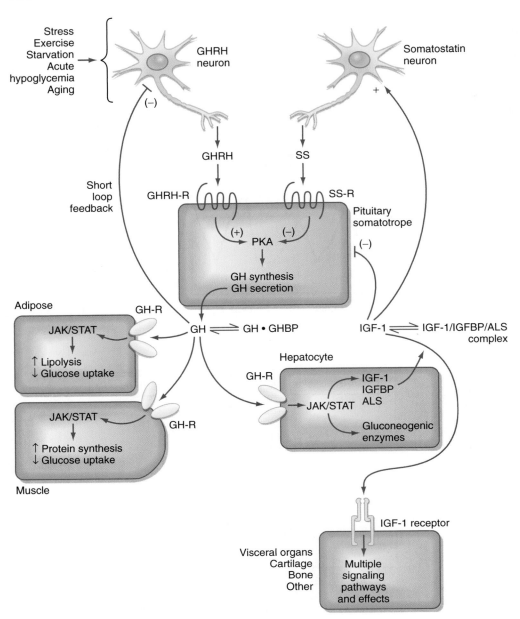

● **Figure 40-17.** Hypothalamic-pituitary-liver axis. ALS, acid labile subunit; GHBP, growth hormone–binding protein; GHRH, growth hormone–releasing hormone; IGFBP, insulin-like growth factor–binding protein; IGF-I, insulin-like growth factor I; SS, somatostatin. (From Porterfield SP, White BA: Endocrine Physiology, 3rd ed. Philadelphia, Mosby, 2007.)

GH secretion, like that of ACTH, shows prominent diurnal rhythms, with peak secretion occurring in the early morning just before awakening. Its secretion is stimulated during deep, slow-wave sleep (stages III and IV). GH secretion is lowest during the day. This rhythm is entrained to sleep-wake patterns rather than light-dark patterns, so a phase shift occurs in people who work night shifts. As is typical of anterior pituitary hormones, GH secretion is pulsatile. Levels of GH in serum vary widely (0 to 30 ng/mL, with most values usually falling between 0 and 3). Because of this marked variation, serum GH values are of minimal clinical value unless the sampling time is known. Frequently, rather than measuring GH, the clinician measures IGF-I because its secretion is regulated by GH and IGF-I has a relatively long circulating half-life that minimizes pulsatile and diurnal changes in secretion.

GH secretion is also regulated by several different physiological states. GH is classified as one of the **"stress" hormones** and is increased by neurogenic and physical stress. It promotes lipolysis, increases protein synthesis, and antagonizes the ability of insulin to reduce blood glucose levels. It is not surprising, therefore, that acute hypoglycemia is a stimulus for GH secretion, and GH is classified as a **hyperglycemic hormone.** A rise in the serum concentration of some amino acids also stimulates GH secretion. In contrast, an increase in blood glucose or free fatty acids inhibits secretion of GH. Obesity also inhibits GH secretion, in

● **Figure 40-18.** Biological actions of GH. The effects on linear growth, organ size, and lean body mass are at least partly mediated by insulin-like growth factors (IGFs) (somatomedins) produced in the liver and in the GH target tissues as well. IGFBP, insulin-like growth factor–binding protein.

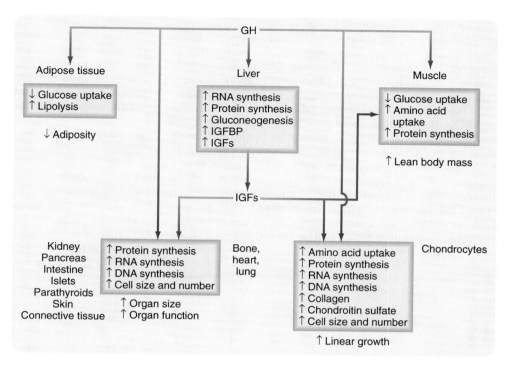

part because of insulin resistance (relative hyperglycemia) and increased circulating free fatty acids. Conversely, exercise and starvation stimulate GH secretion. Other hormones that regulate GH secretion include estrogen, androgens, and thyroid hormone, which enhance GH and IGF-I secretion, as well as bone maturation.

Direct versus Indirect Actions of Growth Hormone. GH acts directly on the liver, muscle, and adipose tissue to regulate energy metabolism (Fig. 40-18). It shifts metabolism to lipid use for energy, thereby conserving carbohydrates and proteins. GH is a **protein anabolic hormone** that increases cellular amino acid uptake and incorporation into protein, and it represses proteolysis. Consequently, it produces nitrogen retention (positive nitrogen balance) and decreases urea production. The muscle wasting that occurs concomitant with aging has been proposed to be caused, at least in part, by the decrease in GH secretion that occurs with aging.

GH is a **lipolytic** hormone. It activates hormone-sensitive lipase and therefore mobilizes neutral fats from adipose tissue. As a result, serum fatty acid levels rise after GH administration, more fats are used for energy production, and fatty acid uptake and oxidation increase in skeletal muscle and liver. GH can be ketogenic as a result of the increase in fatty acid oxidation (the ketogenic effect of GH is not seen when insulin levels are normal). If insulin is given along with GH, the lipolytic effects of GH are abolished.

GH alters carbohydrate metabolism. Many of its actions may be secondary to increased fat mobilization and oxidation. (Remember, an increase in serum free fatty acids inhibits uptake of glucose in skeletal

muscle and adipose tissue.) After administration of GH, blood glucose rises. The hyperglycemic effects of GH are mild and slower than those of glucagon and epinephrine. The increase in blood glucose results in part from decreased glucose uptake and use in skeletal muscle and adipose tissue. Liver glucose output increases, and this is probably not a result of glycogenolysis. In fact, glycogen levels can rise after administration of GH. However, the increase in fatty acid oxidation and hence the rise in liver acetyl coenzyme A (acetyl CoA) stimulate gluconeogenesis, followed by increased glucose production from substrates such as lactate and glycerol.

GH antagonizes the action of insulin at the postreceptor level in skeletal muscle and adipose tissue (but not the liver). **Hypophysectomy** (removal of the pituitary gland) can improve diabetic management because GH, like cortisol, decreases insulin sensitivity. Because GH produces **insulin insensitivity,** it is considered a **diabetogenic hormone.** When secreted in excess, GH can cause diabetes mellitus, and the insulin levels necessary to maintain normal metabolism increase. Excessive insulin secretion resulting from an excess of GH can cause damage to pancreatic beta cells. In the absence of GH, insulin secretion declines. Thus, normal levels of GH are required for normal pancreatic function and insulin secretion.

Indirect Effects of Growth Hormone on Growth. GH increases skeletal and visceral growth; children without GH show growth stunting or dwarfism. GH also promotes cartilage growth, long-bone length, and periosteal growth. Most of these effects are mediated by a group of hormones called **insulin-like growth factors.**

The IGFs are multifunctional hormones that regulate cellular proliferation, differentiation, and metabolism. These protein hormones resemble insulin in structure and function. The two hormones in this family, IGF-I and IGF-II, are produced in many tissues and have autocrine, paracrine, and endocrine actions. IGF-I is the major form produced in most adult tissues, and IGF-II is the major form produced in the fetus. Both hormones are structurally similar to proinsulin, with IGF-I having 42% structural homology with proinsulin. IGFs and insulin cross-react with each other's receptors, and IGFs in high concentration mimic the metabolic actions of insulin. Both IGF-I and IGF-II act through type I IGF receptors, which are similar to insulin and EGF receptors and contain intrinsic tyrosine kinase. However, IGF-II also binds to the type II IGF/mannose-6-phosphate receptor. This receptor does not resemble the insulin receptor and does not have intrinsic tyrosine kinase activity. Binding to these receptors probably facilitates internalization and degradation of IGF. IGFs stimulate glucose and amino acid uptake and protein and DNA synthesis. They were initially called **somatomedins** because they mediate GH (somatotro-

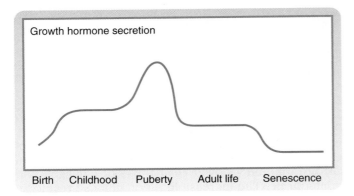

● **Figure 40-19.**   Lifetime pattern of GH secretion. GH levels are higher in children than in adults, with a peak period during puberty. GH secretion declines with aging.

▶ IN THE CLINIC

When ample supplies of nutrients are available, high serum amino acid levels stimulate GH and insulin secretion, and high serum glucose levels stimulate insulin secretion. The high serum GH, insulin, and nutrient supply stimulate IGF production, and these conditions are appropriate for growth. However, if the diet is high in calories but low in amino acids, the hormonal response is different. Whereas high carbohydrate availability results in high insulin availability, low serum amino acid levels inhibit GH and IGF production. These conditions allow dietary carbohydrates and fats to be stored, but conditions are unfavorable for tissue growth. On the other hand, during fasting, when the availability of nutrients decreases, serum GH levels rise and serum insulin levels fall (because of hypoglycemia). IGF production is low, and the conditions are not favorable for growth. In these circumstances, the rise in GH secretion is beneficial because it promotes fat mobilization while minimizing tissue protein loss. In the absence of insulin, peripheral tissue glucose use decreases, thereby conserving glucose for essential tissues such as the brain (Fig. 40-20).

▶ IN THE CLINIC

GH is necessary for growth before adulthood. Deficiencies can produce dwarfism, and excesses can produce gigantism. Normal growth requires not only normal levels of GH but also normal levels of thyroid hormones, insulin, and sex steroids.

Dwarfism. If GH deficiency occurs before puberty, growth is severely impaired. Individuals with this condition are relatively well proportioned and have normal intelligence. If the anterior pituitary deficiency is limited to GH, they can have a normal life span. They are sometimes "pudgy" because they lose GH-induced lipolysis. If they have **panhypopituitary dwarfism** (all anterior pituitary hormones are deficient), with a deficiency of gonadotropins, they may not mature sexually and remain infertile. People with dwarfism show few metabolic abnormalities other than a tendency toward hypoglycemia, insulinopenia, and increased insulin sensitivity. There are multiple potential sites of impairment. GH secretion may be reduced, GH-stimulated IGF production may decrease, or IGF action may be deficient. **Laron dwarfs** are resistant to GH because of a genetic defect in expression of the GH receptor such that the response to GH is impaired. Thus, although serum GH levels are normal to high, Laron dwarfs do not produce IGFs in response to GH. Treating patients afflicted by Laron dwarfism with GH will not correct the growth deficiency. The **African pygmy** represents another example of abnormal growth. Individuals with this condition have normal serum GH levels, but they do not exhibit the normal rise in IGF that occurs at puberty. They also may have a partial defect in GH receptors because IGF-I levels do not rise normally after GH is administered. However, IGF-II levels are normal. Unlike Laron dwarfs, they do not totally lack the IGF response to GH.

GH deficiency in adults is becoming recognized as a pathological syndrome. If the GH deficiency occurs after the epiphyses close, growth is not impaired. GH deficiency is one of many possible causes of hypoglycemia. Recent studies have shown that extended deficiencies of GH lead to changes in body composition. The percentage of body weight that is fat increases, whereas the percentage that is protein decreases. In addition, muscle weakness and early exhaustion are symptoms of GH deficiency. Because the muscle loss that occurs with aging may result from an age-related decline in GH production (Fig. 40-19), GH is being used experimentally in elderly people to delay the physical decline associated with aging. The efficacy of this treatment in humans has not been established.

● **Figure 40-20.** Complementary regulation of GH and insulin
secretion coordinates availability of
nutrients with anabolism and either
caloric storage or mobilization. Note
that both hormones are increased
by protein and that both stimulate
protein synthesis.

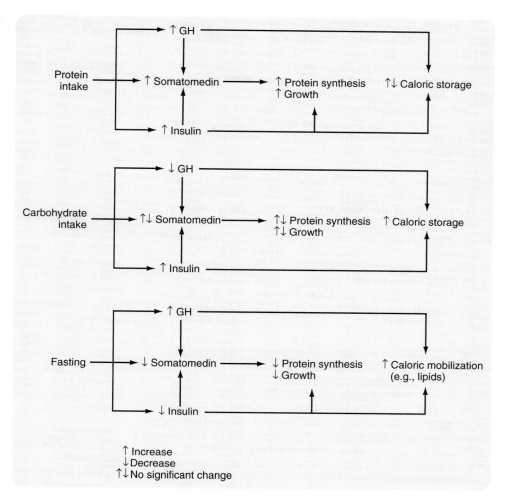

pin) action on cartilage and bone growth. IGFs have
many other actions, and GH is not the only regulator
of IGF formation. Initially, IGFs were thought to be
produced in the liver in response to a GH stimulus. It
is now known that IGFs are produced in many tissues,
and many actions are autocrine or paracrine. The liver
is probably the predominant source of circulating IGFs
(Fig. 40-18).

Essentially all circulating IGFs are transported in
serum bound to **insulin-like growth factor–binding
proteins (IGFBPs).** IGFBPs bind to IGFs and then associate with another protein called **acid labile subunit
(ALS).** GH stimulates the hepatic production of IGF-I,
IGFBPs, and ALS. The IGFBP/ALS/IGF-I complex mediates transport and bioavailability of IGF-I. Although
IGFBPs generally inhibit IGF action, they greatly
increase the biological half-life of IGFs (up to 12 hours).
IGFBP proteases degrade IGFBP and play a role in
locally generating free (i.e., active) IGFs. This is of
interest in the context of IGF-responsive cancers (e.g.,
prostate cancer), which may overexpress one or more
IGFBP proteases.

Although GH is an effective stimulator of IGF production, the correlation between GH and IGF-I is greater
than the correlation between GH and IGF-II. During

puberty, when GH levels increase (Fig. 40-19), IGF-I
levels increase in parallel. Insulin also stimulates IGF
production, and GH cannot stimulate IGF production
in the absence of insulin. Starvation effectively inhibits
IGF secretion, even when GH levels are high. PRL or
hPL can increase IGF-II secretion in the fetus, and IGF-II
is considered a fetal growth regulator. Although GH is
a primary stimulus for IGF production in the liver,
parathyroid hormone (PTH) and estradiol are more
effective stimuli for osteoblastic IGF-I production.

IGFs are mitogenic and have profound effects on
bone and cartilage. They stimulate the growth of
bones, cartilage, and soft tissue and regulate all aspects
of the metabolism of chondrocytes, which are the car-
tilage-forming cells. Although appositional growth of
long bones continues after closure of the epiphyses,
growth in length ceases. IGFs stimulate osteoblast replication and the synthesis of collagen and bone matrix.
Serum IGF levels correlate well with growth in
children.

The Lactotrope

The lactotrope produces the hormone **prolactin,**
which is a 199–amino acid, single-chain protein. PRL
is structurally related to GH and hPL (see Chapter 43).

Like GH, the PRL receptor is a member of the cytokine family coupled to the JAK/STAT signaling pathways. Because the primary action of PRL in humans is related to breast development and function during pregnancy and lactation, the regulation and actions of prolactin will be discussed in detail in Chapter 43.

In the context of the pituitary gland, it should be appreciated that the lactotrope differs from the other endocrine cell types of the adenohypophysis in two major ways:

1. The lactotrope is not part of an endocrine axis. This means that PRL acts directly on nonendocrine cells (primarily of the breast) to induce physiological changes.
2. Production and secretion of PRL are predominantly under inhibitory control by the hypothalamus. Thus, disruption of the pituitary stalk and the hypothalamohypophyseal portal vessels (e.g., secondary to surgery or physical trauma) results in an increase in PRL levels but a decrease in ACTH, TSH, FSH, LH, and GH.

PRL circulates unbound to serum proteins and thus has a relatively short half-life of about 20 minutes. Normal basal serum concentrations are similar in men and women. Release of PRL is normally under tonic inhibition by the hypothalamus. This is exerted by dopaminergic tracts that secrete **dopamine** in the median eminence. There is also evidence for the existence of a **prolactin-releasing factor (PRF).** The exact nature of this compound is not known, although many factors, including TRH and hormones in the glucagon family (secretin, glucagon, VIP, and gastric inhibitory polypeptide [GIP]) can stimulate the release of PRL.

PRL is one of the many hormones released in response to **stress.** Surgery, fear, stimuli causing arousal, and exercise are all effective stimuli. As is the case with GH, sleep increases PRL secretion, and PRL has a pronounced sleep-associated diurnal rhythm. However, unlike GH, the rise in sleep-associated PRL is not associated with a specific sleep phase. Drugs that interfere with the synthesis or action of dopamine increase PRL secretion. Many commonly prescribed antihypertensive drugs and tricyclic antidepressants are dopamine inhibitors. Bromocriptine is a dopamine agonist that can be used to inhibit PRL secretion. Somatostatin, TSH, and GH also inhibit PRL secretion.

■ KEY CONCEPTS

1. The pituitary gland (also called the hypophysis) is composed of epithelial tissue (the adenohypophysis or anterior lobe) and neural tissue (the neurohypophysis or posterior lobe).

2. Magnocellular hypothalamic neurons in the paraventricular and supraoptic nuclei project axons down the infundibular stalk and terminate in the pars nervosa. The pars nervosa is a neurovascular organ in which neurohormones are released and diffuse into the vasculature.

3. Two neurohormones, ADH and oxytocin, are synthesized in the hypothalamus in the magnocellular neuronal cell bodies. ADH and oxytocin are transported intraaxonally down the hypothalamohypophyseal tracts to the pars nervosa. Stimuli perceived by the cell bodies and dendrites in the hypothalamus control the release of ADH and oxytocin at the pars nervosa.

4. The adenohypophysis secretes several tropic hormones that are part of the endocrine axes. An endocrine axis includes the hypothalamus, the pituitary, and a peripheral endocrine gland. The set point of an axis is largely controlled by negative feedback of the peripheral hormone on the pituitary and hypothalamus.

5. The adenohypophysis contains five endocrine cell types: corticotropes, thyrotropes, gonadotropes, somatotropes, and lactotropes. Corticotropes secrete ACTH, thyrotropes secrete TSH, gonadotropes secrete FSH and LH, somatotropes secrete GH, and lactotropes secrete PRL.

6. The hypothalamus regulates the anterior pituitary by secreting releasing hormones. These small peptides are carried via the hypophyseal portal system to the anterior pituitary, where they control synthesis and release of the pituitary hormones ACTH, TSH, FSH, LH, and GH. PRL secretion is inhibited by the hypothalamus through the catecholamine dopamine.

7. GH stimulates growth primarily through regulation of the growth-promoting hormones IGF-I and IGF-II. GH raises blood glucose levels by decreasing peripheral tissue utilization and is protein anabolic and lipolytic.

8. PRL initiates and maintains lactation.

CHAPTER 41

The Thyroid Gland

The thyroid gland produces the prohormone tetraiodothyronine (T_4) and the active hormone triiodothyronine (T_3). Synthesis of T_4 and T_3 requires iodine, which can be a limiting factor in some parts of the world. Much of T_3 is also made by peripheral conversion of T_4 to T_3, primarily through a nuclear receptor that regulates gene expression. T_3 is critical for normal brain development and has broad effects on metabolism and cardiovascular function in adults.

ANATOMY AND HISTOLOGY OF THE THYROID GLAND

The thyroid gland is composed of a right lobe and a left lobe that sit anterolateral to the trachea (Fig. 41-1). Normally, the lobes of the thyroid gland are connected by a midventral isthmus. The thyroid gland receives a rich blood supply. It is drained by three sets of veins on each side: the superior, middle, and inferior thyroid veins. The thyroid gland receives sympathetic innervation that is vasomotor but not secretomotor.

The functional unit of the thyroid gland is the **thyroid follicle,** a spherical structure about 200 to 300 μm in diameter that is surrounded by a single layer of thyroid epithelial cells (Fig. 41-2). The epithelium sits on a basal lamina, the outermost structure of the follicle, and is surrounded by a rich capillary supply. The apical side of the follicular epithelium faces the lumen of the follicle. The follicular lumen itself is filled with **colloid,** which is composed of **thyroglobulin;** thyroglobulin is secreted and iodinated by the thyroid epithelial cells. The size of the epithelial cells and the amount of colloid are dynamic features that change with activity of the gland. The thyroid gland contains another type of cell in addition to follicular cells. Scattered within the gland are **parafollicular cells** called **C cells.** These cells are the source of the polypeptide hormone **calcitonin,** which is discussed in Chapter 39.

PRODUCTION OF THYROID HORMONES

The secretory products of the thyroid gland are **iodothyronines** (Fig. 41-3), a class of hormones formed by the coupling of two iodinated tyrosine molecules. Approximately 90% of the thyroid's output is **3,5,3′,5′-tetraiodothyronine (thyroxine, or T_4).** T_4 is primarily a prohormone. About 10% is **3,5,3′-triiodothyronine (T_3),** which is the active form of thyroid hormone. Less than 1% of thyroid output is **3,3′,5′-triiodothyronine (reverse T_3, or rT_3),** which is inactive. Normally, these three hormones are secreted in the same proportions as they are stored in the gland.

Because the primary product of the thyroid gland is T_4, yet the active form of thyroid hormone is T_3, the thyroid axis relies heavily on **peripheral conversion** through the action of **thyronine-specific deiodinases** (Fig. 41-3). Most conversion of T_4 to T_3 by **type 1 deiodinase** occurs in tissues with high blood flow and rapid exchanges with plasma, such as the liver, kidneys, and skeletal muscle. This process supplies circulating T_3 for uptake by other tissues in which local T_3 generation is too low to provide sufficient thyroid hormone. Type 1 deiodinase is also expressed in the thyroid (again, where T_4 is abundant) and has relatively low affinity (i.e., a K_m of 1 μM) for T_4. Levels of type 1 deiodinase are paradoxically increased in hyperthyroidism and contribute to the elevated circulating T_3 levels in this disease.

The brain maintains constant intracellular levels of T_3 by a high-affinity deiodinase called **type 2 deiodinase** that is expressed in glial cells in the central nervous system. Type 2 deiodinase has a K_m of 1 nM and maintains intracellular concentrations of T_3 even when free T_4 falls to low levels. Type 2 deiodinase is also present in the thyrotropes of the pituitary. In the pituitary, type 2 deiodinase acts as a "thyroid axis sensor" that mediates the ability of circulating T_4 to feed back on secretion of thyroid-stimulating hormone (TSH) (see later). Expression of type 2 deiodinase is increased during hypothyroidism, which helps maintain constant T_3 levels in the brain.

There is also an "inactivating" deiodinase called **type 3 deiodinase.** Type 3 deiodinase is a high-affinity, inner ring deiodinase that converts T_4 to the inactive rT_3. Type 3 deiodinase is increased during hyperthyroidism, which helps blunt the overproduction of T_4. All forms of iodothyronines are eventually further deiodinated to noniodinated thyronine.

Iodide Balance

Because of the unique role of iodide in thyroid physiology, a description of thyroid hormone synthesis requires some understanding of iodide turnover

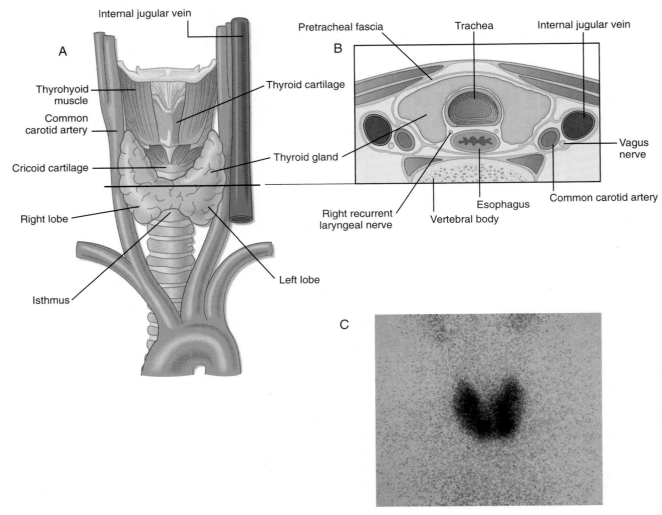

● **Figure 41-1.**   **A** and **B,** Anatomy of the thyroid gland. **C,** Image of pertechnetate uptake by a normal thyroid gland. (Modified from Drake RL et al: Gray's Anatomy for Students. Philadelphia, Churchill Livingstone, 2005.)

(Fig. 41-4). An average of 400 μg of iodide per person is ingested daily in the United States versus a minimum daily requirement of 150 μg for adults, 90 to 120 μg for children, and 200 μg for pregnant women. In the steady state, virtually the same amount, 400 μg, is excreted in urine. Iodide is actively concentrated in the thyroid gland, salivary glands, gastric glands, lacrimal glands, mammary glands, and choroid plexus. About 70 to 80 μg of iodide is taken up daily by the thyroid gland from a circulating pool that contains approximately 250 to 750 μg of iodide. The total iodide content of the thyroid gland averages 7500 μg, virtually all of which is in the form of iodothyronines. In the steady state, 70 to 80 μg of iodide, or about 1% of the total, is released from the gland daily. Of this amount, 75% is secreted as thyroid hormone and the remainder as free iodide. The large ratio (100 : 1) of iodide stored in the form of hormone to the amount turned over daily protects the individual from the effects of iodide defi-

ciency for about 2 months. Iodide is also conserved by a marked reduction in the renal excretion of iodide as its concentration in serum falls.

Overview of Thyroid Hormone Synthesis

To understand thyroid hormone synthesis and secretion, one must appreciate the directionality of each process as it relates to the polarized thyroid epithelial cell (Fig. 41-5). Synthesis of thyroid hormone requires two precursors: iodide and thyroglobulin. Iodide is transported across cells from the basal (vascular) side to the apical (follicular luminal) side of the thyroid epithelium. Amino acids are assembled by translation into thyroglobulin, which is then secreted from the apical membrane into the follicular lumen. Thus, synthesis involves a basal-to-apical movement of precursors into the follicular lumen (Fig. 41-5, *blue arrows*). Actual synthesis of iodothyronines occurs enzymatically in the follicular lumen close to the apical

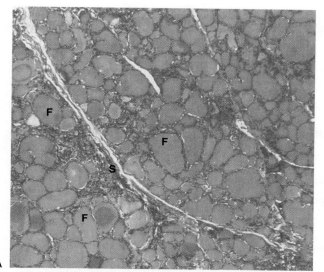

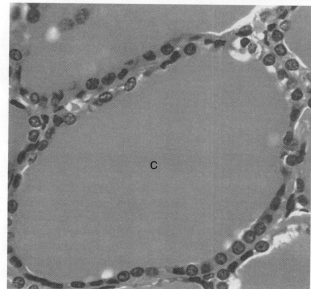

● **Figure 41-2.** Histology of the thyroid gland at low **(upper panel)** and high **(lower panel)** magnification. C, colloid; F, thyroid follicles; S, connective tissue septa. (From Young B et al: Wheater's Functional Histology, 5th ed. Philadelphia, Churchill Livingstone, 2006.)

Synthesis of Iodothyronines within a Thyroglobulin Backbone

Iodide is actively transported into the gland against chemical and electrical gradients by a **2Na$^+$-1I$^-$ symporter) (NIS)** located in the basolateral membrane of thyroid epithelial cells. Normally, a thyroid-plasma free iodide ratio of 30 is maintained. This so-called **iodide trap** requires the generation of energy by oxidative phosphorylation and displays saturation kinetics. NIS is highly expressed in the thyroid gland, but it is also expressed at lower levels in the placenta, salivary glands, and actively lactating breast. One iodide ion is transported uphill against an iodide gradient while two sodium ions move down the electrochemical gradient from extracellular fluid into the thyroid cell. The energy source for this secondary active transporter is provided by Na$^+$,K$^+$-ATPase in the plasma membrane. Expression of the NIS gene is inhibited by iodide and stimulated by TSH. Numerous inflammatory cytokines also suppress NIS gene expression. A reduction in dietary iodide intake depletes the circulating iodide pool and greatly enhances the activity of the iodide trap. When dietary iodide intake is low, the percentage of thyroid uptake of iodide can reach 80% to 90%.

The steps in thyroid hormone synthesis are shown in Figure 41-6. After entering the gland, iodide rapidly moves to the apical plasma membrane of epithelial cells. From there, iodide is transported into the lumen of the follicles by a sodium-independent iodide/chloride transporter named **pendrin.** Iodide is immediately oxidized to iodine and incorporated into tyrosine molecules (Fig. 41-5). The iodinated tyrosine molecules are not free in solution (Fig. 41-6) but are incorporated by peptide linkages within the protein **thyroglobulin.** Thyroglobulin is continually exocytosed into the follicular lumen and is **iodinated** to form both **monoiodotyrosine (MIT)** and **diiodotyrosine (DIT)** (see Fig. 41-6). After iodination, two DIT molecules are **coupled** to form **T$_4$,** or one MIT molecule and one DIT molecule are coupled to form **T$_3$.** Coupling also occurs between iodinated tyrosines that remain part of the primary structure of thyroglobulin. This entire sequence of reactions is catalyzed by **thyroid peroxidase (TPO),** an enzyme complex that spans the apical membrane. The immediate oxidant (electron acceptor) for the reaction is hydrogen peroxide (H$_2$O$_2$). The mechanism whereby H$_2$O$_2$ is generated in the thyroid gland involves **NADPH oxidase,** which is also localized to the apical membrane.

When the availability of iodide is restricted, the formation of T$_3$ is favored. Because T$_3$ is three times as potent as T$_4$, this response provides more active hormone per molecule of organified iodide. The proportion of T$_3$ is also increased when the gland is hyperstimulated by TSH or other activators.

Secretion of Thyroid Hormones

Once thyroglobulin has been iodinated, it is stored in the lumen of the follicle as colloid (Fig. 41-2). Release of T$_4$ and T$_3$ into the bloodstream requires binding of thyroglobulin to the receptor **megalin,** followed by endocytosis and lysosomal degradation of thyroglobu-

membrane of the epithelial cells (see later). Secretion involves receptor-mediated endocytosis of iodinated thyroglobulin and apical-to-basal movement of the endocytic vesicles and their fusion with lysosomes. Thyroglobulin is then enzymatically degraded, which results in the release of thyroid hormones from the thyroglobulin peptide backbone. Finally, thyroid hormones move across the basolateral membrane, probably through a specific transporter, and ultimately into blood. Thus, secretion involves apical-to-basal movement (Fig. 41-5, *red arrows*). There are also scavenger pathways within the epithelial cell that reuse iodine and amino acids after enzymatic digestion of thyroglobulin (Fig. 41-5, *white arrows*).

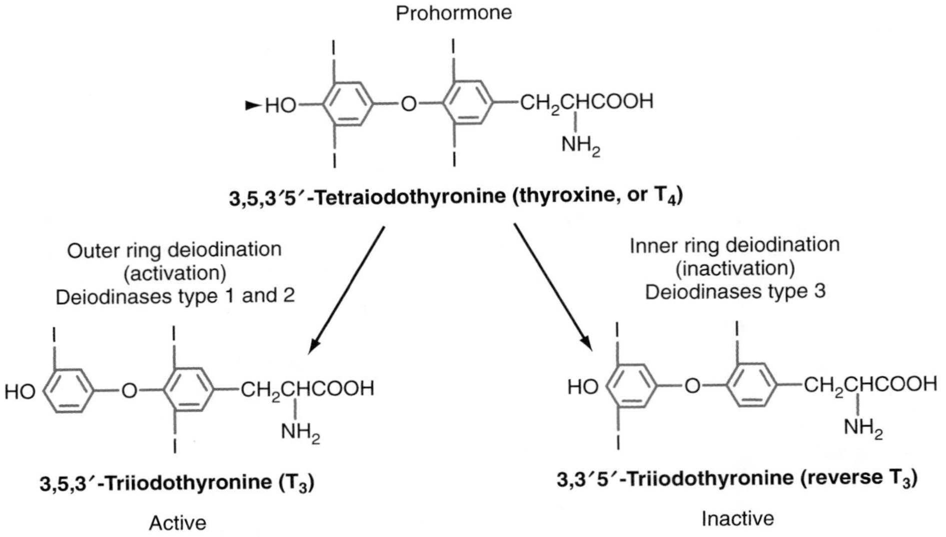

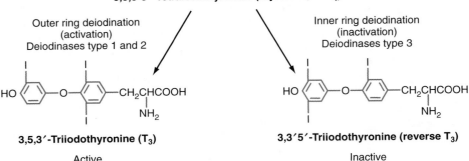

● **Figure 41-3.** Structure of the iodothyronines T$_4$, T$_3$, and reverse T$_3$.

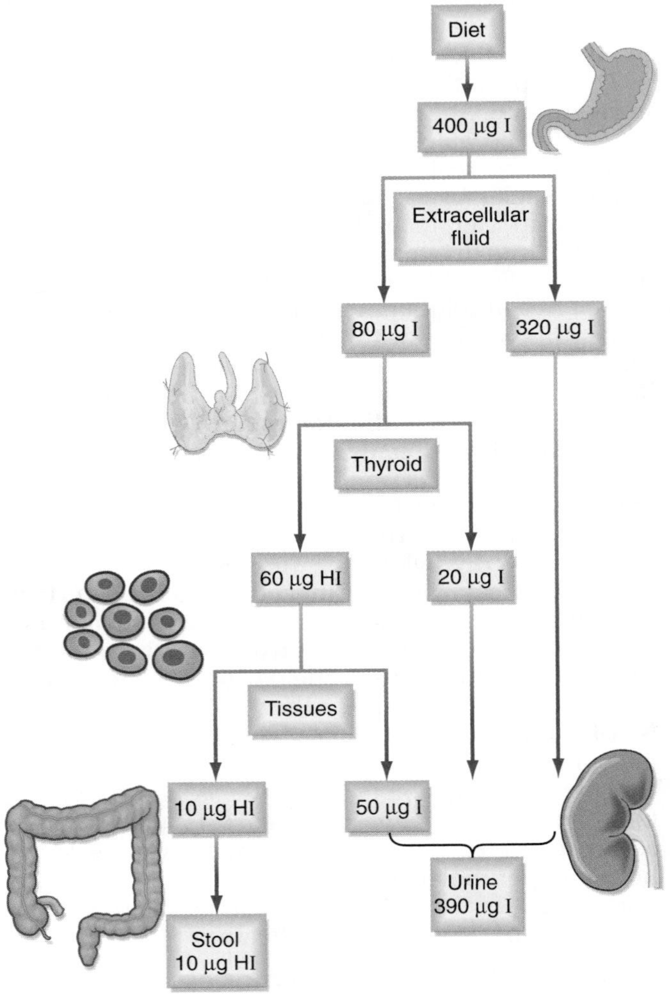

Prohormone

3,5,3′5′-Tetraiodothyronine (thyroxine, or T$_4$)

Outer ring deiodination
(activation)
Deiodinases type 1 and 2

Inner ring deiodination
(inactivation)
Deiodinases type 3

3,5,3′-Triiodothyronine (T$_3$)
Active

3,3′5′-Triiodothyronine (reverse T$_3$)
Inactive

Diet

400 μg I

Extracellular
fluid

80 μg I   320 μg I

Thyroid

60 μg HI   20 μg I

Tissues

10 μg HI   50 μg I

Stool
10 μg HI

Urine
390 μg I

● **Figure 41-4.** Iodine distribution and turnover in humans. HI = hormone-associated iodine.

● AT THE CELLULAR LEVEL

Several transporters mediate transport of thyroid hormones across cell membranes. Thyroid hormone transporters include sodium/taurocholate-cotransporting polypeptides (NCTPs), organic anion–transporting polypeptides (OATPs), L-type amino acid transporters (LATs), and the monocarboxylate transporters (MCTs). These transporters show specificity with respect to T$_4$ versus T$_3$ binding and cell-specific expression. Recently, mutations in MCT8 have been linked to human disease that may be due to an intracellular deficit of thyroid hormone, elevated T$_3$ levels, and severe psychomotor retardation.

lin (Fig. 41-7; also see Fig. 41-5). Enzymatically released T$_4$ and T$_3$ then leave the basal side of the cell and enter the blood.

The MIT and DIT molecules, which also are released during proteolysis of thyroglobulin, are rapidly deiodinated within the follicular cell by the enzyme **intrathyroidal deiodinase** (Fig. 41-5; white arrows). This deiodinase is specific for MIT and DIT and cannot utilize T$_4$ and T$_3$ as substrates. The iodide is then recycled into synthesis of T$_4$ and T$_3$. Amino acids from the digestion of thyroglobulin reenter the intrathyroidal amino acid pool and can be reused for protein synthesis (Fig. 41-5, *white arrows*). Only minor amounts of intact thyroglobulin leave the follicular cell under normal circumstances.

TRANSPORT AND METABOLISM OF THYROID HORMONES

Secreted T$_4$ and T$_3$ circulate in the bloodstream almost entirely bound to proteins. Normally, only about 0.03% of total plasma T$_4$ and 0.3% of total plasma T$_3$ exist in

● **Figure 41-5.** Synthesis *(blue arrows)* and secretion *(red arrows)* of thyroid hormones by the thyroid epithelial cell. White arrows denote pathways involved in the conservation of iodine and amino acids.

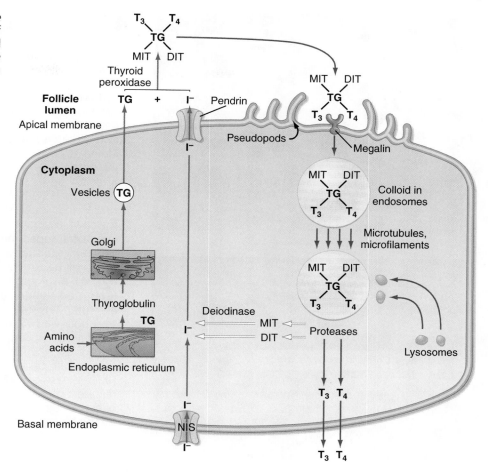

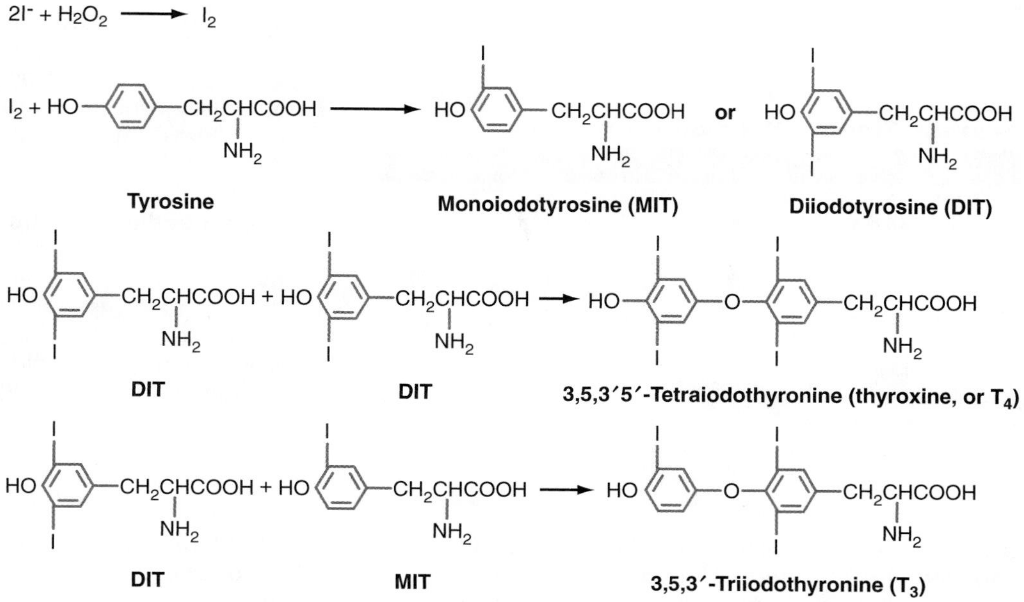

● **Figure 41-6.** Reactions involved in the generation of iodide, MIT, DIT, T_3, and T_4.

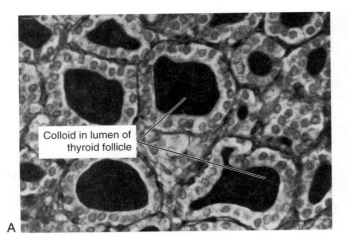

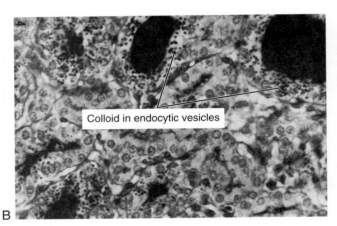

● **Figure 41-7.** Before **(A)** and minutes after **(B)** rapid induction of thyroglobulin endocytosis by TSH. (From Wollman SH et al: J Cell Biol 21:191, 1964.)

● **Table 41-1.**
Average Thyroid Hormone Turnover

	T_4	T_3	rT_3
Daily production (μg)	90	35	35
From thyroid (%)	100	25	5
From T_4 (%)	—	75	95
Extracellular pool (μg)	850	40	40
Plasma concentration			
Total (μg/dL)	8.0	0.12	0.04
Free (ng/dL)	2.0	0.28	0.20
Half-life (days)	7	1	0.8
Metabolic clearance (L/day)	1	26	77
Fractional turnover per day (%)	10	75	90

> ### IN THE CLINIC
>
> Because of its ability to **trap** and incorporate iodine into thyroglobulin (called **organification**), the activity of the thyroid can be assessed by **radioactive iodine uptake (RAIU)**. In this test a tracer dose of ^{123}I is administered and RAIU is measured by placing a gamma detector on the neck at 4 to 6 hours and at 24 hours. In the United States, where the diet is relatively rich in iodine, RAIU is about 15% after 6 hours and 25% after 24 hours (Fig. 41-8). Abnormally high RAIU (>60%) after 24 hours indicates hyperthyroidism. Abnormally low RAIU (<5%) after 24 hours indicates hypothyroidism. In individuals with extreme chronic stimulation of the thyroid (Graves' disease–associated thyrotoxicosis), iodide is trapped, organified, and released as hormone very rapidly. In these cases of elevated turnover, 6-hour RAIU will be very high, but 24-hour RAIU will be lower (Fig. 41-8). A number of anions, such as thiocyanate (CNS^-), perchlorate ($HClO_4^-$), and pertechnetate (TcO_4^-), are competitive or noncompetitive inhibitors of iodide transport via NIS. If iodide cannot be rapidly incorporated into tyrosine **(organification defect)** after its uptake by the cell, administration of one of these anions will, by blocking further iodide uptake, cause rapid release of iodide from the gland (Fig. 41-8). This release occurs as a result of the high thyroid-plasma concentration gradient.
>
> The thyroid can be imaged with a rectilinear scanner or gamma camera after the administration of a tracer, ^{123}I, ^{131}I, or the iodine-mimic pertechnetate (^{99m}Tc). Imaging can display the size and shape of the thyroid (Fig. 41-1, *C*), as well as heterogeneities of active versus inactive tissue within the thyroid gland. Such heterogeneities are often due to the development of **thyroid nodules,** which are regions of enlarged follicles with evidence of regressive changes—indicative of cycles of stimulation and involution. Particular **"hot" nodules** (i.e., nodules that display high RAIU on imaging) are not usually cancerous but may lead to thyrotoxicosis (hyperthyroidism—see later). **"Cold" nodules** are 10 times more likely to be cancerous than "hot" nodules. Such nodules can be sampled for pathological analysis by **fine-needle aspiration biopsy.**
>
> The thyroid can also be imaged by **ultrasonography,** which is superior in resolution to RAIU imaging. Ultrasonography is used to guide the physician during fine-needle aspiration biopsy of a nodule. The highest resolution of the thyroid is achieved with **magnetic resonance imaging (MRI).**

the free state (Table 41-1). Free T_3 is biologically active and mediates the effects of thyroid hormone on peripheral tissues, in addition to exerting negative feedback on the pituitary and hypothalamus (see later). The major binding protein is **thyroxine-binding globulin (TBG).** TBG is synthesized in the liver and binds one molecule of T_4 or T_3.

About 70% of circulating T_4 and T_3 is bound to TBG; 10% to 15% is bound to another specific thyroid-binding protein called **transthyretin (TTR). Albumin** binds 15% to 20%, and 3% is bound to lipoproteins. Ordinarily, only alterations in TBG concentration significantly affect total plasma T_4 and T_3 levels. Two important biological functions have been ascribed to

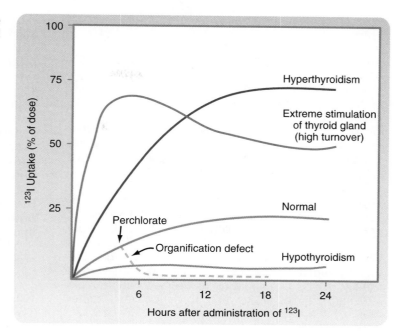

● **Figure 41-8.** Thyroid gland iodothyronine uptake curves for normal, hypothyroid, hyperthyroid, and defective organification states.

TBG. First, it maintains a large circulating reservoir of T_4 that buffers any acute changes in thyroid gland function. Second, binding of plasma T_4 and T_3 to proteins prevents the loss of these relatively small hormone molecules in urine and thereby helps conserve iodide. TTR, in particular, provides thyroid hormones to the central nervous system.

PHYSIOLOGICAL EFFECTS OF THYROID HORMONE

Thyroid hormone acts on essentially all cells and tissues, and imbalances in thyroid function constitute some of the most common endocrine diseases. Thyroid hormone has many direct actions, but it also acts in more subtle ways to optimize the actions of several other hormones and neurotransmitters.

Cardiovascular Effects

Perhaps the most clinically important actions of thyroid hormone are those on cardiovascular physiology. T_3 increases cardiac output, thereby ensuring sufficient delivery of O_2 to tissues (Fig. 41-9). The resting heart rate and stroke volume are increased. The speed and force of myocardial contractions are enhanced (positive chronotropic and inotropic effects, respectively), and the diastolic relaxation time is shortened (positive lusitropic effect). Systolic blood pressure is modestly augmented and diastolic blood pressure is decreased. The resultant widened pulse pressure reflects the combined effects of the increased stroke volume and the reduction in total peripheral vascular resistance secondary to blood vessel dilation in skin, muscle, and heart. These effects, in turn, are partly due to the increase in tissue production of heat and CO_2 that thyroid hormone induces (see later). In addition, however, thyroid hormone decreases systemic

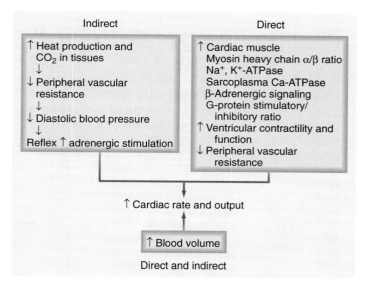

● **Figure 41-9.** Mechanisms by which thyroid hormone increases cardiac output. The indirect mechanisms are probably quantitatively more important.

vascular resistance by dilating resistance arterioles in the peripheral circulation. Total blood volume is increased by activating the renin-angiotensin-aldosterone axis and thereby increasing renal tubular sodium reabsorption (see Chapter 33).

The cardiac inotropic effects of T_3 are indirect, via enhanced responsiveness to catecholamines (see Chapter 42), and direct (Fig. 41-9). Myocardial calcium uptake is increased, which enhances contractile force. Thyroid hormone inhibits expression of the **Na⁺-Ca⁺⁺ antiporter,** thereby increasing intramyocellular $[Ca^{++}]$. T_3 increases the velocity and strength of myocardial contraction. It also increases **ryanodine Ca⁺⁺ channels**

IN THE CLINIC

Thyroid hormone levels in the normal range are necessary for optimum cardiac performance. A deficiency of thyroid hormone in humans reduces stroke volume, left ventricular ejection fraction, cardiac output, and the efficiency of cardiac function. The latter defect is shown by the fact that the stroke work index [(stroke volume/left ventricular mass) × peak systolic blood pressure] is decreased even more than myocardial oxidative metabolism is. The rise in systemic vascular resistance may contribute to this cardiac debility. In contrast, excess thyroid hormone enhances cardiac output and increases the uncoupling proteins UCP-2 and UCP-3 in cardiac muscle; these proteins uncouple ATP production from O_2 utilization during the β oxidation of free fatty acids. This can cause high-output cardiac failure. When **hyperthyroidism** develops in aging individuals, the cardiac effects of thyroid hormone may include rapid atrial arrhythmias, flutter, and fibrillation (see Chapter 15).

in the sarcoplasmic reticulum, which promotes release of Ca^{++} from the sarcoplasmic reticulum during systole. **Sarcoplasmic reticulum Ca^{++}-ATPase (SERCA)** is increased by T_3, and as a result, sequestration of calcium during diastole is facilitated and the relaxation time is shortened.

Effects on Basal Metabolic Rate

Thyroid hormones increase the **basal rate of oxygen consumption** and **heat production** (e.g., **basal metabolic rate**). As mentioned earlier, thyroid hormone increases the expression of mitochondrial **uncoupling proteins** (UCPs). This action is demonstrated in all tissues except the brain, gonads, and spleen. Glucose and fatty acid uptake and oxidation are increased overall, as are lactate-glucose and fatty acid–triglyceride recycling. Thyroid hormone does not augment diet-induced O_2 utilization, and it may not change the efficiency of energy use during exercise.

Thermogenesis must also increase concomitantly with O_2 use. Thus, changes in body temperature parallel fluctuations in availability of thyroid hormone. The potential increase in body temperature, however, is moderated by a compensatory increase in heat loss through appropriate thyroid hormone–mediated increases in **blood flow, sweating,** and **ventilation.** Hyperthyroidism is accompanied by heat intolerance, whereas hypothyroidism is accompanied by cold intolerance.

Increased O_2 use ultimately depends on an increased supply of substrates for oxidation. T_3 augments glucose absorption from the gastrointestinal tract and increases glucose turnover (glucose uptake, oxidation, and synthesis). In adipose tissue, thyroid hormone induces enzymes for the synthesis of fatty acids, acetyl-CoA carboxylase, and fatty acid synthase and enhances lipolysis by increasing the number of β-adrenergic receptors (see later). Thyroid hormone also enhances the clearance of chylomicrons. Thus, lipid turnover

(FFA release from adipose tissue and oxidation) is augmented.

Protein turnover (release of muscle amino acids, protein degradation and, to a lesser extent, protein synthesis and urea formation) is also increased. T_3 potentiates the respective stimulatory effects of epinephrine, norepinephrine, glucagon, cortisol, and growth hormone on gluconeogenesis, lipolysis, ketogenesis, and proteolysis of the labile protein pool. The overall metabolic effect of thyroid hormone has been aptly described as accelerating the response to starvation. In addition, thyroid hormone stimulates the synthesis of cholesterol, but more so its oxidation and biliary secretion. The net effect is a decrease in the body pool and plasma levels of total and low-density lipoprotein cholesterol.

The metabolic clearance of adrenal and gonadal steroid hormones, some B vitamins, and certain administered drugs is also increased by thyroid hormone.

Respiratory Effects

Thyroid hormone stimulates O_2 utilization and also enhances O_2 supply. Appropriately, T_3 increases the **resting respiratory rate, minute ventilation,** and the **ventilatory response** to hypercapnia and hypoxia. These actions maintain a normal arterial PO_2 when O_2 utilization is increased and a normal PCO_2 when CO_2 production is increased. Additionally, the hematocrit increases slightly and thereby enhances the O_2-carrying capacity. This increase in red blood cell mass results from stimulation of **erythropoietin production by the kidney.**

Skeletal Muscle Effects

Normal function of skeletal muscles also requires optimal amounts of thyroid hormone. This requirement may be related to the regulation of energy production and storage. Glycolysis and glycogenolysis are increased and glycogen and creatine phosphate are reduced by an excess of T_4 and T_3. The inability of muscle to take up and phosphorylate creatine leads to increased urinary excretion of creatine.

Effects on the Autonomic Nervous System and Catecholamine Action

There is synergism between catecholamines and thyroid hormones. Thyroid hormones are synergistic with catecholamines in increasing the metabolic rate, heat production, heart rate, motor activity, and excitation of the central nervous system. T_3 may enhance sympathetic nervous system activity by increasing the number of β-adrenergic receptors in heart muscle and the generation of intracellular second messengers, such as cAMP.

Effects on Growth and Maturation

Another major effect of thyroid hormone is to promote growth and maturation. A small but crucial amount of thyroid hormone crosses the placenta, and the fetal thyroid axis becomes functional at midgestation. Thyroid hormone is extremely important for normal neurological development and proper bone formation in the fetus. In infants, insufficient fetal thyroid hormone causes cretinism, characterized by irreversible mental retardation and short stature (see later).

Effects on Bone, Hard Tissue, and Dermis

Thyroid hormone stimulates endochondral ossification, linear growth of bone, and maturation of the epiphyseal bone centers. T_3 enhances the maturation and activity of chondrocytes in the cartilage growth plate, in part by increasing local growth factor production and action. Although thyroid hormone is not required for linear growth until after birth, it is essential for normal maturation of growth centers in the bones of the developing fetus. T_3 also stimulates adult bone remodeling.

The progression of tooth development and eruption depends on thyroid hormone, as does the normal cycle of growth and maturation of the epidermis, its hair follicles, and nails. The normal degradative processes in these structural and integumentary tissues are also stimulated by thyroid hormone. Thus, either too much or too little thyroid hormone can lead to hair loss and abnormal nail formation.

Thyroid hormone alters the structure of subcutaneous tissue by inhibiting the synthesis and increasing the degradation of mucopolysaccharides (glycosaminoglycans) and fibronectin in the extracellular connective tissue.

Effects on the Nervous System

Thyroid hormone regulates the timing and pace of development of the central nervous system. Thyroid hormone deficiency in utero and in early infancy decreases growth of the cerebral and cerebellar cortex, proliferation of axons and branching of dendrites, synaptogenesis, myelinization, and cell migration. Irreversible brain damage results when thyroid hormone deficiency is not recognized and treated promptly after birth. The structural defects just described are paralleled by biochemical abnormalities. Decreased thyroid hormone levels reduce cell size, RNA and protein content, tubulin- and microtubule-associated protein, protein and lipid content of myelin, local production of critical growth factors, and rates of protein synthesis.

Thyroid hormone also enhances wakefulness, alertness, responsiveness to various stimuli, auditory sense, awareness of hunger, memory, and learning capacity. In addition, normal emotional tone depends on proper thyroid hormone availability. Furthermore, the speed and amplitude of peripheral nerve reflexes are increased by thyroid hormone, as is motility of the gastrointestinal tract.

Effects on Reproductive Organs and Endocrine Glands

In both women and men, thyroid hormone plays an important, permissive role in the regulation of reproductive function. The normal ovarian cycle of follicular development, maturation, and ovulation, the homologous testicular process of spermatogenesis, and maintenance of the healthy pregnant state are all disrupted by significant deviations in thyroid hormone levels from the normal range. In part, these deleterious effects may be caused by alterations in the metab-

▶ IN THE CLINIC

Hypothyroidism refers to insufficient production of thyroid hormones and can occur as primary, secondary, or tertiary endocrine disease (see Chapter 40). In primary hypothyroidism, T_4 and T_3 levels are abnormally low, and TSH is high (see later). In secondary and tertiary hypothyroidism, both thyroid hormones and TSH are low. The response of TSH levels to synthetic TRH can be used to distinguish between pituitary and hypothalamic disease.

Hypothyroidism in the fetus or early childhood leads to **cretinism.** Affected individuals have severe mental retardation, short stature with incomplete skeletal development, coarse facial features, and a protruding tongue. The most common cause of hypothyroidism in children is iodide deficiency. Iodide is not plentiful in the environment, and deficiency of iodide is a major cause of hypothyroidism in certain mountainous regions of South America, Africa, and Asia. This tragic form of **endemic cretinism** can easily be prevented by public health programs that add iodide to table salt or that provide yearly injections of a slowly absorbed iodide preparation. **Congenital defects** are a less common cause of neonatal/child hypothyroidism. In most cases, the thyroid gland simply does not develop **(thyroid gland dysgenesis).** Less frequent causes of childhood hypothyroidism are mutations in genes involved in thyroid hormone production (e.g., genes for NIS, TPO, thyroglobulin, and pendrin) and blocking antibodies to the TSH receptor. The severity of the neurological and skeletal defects is closely linked to the time of diagnosis and thyroid hormone (T_4) replacement treatment, with early treatment resulting in a normal IQ and subtle neurological deficits. Hypothyroid babies usually appear normal at birth because of maternal thyroid hormones. However, in geographical areas of endemic iodide deficiency, even the mother may be somewhat hypothyroid and unable to make up for the fetal defects. Alternatively, maternal hypothyroidism can cause mild mental retardation in euthyroid fetuses. **Neonatal screening** (T_4 or TSH levels) has played a major role in the prevention of severe cretinism. If hypothyroidism at birth remains untreated for only 2 to 4 weeks, the central nervous system will not mature normally in the first year of life. Developmental milestones such as sitting, standing, and walking will be late, and severe irreversible mental retardation can result.

Hypothyroidism in adults who are not iodide deficient most often results from idiopathic atrophy of the gland, which is thought to be preceded by a chronic autoimmune inflammatory reaction. In this form of **lymphocytic thyroiditis (Hashimoto's disease),** the antibodies that are produced may block hormone synthesis or growth of the thyroid gland, or they may have cytotoxic properties. Other causes of hypothyroidism include iatrogenic causes (e.g., radiochemical damage or surgical removal for treatment of hyperthyroidism), nodular goiters, and pituitary or hypothalamic disease.

> **IN THE CLINIC—cont'd**
>
> The clinical picture of hypothyroidism in adults is in many respects the exact opposite of that seen in hyperthyroidism. The lower than normal metabolic rate leads to weight gain without an appreciable increase in caloric intake. The decreased thermogenesis lowers body temperature and causes intolerance to cold, decreased sweating, and dry skin. Adrenergic activity is decreased, and therefore bradycardia may occur. Movement, speech, and thought are all slowed, and lethargy, sleepiness, and lowering of the upper eyelids (ptosis) occur. An accumulation of mucopolysaccharides—extracellular matrix—in tissues also causes an accumulation of fluid. This nonpitting **myxedema** produces puffy features; an enlarged tongue; hoarseness; joint stiffness; effusions in the pleural, pericardial, and peritoneal spaces; and pressure on peripheral and cranial nerves, entrapped by excess ground substance, with consequent thyroid dysfunction. Constipation, loss of hair, menstrual dysfunction, and anemia are other signs. In adults lacking thyroid hormone, positron emission tomography demonstrates a generalized reduction in cerebral blood flow and glucose metabolism. This abnormality may explain the psychomotor retardation and depressed affect of hypothyroid individuals.
>
> Replacement therapy with T_4 is curative in adults. T_3 is not needed because it will be generated intracellularly from the administered T_4. Furthermore, giving T_3 raises plasma T_3 to nonphysiological levels.

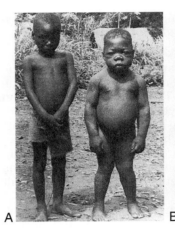
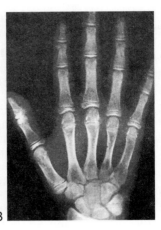
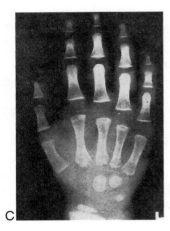

● **Figure 41-10.** **A,** Normal 6-year-old child _(left)_ and a congenitally hypothyroid 17-year-old child _(right)_ from the same village in an area of endemic cretinism. Note especially the short stature, obesity, malformed legs, and dull expression of the mentally retarded hypothyroid child. Other features are a prominent abdomen, a flat broad nose, a hypoplastic mandible, dry scaly skin, delayed puberty, and muscle weakness. (From Delange FM. In Braverman LE, Utiger RD [eds]: Werner and Ingbar's The Thyroid, 7th ed. Philadelphia, Lippincott-Raven, 1996.) X-ray films of the hand of a normal 13-year-old child **(B)** and that of a 13-year-old child suffering from hypothyroidism **(C).** Note that the child with hypothyroidism has a marked delay in development of the small bones of the hands, in growth centers at either end of the fingers, and in the growth center of the distal end of the radius. (**B,** From Tanner JM et al: Assessment of Skeletal Maturity and Prediction of Adult Height (TW2 Method). New York, Academic Press, 1975; **C,** from Andersen HJ. In Gardner LI [ed]: Endocrine and Genetic Diseases of Childhood and Adolescence. Philadelphia, Saunders, 1975.)

olism or availability of steroid hormones. For example, thyroid hormone stimulates hepatic synthesis and release of sex steroid–binding globulin.

Thyroid hormone also has significant effects on other parts of the endocrine system. Pituitary production of growth hormone is increased by thyroid hormone, whereas that of prolactin is decreased. Adrenocortical secretion of cortisol (see Chapter 42), as well as metabolic clearance of this hormone, is stimulated, but plasma free cortisol levels remain normal. The ratio of estrogens to androgens (see Chapter 43) is increased in men (in whom breast enlargement may occur with hyperthyroidism). Decreases in both parathyroid hormone and 1,25-$(OH)_2$-vitamin D production are compensatory consequences of the effects of thyroid hormone on bone resorption (see Chapter 39).

Kidney size, renal plasma flow, glomerular filtration rate, and transport rates for a number of substances are also increased by thyroid hormone.

Mechanism of Thyroid Hormone Action

Free T_4 and T_3 enter cells by a carrier-mediated, energy-dependent process. Transport of T_4 is rate limiting for the intracellular production of T_3. Within the cell, most, if not all of the T_4 is converted to T_3 (or rT_3). Many, but not all T_3 actions are mediated through its binding to one of the members of the **thyroid hormone receptor (TR) family** (Fig. 41-10, _A_). The TR family

belong to the nuclear hormone receptor superfamily of transcription factors (see also Chapters 3 and 39).

REGULATION OF THYROID FUNCTION

The most important regulator of thyroid gland function and growth is the hypothalamic-pituitary **thyroid-releasing hormone–thyroid-stimulating hormone**

● AT THE CELLULAR LEVEL

In humans there are two TR genes, **THRA** and **THRB,** located on chromosomes 17 and 3, respectively, that encode the classic nuclear thyroid hormone receptors. THRA encodes **TRα,** which is alternatively spliced to form two main isoforms. **TR$_{\alpha-1}$** is a bona fide TR, whereas the other isoform does not bind T$_3$. THRB encodes **TR$_{\beta-1}$** and **TR$_{\beta-2}$,** both of which are high-affinity receptors for T$_3$. The tissue distribution of TR$_{\alpha-1}$ and TR$_{\beta-1}$ is widespread. TR$_{\alpha-1}$ is especially expressed in cardiac and skeletal muscle, and TR$_{\alpha-1}$ is the dominant TR that transduces thyroid hormone action on the heart. By contrast, TR$_{\beta-1}$ is expressed more in the brain, liver, and kidney. TR$_{\beta-2}$ expression is restricted to the pituitary and critical areas of the hypothalamus, as well as the cochlea and retina. T$_3$-bound TR$_{\beta-2}$ is responsible for inhibiting expression of the prepro-TRH gene in the paraventricular neurons of the hypothalamus and the β subunit TSH gene in pituitary thyrotropes. Thus, the negative-feedback effects of thyroid hormone on both TRH and TSH secretion are largely mediated by TR$_{\beta-2}$. T$_3$ also down-regulates TR$_{\beta-2}$ gene expression in the pituitary gland.

The unliganded form of the TR-RXR dimer interacts with several corepressor proteins, including **NCoR, SMRT,** and **Alien.** On hormone binding, corepressors are released, and coactivators are recruited to the hormone-receptor complex. The two major coactivator proteins are the **SRC family** (SRC-1, SRC-2, and SRC-3) and the **DRIP-TRAP complex.**

An understanding of TR subtypes and tissue expression is of more than academic interest because inactivating mutant genes have increasingly been found to be causes of clinical syndromes manifested by **resistance to thyroid hormone (RTH syndrome).** The most common mutations occur in the TR$_{\beta-2}$ subtype. In these patients there is incomplete negative thyroid hormone feedback at the hypothalamic-pituitary level. Thus, T$_4$ levels are elevated, but TSH is not suppressed. When the resistance is purely at the hypothalamic-pituitary level, the patient may exhibit signs of hyperthyroidism because of the excess effects of high thyroid hormone levels on peripheral tissue, particularly on the heart through TR$_{\alpha-1}$. These individuals have clinical signs such as goiter, short stature, decreased weight, tachycardia, hearing loss, monochromatic vision, and decreased IQ.

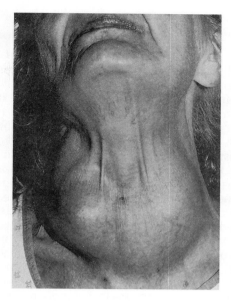

● **Figure 41-11.** The thyroid gland is located in the anterior aspect of the neck, where it is easily visualized and palpated when enlarged (goiter).

entry of glucose into the hexose monophosphate shunt pathway, which generates the NADPH that is needed for the peroxidase reaction. In addition, TSH stimulates the proteolysis of thyroglobulin and release of T$_4$ and T$_3$ from the gland. Intermediate effects of TSH on the thyroid gland occur after a delay of hours to days and involve protein synthesis and the expression of numerous genes, including those encoding NIS, thyroglobulin, TPO, and megalin. Sustained TSH stimulation leads to the long-term effects of hypertrophy and hyperplasia of follicular cells. Capillaries proliferate, and thyroid blood flow increases. These actions, which underlie the growth-promoting effects of TSH on the gland, are supported by the local production of growth factors. A noticeably enlarged thyroid gland is called a goiter (Fig. 41-11). One form of goiter is due to lack of adequate iodine in the diet, which results in low thyroid hormone and elevated TSH levels.

Regulation of thyroid hormone secretion by TSH is under exquisite negative-feedback control (see Chapter 40). Circulating thyroid hormones act on the pituitary gland to decrease TSH secretion, primarily by repressing TSH β subunit gene expression. The pituitary gland expresses the high-affinity type 2 deiodinase. Thus, small changes in free T$_4$ in blood result in significant changes in intracellular T$_3$ in the pituitary thyrotrope. Because the diurnal variation in TSH secretion is small, thyroid hormone secretion and plasma concentrations are relatively constant. Only small nocturnal increases in secretion of TSH and release of T$_4$ occur. Thyroid hormones also feed back on hypothalamic thyroid-releasing hormone (TRH)-secreting neurons. In these neurons, T$_3$ inhibits expression of the prepro-TRH gene. Another important regulator of thyroid gland function is iodide itself, which has a biphasic action. At relatively low levels of iodide intake, the rate of

axis (see Chapter 40, Fig. 40-13). TSH stimulates every aspect of thyroid function. TSH has immediate, intermediate, and long-term actions on the thyroid epithelium. Immediate actions of TSH include induction of pseudopod extension, endocytosis of colloid, and the formation of colloid droplets in the cytoplasm, which represent thyroglobulin within endocytic vesicles (see Fig. 41-7). Shortly thereafter, iodide uptake and TPO activity increase. Concurrently, TSH also stimulates

> ▶ **IN THE CLINIC**

Graves' disease is the most common form of **hyperthyroidism.** It occurs most frequently between the ages of 20 and 50 and is 10 times more common in women than in men. Graves' disease is an autoimmune disorder in which autoantibodies are produced against the TSH receptor. The nature of the specific autoantibodies depends on the epitope that they are directed against. The most critical type is called the **thyroid-stimulating immunoglobulin (TSI).** The hyperthyroidism is often accompanied by a diffuse goiter as a result of hyperplasia and hypertrophy of the gland. The follicular epithelial cells become tall columnar cells, and the colloid shows a scalloped periphery indicative of rapid turnover.

The primary clinical state found in Graves' disease is **thyrotoxicosis**—the state of excessive thyroid hormone in blood and tissues. A patient with thyrotoxicosis presents one of the most striking pictures in clinical medicine. The large increase in metabolic rate is accompanied by the highly characteristic combination of weight loss despite increased intake of food. The increased heat production causes discomfort in warm environments, excessive sweating, and greater intake of water. The increase in adrenergic activity is manifested by a rapid heart rate, hyperkinesis, tremor, nervousness, and a wide-eyed stare. Weakness is caused by a loss of muscle mass, as well as by an impairment in muscle function. Other symptoms include a labile emotional state, breathlessness during exercise, and difficulty swallowing or breathing because of compression of the esophagus or trachea by the enlarged thyroid gland (goiter). The most common cardiovascular sign is sinus tachycardia. There is increased cardiac output associated with a widened pulse pressure secondary to a positive inotropic effect coupled with a decrease in vascular resistance. A major clinical sign in Graves' disease is **exophthalmos** (abnormal protrusion of the eyeball) and **periorbital edema** as a result of recognition by the anti-TSH receptor antibodies of a similar epitope within the orbital cells (probably fibroblasts). Graves' disease is diagnosed by an elevated serum free and total T_4 or T_3 level (i.e., thyrotoxicosis) and the clinical signs of diffuse goiter and ophthalmopathy. In most cases, uptake of iodine or pertechnetate by the thyroid is excessive and diffuse. Serum TSH levels are low because the hypothalamus and the pituitary gland are inhibited by the high levels of T_4 and T_3. Assay of TSH levels and for the presence of circulating TSI will distinguish Graves' disease (a primary endocrine disorder) from a rare adenoma of the pituitary thyrotrophs (a secondary endocrine disease). The latter condition generates elevated TSH levels, unaccompanied by TSI.

Treatment of Graves' disease is usually removal of the thyroid tissue, followed by lifelong replacement therapy with T_4. Thyroid tissue can be ablated by either the radiation effects of ^{131}I or surgery. Surgical removal of the gland rarely but potentially precipitates massive release of hormone that causes **thyroid storm,** which causes death in 30% of patients, primarily as a result of cardiac failure and arrhythmia. An alternative to removal of thyroid tissue is administration of **antithyroid drugs** that inhibit TPO activity.

thyroid hormone synthesis is directly related to the availability of iodide. However, if the intake of iodide exceeds 2 mg/day, the intraglandular concentration of iodide reaches a level that suppresses NADPH oxidase activity and the NIS and TPO genes and thereby the mechanism of hormone biosynthesis. This autoregulatory phenomenon is known as the **Wolff-Chaikoff effect.** As the intrathyroidal iodide level subsequently falls, NIS and TPO genes are derepressed and the production of thyroid hormone returns to normal. In unusual instances, the inhibition of hormone synthesis by iodide can be great enough to induce thyroid hormone deficiency. The temporary reduction in hormone synthesis by excess iodide can also be used therapeutically in hyperthyroidism.

Thyroid hormones increase O_2 utilization, energy expenditure, and heat production. Therefore, it is logical to expect that the availability of active thyroid hormone correlates with changes in the body's caloric and thermal status. In fact, ingestion of excess calories, particularly in the form of carbohydrate, increases the production and plasma concentration of T_3, as well as the individual's metabolic rate, whereas prolonged fasting leads to corresponding decreases. Because most T_3 arises from circulating T_4 (Table 41-1), peripheral mechanisms are important in mediating these changes. However, starvation also gradually lowers T_4 levels in humans.

■ **KEY CONCEPTS**

1. The thyroid gland is situated in the ventral aspect of the neck and is composed of right and left lobes anterolateral to the trachea and connected by an isthmus.

2. The thyroid gland is the source of tetraiodothyronine (thyroxine, T_4) and triiodothyronine (T_3).

3. The basic endocrine unit in the gland is a follicle that consists of a single spherical layer of epithelial cells surrounding a central lumen that contains colloid or stored hormone.

4. Iodide is taken up into thyroid cells by a sodium-iodide symporter in the basolateral plasma membrane.

5. T_4 and T_3 are synthesized from tyrosine and iodide by the enzyme complex thyroid peroxidase. Tyrosine is incorporated in peptide linkages within the protein thyroglobulin. After iodination, two iodotyrosine molecules are coupled to yield the iodothyronines.

6. Secretion of stored T_4 and T_3 requires retrieval of thyroglobulin from the follicle lumen by endocytosis. To support hormone synthesis, iodide is conserved by recycling the iodotyrosine molecules that escape coupling within thyroglobulin.

7. More than 99.5% of T_4 and T_3 circulates bound to the following proteins: thyroid-binding globulin (TBG), transthyretin, and albumin. Only the free fractions of T_4 and T_3 are biologically active.

8. T_4 functions largely as a prohormone whose disposition is regulated by three types of deiodinases. Monodeiodination of the outer ring yields 75% of the daily production of T_3, which is the principal active hormone. Alternatively, monodeiodination of the inner ring yields reverse T_3, which is biologically inactive. Proportioning of T_4 between T_3 and reverse T_3 regulates the availability of active thyroid hormone.

9. T_3 and, to a much lesser extent, T_4 bind to thyroid hormone receptor (TR) subtypes linked to thyroid regulatory elements (TREs) in target DNA molecules. As a result, induction or repression of gene expression increases or decreases a large number of enzymes, as well as structural and functional proteins.

10. Thyroid hormone increases and is a major regulator of the basal metabolic rate. Additional important actions of thyroid hormone are to increase the heart rate, cardiac output, and ventilation and to decrease peripheral resistance. The corresponding increase in heat production leads to increased sweating. Substrate mobilization and disposal of metabolic products are enhanced.

11. Other thyroid hormone effects on the central nervous system and skeleton are crucial to normal growth and development. In the absence of the hormone, brain development is retarded and cretinism results. The stature shortens and the bones fail to mature. In adults, thyroid hormone increases rates of bone resorption and degradation of skin and hair.

12. Thyrotropin (TSH) acts on the thyroid gland via its plasma membrane receptor and cAMP to stimulate all steps in the production of T_4 and T_3. These steps include iodide uptake, iodination and coupling, and retrieval from thyroglobulin. TSH also stimulates glucose oxidation, protein synthesis, and growth of epithelial cells.

CHAPTER 42

The Adrenal Gland

In adults, the adrenal glands emerge as fairly complex endocrine structures that produce two structurally distinct classes of hormones: steroids and catecholamines. The catecholamine hormone **epinephrine** acts as a rapid responder to stresses such as hypoglycemia and exercise to regulate multiple parameters of physiology, including energy metabolism and cardiac output. Stress is also a major secretagogue of the longer-acting steroid hormone **cortisol,** which regulates glucose utilization, immune and inflammatory homeostasis, and numerous other processes. In addition, the adrenal glands regulate salt and volume homeostasis through the steroid hormone **aldosterone.** Finally, the adrenal gland secretes large amounts of the androgen precursor **dehydroepiandrosterone sulfate (DHEAS),** which plays a major role in fetoplacental estrogen synthesis and as a substrate for peripheral androgen synthesis in women.

ANATOMY

The **adrenal glands** are bilateral structures located immediately above the kidneys (*ad,* near; *renal,* kidney) (Fig. 42-1). In humans, they are also referred to as the **suprarenal glands** because they sit on the superior pole of each kidney. The adrenal glands are similar to the pituitary in that they are derived from both neuronal tissue and epithelial (or epithelial-like) tissue. The outer portion of the adrenal gland, called the **adrenal cortex** (Fig. 42-2), develops from mesodermal cells in the vicinity of the superior pole of the developing kidney. These cells form cords of epithelial endocrine cells. The cells of the cortex develop into steroidogenic cells (see Chapter 37). In adults, the adrenal cortex is composed of three zones—the **zona glomerulosa,** the **zona fasciculata,** and the **zona reticularis**—that produce mineralocorticoids, glucocorticoids, and adrenal androgens, respectively (Fig. 42-2, *B*).

Soon after the cortex forms, neural crest–derived cells associated with the sympathetic ganglia, called **chromaffin cells,** migrate into the cortex and become encapsulated by cortical cells. Thus, the chromaffin cells establish the inner portion of the adrenal gland, which is called the **adrenal medulla** (Fig. 42-2). The chromaffin cells of the adrenal medulla have the potential to develop into postganglionic sympathetic neurons. They are innervated by cholinergic preganglionic sympathetic neurons and can synthesize the catecholamine neurotransmitter **norepinephrine** from tyrosine. The enzyme phenylethanolamine *N*-methyl transferase adds a methyl group to norepinephrine to produce the catecholamine hormone **epinephrine,** which is the primary hormonal product of the adrenal medulla (Fig. 42-2, *B*).

ADRENAL MEDULLA

Instead of being secreted near a target organ and acting as neurotransmitters, adrenomedullary catecholamines are secreted into blood and act as hormones. About 80% of the cells of the adrenal medulla secrete **epinephrine,** and the remaining 20% secrete **norepinephrine.** Although circulating epinephrine is derived entirely from the adrenal medulla, only about 30% of the circulating norepinephrine comes from the medulla. The remaining 70% is released from postganglionic sympathetic nerve terminals and diffuses into the vascular system. Because the adrenal medulla is not the sole source of catecholamine production, this tissue is not essential for life.

Synthesis of Epinephrine

The enzymatic steps in the synthesis of epinephrine are shown in Figure 42-4. Synthesis begins with transport of the amino acid **tyrosine** into the chromaffin cell cytoplasm and the subsequent hydroxylation of tyrosine by the rate-limiting enzyme **tyrosine hydroxylase** to produce **dihydroxyphenylalanine (DOPA).** DOPA is converted to **dopamine** by a cytoplasmic enzyme, aromatic amino acid decarboxylase, and is then transported into the secretory vesicle (also called the **chromaffin granule**). Within the granule, dopamine is completely converted to **norepinephrine** by the enzyme dopamine β-hydroxylase. In most adrenomedullary cells, essentially all of the norepinephrine diffuses out of the chromaffin granule by facilitated transport and is methylated by the cytoplasmic enzyme **phenylethanolamine-*N*-methyltransferase (PNMT)** to form epinephrine. Epinephrine is then transported back into the granule.

Secretion of epinephrine and norepinephrine from the adrenal medulla is regulated primarily by descending sympathetic signals in response to various forms of stress, including exercise, hypoglycemia, and hemor-

● **Figure 42-1.** The adrenal glands sit on the superior poles of the kidneys and receive a rich arterial supply from the inferior, middle, and superior suprarenal arteries. The adrenals are drained by a single suprarenal vein. (Modified from Drake RL et al: Gray's Anatomy for Students. Philadelphia, Churchill Livingstone, 2005.)

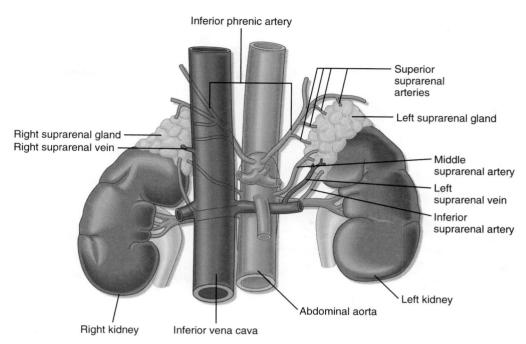

AT THE CELLULAR LEVEL

The high local concentration of cortisol in the medulla is maintained by the vascular configuration within the adrenal gland. The outer connective tissue capsule of the adrenal gland is penetrated by a rich arterial supply coming from three main arterial branches (i.e., the inferior, middle, and superior suprarenal arteries; Fig. 42-1). These give rise to two types of blood vessels that carry blood from the cortex to the medulla (Fig. 42-3): (1) relatively few medullary arterioles, which provide high oxygen- and nutrient-laden blood directly to the medullary chromaffin cells, and (2) relatively numerous cortical sinusoids, into which cortical cells secrete steroid hormones (including cortisol). Both vessel types fuse to give rise to the medullary plexus of vessels that ultimately drains into a single suprarenal vein. Thus, secretions of the adrenal cortex percolate through the chromaffin cells and bathe them in high concentrations of cortisol before leaving the gland and entering the inferior vena cava. Cortisol inhibits neuronal differentiation of the medullary cells, so they fail to form dendrites and axons. Additionally, cortisol induces expression of the enzyme **phenylethanolamine-*N*-methyltransferase (PNMT),** which converts norepinephrine to epinephrine (Fig. 42-4). Glucocorticoid receptor (see later) knockout mice have an enlarged cortex, but the size of the medulla is decreased and PNMT activity is undetectable.

rhagic hypovolemia (Fig. 42-5). The primary autonomic centers that initiate sympathetic responses reside in the hypothalamus and brainstem, and they receive input from the cerebral cortex, the limbic system, and other regions of the hypothalamus and brainstem.

The chemical signal for secretion of catecholamine from the adrenal medulla is **acetylcholine (ACh),** which is secreted from **preganglionic sympathetic neurons** and binds to **nicotinic receptors** on chromaffin cells (Fig. 42-5). ACh increases the activity of the rate-limiting enzyme tyrosine hydroxylase in chromaffin cells (Fig. 42-4). It also increases the activity of dopamine β-hydroxylase and stimulates exocytosis of the chromaffin granules. Synthesis of epinephrine and norepinephrine is closely coupled to secretion so that levels of intracellular catecholamines do not change significantly, even in the face of changing sympathetic activity.

Mechanism of Action of Catecholamines

Adrenergic receptors are generally classified as α- and **β-adrenergic receptors,** with the α-adrenergic receptors further divided into α_1 and α_2 **receptors** and the β-adrenergic receptors divided into β_1, β_2, and β_3 **receptors** (Table 42-1). These receptors can be characterized according to (1) Relative potency of endogenous and pharmacological agonists and antagonists. Epinephrine and norepinephrine are potent agonists for α receptors and for β_1 and β_3 receptors, whereas epinephrine is more potent than norepinephrine for β_2 receptors. A large number of synthetic selective and nonselective adrenergic agonists and antagonists now exist. (2) Downstream signaling pathways. Table 42-1 shows the primary pathways that are coupled to the different adrenergic receptors. This is an oversimplification because differences in signaling pathways for a given receptor have been linked to the duration of agonist exposure and cell type. (3) Location and relative density of receptors. Importantly, different receptor types predominate in different tissues. For example, although both α and β receptors are expressed by pancreatic islet beta cells, the predominant response to a sympathetic discharge is mediated by α_2 receptors.

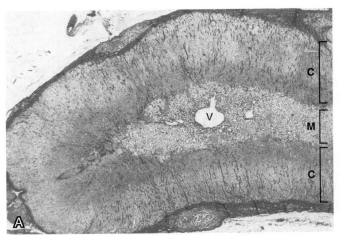

● **Figure 42-2.** Histology of the adrenal gland. **A,** Low magnification illustrating the outer cortex (C) and inner medulla (M; note the central vein [V]). **B,** Higher magnification clearly illustrating the zonation of the cortex. The corresponding endocrine function and the different zones of the cortex and the medulla are noted. (From Young B et al: Wheater's Functional Histology, 5th ed. Philadelphia, Churchill Livingstone, 2006.)

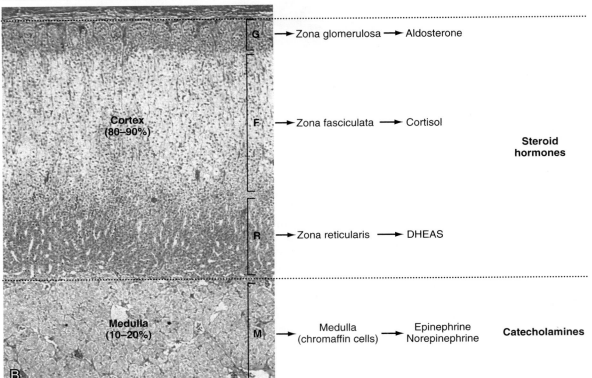

Table 42-1. Adrenergic Receptors

Receptor Type	Primary Mechanism of Action	Examples of Tissue Distribution	Examples of Action
α_1	↑ IP_3 and Ca^{++}, DAG	Sympathetic postsynaptic nerve terminals	Increase vascular smooth muscle contraction
α_2	↓ cAMP	Sympathetic presynaptic nerve terminals; beta cell of pancreatic islets	Inhibit norepinephrine release; inhibit insulin release
β_1	↑ cAMP	Heart	Increase cardiac output
β_2	↑ cAMP	Liver; smooth muscle of vasculature, bronchioles, and uterus	Increase hepatic glucose output; decrease contraction of blood vessels, bronchioles, and uterus
β_3	↑ cAMP	Liver; adipose tissue	Increase hepatic glucose output; increase lipolysis

DAG, diacylglycerol.

● **Figure 42-3.** Blood flow through the adrenal gland. Capsular arteries give rise to sinusoidal vessels that carry blood centripetally through the cortex to the medulla. (Modified from Young B et al: Wheater's Functional Histology, 5th ed. Philadelphia, Churchill Livingstone, 2006.)

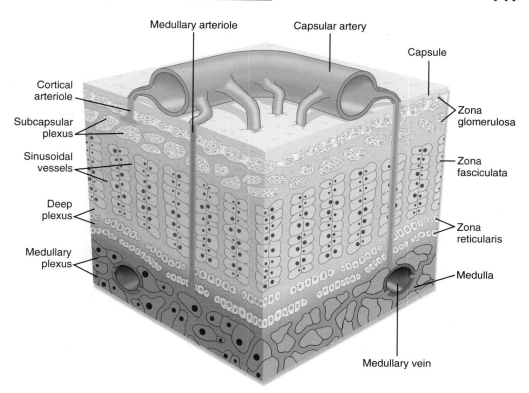

Physiological Actions of Adrenomedullary Catecholamines

Because the adrenal medulla is directly innervated by the autonomic nervous system, adrenomedullary responses are very rapid. Furthermore, because of the involvement of several centers in the central nervous system (CNS), most notably the cerebral cortex, adrenomedullary responses can precede onset of the actual stress (i.e., they can be anticipated) (Fig. 42-5). In many cases, the adrenomedullary output, which is primarily epinephrine, is coordinated with sympathetic nervous activity, as determined by the release of norepinephrine from postganglionic sympathetic neurons. However, some stimuli (e.g., hypoglycemia) evoke a stronger adrenomedullary than sympathetic nervous response, and vice versa.

Many organs and tissues are affected by a sympathoadrenal response (Table 42-2). An informative example of the major physiological roles of catecholamines is the sympathoadrenal response to exercise. Exercise is similar to the **"fight or flight" response,** but without the subjective element of fear, and involves a greater adrenomedullary response (i.e., endocrine role of epinephrine) than a sympathetic nervous response (i.e., neurotransmitter role of norepinephrine). The overall goal of the sympathoadrenal system during exercise is to meet the increased energy demands of skeletal and cardiac muscle while maintaining sufficient oxygen and glucose supply to the brain. The response to exercise includes the following major physiological actions of epinephrine (Fig. 42-6):

1. Increased blood flow to muscles is achieved by the integrated action of norepinephrine and

● **Table 42-2.**
Some Actions of Catecholamine Hormones

β: Epinephrine > Norepinephrine	α: Norepinephrine > Epinephrine
↑ Glycogenolysis	↑ Gluconeogenesis (α_1)
↑ Gluconeogenesis (β_2)	↑ Glycogenolysis (α_1)
↑ Lipolysis (β_3) (β_2)	
↑ Calorigenesis (β_1)	
↓ Glucose utilization	
↑ Insulin secretion (β_2)	↓ Insulin secretion (α_2)
↑ Glucagon secretion (β_2)	
↑ Muscle K$^+$ uptake (β_2)	↑ Cardiac contractility (α_1)
↑ Cardiac contractility (β_1)	
↑ Heart rate (β_1)	
↑ Conduction velocity (β_1)	
↑ Arteriolar dilation: ↓ BP (β_2) (muscle)	↑ Arteriolar vasoconstriction; ↑ BP (α_1) (splanchnic, renal, cutaneous, genital)
↑ Muscle relaxation (β_2)	↑ Sphincter contraction (α_1)
Gastrointestinal	Gastrointestinal
Urinary	Urinary
Bronchial	↑ Platelet aggregation (α_2)
	↑ Sweating ("adrenergic")
	↑ Dilation of pupils (α_1)

BP, blood pressure.

epinephrine on the heart, veins and lymphatics, and nonmuscular (e.g., splanchnic) and muscular arteriolar beds.

2. Epinephrine promotes glycogenolysis in muscle. Exercising muscle can also utilize free fatty acids

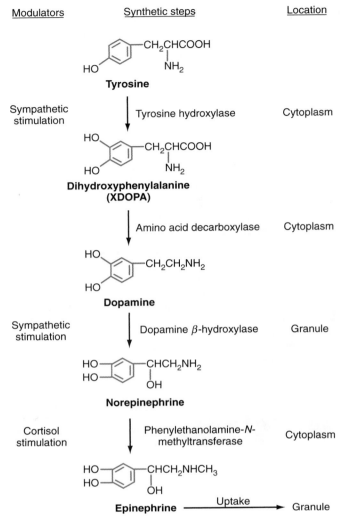

Modulators	Synthetic steps	Location

Tyrosine

Sympathetic stimulation — Tyrosine hydroxylase — Cytoplasm

Dihydroxyphenylalanine (XDOPA)

Amino acid decarboxylase — Cytoplasm

Dopamine

Sympathetic stimulation — Dopamine β-hydroxylase — Granule

Norepinephrine

Cortisol stimulation — Phenylethanolamine-*N*-methyltransferase — Cytoplasm

Epinephrine — Uptake — Granule

● **Figure 42-4.** Steps in the synthesis of catecholamines.

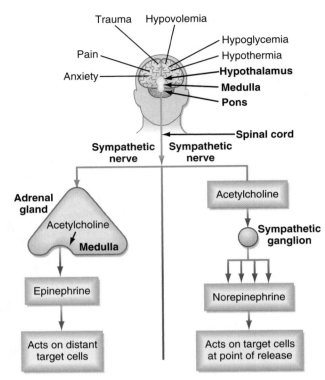

● **Figure 42-5.** Stimuli that enhance the secretion of catecholamines.

(FFAs), and epinephrine and norepinephrine promote lipolysis in adipose tissue. The actions just described increase circulating levels of lactate and glycerol, which can be used by the liver as gluconeogenic substrates to increase glucose. Epinephrine increases blood glucose by increasing hepatic glycogenolysis and gluconeogenesis. The promotion of lipolysis in adipose tissue is also coordinated with an epinephrine-induced increase in hepatic ketogenesis. Finally, the effects of catecholamines on metabolism are reinforced by the fact that they stimulate glucagon secretion (β_2 receptors) and inhibit insulin secretion (α_2 receptors). Efficient production of ATP during normal exercise (i.e., a 1-hour workout) also requires efficient exchange of gases with an adequate supply of oxygen to exercising muscle. Catecholamines promote this by relaxation of bronchiolar smooth muscle.

3. Catecholamines decrease energy demand by visceral smooth muscle. In general, a sympathoadrenal response decreases overall motility of the smooth muscle in the gastrointestinal (GI) and urinary tracts, thereby conserving energy where it is not needed.

Metabolism of Catecholamines

Two primary enzymes are involved in the degradation of catecholamines: **monoamine oxidase (MAO)** and **catechol-*O*-methyltransferase (COMT)** (Fig. 42-7). The neurotransmitter norepinephrine is degraded by MAO and COMT after uptake into the presynaptic terminal. This mechanism is also involved in the catabolism of circulating adrenal catecholamines. However, the predominant fate of adrenal catecholamines is methylation by COMT in nonneuronal tissues such as the liver and kidney. Urinary **vanillylmandelic acid (VMA)** and **metanephrine** are sometimes used clinically to assess the level of catecholamine production in a patient. Much of the urinary VMA and metanephrine is derived from neuronal rather than adrenal catecholamines.

ADRENAL CORTEX

Zona Fasciculata

The zona fasciculata produces the glucocorticoid hormone **cortisol.** This zone is an actively steroidogenic tissue composed of straight cords of large cells. These cells have a "foamy" cytoplasm because they are filled with lipid droplets that represent stored cholesterol esters. These cells make some cholesterol de novo but also import cholesterol from blood in the form of low-density lipoprotein (LDL) and high-density

● **Figure 42-6.** Some of the individual actions of catecholamines that contribute to the integrated sympathoadrenal response to exercise. (Modified from Porterfield SP, White BA: Endocrine Physiology, 3rd ed. Philadelphia, Mosby, 2007.)

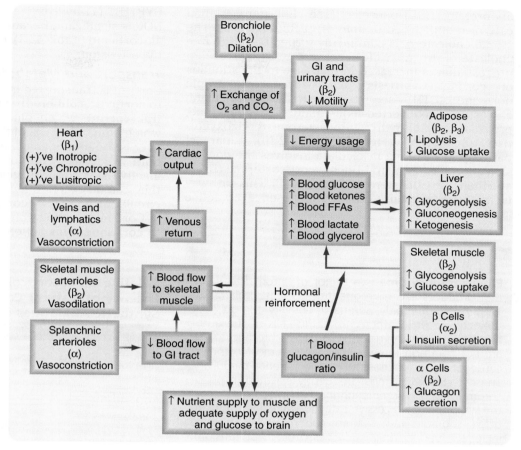

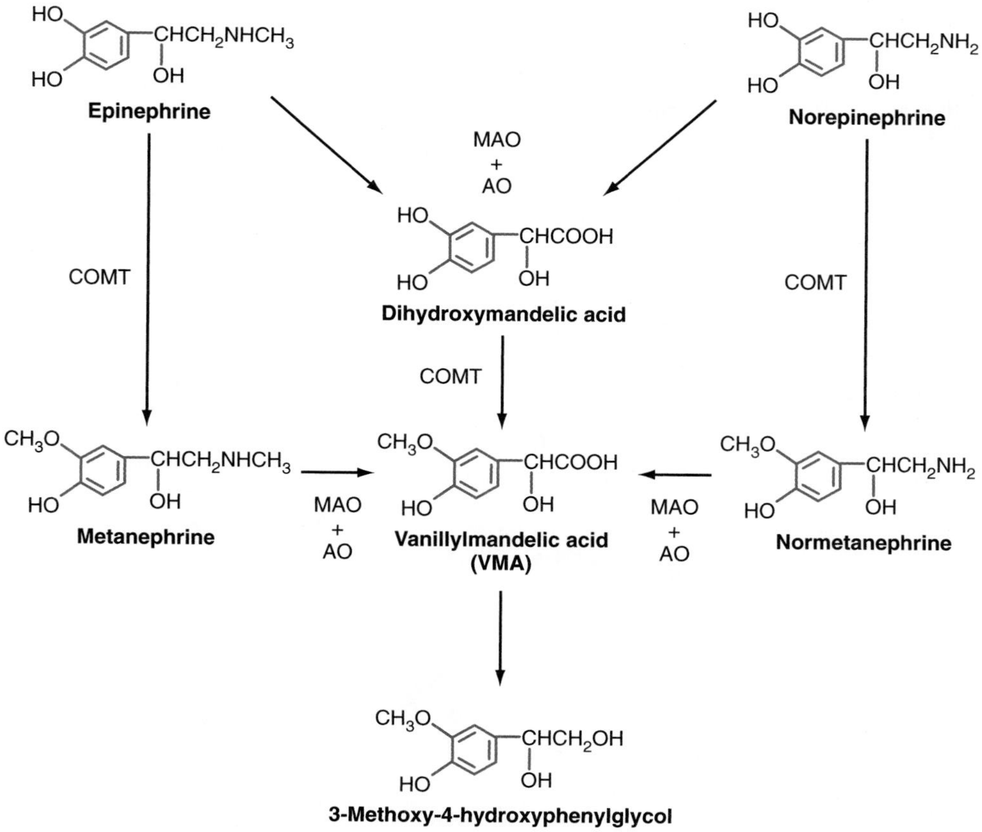

● **Figure 42-7.** Degradative metabolism of catecholamines. MAO stimulates deamination; COMT stimulates methylation.

lipoprotein (HDL) particles. Free cholesterol is then esterified and stored in lipid droplets (Fig. 42-8). The stored cholesterol is continually turned back into free cholesterol by a **cholesterol ester hydrolyase,** a process that is increased in response to the stimulus of cortisol synthesis (e.g., adrenocorticotropic hormone [ACTH]—see later). In the zona fasciculata, cholesterol is converted sequentially to pregnenolone, progesterone, 17-hydroxyprogesterone, 11-deoxycortisol, and cortisol (Figs. 42-9 and 42-10). A parallel pathway in the zona fasciculata involves the conversion of progesterone to 11-deoxycorticosterone (DOC) and then to corticosterone (Fig. 42-10, *C*). This pathway is minor in humans, but in the absence of active CYP11B1 (11-hydroxylase activity), the production of DOC is significant. Because DOC acts as a weak mineralocorticoid (Table 42-3), elevated levels of DOC cause hypertension.

Transport and Metabolism of Cortisol

Cortisol is transported in blood predominantly bound to **corticosteroid-binding globulin [CBG]** (also called **transcortin**), which binds about 90%, and albumin, which binds 5% to 7% of the circulating hormone. The liver is the predominant site of steroid inactivation. It both inactivates cortisol and conjugates active and inactive steroids with glucuronide or sulfate so that they can be excreted more readily by the kidney. The circulating half-life of cortisol is about 70 minutes.

Cortisol is reversibly inactivated by conversion to **cortisone.** This action is catalyzed by the enzyme

---

> ### IN THE CLINIC
>
> **Pheochromocytoma** is a tumor of chromaffin tissue that produces excessive quantities of catecholamines. These are commonly adrenal medullary tumors, but they can occur in other chromaffin cells of the autonomic nervous system. Although pheochromocytomas are not common tumors, they are the most common cause of hyperfunctioning of the adrenal medullary. The catecholamine most frequently elevated in pheochromocytoma is norepinephrine. For unknown reasons, the symptoms of excessive catecholamine secretion are often sporadic rather than continuous. Symptoms include hypertension, headaches (from hypertension), sweating, anxiety, palpitations, and chest pain. In addition, patients with this disorder may show orthostatic hypotension (despite the tendency for hypertension). This occurs because hypersecretion of catecholamines can decrease the postsynaptic response to norepinephrine as a result of down-regulation of the receptors (see Chapter 3). Consequently, the baroreceptor response to blood shifts that occurs on standing is blunted.

● **Table 42-3.**

Relative Glucocorticoid and Mineralocorticoid Potency of Natural Corticosteroids and Some Synthetic Analogues in Clinical Use*

	Glucocorticoid	Mineralocorticoid
Corticosterone	0.5	1.5
Prednisone (1.2 double bond)	4	<0.1
6α-Methylprednisone (Medrol)	5	<0.1
9α-Fluoro-16α-hydroxyprednisolone (triamcinolone)	5	<0.1
9α-Fluoro-16α-methylprednisolone (dexamethasone)	30	<0.1
Aldosterone	0.25	500
Deoxycorticosterone	0.01	30
9α-Fluorocortisol	10	500

*All values are relative to the glucocorticoid and mineralocorticoid potencies of cortisol, which have each been set at 1.0 arbitrarily. Cortisol actually has only 1/500 the potency of the natural mineralocorticoid aldosterone.

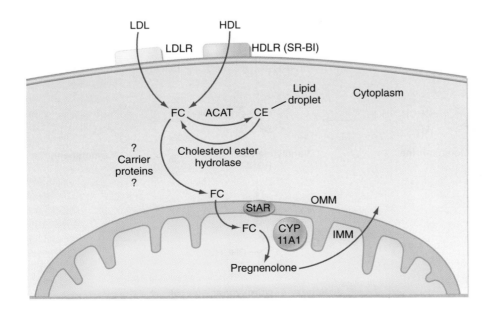

● **Figure 42-8.** Events involved in the first reaction in the steroidogenic pathway (conversion of cholesterol to pregnenolone) in zona fasciculata cells. ACAT, acyl CoA : cholesterol acyltransferase; CE, cholesterol esters; FC, free cholesterol; HDLR, high-density lipoprotein receptor (also called the scavenger receptor BI [SR-BI]); IMM, inner mitochondrial membrane; LDLR, low-density lipoprotein receptor; OMM, outer mitochondrial membrane; StAR, steroidogenic acute regulatory protein. (Modified from Porterfield SP, White BA: Endocrine Physiology, 3rd ed. Philadelphia, Mosby, 2007.)

● AT THE CELLULAR LEVEL

Free cholesterol is modified by five reactions within a steroidogenic pathway to form cortisol (Fig. 42-8). However, cholesterol is stored in the cytoplasm, and the first enzyme of the pathway, CYP11A1, is located on the inner mitochondrial membrane (Fig. 42-9). Thus, the rate-limiting reaction in steroidogenesis is the transfer of cholesterol from the outer to the inner mitochondrial membrane. Although several proteins appear to be involved, one protein, called **steroidogenic acute regulatory protein (StAR protein),** is indispensable in the process of transporting cholesterol to the inner

mitochondrial membrane (Fig. 42-8). StAR protein is short-lived and rapidly activated posttranslationally (phosphorylation) and transcriptionally by pituitary tropic hormones. In patients with inactivating mutations in StAR protein, cells of the zona fasciculata become excessively laden with lipid ("lipoid") because cholesterol cannot be accessed by CYP11A1 within the mitochondria and used for cortisol synthesis. Moreover, these individuals cannot form sex steroid hormones. The placenta does not express StAR, so these individuals have normal placental steroid production in utero.

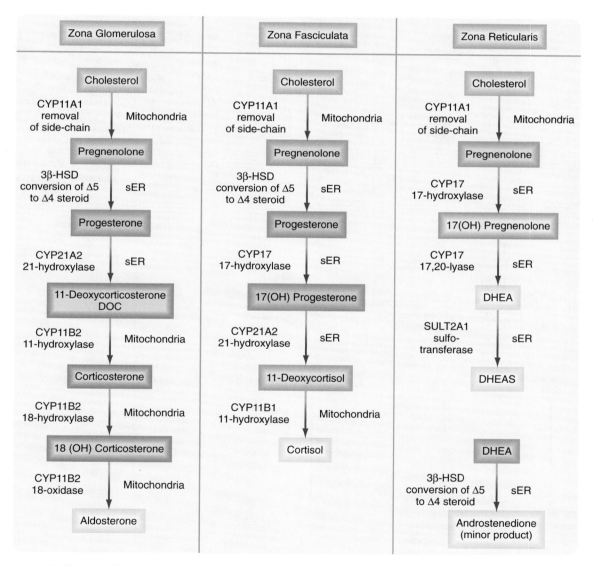

● **Figure 42-9.** Summary of the steroidogenic pathways for each of the three zones of the adrenal cortex. The enzymatic reactions are color-coded across zones. sER, smooth endoplasmic reticulum. (Modified from Porterfield SP, White BA: Endocrine Physiology, 3rd ed. Philadelphia, Mosby, 2007.)

AT THE CELLULAR LEVEL

Steroidogenic enzymes fall into two superfamilies. Most belong to the **cytochrome P-450 monooxidase gene family** and are thus referred to as **CYPs**. These enzymes are located either in the inner mitochondrial matrix, where they use molecular oxygen and a flavoprotein electron donor, or in the smooth endoplasmic reticulum, where they use a different flavoprotein for electron transfer. Different CYP enzymes act as hydroxylases, lyases (desmolases), oxidases, or aromatases. Two of these enzymes have multiple functions. CYP17 has both a 17-hydroxylase function and a 17,20-lyase (desmolase) function. CYP11B2, also called aldosterone synthase, has three functions: 11-hydroxylase, 18-hydroxylase, and 18-oxidase.

The other enzymes involved in steroidogenesis belong to three **hydroxysteroid dehydrogenase** (HSD) families. **3β-HSDs** have two isoforms that convert the hydroxyl group on carbon 3 of the cholesterol ring to a ketone and shift the double bond from the 5-6 (**Δ5**) position to the 4-5 (**Δ4**) position. All active steroid hormones must be converted to Δ4 structures by 3β-HSD. The **17β-HSDs** have at least five members and can act as either oxidases or reductases. 17β-HSDs primarily act on sex steroids and can be activating or deactivating. Finally, the **11β-HSDs** have two isoforms that catalyze the interchange between cortisol (active) and cortisone (inactive).

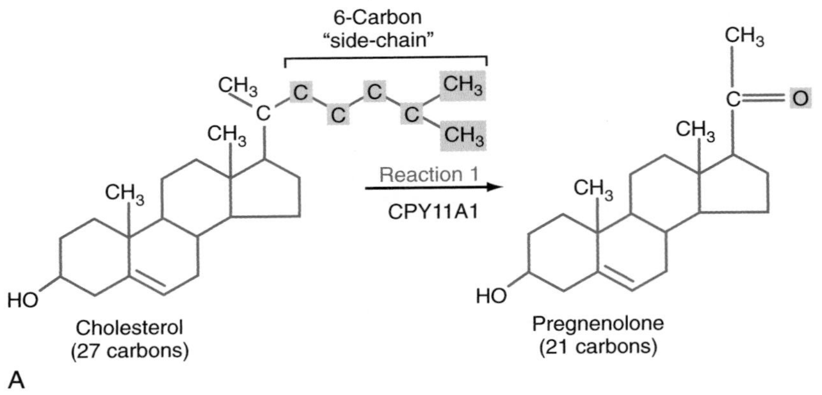

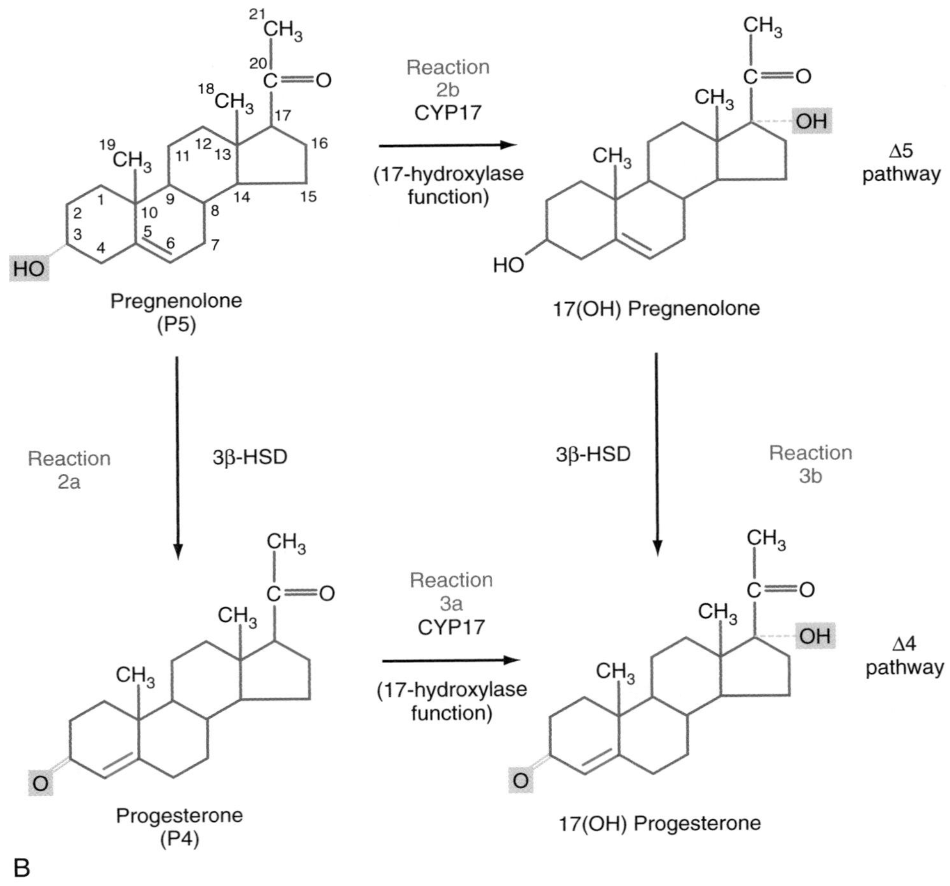

Figure 42-10. **A,** Reaction 1, catalyzed by CYP11A1, in making cortisol. **B,** Reactions 2a/b and reactions 3a/b, involving CYP17 (17-hydroxylase function) and 3β-hydroxysteroid dehydrogenase (3β-HSD), in making cortisol. This figure shows the Δ5 versus Δ4 pathway. **C,** Reactions 4 and 5, involving CYP21B and CYP11B1, in which the last two steps in the synthesis of cortisol are carried out. Also shown is the minor pathway leading to the synthesis of corticosterone in the zona fasciculata. (Modified from Porterfield SP, White BA: Endocrine Physiology, 3rd ed. Philadelphia, Mosby, 2007.)

● **Figure 42-10—cont'd.**

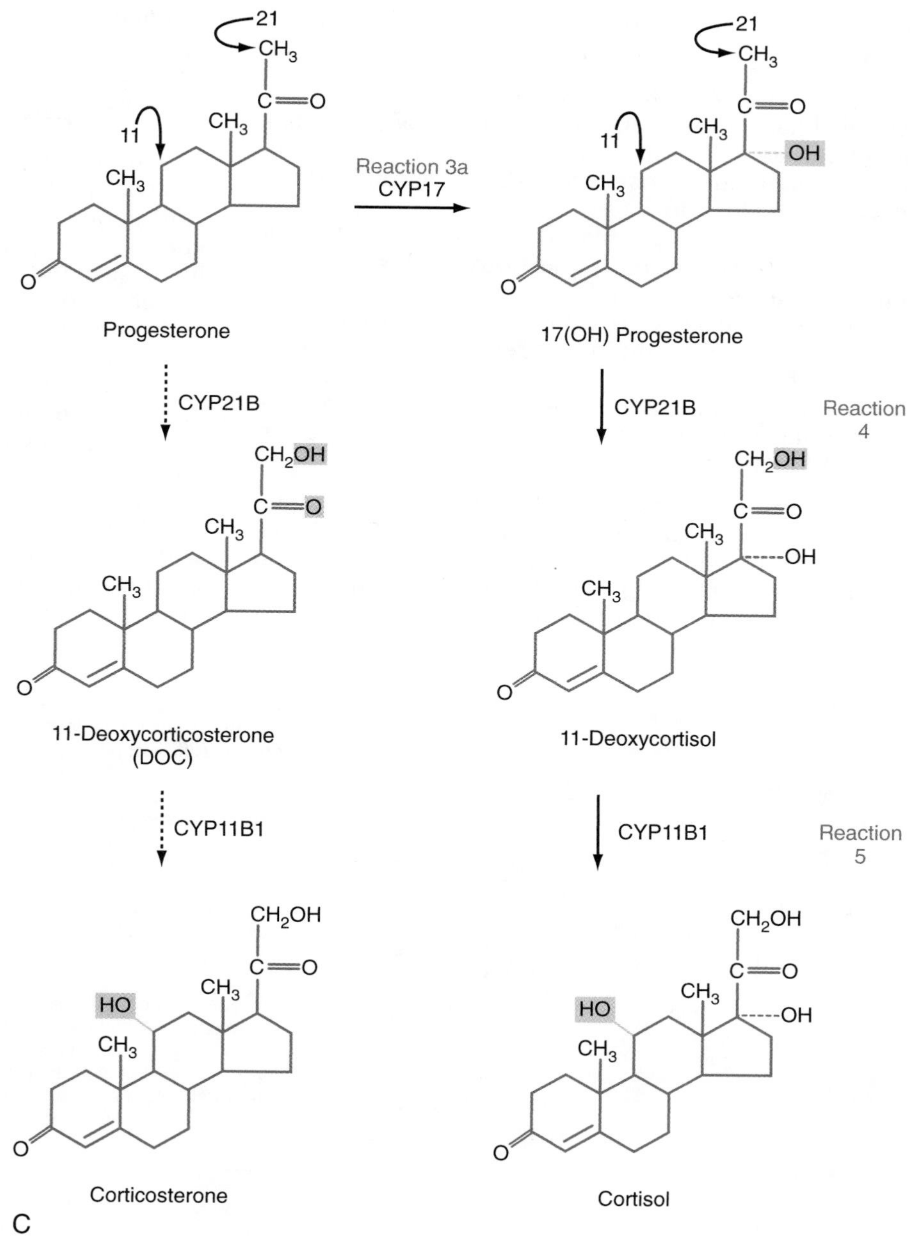

Progesterone

Reaction 3a
CYP17

17(OH) Progesterone

CYP21B

CYP21B   Reaction 4

11-Deoxycorticosterone (DOC)

11-Deoxycortisol

CYP11B1

CYP11B1   Reaction 5

Corticosterone

Cortisol

C

11β-hydroxysteroid dehydrogenase type 2 (11β-HSD2). The inactivation of cortisol by 11β-HSD2 is reversible in that another enzyme, **11β-HSD1,** converts cortisol back to cortisol. This conversion occurs in tissues expressing the glucocorticoid receptor (GR), including liver, adipose tissue, and the CNS, as well as in skin (which is why cortisone-based creams can be applied to skin to stop inflammation).

Mechanism of Action of Cortisol
Cortisol acts primarily through the **glucocorticoid receptor,** which regulates gene transcription (see Chapter 3). In the absence of hormone, the GR resides in the cytoplasm in a stable complex with several **molecular chaperones,** including heat shock proteins

and cyclophilins. Cortisol-GR binding promotes dissociation of the chaperone proteins, followed by

1. Rapid translocation of the cortisol-GR complex into the nucleus
2. Dimerization and binding to **glucocorticoid response elements (GREs)** near the basal promoters of cortisol-regulated genes
3. Recruitment of **coactivator proteins** and assembly of general transcription factors leading to increased transcription of the targeted genes.

Glucocorticoids can also repress gene transcription. In some cases, the GR interacts with other transcription factors, such as the proinflammatory NF-κB transcription factor, and interferes with their ability to activate gene expression. In other cases, GR binds to "negative GREs" and recruits corepressor proteins.

Physiological Actions of Cortisol

Cortisol has a broad range of action and is often characterized as a "stress hormone." In general, cortisol maintains blood glucose levels, CNS function, and cardiovascular function during fasting and increases blood glucose during stress at the expense of muscle protein. Cortisol protects the body against the self-injurious effects of unbridled inflammatory and immune responses. Cortisol also partitions energy to cope with stress by inhibiting reproductive function. As stated later, cortisol has several other effects on bone, skin, connective tissue, the GI tract, and the developing fetus that are independent of its stress-related functions.

Metabolic Actions. As the term glucocorticoid implies, cortisol is a steroid hormone from the adrenal cortex that regulates blood glucose. It increases blood glucose by stimulating gluconeogenesis (Fig. 42-11). Cortisol enhances gene expression of the hepatic gluconeogenic enzymes phosphoenolpyruvate carboxykinase (PEPCK), fructose-1,6-bisphosphatase, and glucose-6-phosphatase (G6Pase). Cortisol also decreases GLUT4-mediated glucose uptake in skeletal muscle and adipose tissue. During the interdigestive period (low insulin-glucagon ratio), cortisol promotes glucose sparing by potentiating the effects of catecholamines on lipolysis, thereby making FFAs available as energy sources. Cortisol inhibits protein synthesis and increases proteolysis, especially in skeletal muscle, thereby providing a rich source of carbon for hepatic gluconeogenesis.

Figure 42-11 also contrasts the normal role of cortisol in response to stress and the effects of **chronically elevated cortisol** as a result of pathological conditions. As discussed later, there are important differences in the overall metabolic effects of cortisol between these two states, particularly with respect to lipid metabolism. During stress, cortisol synergizes with catecholamines and glucagon to promote a lipolytic, gluconeogenic, ketogenic, and glycogenolytic metabolic response while synergizing with

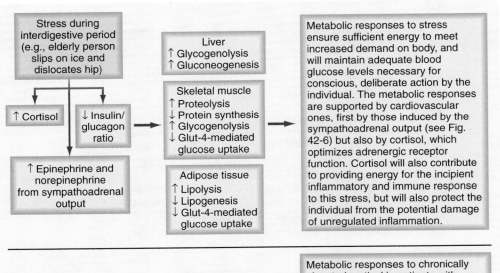

● **Figure 42-11.** Metabolic actions of cortisol (integrated with catecholamines and glucagon) in response to stress **(upper panel)** and contrasted to the actions of chronically elevated cortisol (integrated with insulin) in an otherwise healthy individual **(lower panel).** (Modified from Porterfield SP, White BA: Endocrine Physiology, 3rd ed. Philadelphia, Mosby, 2007.)

catecholamines to promote an appropriate cardiovascular response. During chronically elevated cortisol secondary to pathological overproduction, cortisol synergizes with insulin in the context of elevated levels of glucose (from increased appetite) and hyperinsulinemia (from elevated glucose and glucose intolerance) to promote lipogenesis and truncal (abdominal, visceral) adiposity.

Cardiovascular Actions. Cortisol reinforces its effects on blood glucose by its positive effects on the cardiovascular system. Cortisol has permissive actions on catecholamines and thereby contributes to cardiac output and blood pressure. Cortisol stimulates **erythropoietin** synthesis and hence increases red blood cell production. Anemia occurs when cortisol is deficient, and polycythemia occurs when cortisol levels are excessive.

Antiinflammatory and Immunosuppressive Actions. Inflammation and immune responses are often part of the response to stress. However, inflammation and immune responses have the potential for significant harm and may cause death if they are not held in homeostatic balance. As a stress hormone, cortisol plays an important role in maintaining immune homeostasis. Cortisol, along with epinephrine and norepinephrine, represses the production of proinflammatory cytokines and stimulates the production of antiinflammatory cytokines

The inflammatory response to injury consists of local dilation of capillaries and increased capillary permeability with resultant local edema and accumulation of white blood cells. These steps are mediated by prostaglandins, thromboxanes, and leukotrienes. Cortisol inhibits **phospholipase A$_2$**, a key enzyme in prostaglandin, leukotriene, and thromboxane synthesis. Cortisol also stabilizes lysosomal membranes, thereby decreasing release of the proteolytic enzymes that augment local swelling. In response to injury, leukocytes normally migrate to the site of injury and leave the vascular system. These effects are inhibited by cortisol, as is the phagocytic activity of neutrophils, although release of neutrophils from bone marrow is stimulated. Analogues of glucocorticoid are frequently used pharmacologically because of their antiinflammatory properties.

Cortisol inhibits the immune response, and for this reason glucocorticoid analogues have been used as **immunosuppressants** in organ transplants. High cortisol levels decrease the number of circulating T lymphocytes (particularly helper T lymphocytes) and reduce their ability to migrate to the site of antigenic stimulation. Glucocorticoids promote atrophy of the thymus and other lymphoid tissue. Although corticosteroids inhibit cellular-mediated immunity, antibody production by B lymphocytes is not impaired.

Effects of Cortisol on the Reproductive Systems. Reproduction exacts a considerable anabolic cost on the organism. In humans, reproductive behavior and function are dampened in response to stress. Cortisol decreases the function of the reproductive axis at the hypothalamic, pituitary, and gonadal levels.

Effects of Cortisol on Bone. Glucocorticoids increase bone resorption. They have multiple actions that alter bone metabolism. Glucocorticoids decrease intestinal Ca^{++} absorption and renal Ca^{++} reabsorption. Both mechanisms serve to lower serum [Ca^{++}]. As serum [Ca^{++}] drops, secretion of parathyroid hormone (PTH) increases, and PTH mobilizes Ca^{++} from bone by stimulating resorption of bone. In addition to this action, glucocorticoids directly inhibit osteoblast bone-forming functions (see Chapter 39). Although glucocorticoids are useful for treating the inflammation associated with arthritis, excessive use will result in bone loss (osteoporosis).

Actions of Cortisol on Connective Tissue. Cortisol inhibits fibroblast proliferation and collagen formation. In the presence of excessive amounts of cortisol, the skin thins and is more readily damaged. The connective tissue support of capillaries is impaired, and capillary injury, or bruising, is increased.

Actions of Cortisol on the Kidney. Cortisol inhibits the secretion and action of antidiuretic hormone (ADH), and thus it is an ADH antagonist. In the absence of cortisol, the action of ADH is potentiated, which makes it difficult to increase free water clearance in response to a water load and increases the likelihood of water intoxication. Although cortisol binds to the mineralocorticoid receptor with high affinity, this action is normally blocked by inactivation of cortisol to cortisone by the enzyme 11β-HSD2. However, the mineralocorticoid activity (i.e., renal Na$^+$ and H$_2$O retention, K$^+$ and H$^+$ excretion) of cortisol depends on the relative amount of cortisol (or synthetic glucocorticoids) and the activity of 11β-HSD2. Certain agents (such as compounds in black licorice) inhibit 11β-HSD2 and thereby increase the mineralocorticoid activity of cortisol. Cortisol increases the glomerular filtration rate by both increasing cardiac output and acting directly on the kidney.

Actions of Cortisol on Muscle. When cortisol levels are excessive, muscle weakness and pain are common symptoms. The weakness has multiple origins. In part, it is a result of the excessive proteolysis that cortisol produces. High cortisol levels can result in hypokalemia (via mineralocorticoid actions), which can produce muscle weakness because it hyperpolarizes and stabilizes the muscle cell membrane and thus makes stimulation more difficult.

Actions of Cortisol on the Gastrointestinal Tract. Cortisol exerts a trophic effect on the GI mucosa. In the absence of cortisol, GI motility decreases, GI mucosa degenerates, and GI acid and enzyme production decreases. Because cortisol stimulates appetite, hypercortisolism is frequently associated with weight gain. The cortisol-mediated stimulation of gastric acid and pepsin secretion increases the risk for development of ulcers.

Psychological Effects of Cortisol
Psychiatric disturbances are associated with either excessive or deficient levels of corticosteroids.

Excessive corticosteroids can initially produce a feeling of well-being, but continued excessive exposure eventually leads to emotional lability and depression. Frank psychosis can occur with either excessive or deficient hormone. Cortisol increases the tendency for insomnia and decreases rapid eye movement (REM) sleep. People who are deficient in corticosteroids tend to be depressed, apathetic, and irritable.

Effects of Cortisol during Fetal Development

Cortisol is required for normal development of the CNS, retina, skin, GI tract, and lungs. The best studied system is the lungs, in which cortisol induces differentiation and maturation of type II alveolar cells. During late gestation these cells produce surfactant, which reduces surface tension in the lungs and thus allows the onset of breathing at birth.

Regulation of Cortisol Production

Cortisol production by the zona fasciculata is regulated by a standard hypothalamic-pituitary-adrenal axis involving corticotropin-releasing hormone (CRH), ACTH, and cortisol (see Chapter 40). The hypothalamus and pituitary stimulate cortisol production, and cortisol negatively feeds back on the hypothalamus and pituitary to maintain its set point. Both neurogenic (e.g., fear) and systemic (e.g., hypoglycemia, hemorrhage, cytokines) forms of stress stimulate release of CRH. CRH is also under strong diurnal rhythmic regulation emerging from the suprachiasmatic nucleus such that cortisol levels surge during the early predawn and morning hours and then continually decline throughout the day and evening. CRH acutely stimulates release of ACTH and chronically increases proopiomelanocortin (POMC) gene expression and corticotrope hypertrophy and proliferation. Some parvicellular neurons coexpress CRH and ADH, which potentiates the actions of CRH.

ACTH binds to the **melanocortin 2 receptor (MC2R)** located on cells in the zona fasciculata (Fig. 42-12). The effects of ACTH can be subdivided into three phases:

1. The acute effects of ACTH occur within minutes. Cholesterol is rapidly mobilized from lipid droplets by posttranslational activation of cholesterol ester hydrolase and transported to the outer mitochondrial membrane. ACTH both rapidly increases steroidogenic acute regulatory (StAR) protein gene expression and activates StAR protein through protein kinase A (PKA)-dependent phosphorylation. Collectively, these acute actions of ACTH increase pregnenolone levels.
2. The chronic effects of ACTH occur over a period of several hours. These effects involve increasing transcription of the genes encoding the steroidogenic enzymes and their coenzymes. ACTH also increases expression of the LDL receptor and scavenger receptor BI (SR-BI; the HDL receptor).
3. The trophic actions of ACTH on the zona fasciculata and zona reticularis occur over a period of weeks and months. This effect is exemplified by atrophy of the zona fasciculata in patients receiving therapeutic (i.e., supraphysiological) levels of glucocorticoid analogues for at least 3 weeks. Under these conditions, the exogenous corticosteroids completely repress CRH and ACTH production, thereby resulting in atrophy of the zona fasciculata and a decline in endogenous cortisol production (Fig. 42-13). At the end of therapy, these patients need to be slowly weaned off exogenous glucocorticoids to allow the hypothalamic-pituitary-adrenal axis to reestablish itself and the zona fasciculata to enlarge and produce adequate amounts of cortisol.

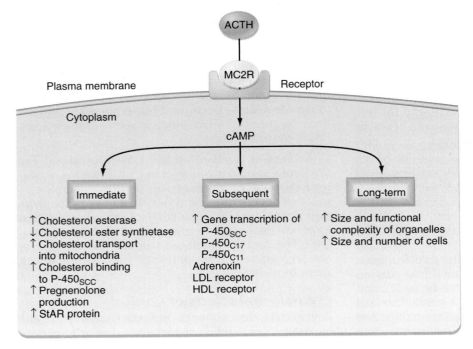

● **Figure 42-12.** Overview of the actions of ACTH on target adrenocortical cells. Note that the major second messenger, cAMP, activates immediate protein mediators and also induces the production of later protein mediators. HDL, high-density lipoprotein; LDL, low-density lipoprotein.

Cortisol inhibits both POMC gene expression at the corticotropes and pro-CRH gene expression at the hypothalamus. However, intense stress can override the negative-feedback effects of cortisol at the hypothalamus and reset the "set point" at a higher level.

Zona Reticularis

The innermost zone, the zona reticularis, begins to appear after birth at about 5 years of age. Adrenal androgens, especially DHEAS, the main product of the zona reticularis, become detectable in the circulation at about 6 years of age. This onset of adrenal androgen production is called **adrenarche,** and it contributes to the appearance of axillary and pubic hair at about age 8. DHEAS levels continue to increase, peak during the mid-twenties, and then progressively decline with age.

Androgen Synthesis by the Zona Reticularis

The zona reticularis differs from the zona fasciculata in several important ways with respect to steroidogenic enzyme activity (Fig. 42-9). First, 3β-HSD is expressed at much lower levels in the zona reticularis

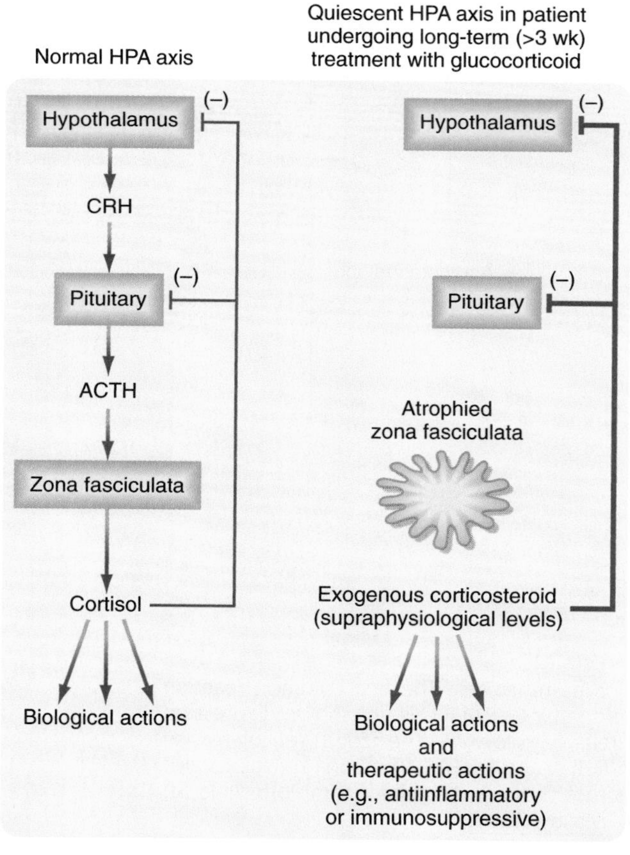

● **Figure 42-13.** Comparison of a normal hypothalamic-pituitary-adrenal (HPA) axis to a quiescent HPA axis in individual receiving exogenous glucocorticoid therapy. The latter causes the zona fasciculata to atrophy after 3 weeks, thus requiring a careful withdrawal regimen to allow rebuilding of the adrenal tissue before total cessation of exogenous corticosteroid administration. (Modified from Porterfield SP, White BA: Endocrine Physiology, 3rd ed. Philadelphia, Mosby, 2007.)

than in the zona fasciculata; thus, the "Δ5 pathway" predominates in the zona reticularis. Second, the zona reticularis expresses cofactors or conditions that enhance the 17,20-lyase function of CYP17, thereby generating the 19-carbon androgen precursor molecule **dehydroepiandrosterone (DHEA)** from 17-hydroxypregnenolone. Additionally, the zona reticularis expresses **DHEA sulfotransferase (SULT2A1 gene),** which converts DHEA into **DHEAS** (Fig. 42-14). A limited amount of the Δ4 androgen **androstenedione** is also made in the zona reticularis. Although small amounts of potent androgens (e.g., testosterone) or 18-carbon estrogens are normally produced by the human adrenal cortex, most active sex steroids are produced primarily from peripheral conversion of DHEAS and androstenedione.

Metabolism and Fate of DHEAS and DHEA

DHEAS can be converted back to DHEA by peripheral **sulfatases,** and DHEA and androstenedione can be converted to active androgens (testosterone, dihydrotestosterone) peripherally in both sexes. DHEA binds to albumin and other globulins in blood with low affinity, so it is excreted efficiently by the kidney. The half-life of DHEA is 15 to 30 minutes. In contrast, DHEAS binds to albumin with very high affinity and has a half-life of 7 to 10 hours.

Physiological Actions of Adrenal Androgens

In men, the contribution of adrenal androgens to active androgens is negligible. However, in women, the adrenal contributes to about 50% of circulating active androgens, which are required for the growth of axillary and pubic hair and for libido.

Apart from providing androgen precursors, it is not clear what other role or roles, if any, that the zona reticularis plays in adult humans. DHEAS is the most abundant circulating hormone in young adults. It increases steadily until it peaks in the mid-twenties and then steadily declines thereafter. Thus, there has been considerable interest in the possible role of DHEAS in the aging process. However, the function of this abundant steroid in young adults and the potential impact of its gradual disappearance on aging are still poorly understood. It should be noted that the age-related decline in DHEA and DHEAS has led to the popular use of these steroids as dietary supplements, even though recent studies indicate no beneficial effects.

▷ IN THE CLINIC

During adrenal androgen excess (e.g., adrenal tumor, Cushing's syndrome, congenital adrenal hyperplasia), **masculinization of women** can occur. This involves masculinization of the external genitalia (e.g., enlarged clitoris) in utero and excessive facial and body hair (called **hirsutism**) and acne in adult women. Excessive adrenal androgens also appear to play a role in ovarian dysovulation (i.e., polycystic ovarian syndrome).

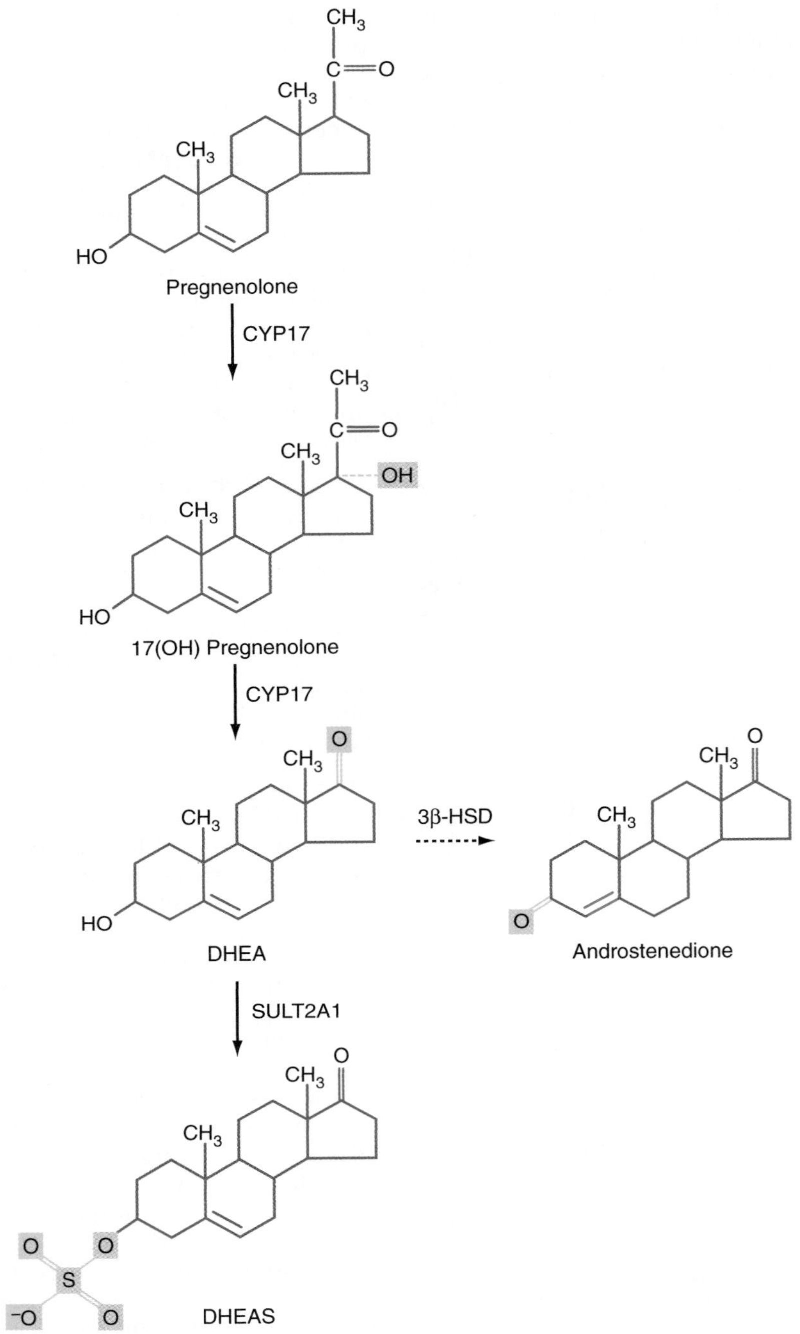

● **Figure 42-14.** Steroidogenic pathways in the zona reticularis. The first common reaction in the pathway, conversion of cholesterol to pregnenolone by CYP11A1, is not shown. Expression of 3β-hydroxysteroid dehydrogenase (3β-HSD) is relatively low in the zona reticularis, so androstenedione is a minor product in comparison to DHEA and DHEAS. The zona reticularis also makes a small amount of testosterone and estrogens (not shown). (Modified from Porterfield SP, White BA: Endocrine Physiology, 3rd ed. Philadelphia, Mosby, 2007.)

● **Figure 42-15.** The "loophole" in the hypothalamic-pituitary-adrenal axis. ACTH stimulates the production of both cortisol and adrenal androgens, but only cortisol negatively feeds back on ACTH and CRH. Thus, if cortisol production is blocked (i.e., CYP11B1 deficiency), ACTH levels increase, along with adrenal androgens. (Modified from Porterfield SP, White BA: Endocrine Physiology, 3rd ed. Philadelphia, Mosby, 2007.)

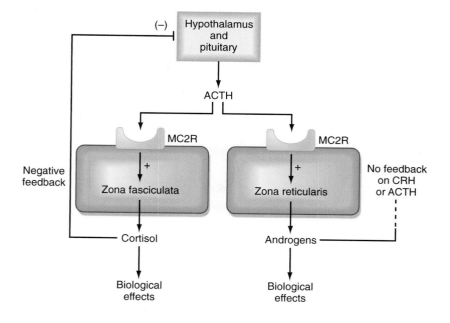

IN THE CLINIC

A crucial clinical aspect of regulation of the zona reticularis is that neither adrenal androgens nor their more potent metabolites (e.g., testosterone, dihydrotestosterone, estradiol-17β) negatively feed back on ACTH or CRH (Fig. 42-15). This means that an enzymatic defect associated with the synthesis of cortisol (e.g., CYP21B deficiency) is associated with a dramatic increase in both ACTH (no negative feedback from cortisol) and adrenal androgens (because of the elevated ACTH). It is this "loophole" in the hypothalamic-pituitary-adrenal axis that gives rise to congenital adrenal hyperplasia.

Regulation of Zona Reticularis Function

ACTH is the primary regulator of the zona reticularis. Both DHEA and androstenedione display the same diurnal rhythm as cortisol (DHEAS does not because of its long circulating half-life). Moreover, the zona reticularis shows the same atrophic changes as the zona fasciculata in conditions typified by little or no ACTH. However, other factors must regulate adrenal androgen function. Adrenarche occurs in the face of constant ACTH and cortisol levels, and the rise and decline of DHEAS is not associated with a similar pattern of ACTH or cortisol production. However, the other factors, whether extraadrenal or intraadrenal, remain unknown.

Zona Glomerulosa

The thin, outermost zone of the adrenal, the zona glomerulosa, produces the mineralocorticoid aldosterone, which regulates salt and volume homeostasis (see Chapter 34). The zona glomerulosa is minimally influenced by ACTH. Rather, it is regulated primarily by the renin-angiotensin system, plasma [K⁺], and atrial natriuretic peptide (ANP).

AT THE CELLULAR LEVEL

CYP11B1 and CYP11B2 are located on chromosome 8 in humans, display 95% similarity, and are separated from each other by only about 50 kilobases. This increases the possibility of uneven crossing over during gametogenesis, with the formation of hybrid genes. In one case, the promoter region and 5′ end of the CYP11B1 gene is fused to the 3′ end of the CYP11B2 gene. This arrangement leads to aldosterone synthase being expressed in the zonae fasciculata and reticularis under the control of ACTH. Because aldosterone is no longer under feedback control by the renin-angiotensin system (see Chapter 34), aldosterone levels are high, and hypertension ensues. This form of primary aldosteronism is called glucocorticoid-remediable aldosteronism, and it is inherited in an autosomal dominant manner. This disease can be confirmed by the polymerase chain reaction technique and by measurement of 18-hydroxycortisol and 18-oxicortisol in a 24-hour urine sample. The disease is treated by the administration of glucocorticoid, which suppresses ACTH and thus expression of the hybrid gene.

An important feature in the steroidogenic capacity of the zona glomerulosa is that it does not express CYP17. Therefore, zona glomerulosa cells never make cortisol, nor do they make adrenal androgens in any form. Pregnenolone is converted to progesterone and DOC by 3β-HSD and CYP21, respectively (Fig. 42-16).

A completely unique feature of the zona glomerulosa among the steroidogenic glands is its expression of CYP11B2, which is regulated by different signaling pathways. Furthermore, the enzyme coded by CYP11B2, called **aldosterone synthase,** catalyzes the last three reactions from DOC to aldosterone within the zona glomerulosa. These reactions are 11-hydroxylation of

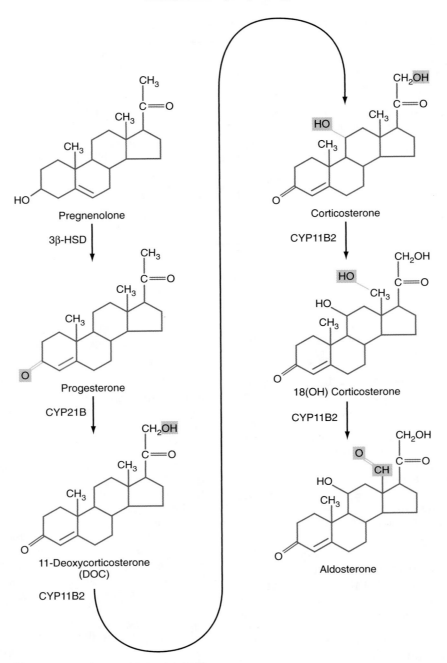

● **Figure 42-16.**   Steroidogenic pathways in the zona glomerulosa. The first common reaction in the pathway, conversion of cholesterol to pregnenolone by CYP11A1, is not shown. Note that the last three reactions are catalyzed by CYP11B2. (Modified from Porterfield SP, White BA: Endocrine Physiology, 3rd ed. Philadelphia, Mosby, 2007.)

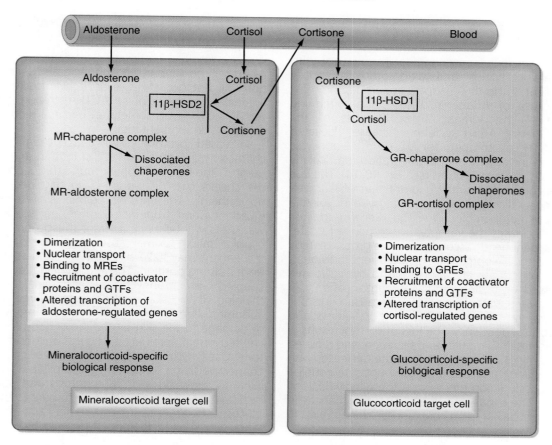

● **Figure 42-17.** The mineralocorticoid receptor (MR) is protected from activation by cortisol by the enzyme 11β-hydroxysteroid dehydrogenase type 2 (11β-HSD2), which converts cortisol to inactive cortisone. Cortisone can be converted back to cortisol in glucocorticoid target cells by the enzyme 11β-HSD type 1. GTF, general transcription factors; MRE, mineralocorticoid response element; GRE, glucocorticoid response element. (Modified from Porterfield SP, White BA: Endocrine Physiology, 3rd ed. Philadelphia, Mosby, 2007.)

DOC to form corticosterone, 18-hydroxylation to form 18-hydroxycorticosterone, and 18-oxidation to form aldosterone (Figs. 42-9 and 42-16).

Transport and Metabolism of Aldosterone
Aldosterone binds to albumin and corticosteroid-binding protein in blood with low affinity and therefore has a biological half-life of about 20 minutes. Almost all aldosterone is inactivated by the liver in one pass, conjugated to a glucuronide group, and excreted by the kidney.

Mechanism of Aldosterone Action
Aldosterone acts much like cortisol (and other steroid hormones) in that its primary mechanism of action is mediated by binding to a specific intracellular receptor (i.e., **mineralocorticoid receptor [MR]**). After dissociation of chaperone proteins, nuclear translocation, dimerization, and binding to the mineralocorticoid response element (MRE), the aldosterone-MR complex regulates the expression of specific genes (see Chapter 3). Cortisol binds to the MR and activates the same genes as aldosterone does. However, as discussed earlier, some cells that express MR also express

IN THE CLINIC

Clinical studies in humans have revealed a deleterious effect of aldosterone on cardiovascular function independent of its effects on renal sodium and water reabsorption. Aldosterone has a **proinflammatory, profibrotic effect** on the cardiovascular system and causes left ventricular hypertrophy and remodeling. This effect of aldosterone is associated with increased morbidity and mortality in patients with essential hypertension.

11β-HSD2, which converts cortisol to the inactive steroid cortisone (Fig. 42-17). Cortisone can be converted back to cortisol by 11β-HSD1, which is expressed in several glucocorticoid-responsive tissues, including the liver and skin.

Physiological Actions of Aldosterone
The actions and regulation of aldosterone are discussed in Chapter 34.

Addison's disease is primary adrenal insufficiency, with both mineralocorticoids and glucocorticoids usually being deficient. In North America and Europe, the most prevalent cause of Addison's disease is autoimmune destruction of the adrenal cortex. Because of the cortisol deficiency, ACTH secretion increases. Elevated levels of ACTH can compete for MC1R in melanocytes and cause an increase in skin pigmentation, particularly in skin creases, scars, and gums (see Fig. 40-14). The loss of mineralocorticoids results in contraction of extracellular volume, which produces circulatory hypovolemia and therefore a drop in blood pressure. Because the loss of cortisol decreases the vasopressive response to catecholamines, peripheral vascular resistance drops, thereby facilitating the development of hypotension. Individuals with Addison's disease are also prone to hypoglycemia when stressed or fasting, and water intoxication can develop if excess water is ingested. Because cortisol is important for muscle function, muscle weakness also occurs in cortisol deficiency. The loss of cortisol results in anemia, decreased GI motility and secretion, and reduced iron and vitamin B_{12} absorption. Appetite decreases with cortisol deficiency, and this decreased appetite coupled with the GI dysfunction predisposes these individuals to weight loss. These patients often have disturbances in mood and behavior and are more susceptible to depression.

Adrenocortical hormone excess is termed **Cushing's syndrome.** Pharmacological use of exogenous corticosteroids is now the most common cause of Cushing's syndrome. The next most prevalent cause is ACTH-secreting tumors. The form of Cushing's syndrome caused by a functional pituitary adenoma is called **Cushing's disease.** The fourth most common cause of Cushing's syndrome is primary hypercortisolism resulting from a functional adrenal tumor. If the disorder is primary or if it is a result of corticosteroid treatment, secretion of ACTH will be suppressed and increased skin pigmentation will not occur. However, if hypersecretion of the adrenal is the result of an ACTH-secreting nonpituitary tumor, ACTH levels sometimes become high enough to increase skin pigmentation.

Increased cortisol secretion causes weight gain with a characteristic centripetal fat distribution and a "buffalo hump." The face will appear round (fat deposition), and the cheeks may be reddened, in part because of the polycythemia. The limbs will be thin as a result of skeletal muscle wasting (from increased proteolysis), and muscle weakness will be evident (from muscle proteolysis and hypokalemia). Proximal muscle weakness is apparent, so the patient may have difficulty climbing stairs or rising from a sitting position. The abdominal fat accumulation, coupled with atrophy of the abdominal muscles and thinning of the skin, will produce a large, protruding abdomen. Purple abdominal striae are seen as a result of damage to the skin by the prolonged proteolysis, increased intraabdominal fat, and loss of abdominal muscle tone. Capillary fragility occurs because of damage to the connective tissue supporting the capillaries. Patients are likely to show signs of osteoporosis and poor wound healing. They have metabolic disturbances that include glucose intolerance, hyperglycemia, and insulin resistance (Fig. 42-11). Prolonged hypercortisolism can lead to manifestations of diabetes mellitus. Because of suppression of the immune system caused by glucocorticoids, patients are more susceptible to infection. The mineralocorticoid activities of glucocorticoids and the possible increase in aldosterone secretion produce salt retention and subsequent water retention that result in hypertension. Excessive androgen secretion in women can produce hirsutism, male pattern baldness, and clitoral enlargement (adrenogenital syndrome).

Any enzyme blockage that decreases cortisol synthesis will increase ACTH secretion and produce adrenal hyperplasia. The most common form of congenital adrenal hyperplasia occurs as a result of deficiency of the enzyme **21-hydroxylase (CYP21).** These individuals cannot produce normal quantities of cortisol, **deoxycortisol,** DOC, corticosterone, or aldosterone (Figs. 42-8 and 42-10, C). Because of impaired cortisol production and resultant elevated ACTH levels, steroidogenesis is stimulated, thereby increasing the synthesis products "upstream" of the missing enzyme, as well as products of the zona reticularis. Because the latter include the adrenal androgens, a female fetus will be masculinized. Because they are unable to produce the mineralocorticoids, aldosterone, DOC, and corticosterone, patients with this disorder have difficulty retaining salt and maintaining extracellular volume. Consequently, they are likely to be hypotensive. If the blockage is at the next step, **11β-hydroxylase** (CYP11B1), DOC will be formed and levels of DOC will accumulate (Figs. 42-8 and 42-10, C). Because DOC has significant mineralocorticoid activity and its levels become high, these individuals tend to retain salt and water and become hypertensive.

■ KEY CONCEPTS

1. The adrenal gland is composed of a cortex that is of mesodermal origin and a medulla that is of neuroectodermal origin. The cortex produces steroid hormones, and the medulla produces catecholamines.

2. The rate-limiting enzymes in medullary catecholamine synthesis are tyrosine hydroxylase and dopamine β-hydroxylase, which are induced by sympathetic stimulation, and phenylethanolamine-*N*-methyltransferase, which is induced by cortisol.

3. Catecholamines increase serum glucose and fatty acid levels. They stimulate gluconeogenesis, glycogenolysis, and lipolysis. Catecholamines increase cardiac output but have selective effects on blood flow to different organs.

4. Pheochromocytoma is a tumor of chromaffin tissue that produces excessive quantities of catecholamines. Symptoms of pheochromocytoma are often sporadic and include hypertension, headaches, sweating, anxiety, palpitations, chest pain, and orthostatic hypotension.

5. The adrenal cortex displays clear structural and functional zonation: the zona glomerulosa produces the mineralocorticoid aldosterone, the zona fasciculata produces the glucocorticoid cortisol, and the zona reticularis produces the weak androgens DHEA and DHEAS.

6. Cortisol binds to the glucocorticoid receptor. During stress, cortisol increases blood glucose by increasing gluconeogenesis in the liver and breaking muscle protein down to supply gluconeogenic precursors. Cortisol also decreases glucose uptake by muscle and adipose tissue and has permissive actions on glucagon and catecholamines. Cortisol has multiple effects on other tissue. From a pharmacological point of view, the most important is the immunosuppressive/antiinflammatory effect.

7. Cortisol is regulated by the CRH-ACTH-cortisol axis. Cortisol negatively feeds back at the hypothalamus on both CRH-producing neurons and pituitary corticotropes. CRH is regulated by several forms of stress, including proinflammatory cytokines, hypoglycemia, neurogenic stress, and hemorrhage, and by diurnal input.

8. The adrenal androgens DHEA, DHEAS, and androstenedione are androgen precursors. They can be converted to active androgens peripherally and provide about 50% of circulating androgens in women. In men, the role of adrenal androgens, if any, remains obscure. In women, adrenal androgens promote pubic and axillary hair growth and libido. Excessive adrenal androgens in women can lead to various degrees of virilization and ovarian dysfunction.

9. The zona glomerulosa of the adrenal cortex is the site of aldosterone production. Aldosterone is the strongest naturally occurring mineralocorticoid in humans. It promotes Na^+ and water reabsorption by the distal tubule and collecting duct while promoting renal K^+ and H^+ secretion. Aldosterone promotes Na^+ and water absorption in the colon and salivary glands. It also has a proinflammatory, profibrotic effect on the cardiovascular system and causes left ventricular hypertrophy and remodeling.

10. Major actions of angiotensin II on the adrenal cortex are increased growth and vascularity of the zona glomerulosa, increased StAR and CYP11B2 enzyme activity, and increased aldosterone synthesis.

11. Major stimuli for aldosterone production are a rise in angiotensin II and a rise in serum $[K^+]$. The major inhibitory signal is ANP.

12. Addison's disease is adrenocortical insufficiency. Common symptoms include hypotension, hyperpigmentation, muscle weakness, anorexia, hypoglycemia, and hyperkalemic acidosis.

13. Cushing's syndrome results from hypercortisolemia. If the basis of the disorder is increased pituitary adrenocorticotropin secretion, the disorder is called Cushing's disease. Common symptoms of Cushing's syndrome include centripetal fat distribution, muscle wasting, proximal muscle weakness, thin skin with abdominal striae, capillary fragility, insulin resistance, and polycythemia.

14. Congenital adrenal hyperplasia is caused by a congenital enzyme deficiency that blocks the production of cortisol. The enzyme blockage results in elevated ACTH secretion, which stimulates adrenal cortical growth and secretion of precursors produced before the block. 21-Hydroxylase (CYP21B) deficiency is the most common form.

CHAPTER 43

The Male and Female Reproductive Systems

The two most basic components of the reproductive system are the **gonads** and the **reproductive tract.** The gonads (**testes** and **ovaries**) perform an **endocrine function,** which is regulated within a **hypothalamic-pituitary-gonadal axis.** The gonads are distinct from other endocrine glands in that they also perform an exocrine function (**gametogenesis**). The reproductive tract is involved in several aspects of gamete development, function, and transport and, in women, allows fertilization, implantation, and gestation. Normal gametogenesis in the gonads and the development and physiology of the reproductive tract are absolutely dependent on the endocrine function of the gonads. The clinical ramifications of this hormonal dependence include infertility in the face of low sex hormone production, ambiguous genitalia in dysregulated hormone or receptor expression, and hormone-responsive cancers, especially uterine and breast cancer in women and prostate cancer in men.

THE MALE REPRODUCTIVE SYSTEM

The male reproductive system has evolved for **continuous, life-long gametogenesis,** coupled with occasional **internal insemination** with a **high density of sperm** ($>60 \times 10^6$/mL in 3 to 5 mL of semen). In adult men the basic roles of gonadal hormones are (1) support of gametogenesis (**spermatogenesis**), (2) maintenance of the male reproductive tract and production of semen, and (3) maintenance of secondary sex characteristics and libido. There is no overall cyclicity of this activity in men.

THE TESTIS

Histophysiology

Unlike the ovaries, the testes reside outside the abdominal cavity in the **scrotum** (Fig. 43-1). This location maintains testicular temperature at about 2 degrees lower than body temperature, which is crucial for optimal sperm development. The human **testis** is covered by a connective tissue capsule and is divided into about 300 **lobules** by fibrous septa (Fig. 43-2). Within each lobule are two to four loops of **seminiferous tubules.** Each loop empties into an anastomosing network of tubules called the **rete testis.** The rete testis is continuous with small ducts, the **efferent ductules,** that lead the sperm out of the testis into the head of the **epididymis** on the superior pole of the testis (Fig. 43-2). Once in the epididymis, the sperm pass from the **head,** to the **body,** to the **tail** of the epididymis and then to the **vas (ductus) deferens.** Viable **sperm** can be stored in the tail of the epididymis and the vas deferens for several months.

The presence of the seminiferous tubules creates two compartments within each lobule: an intratubular compartment, which is composed of the **seminiferous epithelium** of the seminiferous tubule, and a peritubular compartment, which is composed of neurovascular elements, connective tissue cells, immune cells, and the **"interstitial cells of Leydig,"** whose main function is to produce **testosterone** (Fig. 43-3).

The Intratubular Compartment

The seminiferous tubule is lined by a complex **seminiferous epithelium** composed of two cell types: **sperm cells** in various stages of **spermatogenesis** and the **Sertoli cell,** which is a "nurse cell" in intimate contact with all sperm cells (Fig. 43-4).

Developing Sperm Cells

Spermatogenesis involves the processes of **mitosis** and **meiosis.** Stem cells, called **spermatogonia,** reside at the basal level of the seminiferous epithelium (Fig. 43-4). Spermatogonia divide mitotically to generate daughter spermatogonia (**spermatocytogenesis**). One or more spermatogonia remain within the stem cell population, firmly adherent to the basal lamina. However, the majority of these daughter spermatogonia enter meiotic division, which results in haploid spermatozoa on completion of meiosis. These divisions are accompanied by **incomplete cytokinesis** such that all daughter cells remain interconnected by a cytoplasmic bridge. This configuration contributes to the synchrony of development of a clonal population of sperm cells. Spermatogonia migrate apically away from the basal lamina as they enter the first meiotic prophase. At this time they are called **primary spermatocytes** (Fig 43-4). During the first meiotic prophase, the hallmark processes of sexual reproduction involving chromosomal reduplication, synapsis, crossing over, and homologous recombination take place. Completion of the first meiotic division gives rise to **secondary spermatocytes,** which quickly (i.e., within

● **Figure 43-1.** Anatomy of the male reproductive system. (Modified from Drake RL et al: Gray's Anatomy for Students. Philadelphia, Churchill Livingstone, 2005.)

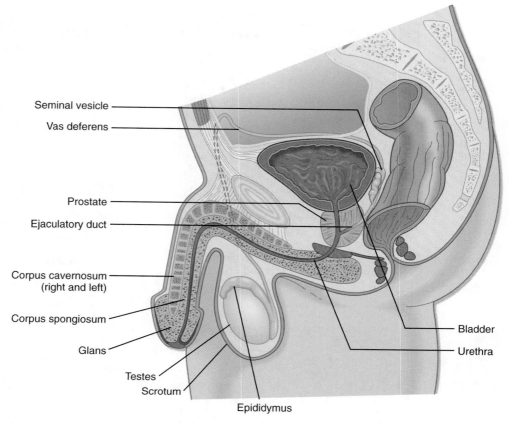

Seminal vesicle

Vas deferens

Prostate

Ejaculatory duct

Corpus cavernosum (right and left)

Corpus spongiosum

Glans

Testes

Scrotum

Epididymus

Bladder

Urethra

● **Figure 43-2.** Anatomy and organization of the testis. (Modified from Drake RL et al: Gray's Anatomy for Students. Philadelphia, Churchill Livingstone, 2005.)

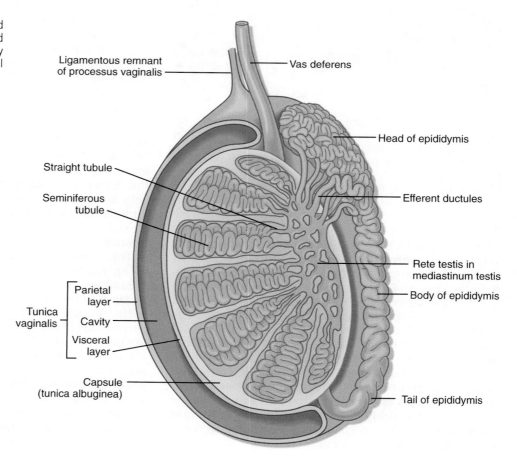

Ligamentous remnant of processus vaginalis

Vas deferens

Straight tubule

Seminiferous tubule

Head of epididymis

Efferent ductules

Rete testis in mediastinum testis

Body of epididymis

Tunica vaginalis

Parietal layer

Cavity

Visceral layer

Capsule (tunica albuginea)

Tail of epididymis

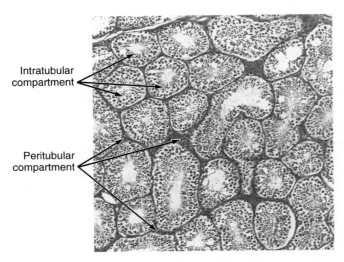

● **Figure 43-3.** Histology of a testicular lobule. (From Young B et al: Wheater's Functional Histology. A Text and Colour Atlas, 5th ed. London, Churchill Livingstone, 2006.)

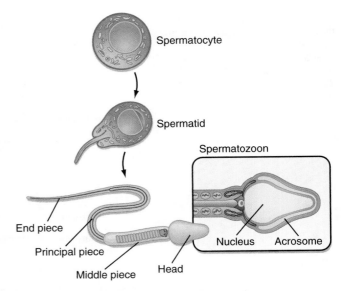

● **Figure 43-5.** Structure of sperm cells during the process of spermatogenesis and spermiogenesis.

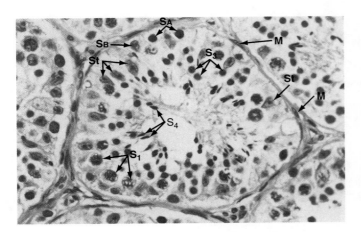

● **Figure 43-4.** Histology of a seminiferous tubule. M, myoid cell just outside the basal lamina; S_1, primary spermatocyte; S_3, spermatid; S_4, mature spermatid or spermatozoon; S_B and S_A, spermatogonia; St, Sertoli cell. (From Young B et al: Wheater's Functional Histology. A Text and Colour Atlas, 5th ed. London, Churchill Livingstone, 2006.)

20 minutes) completes the second meiotic division. The initial products of meiosis are haploid **spermatids** (Fig. 43-4). Spermatids are small, round cells that undergo a remarkable metamorphosis called **spermiogenesis** (Fig. 43-5). The products of spermiogenesis are the streamlined spermatozoa. As the spermatid matures into a **spermatozoon,** the size of the nucleus decreases and a prominent tail is formed. The tail contains microtubular structures that propel sperm, similar to a flagellum. The chromatin material in the sperm nucleus condenses, and most of the cytoplasm is lost. The acrosome is a membrane-enclosed structure on the head of the sperm that acts as a lysosome and contains hydrolytic enzymes that are important for fertilization. These enzymes remain inactive until the acrosomal reaction occurs (see later).

Spermatozoa (Fig. 43-4) are found at the luminal surface of the seminiferous tubule. Release of sperm, or **spermiation,** is controlled by Sertoli cells. The process of spermatogenesis takes about 72 days. A cohort of adjacent spermatogonia enter the process every 16 days so that the process is staggered at one point along a seminiferous tubule. In addition, the process is staggered along the length of a seminiferous tubule (i.e., not all spermatogonia enter the process of spermatogenesis at the same time along the entire length of the tubule or in synchrony with every other tubule; there are about 500 seminiferous tubules per testis; see later). Because the seminiferous tubules within one testis are about 400 m in length, spermatozoa are continually being generated at many sites within the testis at any given time.

The Sertoli Cell

Sertoli cells are the true epithelial cells of the seminiferous epithelium and extend from the basal lamina to the lumen (Fig. 43-4). Sertoli cells surround sperm cells and provide structural support within the epithelium, and they form adhering and gap junctions with all stages of sperm cells. Through the formation and breakdown of these junctions, Sertoli cells guide sperm cells toward the lumen as they advance to later stages of spermatogenesis. Spermiation requires the final breakdown of Sertoli–sperm cell junctions.

Another important structural feature of Sertoli cells is the formation of tight junctions between adjacent Sertoli cells (Fig. 43-6). These Sertoli-Sertoli cell occluding junctions divide the seminiferous epithelium into a basal compartment containing the spermatogonia and early-stage primary spermatocytes and an adluminal compartment containing later-stage primary spermatocytes and all subsequent stages of sperm cells. As early primary spermatocytes move apically from the basal to the adluminal compartment, the tight junctions need to be disassembled and reassembled.

● **Figure 43-6.** Interactions among the various cells of the testis in the hormonal regulation of spermatogenesis. (From Carlson BM: Human Embryology and Developmental Biology. Philadelphia, Mosby, 2004.)

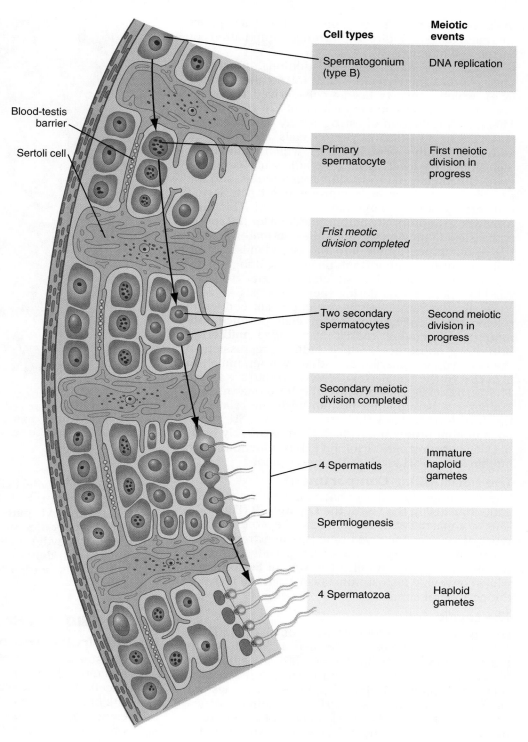

Cell types	Meiotic events
Spermatogonium (type B)	DNA replication
Primary spermatocyte	First meiotic division in progress
Frist meotic division completed	
Two secondary spermatocytes	Second meiotic division in progress
Secondary meiotic division completed	
4 Spermatids	Immature haploid gametes
Spermiogenesis	
4 Spermatozoa	Haploid gametes

Blood-testis barrier

Sertoli cell

These tight junctions form the physical basis for the **blood-testis barrier** (Fig. 43-6), which creates a specialized, immunologically safe microenvironment for developing sperm. By blocking paracellular diffusion, the tight junctions restrict movement of substances between blood and the developing germ cells through a trans–Sertoli cell transport pathway and, in this manner, allow the Sertoli cell to control the availability of nutrients to germ cells.

Healthy Sertoli cell function is essential for sperm cell viability and development. In addition, spermatogenesis is absolutely dependent on testosterone produced by peritubular Leydig cells (see later), yet it is the Sertoli cells that express the **androgen receptor,** not the developing sperm cells. Similarly, the pituitary hormone follicle-stimulating hormone (FSH) is also required for maximal sperm production, and again, it is the Sertoli cell that expresses the **FSH receptor,** not the developing sperm. Thus, these hormones support spermatogenesis indirectly through stimulation of Sertoli cell function.

Sertoli cells have multiple additional functions. They express the enzyme CYP19 (also called aromatase), which converts Leydig cell–derived testosterone to the potent estrogen estradiol-17β (see later). This local production of estrogen may enhance spermatogenesis in humans. Sertoli cells also produce **androgen-binding protein** (ABP), which maintains a high androgen level within the adluminal compartment, the lumens of the seminiferous tubules, and the proximal part of the male reproductive tract. Sertoli cells also produce a large amount of fluid. This fluid provides an appropriate bathing medium for the sperm and assists in moving the immotile spermatozoa from the seminiferous tubule into the epididymis. Sertoli cells perform an important phagocytic function by engulfing **residual bodies,** which represent cytoplasm shed by spermatozoa during spermiogenesis.

Finally, the Sertoli cell has an important endocrine role. During development, Sertoli cells produce **antimüllerian hormone (AMH;** also called **müllerian inhibitory substance**), which induces regression of the embryonic müllerian duct that is programmed to give rise to the female reproductive tract (see later). The Sertoli cells also produce the hormone **inhibin.** Inhibin is a heterodimer protein hormone related to the transforming growth factor-β family. FSH stimulates inhibin production, which then negatively feeds back on gonadotropes to inhibit FSH production. Thus, inhibin keeps FSH levels within a set point.

The Peritubular Compartment

The peritubular compartment contains the primary endocrine cell of the testis, the **Leydig cell** (Fig. 43-7). This compartment also contains the common cell types of loose connective tissue and an extremely rich peritubular capillary network that provides nutrients to the seminiferous tubules (by way of Sertoli cells) while conveying testosterone away from the testes to the peripheral circulation.

The Leydig Cell

Leydig cells are steroidogenic stromal cells. These cells synthesize cholesterol de novo, as well as acquire it through low-density lipoprotein (LDL) receptors and high-density lipoprotein (HDL) receptors (also called scavenger receptor BI [SR-BI]), and store cholesterol as cholesterol esters, as described for adrenocortical cells (see Chapter 42). Free cholesterol is generated by a cholesterol ester hydrolase and transferred to the outer mitochondrial membrane and then to the inner mitochondrial membrane in a steroidogenic acute regulatory (StAR) protein–dependent manner. As in all steroidogenic cells, cholesterol is converted to pregnenolone by CYP11A1. Pregnenolone is then processed to progesterone, 17-hydroxyprogesterone, and androstenedione by 3β-hydroxysteroid dehydrogenase **(3β-HSD)** and **CYP17** (Fig. 43-8). Recall from Chapter 42 that CYP17 is a bifunctional enzyme with **17-hydroxylase activity** and **17,20-lyase activity.** CYP17 displays a robust level of both activities in the Leydig cell. In

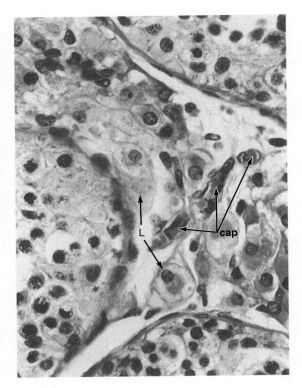

● **Figure 43-7.** Histology of the peritubular space containing Leydig cells (L) and richly vascularized by peritubular capillaries (cap). (Modified from Young B et al: Wheater's Functional Histology. A Text and Colour Atlas, 5th ed. London, Churchill Livingstone, 2006.)

this respect the Leydig cell is similar to the zona reticularis cell, except that it expresses a higher level of 3β-HSD, so the **Δ4 pathway** is ultimately favored. Another major difference is that the Leydig cell expresses a Leydig cell–specific isoform of **17β-hydroxysteroid dehydrogenase (17β-HSD type 3),** which converts **androstenedione** to **testosterone** (Fig. 43-8).

FATES AND ACTIONS OF ANDROGENS

Intratesticular Androgen

The testosterone produced by Leydig cells has several fates and multiple actions. Because of the proximity of Leydig cells to the seminiferous tubules, significant amounts of testosterone diffuse into the seminiferous tubules and become concentrated within the adluminal compartment by ABP (Fig. 43-8). Testosterone levels within the seminiferous tubules that are greater than 100 times more concentrated than circulating testosterone levels are absolutely required for normal spermatogenesis. As mentioned earlier, Sertoli cells express the enzyme **CYP19 (aromatase),** which converts a small amount of testosterone into the highly potent estrogen **estradiol-17β.** Human sperm cells express at least one isoform of the **estrogen receptor,** and there is some evidence from aromatase-deficient men that this locally produced estrogen optimizes spermatogenesis in humans.

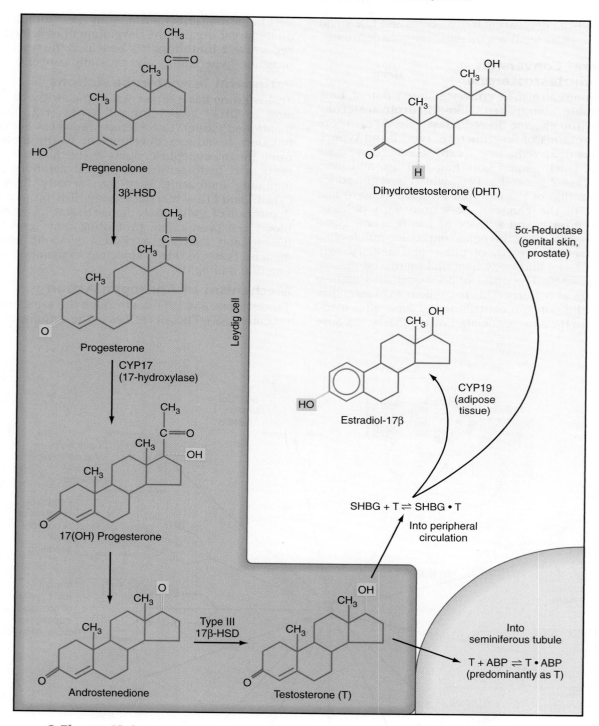

● **Figure 43-8.** Steroidogenic pathway in Leydig cells (the first step of converting cholesterol to pregnenolone is omitted). Testosterone is sequestered by binding to androgen-binding protein (ABP) within the seminiferous tubules or circulates within the peripheral circulation bound to sex hormone–binding globulin (SHBG) and can be peripherally converted to dihydrotestosterone or estradiol-17β. (Modified from Porterfield SP, White BA: Endocrine Physiology, 3rd ed. Philadelphia, Mosby, 2007.)

Peripheral Conversion to Estrogen

In several tissues (especially adipose tissue), testosterone is converted to estrogen (Fig. 43-8). Studies involving men with aromatase deficiency have shown that an inability to produce estrogen results in tall stature because of the lack of epiphyseal closure in long bones and osteoporosis. Thus, peripheral estrogen plays an important role in bone maturation and biology in men. These studies also implicated estrogen in promoting insulin sensitivity, improving lipoprotein profiles (i.e., increasing HDL, decreasing triglycerides and LDL), and exerting negative feedback on pituitary gonadotropins.

Peripheral Conversion to Dihydrotestosterone

Testosterone can also be converted into a potent, **non-aromatizable androgen, 5α-dihydrotestosterone (DHT),** by the enzyme **5α-reductase** (Fig. 43-8). There are two isoforms of 5α-reductase, type 1 and type 2. Major sites of 5α-reductase 2 expression are the male urogenital tract, genital skin, hair follicles, and liver. 5α-Reductase 2 generates DHT, which is required for masculinization of the external genitalia in utero and for many of the changes associated with puberty, including growth and activity of the prostate gland (see later), growth of the penis, darkening and folding of the scrotum, growth of pubic and axillary hair, growth of facial and body hair, and increased muscle mass (Fig. 43-9). The onset of 5α-reductase 1 expression occurs at puberty. This isozyme is expressed primarily in the skin and contributes to sebaceous gland activity and the acne associated with puberty. Because

DHT has strong growth-promoting (i.e., trophic) effects on its target organs, the development of **selective 5α-reductase 2 inhibitors** has benefited the treatment of prostatic hypertrophy and prostatic cancer.

Peripheral Testosterone Actions

Testosterone has a direct action (i.e., without conversion to DHT) in several cell types (Fig. 43-9). As mentioned earlier, testosterone regulates Sertoli cell function. It induces development of the male tract from the mesonephric duct in the absence of 5α-reductase. Testosterone has several metabolic effects, including increasing very low density lipoprotein (VLDL) and LDL while decreasing HDL, promoting the deposition of abdominal adipose tissue, increasing red blood cell production, promoting bone growth and health, and exerting a protein anabolic effect on muscle. Testosterone is sufficient to maintain erectile function and libido.

Mechanism of Androgen Action

Testosterone and DHT act through the same androgen receptor (AR). The AR resides in the cytoplasm bound

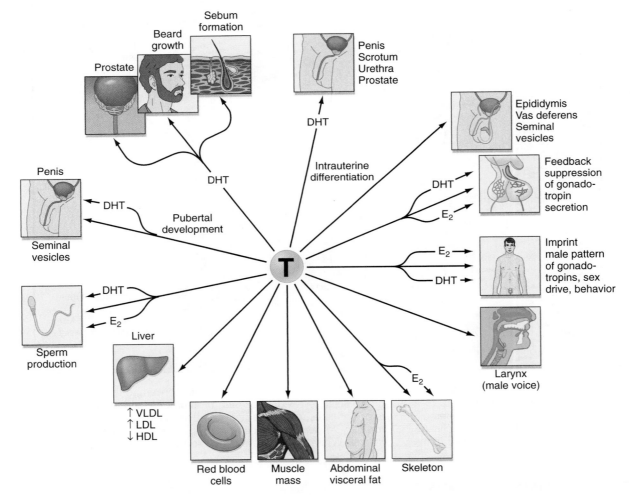

● **Figure 43-9.** Spectrum of effects of testosterone (T). Note that some effects result from the action of testosterone itself, whereas others are mediated by dihydrotestosterone (DHT) and estradiol (E₂) after they are produced from testosterone. VLDL, LDL, HDL, very-low-density, low-density, and high-density lipoproteins, respectively.

to chaperone proteins in the absence of ligand. Testosterone-AR binding or DHT-AR binding causes dissociation of the chaperone proteins, followed by nuclear translocation of the androgen-AR complex, dimerization, binding to an **androgen response element (ARE),** and recruitment of coactivator proteins and general transcription factors to the vicinity of a specific gene's promoter. It remains unclear how testosterone and DHT differ in their ability to activate the AR in the context of different cell types, although the presence of different coactivator proteins in different cell types is probably involved.

Transport and Metabolism of Androgens

As testosterone enters the peripheral circulation, it binds to and quickly reaches equilibrium with serum proteins. About 60% of circulating testosterone is bound to sex hormone–binding globulin (SHBG), 38% is bound to albumin, and about 2% remains as "free" hormone. Testosterone and its metabolites are primarily excreted in urine. Approximately 50% of excreted androgens are found as **urinary 17-ketosteroids,** with most of the remainder being conjugated androgens or diol or triol derivatives. Only about 30% of the 17-ketosteroids in urine are from the testis; the rest are produced from adrenal androgens. Androgens are conjugated with glucuronate or sulfate in the liver, and these **conjugated steroids** are excreted in urine.

HYPOTHALAMIC-PITUITARY-TESTICULAR AXIS

The testis is regulated by an endocrine axis (Fig. 43-10) involving parvicellular hypothalamic **gonadotropin-** releasing hormone (GnRH) neurons and pituitary gonadotropes that produce both luteinizing hormone (LH) and follicle-stimulating hormone (FSH).

Regulation of Leydig Cell Function

The Leydig cell expresses the **LH receptor,** which acts on Leydig cells much like adrenocorticotropic hormone (ACTH) does on zona fasciculata cells in the adrenal cortex (see Chapter 42). Rapid effects include hydrolysis of cholesterol esters and new expression of StAR protein. Less acute effects include an increase in steroidogenic enzyme gene expression and expression of the LDL receptor and SR-BI (the HDL receptor). Over the long term, LH promotes Leydig cell growth and proliferation.

Testosterone negatively feeds back on LH production by the pituitary gonadotrope as testosterone and its metabolites, DHT, and estradiol-17β. All three steroid hormones inhibit the expression of LH-β and the GnRH receptor. These steroids also inhibit the release of GnRH by the hypothalamic neurons (Fig. 43-10).

Regulation of Sertoli Cell Function

The Sertoli cell is stimulated by both testosterone and FSH. In addition to stimulating the synthesis of proteins involved in the "nurse cell" aspect of Sertoli cell function (e.g., ABP), FSH stimulates synthesis of the dimeric protein **inhibin.** Inhibin is induced by FSH and negatively feeds back on the gonadotrope to selectively inhibit FSH production (Fig. 43-10).

THE MALE REPRODUCTIVE TRACT

Once spermatozoa emerge from the efferent ductules, they leave the gonad and enter the male reproductive

● **Figure 43-10.** The hypothalamic-pituitary-testicular axis. Abbreviations as in other figures.

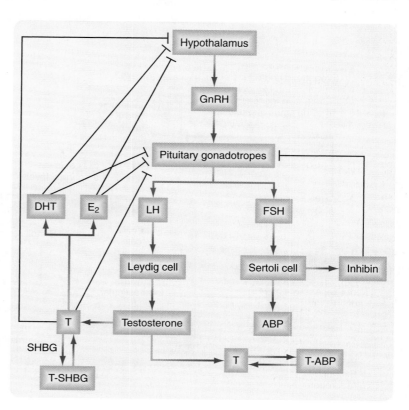

⬤ AT THE CELLULAR LEVEL

There is an important "loophole" in the male reproductive axis that is based on the fact that intratesticular levels of testosterone need to be greater than 100-fold higher than circulating levels of the hormone to maintain normal rates of spermatogenesis; however, it is the circulating levels of testosterone that provide the negative feedback to the pituitary and hypothalamus. This means that exogenous administration of testosterone can raise circulating levels sufficient to inhibit LH but not sufficient to accumulate in the testis at the required concentration for normal spermatogenesis. However, the decreased LH levels will diminish intratesticular production of testosterone by Leydig cells, which results in reduced levels of spermatogenesis (Fig. 43-11). This "loophole" is currently being investigated as a possible strategy for developing a **male oral contraceptive.** It is also the basis for **sterility** in some cases of **steroid abuse** in men.

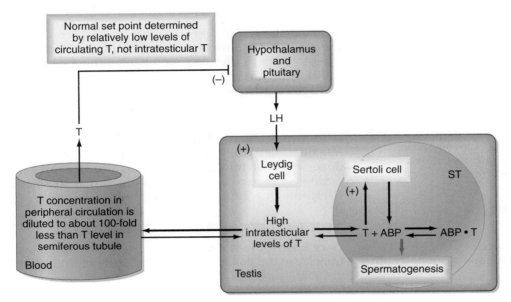

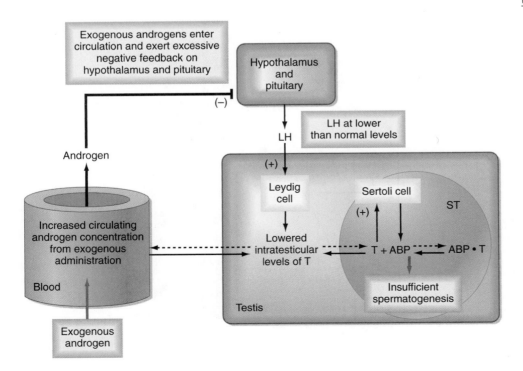

⬤ **Figure 43-11.** The difference in intratesticular testosterone versus circulating testosterone concentrations and its importance in the hypothalamic-pituitary-testis axis. **Upper panel,** Feedback loop in a normal adult man. **Lower panel,** Administration of testosterone (or an androgenic analogue) increases circulating testosterone (androgen) levels, which in turn increase negative feedback on release of LH. Decreased LH levels diminish Leydig cell activity and intratesticular production of androgen. Lowered intratesticular testosterone levels result in reduced sperm production and can cause infertility. Note that the inhibin feedback loop has been omitted from this diagram. (Modified from Porterfield SP, White BA: Endocrine Physiology, 3rd ed. Philadelphia, Mosby, 2007.)

tract (Fig. 43-1). The segments of the tract are as follows: the **epididymis** (**head, body,** and **tail**), the **vas deferens,** the **ejaculatory duct,** the prostatic urethra, the membranous urethra, and the penile urethra. Unlike the female tract, there is a **contiguous lumen** from the seminiferous tubule to the end of the male tract (i.e., the tip of the penile urethra), and the male reproductive tract connects to the **distal urinary tract** (i.e., **male urethra**). In addition to conveying sperm, the primary functions of the male reproductive tract are as follows:

1. *Sperm maturation.* Sperm spend about a month in the epididymis, where they undergo further maturation. The epithelium of the epididymis is secretory and adds numerous components to the seminal fluid. Spermatozoa that enter the head of the epididymis are weakly motile but are strongly unidirectionally motile by the time that they exit the tail. Spermatozoa also undergo the process of **decapacitation,** which involves changes in the cell membrane to prevent spermatozoa from undergoing the acrosome reaction before contact with an egg (see later). Sperm become capacitated by the female reproductive tract within the oviduct. The function of the epididymis is dependent on luminal testosterone-ABP complexes that come from the seminiferous tubules and on testosterone from blood.

2. *Sperm storage and emission.* Sperm are stored in the tail of the epididymis and vas deferens for several months without loss of viability. The primary function of the vas deferens, besides providing a storage site, is to propel sperm during sexual intercourse into the male urethra. The vas deferens has a very thick muscularis that is richly innervated by sympathetic nerves. Normally in response to repeated tactile stimulation of the penis during coitus, the muscularis of the vas deferens receives bursts of sympathetic stimulation that cause peristaltic contractions. Emptying of the contents of the vas deferens into the prostatic urethra is called **emission.** Emission immediately precedes **ejaculation,** which is the propulsion of semen out of the male urethra (see later).

3. *Production and mixing of sperm with seminal contents.* During emission, contraction of the vas deferens coincides with contraction of the muscular coats of the two accessory sex glands, the **seminal vesicles** (right and left) and the **prostate gland** (which surrounds the prostatic urethra). At this point, sperm become mixed with all the components of **semen.** The seminal vesicles secrete approximately 60% of the volume. These glands are the primary source of **fructose,** a critical nutrient for sperm. The seminal vesicles also secrete **semenogelins,** which induce coagulation of semen immediately after ejaculation. The alkaline secretions of the prostate, which make up about 30% of the volume, are high in **citrate, zinc, spermine,** and **acid phosphatase. Prostate-specific antigen (PSA)** is a serine protease that liquefies coagulated semen after a few minutes. PSA can be detected in blood

under conditions of prostatic infection, benign prostatic hypertrophy, and prostatic carcinoma and is currently used as one indicator of prostatic health. The predominant buffers in semen are phosphate and bicarbonate. A third accessory gland, the **bulbourethral glands** (also called Cowper's glands), empty into the penile urethra in response to sexual excitement before emission and ejaculation. This secretion is high in mucus, which lubricates, cleanses, and buffers the urethra. Average sperm counts are between 60 to 100 million/mL semen. Men with sperm counts below 20 million/mL, less than 50% motile sperm, or less than 60% normally conformed sperm are usually infertile.

4. *Erection and ejaculation.* Emission and ejaculation occur during coitus in response to a reflex arc that involves sensory stimulation from the penis (via the pudendal nerve) followed by sympathetic motor stimulation to the smooth muscle of the male tract and somatic motor stimulation to the musculature associated with the base of the penis. However, for sexual intercourse to occur in the first place, the man has to achieve and maintain an **erection** of the **penis.** The penis has evolved as an intromittent organ designed to separate the walls of the vagina, pass through the potential space of the vaginal lumen, and deposit semen at the distal end of the vaginal lumen near the cervix. This process of **internal insemination** can be performed only if the penis is stiffened from the process of erection.

Erection is a neurovascular event. The penis is composed of three erectile bodies: two **corpora cavernosa** and one **corpus spongiosum** (Fig. 43-12, *A*). The penile urethra runs through the corpus spongiosum. These three bodies are composed of **erectile tissue**—an anastomosing network of potential **cavernous vascular spaces** lined with continuous endothelia within a loose connective tissue support. During the **flaccid state,** blood flow to the cavernous spaces is minimal (Fig. 43-12, *A*). This is due to vasoconstriction of the vasculature (called the helicine arteries) and shunting of blood flow away from the cavernous spaces. In

> ### ▶ IN THE CLINIC
>
> An inability to achieve or maintain an erection is termed **erectile dysfunction (ED)** and is one cause of infertility. Multiple factors can lead to ED, including insufficient androgen production; neurovascular damage (e.g., from diabetes mellitus, spinal cord injury); structural damage to the penis, perineum, or pelvis; psychogenic factors (e.g., depression, performance anxiety); and prescribed medications and recreational drugs, including alcohol and tobacco. A major development in the treatment of some forms of erectile dysfunction is the use of selective cGMP phosphodiesterase inhibitors (e.g., **Viagra**), which assist in the maintenance of an erection (Fig. 43-12, *B*).

response to sexual arousal, the parasympathetic cavernous nerves innervating the vascular smooth muscle of the helicine arteries release nitric oxide (NO). NO activates guanylyl cyclase, thereby increasing cGMP, which decreases intracellular $[Ca^{++}]$ and causes muscular relaxation (Fig. 43-12, *B*). The vasodilation allows blood to flow into the cavernous spaces to induce engorgement and erection. It also presses on veins in the penis and reduces venous drainage (Fig. 43-12, *B*).

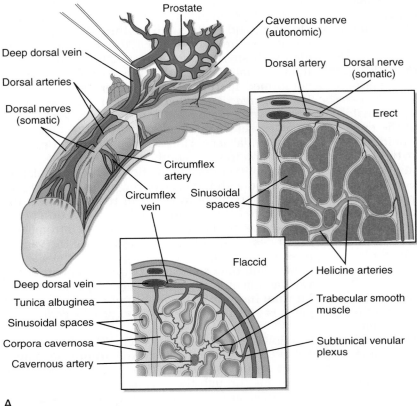

A

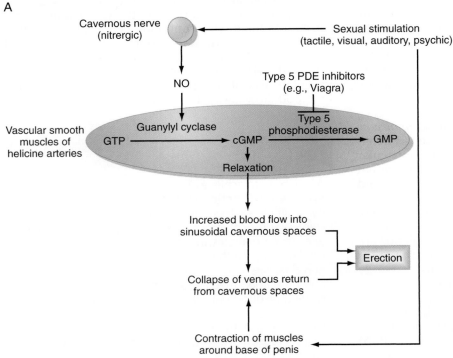

B

● **Figure 43-12.** **A,** Arrangement of the vasculature and cavernous tissue within the penis. During the flaccid state, blood flow into the cavernous spaces is limited by contraction of the helicine arteries. (From Bhasun S et al. In Larsen P et al [eds]: Williams Textbook of Endocrinology, 10th ed. Philadelphia, Saunders, 2003.) **B,** Outline of neurovascular events leading to penile erection.

ANDROPAUSE

There is no distinct **andropause** in men. However, as men age, gonadal sensitivity to LH decreases and androgen production drops. As this occurs, serum LH and FSH levels rise. Although sperm production typically begins to decline after 50 years of age, many men can maintain reproductive function and spermatogenesis throughout life.

THE FEMALE REPRODUCTIVE SYSTEM

The female reproductive system is composed of the gonads, called **ovaries,** and the female reproductive tract, which includes the **oviducts, uterus, cervix, vagina,** and **external genitalia.**

THE OVARY

The ovary is located within a fold of peritoneum called the **broad ligament,** usually close to the lateral wall of the pelvic cavity (Fig. 43-13). Because the ovary extends into the peritoneal cavity, ovulated eggs briefly reside within the peritoneal cavity before they are captured by the oviducts.

The ovary is divided into an outer cortex and inner medulla (Fig. 43-14). Neurovascular elements innervate the medulla of the ovary. The cortex of the ovary is composed of a densely cellular stroma. Within this stroma reside the **ovarian follicles** (Fig. 43-14), which

contain a primary oocyte surrounded by follicle cells. The cortex is covered by a connective tissue capsule, the tunica albuginea, and a layer of simple epithelium consisting of **ovarian surface epithelial cells.** There are no ducts emerging from the ovary to convey its gametes to the reproductive tract. Thus, the process of ovulation involves an inflammatory event that erodes the wall of the ovary. After ovulation, the ovarian surface epithelial cells rapidly divide to repair the wall.

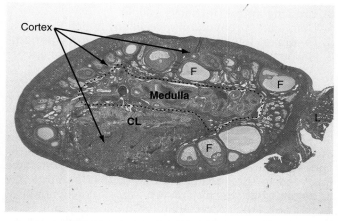

● **Figure 43-14.** Histology of the ovary. CL, corpus luteum; F, follicle; (Modified from Young B et al: Wheater's Functional Histology. A Text and Colour Atlas, 5th ed. London, Churchill Livingstone, 2006.)

● **Figure 43-13.** Anatomy of the female reproductive system. (Modified from Drake RL et al: Gray's Anatomy for Students. Philadelphia, Churchill Livingstone, 2005.)

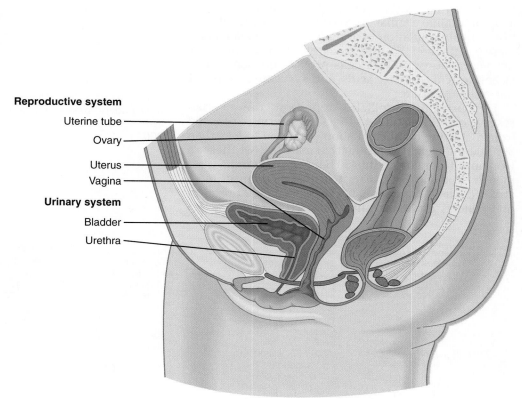

Reproductive system
Uterine tube
Ovary
Uterus
Vagina

Urinary system
Bladder
Urethra

Growth, Development, and Function of the Ovarian Follicle

The ovarian follicle is the functional unit of the ovary, and it performs both gametogenic and endocrine functions. A histological section of the ovary from a premenopausal cycling woman contains follicular structures at many different stages of development. The life history of a follicle can be divided into the following stages:

1. Resting primordial follicle
2. Growing preantral (primary and secondary) follicle
3. Growing antral (tertiary) follicle
4. Dominant (preovulatory, graafian) follicle
5. Dominant follicle within the periovulatory period
6. Corpus luteum (of menstruation or of pregnancy)
7. Atretic follicles

Resting Primordial Follicle

Growth and Structure. Resting primordial follicles (Fig. 43-15) represent the earliest and simplest follicular structure in the ovary. Primordial follicles appear during midgestation through the interaction of gametes and somatic cells. Primordial germ cells that have migrated to the gonad continue to divide mitotically as oogonia until the fifth month of gestation in humans. At this point the approximately 7 million oogonia enter the process of meiosis and become **primary oocytes.** During this time the primary oocytes become surrounded by a simple epithelium of somatic **follicle cells,** thereby creating the primordial follicles (Fig. 43-15). The follicle cells establish **gap junctions** with each other and the oocyte. The follicle cells themselves represent a true avascular epithelium surrounded by a basal lamina. Similar to Sertoli cell–sperm interactions, a subpopulation of granulosa cells remains intimately attached to the oocytes throughout their development. Granulosa cells provide nutrients such as amino acids, nucleic acids, and pyruvate to support oocyte maturation.

The primordial follicles represent the ovarian reserve of follicles (Fig. 43-16). This reserve is reduced from a starting number of about 7 million to less than 300,000 follicles at reproductive maturity. Of these, a woman will ovulate about 450 between menarche (first menstrual cycle) and menopause (cessation of menstrual cycles). At menopause, less than 1000 primordial follicles are left in the ovary. Primordial follicles

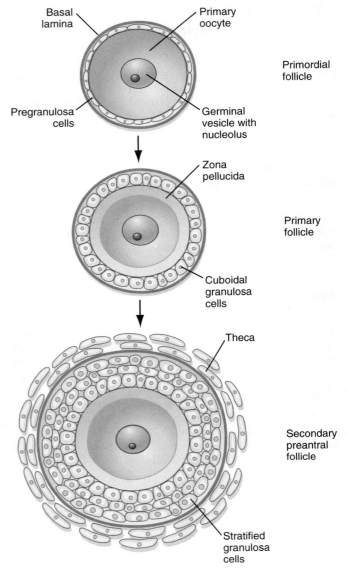

● **Figure 43-15.** Development of a primordial follicle up to a secondary, preantral follicle. (Modified from Porterfield SP, White BA: Endocrine Physiology, 3rd ed. Philadelphia, Mosby, 2007.)

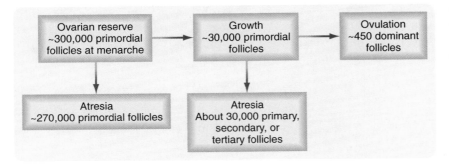

● **Figure 43-16.** Fate of ovarian follicles. (Modified from Porterfield SP, White BA: Endocrine Physiology, 3rd ed. Philadelphia, Mosby, 2007.)

are lost primarily from death as a result of follicular atresia. However, a small subset of primordial follicles will enter follicular growth in waves. Because the ovarian follicular reserve represents a fixed, finite number, the rate at which resting primordial follicles die or begin to develop (or both) will determine the reproductive life span of a woman. Age at the onset of menopause has a strong genetic component but is also influenced by environmental factors. For example, cigarette smoking significantly depletes the ovarian reserve. An overly rapid rate of atresia or development will deplete the reserve and give rise to premature ovarian failure.

Pituitary gonadotropins maintain a normal ovarian reserve by promoting the general health of the ovary. However, the rate at which resting primordial follicles enter the growth process appears to be independent of pituitary gonadotropins. The decision of a resting follicle to enter the early growth phase is primarily dependent on intraovarian paracrine factors that are produced by both the follicle cells and oocytes.

The Gamete. In primordial follicles, the gamete is derived from oogonia that have entered the first meiotic division; such oogonia are referred to as primary oocytes. Primary oocytes progress through most of prophase of the first meiotic division (termed prophase I) over a 2-week period and then arrest in the **diplotene** stage. This stage is characterized by the decondensation of chromatin, which supports the transcription needed for oocyte maturation. Meiotic arrest at this stage, which may last for up to 50 years, appears to be due to "maturational incompetence," or lack of the cell cycle proteins needed to support the completion of meiosis. The nucleus of the oocyte, called the **germinal vesicle,** remains intact at this stage.

Growing Preantral Follicles

Growth and Structure. The first stage of follicular growth is **preantral,** which refers to the development that occurs before the formation of a fluid-filled **antral cavity.** One of the first visible signs of follicle growth is the appearance of cuboidal granulosa cells. At this point the follicle is referred to as a **primary follicle** (Fig. 43-15). As granulosa cells proliferate, they form a multilayered (i.e., stratified) epithelium around the oocyte. At this stage the follicle is referred to as a **secondary follicle** (Fig. 43-15).

Once a secondary follicle acquires three to six layers of granulosa cells, it secretes paracrine factors that induce nearby stromal cells to differentiate into epithelioid **thecal cells.** Thecal cells form a flattened layer of cells around the follicle. Once a thecal layer forms, the follicle is referred to as a **mature preantral follicle** (Fig. 43-15). In humans it takes several months for a primary follicle to reach the mature preantral stage.

Follicular development is associated with an inward movement of the follicle from the outer cortex to the inner cortex, closer to the vasculature of the ovarian medulla. Follicles release angiogenic factors that induce the development of one to two arterioles that form a vascular wreath around the follicle.

The Gamete. During the preantral stage, the oocyte begins to grow and produce cellular and secreted proteins. The oocyte initiates secretion of extracellular matrix glycoproteins, called **ZP1, ZP2,** and **ZP3,** that form the **zona pellucida** (Fig. 43-15). The zona pellucida increases in thickness and provides a species-specific binding site for sperm during fertilization (see later). Importantly, granulosa cells and the oocyte maintain gap junctional contact via cellular projections through the zona pellucida. The oocyte also continues to secrete paracrine factors that regulate follicle cell growth and differentiation.

Endocrine Function. Granulosa cells express the **FSH receptor** during this period, but they are primarily dependent on factors from the oocyte to grow. They do not produce ovarian hormones at this early stage of follicular development. The newly acquired thecal cells are analogous to testicular Leydig cells in that they reside outside the epithelial "nurse" cells, express the **LH receptor,** and produce **androgens.** The main difference between Leydig cells and thecal cells is that thecal cells do not express high levels of 17β-HSD. Thus, the major product of theca cells is **androstenedione,** as opposed to testosterone. Androstenedione production at this stage is minimal.

Growing Antral Follicles

Growth and Structure. Mature preantral follicles develop into **early antral follicles** (Fig. 43-17) over a period of about 25 days, during which they grow from a diameter of about 0.1 mm to a diameter of 0.2 mm. Once the granulosa epithelium increases to six to seven layers, fluid-filled spaces appear between cells and coalesce into the **antrum.** Over a period of about 45 days, this wave of small antral follicles will continue to grow to large, recruitable antral follicles that are 2 to 5 mm in diameter. This period of growth is characterized by about a 100-fold increase in granulosa cells (from about 10,000 to 1,000,000 cells). It is also characterized by swelling of the antral cavity, which increasingly divides the granulosa cells into two discrete populations (Fig. 43-17).

Mural granulosa cells (also called the **stratum granulosum**) form the outer wall of the follicle. The basal layer is adherent to the basal lamina and in close proximity to the outer-lying thecal layers. Mural granulosa cells become highly steroidogenic and remain in the ovary after ovulation to differentiate into the corpus luteum.

Cumulus cells are the inner cells that surround the oocyte (they are also referred to as **the cumulus oophorus** and **corona radiata**). The innermost layer of cumulus cells maintains gap and adhesion junctions with the oocyte. Cumulus cells are released with the oocyte (collectively referred to as the **cumulus-oocyte complex**) during the process of ovulation. Cumulus cells are crucial for the ability of the fimbriated end of the oviduct to "capture" and move the oocyte by a ciliary transport mechanism along the length of the oviduct to the site of fertilization (see later).

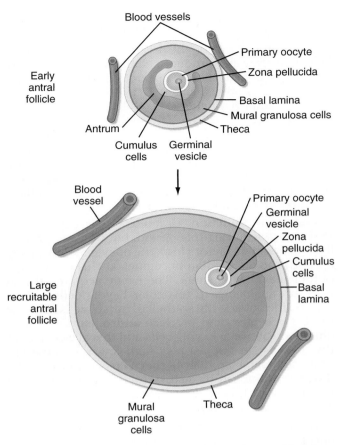

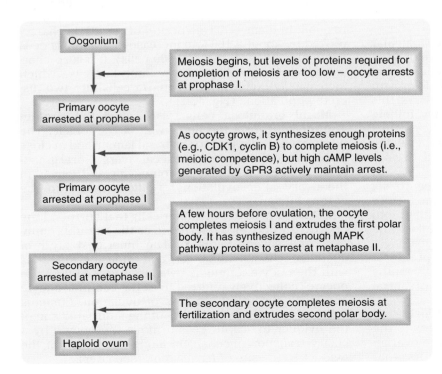

Early antral follicles are dependent on pituitary FSH for normal growth. Large antral follicles become highly dependent on pituitary FSH for their growth and sustained viability. As discussed later, 2- to 5-mm follicles are recruited to enter a rapid growth phase via the transient increase in FSH that occurs toward the end of the previous menstrual cycle.

The Gamete. The oocyte grows rapidly in the early stages of antral follicles—growth then slows in larger follicles. During the antral stage, the oocyte synthesizes sufficient amounts of cell cycle components so that it becomes competent to complete meiosis I at ovulation (note that the human egg arrests after ovulation at a second point, metaphase II, until it is fertilized by sperm). Thus, in early primary and secondary follicles, the oocyte fails to complete meiosis I because of a dearth of specific meiosis-associated proteins. However, larger antral follicles gain **meiotic competence** but still maintain **meiotic arrest** until the midcycle LH surge. Meiotic arrest is achieved by maintenance of elevated cAMP levels in the mature oocyte (Figs. 43-18 and 43-19).

Endocrine Function. The thecal cells of large antral follicles produce significant amounts of androstenedione and testosterone. Androgens are converted to estradiol-17β by the granulosa cells (see later). However, at this stage, FSH stimulates the proliferation of granulosa cells and induces the expression of CYP19 (aromatase) required for the synthesis of estrogen. Additionally, the mural granulosa cells of the large antral follicles produce increasing amounts of **inhibin B** during the early follicular phase. Low levels of estrogen and inhibin negatively feed back on FSH secretion, thereby contributing to selection of the follicle with the most FSH-responsive cells.

● **Figure 43-17.** Development of an early antral follicle to a mature preovulatory follicle. (Modified from Porterfield SP, White BA: Endocrine Physiology, 3rd ed. Philadelphia, Mosby, 2007.)

● **Figure 43-18.** Events involved in meiotic arrest and maturation of the oocyte. MAPK, mitogen-activated protein kinase. (Modified from Porterfield SP, White BA: Endocrine Physiology, 3rd ed. Philadelphia, Mosby, 2007.)

Dominant Follicle

Growth and Structure. At the end of a previous menstrual cycle, a crop of large (2 to 5 mm) antral follicles (Fig. 43-17) are **recruited** to begin rapid, gonadotropin-dependent development. The total number of recruited follicles in both ovaries can be as high as 20 in a younger woman (<33 years old) but rapidly declines at older ages. The number of recruited folli-

cles is reduced to the **prolifera quota** (one in humans) by the process of selection. As FSH levels decline, the rapidly growing follicles progressively undergo atresia until one follicle is left. Generally, the largest follicle with the most FSH receptors of the recruited crop becomes the **dominant follicle.** Selection occurs during the early follicular phase. By midcycle, the dominant follicle becomes a large **preovulatory follicle** that is 20 mm in diameter and contains about 50 million granulosa cells by the midcycle gonadotropin surge.

The Gamete. The oocyte is competent to complete meiosis I but remains arrested in the dominant follicle until the LH surge. Growth of the oocyte continues, but at a slower rate, until the oocyte reaches a diameter of about 140 μm by ovulation.

Endocrine Function. The newly selected follicle emerges for the first time during its development as a significant steroidogenic "gland." Ovarian steroidogenesis requires both theca and granulosa cells (Fig. 43-20). As discussed earlier, thecal cells express **LH receptors** and produce androgens. Basal levels of LH stimulate the expression of steroidogenic enzymes, as well as the **LDL receptor** and **HDL receptor (SR-B1)**, in the theca. Thecal cells show robust expression of **CYP11A1** (side chain cleavage enzyme), **3β-HSD,** and **CYP17** with both 17-hydroxylase activity and 17,20-lyase activity. Androgens (primarily **androstenedione** but also some **testosterone**) released from the theca diffuse into the mural granulosa cells or enter the vasculature surrounding the follicle.

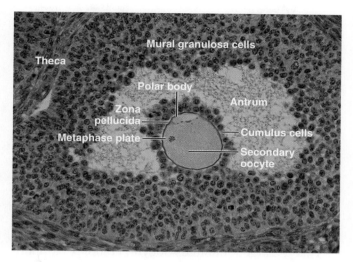

● **Figure 43-19.** Histology of an abnormal, unovulated secondary oocyte in a medium-sized antral follicle from a GPR3 knockout mouse. (Modified from Mehlmann LM et al: Science 306:1947, 2004, with permission.)

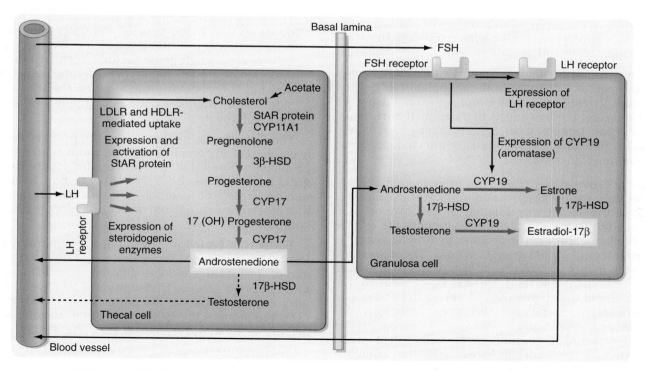

● **Figure 43-20.** Two-cell model for steroidogenesis in the dominant follicle. (Modified from Porterfield SP, White BA: Endocrine Physiology, 3rd ed. Philadelphia, Mosby, 2007.)

The mural granulosa cells of the selected follicle have a high number of **FSH receptors** and are very sensitive to FSH, which up-regulates **CYP19 (aromatase)** gene expression and activity (Fig. 43-20). CYP19 converts androstenedione to the weak estrogen **estrone** and converts testosterone to the potent estrogen **estradiol-17β.** Granulosa cells express activating isoforms of **17β-HSD,** which ultimately drives steroidogenesis toward the production of estradiol-17β. In addition, FSH induces the expression of inhibin B during the follicular phase.

Importantly, FSH also induces the expression of LH receptors in mural granulosa cells during the second half of the follicular phase (Fig. 43-20). Thus, mural granulosa cells become responsive to both gonadotropins, which allows these cells to maintain high levels of CYP19 in the face of declining FSH levels. Acquisition of LH receptors also ensures that mural granulosa cells respond to the LH surge.

The Dominant Follicle during the Periovulatory Period

The **periovulatory period** is defined as the time from the onset of the LH surge to expulsion of the cumulus-oocyte complex out of the ovary (i.e., ovulation). This process lasts for 32 to 36 hours in women. Starting at the same time and superimposed on the process of ovulation is a change in the steroidogenic function of theca and mural granulosa cells. This process is called **luteinization** and culminates in the formation of a **corpus luteum** that is capable of producing high amounts of **progesterone,** along with estrogen, within a few days after ovulation. Thus, the LH surge induces the onset of complex processes during the periovulatory period that complete the gametogenic function of the ovary for a given month and switches the endocrine function to prepare the female reproductive tract for implantation and gestation.

Growth and Structure. The LH surge induces dramatic structural changes in the dominant follicle that involves its rupture, ovulation of the cumulus-oocyte complex, and the biogenesis of a new structure called the **corpus luteum** from the remaining thecal and mural granulosa cells. Major structural changes occur during this transition:

1. Before ovulation, the large preovulatory follicle presses against the ovarian surface and generates a poorly vascularized bulge of the ovarian wall called the **stigma.** The LH surge induces the release of inflammatory cytokines and hydrolytic enzymes from the theca and granulosa cells. These secreted components lead to breakdown of the follicle wall, tunica albuginea, and surface epithelium in the vicinity of the stigma (Fig. 43-21). At the end of this process, the antral cavity becomes continuous with the peritoneal cavity.
2. The attachment of the cumulus cells to the mural granulosa cells degenerates, and the cumulus-oocyte complex becomes free-floating within the antral cavity (Fig. 43-21). Cumulus cells also respond to the LH surge by secreting hyaluronic acid and

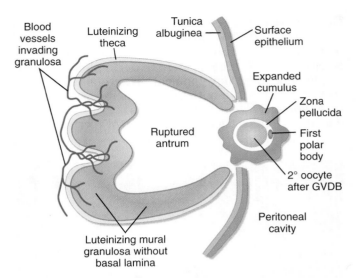

● **Figure 43-21.** Ovulation. (Modified from Porterfield SP, White BA: Endocrine Physiology, 3rd ed. Philadelphia, Mosby, 2007.)

other extracellular matrix components. These substances enlarge the entire cumulus-oocyte complex, a process called **cumulus expansion** (Fig. 43-21). This enlarged cumulus-oocyte complex is more easily captured and transported by the oviduct. The expanded cumulus also makes the cumulus-oocyte complex easier for spermatozoa to find. Sperm express a **membrane hyaluronidase** that allows them to penetrate the expanded cumulus. The cumulus-oocyte complex is released through the ruptured stigma in a slow, gentle process.

3. The basal lamina of mural granulosa cells is broken down so that blood vessels and outer-lying theca cells can push into the granulosa cells. Granulosa cells secrete **angiogenic factors,** such as vascular endothelial growth factor (VEGF), angiopoietin 2, and basic fibroblast growth factor (bFGF), which significantly increase the blood supply to the new corpus luteum.

The Gamete. Before ovulation, the primary oocyte is competent to complete meiosis, but it is arrested in prophase I. The LH surge induces the oocyte to progress to metaphase II (Fig. 43-18). The oocyte subsequently arrests at metaphase II until fertilization. LH receptors are present on mural granulosa cells, not cumulus cells.

Endocrine Function. Both theca and mural granulosa cells express LH receptors at the time of the LH surge. The LH surge induces differentiation of the granulosa cells—a process that continues for several days after ovulation. During the periovulatory period, the LH surge induces the following shifts in steroidogenic activity of the mural granulosa cells (Fig. 43-22):

1. _Transient inhibition of CYP19 expression and, consequently, estrogen production._ The rapid decline in estrogen helps turn off the positive feedback on LH secretion.

● **Figure 43-22.** Steroidogenic pathways in the corpus luteum. (Modified from Porterfield SP, White BA: Endocrine Physiology, 3rd ed. Philadelphia, Mosby, 2007.)

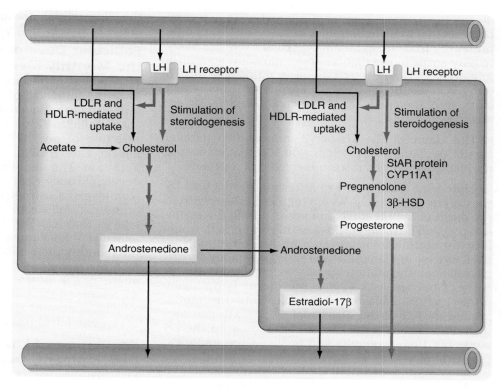

2. *Breakdown of the basal lamina and vascularization of the granulosa cells.* This makes LDL and HDL cholesterol accessible to these cells for steroidogenesis. The LH surge also increases expression of the LDL receptor and HDL receptor (SR-BI) in granulosa cells.

3. *Increased expression of StAR protein, CYP11A1 (side chain cleavage enzyme), and 3β-HSD.* Because CYP17 activity, especially its 17,20-lyase function, is largely absent in granulosa cells, these cells begin to secrete progesterone, and progesterone levels gradually increase over the next week.

The Corpus Luteum

Growth and Structure. After ovulation, the remnant of the antral cavity fills with blood from damaged blood vessels in the vicinity of the stigma. This gives rise to a **corpus hemorrhagicum** (Fig. 43-23). Within a few days, red blood cells and debris are removed by macrophages, and fibroblasts fill in the antral cavity with a hyaline-like extracellular matrix. In the mature **corpus luteum,** the granulosa cells, now called **granulosa lutein cells,** enlarge and become filled with lipid (cholesterol esters). The enlarged granulosa lutein cells collapse into and partially fill in the old antral cavity. Proliferation of these cells is very limited. The theca, along with blood vessels, mast cells, macrophages, leukocytes, and other resident connective tissue cells, infiltrate the granulosa layer at multiple sites.

The human corpus luteum is programmed to live for 14 days, plus or minus 2 days **(corpus luteum of menstruation),** unless "rescued" by the LH-like hormone **human chorionic gonadotropin (hCG),**

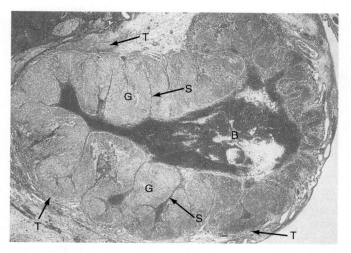

● **Figure 43-23.** Histology of an early corpus luteum, called a corpus hemorrhagicum. B, blood clot in the former antral space; G, luteinized granulosa cells; S, septa of connective tissue cells and blood vessels within the granulosa layer; T, luteinized theca cells. (From Young B et al: Wheater's Functional Histology. A Text and Colour Atlas, 5th ed. London, Churchill Livingstone, 2006.)

which originates from an implanting embryo. If rescued, the **corpus luteum of pregnancy** will remain viable during the pregnancy (usually about 9 months). The mechanism by which the corpus luteum of menstruation regresses in 14 days is not fully understood. Regression appears to involve release of the **prostaglandin PGF$_{2α}$** from both granulosa lutein cells and the uterus in response to declining levels of progesterone during the second week of the luteal phase. Several paracrine factors (endothelin, monocyte chemotactic protein-1) from immune and vascular cells are likely to play a role in the demise and removal of granulosa lutein cells. The corpus luteum is ultimately turned into a scar-like body called the **corpus albicans,** which sinks into the medulla of the ovary and is slowly absorbed.

The Gamete. The LH surge induces two parallel events, ovulation and luteinization. If ovulation occurs normally, the corpus luteum is devoid of a gamete.

Endocrine Function. Progesterone production by the corpus luteum (Fig. 43-22) increases steadily from the onset of the LH surge and peaks during the midluteal phase. The main purpose of this timing is to transform the uterine lining into an adhesive and supportive structure for implantation and early pregnancy. As discussed later, the midluteal phase is synchronized with early embryogenesis so that the uterus is optimally primed when a blastocyst tumbles into the uterus around day 22 of the menstrual cycle. Estrogen production transiently decreases in response to the LH surge but then rebounds and peaks at the midluteal phase.

Luteal hormonal output is absolutely dependent on basal LH levels (Fig. 43-22). In fact, progesterone output is closely correlated with the pulsatile pattern of LH release in women. Both FSH and LH are reduced to basal levels during the luteal phase by negative feedback from progesterone and estrogen. In addition, granulosa lutein cells secrete **inhibin A,** which selectively represses FSH secretion. The elevated estrogen levels at the midluteal phase may be responsible for the decrease in sensitivity of the corpus luteum to LH, so progesterone and estrogen levels decline during the second half of the luteal phase unless an increase in circulating LH-like activity (i.e., in the form of hCG) compensates for the decreased sensitivity to LH.

The corpus luteum must generate large amounts of progesterone to support implantation and early pregnancy. Accordingly, the life of the corpus luteum is very regular, and a shortened luteal phase typically leads to infertility. The quality of the corpus luteum is largely dependent on the size and health of the dominant follicle from which it developed, which in turn is dependent on normal hypothalamic and pituitary stimulation during the follicular phase. Numerous factors that perturb hypothalamic and pituitary output during the follicular phase, including heavy exercise, starvation, high prolactin levels, and abnormal thyroid function, can lead to **luteal phase deficiency** and **infertility.**

Atretic Follicles

Follicular atresia refers to the demise of an ovarian follicle. During atresia, the granulosa cells and oocytes undergo **apoptosis.** The thecal cells typically persist and repopulate the cellular stroma of the ovary. The thecal cells retain LH receptors and the ability to produce androgens and are collectively referred to as the **"interstitial gland"** of the ovary. Follicles can undergo atresia at any time during development.

Follicular Development with Respect to the Monthly Menstrual Cycle

The first half of the monthly menstrual cycle is referred to as the **follicular phase** of the ovary and is characterized by the recruitment and growth of 15 to 20 large antral follicles (2 to 5 mm in diameter), followed by selection of one of these follicles as the dominant follicle and growth of the dominant follicle until ovulation. The dominant follicle must contain a fully developed oocyte and somatic follicle cells that secrete high levels of estrogen. It takes several months for a primordial follicle to reach the size of a large antral follicle that can be recruited. Therefore, much of follicular development occurs independently of the monthly menstrual cycle. The second half of the monthly menstrual cycle is referred to as the **luteal phase** of the ovary and is dominated by hormonal secretions of the corpus luteum. Nevertheless, small follicles continue to develop within the ovarian stroma during the luteal phase.

Regulation of Late Follicular Development, Ovulation, and Luteinization: The Human Menstrual Cycle

As stated earlier, late follicular development and luteal function are absolutely dependent on normal hypothalamic and pituitary function. As in the male, hypothalamic neurons secrete GnRH in a pulsatile manner. GnRH, in turn, stimulates LH and FSH production by pituitary gonadotropes. A high frequency of GnRH pulses (1 pulse per 60 to 90 minutes) selectively promotes LH production, whereas a slow frequency promotes FSH production. A major difference between the male and female reproductive axes is the midcycle gonadotropin surge, which is dependent on a constant, high level of estrogen coming from the dominant follicle.

A highly dynamic "conversation" occurs among the ovary, pituitary, and hypothalamus in which the events of the menstrual cycle are orchestrated, beginning with the ovary at the end of the luteal phase of a previous, nonfertile cycle (Fig. 43-24):

Event 1: In the absence of fertilization and implantation, the corpus luteum regresses and dies (called **luteolysis**). This leads to a dramatic decline in levels of progesterone, estrogen, and inhibin A by day 24 of the menstrual cycle.

Event 2: The gonadotrope perceives the end of luteal function as a release from negative feedback. This permits a rise in FSH about 2 days before the onset of menstruation. The basis for the selective increase in FSH is incompletely understood, but it may be due to the slow frequency of GnRH pulses during the luteal phase, which in turn is due to high progesterone levels.

Event 3: The rise in FSH levels recruits a crop of large (2 to 5 mm) antral follicles to begin rapid, highly gonadotropin-dependent growth. These follicles produce low levels of estrogen and inhibin B.

● **Figure 43-24.** The human menstrual cycle, with emphasis on the "dialogue" between ovary and pituitary gonadotropes.

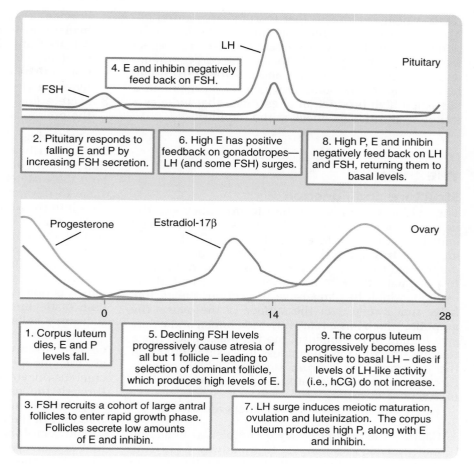

Event 4: The gonadotrope responds to the slowly rising levels of estrogen and inhibin B by decreasing FSH secretion. Loss of high levels of progesterone and estrogen causes an increase in the frequency of GnRH pulses, thereby selectively increasing LH synthesis and secretion by the gonadotrope. Thus, the LH/FSH ratio slowly increases throughout the follicular phase.

Event 5: The ovary's response to declining FSH levels is follicular atresia of all of the recruited follicles, except for one dominant follicle. Thus, the process of selection is driven by an extreme dependency of follicles on FSH in the face of declining FSH secretion. Usually, only the largest follicle with the most FSH receptors and best blood supply can survive. This follicle produces increasing amounts of estradiol-17β and inhibin B. FSH also induces the expression of LH receptors in the mural granulosa cells of the dominant follicle.

Event 6: Once the dominant follicle causes circulating estrogen levels to exceed 200 pg/mL for about 50 hours in women, estrogen exerts a positive feedback on the gonadotrope to produce the midcycle LH surge. This is enhanced by the small amount of progesterone secreted at midcycle. The exact mechanism of the positive feedback is unknown, but it occurs largely at the level of the pituitary. **GnRH receptors** and the sensitivity to GnRH signaling

increase dramatically in the gonadotropes. The hypothalamus contributes to the gonadotropin surge by increasing the frequency of GnRH pulses and the secretion of a small amount of progesterone.

Event 7: The LH surge drives meiotic maturation, ovulation, and differentiation of granulosa cells into progesterone-producing cells.

Event 8: Rising levels of progesterone, estrogen, and inhibin A by the mature corpus luteum negatively feed back on the pituitary gonadotrope. Even though estrogen levels exceed the 200-pg/mL threshold for positive feedback, the high progesterone levels block any positive feedback. Consequently, both FSH and LH levels decline to basal levels.

Event 9: Basal levels of LH (but not FSH) are absolutely required for normal corpus luteum function. However, the corpus luteum becomes progressively insensitive to LH signaling and will die unless LH-like activity (i.e., hCG from an implanted embryo) increases. In a nonfertile cycle, the corpus luteum of menstruation will regress in 14 days, and progesterone and estrogen levels will start to decline by about 10 days, thereby cycling back to event 1.

From this sequence of events it is evident that the ovary is the primary clock for the menstrual cycle. The timing of the two main pituitary-based events—

the transient rise in FSH that recruits large antral follicles and the LH surge that induces ovulation—is determined by two ovarian events. These are respectively the highly regular life span of the corpus luteum and its demise after 14 days and growth of the dominant follicle to the point at which it can maintain a sustained high production of estrogen that induces a switch to positive feedback at the pituitary.

THE OVIDUCT

Structure and Function

The **oviducts** (also called the **uterine tubes** and the **fallopian tubes)** are muscular tubes with the distal ends close to the surface of each ovary and the proximal ends traversing the wall of the uterus. The oviducts are divided into four sections (going from distal to proximal): the **infundibulum,** or open end of the oviduct, which has finger-like projections called **fimbriae** that sweep over the surface of the ovary; the **ampulla,** which has a relatively wide lumen and extensive folding of the mucosa; the **isthmus,** which has a relatively narrow lumen and less mucosal folding; and the **intramural** or **uterine segment,** which extends through the uterine wall at the superior corners of the uterus (Fig. 43-25).

The main functions of the oviducts are to

1. Capture the cumulus-oocyte complex at ovulation and transfer the complex to a midway point (the **ampullary-isthmus junction**), where fertilization takes place. Oviductal secretions coat and infuse the cumulus-oocyte complex and may be required for viability and fertilizability.

2. Provide a site for sperm storage. Women who ovulate up to 5 days after sexual intercourse can get pregnant. Sperm remain viable by adhering to the epithelial cells lining the isthmus. The secretions of the oviduct also induce capacitation and hyperactivity of sperm.

3. Secrete fluids that provide nutritional support to the preimplantation embryo.

The timing of movement of the embryo into the uterus is critical because the uterus has an implantation window of about 3 days. The oviduct needs to hold the early embryo until it reaches the blastocyst stage (5 days after fertilization) and then allow it to pass into the uterine cavity.

The wall of the oviduct is composed of a mucosa (called the **endosalpinx**), a two-layered muscularis (called the **myosalpinx**), and an outer-lying connective tissue (the **perisalpinx**). The endosalpinx is thrown into many folds, almost to the extent that the lumen is obliterated, and is lined by a simple epithelium made up of two cell types: **ciliated cells** and **secretory cells.** The cilia are most numerous at the infundibular end and propel the cumulus-oocyte complex toward the uterus. The cilia on the fimbriae are the sole mechanism for transport of the ovulated cumulus-oocyte complex. Once the complex passes through the ostium of the oviduct and enters the ampulla, it is moved by both cilia and peristaltic contractions of the muscularis.

The secretory cells produce a protein-rich mucus that is conveyed along the oviduct to the uterus by the cilia. This ciliary-mucus escalator maintains a healthy epithelium, moves the cumulus-oocyte complex toward the uterus, and may provide directional cues for swimming sperm. Movement of the

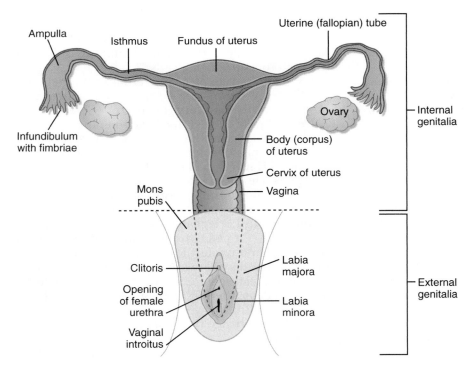

● **Figure 43-25.** Schematic of the female reproductive system. (Modified from Porterfield SP, White BA: Endocrine Physiology, 3rd ed. Philadelphia, Mosby, 2007.)

cumulus-oocyte complex slows at the ampullary-isthmus junction, where fertilization normally takes place. This appears to be due, in part, to thick mucus produced by the isthmus and increased tone of the muscularis of the isthmus. The composition of oviductal secretions is complex and includes growth factors, enzymes, and oviduct-specific glycoproteins. Note that the clinical process of in vitro fertilization has shown that secretions of the oviduct are not absolutely necessary for fertility. However, normal oviductal function is absolutely required for both fertilization and implantation after in vivo insemination. Normal oviductal function also minimizes the risk of **ectopic implantation** and **pregnancy.**

Hormonal Regulation during the Menstrual Cycle

In general, estrogen secreted during the follicular phase increases epithelial cell size and height in the endosalpinx. Estrogen increases blood flow to the lamina propria of the oviducts, promotes the production of oviduct-specific glycoproteins (whose functions are poorly understood), and increases ciliogenesis throughout the oviduct. Estrogen promotes the secretion of thick mucus in the isthmus and increases the tone of the muscularis of the isthmus, thereby keeping the cumulus-oocyte complex at the ampullary-isthmus junction for fertilization. High progesterone, along with estrogen, during the early luteal to midluteal phase decreases epithelial cell size and function. Progesterone promotes deciliation. It also decreases the secretion of thick mucus and relaxes the tone in the isthmus. In addition, it should be noted that oviductal epithelial cells express the LH receptor, which may synergize with estrogen to optimize oviductal function during the periovulatory period.

THE UTERUS

Structure and Function

The **uterus** is a single organ that sits in the midline of the pelvic cavity between the bladder and the rectum (Fig. 43-13). The mucosa of the uterus is called the **endometrium;** the three-layered, thick muscularis is called the **myometrium;** and the outer connective tissue and serosa are called the **perimetrium.** The parts of the uterus are (1) the **fundus,** which is the portion that rises superiorly from the entrance of the oviducts; (2) the **body** of the uterus, which makes up most of the uterus; (3) the **isthmus,** a short narrowed part of the body at its inferior end; and (4) the **cervix,** which extends into the **vagina** (Figs. 43-13 and 43-25). Because the cervical mucosa is distinct from the rest of the uterus and does not undergo the process of menstruation, it will be discussed separately later.

The established functions of the uterus are all related to fertilization and pregnancy (see later). The main functions of the uterus are to

1. Assist the movement of sperm from the vagina to the oviducts.

2. Provide a suitable site for attachment and implantation of the blastocyst, including a thick, nutrient-rich stroma.
3. Limit the invasiveness of the implanting embryo so that it stays in the endometrium and does not reach the myometrium.
4. Provide a maternal side of the mature placental architecture. This includes the basal plate, to which the fetal side attaches, and large intervillous spaces that become filled with maternal blood after the first trimester.
5. Grow and expand with the growing fetus so that the fetus develops within an aqueous, nonadhesive environment.
6. Provide strong muscular contractions to expel the fetus and placenta at term.

To understand the function of the uterus and uterine changes during nonfertile menstrual cycles, the fine structure of the endometrium and the relationship of uterine blood supply to the endometrium will be reviewed (Fig. 43-26). The luminal surface of the endometrium is covered with a simple cuboidal/columnar epithelium. The epithelium is continuous with mucosal glands (called **uterine glands**) that extend deep into the endometrium. The mucosa is vascularized by **spiral arteries,** which are branches of the **uterine artery** that run through the myometrium. The terminal arterioles of the spiral arteries project just beneath the surface epithelium. These arterioles give rise to a subepithelial plexus of capillaries and venules that have ballooned, thin-walled segments called **venous lakes** or **lacunae.** The lamina propria itself is densely cellular. The stromal cells of the lamina propria play important roles during both pregnancy and menstruation.

About two thirds of the luminal side of the endometrium is lost during menstruation and is called the **functional zone** (also called the **stratum functionalis**) (Fig. 43-26). The basal third of the endometrium that remains after menstruation is called the **basal zone** (also called the **stratum basale**). The basal zone is fed by straight arteries that are separate from the spiral arteries, and it contains all the cell types of the endometrium (i.e., epithelial cells from the remaining tips of glands, stromal cells, and endothelial cells).

HORMONAL REGULATION OF THE UTERINE ENDOMETRIUM DURING THE MENSTRUAL CYCLE

Proliferative Phase

Monthly oscillations in ovarian steroids induce the uterine endometrium to enter different stages. At the time of selection of the dominant follicle and its production of estrogen, the uterine endometrium is just ending menstruation. The stratum functionalis has been shed, and only the stratum basale remains (Fig. 43-27). The rising levels of estrogen during the mid to late follicular phase of the ovary induce the **proliferative phase** of the uterine endometrium. Estrogen induces all cell

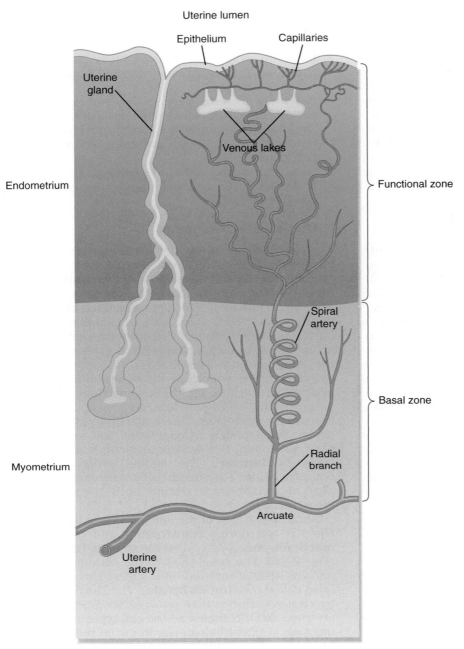

● **Figure 43-26.** Diagram of the organization of glands and blood flow within the uterine endometrium. (From Straus III. In Yen SSC et al [eds]: Reproductive Endocrinology, 4th ed. Philadelphia, Saunders, 1999.)

types in the stratum basale to grow and divide. In fact, the definition of an **"estrogenic"** compound has historically been one that is **"uterotropic."** Estrogen increases cell proliferation directly through its cognate receptors (ER-α and ER-β), which regulate gene expression (Fig. 43-28). Estrogen also controls uterine growth indirectly through the local production of growth factors. In addition, estrogen induces the expression of progesterone receptors, thereby "priming" the uterine endometrium so that it can respond to progesterone during the luteal phase of the ovary.

Secretory Phase

By ovulation, the thickness of the stratum functionalis has been reestablished under the proliferative actions of estradiol-17β (Fig. 43-27). After ovulation, the corpus luteum produces high levels of progesterone, along with estradiol-17β. The luteal phase of the ovary switches the proliferative phase of the uterine endometrium to the **secretory phase.** In general, progesterone inhibits further endometrial growth and induces the differentiation of epithelial and stromal cells. Progesterone induces the uterine glands to secrete a nutrient-rich product that supports blastocyst viability. As the secretory phase proceeds, the mucosal uterine glands become corkscrewed and sacculated (Fig. 43-27). Progesterone also induces changes in adhesivity of the surface epithelium, thereby generating the "window of receptivity" for implantation of an embryo (see later). Additionally, progesterone

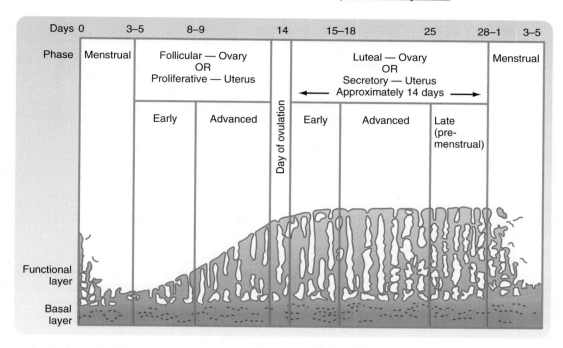

● **Figure 43-27.** The menstrual cycle of the uterine endometrium. (Modified from Porterfield SP, White BA: Endocrine Physiology, 3rd ed. Philadelphia, Mosby, 2007.)

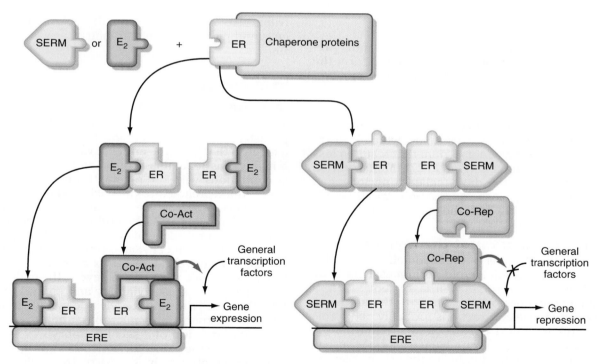

● **Figure 43-28.** Molecular mechanism by which the estrogen receptor (ER) regulates gene expression. **Left,** Estradiol-17β binds to the ER and changes its conformation so that it binds as a dimer to estrogen-response element (ERE) and recruits coactivator proteins (Co-Act), which leads to stimulation of gene expression. **Right,** Selective estrogen receptor modulators (SERMs), such as tamoxifen in the breast, alter ER conformation so that it recruits corepressor proteins (Co-Rep), thereby inhibiting gene expression. In this case the SERM acts as an ER antagonist, but in some tissues, the same SERM can act as an ER agonist. (Modified from Porterfield SP, White BA: Endocrine Physiology, 3rd ed. Philadelphia, Mosby, 2007.)

● AT THE CELLULAR LEVEL

Progesterone opposes the proliferative actions of estradiol-17β and down-regulates the estrogen receptor (ER). Progesterone also induces **inactivating isoforms of 17β-HSD,** thereby converting the active estradiol-17β into the inactive estrone. This opposition of the mitogenic actions of estradiol-17β by progesterone is important to protect the uterine endometrium from estrogen-induced uterine cancer. In contrast, the administration of **"unopposed estrogen"** to women significantly increases the risk for uterine cancer.

Drugs called **selective estrogen receptor modulators (SERMs)** have been developed that inhibit ER function in a tissue-specific manner (Fig. 43-28). For example, the SERM **tamoxifen** is used as an ER antagonist for the treatment of breast cancer (whose early progression is promoted by estrogen). Binding of SERM to the ER induces conformational changes that allow corepressors to bind to the ER or promote degradation of the ER (or both; Fig. 43-28). Because tamoxifen has some uterotropic activity (i.e., makes uterine endometrial tissue grow), newer SERMs such as **raloxifene** have been developed to have ER antagonist activity on the breast, beneficial ER agonist activity on bone (see later), and no activity or ER antagonistic activity on the uterine endometrium.

▶ IN THE CLINIC

Disorders of menstruation are relatively common and include **menorrhagia** (heavy menstrual flow leading to loss of more than 80 mL of blood), **metrorrhagia** (irregular and sometimes prolonged menstrual flow between normal periods), and **dysmenorrhea** (painful periods). The existence of a few, irregular periods, called **oligomenorrhea,** and the absence of periods, called **amenorrhea,** are often due to dysfunction of the hypothalamic-pituitary-ovarian axis, as opposed to local pelvic pathophysiology.

Because endometrial tissue is naturally sloughed in fragments that contain viable cells, endometrial tissue occasionally gains access to other parts of the female tract (e.g., oviducts, ovary), as well as the lower part of the abdomen and associated structures (e.g., rectum, bladder). These implants give rise to **endometriosis**—a foci of hormonally responsive endometrial tissue outside the uterus. The spread of endometriosis may be due to reflux of menstrual tissue into the oviducts or movement of tissue through lymphatics, or both. Endometriosis frequently exhibits cyclic bleeding and is associated with infertility, pain on defecation, pain on urination, pain with sexual intercourse, or generalized pelvic pain.

promotes the differentiation of stromal cells into **"predecidual cells,"** which must be prepared to form the decidua of pregnancy or to orchestrate menstruation in the absence of pregnancy.

Menstrual Phase

In a nonfertile cycle, death of the corpus luteum results in sudden withdrawal of progesterone, which leads to changes in the uterine endometrium that result in loss of the lamina functionalis (Fig. 43-27). **Menstruation** normally lasts for 4 to 5 days (called a **period**), and the volume of blood loss ranges from 25 to 35 mL. Menstruation coincides with the early follicular phase of the ovary.

Hormonal Regulation of the Myometrium

The smooth muscle cells of the myometrium are also responsive to changes in steroid hormones. Peristaltic contractions of the myometrium favor movement of the luminal contents from the cervix to the fundus at ovulation, and these contractions probably play a role in rapid, bulk transport of ejaculated sperm from the cervix to the oviducts. During menstruation, contractions propagate from the fundus to the cervix, thereby promoting expulsion of sloughed stratum functionalis. The size and number of smooth muscle cells are determined by estrogen and progesterone. Healthy, cycling women maintain a robust myometrium, whereas the myometrium progressively thins in postmenopausal women. The most drastic changes are seen during pregnancy, when the smooth muscle cells increase from 50 to 500 μm in length. The pregnant myome-

trium also has a greater number of smooth muscle cells and more extracellular matrix.

THE CERVIX

Structure and Function

The cervix is the inferior extension of the uterus that projects into the vagina (Figs. 43-13 and 43-25). It has a mucosa that lines the **endocervical canal,** which has a highly elastic lamina propria and a muscularis that is continuous with the myometrium. The part of the cervix that extends into the vaginal vault is called the **ectocervix,** whereas the part surrounding the endocervical canal is called the **endocervix.** The openings of the endocervical canal at the uterus and vagina are called the **internal cervical os** and the **external cervical os,** respectively. The cervix acts as a gateway to the upper female tract—at midcycle, the endocervical canal facilitates sperm viability and entry. During the luteal phase, the endocervical canal impedes the passage of sperm and microbes, thereby inhibiting **superimplantation** of a second embryo or ascending infection into the placenta, fetal membranes, and fetus. The cervix physically supports the weight of the growing fetus. At term, **cervical softening and dilation** allow passage of the newborn and placenta from the uterus into the vagina.

Hormonal Regulation of Cervical Mucus during the Menstrual Cycle

The endocervical canal is lined by a simple columnar epithelium that secretes **cervical mucus** in a hormonally responsive manner. Estrogen stimulates the production of a copious quantity of thin, watery, slightly alkaline mucus that is an ideal environment for sperm. Progesterone stimulates the production of a scant, viscous, slightly acidic mucus that is hostile to sperm. During the normal menstrual cycle, the conditions of the cervical mucus are ideal for sperm penetration and viability at the time of ovulation.

THE VAGINA

Structure and Function

The vagina is one of the copulatory structures in women and acts as the birth canal (Figs. 43-13 and 43-25). Its mucosa is lined by a nonkeratinized, stratified squamous epithelium. The mucosa has a thick lamina propria enriched with elastic fibers and is well vascularized. There are no glands in the vagina, so lubrication during intercourse comes from (1) cervical mucus (especially with intercourse that occurs midcycle), (2) a transudate (i.e., ultrafiltrate) from the blood vessels of the lamina propria, and (3) the vestibular glands. The mucosa is surrounded by a relatively thin (i.e., relative to the uterus and cervix), two-layered muscularis and an outer connective tissue. The vaginal wall is innervated by branches of the pudendal nerve, which contribute to sexual pleasure and orgasm during intercourse.

Hormonal Regulation during the Menstrual Cycle

The superficial cells of the vaginal epithelium are continually desquamating, and the nature of these cells is influenced by the hormonal environment. Estrogen stimulates proliferation of the vaginal epithelium and increases its glycogen content (referred to as **"cornification"**—but in humans, true cornification or keratinization does not occur). The glycogen is metabolized to lactic acid by commensal lactobacilli, thereby maintaining an acidic environment. This inhibits infection by noncommensal bacteria and fungi. Progesterone increases the desquamation of epithelial cells.

THE EXTERNAL GENITALIA

Structure and Function

The female external genitalia are surrounded by the **labia majora** (homologues of the scrotum) laterally and the **mons pubis** anteriorly (Fig. 43-25). The **vulva** collectively refers to an area that includes the labia majora and the mons pubis, plus the **labia minora,** the **clitoris,** the **vestibule of the vagina,** the **vestibular bulbs** (glands), and the **external urethral orifice.** The vulva is also referred to as the **pudendum** by clinicians. The structures of the vulva serve the functions of sexual arousal and climax, directing the flow of urine, and partially covering the opening of the vagina, thereby inhibiting the entry of pathogens.

The clitoris is the embryological homologue of the penis and is composed of two **corpora cavernosa,** which attach the clitoris to the ischiopubic rami, and a **glans.** These structures are composed of erectile tissue and undergo the process of erection in essentially the same manner as the penis. Unlike the penis, clitoral tissue is completely separate from the urethra. Thus, the clitoris is involved in sexual arousal and climax at orgasm. The vagina is likewise involved in sexual satisfaction but also serves as the copulatory organ and birth canal.

Hormonal Regulation during the Menstrual Cycle

The structures of the vulva do not show marked changes during the menstrual cycle. However, the health and function of these structures are dependent on hormonal support. The external genitalia and vagina are responsive to androgens (testosterone and dihydrotestosterone) and estrogen. Androgens also act on the central nervous system (CNS) to increase libido in women.

BIOLOGY OF ESTRADIOL-17β AND PROGESTERONE

Biological Effects of Estrogen and Progesterone

Estradiol-17β and progesterone fluctuate during the menstrual cycle, and they have multiple effects that can be categorized according to whether they are directly related to the reproductive system or not. Both hormones have profound effects on the ovary, oviduct, uterus, cervix, vagina, and external genitalia and on the hypothalamus and pituitary. Estrogen and progesterone also have important effects on nonreproductive tissues, including the following:

Bone: Estrogen is required for closure of the epiphyseal plates of long bones in both sexes. Estradiol-17β has a **bone anabolic** and **calciotropic effect** (see Chapter 39). It stimulates intestinal Ca^{++} absorption. Estradiol-17β is also one of the most potent regulators of osteoblast and osteoclast function. Estrogen promotes the survival of osteoblasts and apoptosis of osteoclasts, thereby favoring bone formation over resorption.

Liver: The overall effect of estradiol-17β on the liver is to improve circulating lipoprotein profiles. Estrogen increases expression of the LDL receptor, thereby increasing clearance of cholesterol-rich LDL particles by the liver. Estrogen also increases circulating levels of HDL. Estrogen regulates the hepatic production of several transport proteins, including cortisol-binding protein, thyroid hormone–binding protein, and SHBG.

Cardiovascular organs: Premenopausal women have significantly less cardiovascular disease than men or postmenopausal women do. Estrogen promotes vasodilation through increased production of **nitric oxide,** which relaxes vascular smooth muscle and inhibits platelet activation. Single-nucleotide polymorphisms in the estrogen receptor have been associated with increased cardiovascular disease.

784   *Berne and Levy Physiology*

Integument: Estrogen and progesterone maintain a healthy, smooth skin with normal epidermal and dermal thickness. Estrogen stimulates proliferation and inhibits apoptosis of keratinocytes. In the dermis, estrogen and progesterone increase collagen synthesis and inhibit (along with progesterone) the breakdown of collagen by suppressing matrix metalloproteinases. Estrogen also increases glycosaminoglycan production and deposition in the dermis and promotes wound healing.

CNS: Estrogen is neuroprotective—that is, it inhibits neuronal cell death in response to hypoxia or other insults. Estrogen's positive effects on angiogenesis may account for some of the beneficial and stimulant-like actions of estrogen on the CNS. Progesterone acts on the hypothalamus to increase the set point for thermoregulation, thereby elevating body temperature approximately 0.5°F. This is the basis for using body temperature measurements to determine whether ovulation has occurred. Progesterone is a CNS depressant. Loss of progesterone on demise of the corpus luteum of menstruation is the basis for **premenstrual dysphoria (premenstrual syndrome [PMS]).** Progesterone also acts on the brainstem to sensitize the ventilatory response to P_{CO_2} so that ventilation increases and P_{CO_2} decreases.

Adipose tissue: Estrogen decreases adipose tissue by decreasing lipoprotein lipase activity and increasing hormone-sensitive lipase (i.e., it has a lipolytic effect). Loss of estrogen results in the accumulation of adipose tissue, especially in the abdomen.

Transport and Metabolism of Ovarian Steroids

Steroid hormones are slightly soluble in blood and are bound to plasma proteins. Approximately 60% of the estrogen is transported bound to **sex hormone–binding globulin,** 20% is bound to albumin, and 20% is in the free form. Progesterone binds primarily to **cortisol-binding globulin (transcortin)** and albumin.

Because it has relatively low binding affinity for these proteins, its circulating half-life is about 5 minutes.

Although the ovary is the primary site of estrogen production, peripheral aromatization of androgens to estrogens can generate locally high levels of estradiol-17β in some tissues. Peripheral conversion of adrenal and ovarian androgens serves as an important source of estrogen after menopause (see later). The fact that CYP19 (aromatase) is expressed in the breast is the basis for the use of **aromatase inhibitors** in the treatment of estrogen-dependent breast cancer in postmenopausal women.

Estrogens and progestins are degraded in the liver to inactive metabolites, conjugated with sulfate or glucuronide, and excreted in urine. Major metabolites of estradiol include estrone, estriol, and catecholestrogens (2-hydroxyestrone and 2-methoxyestrone). The major metabolite of progesterone is pregnanediol, which is conjugated with glucuronide and excreted in urine.

ONTOGENY OF THE REPRODUCTIVE SYSTEMS

Unlike most other organ systems, the reproductive systems undergo significant changes in their activity during the life span of a man or woman (Fig. 43-29). Development of the reproductive systems occurs in utero and results in female or male fetuses. After birth and during infancy, the reproductive systems are largely quiescent. At puberty, the hypothalamic-pituitary-gonadal axes "wake up," and the gonads begin producing sex steroids, which in turn induce the sexually dimorphic changes in appearance and behavior associated with men and women. The reproductive life span of women is set by their ovarian reserve and degree of follicular development (see earlier) and ends at menopause, usually in the fifth decade of life. The loss of estrogen production by the ovaries has a clear clinical impact on many postmenopausal women. Men

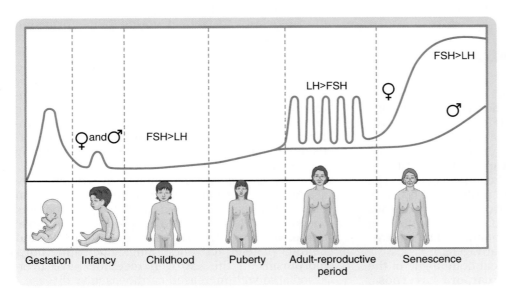

● **Figure 43-29.** Pattern of gonadotropin secretion throughout life. Note the transient peaks during gestation and early infancy and the low levels thereafter in childhood. Women subsequently have monthly cyclic bursts, with luteinizing hormone (LH) exceeding follicle-stimulating hormone (FSH); men do not. Both genders show increased gonadotropin production after 50 years of age, with FSH exceeding LH.

Gestation   Infancy   Childhood   Puberty   Adult-reproductive period   Senescence continue to produce sperm throughout life but can experience a decline in androgen production (andropause), which is associated with its own clinical sequelae.

PREGNANCY

The reproductive system of women undergoes dramatic changes during pregnancy. The production of gonadotropin and gonadal steroids is switched from the maternal hypothalamic-pituitary-ovarian axis, which is strongly repressed during pregnancy, to the fetal placenta. Indeed, it is the endocrine function of fetal placental tissue that (1) maintains a quiescent gravid uterus, (2) alters maternal physiology to ensure fetal nutrition in utero, (3) alters maternal pituitary function and mammary gland development to ensure ongoing fetal nutrition after birth, and (4) determines the time of labor and delivery (also called **parturition**). The placenta also plays an important role in fetal testosterone production and male differentiation of the reproductive system before the fetal hypothalamus and pituitary develop into a functional axis.

Fertilization, Early Embryogenesis, Implantation, and Placentation
Synchronization with Maternal Ovarian and Reproductive Tract Function

Fertilization, early embryogenesis, implantation, and early gestation are all synchronized with the human menstrual cycle (Fig. 43-30). Just before ovulation, the ovary is in the late follicular stage and produces high levels of estrogen. Estrogen promotes growth of the uterine endometrium and induces expression of the progesterone receptor. Estrogen ultimately induces the LH surge, which in turn induces meiotic maturation of the oocyte and ovulation of the cumulus-oocyte complex.

The events between fertilization and implantation take about 6 days to complete, so implantation occurs at about day 22 of the menstrual cycle. At this time the ovary is in the midluteal phase and secreting large amounts of progesterone. Progesterone stimulates secretion from the uterine glands, which provide nutrients to the embryo. This is referred to as histiotropic nutrition and is an important mode of maternal-to-fetal transfer of nutrients for about the first trimester of pregnancy, after which it is replaced by hemotropic nutrition (see later). Progesterone inhibits myometrial contraction and prevents the release of paracrine factors (e.g., cytokines, prostaglandins, chemokines, and vasoconstrictors) that lead to menstruation. Progesterone induces the **"window of receptivity"** in the uterine endometrium, which exists from about day 20 to day 24 of the menstrual cycle. This receptive phase is associated with increased adhesivity of the endometrial epithelium and involves the formation of cellular extensions, called **pinopodes,** on the apical surface of endometrial epithelia, along with increased expression of adhesive proteins (e.g., integrins, cadherins) and decreased expression of antiadhesive proteins (e.g., mucins) in the apical cell membrane.

When a fertilized egg implants in the uterus, the uterine endometrium is at its full thickness, is actively secreting, and is capable of tightly adhering to the implanting embryo.

Fertilization

Fertilization accomplishes both recombination of genetic material to form a new, genetically distinct organism and initiation of events that begin embryonic development. Several steps must occur to achieve successful (unassisted) fertilization (Fig. 43-31), including the following:

Step 1: Penetration of the expanded cumulus by the sperm. This involves digestion of the extracellular matrix of the cumulus by a membrane hyaluronidase, PH-20.

Step 2: Penetration of the zona pellucida by the sperm. This involves binding of the sperm to the zona protein ZP3 (step 2a), which induces the release of acrosomal enzymes (called the **acrosomal reaction** (step 2b). The sperm secondarily bind to another zona protein, ZP2 (step 2c), as the zona pellucida is digested and the sperm swims through to the egg (step 2d).

Step 3: Fusion of the sperm and egg membrane takes place.

Step 4: A Ca^{++} signaling cascade (see Chapter 3) occurs.

Step 5: The signaling cascade activates the exocytosis of enzyme-filled vesicles, called **cortical granules,** that reside in the outermost, or cortical, region of the unfertilized egg. The enzymes contained in the cortical granules are released to the outside of the egg upon exocytosis. These enzymes modify both ZP2 and ZP3 of the zona pellucida such that ZP2 can no longer bind acrosome-reacted sperm and ZP3 can no longer bind capacitated, acrosome-intact sperm. Thus, only one sperm usually enters the egg. Occasionally, more than one sperm does enter the egg. This results in a **triploid** cell that is unable to develop further. Therefore, prevention of polyspermy is critical for normal development of the fertilized egg.

Step 6: The entire sperm enters the egg during fusion. The flagellum and mitochondria disintegrate, so most of the mitochondrial DNA in cells is maternally derived. Once inside the egg, decondensation of the sperm DNA occurs. A membrane, called the pronucleus, forms around the sperm DNA as the newly activated egg completes the second meiotic division.

In mammalian eggs, a large initial release of Ca^{++} is followed by a series of subsequent, smaller Ca^{++} oscillations that can last for hours. A major consequence of this signaling pathway is that it "wakes up" the metabolically quiescent egg so that it can resume meiosis and begin embryonic development. This process is called **egg activation.**

The activated egg completes the second meiotic division as the sperm DNA decondenses and a pronucleus

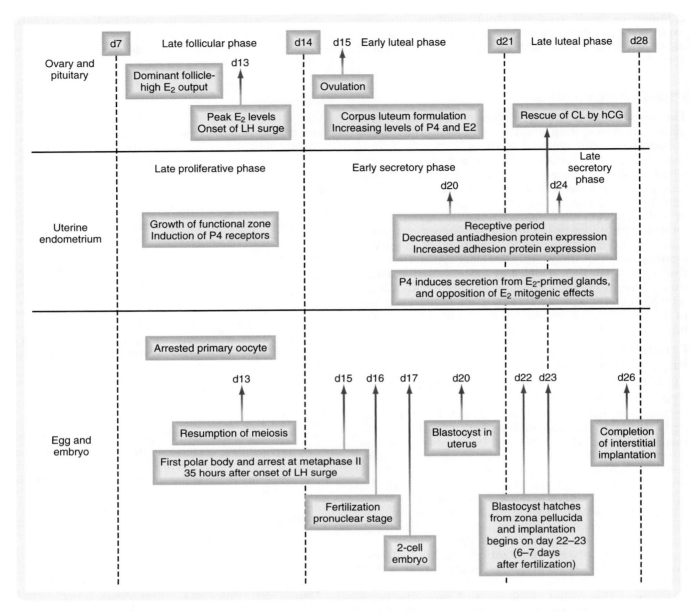

● **Figure 43-30.**   Synchronization of events of the menstrual cycle (ovary and endometrium) with fertilization, early development in the oviduct, and implantation in the uterus. E$_2$, estradiol. (Modified from Porterfield SP, White BA: Endocrine Physiology, 3rd ed. Philadelphia, Mosby, 2007.)

forms around it (Fig. 43-32). Once the egg has completed meiosis, a pronucleus forms around the female chromosomes as well. A **centrosome,** contributed by the sperm, becomes a microtubule organizing center from which microtubules extend until they contact the female pronucleus. The male and female DNA replicate as the two pronuclei are pulled together. Once the pronuclei contact each other, the nuclear membranes break down, the chromosomes align on a common metaphase plate, and the first cleavage occurs.

Early Embryogenesis and Implantation
Fertilization typically occurs on day 16 to 17 of the menstrual cycle, and implantation occurs about 6 days

later. Thus, the first week of embryogenesis takes place within the lumens of the oviduct and uterus. For most of this time, the embryo remains encapsulated by the zona pellucida. The first two cleavages take about 2 days, and the embryo reaches a 16-cell **morula** by 3 days. The outer cells of the morula become tightly adhesive with each other and begin transporting fluid into the embryonic mass. During days 4 and 5, the transport of fluid generates a cavity, called the blastocyst cavity, and the embryo is now called a **blastocyst** (Fig. 43-33). The blastocyst is composed of two subpopulations of cells: an eccentric **inner cell mass** and an outer, epithelial-like layer of **trophoblasts.** The region of the trophoblast layer immediately adjacent

● **Figure 43-31.** Events involved in fertilization (see text for details). (Modified from Porterfield SP, White BA: Endocrine Physiology, 3rd ed. Philadelphia, Mosby, 2007.)

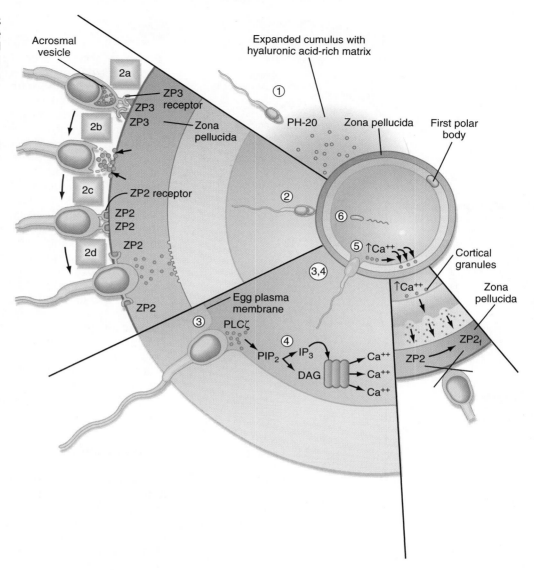

to the inner cell mass is referred to as the **embryonic pole,** and it is this region that attaches to the uterine endometrium at implantation (Fig. 43-33).

The embryo resides within the oviduct during the first 3 days and then enters the uterus. By 5 to 6 days of development, the trophoblasts of the blastocyst secrete proteases that digest the outer-lying zona pellucida. At this point, corresponding to about day 22 of the menstrual cycle, the **"hatched" blastocyst** is able to adhere to and implant into the receptive uterine endometrium (Fig. 43-33).

At the time of attachment and implantation, the trophoblasts differentiate into two cell types: an inner layer of **cytotrophoblasts** and an outer layer of multinuclear/multicellular **syncytiotrophoblasts** (Fig. 43-33). The cytotrophoblasts initially provide a feeder layer of continuously dividing cells. Syncytiotrophoblasts initially perform three general types of function: adhesive, invasive, and endocrine. Syncytiotrophoblasts express adhesive surface proteins (i.e., cadherins and integrins) that bind to uterine surface epithelia

and, as the embryo implants, to components of the uterine extracellular matrix. In humans, the embryo completely burrows into the superficial layer of the endometrium (Fig. 43-33). This mode of implantation, called **interstitial implantation,** is the most invasive among placental mammals. Invasive implantation involves adhesion-supported migration of syncytiotrophoblasts into the endometrium, along with the breakdown of extracellular matrix by the secretion of matrix metalloproteinases and other hydrolytic enzymes.

The endocrine function begins with the onset of implantation, when syncytiotrophoblasts start secreting the LH-like protein **human chorionic gonadotropin,** which maintains the viability of the corpus luteum and thus progesterone secretion. Syncytiotrophoblasts also become highly steroidogenic. By 10 weeks, the syncytiotrophoblasts acquire the ability to make progesterone at sufficient levels to maintain pregnancy independently of a corpus luteum. Syncytiotrophoblasts produce several other hormones, as well as enzymes that modify hormones.

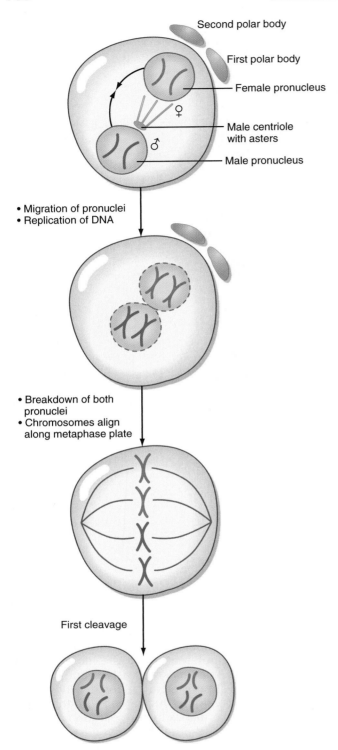

Second polar body

First polar body

Female pronucleus

♀

Male centriole
with asters

♂

Male pronucleus

• Migration of pronuclei
• Replication of DNA

• Breakdown of both
  pronuclei
• Chromosomes align
  along metaphase plate

First cleavage

● **Figure 43-32.**   Overview of genetic events after fertilization up to the first embryonic cleavage. (Modified from Porterfield SP, White BA: Endocrine Physiology, 3rd ed. Philadelphia, Mosby, 2007.)

As implantation and placentation progress, syncytiotrophoblasts take on the important functions of phagocytosis (during histiotropic nutrition) and bidirectional placental transfer of gases, nutrients, and wastes. Exchange across the syncytiotrophoblasts

> ## ▶ IN THE CLINIC
>
> **Placenta accreta** is destruction of the endometrium and adherence of the placenta to the myometrium, a condition associated with potentially life-threatening postpartum hemorrhage. The decidual response occurs only in the uterus. Thus, the highly invasive nature of the human embryo poses considerable risk to the mother in the case of **ectopic implantation.** Ectopic implantation refers to the implantation of an embryo at a site other than the uterus, and an **ectopic pregnancy** refers to a developing embryo at a site of ectopic implantation. Most ectopic pregnancies (>90%) occur within the oviducts (called **tubal pregnancies**), but they can also occur in the ovary and abdominal cavity. Implantation in the oviducts is often associated with long-term infection and inflammation (called **pelvic inflammatory disease**) and obstruction of the tube. In a tubal pregnancy, the highly invasive nature of the human syncytiotrophoblast, which is normally moderated by the uterine decidual response, usually leads to burrowing of the implanted embryo through the wall of the oviduct. Although abdominal pregnancies can proceed to term, undetected oviductal pregnancies usually lead to rupture of the oviductal wall. The resulting internal hemorrhage can be catastrophic to the mother and requires immediate surgical intervention.

involves diffusion (e.g., gases), facilitated transport (e.g., GLUT1-mediated transfer of glucose), active transport (e.g., amino acids by specific transporters), and pinocytosis/transcytosis (e.g., of iron-transferrin complexes).

There is also a maternal response to implantation that involves transformation of the endometrial stroma. This response, called **decidualization,** involves an enlargement of stromal cells as they become lipid- and glycogen-filled decidual cells (at this time, the endometrium is referred to as the **decidua**). The decidua forms an epithelial-like sheet with adhesive junctions that inhibit migration of the implanting embryo. The decidua also secretes factors, such as **tissue inhibitors of metalloproteinases (TIMPs),** that moderate the activity of syncytiotrophoblast-derived hydrolytic enzymes in the endometrial matrix. Consequently, decidualization allows regulated invasion during implantation. Normally, the implanting embryo and placenta do not extend to and involve the myometrium.

Placental Endocrinology

Human Chorionic Gonadotropin. The first hormone produced by syncytiotrophoblasts is **hCG.** hCG is structurally related to the pituitary glycoprotein hormones (see Chapter 40). As such, hCG is composed of a common **α-glycoprotein subunit (α-GSU)** and a **hormone-specific β subunit (β-hCG).** Antibodies used to detect hCG (i.e., in laboratory assays and over-the-counter pregnancy tests) are designed to specifically detect the β subunit. hCG is most similar to LH and

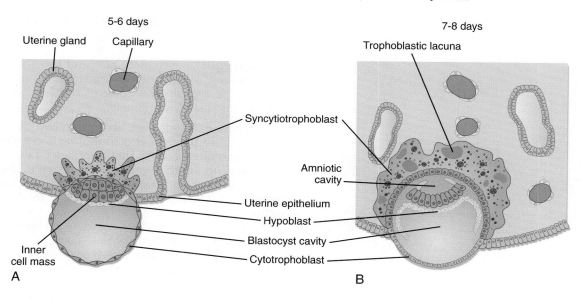

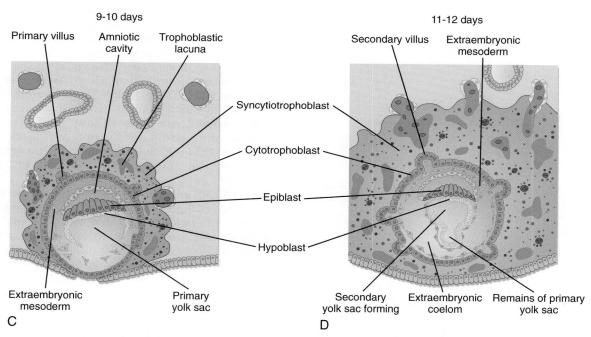

● **Figure 43-33.** Events involved in early embryonic implantation. (From Carlson BM: Human Embryology and Developmental Biology. Philadelphia, Mosby, 2004.)

binds with high affinity to the LH receptor. The β subunit of hCG is longer than that of LH and contains more sites for **glycosylation,** which greatly increases the half-life of hCG to 24 to 30 hours. The stability of hCG allows it to rapidly accumulate in the maternal circulation such that hCG is detectable within maternal serum within 24 hours of implantation. Serum hCG levels double every 2 days for the first 6 weeks and peak at about 10 weeks. Serum hCG then declines to a constant level at about 50% of the peak value (Fig. 43-34, *A*).

The primary action of hCG is to stimulate LH receptors on the corpus luteum. This prevents luteolysis and maintains a high level of luteal-derived progester-one production during the first 10 weeks. The rapid increase in hCG is responsible for the nausea of **"morning sickness"** associated with early pregnancy. A small amount (i.e., 1% to 10%) of hCG enters the fetal circulation. hCG stimulates fetal Leydig cells to produce testosterone before the fetal gonadotropic axis is fully mature. hCG also stimulates the fetal adrenal cortex (see later) during the first trimester.

Progesterone. The placenta produces a high amount of **progesterone,** which is absolutely required to maintain a quiescent myometrium and a pregnant uterus. Progesterone production by the placenta is largely unregulated—the placenta produces as much proges-

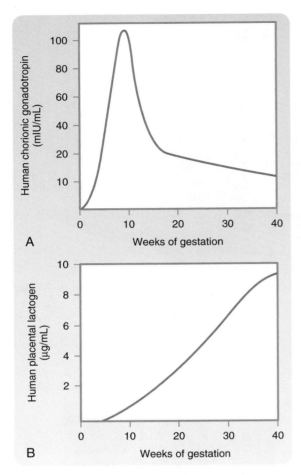

● **Figure 43-34.** Circulating levels of human chorionic gonadotropin and human placental lactogen in maternal blood during pregnancy. (Modified from Porterfield SP, White BA: *Endocrine Physiology*, 3rd ed. Philadelphia, Mosby, 2007.)

terone as the supply of cholesterol and the levels of CYP11A1 and 3β-HSD allow (Fig. 43-35). Notably, placental steroidogenesis differs from that in the adrenal cortex, ovaries, and testis in that cholesterol is transported into the placental mitochondria by a mechanism that is independent of **StAR protein.** Thus, this first step in steroidogenesis is not a regulated, rate-limiting step in the placenta as it is in other steroidogenic glands. This means that fetuses with an inactivating mutation in StAR protein will develop **lipoid congenital adrenal hyperplasia** (see Chapter 42) and **hypogonadism** but will have normal progesterone levels produced by their placenta. Progesterone production by the placenta does not require fetal tissue. Consequently, progesterone levels are largely independent of fetal health and cannot be used as a measure of fetal health. Maternal progesterone levels continue to increase throughout pregnancy.

Progesterone is released primarily into the maternal circulation and is required for implantation and maintenance of pregnancy. Progesterone also has several effects on maternal physiology and induces

breast growth and differentiation. The switch from corpus luteum–derived progesterone to placental-derived progesterone (referred to as the **luteal-placental shift**) is complete at about the eighth week of pregnancy. Progesterone (and pregnenolone) are used by the transitional zone of the fetal cortex to make cortisol late in pregnancy.

Estrogen. Estrogens are also produced by the syncytiotrophoblasts. Syncytiotrophoblasts are similar to ovarian granulosa cells in that they lack CYP17 and are dependent on another cell type to provide 19-carbon androgens for aromatization (Fig. 43-36). The ancillary, androgen-producing cell resides in the **fetal adrenal cortex.**

The fetal adrenal cortex contains an outer **definitive zone,** a middle **transitional zone,** and an inner **fetal zone.** The definitive and transitional zones give rise to the zona glomerulosa and zona fasciculata, respectively. Aldosterone synthesis is initiated close to parturition. Synthesis of cortisol begins at about 6 months and increases during late gestation. The fetal zone is the predominant portion of the adrenal cortex in the fetus; it constitutes as much as 80% of the bulk of the large fetal adrenal and is the site of most fetal adrenal steroidogenesis. The fetal zone strongly resembles the zona reticularis in that it expresses little or no 3β-HSD (Fig. 43-36). The fetal zone primarily releases the sulfated form of the inactive androgen **dehydroepiandrosterone sulfate** (DHEAS) throughout most of gestation. Production of DHEAS from the fetal adrenal is absolutely dependent on fetal ACTH from the fetal pituitary by the end of the first trimester.

The DHEAS released from the fetal zone has two fates. First, DHEAS can go directly to the syncytiotrophoblast, where it is desulfated by a placental **steroid sulfatase** and used as a 19-carbon substrate for the synthesis of estradiol-17β and estrone (Fig. 43-36). The second fate of DHEAS is **16-hydroxylation** in the fetal liver by the enzyme CYP3A7. 16-Hydroxyl-DHEAS is then converted by syncytiotrophoblasts to the major estrogen of pregnancy, called **estriol** (Fig. 43-36).

Maternal estrogen levels increase throughout pregnancy. Because estrogen production is dependent on a healthy fetus, estriol levels can be used to assess fetal health. The collective term used for the placental syncytiotrophoblasts and fetal organs in the context of estrogen production is the **fetoplacental unit.** Estrogens increase uteroplacental blood flow, enhance LDL receptor expression in syncytiotrophoblasts, and induce several components (e.g., prostaglandins, oxytocin receptors) involved in parturition. Estrogens increase breast growth directly and indirectly through the stimulation of maternal pituitary prolactin production. Estrogens also increase lactotrope size and number, thereby increasing overall pituitary mass by more than twofold by term. Estrogens also affect several aspects of maternal physiology.

Human Placental Lactogen. Human placental lactogen (hPL), also called **human chorionic somatomam-**

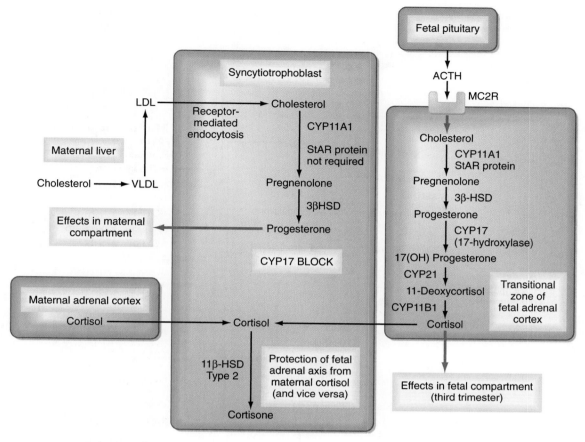

● **Figure 43-35.** Production of progesterone and inactivation of cortisol by syncytio-trophoblast. (Modified from Porterfield SP, White BA: Endocrine Physiology, 3rd ed. Philadelphia, Mosby, 2007.)

motropin (hCS), is a 191–amino acid protein hormone produced in the syncytiotrophoblast that is structurally similar to growth hormone (GH) and prolactin (PRL). Its function overlaps those of both GH and PRL. It can be detected within the syncytiotrophoblast by 10 days after conception and in maternal serum by 3 weeks of gestation (Fig. 43-34). Maternal serum levels rise progressively throughout the remainder of the pregnancy. The quantity of hormone produced is directly related to the size of the placenta such that as the placenta grows during gestation, hPL secretion increases. As much as 1 g/day of hPL can be secreted late in gestation.

Like GH, hPL is protein anabolic and lipolytic. Its antagonistic action to insulin is the major basis for the diabetogenicity of pregnancy. Like PRL, it stimulates mammary gland growth and development. Mammary gland development in pregnancy results from the actions of hPL, PRL, estrogens, and progestins. hPL inhibits maternal glucose uptake and use, thereby increasing serum glucose levels. Glucose is a major energy substrate for the fetus, and hPL increases fetal glucose availability.

As with hCG, far less hPL is found in the fetal circulation than in the maternal circulation. This suggests that the hormones may play a more important role in the mother than in the fetus. hPL is not essential for the pregnancy.

Both hPL and PRL act as fetal growth hormones and stimulate production of the fetal growth-promoting hormones insulin-like growth factor I and II (IGF-I and IGF-II). Ironically, fetal GH does not appear to regulate growth, and anencephalic infants and GH-deficient children typically have normal birth weight.

Diabetogenicity of Pregnancy

Pregnancy represents an **insulin-resistant state** (Fig. 43-37). During the last half of pregnancy, when hPL levels are highest, maternal energy metabolism shifts from an anabolic state, in which nutrients are stored, to a catabolic state, sometimes described as **accelerated starvation,** in which maternal energy metabolism shifts toward fat utilization with sparing of glucose. As maternal use of glucose for energy decreases, lipolysis increases and fatty acids become major energy sources. The peripheral responsiveness to insulin decreases and pancreatic insulin secretion increases. Beta cell hyperplasia occurs in pregnancy. Although this does not usually lead to a clinical condition, pregnancy aggravates existing diabetes mellitus, and diabetes can develop for the first time in pregnancy. If the diabetes resolves spontaneously with delivery, the

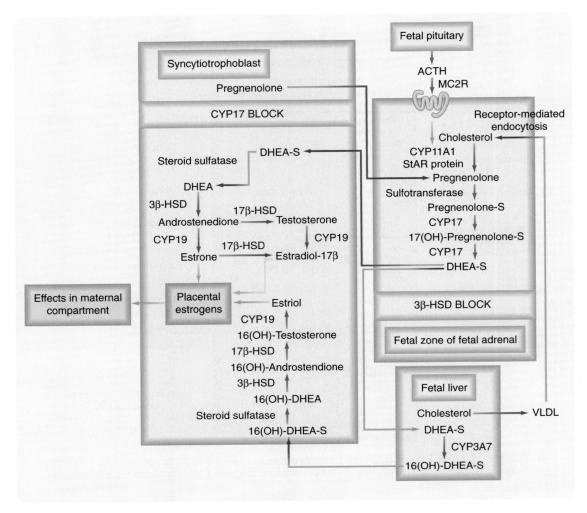

● **Figure 43-36.** Estrogen biosynthesis by the fetoplacental unit. ACTH, adrenocorticotropic hormone; DHEA, dehydroepiandrostenedione; DHEA-S, dehydroepiandrostenedione sulfate; 3β-HSD, 3β-hydroxysteroid dehydrogenase; 17β-HSD, 17β-hydroxysteroid dehydrogenase; MC2R, melanocortin-2 receptor (ACTH receptor); 16(OH)-, 16-hydroxy-; StAR protein, steroidogenic acute regulatory protein; VLDL, very low density lipoproteins. (Modified from Porterfield SP, White BA: *Endocrine Physiology,* 3rd ed. Philadelphia, Mosby, 2007.)

condition is referred to as **gestational diabetes.** Other hormones contributing to the diabetogenicity of pregnancy are estrogens and progestins because both these hormones decrease insulin sensitivity.

Parturition

Human pregnancy lasts an average of 40 weeks from the beginning of the last menstrual period (gestational age). This corresponds to an average fetal age of 38 weeks. **Parturition** is the process whereby uterine contractions lead to childbirth. **Labor** consists of three stages: strong uterine contractions that force the fetus against the cervix, with dilation and thinning of the cervix (several hours); delivery of the fetus (less than 1 hour); and delivery of the placenta, along with contractions of the myometrium to halt bleeding (less than 10 minutes).

Control of parturition in humans is complex, and the exact mechanisms underlying its control are not well understood.

Placental CRH and the Fetal Adrenal Axis

The placenta produces **corticotropin-releasing hormone (CRH),** which is identical to the 41–amino acid peptide produced by the hypothalamus. Placental CRH production and maternal serum CRH levels increase rapidly during late pregnancy and labor. Moreover, circulating CRH is either in the form of free CRH, which is bioactive, or complexed to a CRH-binding protein. Maternal levels of CRH-binding protein plummet during late pregnancy and labor, so free CRH levels increase. Placental CRH also accumulates in the fetal circulation and stimulates fetal ACTH secretion. ACTH stimulates both fetal adrenal cortisol production and fetoplacental estrogen production. In contrast to the inhibitory effect of cortisol on hypothalamic CRH production, cortisol stimulates placental CRH production. This establishes a self-amplifying positive feedback. CRH itself promotes myometrial contractions by sensitizing the uterus to prostaglandins and

● **Figure 43-37.** Overview of energy use by the maternal and fetal compartments. (Modified from Porterfield SP, White BA: Endocrine Physiology, 3rd ed. Philadelphia, Mosby, 2007.)

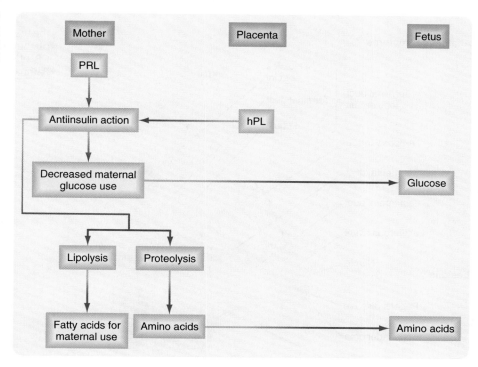

oxytocin (see later). Estrogens also directly and indirectly stimulate myometrial contractility. Moreover, this model correlates the onset of parturition with cortisol-induced maturation of fetal systems, including the lungs and gastrointestinal tract.

Estrogen and Progesterone Secretion

Although a rise in maternal serum estrogen and a drop in progesterone levels occur late in gestation in some species, no change in the ratio of the two hormones is seen in human serum. However, "functional" progesterone withdrawal involving changes in uterine progesterone receptor and progesterone metabolism has been proposed.

Oxytocin

Oxytocin is secreted from the pars nervosa of the pituitary gland (see Chapter 40). Oxytocin, which stimulates powerful uterine contractions, plays a major role in parturition. Oxytocin is released in response to stretch of the cervix through a neuroendocrine reflex, and it stimulates uterine contractions and thereby facilitates delivery. Oxytocin can be used to induce parturition, and uterine sensitivity to oxytocin increases before parturition. Because maternal serum oxytocin levels do not increase until after parturition has begun, oxytocin is not thought to initiate parturition. However, progesterone inhibits and estrogen stimulates the synthesis of oxytocin receptors, and although maternal serum progesterone levels do not decrease immediately before human parturition, estrogen levels rise and oxytocin receptor synthesis increases.

Prostaglandins

Prostaglandins and other cytokines increase uterine motility, and levels of these compounds increase during parturition, thereby facilitating delivery. Their exact role in the initiation of parturition is not known. Prostaglandin levels in amnionic fluid, fetal membranes, and uterine decidua increase before the onset of labor. The prostaglandins $F_{2\alpha}$ and E_2 increase uterine motility. Large doses of these compounds have been used to induce labor. Because estrogens stimulate prostaglandin synthesis in the uterus, amnion, and chorion, the rising estrogen levels late in gestation can increase uterine prostaglandin formation before parturition.

Uterine Size

Uterine size is thought to be a factor regulating parturition because stretch of smooth muscle, including the uterus, increases muscle contraction. In addition, uterine stretch stimulates uterine prostaglandin production. Multiple births generally occur prematurely. The tendency for early delivery can be a result of increased uterine size, increased fetal production of chemicals stimulating delivery, or both.

MAMMOGENESIS AND LACTATION

Structure of the Mammary Gland

The **mammary gland** is composed of about 20 lobes, each with an excretory **lactiferous duct** that opens at the nipple (Fig. 43-38). The lobes, in turn, are composed of several lobules that contain secretory

Anatomic Structures

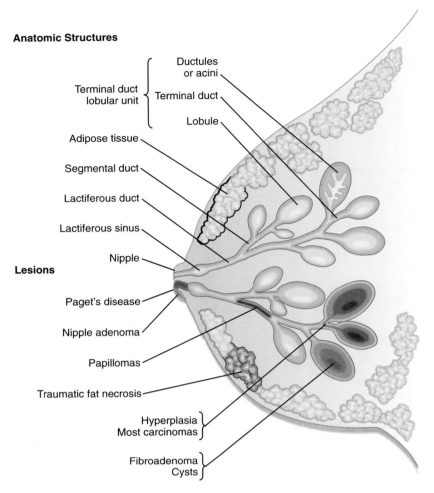

● **Figure 43-38.** Diagram of the structure of the breast, along with some pathological conditions of the breast and where they occur. (From Crum CP et al. In Kumar V et al [eds]: Robbins Basic Pathology, 7th ed. Philadelphia, Saunders, 2003.)

Ductules or acini

Terminal duct lobular unit — Terminal duct

Lobule

Adipose tissue

Segmental duct

Lactiferous duct

Lactiferous sinus

Nipple

Lesions

Paget's disease

Nipple adenoma

Papillomas

Traumatic fat necrosis

Hyperplasia Most carcinomas

Fibroadenoma Cysts

structures called **alveoli** and the terminal portions of the ducts. The epithelium of the alveoli and ducts is a simple one, except for the presence of a **myoepithelial cell** layer on the basal side of the epithelium (but apical to the basal lamina). Myoepithelial cells are stellate, smooth muscle–like cells, and contraction of these cells in response to a stimulus (see later) expels milk from the lumens of the alveoli and ducts. Lobes and lobules are supported within a connective tissue matrix. The other major tissue component of the breast is adipose tissue. The lactiferous ducts empty at the **nipple,** which is a highly innervated, hairless protrusion of the breast designed for suckling by an infant. The nipple is surrounded by a pigmented, hairless areola that is lubricated by sebaceous glands. Protrusion of the nipple, called **erection,** is mediated by sympathetic stimulation of smooth muscle fibers in response to suckling and other mechanical stimulation, erotic stimulation, and cold.

Hormonal Regulation of Mammary Gland Development

At puberty, estrogen increases ductal growth and branching. With onset of the luteal phases of the ovary, progesterone and estrogen induce ductal growth and the formation of rudimentary alveoli. During nonpreg-

nant cycles, the breasts develop somewhat and then regress. Estrogen also increases the deposition of adipose tissue, which makes a major contribution to the size and overall form of the breasts. Adipose tissue expresses CYP19, so accumulation of this tissue in the breast increases the local production of estrogens from circulating androgens.

Breast development is facilitated by pregnancy, during which extensive ductal growth and branching and lobuloalveolar development occur. The parenchymal growth of the breast during development occurs at the expense of stroma, which is degraded to make room for enlarging lobuloalveolar structures. Several placental hormones stimulate breast development, including **estrogen, progesterone, placental lactogen,** and a **growth hormone variant (GH-V).** Estrogen acts on the breast both directly and indirectly through increasing maternal pituitary PRL. Estrogen increases PRL secretion from pituitary lactotropes. Estrogen also stimulates lactotrope hypertrophy and proliferation, which accounts for the twofold increase in pituitary volume during pregnancy in humans. Although epithelial cells express genes encoding milk protein and enzymes involved in milk production, progesterone inhibits the onset of milk production and secretion **(lactogenesis).**

After parturition, the human breast produces **colostrum,** which is enriched with antimicrobial and antiinflammatory proteins. In the absence of placental progesterone, normal breast milk production occurs within a few days. The lobuloalveolar structures produce milk, which is subsequently modified by the ductal epithelium. Lactogenesis and maintenance of milk production **(galactopoiesis)** require stimulation by pituitary PRL in the presence of normal levels of other hormones, including insulin, cortisol, and thyroid hormone. Although placental estrogen stimulates PRL secretion during pregnancy, the stimulus for PRL secretion during the nursing period is suckling by the infant (Fig. 43-39). Levels of PRL are directly correlated with the frequency and duration of suckling at the nipple. The link between suckling at the nipple and PRL secretion involves a neuroendocrine reflex in which dopamine secretion at the median eminence is inhibited (the PRL release inhibitory factor; see Chapter 40). It is also possible that suckling increases the secretion of unidentified PRL-releasing hormones.

PRL also inhibits release of GnRH, and consequently, nursing can be associated with **lactational amenorrhea** (Fig. 43-39). This effect of prolactin has been called "nature's contraceptive," and it may play a role in spacing out pregnancies. However, only regular nursing over a 24-hour period is sufficient to induce a PRL-induced anovulatory state in the mother. Thus, lactational amenorrhea is not an effective or reliable form of birth control for most women. The inhibition of GnRH by high levels of PRL is important clinically. A **prolactinoma** is the most common form of hormone-secreting pituitary tumor, and **hyperprolactinemia** is a significant cause of infertility in both sexes. Hyperprolactinemia can likewise be associated with **galactorrhea,** or the inappropriate flow of breast milk, in men and women.

Suckling at the nipple also stimulates the release of **oxytocin** from the pars nervosa (see Chapter 40) through a neuroendocrine reflex (Fig. 43-39). Contraction of myoepithelial cells induces **milk let-down,** or expulsion of milk from the alveolar and ductal lumens. Thus, the nursing infant does not gain milk by applying negative pressure to the breast from suckling. Rather, milk is actively ejected through a neuroendocrine reflex. Oxytocin release and milk let-down can be induced by psychogenic stimuli, such as the mother hearing a baby crying on television or thinking about her baby. Such psychogenic stimuli do not affect PRL release.

IN THE CLINIC

There are multiple behavioral methods of contraception. Total abstinence is the best way to avoid getting pregnant. Other methods include the rhythm method, which relies on abstinence from sexual intercourse during fertile periods around the time of ovulation. The fertile period extends from 3 to 4 days before the time of ovulation until 3 to 4 days afterward. A second method is withdrawal before ejaculation, **coitus interruptus.** Both these methods have higher failure rates (20% to 30%) than **barrier methods** (2% to 12%), **intrauterine devices (IUDs)** (<2%), and **oral contraceptives** (<1%) do. Barriers such as **condoms** or **diaphragms** are more effective when used with **spermicidal jellies.** Of all methods, only condoms provide effective protection from sexually transmitted diseases in sexually active individuals. IUDs are relatively effective. They prevent implantation by locally producing an inflammatory response in the endometrium. Some forms of IUDs contain copper, zinc, or progestins, which inhibit sperm transport or viability in the female reproductive tract.

Oral contraceptives have been marketed in the United States since the early 1960s. The doses of steroids used today are many-fold lower than those used 35 years ago. Properly used, oral contraceptives have a low failure rate. Many forms of oral contraceptives are marketed today. The trend over the years has been to decrease the dosage of steroids used because the side effects are dose dependent. All oral steroidal contraceptives contain either a combination of an estrogen and a progestin or a progestin alone. Oral contraceptives work through multiple mechanisms. Most block the LH surge that triggers ovulation. However, some pills, such as the progestin-only mini-pill, do not prevent LH surges. Fertility is also blocked by changing the nature of cervical mucus, by altering endometrial development, and by regulating fallopian tube motility. Because these contraceptives suppress FSH, they impair early follicular development.

Emergency contraception involves hormonal treatment designed to inhibit or delay ovulation, inhibit corpus luteum function, disrupt the function of the oviducts and uterus, or any combination of these mechanisms. For example, candidates for emergency contraception include women who are sexually assaulted or who experienced failure of a barrier method (e.g., ruptured condom). There are more than 20 types of commercially available "morning after" pills. The currently preferred medication is **levonorgestrel (Plan B),** which is a synthetic progestin-only pill. The efficacy of the pill is inversely correlated with the time that it is taken after intercourse. The exact mechanism of action is not known. Treatment has no effect if implantation has occurred.

Medical (hormonal) termination of pregnancy **(abortion)** can be achieved up to 49 days of gestation by the administration of **mifepristone (RU-486),** a **progesterone receptor antagonist** that induces collapse of the pregnant endometrium. Mifepristone is followed 48 hours later by the ingestion or vaginal insertion of a synthetic **prostaglandin E** (e.g., misoprostol), which induces myometrial contractions.

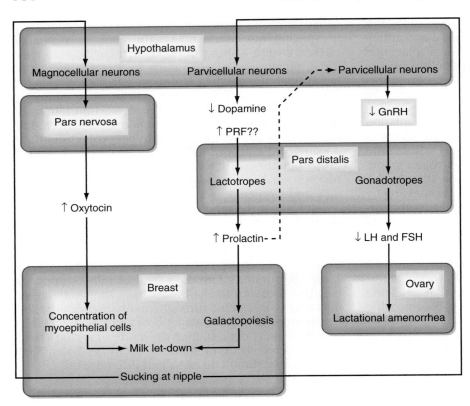

● **Figure 43-39.** Neuroendocrine reflex caused by suckling at the nipple and leading to secretion of oxytocin and prolactin. In turn, these hormones induce continued milk production (galactopoiesis) and milk let-down. Prolactin also induces lactational amenorrhea. (Modified from Porterfield SP, White BA: Endocrine Physiology, 3rd ed. Philadelphia, Mosby, 2007.)

MENOPAUSE

Though related to the depletion of ovarian follicles, the causes and process of **menopause** are poorly understood. Age-related changes in the CNS, including critical patterns of GnRH secretion, precede follicular depletion and may play an important role in menopause. Because follicles do not develop in response to LH and FSH secretion, estrogen and progesterone levels drop. Loss of the negative-feedback inhibition of estrogen on GnRH and LH/FSH results in a marked rise in serum LH and FSH. FSH levels rise more than LH levels. This could result from loss of ovarian inhibin.

Menopause typically occurs between 45 and 55 years of age. It extends over a period of several years. Initially, the cycles become irregular and are periodically anovulatory. The cycles tend to shorten, primarily in the follicular phase. Eventually, the woman ceases to cycle altogether. Serum estradiol levels drop to about a sixth the mean levels for younger cycling women, and progesterone levels drop to about a third those in the follicular phase of younger women. Production of these hormones does not cease entirely, but the primary source of these hormones in postmenopausal women becomes the adrenal, although interstitial cells of the ovarian stroma continue to produce some steroids. Most circulating estrogens are now produced peripherally from androgens. Because estrone is the primary estrogen produced in adipose tissue, it becomes the predominant estrogen in postmenopausal women.

Most of the symptoms associated with menopause result from **estrogen deficiency.** The vaginal epithelium atrophies and becomes dry, and bone loss is accelerated and may lead to osteoporosis. The incidence of coronary artery disease increases markedly after menopause. **Hot flashes** result from periodic increases in core temperature, which produces peripheral vasodilation and sweating. Hot flashes are thought to be linked to increases in LH release and are probably associated not with the pulsatile rise in LH secretion but rather with central mechanisms controlling GnRH release. Hot flashes typically subside within 1 to 5 years of the onset of menopausal symptoms.

■ KEY CONCEPTS

1. The reproductive systems are composed of gonads, an internal reproductive tract with associated glands, and external genitalia. Mammary glands are accessory reproductive glands in women.

2. Gonads have two main functions: production of gametes and production of hormones. Hormones (primarily sex steroids) are absolutely necessary for normal function of the reproductive system, and their production is regulated by a hypothalamic-pituitary-gonadal axis.

3. Seminiferous tubules in the testis contain Sertoli cells and developing sperm cells.

4. Spermatogenesis refers to the progression of sperm cells from spermatogonia through the pro-

cesses of meiosis and spermiogenesis to form mature spermatozoa.

5. Testosterone and pituitary FSH are required for normal sperm production. Only Sertoli cells express the androgen receptor and the FSH receptor, so these hormones regulate spermatogenesis indirectly through their actions on Sertoli cells. Sertoli cells produce the hormone inhibin, which negatively feeds back on pituitary FSH production.

6. Sertoli cells have many functions, including the production of androgen-binding protein (ABP) and fluid and creation of the blood-testis barrier.

7. Leydig cells are stromal cells that reside outside the seminiferous tubules. They respond to LH by producing testosterone.

8. Testosterone is an active androgen. It can be converted peripherally to DHT, which is more active in certain tissues (e.g., prostate), or to estradiol.

9. Leydig cells are regulated within a hypothalamic-pituitary-testicular axis. The hypothalamus produces GnRH, which stimulates pituitary gonadotropes to secrete LH and FSH. Testosterone, DHT, and estradiol negatively feed back at the pituitary and hypothalamus and inhibit LH more than FSH secretion. Inhibin from the Sertoli cells selectively inhibits FSH.

10. Testosterone, DHT, and estradiol have numerous actions on the male reproductive tract, external genitalia, and male secondary sex characteristics, as well as on other organ systems (e.g., blood cell production, lipoprotein production, bone maturation).

11. The male tract includes tubal structures (epididymis, ductus deferens, and male urethra), accessory sex glands (seminal vesicles, prostate), and the penis. The seminal vesicles and the prostate produce most of the ejaculate, which nourishes, buffers, and protects sperm.

12. Penile erection involves a complex neurovascular response leading to engorgement of the erectile tissue within the penis base and shaft with blood.

13. The follicle is the functional unit of the ovary. Follicles contain epithelial cells (granulosa and cumulus) and outer stromal cells (thecal). All these cells surround a primary oocyte that remains arrested in the first meiotic prophase until just before ovulation.

14. Follicles develop from the smallest (primordial) to a large antral follicle over a period of months. The latter part of follicular development requires gonadotropins.

15. The menstrual cycle refers to an approximately 28-day cycle that is driven by the following ovarian events: development of one large antral follicle to a preovulatory follicle (the follicular phase), ovulation, and the formation and death of a corpus luteum of menstruation (the luteal phase).

16. The follicular phase of the ovary corresponds to the menstrual and proliferative phases of the uterine endometrium. The luteal phase of the ovary corresponds to the secretory phase of the uterine endometrium.

17. One dominant follicle is selected per menstrual cycle—usually the largest follicle with the most FSH receptors.

18. High levels of estradiol occur around midcycle and exert positive feedback on gonadotropin secretion. This induces the LH (and a smaller FSH) surge. The midcycle gonadotropin surge induces (a) meiotic maturation of the primary oocyte so that it progresses to a secondary oocyte (with one polar body) arrested at metaphase of the second meiotic division, (b) breakdown of the ovarian and follicular wall so that the oocyte-cumulus complex is extruded (called ovulation), and (c) differentiation of the remaining follicular cells into a corpus luteum. The corpus luteum produces high levels of progesterone, estradiol, and inhibin.

19. If pregnancy does not occur, the corpus luteum will die in 14 days. This constitutes the luteal phase of the menstrual cycle.

20. The oviducts capture the ovulated cumulus-oocyte complex and transport it medially into the oviduct and toward the uterus. Estrogen promotes ciliation and transport; progesterone inhibits transport.

21. The uterine mucosa, called the endometrium, is the normal site of embryonic implantation. The mucosa is increased in thickness in preparation for implantation and is sloughed away if no pregnancy occurs.

22. During the mid to late follicular phase (days 6 to 14 of the menstrual cycle), the ovary produces estradiol, which induces all cells of the endometrium to proliferate (called the proliferative phase of the uterus).

23. After ovulation, the ovary enters the luteal phase (days 16 to 28) and produces progesterone. Progesterone stimulates secretion from the uterine glands (called the secretory phase of the uterus).

24. In the absence of an implanting embryo, the corpus luteum dies, progesterone production ceases, and the uterine endometrium is sloughed (called the menstrual phase, or period, of the uterus—this corresponds to days 1 to 5 of the follicular phase of the ovary).

25. The cervix is the lower portion of the uterus. Cervical mucus is hormonally regulated so that at midcycle in response to estrogen, cervical mucus

promotes entry of sperm into the uterus from the vagina. During the luteal phase in response to progesterone, cervical mucus becomes thick and poses a barrier to entry of sperm and microbes into the uterus.

26. Fertilization is a complex series of events that occur in the oviduct and lead to penetration of the oocyte by sperm.

27. Early embryogenesis (up to day 6 after fertilization) occurs in the oviduct and gives rise to a blastocyst that hatches from the zona pellucida.

28. The placenta develops from the outer, extraembryonic trophoblast. The endocrine function of the placenta includes the production of hCG, progesterone, estrogens, and placental lactogen. Estrogen production requires placental cells (syncytiotrophoblasts), as well as the fetal adrenal and liver—collectively called the fetoplacental unit.

29. Pregnancy and the hormones of pregnancy induce major changes in maternal physiology, including an increase in insulin resistance, an increase in the use of free fatty acids by the mother, and development of the mammary glands. Mammary gland development (but not lactation) is promoted by estrogen, progesterone, and placental lactogen, but also by maternal pituitary prolactin, whose secretion is stimulated by placental estrogens.

30. Oxytocin is a pituitary hormone that promotes the contraction of certain smooth muscles, including myometrial contractions during labor and myoepithelial contractions in the breasts that lead to let-down of milk in response to suckling.

31. Menopause results from exhaustion of the ovarian reserve and is characterized by low ovarian hormone and elevated gonadotropin levels.

Note: Page numbers followed by *f* and *t* indicate figures and tables, respectively. Numbers followed by *b* indicate boxed information (i.e., "In the Clinic" and "At the Cellular Level"). Footnotes are indicated by *n*.